TEL. 01803 656700

Visit our website

to find out about other books from Churchill Livingstone
and our sister companies in Harcourt Health Sciences

Register free at
www.harcourt-international.com

and you will get

- **the latest information on new books, journals and electronic products in your chosen subject areas**

- **the choice of e-mail or post alerts or both, when there are any new books in your chosen areas**

- **news of special offers and promotions**

- **information about products from all Harcourt Health Sciences companies including W. B. Saunders, Churchill Livingstone, and Mosby**

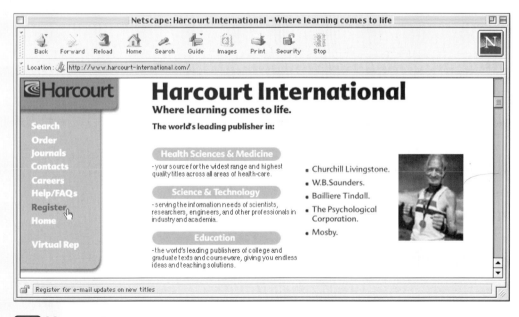

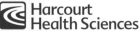

SECOND EDITION

CLINICAL ULTRASOUND
a comprehensive text

Ultrasound in Obstetrics and Gynaecology

VOLUME 3

This title is a self-contained work entitled *Ultrasound in Obstetrics and Gynaecology*. Additionally, it forms an integral part of *Clinical Ultrasound: a comprehensive text* together with its companion title, *Abdominal and General Ultrasound*, which may also be purchased seperately.

Commissioning Editor Michael J Houston
Project Development Manager Paul Fam
Project Manager Rolla Couchman
Production Manager Helen Sofio
Designer Sarah Russell
Illustration Manager Mick Ruddy
Illustrator Jenni Miller

SECOND EDITION

CLINICAL ULTRASOUND
a comprehensive text

Ultrasound in Obstetrics and Gynaecology

VOLUME 3

Edited by

Keith C Dewbury BSc MBBS FRCR
Consultant Radiologist, Southampton General Hospital, Southampton, United Kingdom

Hylton B Meire FRCR
Consultant Radiologist, King's College Hospital, London, United Kingdom

David O Cosgrove MA MSc FRCR FRCP
Professor of Clinical Ultrasound, Department of Imaging, Hammersmith Hospital, London, United Kingdom

Pat Farrant DCRR DMU
Superintendent Research Sonographer, King's College Hospital, London, United Kingdom

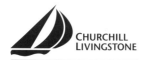

CHURCHILL
LIVINGSTONE

LONDON EDINBURGH NEW YORK PHILADELPHIA ST LOUIS SYDNEY TORONTO 2001

CHURCHILL LIVINGSTONE
An imprint of Harcourt Publishers Limited

First edition published 1993
          reprinted 1993
          reprinted 1994 (twice)
          reprinted 1995
Second edition published 2001

ISBN 0 443 06152 1 (volumes 1 & 2)
ISBN 0 443 06154 8 (volume 3)
ISBN 0 443 06350 8 (3 volume set)

British Library Cataloguing in Publication Data
A catalogue record for this book is available from the British Library

Library of Congress Cataloging in Publication Data
A catalog record for this book is available from the Library of Congress

Note
Medical knowledge is constantly changing. As new information
becomes available, changes in treatment, procedures, equipment and
the use of drugs become necessary. The editors, contributors and the
publishers have taken care to ensure that the information given in this
text is accurate and up to date. However, readers are strongly advised
to confirm that the information, especially with regard to drug usage,
complies with the latest legislation and standards of practice.

The
publisher's
policy is to use
**paper manufactured
from sustainable forests**

Typeset by Expo Holdings, Malaysia
Printed in the UK by Polestar Wheatons, Exeter

Preface

In the years since the publication of the first edition of this book, the subject of ultrasound has advanced at a dizzying pace, one that could not have been foreseen when we worked on the original edition. Not only have advances concerned technical aspects – harmonic imaging, 3D, power Doppler, contrast agents – which are in the process of rewriting the methodology of ultrasound, but they have also affected the clinical practice of ultrasound where we have seen marked improvements in techniques, understanding and appreciation of the method. Far from being replaced by alternative tomographic techniques, ultrasound has gone from strength to strength as a diagnostic tool to the point where it is now the fastest growing imaging modality. It has consolidated its role in classic applications remaining paramount in obstetrics and in cardiac imaging. It is the primary method for small parts imaging and for biopsy guidance and is carving out new roles in musculoskeletal and vascular investigations. Some of the impetus behind this has been the downward pressure on medical spending – ultrasound is still the most cost-effective way to investigate many medical and surgical problems.

In preparing this new edition – no mean task! – we have tried to retain the basic material that made the first edition useful as a reference and basic learning text, and have tried to provide a systematic description of the proven applications of ultrasound to act as a guide in day-to-day practice. Keeping this balance between the routine and the provisional is sometimes difficult for enthusiasts in a discipline and we crave the reader's indulgence if occasionally we have allowed exciting innovations too prominent a description.

Our great indebtedness to the numerous contributors is obvious and we would like to extend to these experts our most sincere thanks for their patience and labour. The project could not have been completed without the endless support of the publishing team at Harcourt: Michael Houston, who was responsible for cajoling us into taking up the editorial pen again and oversaw the entire effort, Paul Fam and Rolla Couchman who worked with us and our contributors on a weekly and sometimes daily basis keeping the project to schedule and coping with the inevitable technical difficulties that beset such an endeavour.

Pat Farrant was inadequately noted as an assistant editor in the first edition: here she has rightly been recognised as the full editor that she always was.

We all extend our thanks to our colleagues and families who supported us with encouragement and patience, indulging the many hours of time we stole from other activities. We sincerely hope that the result is as useful as before.

Hylton Meire
David Cosgrove
Keith Dewbury
Pat Farrant
2000

Preface to the first edition

Most textbooks, at least in the field of diagnostic imaging, stem from the wish of the authors or editors to make their special expertise more widely available. The origin of *Clinical Ultrasound* is rather unusual in that it is a response to a proposal by the publishers, Churchill Livingstone, that the time was right for a comprehensive ultrasound textbook with a strong clinical content.

At first approach, we have to confess to having been sceptical of the need for such a textbook and we were most reluctant to embark on such a monumental task but, as we began to review the field, it was possible to envisage it being broken down into more manageable components. It was also clear that there really was no comprehensive textbook on the market, all of the available books concentrated on a particular application or body region.

An initial hurdle was to secure the editorship of Dr Peter Wilde to oversee the cardiology section; initially Peter was as reluctant as the rest of us, having heavy commitments on his hands but, fired by the prospect of a comprehensive and strongly clinical reference work, he was persuaded. The cardiology section has been completely under his editorship, though it adheres to the general format and goals of the entire book.

For the remaining large sections, a decisive influence in our agreeing to proceed was the fact that Pat Farrant was enthusiastic, something she may have come to regret as time went by! Pat agreed to take control of the massive task of handling all of the editing and advising that underlay the organising of the extensive text and innumerable figures together with their orientation diagrams, keeping track of where alterations had to be entered, checking that tables referred to in the text were, in fact, contained in the chapter or appendix and generally managing the entire process of creation and collation which extended to double the 18 months that we had originally anticipated. However, that was not all for, as we got further into the project, Pat was also called upon to contribute large portions of chapters that had somehow fallen by the wayside and her input into almost every section has been absolutely invaluable. It was in the knowledge that she would give this kind of support that we entered the 'battle'. None of us foresaw just how protracted a battle it would become nor how large Pat's contribution would turn out to be – 'siege' would have been a more apposite term!

We would also like to thank our families and friends who have borne with us during the past three stressful years. Special thanks are due to Christine Dewbury and Gill Meire for their continuing support and encouragement, and for hosting so many editorial meetings.

From this explanation, our intentions should be clear. We have aimed to provide an up-to-date textbook on clinical diagnostic ultrasound that would cover the entire gamut of its applications, both imaging and Doppler. Because of its clinical basis, the physics of ultrasound does not feature as a formal topic, though its important practical consequences and implications, especially in newer, less familiar areas such as Doppler, are covered.

Diagnostic ultrasound has become so extensive that, inevitably, this had to be a large book and a small team of specialists could not hope to cover the entire field. Therefore, we commissioned a large number of contributing authors from Europe and the Americas, most well known experts in their own areas. We stand to lose friends however, because we have exercised strong editing rights in the interests of maintaining a uniform style – we hope our loyal contributors will feel that our sometimes heavy alterations have contributed to the overall quality of the book and will not take offence that we have freely altered their prose and even sometimes substituted scans that seemed clearer or that made the intended point better.

With respect to the division of material through the book, the separation of cardiology from the other applications already referred to, made it obvious that this should form a separate volume that is available on its own. Obstetrics and Gynaecology formed a second distinct section and so we have arranged that this also be a separate volume with its own page numbering and index. The other two volumes, which contain the remaining applications (abdominal, small parts, vascular, miscellaneous), are offered together as two sections of a single book: pages are numbered through and they have been indexed together in the expectation that few users will need only one of the pair.

We hope that *Clinical Ultrasound* will become a reference work for all who use ultrasound in their clinical practice and that users will find in it comprehensive answers to their everyday needs. It should provide critical information in a form that is easy to look up, as well as form the basis for specialist training.

Hylton Meire
David Cosgrove
Keith Dewbury.
1992

Terminology and scan position indicators

The aim of this book is to serve as a reference text and as an aid to education and teaching. During the editorial process it was clear to us that the terminology used to describe ultrasound appearances is extremely diverse, confusing and occasionally inaccurate. We have therefore unified the terminology in *Clinical Ultrasound*. In doing this we have considered the two main interactions between the ultrasound beam and the tissue; namely reflective and attenuation.

Meaningless terms such as 'sonolucent' and 'echo dense' have been eradicated. We also considered the use of the prefixs 'hyper-' and 'hypo-' a source of confusion and found several instances where the secretaries typing the manuscript had confused the two.

Where backscattered amplitude is being discussed the ultrasound appearances are described as of reduced, normal or increased reflectivity (by inference compared with that which would normally be expected).

The above features of *Clinical Ultrasound* have been incorporated in an attempt to make these volumes more valuable and easier to understand, and it is hoped that the terminology we have used will encourage readers to consider more carefully the terminology they use to describe their own ultrasound findings.

The relatively small field of view of modern ultrasound scanners, and the infinitely variable planes of imaging, sometimes lead to difficulties in interpreting the anatomy and orientation of an ultrasound image. Rather than using extensive free narrative to describe the positions from which images have been obtained we have used a system of body markers on which the position of the scans has been indicated. When referring to these the reader should be aware that the scans indicating a lateral area of contact do not necessarily imply that the patient was moved into an oblique or decubitus position, but simply that the transducer was located on a lateral aspect of the patient.

The orientation of the conventional extracavitory images included in this book has generally been adjusted such that longitudinal scans are viewed as if from the patient's rightside and transverse scans as if from the patient's feet. Unfortunately there is no stanadardisation for the orientation of intracavitory images and, in general, these have been displayed with the orientation unaltered from that supplied by the individual authors. We have not attempted to verify the position of the transducer or the orientation of the image for intracavitory scans as these should be clear from the accompanying text in each case.

Hylton Meire
David Cosgrove
Keith Dewbury
Pat Farrant

Contributors

Douglas G Altman BSc DSc
Director, ICRF Medical Statistics Group
Centre for Statistics on Medicine
Institute of Health Sciences
Oxford
United Kingdom

Heather Andrews MBBS DMRD MRCP FRCR
Consultant Radiologist
Ultrasound Department
Bristol Royal Infirmary
Bristol
United Kingdom

Carol B Benson MD
Associate Professor of Radiology
Harvard Medical School
Director of Ultrasound
Department of Radiology
Brigham & Women's Hospital
Boston
Massachusetts
USA

Lyn S Chitty PhD MRCOG
Senior Lecturer and Consultant in Genetics
  and Fetal Medicine
Department of Obstetrics and Gynaecology
Institute of Child Health and University College Hospital
London
United Kingdom

David Churchill MB ChB MD MRCOG
Consultant Obstetrician
Department of Obstetrics
Good Hope Hospital
Sutton Coldfield
United Kingdom

Anna P Cockell MRCOG MD
Consultant in Genetics and Fetal Medicine
Fetal Medicine Unit
Institute of Child Health and University College Hospital
London
United Kingdom

Glyn Constantine BSc MBChB(Hons) MRCP FRCOG
Consultant in Obstetrics and Gynaecology
Department of Obstetrics and Gynaecology
Good Hope Hospital
Sutton Coldfield
United Kingdom

David O Cosgrove MA MSc FRCR FRCP
Professor of Clinical Ultrasound
Department of Imaging
Hammersmith Hospital
London
United Kingdom

Peter M Doubilet MD PhD
Associate Professor of Radiology
Harvard Medical School
Vice-chairman of Radiology
Department of Radiology
Brigham and Women's Hospital
Boston
Massachusetts
USA

Sturla H Eik-Nes MD PhD
Professor of Obstetrics
Department of Obstetrics and Gynaecology
National Centre for Fetal Medicine
University Hospital of Trondheim
Trondheim
Norway

Alison Fowlie FRCOG
Consultant Obstetrician and Gynaecologist
Department of Obstetrics and Gynaecology
Derby City General Hospital
Derby
United Kingdom

Andrew M Fried MD
Professor of Diagnostic Radiology
Department of Diagnostic Radiology
University of Kentucky Medical Center
Lexington
Kentucky
USA

John L Gibbs FRCP
Consultant Paediatric Cardiologist
Department of Paediatric Cardiology
Leeds General Infirmary
Leeds
United Kingdom

David R Griffin FRCOG
Consultant Obstetrician and Gynaecologist
Department of Obstetrics and Gynaecology
Watford General Hospital
Watford
United Kingdom

Eric R M Jauniaux MD PhD
Reader in Obstetrics and Fetal Medicine
Department of Obstetrics and Gynaecology
University College London Medical School
London
United Kingdom

Olujimi A Jibodu MBBS MRCOG
Associate Specialist in Obstetrics and Gynaecology
Department of Obstetrics and Gynaecology
Derby City Hospital
Derby
United Kingdom

Phillipa M Kyle MBChB MRCOG MD
Consultant in Maternal and Fetal Medicine
Fetal Medicine Unit
St Michael's Hospital
Bristol
United Kingdom

Josephine M McHugo FRCR FRCP FRCPCH
Honorary Senior Lecturer
Birmingham University
Consultant Radiologist
Birmingham Women's Hospital
Birmingham
United Kingdom

Karel Marsál MD PhD
Professor of Obstetrics and Gynaecology
Department of Obstetrics and Gynaecology
University Hospital of Lund
Malmö
Sweden

Ian G Parkin MBChB
Clinical Anatomist
Department of Anatomy
University of Cambridge
Cambridge
United Kingdom

John H Parsons MB ChB MRCOG DA
Senior Lecturer and Honorary Consultant
King's College School of Medicine and Dentistry
London
United Kingdom

Charles H Rodeck FMBBS BSc DSc(Med) FRCOG
  FRCPath FMedSci
Professor and Head
Department of Obstetrics and Gynaecology
University College London
London
United Kingdom

Christopher Steer MD FRCOG
Consultant Obstetrician and Gynaecologist
Department of Obstetrics and Gynaecology
Farnborough Hospital
Orpington
United Kingdom

Peter Twining FRCR BSc BS MB
Consultant Radiologist
Department of Radiology
Queen's Medical Centre
Nottingham
United Kingdom

Janet I Vaughan MBBS FRANZCOG MRCOG
COGU DDU
Associate Professor of Maternal Fetal Medicine
Department of Ultrasound and Fetal Medicine
King George V Hospital
Sydney
New South Wales
Australia

Michael J Weston MBChB MRCP FRCR
Consultant Radiologist
Ultrasound Department
St James' University Hospital
Leeds
United Kingdom

Martin J Whittle MD FRCOG FRCP(Glas)
Professor of Fetal Medicine
Academic Department of Obstetrics and Gynaecology
Birmingham Women's Hospital
Birmingham
United Kingdom

Contents

1

Pelvic anatomy

David O Cosgrove and Nayna Patel

Introduction

Because the skeleton forms the framework to which the viscera are attached it determines the general anatomy of the pelvis and so needs to be understood, although it is itself not well visualised on ultrasound. In the following description the anatomy is described as viewed from within the pelvis, corresponding to the ultrasound point of view.[1–8]

The bony pelvis

The lateral elements, the paired hip bones or coxae (which bear the acetabula laterally), articulate with the wings of the sacrum posteriorly (Figs 1.1 and 1.2). Anteriorly each gives rise to two band-like bones, the superior and inferior pubic rami, which curve anteromedially to fuse in front as the pubic bones, the right and left articulating in the midline at the pubic symphysis. The spaces between the pubic rami, the obturator foramina, are covered by a fibrous membrane. Overall this complex forms a complete bony ring known as the true pelvis.

Superior to the pelvis the iliac bones, arising from the hip bones, form the iliac fossae. They also articulate with the sacrum posteromedially, but are unattached anteriorly and superiorly so that this upper part of the pelvis forms an incomplete bowl, known as the false pelvis: this space is actually the lowest part of the abdomen. The inlet to the true pelvis is marked by a prominent curved thickening of the hip bone, the arcuate line or iliopubic eminence. Whereas the inlet to the true pelvis faces anteriorly, its outlet faces posteriorly; the change in direction of about 60° occurs because of the steep angulation of the sacrum on the lower lumbar vertebrae.

Pelvic muscles

All the muscles are paired; those in the true pelvis fall into two groups, lateral and medial. The obturator interni are the major lateral muscles; they arise from the membranes covering the obturator fossae and the surrounding bones, and form sheets a few millimetres thick that pass postero-inferiorly to leave the pelvis, their tendons angling laterally and attaching to the upper femora. They are seen on ultrasound as echo-poor strips forming the pelvic side walls (Fig. 1.3). Superior to the obturator internus lie the pyriformis muscles, forming transverse-lying strips that leave the pelvis laterally. They are pararectal in position and, being situated high in the pelvis, are difficult to image on ultrasound, requiring scans with a marked cephalad angulation.

The medial groups form the levator ani muscles (Fig. 1.3). Each is a curved sheet originating from the upper margin of the true pelvis and curving postero-medially to fuse with its opposite number in the midline to form a hammock-shaped muscular bowl (known as the 'pelvic sling') that closes the pelvic outlet.[9] Midline perforations transmit the urethra, vagina and rectum. Each levator ani muscle is composed of two portions: one, the iliococcygeus, originating from the medial surface of the obturator internus muscle, has a mainly posteromedial lie, whereas the other, the pubococcygeus, taking origin from the inner surface of the pubic bone, passes posteriorly to the coccyx itself. This portion forms an anteroposterior-lying band lying close to the midline; it is extremely variable, being rudimentary in some subjects and easily visualised in others.

The muscles of the false pelvis are the iliacus, which arises from the entire iliac fossa, and the psoas, which arises from the lumbar vertebrae and passes inferiorly to lie on the anteromedial surface of the iliacus. Together the fused iliopsoas muscles pass inferiorly immediately above and lateral to the brim of the true pelvis. Each passes under its respective inguinal ligament to attach to the lesser trochanter of the femora.

Vessels

The common iliac arteries, formed at the level of L5 by the division of the aorta, enter the false pelvis by crossing the iliopsoas muscles as they diverge from the midline. At the level of the lower end of the sacroiliac joints each divides into external and internal iliac branches. The former continue the inferior course, often swinging anteriorly also, to leave the pelvis by crossing under the inguinal ligament, where they lie medial to the iliopsoas muscles. They supply the leg and may be visualised by scanning across the pelvis using the filled bladder as a window (Fig. 1.4). All of the blood supply to the pelvic muscles and viscera comes from the internal iliac arteries. They form short trunks which soon divide into anterior and posterior main branches of equal size. These in turn rapidly break up into numerous smaller branches that supply individual pelvic viscera. Important branches are the rectal and vesical arteries. In gynaecology the uterine branches are of major importance: they pass medially from the pelvic side walls and run to the lateral borders of the cervix. Here each divides into a descending vaginal branch and a larger, uterine branch that ascends along the lateral margin of the uterus, supplying it by curving branches known as arcuate arteries. The terminal portions of the main trunks continue along the uterine (fallopian) tubes, each ending in a small ovarian branch. In contrast, the main ovarian arteries are abdominal vessels, arising directly from the aorta at renal level; thus the ovaries have a dual supply.

Pelvic viscera

The pelvic viscera are cradled in the musculoskeletal framework (Fig. 1.5). Anteriorly the bladder lies on the

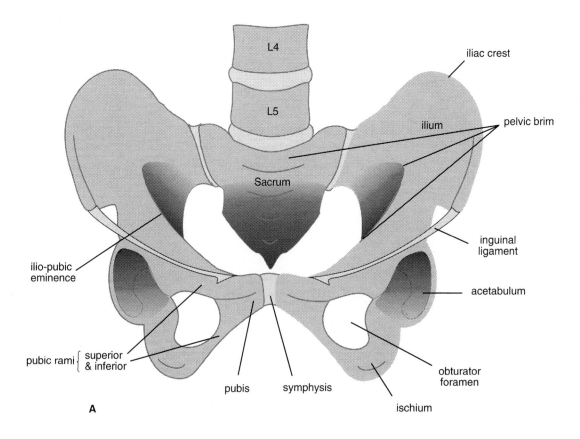

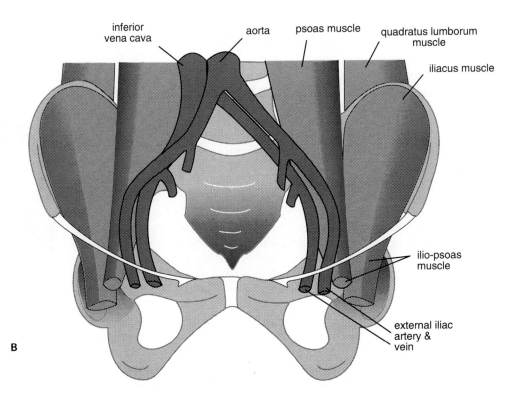

Fig. 1.1 The pelvic skeleton. Diagrams of the bony skeleton **A**: to show the pelvic brim and **B**: with the muscles of the false pelvis (iliopsoas) as well as the major vessels added.

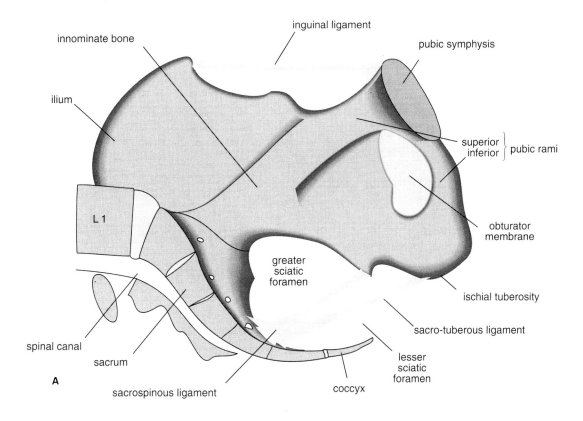

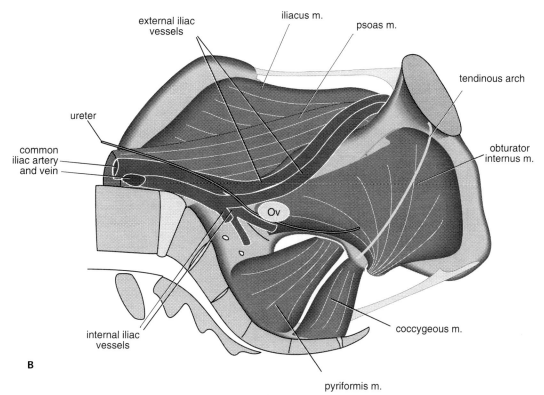

Fig. 1.2 The pelvic side wall. A: Bones and ligaments of the left pelvic side wall in a hemipelvis viewed from the right. **B:** With side wall muscles and major blood vessels superimposed. Note the position of the ovary (Ov) in the fossa delineated by the external and internal iliac vessels; the ureter lies close by. **C:** With the iliococcygeus and pubococcygeus portions of the levator ani muscles added. (*Fig. 1.2C, see overleaf*)

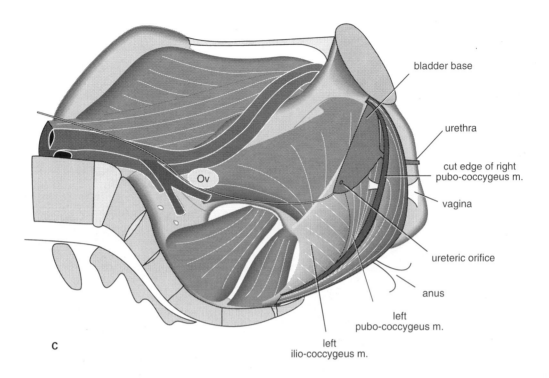

bladder base

urethra

cut edge of right
pubo-coccygeus m.

vagina

ureteric orifice

anus

left
pubo-coccygeus m.

left
ilio-coccygeus m.

Ov

c

Fig. 1.2C

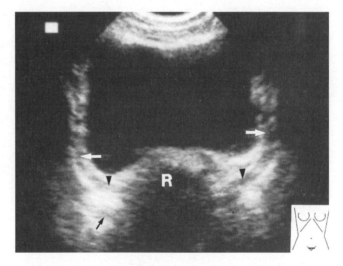

Fig. 1.3 The muscles of the pelvis. Seen in transverse section the
obturator internus muscles (white arrows) form echo-poor
anteroposterior strips against the pelvic side walls. The iliococcygeus
portions of the levator ani muscles (arrowheads) can often be discerned
arising from their medial surfaces and passing posteriorly towards the
midline. In this subject the right pyriformis muscle is also demonstrated
(black arrow). R – rectum.

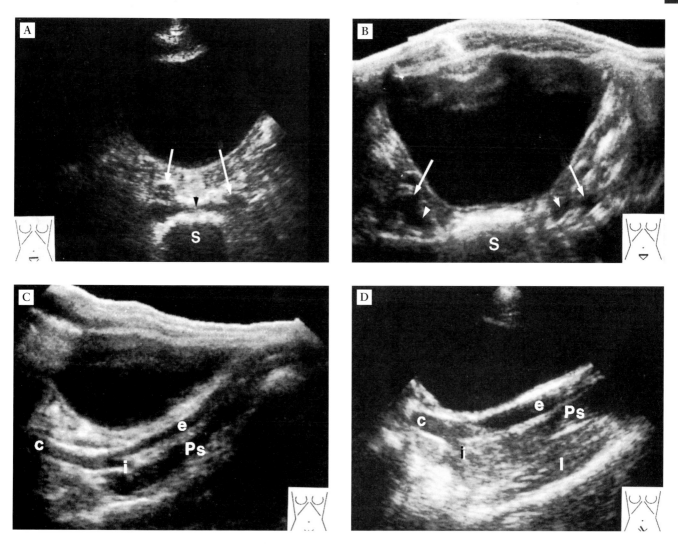

Fig. 1.4 Arteries of the pelvis. A: Transverse section at the pelvic brim shows the junction of the common iliac veins (arrowhead) to form the inferior vena cava. The common iliac arteries (arrows) lie anterolaterally. S – spine. **B:** Transverse section slightly further inferiorly shows the common iliac veins (arrowheads) and arteries (arrows). **C and D:** Oblique longitudinal sections in the iliac fossae along the line of the iliac artery show the division of the common (c) into internal (i) and external (e) arterial branches. The arteries lie on the psoas (Ps) and iliacus (I) muscles.

levator ani muscles, the urethra passing through a foramen between them. The ureters, having entered the pelvis by crossing medial to the common iliac artery and vein, curve inferiorly around the pelvic side wall and then pass medially to enter the bladder base. The undilated ureters are rarely visualised on ultrasound, but the position of the ureterovesical junctions can be identified by the intermittent echoes from the jets of urine emptied into the bladder by ureteric peristalsis (Fig. 1.6). The uterus lies immediately posterior to the bladder, its anterior surface lying in contact with the bladder base and its posterior wall, whereas the rectum lies posteriorly. Gaps between the left and right levator ani muscles in the midline transmit the vagina and anus.

Uterus

The uterus, a pear-shaped muscular structure, is divided into the cervix inferiorly and the body and domed fundus superiorly (Fig. 1.7). Since it is composed mainly of muscle, the uterus returns low level echoes, somewhat higher than those from the pelvic musculature (Fig. 1.8). The endometrium, on the other hand, with its complex tubular structure on microscopy, gives rise to higher-amplitude echoes. Between the endometrium and the myometrium a fine echo-poor line, the transitional zone, is usually visible. This has been attributed to the deepest, more vascular layer of the myometrium; alternatively, it may represent the outer layer of the endometrium, i.e. the non-deciduous portion.

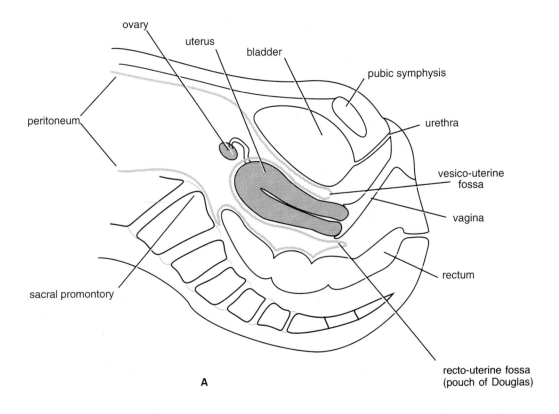

ovary

uterus

bladder

pubic symphysis

peritoneum

urethra

vesico-uterine fossa

vagina

rectum

sacral promontory

recto-uterine fossa (pouch of Douglas)

A

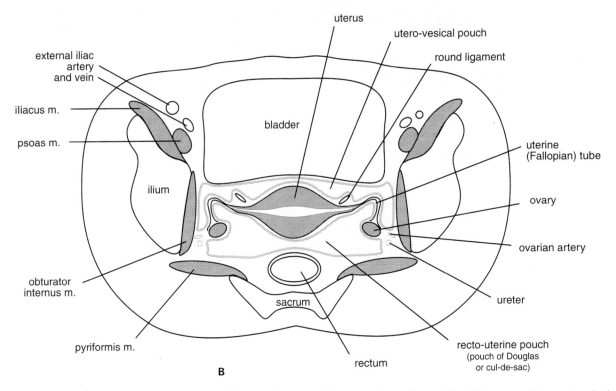

uterus

utero-vesical pouch

external iliac artery and vein

round ligament

iliacus m.

bladder

psoas m.

uterine (Fallopian) tube

ilium

ovary

ovarian artery

obturator internus m.

ureter

pyriformis m.

sacrum

recto-uterine pouch (pouch of Douglas or cul-de-sac)

rectum

B

Fig. 1.5 Viscera of the pelvis – sectional anatomy. A: Midline sagittal section of the uterus with a filled bladder. (The ovary and its associated tube are not likely to be visualised in a sagittal section and are depicted for orientation.) **B:** Mid-pelvic transverse section. The peritoneum is indicated as a grey line.

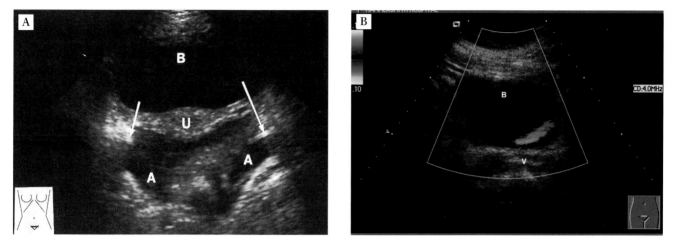

Fig. 1.6 Position of the ureters. A: The normal ureters are rarely identified on ultrasound but the strong echoes from a ureteric stent are obvious (arrows). This patient also had ascites (A). U – uterus, B – bladder. **B:** The jet in the bladder, seen as the flame-shaped colour Doppler signal, indicates the position of the ureterovesical junction; it lies close to the vaginal vault cervix (V), a fact that accounts for the high risk of ureteric obstruction in cervical carcinoma.

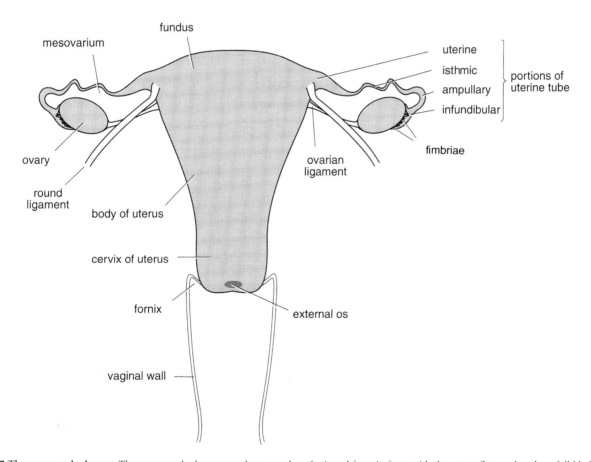

Fig. 1.7 The uterus and adnexae. The uterus and adnexae are drawn as though viewed from in front with the uterus flattened, as by a full bladder for a transabdominal scan.

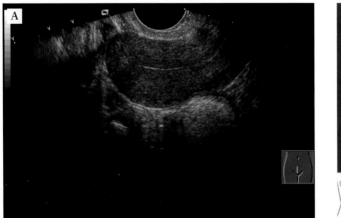
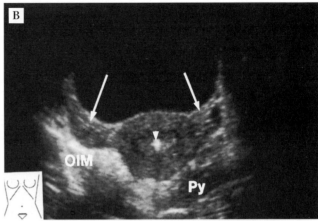

Fig. 1.8 The uterus. A: Longitudinal trans-vaginal and **B:** transverse transabdominal sections. The myometrium is a little more reflective than the pelvic muscles (Py – pyriformis muscle, OIM – obturator internus muscle) and about the same as the ovaries (arrows). The endometrial echo intensity depends on the stage of the menstrual cycle – in this subject, scanned towards the end of the follicular phase, the endometrium is thick and reflective. Note also the very intense echoes from the intra-uterine contraceptive device (arrowhead).

The uterine cavity is usually empty and is seen only as a strong central interface, sometimes called the cavitary echo; it should be straight or smoothly curved. A trace of endometrial fluid may be detected at the time of ovulation, perhaps representing secretions in response to hormone changes.[10] This fluid amounts to no more than a slight separation of the endometrial layers and is transient, disappearing over the next 24 hours. During menstruation the shed endometrium may be visualised in the cavity as a

fluid space a millimetre or so in thickness; there may also be menstrual fluid within the vagina, though this is often obscured by the intense echoes from a tampon. The menstrual fluid normally clears within a few days.

The uterus measures approximately 6 cm in length by 4 cm anteroposteriorly and 5 cm transversely, but there are marked functional changes (Fig. 1.9).[11] In the prepubertal child all dimensions are smaller but the cervix is disproportionately larger, occupying up to one-half the

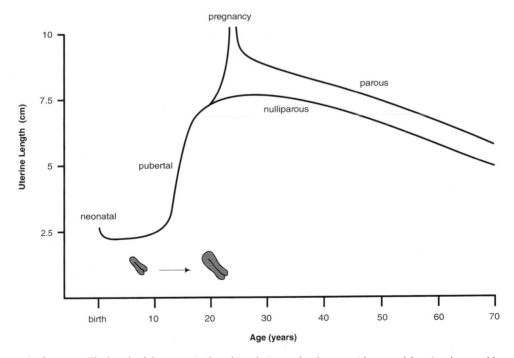

Fig. 1.9 Age changes in the uterus. The length of the uterus is plotted in relation to the changes with age and functional status. Note the relatively large cervix before puberty and the permanent increase in length following a pregnancy.

size of the uterus (see vol 2., Ch. 50).[12,13] (An exception is the neonate, where the uterus may be large and have an active endometrium in response to the high maternal hormone levels during pregnancy.) At puberty the body and fundus enlarge more than the cervix, to reach the adult proportions in which the cervix occupies about one-third of the uterus. The uterus never completely regresses from the dramatic hypertrophy in pregnancy, so that the parous uterus measures up to 7 cm in length. After the menopause it gradually atrophies while retaining the adult proportions.[14]

The degree of bladder filling alters the lie of the uterus: when empty, as is usual for trans-vaginal scanning, the uterus is angled forwards from the lie of the vagina, whereas a full bladder straightens the uterus. The body and fundus of the uterus very often lie to one side of the midline, sometimes markedly so, though the cervix always remains a midline structure.

Extending laterally from the cornua of the fundus of the uterus are the paired uterine ('fallopian') tubes; these fine tortuous structures with a lumen of about a millimetre in diameter are too small to be visualised reliably on transabdominal ultrasound, though they are sometimes demonstrated with the superior resolution of trans-vaginal scanning, and the lumen is well outlined on contrast salpingography[15] (see Ch. 5). The lateral, fimbriated end of each tube opens directly into the peritoneum in the immediate vicinity of its respective ovary, to which it is attached by one of the fimbria.

Minor variations in uterine position are normal. For example, the fundus of the uterus may be tipped posteriorly, either by flexion at the lower segment of the uterus or by rotation around the vaginal vault (retroversion) (Fig. 1.10). Both produce confusing appearances, particularly on transabdominal scanning, when the deeper portions of the fundus are difficult to delineate and may even appear to be abnormal because of shadowing from the intervening body and cervix. It is not usually possible with ultrasound to distinguish between retroversion and retroflexion, so the general term 'retropositioned' is often used.

On trans-vaginal scans all these features are more easily observed because of the higher resolution obtained (Fig. 1.8A, Fig. 1.10A).[16] However, the most immediately obvious difference from transabdominal scans is the position of the uterus: as trans-vaginal scanning is performed with the bladder empty (in order to keep the pelvic viscera as close as possible to the probe) the uterus is usually anteflexed, so that the fundus comes to lie anterior to the cervix. When imaged from below the cervix is encountered first, in either longitudinal or transverse section, depending on probe orientation. As the transducer is advanced into the posterior fornix of the vagina the body and fundus of the uterus come into view. Commonly the entire length of the uterus can be imaged in one plane, although when it is sharply angled the tomogram may pass through the upper part of the uterus alone, or vice versa. Initially these

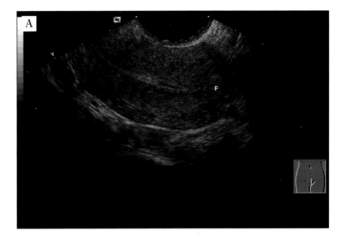

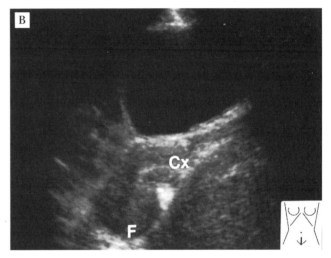

Fig. 1.10 **Retropositioned uterus. A:** on a trans-vaginal scan the appearance is a left-right mirror image of the more usual arrangement where the fundus lies superiorly. **B:** in a transabdominal scan the appearance may be more confusing because the uterine fundus lies further posteriorly than usual and thus may be difficult to evaluate. Cx – cervix; F – fundus.

relationships are confusing: together with the greater detail obtainable the operator may be disorientated, although the true anatomical content is similar but superior to that obtained on transabdominal scanning. A further confusing feature is the prominence of the pelvic veins, which are compressed by the full bladder in transabdominal scans: they are seen as tortuous channels around the uterus and adnexae, in which flowing 'particles' may be visualised, though often the flow velocity is too low for Doppler detection.

Endometrium

The appearance of the endometrium also varies throughout the menstrual cycle,[11] acting as an indicator of oestrogenic and progestogenic stimulation (Fig. 1.11).

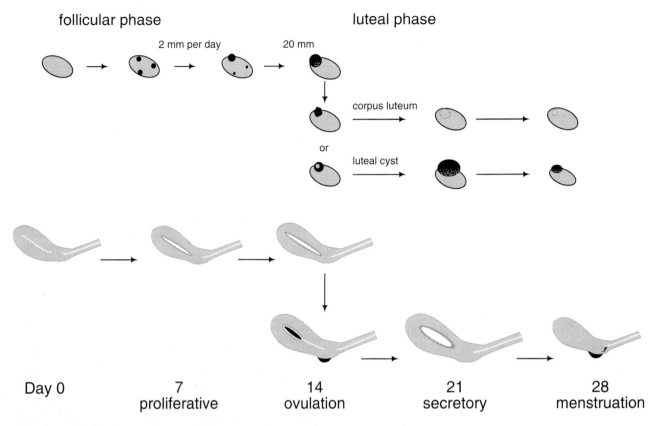

follicular phase

luteal phase

2 mm per day

20 mm

corpus luteum

or

luteal cyst

Day 0 | 7 proliferative | 14 ovulation | 21 secretory | 28 menstruation

Fig. 1.11 Cyclical changes in the ovaries and uterus.

After menstruation, when the majority of the endometrium (the decidual inner layer) has been shed, no endometrial layer is visualised, only a fine cavitary line being demonstrable (Fig. 1.8A, Fig. 1.12). As it thickens in the proliferative phase of the cycle the endometrium becomes more prominent, though it remains relatively echo poor. Through the second, secretory, phase the endometrium continues to thicken, but also becomes more reflective; presumably the strong echoes are caused by the multiple tissue/fluid interfaces as the glands become tortuous and fill with mucin. Towards the end of the cycle the endometrium, measured as the double thickness of the echogenic layers, reaches up to 10 mm.[17] It may have a lower attenuation (probably because of its high fluid content), which may be especially apparent on transverse sections as a bright band over the deeper tissues. The margin between the endometrium and the myometrium may cast an edge shadow, again more obvious on transverse sections.

Following the menopause the endometrium is inactive, though it may remain as a thin layer (<5 mm) for a year or so after the last menstrual period. In taking this double-layer measurement any endometrial fluid is excluded. An inactive endometrium is also characteristic of any condition in which ovulation is suppressed, such as when the contraceptive pill is used and, contrariwise, the post-menopausal endometrium may be prominent in women taking hormone replacement therapy. On the other hand, drugs that have oestrogenic actions, such as tamoxifen, cause the endometrium to thicken, though the changes in this case seem to affect the deepest layers of the myometrium as much as the endometrium.[18,19]

Ovaries

The ovaries are typically oval structures measuring some $4 \times 2 \times 1$ cm (Fig. 1.8B). In practice their shape varies widely from spherical to linear, in addition to the striking functional alterations associated with ovulation.[20] Because of this variation, ovarian size is better evaluated as a volume, closely approximated in millilitres by taking one-half of the product of the three diameters in centimetres. For this measurement any cysts larger than 1 cm in diameter are excluded. The normal volume ranges up to 14 ml at or soon after puberty, and then progressively decreases to about 2.5 ml at the menopause and 0.5 ml by 10 years post-menopause. The two ovaries should be approximately equal in volume: neither should be more than twice the volume of the other. Classically they lie against the pelvic side wall muscles in close proximity to the iliac vessels, but their mobility leads to great variation in their

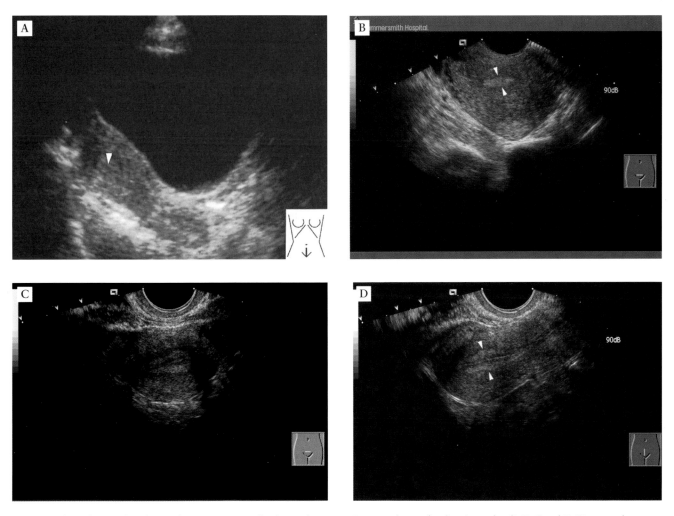

Fig. 1.12 The endometrial cycle. A: After menstruation the thin endometrium is seen only as a fine line (arrowhead). **B, C** and **D:** Hypertrophy through the proliferative and secretory phases of the cycle results in an increase in both thickness and reflectivity (arrowheads) to a maximum double thickness of some 20 mm.

positions (Fig. 1.13). In longitudinal sections they may indent the posterior surface of a well filled bladder.

The ovaries are uniform in texture at the beginning of the cycle (Fig. 1.8B) but soon thereafter the developing follicles can be observed within them (Figs 1.11 and 1.14); initially there are several, but by about the end of the first week one follicle dominates and enlarges progressively at approximately 1 mm per day to reach a diameter of some 20–25 mm by mid-cycle. The follicles are echo-free apart from a few low-level echoes representing the cumulus ovarii that is sometimes visualised on trans-vaginal scanning shortly before ovulation. After ovulation a small amount of free fluid may be detectable in the pouch of Douglas.

The corpus luteum that develops from the follicle forms a mass of about a centimetre in diameter; usually its reflectivity is very similar to that of the normal ovary (Fig. 1.15), but when it forms as a cyst it may be much larger and very obvious. Its irregular walls and low-level

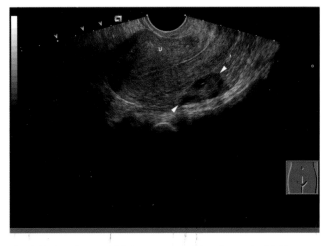

Fig. 1.13 Ectopic ovary. Their mesentery makes the ovaries highly mobile and they may be encountered in unexpected positions, e.g. in the pouch of Douglas, as in this example (arrowheads). U – uterus.

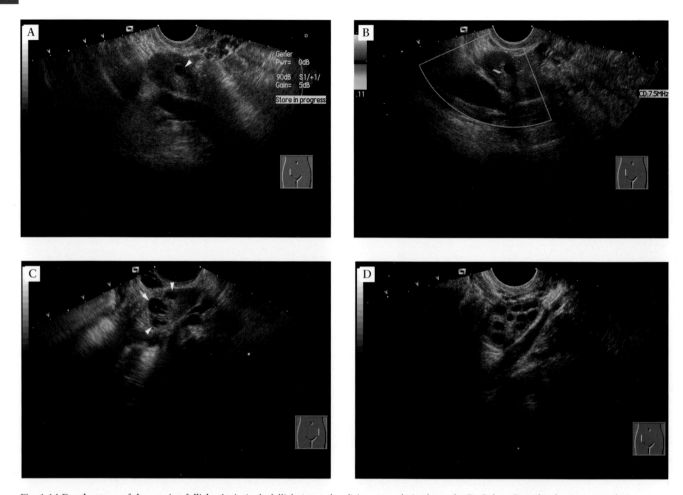

Fig. 1.14 Development of the ovarian follicle. A: A single follicle (arrowhead) is seen early in the cycle. **B:** Colour Doppler demonstrates the moderate vascularity of the ovary. **C:** Several smaller follicles (arrowheads) as well as the dominant follicle (arrow) are seen. **D:** Numerous follicles are sometimes seen as a normal variant, a pattern that also occurs in the stimulated ovary.

internal echoes (possibly due to haemorrhage) may be a cause for concern, and in addition are typically very vascular, with low-impedance signals that can seem suspicious. However, unless a pregnancy occurs the corpus luteum involutes toward the end of the cycle so that, where there is real diagnostic difficulty, a repeat scan after 2 or 6 weeks (i.e. in the follicular phase of the cycle) will usually resolve the dilemma.

The scarred corpora lutea form còrpora albicans, which are usually not apparent on ultrasound, although on high-resolution trans-vaginal studies they form small reflective foci.[21] If a pregnancy ensues the corpus luteum hypertrophies, producing sufficient progesterone to maintain the early pregnancy until 15 weeks, when the placenta takes over progesterone secretion and the corpus luteum atrophies.

The menopause occurs when the supply of ova is exhausted and the pituitary FSH can no longer stimulate an ovarian cycle. The ovaries subsequently atrophy, so that the post-menopausal ovary usually measures 2.0–2.5 ml (upper limit 4 ml) in volume; their symmetry should be maintained, but they may be impossible to locate.

Anomalies

Apart from their variable positions (Fig. 1.13), the ovaries are not subject to anomalies. However, the uterus frequently reveals evidence of its complex embryology from fusion of the paired Müllerian ducts.[22] Complete failure of fusion results in duplication of the uterus, cervix, and occasionally even also of the vagina. This extreme form, the 'didelphic uterus', is rare but minor fusion failures are common, for example where the upper part of the fundus of the uterus has a notch, or where a muscular septum extends inferiorly from the fundus, partially dividing the cavity. On ultrasound these may be evidenced by a widening in the transverse plane of the uterus, and in particular of the endometrial line and, in the more marked variants, in the appearance of two endometrium-lined cavities lying side by side at the upper part of the uterus (Fig. 1.16).

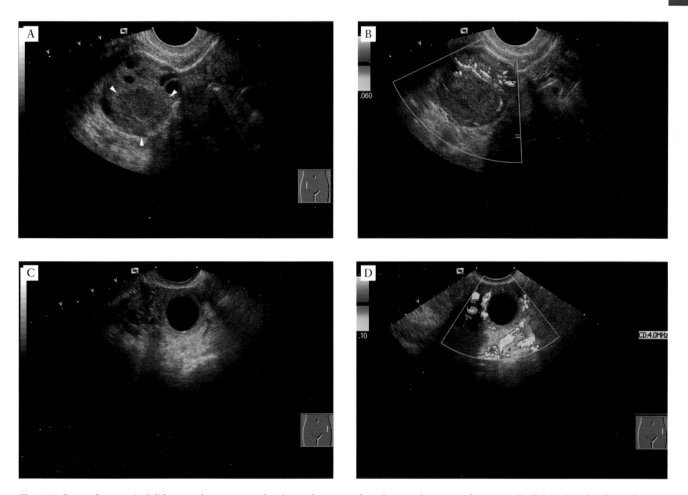

Fig. 1.15 Corpus luteum. **A:** Solid corpus luteum (arrowheads), with very similar echoes to the surrounding ovary. **B:** Colour Doppler shows the increase in vascularity of the surrounding ovary. These changes should settle within 2 weeks. **C:** The corpus luteum may be cystic with a simple appearance, as in this example, or have a complex appearance. **D:** Colour Doppler reveals the neovascularisation.

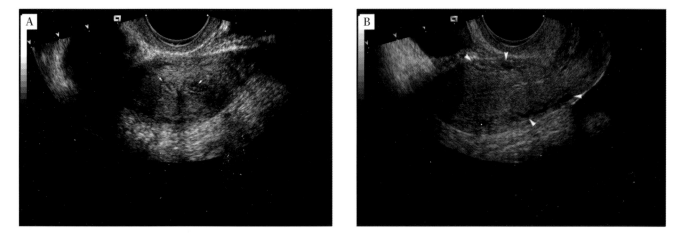

Fig. 1.16 Bicornuate uterus. **A:** A transverse section through the body of the uterus shows the two separate cornua (arrowheads). **B:** In longitudinal section a bicornuate uterus may be difficult to detect. Note the prominent (but normal) uterine veins in the superficial portions of the myometrium (arrowheads). In this patient the left kidney was absent, with compensatory hypertrophy on the right: anomalies of the renal tract are commonly associated with fusion failures of the uterus.

They are better delineated with saline infusion into the uterine cavity,[23] but full evaluation of these anomalies requires a conventional salpingogram.

REFERENCES

1. Netter F. Atlas of Human Anatomy. West Caldwell, New Jersey: Ciba-Geigy, 1989
2. Sanders R C, James A E, eds. The principles and practice of ultrasonography in obstetrics and gynaecology, 3rd edn. Norwalk, Connecticut: Appleton-Century Crofts, 1990
3. Schneck C D. The anatomical basis of abdomino-pelvic sectional imaging. Clin Diagn Ultrasound 1983; 11: 13–41
4. Athey P A, Hadlock F P. Ultrasound in obstetrics and gynaecology, 2nd edn. St Louis: Mosby, 1985
5. Gratton D, Harrington C, Holt S C, Lyons E A. Normal pelvic anatomy using transvaginal scanning. Obstet Gynecol Clin North Am 1991; 18: 693–711
6. Dodson M G, Deter R L. Definition of anatomical planes for use in transvaginal sonography. JCU 1990; 18: 239–242
7. Guy R L, King E, Ayers A B. The role of transvaginal ultrasound in the assessment of the female pelvis. Clin Radiol 1988; 39: 669–672
8. Lenck L C, Vanneuville G. [Schematic sections of the female pelvis]. Rev Fr Gynecol Obstet 1995; 90: 465–470
9. DeLancey J O. The anatomy of the pelvic floor. Curr Opin Obstet Gynecol 1994; 6: 313–316
10. Hansmann M, Hackeloer B-J, Staudach A. Ultrasound diagnosis in obstetrics and gynaecology. Berlin: Springer Verlag, 1985
11. Forrest T S, Elyaderans M K, Muilenberg R I. Cyclical endometrial changes: US assessment with histological correlation. Radiology 1988; 167: 233–237
12. Teele R L, Share J C. Ultrasonography of the female pelvis in childhood and adolescence. Radiol Clin North Am 1992; 30: 743–758
13. States L J, Bellah R D. Imaging of the pediatric female pelvis. Semin Roentgenol 1996; 31: 312–329
14. Sladkevicius P, Valentin L, Marsal K. Transvaginal gray-scale and Doppler ultrasound examinations of the uterus and ovaries in healthy postmenopausal women. Ultrasound Obstet Gynecol 1995; 6: 81–90
15. Ayida G, Harris P, Kennedy S, Seif M, Barlow D, Chamberlain P. Hysterosalpingo-contrast sonography (HyCoSy) using Echovist-200 in the outpatient investigation of infertility patients. Br J Radiol 1996; 69: 910–913
16. Tessler F N, Schiller V L, Perrella R R, Sutherland M L, Grant E G. Transabdominal versus endovaginal pelvic sonography: prospective study. Radiology 1989; 170: 553–556
17. Malpani A, Singer J, Wolverson M K, Merenda G. Endometrial hyperplasia: value of endometrial thickness in ultrasonographic diagnosis and clinical significance. JCU 1990; 18: 173–177
18. Willen R, Lindahl B, Andolf E, Ingvar C, Liedman R, Ranstam J. Histopathologic findings in thickened endometria, as measured by ultrasound in asymptomatic, postmenopausal breast cancer patients on various adjuvant treatment including tamoxifen. Anticancer Res 1998; 18: 667–676
19. Kedar R, Bourne T, Pwowles T et al. Effects of tamoxifen on uterus and ovaries of postmenopausal women in a randomised breast cancer. Lancet 1994; 343: 1318–1321
20. Fleischer A C, Wentz A C, Jones H W. Ultrasound evaluation of the ovary. In: Ultrasonography in Obstetrics and Gynaecology. Philadelphia: WB Saunders, 1988
21. Kupfer M C, Ralls P W, Fu Y S. Transvaginal sonographic evaluation of multiple peripherally distributed echogenic foci of the ovary: prevalence and histologic correlation. AJR 1998; 171: 483–486
22. Letterie G S, Haggerty M, Lindee G. A comparison of pelvic ultrasound and magnetic resonance imaging as diagnostic studies for mullerian tract abnormalities. Int J Fertil Menopaus Stud 1995; 40: 34–38
23. Perrot N, Frey I, Bigot J M. Ultrasono-hysterography: techniques and indications. J Radiol 1996; 77: 687–690

Uterine pathology

Heather Andrews

Introduction

Ultrasound is the initial and often the only method of imaging for uterine pathology. The examination is generally performed either transabdominally and or trans-vaginally, although in certain patients, where it is impossible to perform a trans-vaginal examination a trans-perineal or trans-labial approach may be helpful. A combination of transabdominal (TAS) and trans-vaginal scanning (TVS), together with Doppler studies where appropriate, provides excellent visualisation of the uterus. Frequently no further investigation will be required. However, in specific clinical situations, such as the investigation and staging of uterine and cervical carcinomas, MRI provides more information than ultrasound.

The use of a high-frequency trans-vaginal probe (5–10 MHz) improves resolution at the expense of limited depth penetration, which precludes visualisation of more distant structures. Large pelvic masses, such as uterine fibroids, may prevent adequate visualisation of the uterus and adnexae and transabdominal scanning may be needed. Conversely, when it is necessary to obtain exquisite detail of the endometrial cavity, for instance when a very small endometrial polyp is being sought, then the trans-vaginal approach is superior. It is seldom possible to image satisfactorily a retroverted uterus transabdominally, but the trans-vaginal approach allows excellent visualisation as the probe may be directed posteriorly.

Doppler provides additional information on the uterine and pelvic vasculature. Colour Doppler indicates the general distribution of the vessels and the resistance to flow in the uterine arteries can be assessed with spectral Doppler. The information complements the morphological assessment of the uterus with B-mode and should not be used in isolation, as similar spectral abnormalities are seen with widely differing pathologies.

Whether the examination is carried out transabdominally or trans-vaginally uterine position, size, irregularity of outline and texture should be routinely assessed. The position of a normal uterus depends on the degree of bladder filling and/or loading of the sigmoid colon. Focal myometrial abnormalities should be sought, measured and recorded. The peripherally arranged uterine blood vessels, which may appear as small anechoic collections, should not be mistaken for focal myometrial abnormalities. Particular attention should be paid to the endometrial cavity/stripe, whose layers are measured together, and to focal endometrial abnormalities. The endometrial thickness varies with the stage of the menstrual cycle.

The transabdominal scan can be extended to the upper abdomen where appropriate. When a large pelvic mass is found the kidneys should be examined for hydronephrosis caused by ureteric obstruction due to external ureteric compression or to malignant invasion of the ureter. The upper abdomen may also be examined for metastatic disease, particularly in the liver, but also for abdominal lymphadenopathy and generalised ascites.

In the elderly patient in whom it proves impossible to obtain either a bladder scan or in whom trans-vaginal examination cannot be tolerated, trans-perineal or trans-labial sonography may be a useful alternative.

Other imaging modalities

Magnetic resonance imaging (MRI)

MRI has an important role in the investigation of uterine pathology. Congenital abnormalities and fibroids are well visualised. Cervical and endometrial carcinoma may be diagnosed, staged and followed up to assess recurrence. Normal uterine anatomy is best demonstrated on MRI, with exquisite detail of the zonal architecture of the uterus on T_2-weighted images. The endometrium is seen as a high signal stripe, in contrast to the low signal of the inner myometrium. The outer myometrium is of medium signal.

Computed tomography (CT)

TVS and MRI have gradually replaced CT in the investigation of uterine and other gynaecological pathology, although CT is of great value in the assessment of lymphadenopathy, particularly when assessing for recurrence in patients with pelvic malignancy.

Hysterosalpingography (HSG)/sonohysterography

Both these invasive techniques demonstrate intracavity pathology. HSG is important in the diagnosis of congenital and acquired abnormalities of the uterus and fallopian tubes, but uses ionising radiation and contrast media. Sonohysterography provides similar information without the hazard of ionising radiation. Instillation of saline into the uterine cavity under trans-vaginal ultrasound control gives excellent visualisation of the intracavity anatomy and of any pathology, together with assessment of tubal patency.

Hysteroscopy

Fibre-optic hysteroscopy allows a panoramic endoscopic view of the cervical canal and endometrial cavity. This procedure and sonohysterography have similar diagnostic accuracies, but hysterography has the significant advantage of a therapeutic capability and, together with blind endometrial biopsy, has largely replaced the use of dilatation and curettage. Hysteroscopy is performed under local anaesthetic as an outpatient procedure and is generally used for the investigation of abnormal uterine bleeding and infertility problems. Carbon dioxide insufflation into the uterine cavity allows inspection, diagnosis and treatment of intracavity lesions. Cavity lesions such as polyps and sub-mucosal fibroids may be removed either with a cutting loop resecting hysteroscope or by laser ablation.

At present, when diagnostic accuracy, ease of use and cost are considered, ultrasound is overall the primary diagnostic tool in the female pelvis. In future, when MRI becomes cheaper, it will play a greater role in gynaecological imaging. However, developments in ultrasound technology, with further refinements of Doppler techniques and the development of 3D ultrasound, will further enhance the present pre-eminent role of ultrasound in gynaecological imaging.

Abnormal bleeding

Defined as any non-cyclical genital tract bleeding, abnormal bleeding may occur at mid-cycle in normal or anovulatory cycles; however, it rarely persists for more than 2–3 cycles. Irregular bleeding is often dysfunctional in nature, but may result from pelvic pathology.

Classification of abnormal uterine bleeding

Menorrhagia: heavy menstrual periods, defined as a measured menstrual loss of more than 80 ml per cycle.

Dysfunctional uterine bleeding (DUB): irregular or non-cyclical uterine bleeding, often heavy, that results from endogenous or exogenous hormonal fluctuations such as anovulation or hormone replacement therapy (HRT).

Inter-menstrual bleeding (IMB): bleeding between periods, usually caused by uterine pathology, most commonly an endometrial polyp.

Post-coital bleeding (PCB): bleeding following intercourse; it generally results from cervicitis or vaginal wall pathology.

Post-menopausal bleeding (PMB): bleeding that commences more than a year after the last period.

The causes of menorrhagia fall into four categories: pelvic pathology, dysfunctional uterine bleeding, bleeding disorders and general medical disorders. Thus, many patients complaining of menorrhagia presenting for ultrasound will have an entirely normal examination. The commonest gynaecological causes of menorrhagia are fibroids, adenomyosis and endometrial polyps.

Abnormal vaginal bleeding (syn. abnormal uterine bleeding)

Although most abnormal vaginal bleeding is of uterine origin, it may also emanate from the cervix and vagina (Table 2.1). Non-gynaecological causes should also be considered.

Table 2.1 Causes of abnormal bleeding

Uterus
  fibroids
   adenomyosis
   endometrium
    hyperplasia
     polyp
     carcinoma
   pregnancy-related problems
   endometritis
    chronic
     atrophic, post-menopausal
   secondary uterine influences
    exogenous oestrogen production
    HRT, tamoxifen
    ovarian or adrenal tumours
   blood dyscrasias
   anticoagulants
Cervix
  polyp
  chronic cervicitis
  carcinoma
Vagina
  vaginitis
   infection, atrophy, trauma
  carcinoma
Non-gynaecological causes
  haematuria
   rectal bleeding

Hormonal influences on the endometrium

The endometrium is a specialised form of mucous membrane whose sonographic appearance reliably reflects the hormonal status of the patient. The active endometrium measures up to 12 mm in double-layer thickness, although prior to the menarche and after the menopause it is very thin (<3 mm). Hormonal stimulation is provided by naturally secreted oestrogen and progesterone, although exogenously administered hormones produce a similar effect. Oestrogen is responsible for the early proliferative phase of the menstrual cycle, and progesterone for involution in the secretory phase. An inappropriate endometrial pattern not characteristic of either the proliferative or the secretory phase of the cycle suggests ovarian dysfunction or hormonal imbalance. During the later menstrual years modest uterine enlargement occurs, almost certainly due to the effect of oestrogen unopposed by progesterone, and is associated with anovulatory cycles. This slight increase in size should not be considered pathological.

Endometrial atrophy

Endometrial atrophy results from oestrogen deficiency; it is normal in post-menopausal women, and in pre-menopausal women presents as oligomenorrhoea or

Table 2.2 Causes of endometrial atrophy

Endogenous causes
    premature ovarian failure
    perimenopausal period
    menopause
    excessive androgens

Exogenous medications
    oral contraceptive pill (OCP)
    progesterone compounds
        medroxyprogesterone (Depoprovera)
        danazol

Pelvic irradiation

amenorrhoea (Table 2.2). Whatever the cause, sonographically the endometrium appears as a thin white line less than 5 mm thick. It is often too thin to measure accurately.

Endometrial thickening

During childbearing years the normal endometrium measures up to 12 mm; after the menopause it falls to less than 5 mm (double layer). The thicker the endometrium the greater the likelihood of significant pathology (Table 2.3).

Post-menopausal bleeding

The menopause results from a natural fall in endogenous oestrogen levels at an average age of 53 years. Menstruation ceases and the endometrium atrophies. Irregular bleeding is common in the perimenopausal period, i.e. 1 year before and after the menopause. Post-menopausal bleeding (PMB), defined as bleeding from the genital tract at least 1 year after the last menstural period, divides into three groups: 10% have endometrial carcinoma, 10% have significant benign pathology, and the remaining 80% have no significant pathology. Overall the commonest cause of PMB is atrophic endometritis. Investigation depends on trans-vaginal sonographic visualisation of the endometrium with or without biopsy.

Accurate measurement of endometrial thickness is straightforward in the post-menopausal woman as it is not subject to cyclical variation. A thorough survey of the endometrial cavity in both sagittal and axial planes should be made, looking for any disturbance of the texture such as irregularity, cystic change or reflective foci. The sub-endometrial echo-poor halo should be assessed in both axial and sagittal planes. It should be symmetrical and well defined with benign pathology. Asymmetry of the halo or endometrium is highly suggestive of significant pathology, whatever the overall thickness of the endo-metrium.[1] The thickest part of the endometrium (usually towards the uterine fundus) should be measured in the mid-sagittal plane in the section that includes the cervical canal. Both reflective layers are measured, excluding any fluid in the cavity. Several studies have established that in normal post-menopausal women the endometrial thickness does not exceed 5 mm.[2,3] Sonohysterography may be of great value when a focal lesion is identified.

The adnexae should be screened for any ovarian mass, such as an oestrogen-secreting tumour.

Diagnostic difficulties

Accurate measurement of the endometrial thickness is occasionally difficult to obtain, particularly if the uterus lies in an axial position; in such cases it is preferable that no sonographical assessment should be made.[4] Other uterine pathology, especially fibroids, may make identification of the endometrial cavity impossible, either trans-abdominally or trans-vaginally. Sonohysterography or MRI may be of value in difficult cases.

Aetiology (Table 2.4)

Obese women may have endometrial thickening owing to increased amounts of endogenous oestrogen being stored in their body fat, and the endometrial thickness may be directly related to their body mass index.[5] Treatment with

Table 2.3 Causes of endometrial thickening

Secretory phase of normal menstrual cycle
Decidual reaction in early pregnancy
Infections, i.e. endometritis
Endometrial hyperplasia/polyp
Endometrial carcinoma
Increased endogenous oestrogen
    ovarian tumours
    adrenal tumours
Oestrogen-type medications
    hormone replacement therapy (HRT)
    tamoxifen

Table 2.4 Aetiology of endometrial thickening

Uterine
    normal friable atrophic endometrium (commonest cause)
    endometrial hyperplasia/polyp
    endometrial carcinoma

Cervix
    chronic cervicitis
    cervical carcinoma

Vagina
    atrophic vaginitis
    mechanical injury
        ring pessary
        procidentia
    tumour

Non-gynaecological
    urinary tract
    rectal

Table 2.5 Algorithm for management of PMB

Endometrial thickness (mm)	Action
Less than 5	No further action whether bleeding or asymptomatic
5–8	If bleeding, perform biopsy If not bleeding, consider biopsy Interval ultrasound
8	Biopsy regardless of history

exogenous hormones such as HRT and tamoxifen may produce endometrial thickening.

The accuracy of measurement is generally good, and it should be possible to measure endometrial thickness to within 1 mm.[6] Unfortunately, a definitive diagnosis cannot be made with ultrasound alone and, in particular, endometrial carcinoma cannot be excluded.[7] In a study of 1000 women presenting with PMB, using 4 mm as the upper limit of normal, no endometrial carcinomas were missed and two carcinomas measuring 5 mm were identified. The study provided a sensitivity of 96% and a negative predictive value of 97%.[8] In another study of 103 women with PMB the endometrial thickness provided some indication of pathology. Patients with endometrial atrophy had a mean thickness of 6.2 mm, whereas those with endometrial hyperplasia and endometrial carcinoma had mean measurements of 13 and 14 mm, respectively.[9]

Measurements of the uterine artery resistance index have not proved to be reliable in distinguishing between benign and malignant disease.

Some gynaecologists biopsy the endometrium regardless of the sonographically measured endometrial thickness, whereas others use an algorithm similar to that given in Table 2.5. Unfortunately, biopsy either by D&C, using a 2.5 mm plastic endometrial aspiration device (Pipelle) or undertaken at hysteroscopy, may not be entirely satisfactory as it is impossible to sample the entire endometrial cavity. In contrast, a properly conducted ultrasound examination will allow a survey of the whole cavity in most patients.

In summary

A normal post-menopausal patient will have an endometrial thickness of less than 3 mm. In patients receiving HRT a measurement of up to 8 mm is generally regarded as satisfactory. With endometrial hyperplasia or carcinoma an average measurement of 15 mm may be expected.

Medications and the endometrium

Oral contraceptive pill

This is generally a combined oestrogen and progesterone compound taken cyclically. The unstimulated endometrium characteristically appears as a 'single line' which is slightly thicker than that seen in post-menopausal women.[10] There may also be a slight overall increase in uterine size. Ovarian follicular development may occur, typically with multiple small, randomly arranged cysts.

Hormone replacement therapy (HRT)

Women in the western world will spend at least one-third of their lives in a state of relative oestrogen deficiency, and HRT is commonly prescribed as a remedy. HRT alleviates post-menopausal symptoms and, more importantly, reduces the incidence of osteoporosis and the morbidity and mortality of cardiovascular disease. Numerous different formulations are available; most contain oestradiol, the main natural form of oestrogen produced by the ovaries. Oestrogen is an effective agent, but when given alone up to 40% of women will develop endometrial hyperplasia.[11] There is also an increased risk of endometrial carcinoma.[12] In order to protect the patient from these unwanted effects progesterone is normally added to the oestrogen in order to effect endometrial atrophy. There are two main regimens:

1. continuous combined (continuous oestrogen and progesterone to produce permanent amenorrhoea and endometrial atrophy),
2. cyclical/sequential (oestrogen for days 1–25 and progesterone from days 15–25).

On ultrasound the uterus may enlarge[13] and the vascular resistance may fall, with a reduction in the pulsatility index (PI).[14] The two regimens may produce different sonographic appearances. Continuous combined treatment results in an atrophic endometrium (<5 mm thickness) and this does not change through the month (Fig. 2.1A).

Cyclical treatment may cause endometrial thickening (>8 mm in 15%)[15] (Fig. 2.1B), and this may vary by 3 mm through the cycle.[16] Thus, if there is doubt over the measurements the examination should be repeated at a different stage in the cycle, preferably post-bleed.

Tamoxifen

Tamoxifen is the most important non-surgical method of treatment for breast cancer in both pre- and post-menopausal women, producing a significant recurrence-free period and an increase in overall survival time. Its exact mechanism is imprecisely understood owing to the paradoxical nature of its effects. It is a non-steroidal anti-oestrogenic compound which binds to oestrogen receptors in the breast. This antagonistic action is in contrast to its agonistic oestrogen effect on the genital tract.[17] Tamoxifen produces endometrial pathology of a variable nature, both benign and malignant. Endometrial metaplasia, hyperplasia, polyps and carcinoma are histologically recognised. There is a sixfold increase in the instance of endometrial carcinoma in women treated with 40 mg tamoxifen daily

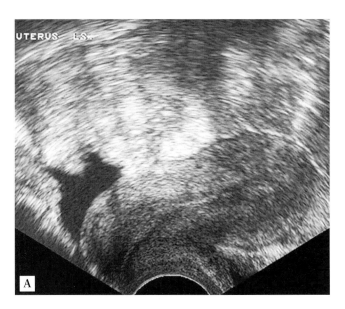 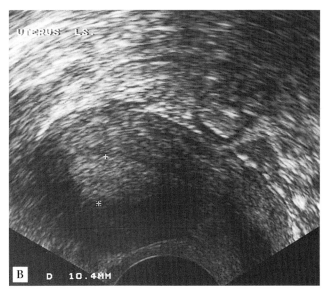

Fig. 2.1 Normal and thickened endometrium. A: Sagittal TVS showing normal endometrial thickness in patient receiving continuous combined HRT. **B:** Sagittal TVS showing thickened endometrium in post-menopausal patient receiving cyclical HRT (10 mm AP).

for 5 years.[19] The effect on the uterus is more marked when treatment is commenced many years after menopause, compared with that begun in the peri-menopausal period. The risk of endometrial carcinoma is cumulative and depends on the dose and length of treatment. Interestingly, HRT does not produce the same response as tamoxifen, perhaps because of endometrial shedding, although it may also be associated with endome-trial carcinoma. More recently it has become recognised that the myometrium also responds to tamoxifen, with the development of subendometrial cysts, which may represent a form of adenomyosis.[20] (Fig. 2.2).

On ultrasound there is moderate generalised increase in uterine size,[21] with a variable increase in myometrial thickness and reflectivity. Polyps may develop in the endometrium (Fig. 2.3) and a central reflective region may be found, often containing cystic areas (Fig. 2.4). Doppler studies may show abnormal blood flow with low-impedance diastolic flow, which is not normally expected following the menopause.

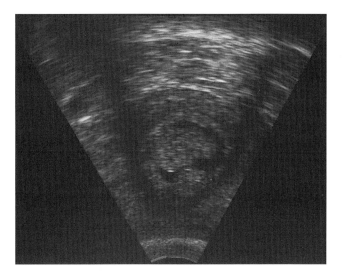

Fig. 2.2 MRI scan of the uterus. T_2-weighted sagittal MRI scan of the uterus, showing marked endometrial hyperplasia with small subendometrial cysts.

Fig. 2.3 Endometrial polyp. Axial TVS of endometrium showing a large tamoxifen-induced polyp outlined with a little fluid.

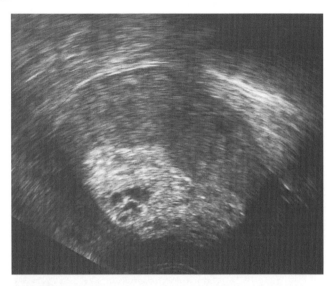

Fig. 2.4 **Tamoxifen associated endometrial appearances.** Sagittal TVS showing a typical tamoxifen-induced central reflective endometrial mass with cystic areas within.

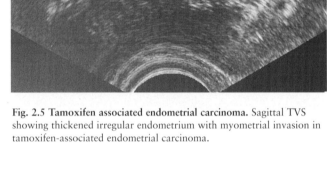

Fig. 2.5 **Tamoxifen associated endometrial carcinoma.** Sagittal TVS showing thickened irregular endometrium with myometrial invasion in tamoxifen-associated endometrial carcinoma.

It may be difficult to determine the nature of the central uterine 'mass' and, if it is thicker than 10 mm, significant pathology may be expected. Sonohysterography demonstrates endometrial polyps and Doppler studies may be useful as the atrophic endometrium is poorly vascularised, in contrast to endometrial carcinomas.

Management of patients with endometrial/myometrial thickening

The management of patients with endometrial or myometrial thickening is difficult. Less than 8% of normal post-menopausal women have an endometrial thickness >10 mm, compared to 50% of women receiving tamoxifen, in whom one-third also have polyps.[17,22,23] At present neither uterine morphology nor Doppler studies allows good enough definition between tamoxifen changes and endometrial carcinoma (Fig. 2.5) and biopsy may be necessary.

Overall, if the endometrium is not thickened no action is required, but if it is >5 mm sonohysterography may be helpful and any abnormalities found should be biopsied. Some authorities suggest that women receiving tamoxifen should have an annual TVS whether they are symptomatic or not.[24–26]

Dysfunctional uterine bleeding

Dysfunctional uterine bleeding (DUB) is a greater diagnostic challenge in the premenopausal woman than in those presenting with post-menopausal bleeding because of the wider range of possible pathologies. Most are of hormonal origin but other pathologies, such as bleeding disorders,

endometritis, adenomyosis and fibroids, must be considered. Sonographically endometrial thickening is found in about one-third of patients with DUB and this may be useful to direct appropriate therapy, progesterone being prescribed for those with thickened endometrium and combined oestrogen and progesterone for those with endometrial thinning.[27]

Endometrial hyperplasia

This common condition presents with abnormal uterine bleeding, most commonly in the late reproductive years. It is usually a response to unopposed or excessive oestrogen, whether endogenous or exogenous in origin (Table 2.6). It is found in up to 10% of all endometrial biopsy specimens.

Histological examination of the endometrium will demonstrate an abnormal proliferation of the endometrial glands and stroma (Fig. 2.6). Dilated glands will produce a cystic appearance (Fig. 2.7).

Three histological forms of hyperplasia are recognised: cystic, adenomatous and atypical. The cystic form, which

Table 2.6 Aetiology of endometrial hyperplasia

Reproductive years
obesity
polycystic ovary syndrome
idiopathic
Perimenopausal
anovulatory cycles
exogenous oestrogens
Post-menopausal
tamoxifen

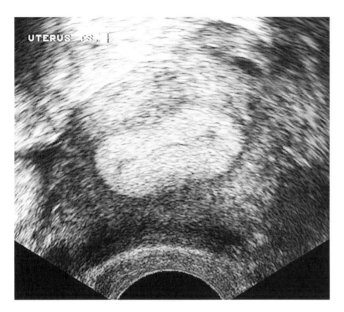

Fig. 2.6 **Endometrail hyperplasia.** Axial TVS showing markedly reflective thickened endometrium due to endometrial hyperplasia (20 mm AP).

Table 2.7 Ultrasound appearances of endometrial hyperplasia

Endometrium
  thickened (usually >1 cm)[29] (Fig. 2.6)
  highly reflective and unchanging through the menstrual cycle
  multiple small cysts in cystic type (Fig. 2.7).

Uterus
  moderate enlargement may occur if the endometrium is very thick

Ovaries
  functional cysts common, often multiple

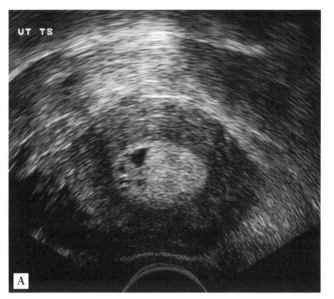

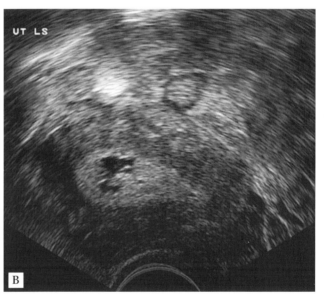

Fig. 2.7 **Cystic endometrial hyperplasia. A:** Axial and **B:** sagittal TV scans demonstrating cystic endometrial hyperplasia.

may produce a cystic appearance on ultrasound, is not considered premalignant, but the other two types are. They cannot be differentiated on ultrasound and the differential diagnosis includes endometrial polyps, endometrial carcinoma and trophoblastic disease.[28] (Table 2.7).

Causes of increased uterine reflectivity (Table 2.8)

Polyps are not true tumours but are merely focal areas of adenomatous or hyperplastic endometrium covered with epithelium; they range in size from 0.5 to 5.0 cm, but are rarely larger than 1 cm.[28,30] They may be single or multiple and may be situated anywhere in the uterine cavity. Although generally sessile, they may be pedunculated and may extrude into the cervical canal or upper vagina. Polyps generally develop in women aged 35–50, being most common in perimenopausal patients. Presentation is with inter-menstrual bleeding, other menstrual problems and vaginal discharge. The true incidence is unknown, as small polyps are often unrecognised at curettage. There is an association with infertility. Polyps are usually benign, particularly in premenstrual women, but are found in some 10% of patients with endometrial cancer, although only 1% undergo malignant change.[31] They are best visualised trans-vaginally, especially if saline is instilled. They are seen as a small, well defined reflective mass (Fig. 2.9), which may be surrounded by fluid, particularly if it secretes serous fluid or bleeds (Fig. 2.10). They may be mobile and may prolapse through the cervical canal (Fig. 2.11), and there is often associated endometrial thickening and hyperplasia (Fig. 2.12). Polyps are commonly multiple (Fig. 2.13).

Table 2.8 Causes of increased uterine reflectivity

Endometrium
    secretory phase of normal menstrual cycle
    HRT in the post-menopausal patient
    endometrial polyp and or hyperplasia
    endometrial carcinoma

Endometrial cavity contents
    haematometra/pyometra
    retained products of conception
    trophoblastic disease

Myometrium
    fibroids
    all causes of uterine calcification
    lipoma/lipomatous degeneration in a fibroid

Vascular calcification
    arcuate arteries (hypertension, renal failure and diabetes mellitus)
      (Fig. 2.8)

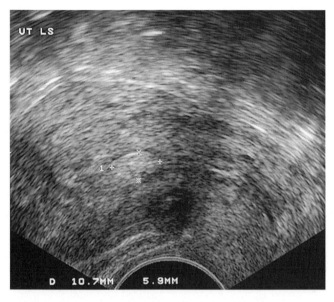

Fig. 2.9 Endometrial polyp. Sagittal TVS showing reflective endometrial polyp lying in the mid-cavity.

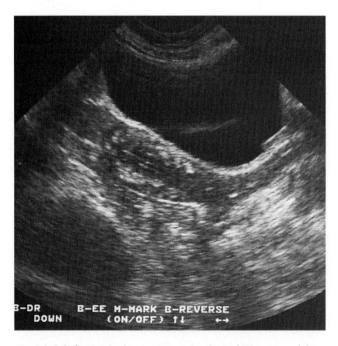

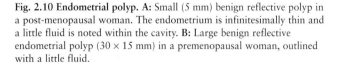

Fig. 2.8 Calcification in the arcuate arteries. Sagittal TA section of the uterus in a post-menopausal woman showing punctate calcification in the uterine arcuate arteries.

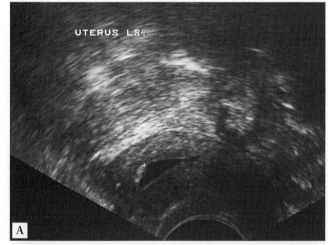

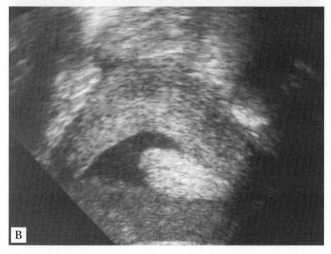

Fig. 2.10 Endometrial polyp. A: Small (5 mm) benign reflective polyp in a post-menopausal woman. The endometrium is infinitesimally thin and a little fluid is noted within the cavity. **B:** Large benign reflective endometrial polyp (30 × 15 mm) in a premenopausal woman, outlined with a little fluid.

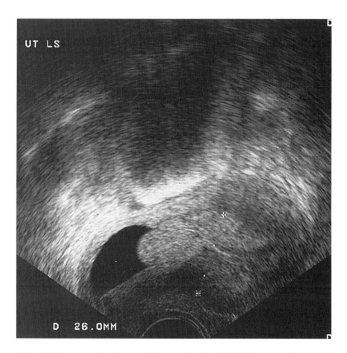

Fig. 2.11 Prolapsed endometrial polyp. Sagittal TVS of uterus showing distended fluid-filled cervical canal containing a reflective prolapsed uterine endometrial polyp.

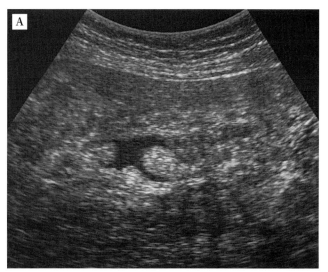

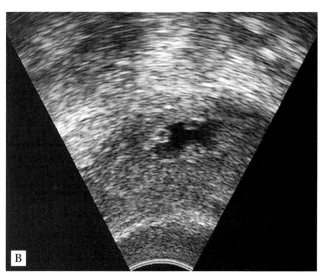

Fig. 2.13 Endometrial polyp. A: Axial TA scan showing multiple reflective polyps outlined with fluid in the endometrial cavity of a fibroid uterus in a premenopausal woman presenting with inter-menstrual bleeding. **B:** Axial TVS of the uterus showing three small, unusual, relatively echo-poor benign polyps within the fluid-filled endometrial cavity in a post-menopausal woman.

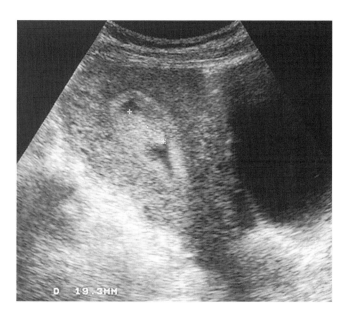

Fig. 2.12 Endometrial polyp with endometrial hyperplasia. Sagittal TA scan of uterus showing 19 mm reflective polyp associated with endometrial hyperplasia.

Polyps may be difficult to distinguish from endometrial carcinoma and hyperplasia, particularly as they may be associated. The blood supply to the polyp via the pedicle can generally be demonstrated with colour Doppler (Fig. 2.14). The examination is best performed early in the menstrual cycle in the proliferative phase, when the thin, relatively less reflective endometrium allows better discrimination between the polyp and normal endometrium. Blood clot may be mistaken, but a polyp will be unchanged at a follow-up examination. A submucosal fibroid may be mistaken for a polyp, but a relatively echo-poor lesion with a broad base continuous with the myometrium with associated acoustic shadowing should suggest the diagnosis (Fig. 2.15). Sonohysterography is the ideal method of diagnosis.[32]

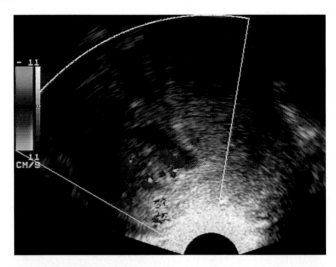

Fig. 2.14 The blood supply to an endometrial polyp. Axial TVS of the uterus showing blood supply to a benign endometrial polyp.

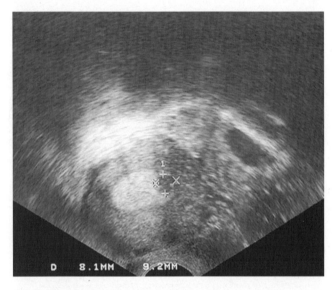

Fig. 2.15 Submucosal fibroid. Axial TVS of the uterus showing a small echo-poor submucosal fibroid in a patient with endometrial hyperplasia.

Carcinoma of the endometrium

The incidence of endometrial cancer is gradually increasing as a result of the ageing population and the many oestrogenic compounds prescribed during a woman's life. It is the fourth commonest female malignancy, with 4000 new cases per annum in the UK. Most patients are post-menopausal: 80% present with post-menopausal bleeding at a peak age incidence of 60 years. The longer the interval between the menopause and the onset of PMB the more likely is the cause to be neoplastic. Histologically 90% are adeno-carcinomas, with a few squamous cell or other unusual tumours, such as mixed Müllerian tumours with both car-cinomatous and sarcomatous elements. The malignancy develops in the glandular element of the endometrium, which produces increased secretions; this may account for the high reflectivity typical of these tumours.

Many predisposing factors have been identified, but a common link is the effect of unopposed oestrogen stimulation on the endometrium. They include a family history of breast and endometrial carcinoma, late menarche and early menopause, nulliparity or low parity, anovulatory conditions (e.g. polycystic ovary syndrome), medications (exogenous oestrogens such as the pill, tamoxifen, HRT), endogenous oestrogens (oestrogen-producing tumours, i.e. granulosa–theca-cell tumour of the ovary), medical conditions (hypertension, diabetes mellitus) and premalignant endometrial pathology (e.g. polyps, hyperplasia).

Endometrium carcinoma has been shown to develop in patients with high oestrogen levels, in apparent contradiction to the higher incidence in post-menopausal patients, who would be expected to have relatively low oestrogen levels. The explanation seems to relate to the even lower levels of progesterone in the post-menopausal period, which allows relative unopposed oestrogen activity.[33] There is some reduction of risk in patients who have taken the oral contraceptive pill.

The ultrasound appearances depend on the timing of presentation. Most present with the disease confined to the endometrium. A few patients present with more advanced disease, often with a pelvic mass. The examination should be performed trans-vaginally, and Doppler studies and sonohysterography may be of value.

In patients with confined disease the uterus is not enlarged but usually endometrial thickening is obvious, with measurements of 15 mm and more (Fig. 2.16). The endometrium is reflective and heterogeneous in texture, with small cystic areas often apparent. There may be fluid in the cavity, and this often reveals the irregularity of the endometrial surface just as is seen on sonohysterography (Fig. 2.17). The endometrial–myometrial junction should be assessed for poor definition and irregularity to determine whether there has been myometrial invasion by the tumour (Fig. 2.18). In practice this is often difficult to assess except in advanced disease. Small cornual carcinomas may be missed unless the cavity is very carefully assessed in both scan planes.

In the presence of more advanced tumours the uterus enlarges and sonographic assessment is more difficult, and the resulting large pelvic mass may be mistaken for uterine fibroids or an ovarian mass. The mass may have a smooth or irregular outline, often with a very heterogenous texture (Fig. 2.19). Cervical invasion produces a stenosis, often complicated by haematometra or pyometra. The intracavitary fluid may outline polypoid tumours (Fig. 2.20). There may be signs of local spread, with invasion of local structures, ascites, lymphadenopathy, and distant spread to the liver.

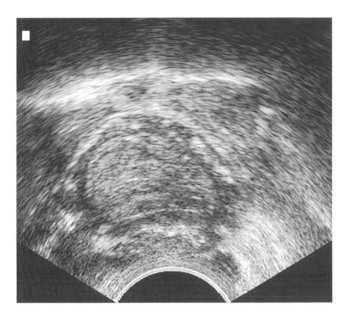

Fig. 2.16 Endometrial carcinoma. Axial TVS of the uterus with reflective cavity mass (20 mm AP) in a post-menopausal patient with endometrial carcinoma. There is no myometrial invasion. Note arcuate artery calcification.

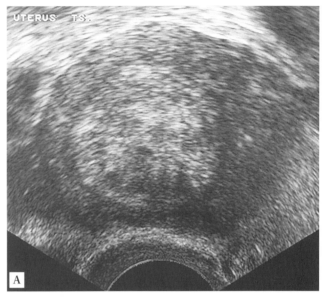

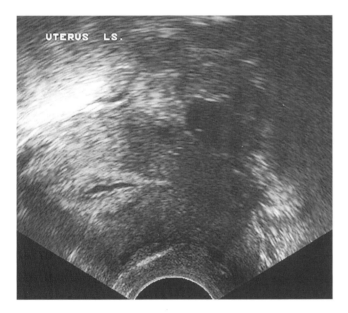

Fig. 2.17 Endometrial carcinoma. Sagittal TVS of uterus showing irregular endometrial thickening with a little cavity fluid in a patient with endometrial carcinoma.

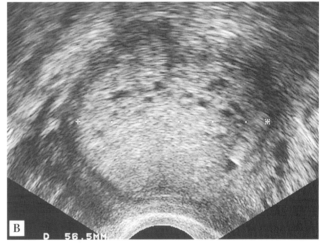

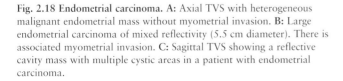

Fig. 2.18 Endometrial carcinoma. A: Axial TVS with heterogeneous malignant endometrial mass without myometrial invasion. **B:** Large endometrial carcinoma of mixed reflectivity (5.5 cm diameter). There is associated myometrial invasion. **C:** Sagittal TVS showing a reflective cavity mass with multiple cystic areas in a patient with endometrial carcinoma.

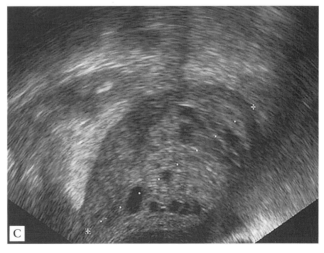

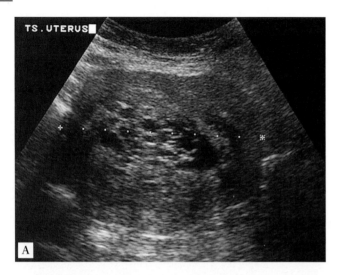

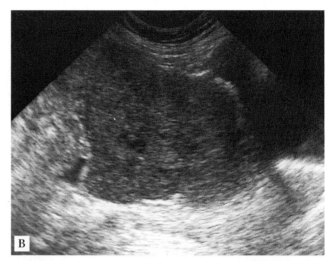

Fig. 2.19 Advanced endometrial carcinoma. A: Axial TA scan showing 9 cm complex endometrial carcinoma. **B:** Sagittal TA scan showing unusual large lobulated solid advanced endometrial carcinoma.

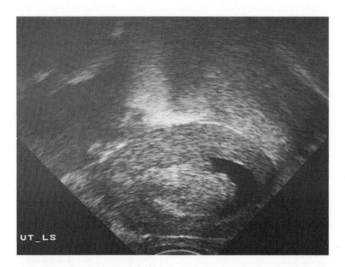

Fig. 2.20 Lobulated endometrial carcinoma. Sagittal TVS showing lobulated endometrial carcinoma outlined with fluid. This appearance is similar to a benign endometrial polyp (see Fig 2.10B).

The premenopausal endometrium is highly vascular, but after the menopause it becomes hypovascular with a concomitant increase in vascular resistance. However, when endometrial pathology such as hyperplasia or carcinoma develops the situation is reversed, and Doppler studies demonstrate low-impedance flow. Tumour angiogenesis results in most endometrial carcinomas being highly vascular, with many abnormal blood vessels coursing through the tumour (Fig. 2.21). The resistance indices reduce in both the intratumoral vessels and in the main uterine arteries, with a PI typically less than 1. In one series the main PI was 0.49, with a range of 0.3–0.92.[34] However, these results are not discriminatory, as similar values may be obtained in some women with HRT or tamoxifen-related endometrial hyperplasia. Thus at present Doppler indices must not be used in isolation, but should be seen as an adjunct to the morphological appearance.

Other investigations

MRI is the investigation of choice for staging endometrial carcinoma, with T_2-weighted images clearly portraying widening of the endometrial cavity (Fig. 2.22). Assessment of the junctional zone is crucial to the staging of early disease. Although this is clearly defined in premenopausal women, after the menopause it may become indistinct. However, an intact transitional zone confirms that the disease is confined to the endometrium and is thus staged as IA. Intravenous contrast agents such as gadolinium produce tumour enhancement and may be useful in assessing the degree of myometrial invasion.[35] Although MRI delineates pathology well, it does not differentiate between endometrial malignancy and hyperplasia; in most instances a histological diagnosis will have been made prior to staging MRI. This modality also demonstrates cervical extension of the tumour, haematometra, parametrial extension, extension to other pelvic organs and lymphadenopathy. The accuracy of MRI in diagnosing myometrial invasion varies between 71 and 97%, and the accuracy in correctly staging endometrial carcinoma varies between 85 and 92%.

CT is not regarded as being as valuable as MRI in staging endometrial carcinoma owing to its inability to differentiate some fibroids from tumour, or to determine the depth of myometrial invasion or to detect rectosigmoid invasion. In particular, CT is unable to differentiate between stage I and stage II disease. However, it is of value in the assessment of recurrent disease in the chest, abdomen and pelvis.

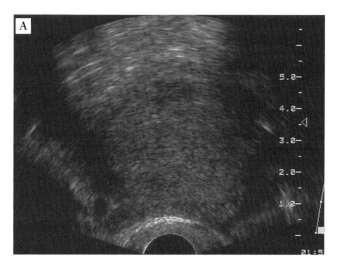

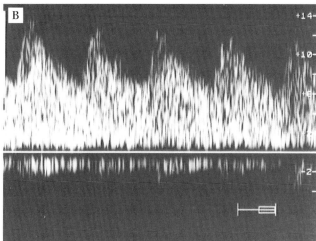

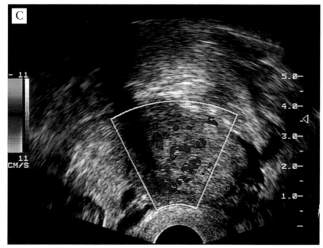

Fig. 2.21 **Endometrial carcinoma vascularity. A,B** and **C:** Large vascular endometrial carcinoma with typical spectral Doppler pattern.

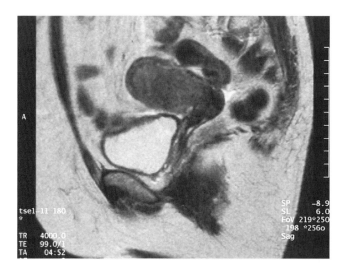

Fig. 2.22 **Myometrial invasion.** Sagittal T$_2$-weighted MRI scan showing large endometrial tumour with myometrial invasion.

Management

The definitive diagnosis is normally made histologically following sonographic or clinical diagnosis. There is a very close correlation between the accuracy of TVS and hysteroscopy in detecting early endometrial carcinoma, with 100% identification at hysteroscopy and a 95.8% identification at TVS.[36] Ultrasound, however, is generally inadequate for accurate staging. These tumours are clinically staged using the classification of the Fédération Internationale de Gynécologie et Obstétrique (Table 2.9).

However, in 20% of patients the stage is underestimated on ultrasound,[37] and so nowadays tumours are staged by MRI. The prognosis depends upon the degree of myometrial invasion and the presence of lymphadenopathy. Assessment of the uterine zonal anatomy is important in staging, and although TVS will demonstrate myometrial invasion, the exquisite detail of uterine anatomy seen on T$_2$-weighted MRI is superior.

Table 2.9 FIGO staging of endometrial carcinoma

Stage	Description
IA	Carcinoma confined to the corpus
IA	The length of the uterine cavity is 8 cm or less
IB	The length of the uterine cavity is greater than 8 cm
II	Carcinoma has involved corpus and cervix but has not extended outside the uterus
III	Carcinoma has extended outside the uterus but not outside the true pelvis
IV	Carcinoma has extended outside the true pelvis, or has obviously involved the mucosa of the bladder or rectum
IVA	Carcinoma has spread to adjacent organs
IVB	Carcinoma has spread to distant organs

Whereas stage IA and IB disease is managed surgically, stage II disease is treated with pre-operative radiotherapy. Stage III and IV disease are treated with DXR only. Surgery involves total abdominal hysterectomy and bilateral salpingo-oophorectomy, with lymph node dissection as required. With stage I disease there is a 95% 5-year survival, which reduces to 50% for stage IV disease. Overall an 85% 5-year survival rate can be expected.[38]

Haematometra and related conditions

Obstruction of the female genital tract may occur at differing levels – usually distal to the introitus, but also at varying levels in the vagina, or more proximally at the level of the cervix. In the child or adolescent obstruction may result from an intact hymen or vaginal obstruction, which may be due to atresia, stenosis or the presence of an obstructing membrane (see Vol. 2, Ch. 50). In adults the obstruction is usually at the cervical level, whatever the cause (Table 2.10). Obstruction leads to an accumulation of fluid, which may be serous (mucus secretion by cervical or vaginal glands) or contain menstrual blood (the commonest) or pus. In the neonate and infant maternal hormonal stimulation of the endometrium means that the cavity fluid will be menstrual blood. Fluid accumulation produces distension of the organs above the level of the obstruction. Coexistent urinary tract anomalies are common in these patients and must always be sought.[39]

Table 2.10 Aetiology of adult cervical obstruction

Fibrotic atrophy in the elderly
Tumour
　cervical, endometrial and vaginal carcinoma
Radiation therapy
　external or intracavity
Trauma
　post-instrumentation
　cervical cone biopsy

The terminology used for these conditions depends on the level of the obstruction and the nature of the contained fluid. When blood is contained the following terms are used:

Haematocolpos – vaginal distension
Haematometrocolpos – vaginal and uterine distension
Haematometra – uterine distension alone
Haematosalpinx – distension of the fallopian tubes.

If the fluid is serous in nature the term hydro- is prefixed, or pyo- if an infection or pus is present.

Presentation is variable, but abdominal pain, pelvic mass, amenorrhoea and urinary obstruction are common presenting features.

A central cystic lower abdominal mass of varying shape, size and reflectivity is apparent on ultrasound. It is often impossible to determine the nature of the fluid, but internal echoes suggest the presence of blood or pus. Multiple, almost confluent, fine low-level echoes similar to those seen with an endometriotic cyst suggest the presence of altered blood. Occasionally this may be highly reflective, and layering may be seen in the fluid. When no internal echoes are present the fluid is likely to be serous. There may be associated ascites.

In *vaginal distension* a large tubular cystic fluid-filled structure is seen low and centrally in the pelvis (Fig. 2.23 a and b). In general the uterine component is relatively small and recognised in continuity with the superior aspect of the mass (Fig. 2.24). Although abdominal sonography allows the diagnosis of vaginal obstruction the precise level and nature of the lesion canot be determined, although the level is usually at the junction of the middle and lower thirds of the vagina. In order to plan reconstructive surgery it is essential to know not only the level of the obstruction, but also its cause. Trans-perineal ultrasound, using a stand-off device, produces very satisfactory images and can be used to evaluate the length of the stenotic segment (usually 1–4 cm), and demonstrates any solid tissue septum extending from the caudal aspect of the distended vagina to the perineum.[40] MRI is frequently employed to produce definitive images of the anatomical abnormality.

In *uterine distension* a fluid-filled central pelvic mass is identified: the normal uterine body cannot be seen. Depending on the the pathology there may be associated distension of the vagina and fallopian tubes. The normal cervix has a relatively fibrous nature and is thus not very distensible, so that it produces an 'hourglass' constriction between the dilated uterus above and the vagina below (Fig. 2.25). The contents of the fluid-filled uterine cavity may be mistaken for retained products of conception. The cervix must be identified so that a distinction may be made between a haematocolpos and a haematometrocolpos.

Haematotrachelos, or distension of the cervix with blood, is rare: it may be congenital or may develop as a

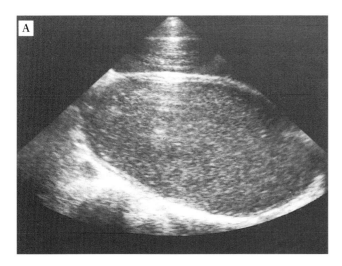

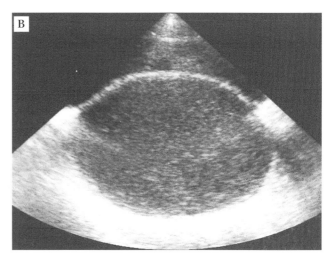

Fig. 2.23 Haematocolpos. A: Sagittal and **B:** axial TA scans in a 15-year-old girl presenting with amenorrhoea. There is a large tubular sausage-shaped structure in the lower pelvis with fairly confluent internal echoes typical of altered blood in a haematocolpos resulting from an intact hymen.

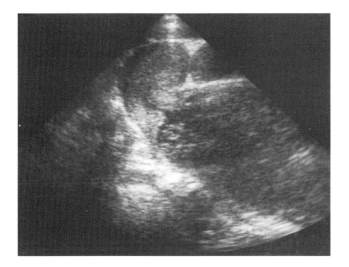

Fig. 2.24 Haematocolpos. Sagittal TA scan of pelvis in same patient as Fig. 2.23, showing haematocolpos with normal uterus at the upper pole of the vaginal mass.

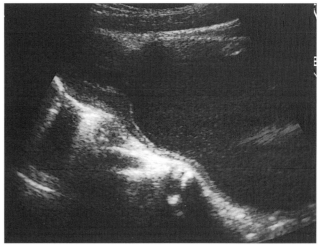

Fig. 2.25 Haematocolpos. Sagittal TA pelvic scan showing hourglass appearance in haematometrocolpos in a 13-year-old with distal vaginal atresia presenting with amenorrhoea.

complication of cervical cone biopsy (Table 2.10) The congenital type is usually associated with vaginal atresia and should be differentiated from a high vaginal septum. Sonographically the normal cervix cannot be identified and the relatively thick-walled cervical canal is distended with blood[41] (Fig. 2.26). It should be noted that a mass in the body of the uterus, such as a pedunculated fibroid or polyp, may protrude into the cervical canal and cause significant distension.

Dilatation of the fallopian tubes is most commonly infective in nature. However, it may rarely result from lower genital tract obstruction and be unilateral or bilateral, depending on the nature of the obstruction. Thus when there is a haematometra the adnexae should be examined for evidence of tubal dilatation. An uncommon cause of unilateral fallopian tube dilatation in the elderly is fallopian tube carcinoma. The ultrasound appearances are characteristic of a hydrosalpinx, with a serpiginous adnexal mass connecting to the uterine cornua. Problems with the diagnosis may be encountered when only one moiety of a uterus didelphys is obstructed. The unobstructed moiety is assumed to be a normal uterus and the obstructed moiety may be mistaken for a cystic adnexal mass.

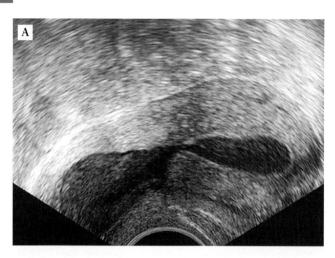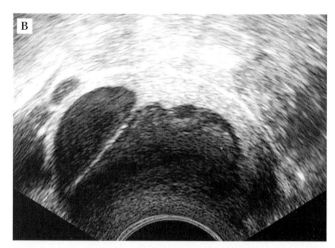

Fig. 2.26 Haematotrachelos and haematometra. A and **B:** Sagittal and axial TV images of the cervix showing haematotrachelos and haematometra in a patient with cervical stenosis. In addition, on the axial view a large fluid distended cervical gland is noted.

Pelvic inflammatory disease (PID)
(Table 2.10)

Endometritis

Endometritis is an acute infective process involving the endometrium and may be acute or chronic (Table 2.11). When associated with PID, endometritis develops as a result of an ascending venereal infection, passing from the vagina to the fallopian tubes and adnexae via the uterine cavity.[42] Normal endometrium is relatively resistant to infection because of the cyclical menstrual shedding and consequent drainage of infected material. The common causal agents are the venereal organisms *Chlamydia trachomatis* and *Neisseria gonorrhoeae*, although less commonly coliforms and staphylococci may be implicated.[43] As a result of the infection, the endometrium becomes oedematous and hyperaemic. Rarely, secondary inflammation of the myometrium causes myometritis.

Table 2.11 Aetiology of endometritis

Ascending infection
   pelvic inflammatory disease
Post-invasive procedure
   cervical biopsy or cautery
   uterine instrumentation
   hysterosalpingogram
   IUCD insertion
   endometrial biopsy
Pregnancy associated
   premature rupture of membranes
   post-abortion
   post-partum
   prolonged labour
Haematogenous spread
   TB

The clinical presentation is very variable, depending on the chronicity of the infection. Abnormal bleeding is unusual, but occasionally there may be hypo- or amenorrhoea. A vaginal discharge may be associated with lower abdominal pain and pyrexia. The diagnosis is made by endometrial biopsy and culture of the organisms.[44] In the long term there may be infertility and, rarely, Asherman's syndrome may develop.

The ultrasound appearances are very variable and are commonly normal. Non-specific abnormalities are an echo-poor moderately enlarged uterus with an indistinct outline,[45] loss of the endometrial–myometrial junction, and an echo-poor myometrium when myometritis develops. The endometrium may be thickened and reflective, with reactive fluid in the cavity (Table 2.12). If the cavity fluid is purulent it may appear very reflective, with multiple internal echoes and intracavitary gas if an anaerobic organism is responsible (Fig. 2.27). There is rarely significant distension of the uterine cavity, as the fluid readily drains through the cervical canal. Other signs of infection, such as free fluid, an adnexal mass or abscesses or a pyosalpinx, should be sought.

In one series 94% of post-menopausal women with significant fluid collections had endometrial or cervical carcinomas (Fig. 2.28).[46]

Uterine fibroids

Fibroids (more correctly, fibroleiomyomas) are the most common uterine tumour, affecting 40% of women over 35.[47] They are nine times more common in women of Afro-Caribbean origin, in whom they tend to be large, multiple, and develop at a relatively early age.[48] Fibroids are benign tumours composed of smooth muscle fibres, very similar to normal myometrium, with a variable fibrous connective tissue element. The fibrous tissue is

Table 2.12 Uterine cavity fluid collections

Infancy and childhood (pre-menarche)
    hydro/haematocolpos
    hydro/haematometrocolpos

Menstrual years
    menstrual fluid
    pregnancy
        normal early pregnancy
        intra-uterine haematoma
        ectopic pregnancy – pseudogestation sac
        retained products of conception
    endometrial pathology
        hyperplasia
        polyp
        carcinoma
    infection, endometritis
    Cervical obstruction

Post-menopausal
    normal (small amount) (Fig. 2.28)
    endometrial pathology (as above)
    cervix – atrophic stenosis
    cervical or endometrial carcinoma

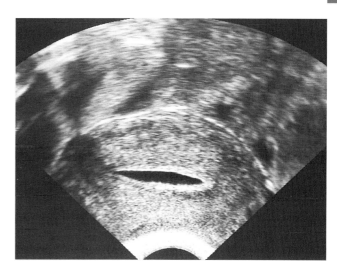

Fig. 2.28 Axial view of the uterus showing a small amount of intracavitary fluid. The endometrium is not thickened.

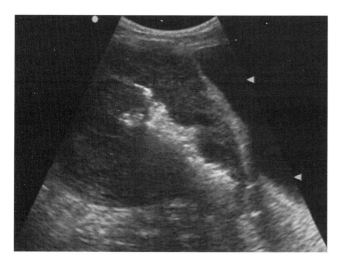

Fig. 2.27 Post-partum endometritis. Sagittal TA scan of the uterus in patient with post-partum endometritis. The uterus is appropriately enlarged and gas is noted in the cavity from a gas-forming organism.

arranged in concentric whorls, which may account for some of the ultrasound appearances. The fibroid is smooth in outline, with only a thin layer of connective tissue separating it from the normal myometrium. As they enlarge they tend to outgrow their blood supply and areas of central necrosis and cystic degeneration may appear. The malignant potential of the fibroid is thought to be very small (around 0.2%). The malignant form is a leiomyosarcoma, but probably most cases arise *de novo*, although many are found in association with fibroids.

The aetiology is unknown, but there is a known association with oestrogens, which stimulate the growth of these tumours. Fibroids are associated with nulliparity, which suggests a relationship with continuous oestrogen stimulation uninterrupted by pregnancy and lactation. Fibroids are also more commonly seen in the obese, and may enlarge in pregnancy or following treatment with tamoxifen. The risk of developing fibroids reduces with increasing parity, use of the oral contraceptive pill and smoking. Although fibroids normally shrink following the menopause, HRT may cause a modest increase in size. The risk factors are thus very similar to those of endometrial carcinoma, i.e. high and unopposed oestrogen levels.[49]

Characteristically fibroids do not develop until after the menarche; they enlarge during the reproductive years and shrink after the menopause. They vary from a few millimetres to 20 cm in size. Their presentation is very variable and does not always relate to size; indeed, very large fibroids may be asymptomatic, whereas small lesions may present with serious menstrual disorders. Menorrhagia, menstrual irregularity and dysmenorrhoea are common presenting features.[50] However, presentation depends on the patient's age, together with the number, site and type of lesion. A pelvic mass, which may be palpable, can produce urinary symptoms by pressure on the bladder. Occasionally a large mass may cause rectal compression and discomfort.

In 98% of patients fibroids are multiple.[51] The majority arise in the uterine body, only 3% developing in the cervix (Fig. 2.29), most commonly in the intramural myometrium, although some migrate into subserosal or submucosal positions (Figs 2.30 and 2.31). The 5% that are submucosal are disproportionally symptomatic, as the increased endometrial surface area may cause menorrhagia. Submucosal fibroids may become polypoid and enlarge the area of the uterine cavity.[48] Pedunculated sub-

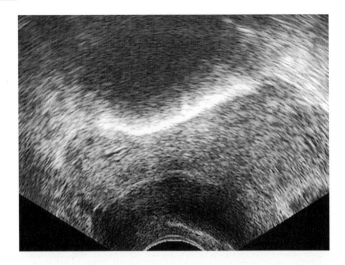

Fig. 2.29 Cervical fibroid. Sagittal TVS of cervix and uterus showing small posterior cervical fibroid.

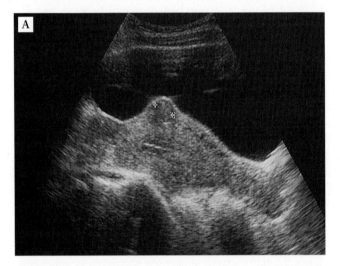

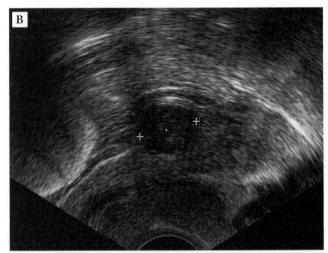

Fig. 2.30 Subserosal fibroids. A: Sagittal TA scan shows a small (13 mm) subserosal anterior fibroid. **B:** Sagittal TVS showing a 21 mm posterior subserosal fibroid.

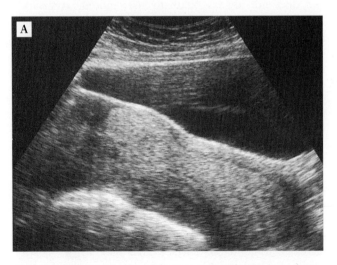

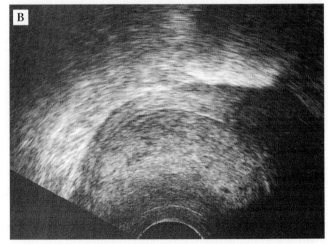

Fig. 2.31 Prolapsed submucosal fibroid. Large prolapsed reflective pedunculated submucosal fibroid distending the cervical canal. **A:** Sagittal TA view, **B:** Axial TV view of cervix.

Table 2.13 Differential diagnosis of uterine enlargement (most commonly oestrogen mediated, with generalised enlargement)

Physiological
    menarche
    late menstrual years
    pregnancy
    post-partum uterus (concealed pregnancy)
Uterine pathology
    fibroid
    adenomyosis
    endometrial/myometrial tumour
    trophoblastic disease
    fluid distension of the uterine cavity
Medications
    oral contraceptive pill
    tamoxifen
    hormone replacement therapy

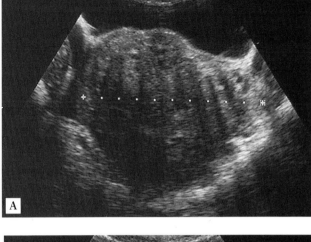

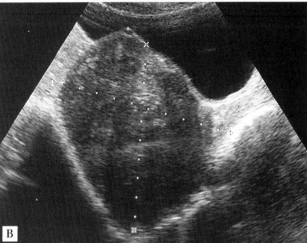

Fig. 2.32 **Large irregular fibroid mass. A:** Axial and **B:** sagittal TA images showing heterogeneous texture and diverging 'Venetian blind' sign.

mucosal fibroids may prolapse through the cervical canal to cause pain, inter-menstrual bleeding and, if very large, uterine invagination. Subserosal fibroids may project anteriorly, posteriorly or laterally from the uterine surface. Laterally projecting fibroids may lie within the layers of the broad ligament and simulate an adnexal mass. Indeed, some fibroids may develop independently within the broad ligaments. Some very superficial subserosal fibroids may become pedunculated and mobile, and may occasionally lie at some distance from the uterine body.

The varied sonographic appearance of fibroids mirrors the variability of their histology. Uterine enlargement is common, particularly in symptomatic patients (Table 2.13). Most fibroids are ovoid or spherical, producing an irregularity of the outline of the uterus which may appear very lobulated and indent the bladder (Fig. 2.32). The uterine cavity may be distorted and appear undulating (Fig. 2.33). The texture of fibroids depends on the relative percentage of smooth muscle and connective tissue within the tumour: they may be echo poor, highly reflective or isoreflective with the myometrium. In some patients a combination of all these appearances may be present (Fig. 2.34). Acoustic shadowing may produce the characteristic 'Venetian blind' appearance when the fibrous tissue produces diverging linear bands of shadowing (Fig. 2.32A). Calcification is often present. The common punctate form (Fig. 2.35) is most marked in older patients, in whom the calcification can be very dense and prevent through transmission of the ultrasound beam, making it impossible to perform a satisfactory sonographic study; an abdominal radiograph is therefore required. Circumferential rim calcification is also common, especially following degeneration and subsequent necrosis (Fig. 2.36). Central cystic areas may follow necrosis. They

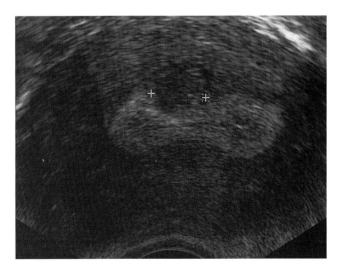

Fig. 2.33 **Fibroid distorting the uterine cavity.** Axial TVS showing a small (12 mm) submucosal fibroid producing an undulating endometrial sign.

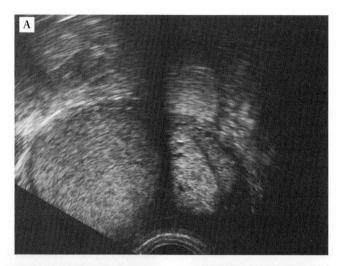

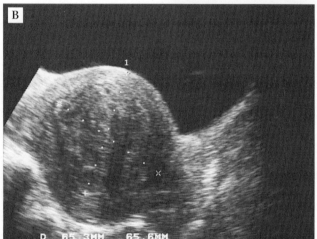

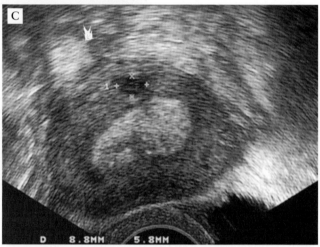

Fig. 2.34 Varying appearances seen in fibroids. A: Axial TVS of uterus showing reflective left-sided fibroid (note thickened endometrium). **B:** Sagittal TA scan shows a single 6.5 cm fibroid of mixed reflectivity. **C:** Axial TVS shows a small echo-poor intramyometrial fibroid.

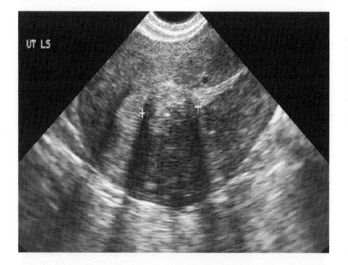

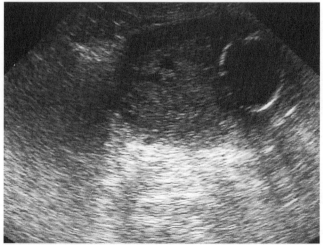

Fig. 2.35 Punctate calcification in a fibroid. Axial TVS shows a small (15 mm) submucosal fibroid with punctate calcification.

Fig. 2.36 Rim calcification in a fibroid. Axial TA scan shows circumferential rim calcification in a fibroid.

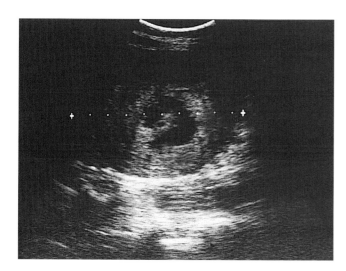

Fig. 2.37 Fibroid with cystic degeneration. Sagittal TA scan showing cystic degeneration of a fibroid in pregnancy.

may be irregular or smooth in outline, with occasional septa, fluid–fluid levels and solid inclusions (Fig. 2.37). A large fibroid uterus may compress the bladder and the ureters, and so when a large fibroid is found the kidneys should always be examined for hydronephrosis. Generally fibroids are less vascular than the adjacent myometrium (Fig. 2.38). The blood flow characteristics of fibroids are very variable, with a wide spectrum of impedance and velocity values. Larger masses reduce the impedance in the main uterine arteries and the myometrial branches. Thus a low-resistance high-velocity waveform may be expected. However, this finding is of little diagnostic value, as similar findings occur with other uterine pathologies.[52]

There are many potential problems in the ultrasound imaging of fibroids. Identification of the ovaries may be

difficult because of their very high or very low lie in the pelvis when a large mass is present. Determination of whether a large pelvic mass is uterine or ovarian in origin may be difficult or impossible, especially if the bladder cannot be filled sufficiently. A retroverted uterus presents particular problems with visualisation. The posterior position of the fundus and the increased attenuation of the beam owing to the vertical lie of the body of the uterus may simulate the presence of a fundal fibroid on transabdominal examination. Trans-vaginal sonography resolves these problems and demonstrates the uterine outline, the myometrial texture and the normal position of the central endometrial echo.

Subserosal and broad-ligament fibroids can be mistaken for ovarian or other adnexal masses – the ovaries must be separately identified and the trans-vaginal sonographic equivalent of a bimanual pelvic examination may be valuable in this clinical situation: with the operator's hand on the patient's hypogastrium, when the probe is gently manipulated it is possible to demonstrate whether the uterus and the mass move separately. Normally the pelvic organs slide over each other, but a subserosal fibroid will not show this differential movement. Ovarian fibromas may be particularly confusing, as their reflectivity is identical to that of a fibroid. Conversely, cystic uterine fibroids may mimic ovarian cysts and other cystic masses.[53] A bicornuate uterus may give the impression of a normal uterine body with an adjacent fibroid, but the presence of the two central endometrial echo complexes allows differentiation (Fig. 2.39). This problem is compounded in pregnancy, when asymmetrical enlargement of the pregnant and non-pregnant horns is more likely to produce an erroneous diagnosis of a fibroid. The presence

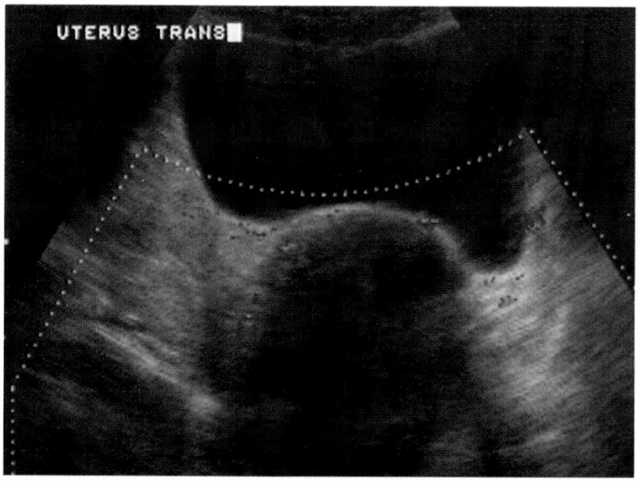

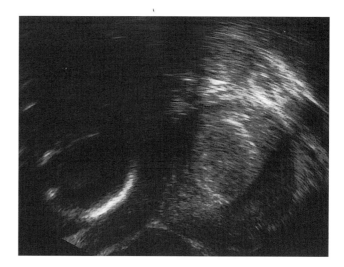

Fig. 2.38 Fibroid blood flow. Axial TA scan showing a large, mainly avascular uterine fibroid with only peripheral blood flow apparent with colour flow Doppler.

Fig. 2.39 Bicornuate uterus mimicking fibroid. Axial TVS of a gravid bicornuate uterus at 14 weeks gestation. The non-pregnant horn mimics a fibroid, but the presence of the desidual reaction allows differentiation.

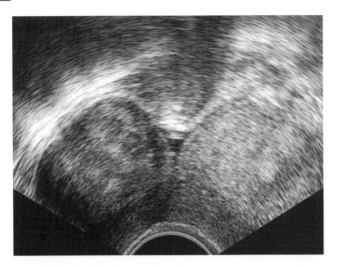

Fig. 2.40 Pedunculated fibroid. Axial TVS of the uterus showing a left-sided pedunculated fibroid separated from the uterine body by a small amount of fluid. Note the difference in texture between the fibroid and the normal uterine body.

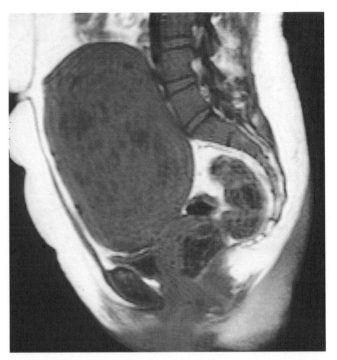

Fig. 2.41 MRI scan of a fibroid. Sagittal T_1-weighted MRI scan of a large uterine fibroid.

of a decidual reaction in the non-pregnant horn should be sought.

Pedunculated fibroids pose a particular diagnostic problem as they may appear entirely separate to the uterine body (Fig. 2.40). Depending on the length of the pedicle, the fibroid may be very mobile and lie outside the true pelvis, even on the opposite side. Colour Doppler may identify the pedicle. Pedunculated fibroids are particularly prone to torsion and degeneration, generally presenting with a painful tender adnexal mass. Doppler studies may reveal absent or reduced flow within the pedicle and/or mass.

Ultrasound fails to demonstrate approximately 22% of fibroids, particularly those smaller than 5 mm.[54] MRI has proved helpful in the assessment of uterine fibroids and its multiplanar imaging clearly demonstrates their size, number and location, as well as the details of their internal architecture (Fig. 2.41). Fibroids are shown as being well defined and of low signal intensity on T_1- and T_2-weighted images. However, necrosis produces high signals on the T_2 images.[55] MRI detects 92% of fibroids, including those as small as 5 mm. When myomectomy is being considered in the subfertile patient a very precise knowledge of the fibroid's anatomy is required, and in this clinical situation MRI is often superior to ultrasound.[56]

Fibroids and adenomyosis may coexist and it may be difficult or impossible to differentiate them on ultrasound; however, MRI may be of value.[57]

Fibroids and pregnancy

Several recent series have contradicted the traditional teaching that fibroids increase in size during pregnancy. Indeed, 78% are unchanged or even decrease in size.[58] The presence of fibroids may be a contributory factor in many complicated pregnancies but conversely, pregnancy may not adversely affect a pre-existing fibroid.

Changes in the uterine blood supply in pregnancy may render a fibroid ischaemic and produce painful acute necrosis and cystic degeneration. Most cases are treated expectantly, but occasionally emergency myomectomy is required.

Fibroids may block the tubal ostia or prevent implantation of the embryo because they distort the uterine cavity. However, a review of 670 patients undergoing surgery for preservation or enhancement of fertility revealed that in only 2% could no other cause for infertility be found.[50]

Spontaneous abortion in the first or second trimester is more common because of abnormal placentation and there is an increased risk of ectopic pregnancy.

Compression effects mainly occur in the third trimester: they lead to fetal compression deformities and malpresentation, and may be particularly important with cervical fibroids. Cavity distortion leads to an increased incidence of placental abruption, antepartum haemorrhage, retained placenta, post-partum haemorrhage and premature rupture of the membranes. When a fibroid lies in the lower uterine segment or cervix normal vaginal delivery may be impossible. All these problems are likely to be exacerbated if there are multiple fibroids.[59,60]

For the most part the ultrasound appearances are very similar to those in the non-pregnant uterus. In pregnancy

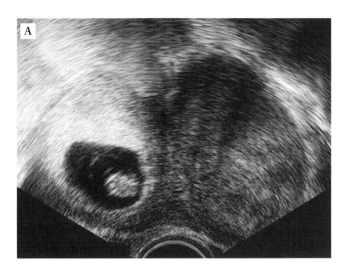

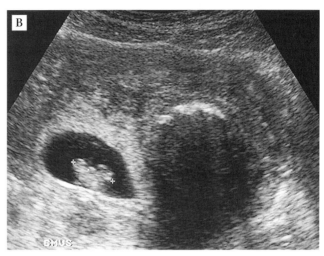

Fig. 2.42 Fibroids and pregnancy. A: Axial TVS of 8-week gestation pregnancy with large associated fibroid. **B:** Sagittal TA scan showing 8-week fetus with a calcified fibroid adjacent to the gestation sac.

the majority of fibroids are echo poor; some are heterogeneous and a few have a highly reflective rim, in part due to calcification which may simulate the appearance of the fetal head or, if incomplete, fetal parts[48] (Fig. 2.42). Cystic degeneration is a common feature.

Braxton Hicks uterine contractions can be distinguished from fibroids by their transient alteration in the myometrial contour and their normal reflectivity. It may be necessary to wait up to 20 minutes for the contraction to pass to confirm that the apparent uterine mass is indeed a Braxton Hicks contraction.

Treatment of fibroids

Ultrasound may also be used to monitor response to treatment, which is not simply indicated by the size of the fibroids. Previously hysterectomy was the only surgical treatment, but myomectomy based on imaging findings may be performed when hysterectomy is undesirable, for example in women wishing to enhance their fertility. Gonadotrophin-releasing hormones (GnRH analogues) are hypo-oestrogenic agents, being derivatives of the hypothalamic hormone LHRH (luteinising hormone-releasing hormone). Their continuous administration suppresses the pituitary–ovarian axis, inducing a pseudomenopause. Typically fibroid volume reduces by 50%; however, once treatment is stopped the fibroids regrow and 80% of patients become symptomatic again.[61] These changes may be monitored with serial ultrasound. Recently the technique of uterine artery embolisation has gained favour for the treatment of fibroids, and although it is too early to assess the results, work in two centres has shown up to a 50% reduction in uterine volume, with significant amelioration of symptoms.[62]

Uterine adenomyosis

Adenomyosis is a common benign condition that often coexists with endometriosis. Histologically endometrial glands and stroma invade the basal layer of the myometrium, causing a reactive proliferation. Up to 20% of hysterectomy specimens show this condition. The typical patient is a middle-aged multiparous woman presenting with menorrhagia and dysmenorrhoea. In contrast, the typical patient with endometriosis is nulliparous, in her 20s or 30s, presenting with infertility.

The disease is usually generalised, although a localised focus may be termed an adenomyoma. Generalised adenomyosis involves the inner two-thirds of the myometrium of the body of the uterus, cervical involvement being very rare. It is said that caesarean section may predispose to adenomyosis because of implantation of the endometrium in the myometrium at the time of surgery. The differential diagnosis includes dysfunctional uterine bleeding and fibroids, which often cannot be differentiated either clinically or sonographically.[63]

Frequently the sonographical appearances will be entirely normal or, if abnormal, may be non-specific. Moderate symmetrical uterine enlargement due to myometrial thickening is found in up to three-quarters of patients. The uterus is generally smooth in outline, often with a normal endometrial and myometrial texture (Fig. 2.43). Occasionally small cystic areas measuring 2–4 mm are apparent (Fig. 2.44). Rarely larger cysts measuring up to 3 cm in diameter may be present[64] (Fig. 2.45). A focal adenomyoma may occasionally be recognised as a small bulge on the uterine surface with or without a change in texture. The myometrium may develop a somewhat coarse and irregular appearance, with areas of

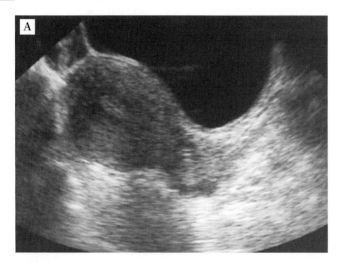

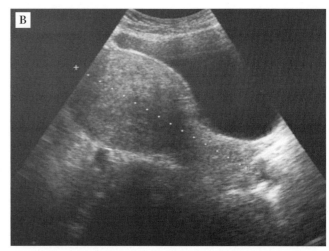

Fig. 2.43 Adenomyosis. A and **B:** Sagittal TA scans of two patients with diffuse adenomyosis. Note the spherical shape of the uterine body and the bland texture.

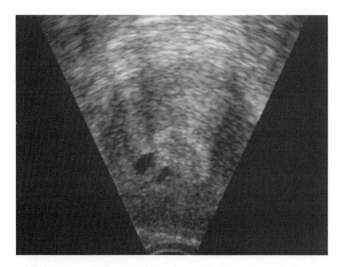

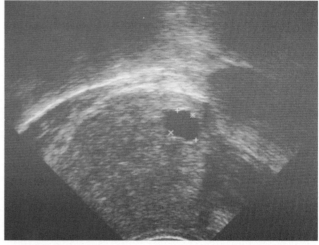

Fig. 2.44 Cystic adenomyosis. Axial TVS showing a small cystic intramyometrial areas of adenomyosis.

Fig. 2.45 Cystic adenomyosis. Axial TV uterine scan with 13 mm area of cystic adenomyosis

increased and decreased reflectivity (Fig. 2.46). Colour Doppler may show areas of increased blood flow adjacent to foci of adenomyosis. A variant of adenomyosis may be seen in patients receiving tamoxifen therapy[65] (Fig. 2.47).

Adenomyosis may coexist with fibroids, in which case a precise diagnosis may be difficult. There may also be evidence of extra-uterine endometriosis, with the presence of single or multiple adnexal endometriotic cysts.

Ultrasound is therefore a poor discriminator in diagnosing adenomyosis. MRI is more valuable, demonstrating both focal and diffuse forms of the disease, particularly on T_2-weighted images.[66] Focal lesions are shown as myometrial masses with ill-defined borders, which may contain small high-signal focal areas of haemorrhage. Diffuse disease may be demonstrated as isointense thick-

ening of the junctional zone. Coincidental endometriomata may be identified. Overall MRI is significantly more reliable in distinguishing between adenomyosis and fibroids than is sonography.[57]

Adenomyomatosis is treated with anti-oestrogens such as GnRH analogues to suppress menstruation.

Asherman's syndrome

Total or partial obliteration of the uterine cavity by adhesions may follow uterine instrumentation. Most (90%) of these adhesions, also known as synechiae, develop as a result of over-zealous curettage following abortion, termination of pregnancy, or in the post-partum period. Less commonly they are caused by myomectomy or caesarean

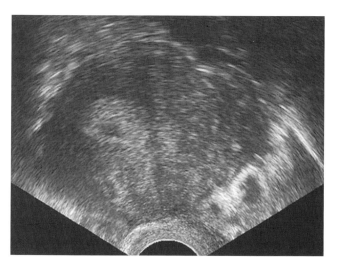

Fig. 2.46 Adenomyosis. Axial TV scan of an irregularly shaped uterus with heterogeneous echo pattern in a patient with adenomyosis. This appearance is very similar to that seen with diffuse uterine fibroids.

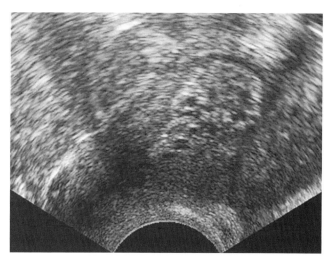

Fig. 2.47 Tamoxifen induced adenomyosis. Sagittal TV uterine scan showing a complex, partly reflective partly cystic central uterine mass, which is a tamoxifen-induced variant of adenomyosis. Normal curettings were obtained in this patient.

section, and occasionally result from endometritis. The hormonal changes of pregnancy produce myometrial softening, which allows the basal layers of the endometrium to be removed by curettage, and this produces scarring. As healing occurs fibrinous bands bridge the apposing endometrial walls. Symptoms and signs are variable but include amenorrhoea, hypomenorrhoea and dysmenorrhoea. Infertility may result from tubal occlusions and implantation problems. Should pregnancy ensue there is an increased risk of early miscarriage and, later, of postpartum haemorrhage and placental retention.

Asymmetrically located single or multiple highly reflective foci in the endometrial cavity or at the endometrial–myometrial junction mark the sites of adhesions (Figs 2.6 and 2.48 A). They measure only a few millimetres across and do not produce acoustic shadowing.[67] These reflective foci are common in older women and are generally asymptomatic and require no further investigation. In the infertile woman the diagnosis may be suspected on ultrasound and require further investigation by hysterosalpingography, sonohysterography or hysteroscopy. Treatment is by division of the adhesions at hysteroscopy. Adhesions straddling the amniotic cavity may be demonstrated in the second and third trimesters of pregnancy as thick membranes producing paired communicating intra-amniotic cavities.[68] (Fig. 2.49)

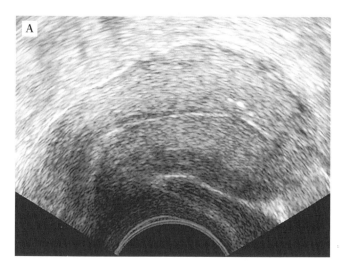

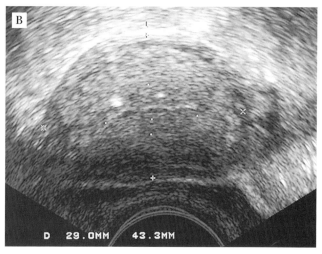

Fig. 2.48 Asherman's syndrome. A: Sagittal and B: axial TV scans of the uterus showing small reflective foci at the endometrial myometrial junction in a patient with Asherman's syndrome.

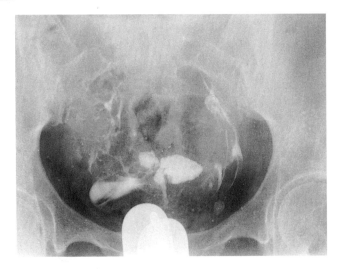

Fig. 2.49 **Uterine adhesions.** HSG demonstrates uterine adhesions.

Unusual uterine tumours

Uterine sarcomas are rare, accounting for less than 3% of all uterine malignancies. The histology is variable but all forms are aggressive. Uterine leiomyosarcoma is the commonest form of genital tract sarcoma and some 10% develop in pre-existing fibroids. Typically they present with post-menopausal bleeding in the sixth decade. The sonographer should be alerted to the diagnosis by a history of rapid uterine growth in a post-menopausal woman. They form bulky uterine masses which may be reflective or complex and cystic in nature (Fig. 2.50). Characteristically the mass distends the endometrial cavity and may protrude through the cervix. Generally areas of haemorrhage and necrosis are found within the mass, rarely with associated calcification. Doppler demonstrates low-impedance flow. These tumours may be indistinguishable from large non-malignant fibroids or large endometrial carcinomas (Fig. 2.51). There may be signs of urinary tract obstruction and of local or distant spread.[69]

Mixed Müllerian sarcomas are mesenchymal uterine tumours that are histologically part carcinoma and part sarcoma. They arise from pluripotential primordial cells in the Müllerian duct system, from which the uterus develops. Aggressive, often rapidly invasive, these endometrial tumours generally show deep myometrial penetration and have usually metastasised to local lymph nodes by the time of diagnosis.[70] Sonographically a large heterogeneous pelvic mass is seen (Fig. 2.52).

Lymphoma may infiltrate the uterine corpus and cervix and is usually a part of a generalised lymphatic disease: primary lymphoma of the genital tract is rare. Ultrasound shows an echo-poor uterine mass which is rarely calcified.[71]

Metastases to the uterus are rare, mainly originating from the breast or stomach,[72] and may be associated with Krukenberg tumours of the ovaries. The endometrium is

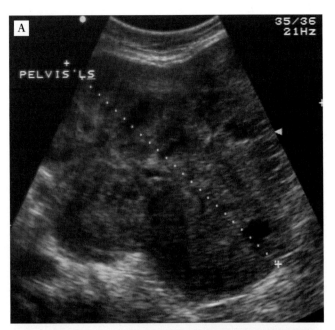

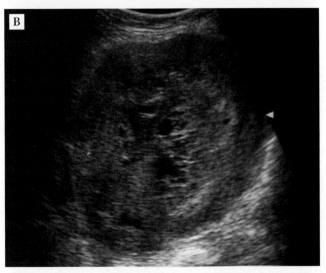

Fig. 2.50 **Leiomyosarcoma. A:** Sagittal and **B:** axial TA scans of a large uterine mass of mixed reflectivity caused by leiomyosarcoma.

more commonly involved than the myometrium. Presentation is generally with abnormal bleeding and pain. The ultrasound appearances are similar to those of endometrial carcinoma, with single or multiple masses of varying reflectivity. Dystrophic calcification may be present.[37]

Primary osteosarcoma is a very rare uterine tumour presenting as a calcified mass,[73] the differential diagnosis of which is fibroid, leiomyosarcoma, metastasis or lymphoma.

All these tumours are rare and usually present with post-menopausal bleeding. Ultrasound confirms the presence of the mass, but staging requires CT or MRI. Generally the diagnosis is only made at histology. Treatment is surgical, radiotherapy being unhelpful. The

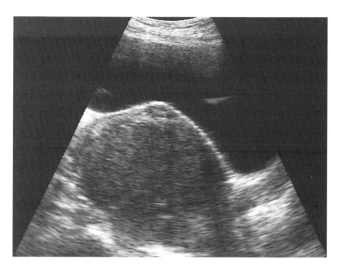

Fig. 2.51 Endometrial sarcoma. Sagittal TA scan showing an echo-poor uterine mass caused by a low-grade endometrial sarcoma. This appearance mimics a fibroid.

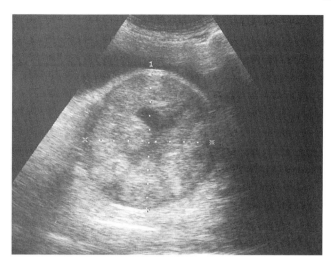

Fig. 2.52 Mixed Müllerian sarcoma. Axial TA scan of a large uterine mass of mixed reflectivity due to a mixed Müllerian sarcoma.

5-year survival is 50%, and when the tumour has spread beyond the uterus the prognosis is poor.

Benign uterine tumours

Lipomas are very rare and form a highly reflective uterine mass, generally in post-menopausal women. They may be mistaken for a fibroid, particularly when lipomatous degeneration of a fibroid is considered (Fig. 2.53). MRI and CT demonstrate the fatty nature of the tumour.[74]

Uterine **arteriovenous malformations** (AVMs) are rare but potentially life threatening, generally presenting with intractable menorrhagia. These congenital or acquired

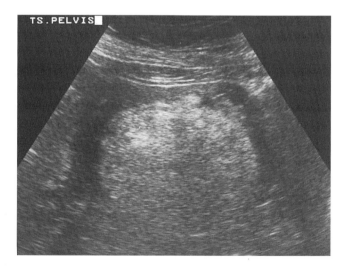

Fig. 2.53 Lipomatous degeneration of a fibroid. Axial TA scan of a large reflective uterine mass due to lipomatous degeneration of a fibroid.

lesions are diagnostically challenging, but may be identified with colour Doppler. Acquired lesions may result from previous pelvic surgery, dilatation and curettage and cervical or endometrial carcinoma. Diagnostic endometrial curettage should be avoided as it may lead to massive haemorrhage, which may require hysterectomy.

Uterine AVMs form complex cystic myometrial lesions which may be pulsatile and may cause uterine enlargement. Multiple vascular spaces may be seen within the lesion, which are easily demonstrated with colour Doppler with high-velocity, low-impedance flow on the spectral trace.[75] The differential diagnosis includes haemangioma and invasive trophoblastic disease.

Cystadenocarcinomas of the fallopian tube are rare, either primary or secondary,[76] and characteristically present with a continuous watery vaginal discharge or, less commonly, with post-menopausal bleeding. The discharge occurs as a result of fluid secretion by the tumour within the affected tube. Ultrasound often demonstrates a cylindrical cystic adnexal mass, separate from the uterus. Multiple small polypoid, moderately reflective masses may be demonstrated projecting into the distended tube, which may be observed periodically to change in shape and size, as fluid is discharged into the uterus. The cystic mass can be mistaken for a simple hydrosalpinx or an ovarian cyst. The tumour spreads in an identical fashion to ovarian carcinoma and indeed, as ovarian carcinoma may metastasise to the tube, it may occasionally be difficult to differentiate the two lesions.

Gestational trophoblastic disease includes incomplete and partial hydatidiform mole, invasive mole and gestational choriocarcinoma. Trophoblastic disease develops in the chorionic villi and is thus always associated with a conceptus, whether livebirth, stillbirth, abortion, ectopic pregnancy, or after termination of pregnancy. The incidence of hydatidiform mole is approximately 1:1500 pregnancies in the UK, but is much more common in southeast Asia. Fifteen percent develop into an invasive mole, in which the trophoblastic tissue invades the myometrium, and 5% become malignant choriocarcinomas.

Gestational trophoblastic tumours are characterised by abundant neoangiogenesis and so are strikingly vascular. Choriocarcinoma is a very fast growing, aggressive tumour, with characteristically early pulmonary metastatic disease. Methotrexate chemotherapy is highly effective, with a cure rate of greater than 95%. The tumour produces a serological marker, human chorionic gonadotrophin (b-HCG), which is used to monitor the progress of the disease. A b-HCG level of less than 1 IU/l excludes the diagnosis. The presenting symptoms and signs are similar to those of early pregnancy, with uterine enlargement, nausea and abnormal uterine bleeding.

No common ultrasound appearance has been described either prior to or after chemotherapy. Changes in uterine morphology are very variable, ranging from relatively small intracavitary masses of mixed reflectivity to large masses extending into the parametrium. When small lesions are present evidence of myometrial invasion should be sought. An additional sonographic feature is the presence of theca luteal cysts within the ovaries. The vascularity of these tumours is apparent on colour and spectral Doppler, which are useful in determining the extent of the tumour. Multiple confluent low-resistance (PI <1) blood vessels are seen. In general, the sonographical appearances and b-HCG levels reflect the severity of the condition.[77] Monitoring the response to treatment with serial Doppler ultrasound and b-HCG levels is an effective non-invasive regimen. Persistent tumour is recognised by abnormal uterine morphology and/or persistent vascularisation on colour Doppler. In one series of 25 patients there was 100% accuracy in predicting local resolution or persistence of disease.[78]

Uterine surgery

Hysterectomy

Hysterectomy is the most common major surgical procedure in women and is most often performed premenopausally for non-malignant disease. The uterus and cervix are removed, sometimes together with the ovaries, by the abdominal or vaginal route. Postoperative ultrasound demonstrates the residual vagina as a blind-ending midline tubular structure (Fig. 2.54). Occasionally small retention cysts are demonstrated in the upper vagina in the region of the vault scar, but these are of no clinical significance. A small post-menopausal uterus, particularly when retroverted, may be difficult to identify on ultrasound: questioning of the patient should ensure that this is not mistaken for absence of the uterus after hysterectomy.

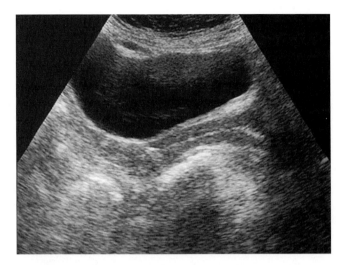

Fig. 2.54 Vaginal stump. Sagittal TA scan showing blind-ending vaginal stump post-hysterectomy.

Subtotal hysterectomy with preservation of the cervix is now rarely performed. The residual cervix is sonographically demonstrated as a rounded soft tissue structure in continuity with the upper vagina (Fig. 2.55). Retention cysts may develop in the cervical stump.

Radical surgery is required for pelvic malignancy: total abdominal hysterectomy and bilateral salpingo-oophorectomy are combined with lymph node dissection and other procedures where necessary. The greater the technical difficulty of the procedure the greater the risk of complication.

A small amount of pelvic fluid is normal in the post-hysterectomy patient, but in approximately one-third a

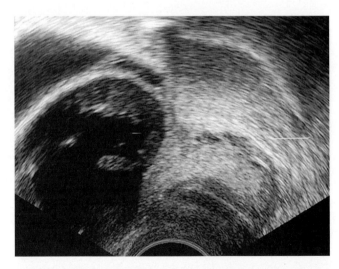

Fig. 2.55 Residual cervix after sub-total hysterectomy. Sagittal TVS in a patient following sub-total hysterectomy. The residual cervix is noted on the right, together with a left-sided complex cystic mass which is typical of a pelvic haematoma.

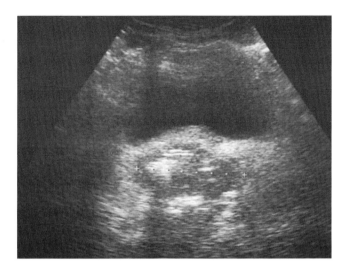

Fig. 2.56 Infected pelvic haematoma. Axial TA scan shows a complex pelvic mass following hysterectomy. There are areas of increased reflectivity within this infected gas-containing pelvic haematoma.

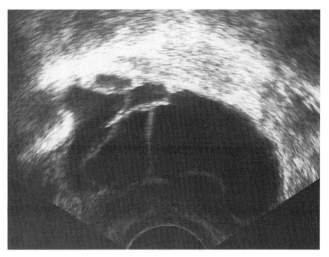

Fig. 2.57 Pelvic lymphocele. Large pelvic lymphocele which developed 10 days post-hysterectomy and subsequently resolved spontaneously.

significant-sized fluid collection will develop and many of these patients will develop a pyrexia.[79] Although the majority of fluid collections lie in the pelvis between the bladder and the rectum, the anterior abdominal wall wound should also be examined. Generally the morbidity and mortality of gynaecological surgery is low, but ureteric damage occurs in 0.5–2.5% of women and thus the kidneys should be examined in all patients with post-hysterectomy complications.

Pelvic haematomas are seen as irregular fluid collections of varying size with a wall of varying thickness. There may be internal echoes (Fig. 2.55), fluid–fluid levels and reflective masses due to clot retraction. The haematoma may become infected and gas may be seen in up to 50% of such cases (Fig. 2.56). Anterior abdominal wall or rectus sheath haematomas are identified as ovoid or plate-like collections close to the wound (see Vol. 2, Ch. 36).

Urinomas, following damage to the ureter, produce focal or free pelvic fluid collections. Lymphoceles (also termed lymphocysts) generally appear within 3 weeks of surgery and present as thin-walled fluid collections. They occur in 1–3% of post-radical hysterectomy patients (Fig. 2.57). Peritoneal inclusion cysts are a long-term consequence of pelvic surgery in which damage to the peritoneum and lymphatic drainage reduces peritoneal fluid absorption, allowing the development of a uni- or multi-locular cyst containing clear fluid (Fig. 2.58). They may also occur in PID and endometritis.

The majority of haematomas resolve spontaneously or, if infected, after a course of antibiotics. Persistent fluid collections can be drained under ultrasound control, either trans-abdominally or trans-vaginally. Damage to the ureters may necessitate percutaneous nephrostomy and ureteric reimplantation.

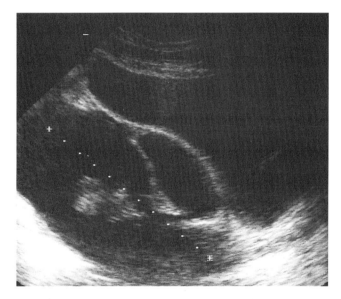

Fig. 2.58 Peritoneal inclusion cyst. 12 cm complex right-sided cystic pelvic mass caused by a peritoneal inclusion cyst following hysterectomy. This appearance persisted for many months.

Endometrial ablation

Endometrial ablation or trans-cervical resection of the endometrium (TCRE) is used as an alternative to hysterectomy or medical therapy to treat dysfunctional uterine bleeding. The endometrium is coagulated or resected using either a heat source or a laser. With a good result the endometrial cavity is reduced to a narrow fibrotic tube (Fig. 2.59), and a good predictor of success is a pre-operative endometrial thickness less than 8 mm. Thus it is preferable to perform the procedure in the early part of the cycle, when the endometrium is at its thinnest.[80]

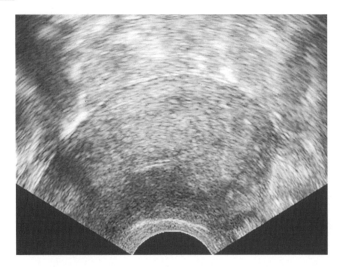

Fig. 2.59 Endometrium after ablation. Sagittal TVS showing a narrowed, poorly visualised uterine cavity following TCRE.

A significant reduction in uterine dimensions can be expected in 50% of patients.[81]

During ablation the basal layer of the endometrium and a few millimetres of myometrium are removed. Immediately after the procedure a small endometrial fluid collection may be apparent in a scarred loculated endometrial cavity (Fig. 2.60). A 3-monthly follow-up ultrasound examination should be performed to look for adhesions and residual endometrium. Occasionally there will be residual irregular pockets of fluid within the cavity.[82] The endometrium has a huge potential for regrowth, which occurs in up to 38% of women. Thus the post-ablation ultrasound appearances are very variable, depending on the relative success of the procedure. If menorrhagia recurs, a second ablation or hysterectomy may be necessary.

Dilatation and curettage

Although a once common procedure in premenstrual women and generally performed for menstrual irregularities, particularly menorrhagia, 'D&C' is becoming less popular as many new techniques are developed. In a D&C the superficial layer of the endometrium is removed and complications are rare. However, if it is carried out in pregnancy the deeper layers of endometrium may be removed inadvertently because the pregnant endometrium is very friable. This may expose small areas of myometrium, allowing the formation of small areas of fibrosis or endometrial adhesions, producing small reflective foci. Occasionally calcification may occur. Such adhesions may be associated with subfertility and treatment by division at hysteroscopy may be effective. In one series of patients with subendometrial reflective foci, 35/80 had had previous uterine instrumentation, compared with 2/174 patients who had not.[83]

Intra-uterine contraceptive device

Intra-uterine contraceptive devices (IUCD/IUD) produce a local foreign body inflammatory response in the endometrium which interferes with the viability of ova and sperm and inhibits implantation. The active agent in many IUCDs is copper (e.g. the Copper 7 and Copper T devices). More recently a new form of IUCD consisting of six copper beads has been developed (Gynaefix). Unusually, the leading edge of this device is embedded in the fundal myometrium at the time of insertion. Another recent development is that of the hormone-releasing IUCD that releases progesterone for up to 5 years. This type of coil leads to endometrial atrophy, which is effective both as a contraceptive and also in the treatment of menstrual

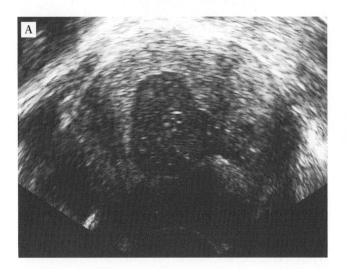
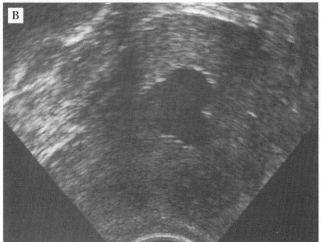

Fig. 2.60 Endometrial fluid collection after ablation. A and **B:** Axial TVS of two patients with irregular distended fluid-filled uterine cavities post TCRE.

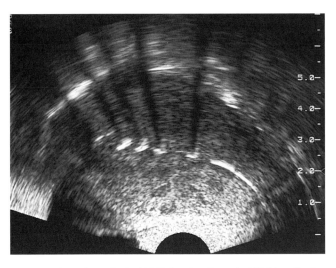

Fig. 2.61 Lippes loop. Sagittal TVS showing the typical highly reflective appearance of a Lippes loop, with all five arms being visualised.

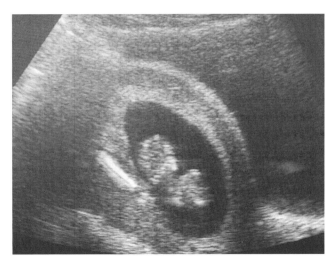

Fig. 2.63 Pregnancy and IUCD. Sagittal TA scan of uterus showing 9-week gestation together with a posterior retained IUCD.

disorders. The serpiginous-shaped Lippes loop device is no longer used but is occasionally seen in patients in whom it has been *in situ* for more than 20 years (Fig. 2.61). Most devices are changed at 5-yearly intervals, provided there are no complications. Trans-vaginal ultrasound is the investigation of choice for imaging an IUCD, both to confirm that it is correctly sited and also to check for complications. IUCD failure rate is of the order of 0.4–2.4/100 woman years. In nearly 80% of failures incorrect placement of the device is responsible[84] (Fig. 2.62).

Complications of IUCD use include perforation, partial or complete, in some 5%. It generally occurs at the time of insertion and the patient presents with pain and bleeding. With modern devices extrusion is rare (0.2%). Pregnancy with a retained coil is recognised in around 1 woman per 100 years[85] (Fig. 2.63) and, not unexpectedly, may occur if

the coil is expelled. PID and consequent infertility result from the coil acting as a nidus for infection. Menorrhagia is presumably caused by endometrial irritation.

Older reports showed that up to 90% of IUCDs were not correctly identified on ultrasound; however, with modern techniques almost all should be satisfactorily identified, particularly if 3D imaging is employed, because this allows simultaneous visualisation of the shaft and arms of the device.[86] A highly reflective intra-uterine structure producing strong acoustic shadowing is seen high and centrally in the uterine cavity, with the most cephalad component lying approximately 1.5 cm from the fundal uterine surface (Fig. 2.64). It should be identified in both the axial and sagittal planes. The strings may be visualised in the cervical canal. If the endometrium is reflective, as is seen during the normal secretory phase of the cycle, the device may be more difficult to visualise. Occasionally it is possible to obtain a frontal view (Fig. 2.65). Copper-containing IUCDs produce strong acoustic shadows: the Gynaefix coil is seen as a row of six spots (Fig. 2.66). Progesterone-containing types, such as the Mirena, are less reflective and may be more difficult to visualise, although strong acoustic shadowing is present (Fig. 2.67).

In partial perforation the device may lie partly within the cavity and partly within the myometrium; wholly within the myometrium; or with partial extrusion through the serosal surface of the uterus (Fig. 2.68). If complete, the device lies in the peritoneum, typically in the pelvis, and is rarely visualised on ultrasound as it will be obscured by bowel gas, although an associated pelvic haematoma may be visible in the acute phase. Perforation of the bladder and colon are rare.[87] If the device is not identified on ultrasound, an abdominal radiograph should be obtained to determine whether there has been expulsion or extrusion.

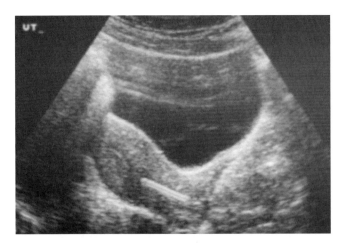

Fig. 2.62 Low-lying IUCD. Sagittal TA scan showing a low-lying IUCD in the lower uterine cavity and cervix.

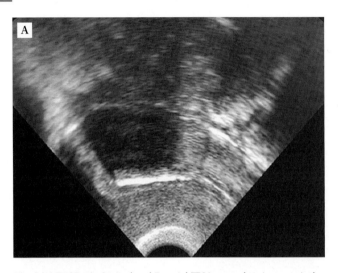

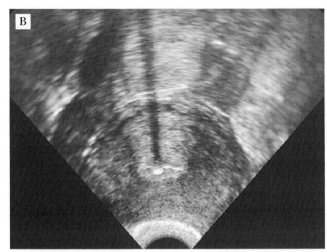

Fig. 2.64 IUCD. A: Sagittal and **B:** axial TV images showing a typical normally sited reflective IUCD with strong acoustic shadowing.

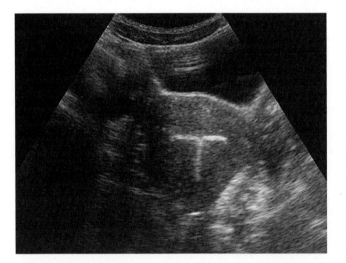

Fig. 2.65 Copper T IUCD. Axial oblique TA scan showing coronal view of Copper T coil.

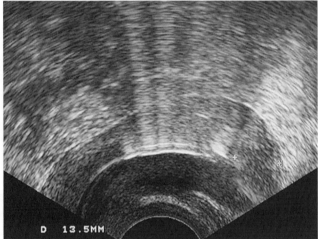

Fig. 2.66 Gynaefix IUCD. Sagittal TVS showing a Gynaefix IUCD.

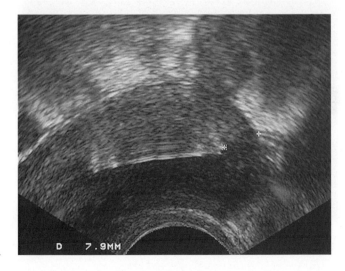

Fig. 2.67 Mirena IUCD. Sagittal TVS of uterus showing Mirena IUCD.

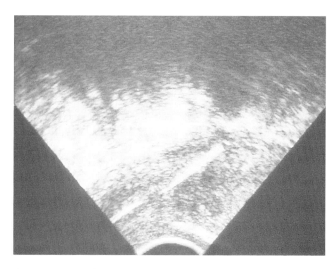

Fig. 2.68 Incorrectly positioned IUCD. Sagittal TVS showing IUCD penetrating the posterior uterine wall following insertion.

Cervical pathology

The cervix may be difficult to visualise because of its deep position on a transabdominal scan; when scanned transvaginally its close proximity to the transducer may place it in the near field. However, with care it should be possible trans-vaginally to identify the internal os, cervical canal and external os.

Benign conditions

Small endocervical (nabothian) cysts develop as a result of chronic cervitis in perimenopausal women and are of no clinical significance.[88] Cervical inflammation leads to the formation of erosions and, once these heal, residual islands of columnar epithelium covered with squamous epithelium continue to secrete mucus. Mucus retention cysts are thus formed. These are easily identified by their position adjacent to the cervical canal. Most are small (0.5–1 cm in diameter), although occasionally large cysts measuring up to 5 cm may be seen (Fig. 2.69). They are frequently multiple and, although usually echo free, may contain debris. Care should be taken not to confuse a nabothian cyst with a small low-lying gestational sac in the cervical canal.

Cervical polyps are common, small benign tumours which are frequently present, particularly in multiparous women, in the perimenopausal years. Although they are said to occur in up to 4% of women, few are identified sonographically unless saline instillation is used. Generally they are asymptomatic but may present with vaginal bleeding or discharge. Occasionally they become very large and may measure several centimetres in diameter. They are generally but not always reflective, and may be mistaken for pedunculated uterine polyps or fibroids. (see Fig. 2.31) Cervical polyps are not known to have malignant potential.

The diagnosis of cervical incompetence is generally made clinically following painless, bloodless miscarriages. Premature dilatation of the cervical canal leads to the expulsion of an intact gestation sac, generally in the second trimester. The incidence is less than 2 per 1000 pregnancies. Although often idiopathic, predisposing factors include previous obstetric and gynaecological trauma, with cone biopsy of the cervix and dilatation and curettage commonly implicated. Congenital genital tract anomalies may also be contributory. Precautionary cervical cerclage may be performed at 12–14 weeks gestation; alternatively it may be preferable to monitor the appearance of the cervix with serial ultrasound examinations.

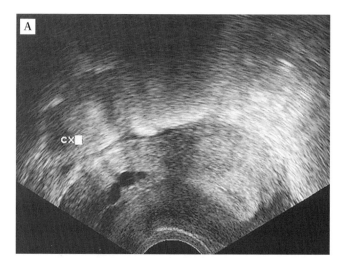
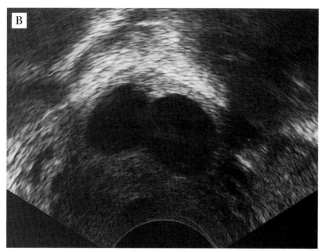

Fig. 2.69 Nabothian cyst. A: Sagittal TVS of cervix and uterus showing multiple small nabothian cysts in the cervix. **B:** Axial scan of cervix showing two large nabothian cysts.

In the non-pregnant patient hysterosalpingography is of value in the assessment of the cervix, which is optimally visualised trans-vaginally, avoiding a full bladder which may stretch the cervix, leading to an over-estimation of cervical length (Figs 2.70 and 2.71). The diagnosis is based on the observation of cervical shortening together with dilation of the internal os. The cervix is examined in the long axis and in the transverse plane at the level of the internal os, the position of which is determined by the transverse course of the uterine arteries.[89]

The mean length of the pregnant cervix at 12–16 weeks gestation in primigravidae is 42 mm, compared to 40 mm in parous women.[89] The relationship of the lower uterine segment to the cervix is normally Y-shaped (Fig. 2.72), whereas in cervical incompetence the lower segment may balloon or funnel into a shortened cervix (Fig. 2.73). If the cervix is less than 3 cm in length and the transverse diameter of the canal is greater than 1 cm, then a diagnosis of cervical incompetence is likely.[90] The dilated cervix may contain membranes, liquor and, occasionally, fetal parts. In very severe cases these may be seen bulging through the external os into the upper vagina. In this situation the differentiation between cervical incompetence and inevitable abortion may be impossible. A small amount of fluid or mucus in the cervical canal, visualised as a thin echo-poor line within the cavity, is a normal finding and is of no clinical significance when the cervix is of normal length.

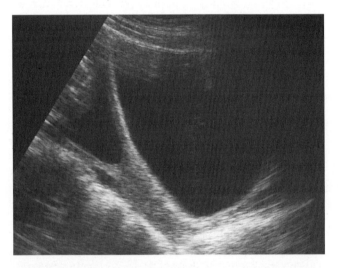

Fig. 2.70 Stretched cervix. Sagittal TA view showing a stretched cervix caused by over-distension of the bladder.

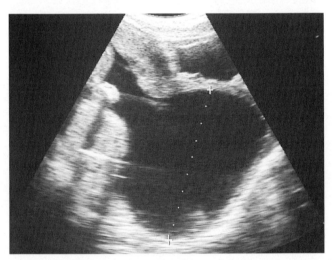

Fig. 2.71 Cervical incompetence. Sagittal TA scan of cervix showing cervical incompetence at 22 weeks gestation. AP dimension of cervix = 9 cm.

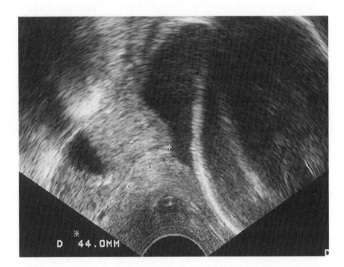

Fig. 2.72 Normal cervix at 26 weeks. Sagittal TVS showing normal cervix at 26 weeks gestation. The cervix measures 4.4 cm.

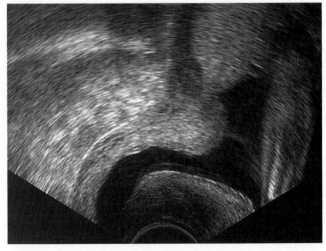

Fig. 2.73 Open cervical canal in cervical incompetence. Sagittal TVS of cervix with entire canal open at 22 weeks gestation.

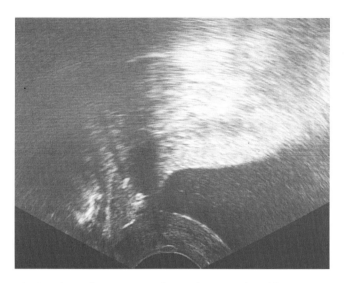

Fig. 2.74 Cervical sutures. Sagittal TVS of cervix with widely open cervical canal to the level of the reflective cervical sutures.

Following the diagnosis, cervical cerclage will usually be performed. This involves trans-vaginal suturing of the ecto-cervix. The suture material is highly reflective and is clearly visible in both transverse and sagittal planes[91] (Fig. 2.74). Cervical cerclage does not alter the configuration of the internal os as the sutures are not placed close to the os. Cervical cerclage allows 85% of patients to deliver normally at full term, following removal of the suture.

Carcinoma of the cervix

Carcinoma of the cervix is the sixth must common female tumour and the second commonest gynaecological tumour, with approximately 4000 new cases per year in the UK. National screening programmes are steadily reducing the incidence of invasive disease by detecting early micro-invasive disease with exfoliative cytology. Ninety per cent of patients with invasive disease present with abnormal bleeding, such as post-coital bleeding, inter-menstrual bleeding, menorrhagia, post-menopausal bleeding or vaginal discharge. In more advanced disease tumour pressure or invasion may produce urinary or rectal symptoms, leg oedema and renal failure. The peak incidence is 40–45 years, but as a result of changing sexual mores more patients now present in their 20s. The disease is rare in the sexually inactive and there is a well-established relationship between frequent coitus at an early age, promiscuity and venereal disease. The human papilloma virus is undoubtedly a causative agent, although the exact mechanism is uncertain. Of patients with invasive disease 40% are dead within 3 years. Low socio-economic class and high parity are also related factors.

The diagnosis is made on clinical grounds, either with local or cone biopsy of the cervix. Ninety per cent are squamous cell carcinomas, arising from the squamous epithelium of the ectocervix, and the remainder are adeno-carcinomas, arising from the columnar epithelium of the endocervical canal. About 20% of the tumours lie within the cervical canal and may not be clinically apparent, only being diagnosed at cone biopsy. Other rare tumours include sarcomas, melanoma, lymphoma and metastases.[55] The prognosis is determined by the stage of the disease and tumour volume at presentation, and falls steeply and progressively. FIGO staging is based on a clinical assessment made at examination under anaesthetic (see Table 2.9).

Ultrasound appearances

Early tumours cannot be detected by ultrasound and with stage I and II tumours the cervix is generally normal in size and texture. Enlargement of the cervix may be the first visible feature, the differential diagnosis being fibroid, lymphoma or sarcoma (Fig. 2.75). Cervical tumours are relatively echo poor compared to normal cervix, and small cystic areas may be apparent if tumour necrosis occurs. In more advanced disease irregularity of the cervical outline is a common feature, suggesting tumour spread into the parametrium, i.e. the tissue lying below the level of the uterine arteries between the cervix and the pelvic side walls. External bladder compression or invasion may be demonstrated with the full bladder technique. The endometrial stripe generally appears normal, but if tumour extends to the cervical canal the endometrial cavity will commonly be distended with blood or pus. Cervical stenosis developing after cone biopsy or radiation therapy may also lead to the development of hydrometra, haematometra or pyometra (Fig. 2.76). Hydro-ureter and hydronephrosis result from ureteral invasion and are all too common in late-stage disease, when regional lymphadenopathy and distant spread may be evident.

Accurate staging is essential before planning therapy. Traditionally this has been done at examination under anaesthetic, but the method is notoriously inaccurate, often resulting in understaging. Therefore, the newer imaging modalities are now regularly employed (Fig. 2.77). Generally, stage I and IIA disease is treated with radical surgery and more advanced disease with radiation therapy. In practical terms it is essential to distinguish between IIA and IIB disease in order to make this crucial management decision. Abdominal ultrasound has no place in the diagnosis of early disease, and is only of value in demonstrating the gross effects of advanced disease, i.e. hydronephrosis or bladder invasion. Until recently CT was the imaging method of choice for staging cervical carcinoma. However, it is unable to distinguish between normal and abnormal cervical tissue, nor can it reliably distinguish between stage IIA and IIB disease, i.e. whether there is parametrial involvement. However, tumour spread to the pelvic side walls and regional lymphadenopathy can

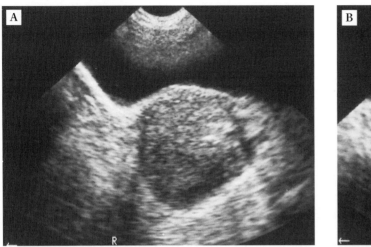
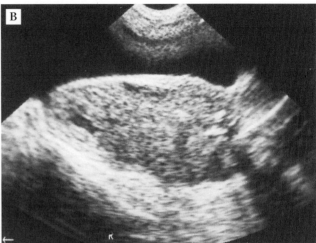

Fig. 2.75 Cervical carcinoma. A: Axial TA scan of a large cervical mass. **B:** Sagittal TA scan of a large cervical mass invading the endometrial cavity.

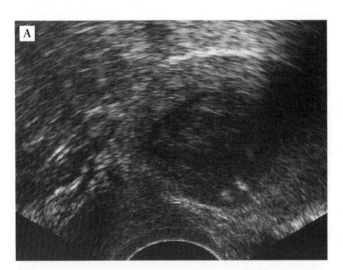
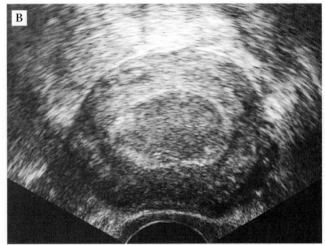

Fig. 2.76 Pyometra. A: Axial and **B:** sagittal views of distended uterine cavity due to a pyometra resulting from DXR treatment of cervical carcinoma.

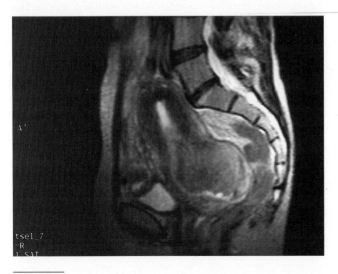

Fig. 2.77 MRI scan of a cervical carcinoma. T$_2$-weighted sagittal MRI scan showing a large cervical carcinoma involving mainly the posterior lip of the cervix.

be clearly demonstrated.[58] MRI has been used to stage cervical carcinoma, with good results.[59] Direct multiplanar imaging has great advantages: the cervix, vagina and uterus are well demonstrated; because of its high signal intensity, cervical tumour can easily be differentiated from normal cervical tissue and tumour volume can be assessed accurately. The presence of a low signal rim around the tumour is completely specific for assigning the disease to stage I or II.

Thus it can be seen that MRI is the chosen method of investigation, whether for staging or for assessing recurrence, as it is superior to CT for tumour assessment and is equivalent in accuracy to CT when assessing for lymphadenopathy.[92]

Vaginal pathology

The diagnosis of vaginal pathology is generally made at clinical examination, but occasionally vaginal abnormalities are diagnosed incidentally at pelvic ultrasound.[93] The vagina is often best imaged transabdominally, as transvaginal assessment is difficult owing to the close proximity of the transducer. The trans-labial or trans-perineal approach, with or without a stand-off device, may be helpful in the young patient or where there is vaginal obstruction. Young girls presenting with delayed puberty should be assessed for uterine absence, haematocolpos due to vaginal obstruction and ovarian pathology.

Developmental anomalies

Vaginal fusion defects obstruct the vagina at varying levels, with two-fifths being high, two-fifths being in the mid part and one-fifth lying low in the vagina. Whatever the level,

the most common presentation is that of amenorrhoea in young adulthood. A pelvic mass may be apparent, which may cause frequency of micturition due to bladder compression. The mass may be sufficiently large to render visualisation of the uterus almost impossible and in this situation MRI may be of value. The differential diagnosis includes other cystic pelvic masses, such as ovarian cysts and haematometra. The presence of an imperforate hymen may produce a similar appearance. Associated urinary tract anomalies such as duplication and ectopia are common and so the kidneys should always be examined.

Vaginal fluid collections

Transient small collections of fluid may be readily identified in the vagina and are most commonly due to menstrual blood. Larger collections of vaginal blood may be seen after abortion and with congenital vaginal obstruction (Fig. 2.78).

In the young child urine may be present in the vagina as a result of vaginal reflux during micturition. Larger pathological collections of urine may be found in the vagina in those suffering from urinary incontinence, or due to continuous leakage of urine into the vagina through a urinary fistula or via an ectopic ureter.[94] Although uncommon, extravaginal fluid collections such as para-urethral cysts and paravaginal haematomas may compress the normal vagina, giving the erroneous impression of a vaginal mass.

Gartner's duct cyst

These cysts arise from vestigial remnants of the mesonephric or Wolffian duct systems which, as the 'so-called' Gartner's ducts, course along the anterolateral outer

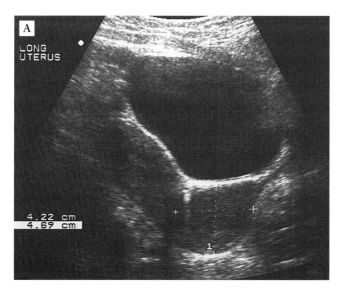
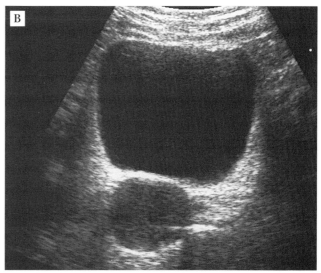

Fig. 2.78 Vaginal obstruction. A: TA scan of proximal haematocolpos due to proximal vaginal septum. **B:** Axial TA scan of haematocolpos.

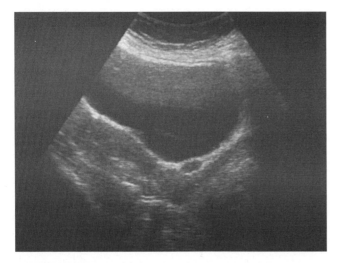

Fig. 2.79 Gartner's cyst. Sagittal TA scan of uterus showing a small Gartner's cyst anterior to the proximal vagina.

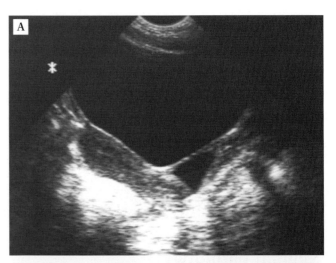

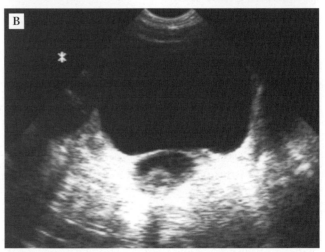

Fig. 2.80 Gartner's cyst. A and B: TA sagittal axial scans showing an anterior Gartner's cyst enveloping the exocervix.

aspects of the vaginal canal[95] (Fig. 2.79). They are usually incidental sonographical findings,[96] and may be single or multiple and, although generally small, may measure up to 10 cm in diameter.[97] Occasionally the cysts communicate with the cervix, or may be large enough to bulge through the introitus.

Sonographically the cysts may be shown to distend the upper vagina and may outline the ectocervix (Fig. 2.80). When large, such a cyst may mimic a hydrocolpos. There is an association with ipsilateral renal agenesis and therefore the urinary tract should always be examined when this diagnosis is made. Asymptomatic cysts do not require treatment but when symptomatic marsupialisation is the treatment of choice.

Vaginal foreign bodies

A foreign body (Table 2.14) may cause vaginitis, presenting with a persistent bloody or serous vaginal discharge. Abdominal ultrasound generally reveals the structure, sometimes together with a fluid collection.

A tampon may be clearly visualised because of the air it contains, which produces a well-defined, highly reflective rectilinear shape lying centrally in the vaginal canal, producing strong acoustic shadowing (Fig. 2.81). There may be indentation of the bladder base. Uterine prolapse may

Table 2.14 Reflective vaginal masses

| Tampon |
| Ring pessary |
| Displaced IUCD |
| Foreign body |
| Calculus |
| Retained air |

be conservatively treated with a ring pessary placed in the vaginal vault. The pessary produces intense acoustic shadowing high in the vagina, with the two lateral margins seen in the axial plane and the superior and inferior margins seen in the sagittal plane (Fig. 2.82).

Vaginal calculi are rare and of varying aetiologies, including ulceration of a bladder calculus through the vesicovaginal septum and calcification of retained foreign bodies. Both congenital and acquired vaginal strictures are said to predispose to the formation of vaginal calculi, as does urinary incontinence. In childhood, ultrasound may be of value in identifying a foreign body.

After instrumentation and sexual intercourse gas may be visible in the vagina. Emphysematous vaginitis is an unusual condition in which gas-filled blebs develop in the submucous layer of the upper vagina. The aetiology is unknown and the condition may occur in association with pregnancy.[98]

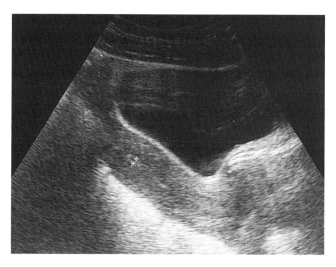

Fig. 2.81 Tampon. Sagittal TA scan of uterus and vagina showing a reflective rectilinear tampon indenting the posterior bladder wall.

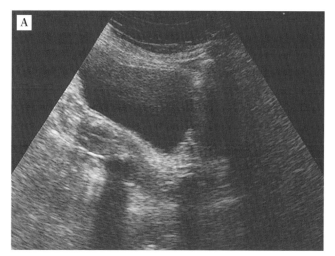

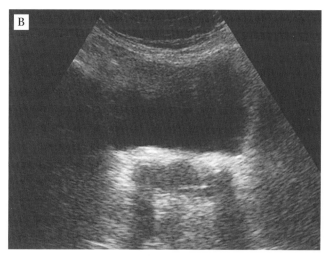

Fig. 2.82 Ring pessary. A: Sagittal and B: axial views of a pessary, shown as two areas of strong acoustic shadowing showing superior and inferior margins on sagittal view and lateral margins on axial view.

Vaginal tumours

Primary vaginal tumours are rare, accounting for only 1–2% of all gynaecological malignancies; most occur in the elderly (Table 2.15). Squamous cell carcinomas account for 80–90%, with adenocarcinomas and melanoma being rare. The very rare sarcomata almost always present in early childhood.

Treatment with diethylstilboestrol for early recurrent miscarriage may be associated with vaginal malignancy in the daughters of these women. Such patients, whose mothers were treated some 40–50 years ago, have a predisposition to develop an unusual, very aggressive clear-cell adenocarcinoma of the upper vagina. Unlike the squamous-cell carcinoma that develops in the sixth and seventh decades of life, the clear-cell carcinoma develops in early adulthood.[99]

Tumours usually present with vaginal bleeding and/or discharge, and are clinically obvious, with a diagnosis made at biopsy. Ultrasound demonstrates the tumour as a solid mass with low-amplitude echoes; 50% develop in the upper third of the vagina and spread in a similar fashion to carcinoma of the cervix. Stage I tumours are confined to the vagina. Stage II tumours extend beyond the vagina but not to the pelvic side walls. Stage III tumours reach the pelvic side walls and stage IV tumours have distant spread. These late-presenting tumours are difficult to treat. Stage I and II tumours may be treated with radical surgery, but generally radiotherapy is used palliatively and the prognosis is poor. Local staging and monitoring of recurrence is performed with CT and MRI. Ultrasound is rarely of value unless a tumour is found incidentally.

Secondary tumours of the vagina are very uncommon and almost all result from local invasion by cervical, vesical or colorectal tumours.

Rhabdomyosarcoma (embryonal sarcoma, sarcoma botryoides)

This is the commonest soft tissue sarcoma of childhood. It is occasionally present at birth but generally presents before the age of 2 years, and almost always before the age of 5 years. Embryonal sarcomas account for 4–8% of all malignant disease in children under 15 years of age, and

Table 2.15 Aetiology of vaginal tumours

Radiation therapy for cervical carcinoma and other pelvic tumours
Mechanical irritation
procidentia
ring pessary
Diethylstilboestrol

18% affect the genitourinary tract.[100] In the female most are vaginal in origin, less commonly arising from the uterus, although extension from one to the other may occur.

A large polypoid mass develops in the vagina, generally attached to the upper vaginal vault or cervix. Protrusion of the mass through the introitus may be the presenting feature. Alternatively, a lower abdominal mass with vaginal bleeding or discharge may alert the clinician to the diagnosis. The tumour may grow very rapidly, with invasion of the para-vaginal tissues, bladder and other pelvic organs. Lymph node and pulmonary metastases are common.

The ultrasound appearances are variable, but in general a large pelvic mass of variable reflectivity is apparent Multiple irregular cystic areas within the mass are common. Secondary features, such as hydro-ureter and hydronephrosis, should be sought, together with evidence of distant spread. Staging by CT and MRI is preferable to ultrasound.

The post-partum uterus

The puerperium is the post-partum period during which the body returns to its prepregnant state. This is usually completed within 6 weeks and in the vast majority of patients is uneventful. Immediately after delivery the uterus weighs approximately 900 g and the fundus is palpable some 12 cm above the symphysis pubis. There is a subsequent rapid reduction in uterine tissue mass, which halves by the end of the first week post-delivery. By 6 weeks the uterus weighs less than 100 g and is only very slightly larger than it was in its prepregnant state. Within 3 days of parturition the superficial layer of decidua becomes necrotic and is shed as the lochia. The restoration of the endometrial covering takes approximately 3 weeks, by which time uterine blood loss has been curtailed.[101]

Ultrasound appearances

Immediately post-partum the uterus is significantly enlarged, with a smooth and globular outline and a longitudinal dimension of approximately 20 cm (Fig 2.83). It is not uncommon for small amounts of air to be seen in the uterine cavity immediately post-partum.[102] A small amount of fluid within the endometrial cavity is a normal finding. There is a steady reduction in uterine size over the next 6 weeks. Fibroids shrink and any areas of necrosis that have developed slowly resolve.

Post-partum complications
Retained products of conception

Incomplete evacuation of the uterus following either vaginal delivery or caesarean section generally presents with excessive bleeding within a few days of delivery, although ocasionally presentation is delayed by some weeks. The uterus does not involute as fast as might normally be expected. This complication is associated with an increased risk of endometritis. Ultrasound shows the uterus to be inappropriately large, with distension of the endometrial cavity by fluid of mixed reflectivity, with varying amounts of fluid and blood clot, membranes and placental tissue (Fig 2.84). It may be impossible to distinguish between blood clot and placental tissue, as both are similarly reflective. Similar appearances may be seen following spontaneous or induced abortion. Where a significant amount of retained products of conception is present,

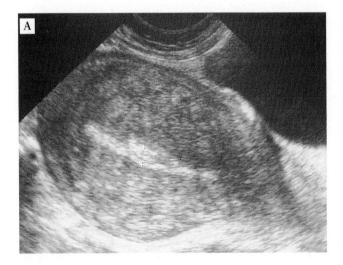
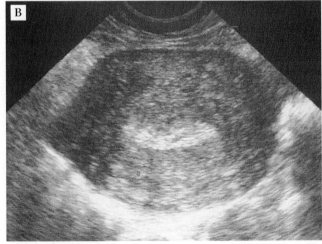

Fig. 2.83 Post-partum uterus. A: Sagittal and B: axial TA views of a normal uterus 5 days postpartum.

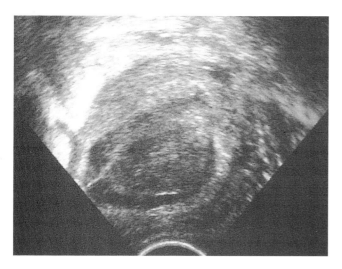

Fig. 2.84 **Retained products of conception.** Axial TVS 6 days post-partum showing retained products of conception.

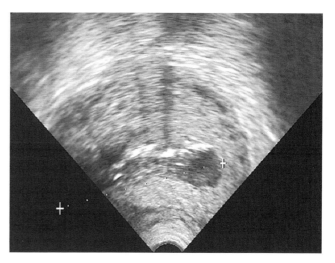

Fig. 2.85 **Post-partum endometritis.** Axial TV view of uterus showing debris and gas due to gas-forming organisms in a patient with post-partum endometritis.

evacuation of the uterus may be performed. When only small amounts of abnormal tissue and fluid are found medical or expectant management is widely accepted, with sonography used to monitor resolution.

Endometritis

Prompt treatment with antibiotics means that serious post-partum infection with either endometritis, myometritis or both is rarely encountered. Generally the patient presents 2–5 days after delivery with uterine tenderness, pyrexia, abnormal bleeding and offensive lochia. Whereas only 2–3% of patients are likely to develop a serious infection after a vaginal delivery, the risk is higher (10–15%) after caesarean section and the incidence is higher when there have been serious lacerations. Streptococci are the commonest organisms. The infection initially involves the endometrium, thereafter spreading rapidly to involve the myometrium and adnexae. Septicaemia may occur if prompt antibiotic treatment is not given.

The ultrasound appearances may be indistinguishable from those of retained products of conception, and thus the diagnosis is generally made on clinical grounds. There may be inappropriate enlargement of the uterus and the myometrium may appear relatively echo poor in severe infection. Varying amounts of tissue, fluid and occasionally gas may be present in the uterine cavity (Fig 2.85).

Paravaginal haematoma

Following complicated vaginal delivery, with or without cervical or vaginal lacerations, damage to the paravaginal venous plexus may cause bleeding and produce a para-

vaginal haematoma. This is visualised as a fluid collection lying lateral to the vagina. Of varying size, the haematoma may compress or deviate the vagina.

Uterine inversion

This is an unusual post-partum complication with an incidence of 1:30 000 deliveries. Complete uterine inversion is diagnosed clinically and is a devastating process which may result in severe shock and death. Partial uterine inversion is less serious and presents with pelvic pain and abnormal bleeding. On ultrasound the uterine fundus is poorly visualised because of the inversion of the uterus upon itself, and the normal midline echo assumes a 'Y' shape. In transverse section a ring shape corresponding to the inverted endometrial cavity is seen. Thus the appearance is reminiscent of the appearances of intestinal intussusception. Treatment is manual decompression of the uterus or, when this fails, emergency hysterectomy.[103]

Caesarean section

The incidence of caesarean section is steadily increasing and is performed in up to 30% of pregnancies, depending on local practice. The uterine incision is either the classic vertical or, more commonly, a horizontal lower segment incision. In the days following operation the incision site is clearly visible on ultrasound as a well defined oval area between the lower uterine segment and the posterior wall of the urinary bladder (Fig 2.86). It produces a slight indentation of the bladder. Suture material appears as small punctate, regularly spaced highly reflective foci, and may be clearly visualised.[104] Within a few weeks, however, the wound heals, the suture material disappears and the

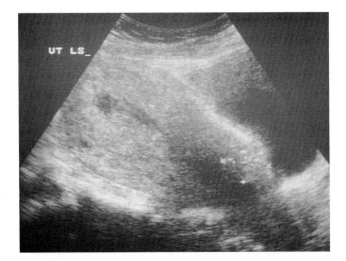

Fig. 2.86 Post-partum uterus with caesarean section scar. Axial TA scan of 5-day post-partum uterus showing caesarean section scar on the lower anterior uterine wall.

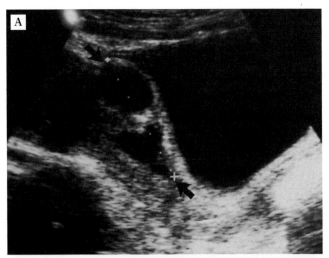

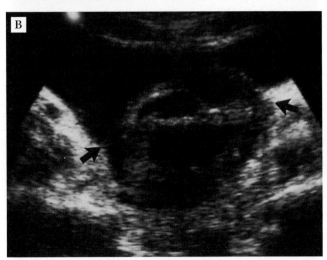

Fig. 2.87 Uterine haematoma. A: longitudinal and **B:** transverse scans of a large haematoma (arrows) involving a previous caesarean scar. This occurred following a normal vaginal delivery

deformity is no longer visualised.[4] In some patients, however, a small step-like deformity of the anterior uterine wall persists and may give rise to an acoustic shadow at the site of the scar. This may cause the erroneous impression of a small fibroid, but the history and the classic site of the scar at the junction of the middle and lower thirds of the uterus should allow confident diagnosis. Vertical uterine scars, however, are more difficult to identify.[105] Postoperatively small, rapidly resolving fluid collections commonly develop adjacent to the uterine incision. Infection and haemorrhage are the commonest postoperative complications and may involve the uterine wound, the anterior abdominal wall, or may develop in the peritoneal, extraperitoneal or paravesical spaces. The so-called 'bladder flap' haematoma develops in relationship to the uterine wound. This occurs when haemostasis is not obtained after closure of the uterine wound, and a retroperitoneal haematoma may form between the anterior uterine wall and posterior bladder wall[106] (Fig 2.87). Fluid collections in the abdominal wound may be localised or may track cephalad in the fascial planes of the anterior abdominal wall. Bleeding at the site of the uterine scar may occur during subsequent pregnancies and result in haematoma formation, dehiscence or uterine rupture. This is most likely to occur after a trial of labour, and is why many authorities recommend a repeat caesarean section in subsequent pregnancies. When a patient undergoing a trial of labour complains of pain and tenderness over a caesarean section scar, an urgent ultrasound scan is needed: it may be possible to demonstrate thinning of the anterior uterine wall or to diagnose a dehiscence.[107] Over half the cases of uterine rupture affect a previous caesarean section scar. Bleeding into the broad ligaments may produce an adnexal mass.

REFERENCES

1 Cecchini S, Ciatta S, Bonardi R, Grazzini G, Mazzota A. Endometrial ultrasonography – an alternative to invasive assessment in women with postmenopausal vaginal bleeding. Tumori 1996; 82: 38–39

2 Granberg S, Karlsson B, Wikland M, Gull B. Transvaginal sonography of uterine and endometrial disorders. In: Fleischer A C, Manning F A, Jeanty P, Romero R, eds. Sonography in obstetrics and gynaecology: principles and practice, 5th edn. Stamford, Conn.: Appleton & Lange, 1996; 851–868

3 Goldstein S R, Nachtigall M, Snyder J R, Nachtigall L. Endometrial assessment by vaginal ultrasonography before endometrial sampling in patients with postmenopausal bleeding. Am J Obstet Gynecol 1990; 163: 119–230

4 Karlsson B, Granberg S, Ridell B, Wikland M. Endometrial thickness as measured by transvaginal sonography: interobserver variation. Ultrasound Obstet Gynecol 1994; 320–325

5 Andolf E, Kahlander K, Aspenberg P. Ultrasonic thickness of the endometrium correlated to body weight in asymptomatic postmenopausal women. Obstet Gynecol 1993; 82: 936–940

6 Delisle M, Villeneuve M, Boulvain M. Measurement of endometrial thickness with transvaginal ultrasonography; is it reproducible? J Ultrasound 1998; 17: 481–486

7 Langer R D, Pierce J J, O'Hanlan K A et al. Transvaginal ultrasonography compared with endometrial biopsy for the detection of endometrial disease. N Engl J Med 1997; 337: 1792–1798

8 Van den Bosch T, Vandendael A, Van Schoubroeck D, Wranz P A B, Lombard C J. Combining vaginal ultrasonography and office endometrial sampling in the diagnosis of endometrial disease in postmenopausal women. Obstet Gynecol 1995; 85: 349–352

9 Fistonic I, Hodek B, Klaric P, Jokanovic L, Grubisic G, Ivicevic-Bakulic T. Transvaginal sonographic assessment of premalignant and malignant changes in the endometrium in postmenopausal bleeding. JCU 1997; 25: 431–435

10 Dodson M L. Transvaginal ultrasound. Edinburgh: Churchill Livingstone, 1991; 83.

11 Clisham P R, Cedars M I, Greendate G et al. Longterm transdermal estradiol therapy: effects on endometrial histology and bleeding patterns. Obstet Gynecol 1992; 79: 196–201

12 Voight L F, Weiss N S, Chu J et al. Progestogen supplementation of exogenous oestrogens and risk of endometrial cancer. Lancet 1991; 338: 274–277

13 Pirhonen J P, Vuento M H, Makinen J I, Salmi T A. Long term effect of hormone replacement therapy on the uterus and uterine circulation. Am J Obstet Gynecol 1993; 168: 620–630

14 Achiron R, Lipitz S, Frenkel Y, Mashiach S. Endometrial blood flow response to estrogen replacement therapy and tamoxifen in asymptomatic, postmenopausal women; a transvaginal Doppler study. Ultrasound Obstet Gynecol 1995; 5: 411–414

15 Lin M C, Gosink B B, Wolf S L et al. Endometrial thickness after menopause: effect of hormone replacement. Radiology 1991; 180: 427–432

16 Levine D, Gosink B B, Johnson L A. Change in endometrial thickness in postmenopausal women undergoing hormone replacement therapy. Radiology 1995; 197: 603–608

17 Lahti E, Blanco G, Kaupilla A, Apaja-Sarkkinen M, Taskinen P J, Laatikainen T. Endometrial changes in postmenopausal breast cancer patients receiving tamoxifen. Obstet Gynecol 1993; 81: 660–664

19 Fornander T, Cedermark B, Mattsson A et al. Adjuvant tamoxifen in early breast cancer: occurrence of now primary cancers. Lancet 1989; i: 117

20 Goldstein S. Unusual ultrasonographic appearance of the uterus in patients receiving tamoxifen. Am J Obstet Gynecol 1994; 170: 447

21 Kedar P R, Bourne T H, Powles T J et al. Effects of tamoxifen on uterus and ovaries of postmenopausal women in a randomised breast cancer prevention trial. Lancet 1994; 343: 1318–1321

22 Achiron R, Lipitz S, Sivan E et al. Changes mimicking endometrial neoplasia in postmenopausal, tamoxifen-treated women with breast cancer: a transvaginal Doppler study. Ultrasound Obstet Gynecol 1995; 6: 116–120

23 Exacoustos E, Zupi E, Cangi B, Chiaretti M, Arduimi D, Romaninis C. Endometrial evaluation in postmenopausal breast cancer patients receiving tamoxifen: an ultrasound, color flow Doppler hysteroscopic and histological study. Obstet Gynecol 1995; 6: 435–442

24 Cohen I, Rosen D J, Shapira J et al. Endometrial change in post-menopausal women treated with tamoxifen for breast cancer. Br J Obstet Gynaecol 1993; 100: 567–570

25 Seoud M A, Johnson J, Weed J C. Gynaecologic tumours in tamoxifen-treated women with breast cancer. Obstet Gynecol 1993; 82: 165–169

26 Uziely B, Levin A, Brufman G et al. The effect of tamoxifen on the endometrium. Breast Cancer Rest Trat 1993; 26: 101–105

27 Lewit N, Thaler I, Rottem S. The uterus: a new look with transvaginal sonography. JCU 1990; 18: 331–336

28 Fleischer A, Gordon A N, Entman S S, Kepple D M. Transvaginal scanning of the endometrium. JCU1990; 18: 337–349

29 Occhipinti K, Kutcher R, Rosenblatt R. Sonographic appearance and significance of arcuate artery calcification. J Ultrasound Med 1991; 10: 97

30 Malpani A, Singer J, Wolverson M K, Merenda G. Endometrial hyperplasia: value of endometrial thickness in ultrasonographic diagnosis and clinical significance. JCU 1990; 18: 173–177

31 Novak's textbook of gynecology, 11th edn. Baltimore: Williams & Wilkins, 1988; 726

32 Syrop C H, Sahakian V. Transvaginal sonographic detection of endometrial polyps with fluid contrast augmentation. Obstet Gynecol 1992; 79: 1041–1043

33 Novak's textbook of gynecology, 11th edn. Baltimore: Williams & Wilkins, 1988: 728–738

34 Bourne T H, Campbell S, Steer CV et al. Detection of endometrial cancer by transvaginal ultrasonography with colour flow imaging and blood flow analysis: a preliminary report. Gynecol Oncol 1991; 40: 253

35 Sironi S, Colombo E, Villa G et al. Myometrial invasion by endometrial carcinoma: assessment with plain and gadolinum enhanced MR imaging. Radiology 1992; 185: 207

36 Rullo S, Piccioni M G, Framarino dei Malatesta M L et al. Sonographic, hysteroscopic, histological correlation in the early diagnosis of endometrial carcinoma. Eur J Gynecol Oncol 1991; 12: 463–469

37 Hrick H, Rubinstein L V, Gherman G M et al. MR imaging evaluation of endometrial carcinoma: results of an NCI cooperative study. Radiology 1991; 179: 829

38 American Cancer Society. Cancer statistics 1996. CA. Cancer J Clin 1996; 46: 5–29

39 Hahn-Pedersen J, Kvist N, Nielson O H. Hydrometrocolpos: current views on pathogenesis and Management. J Urol 1984; 132: 537–540

40 Scanlon K A, Pozniak M A, Fagerholm M, Shapiro S. Value of transperineal sonography in the assessment of vaginal atresia. AJR 1990; 154: 545–548

41 Sherer D M, Beyth Y. Ultrasonic diagnosis and assisted surgical management of haematotrachelos and haematometra due to uterine cervical atresia with associated vaginal agenesis. J Ultrasound Med 1989; 8: 321–323

42 Novak's textbook of gynecology, 11th edn. Baltimore: Williams & Wilkins, 1988: 508

43 Novak's textbook of gynecology, 11th edn. Baltimore: Williams & Wilkins, 1988: 512

44 Novak's textbook of gynecology, 11th edn. Baltimore: Williams & Wilkins, 1988: 383

45 Bowie J D. Ultrasound of gynaecological pelvic masses: the indefinite uterus and other patterns associated with diagnostic error. JCU 1977; 5: 323

46 Breckenridge J W, Kurtz A B, Ritchie W G M, Macht E L. Postmenopausal uterine fluid collection; indicator of carcinoma. AJR 1982; 139: 529–534

47 Gompel C, Silverberg S G. Pathology, gynecology and obstetrics, 2nd edn. Philadelphia: J B Lippincott, 1977

48 Ross R K, Pike M C, Vessey M P, Bull D, Yeates D, Casagrande J T. Risk factors for uterine fibroids: reduced risk associated with oral contraceptives. BMJ 1986; 293: 359–363

49 Vollenhoven B J, Lawrence A S, Healy D L. Uterine fibroids: a clinical review. Br J Obstet Gynaecol 1990; 97: 285–298

50 Buttram V C, Reiter R C. Uterine leiomyomata: etiology, symptomatology and management. Fertil Steril 1981; 36: 433–445

51 Sanders R C, James A E. Principles and practice of ultrasonography in obstetrics and gynecology, 3rd edn. Norwalk, Connecticut: Appleton Century Crofts, 1985; 540–542

52 Sladkericius P, Valentin L, Marsal K. Transvaginal Doppler examination of uteri with myomas. JCU 1996; 24: 135–140

53 Baltarowich O H, Kurtz A B, Pennell R G, Needleman L, Vilaro M M, Goldberg B. Pitfalls in the sonographic diagnosis of uterine fibroids. AJR 1988; 151: 728

54 Gross B H, Silver T M, Jaffe M H. Sonographic features of uterine leiomyomas. J Ultrasound Med 1983; 2: 401–406

55 Hricak H, Finck S, Honda G et al. MR imaging in the evaluation of benign uterine masses. Am J Radiol 1992; 158: 1043

56 Hricak H, Tscholakoff D, Heinrichs L et al. Uterine leiomyomas; correlation of MR, histopathologic findings and symptoms. Radiology 1986; 158: 385–391

57 Ascher S, Arnold L, Patt R et al. Adenomyosis; prospective comparison of MR imaging and transvaginal sonography. Radiology 1994; 190: 803

58 Lev-Toaff A, Coleman B, Arger P. Leiomyomas in pregnancy: sonographic study. Radiology 1987; 164: 683

59 Lev-Toaff A S, Coleman B G, Arger P H, Mintz M C, Arenson R L, Toaff M E. Leiomyomas in pregnancy: sonographic study. Radiology 1987; 164: 375–380

60 Muram D, Gillieson M, Walters J H. Myomas of the uterus in pregnancy: ultrasonographic follow-up. Am J Obstet Gynecol 1980; 138: 16–19

61 Matta W H M, Stabile I, Shaw R W, Campbell S. Doppler assessment of uterine blood flow changes in patients with fibroids receiving the gonadotropin-releasing hormone agonist buserelin. Fertil Steril 1988; 49: 1083

62 Bradley E A, Reidy J F, Forman R G et al. Transcatheter uterine artery embolisation to treat large uterine fibroids. Br J Obstet Gynaecol 1998; 105: 235–240

63 Novak's textbook of gynecology, 11th edn. Baltimore: Williams & Wilkins, 1988; 450–453

64 Iribarne C, Plaza J, De la Fuente P, Garrido C, Garzon A, Olaizola J I. Intramyometrial cystic adenomyosis. JCU 1994; 22: 348–350

65 Goldstein S R. Unusual ultrasound appearance of the uterus in patients receiving tamoxifen. Am J Obstet Gynecol 1994; 170: 447

66 Mark A S, Hrick H, Heinrichs L W et al. Adenomyosis and leiomyoma with MR imaging. Radiology 1987; 163: 527

67 Confino E, Friberg J, Giglia R V, Fleicher N. Sonographic imaging of intrauterine adhesions. Obstet Gynecol 1985; 66: 596–598

68 Smeele B, Wamsteker K, Sarstadt T, Exalto N. Ultrasonic appearance of Asherman's syndrome in the third trimester of pregnancy. JCU 1989; 17: 602–606

69 Hannigan E V, Gomez L G. Uterine leiomyosarcoma: a review of prognostic, clinical and pathologic features. Am J Obstet Gynecol 1979; 134: 557–564

70 Shapiro L G, Hrick H. Mixed Müllerian sarcoma of the uterus: MR imaging findings. AJR 1989; 153: 317–319

71 Malatsky A, Reuter K L, Woda B. Sonographic findings in primary uterine cervical lymphoma. JCU 1991; 19: 62–64

72 Kim S H, Hwang H Y, Choi B I. Case report: uterine metastasis from stomach cancer: radiological findings. Clin Radiol 1990; 42: 285–286

73 Caputo M G, Reuter K L, Reale F. Primary osteosarcoma of the uterus. Br J Radiol 1990; 63: 578–580

74 Jacobs J E, Markowitz S K. CT diagnosis of uterine lipoma. AJR 1988; 150: 1335.

75 Müngen E, Yergök Y Z, Ertekin A A, Ergür R, Uçmakli E, Aytaçlar S. Color Doppler sonographic features of uterine arteriovenous malformations; report of two cases. Ultrasound Obstet Gynecol 1997; 215–219

76 Ajjimakorn S, Bhamarapravati Y. Transvaginal ultrasound and the diagnosis of fallopian tubal carcinoma. JCU 1991; 19: 116–119

77 Woo J S K, Wong L C, Ma H K. Sonographic patterns of pelvic and hepatic lesions in persistent trophoblastic disease. J Ultrasound Med 1985; 4: 189–198

78 Zanetta G, Lissoni A, Colombo M, Marzola M, Cappellini A, Mangioni C. Detection of abnormal intrauterine vascularization by color Doppler imaging: a possible additional aid for the follow up of patients with gestational trophoblastic tumors. Ultrasound Obstet Gynecol 1996; 7: 32–37

79 Toglia M R, Pearlman M D. Pelvic fluid collections following hysterectomy and their relation to febrile morbidity. Obstet Gynecol 1994; 83: 766–770

80 Istre O, Forman A, Bourne T H. The relationship between preoperative endometrial thickness, the anteroposterior diameter of the uterus and clinical outcome following transcervical resection of the endometrium. Ultrasound Obstet Gynecol 1996; 8: 412–416

81 Khasgir G, Mascarenhas L J, Shaxted E J. The role of transvaginal ultrasonography in pre-operative case selection and post-operative follow-up of endometrial resection. Br J Radiol 1993; 66: 600–604

82 Perrella R R, McLucas B, Ragavendra N, Tessler F N, Schiller V L, Grant E G. Sonographic findings after surgical ablation of the endometrium. AJR 1992; 159: 1239–1241

83 Burks D D, Stainken B R, Burkard T K, Balsara Z N. Uterine inner myometrial foci – relationship prior to dilatation and curettage and endocervical biopsy. J Ultrasound Med 1991; 10: 487–492

84 Novak's textbook of gynecology, 11th edn. Baltimore: Williams & Wilkins, 1988; 728–738

85 Lee A, Eppel W, Sam C, Kratochwil J, Deutinger J, Bernaschek G. Intrauterine device localization by three-dimensional transvaginal sonography. Ultrasound Obstet Gynecol 1997; 10: 289–292

86 White R G, Lyons M, McDowell M. Transvaginal ultrasonography and the IUD. Br J Fam Plann 1990; 16: 22–24

87 Caspi B, Rabinerson D, Appleman Z, Kaplan B. Penetration of the bladder by a perforating intrauterine contraceptive device. Ultrasound Obstet Gynecol 1996; 7: 458–460

88 Vogel S T, Slaskyn B S. Sonography of Nabothian cysts. AJR 1980; 138: 927

89 Quinn M J, Farnsworth B, Bisson D, Stirrat G M. Vaginal endosonography

90 Bernstein R L, Lee S H, Crawford N L. Sonographic evaluation of the incompetent cervix. JCU 1981; 9: 417

91 Parulekar S G, Kiwi R. Ultrasound evaluation of sutures following cervical cerclage for incompetent cervix. J Ultrasound Med 1982; 1: 223–228

92 Subak L L, Hrick H, Powell C B et al. Cervical carcinoma: computed tomography and magnetic resonance imaging for pre operative staging. Obstet Gynecol 1996; 86: 43

93 McCarthy S, Taylor K J W. Sonography of vaginal masses. AJR 1983; 140: 1005–1008

94 Whitehouse G H. Gynaecological radiology, Oxford: Blackwell Scientific, 1981; 135

95 Novak's textbook of gynecology, 11th edn. Baltimore: Williams & Wilkins 1988; 135

96 Sheible F W. Ultrasonic features of Gartner's duct cysts. JCU 1987; 6: 438–439

97 Hagspiel K D. Giant gartner's duct cyst: magnetic resonance imaging findings. Abdom Imaging 1995; 20: 566–568

98 Novak's textbook of gynecology, 11th edn. Baltimore: Williams & Wilkins, 1988; 567

99 In utero exposure to diethylstilboestrol. In: Novak's textbook of gynecology; 11th edn. Baltimore: Williams & Wilkins, 1988; Ch. 25

100 McLeod A L, Lewis E. Sonographic evaluation of paediatric rhabdomyosarcoms. J Ultrasound Med 1984; 3: 69–73

101 Turnbull A, Chamberlain G. Obstetrics. Edinburgh: Churchill Livingstone, 1989; 891

102 Wachsberg R H, Kurz A B. Gas within the endometrial cavity at post partum ultrasound: a normal finding after spontaneous vaginal delivery. Radiology 1992; 183: 431–433

103 Gross R C, McGahan J P. Sonographic detection of partial uterine inversion. AJR 1985; 144: 761–762

104 Baker M E, Kay H, Mahony B S D, Cooper C J, Bowie J D. Sonography of the low transverse incision caesarean section: a prospective study. J Ultrasound Med 1988; 7: 389–393

105 Lonky N M, Worthen N, Ross M G. Prediction of caesarean section scars with ultrasound imaging during pregnancy. J Ultrasound Med 1989; 8: 15–19

106 Herzberg B S, Bowie J D, Kliewer M A. Complications of caesarean section: role of transperineal ultrasound. Radiology 1993; 188: 533–536

107 Avrech O M, Weinaub Z, Herman A et al. Ultrasonic antepartum assessment of a classical caesarean uterine scar and diagnosis of dehiscence. Ultrasound Obstet Gynecol 1994; 4: 151–15

The ovaries

Andrew M Fried

Normal appearances

The ovary varies in size and morphology with both the age and physiological status of the patient. Full evaluation of the ovary is best achieved by the combined use of transabdominal and trans-vaginal scanning. The transabdominal route utilises the filled urinary bladder as an acoustic window and provides an overview of both normal structures and pathological processes. When large masses or fluid collections are present this may be particularly important to define the full extent of the abnormality. The trans-vaginal probe can be used in almost all patients who are sexually active or using tampons, and produces excellent detail of pelvic structures close to the transducer.

Technique of examination

Transabdominal scanning

Drinking 1 litre of fluid 1 hour before the examination will generally adequately fill the bladder, which both serves as a window into the pelvis and displaces bowel. A systematic study of the pelvis is then carried out in both sagittal and transverse planes. The sagittal scans begin in the midline and proceed to the pelvic side wall, to include visualisation of the iliopsoas muscle group and/or the bony pelvis. The margin of the bony pelvis is identified as a highly reflective line with no through transmission of sound.

The variable position of the ovaries makes a complete survey of the pelvis necessary, as they may lie anywhere from immediately posterior to the uterus in the *cul de sac* to laterally against the pelvic side wall.

The transverse scans should proceed from the level of the vagina to above the uterine fundus to ensure complete coverage. Again, the pelvic side walls should be reached by lateral angulation of the transducer. It is often useful to place the transducer in a paramedian position and angle through the filled bladder to image the contralateral adnexa; this technique tends to make maximum use of the bladder as an acoustic window, and can be used in both sagittal and transverse scanning.

The overdistended urinary bladder is not only extremely uncomfortable, but can displace pelvic masses out of the pelvis. Sizeable masses may be overlooked if scanning is not taken sufficiently cephalad.

Trans-vaginal scanning

For the trans-vaginal approach the patient should empty her bladder a short time before the examination. A small amount of urine still present in the bladder helps to maximise patient comfort and the range of angulation of the trans-vaginal probe.

Scanning gel is applied to the probe, which is then covered by a protective sheath, usually a condom.

Elevating the patient's pelvis on a cushion provides increased latitude for motion of the probe. In the absence of a gynaecological examination table equipped with stirrups, the patient merely places her heels together and lets her knees fall apart.

Scans are again performed in a systematic fashion in both sagittal and what is now the coronal plane, extending as far toward each pelvic side wall, the sacral hollow and the retropubic space as can comfortably be managed by moving the handle of the probe. The uterus serves as a useful landmark, as do the internal iliac vessels, as the ovary is usually positioned immediately anterior to these vessels.

Size and morphology

The size of the ovary is generally calculated as an approximate volume (of an ellipse) using the formula: length × width × height × 0.5. The ovary tends to be of slightly lower reflectivity than the uterus, with low-level echoes surrounding the follicles of varying sizes that are also often seen. Calculated volumes include the follicles.

In the child under 5 years old the volume of the ovary is generally less than 1 ml, frequently making it difficult to identify. No lower limit of normal has been suggested in the literature, but failure to identify the ovary does not necessarily imply agenesis or dysgenesis.[1,2] In the premenarchal child from approximately 5 to 9 years of age the ovary averages 3.0 ml, and, at menarche, when the average volume is 4.0 ml, the maximum can reach 6.5 ml (Fig. 3.1).

The previously established maximum normal volume of 6.0 ml for the ovary of a menstruating female is now considered too low. In teenagers and young adults the ovary may reach 14 ml in volume and should still be considered

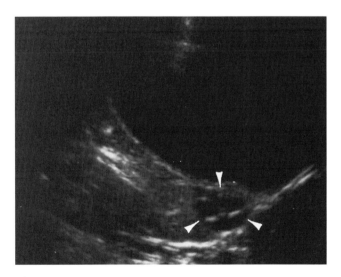

Fig. 3.1 Normal prepubertal ovary. Transabdominal scan of a normal ovary (arrowheads) in a 7-year-old girl. Multiple small follicles are recognisable as echo-free areas without a single dominant developing follicle in this premenarchal subject.

normal.[3–5] A recent study noted an average volume of 9.8 ml for an ovary of a woman in the childbearing years.[6]

In the post-menopausal patient the average volume of a normal ovary has been estimated at 5.8 ml, superseding the previous limit of 2.5 ml.[6,7] It is, however, not uncommon and not necessarily pathological to be unable to image the ovaries in a post-menopausal patient; in one study[8] this occurred in more than a quarter of clinically normal subjects of this age.

Cyclical variations

Although it is possible to detect small follicles in the ovary of a young child they are not commonly seen until at or shortly before menarche. Subsequently, throughout the childbearing years, small round well circumscribed 'cysts' are identified within the ovaries: these are follicles at varying stages of development (Figs 3.2 and 3.3). They

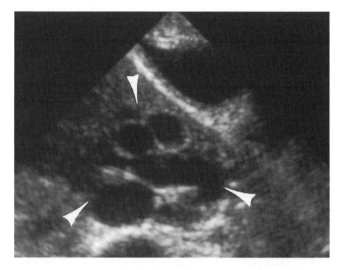

Fig. 3.3 **Normal ovary – trans-vaginal scan.** Multiple follicles are seen in great detail in this scan of a normal adult ovary (arrowheads).

measure 4–5 mm in diameter and commonly remain below 10 mm.

In patients of childbearing age several follicles may be discerned in each ovary at any given time, although there is usually only a single dominant follicle, which enlarges over the course of the first half of the menstrual cycle to reach 20–22 mm in diameter (Figs 3.4 and 3.5). Ovulation generally occurs when the follicle has reached this size, and the timing of planned oocyte retrieval for *in vitro* fertilization is carried out after daily monitoring of follicle size, commencing at about the 9th day of the cycle.[9–11] Identification of the cumulus oophorus as a crescentic

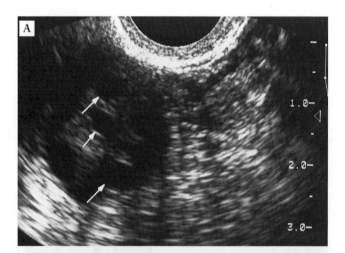

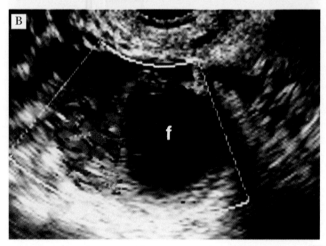

Fig. 3.2 **Normal ovary. A:** Trans-vaginal image of normal adult ovary with multiple small follicles (arrows), none of which is dominant. **B:** Colour flow images of normal ovary with a follicular cyst (f). Note flow throughout the parenchyma.

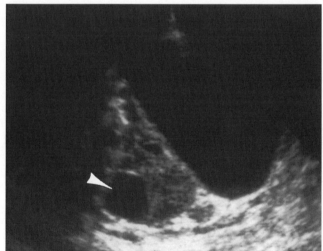

Fig. 3.4 **A dominant follicle.** In this transabdominal view a dominant follicle (arrowhead) is developing and measures approximately 18 mm in maximum diameter. This is within the range of sizes (18–22 mm) at which ovulation will occur.

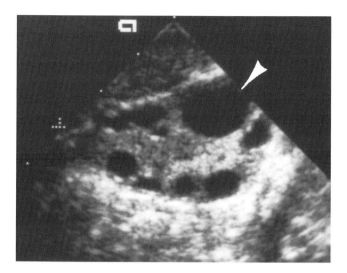

Fig. 3.5 **Dominant follicle – trans-vaginal scan.** Multiple follicles ranging in size from 3 to 8 mm in diameter are seen, with one follicle (arrowhead) measuring 14 mm and destined to be the dominant one.

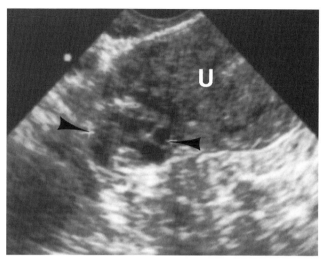

Fig. 3.6 **Normal ovary.** Trans-verse transvaginal scan displays the right ovary (arrowheads) in its most common location immediately adjacent to the lateral aspect of the uterus (U).

reflective focus with an echo-poor centre within the dominant follicle is taken to be a sign of imminent ovulation.[12] Failure to visualise the cumulus is encountered in 50% of women with primary or secondary infertility.

Following ovulation, the follicle shrinks to form a small highly reflective structure representing the corpus luteum. This forms initially with haemorrhage at the time of extrusion of the ovum, and later by deposition of lipid-containing luteal cells.[13] Persistence of the corpus luteum as a recognisable cyst within the postovulatory period is not uncommon, particularly when fertilisation has occurred. The cyst normally regresses spontaneously. The greater anatomical detail that can be achieved using the trans-vaginal approach has led to this becoming the standard method for monitoring patients in infertility programmes. Cyclical changes cease a year or so after the menopause and the finding of cystic enlargement of the ovary in the post-menopausal patient should be viewed with suspicion. However, benign cysts are encountered in the post-menopausal patient and may frequently be followed to spontaneous resolution.[14] Small cysts (less than 3 cm in diameter) are new encountered in up to 15% of post-menopausal ovaries.[15] Simple cysts (without septations or solid internal components) measuring less than 5 cm may be followed sonographically without surgical intervention.[16–19] Cystic masses lying outside these criteria should be removed surgically.

Position

The ovaries most commonly lie lateral to the uterus (usually within a few centimetres) at about the level of the cornua (Fig. 3.6). They are enveloped in the two layers of peritoneum that constitute the broad ligament. Variations

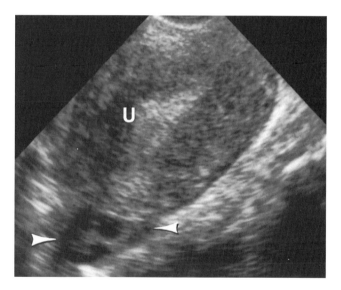

Fig. 3.7 **The normal ovary** (arrowheads) in this sagittal trans-vaginal scan lies posterior to the fundus of the uterus (U). This represents only one of many normal variants.

are, however, frequent and of no clinical significance. It is, for example, not uncommon to find an ovary in the pouch of Douglas, or lying laterally near the pelvic side wall (this latter situation occurs particularly in multiparae, in whom the ligamentous structures may be relatively lax) (Figs 3.7 and 3.8). Ovarian masses, both benign and malignant, may displace the ovary out of the pelvis, as may the enlarging uterus in pregnancy.

A relatively constant relationship of the ovaries is their situation anterior to the internal iliac vessels. These vessels serve as particularly useful landmarks for the location of the ovaries during trans-vaginal scanning, when orien-

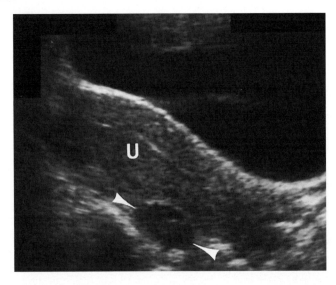

Fig. 3.8 Normal ovary. This ovary (arrowheads) is found in the *cul de sac* posterior to the uterus (U), another common location.

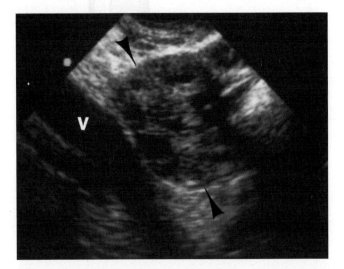

Fig. 3.9 Normal ovary. In this sagittal trans-vaginal scan the ovary (arrowheads) was located by first identifying the internal iliac vessels. The ovary is seen to lie immediately anterior to the internal iliac vein (V).

tation of the scan plane can sometimes be confusing (Fig. 3.9).

Pathological changes

Absence

In patients with Turner's syndrome (45 XO karyotype) ultrasound usually fails to demonstrate the ovaries, in keeping with the pathological descriptions of absent or fibrous streak ovaries. In genetic mosaicism, however, small or near-normal ovaries may be identified. Because of this, the demonstration of ovarian tissue does not exclude

Turner's syndrome.[20] Absence of the ovaries is also a feature of pure gonadal dysgenesis (Swyer's syndrome), but the patient is of normal stature.[21]

Some form of renal anomaly, most commonly a horseshoe kidney,[22] has been identified in a significant proportion of patients with Turner's syndrome (39% in one study); it is therefore important to examine the kidneys at the time of the pelvic examination.

Functional cysts

Follicular cyst

The normal follicle typically reaches a maximum diameter of 22–25 mm at ovulation, and either shrinks dramatically or disappears entirely following extrusion of the ovum. Failure of the follicle to rupture or involute may result in a follicular cyst. Morphologically this remains a simple, sharply marginated cyst with very thin walls; it may reach 4 cm in diameter (Fig. 3.10). Spontaneous regression is usual, and repeating the study 6–8 weeks later will confirm this (Figs 3.11 and 3.12). Haemorrhage into a follicular cyst may result in internal echoes in the form of septa or gravity-dependent particulate debris (Figs 3.13 to 3.15). This does not alter the ultimate outcome.[23,24]

Corpus luteum cyst

Failure of involution of the corpus luteum following ovulation may result in the formation of a corpus luteum cyst, instead of the small highly reflective focus within the ovary which represents the usual residuum. A corpus luteum cyst usually has a thicker wall than a follicular cyst and may grow to 5–10 cm in diameter. It is more likely to produce

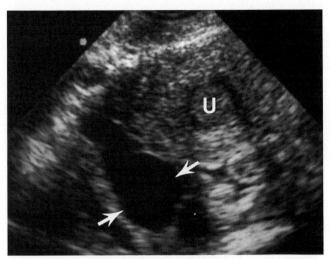

Fig. 3.10 Follicular cyst. The thin-walled cyst (arrows) seen in the right adnexa on trans-vaginal scan in all likelihood represents a follicular cyst in the right ovary and will regress spontaneously. U – uterus.

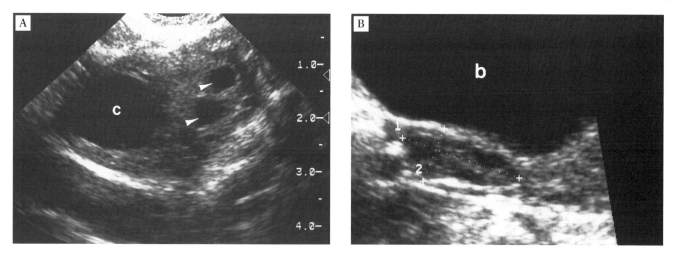

Fig. 3.11 Functional cyst. A: Trans-vaginal scans of ovary with a functional cyst (c) and two small follicles (arrowheads). **B:** Transabdominal scan 7 weeks later; the cyst has regressed spontaneously. Ovary is delineated by calipers. b – urinary bladder.

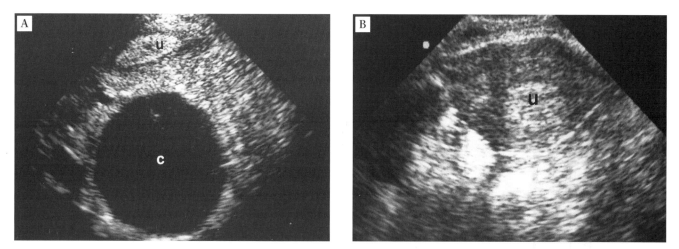

Fig. 3.12 Simple cyst. A: Trans-vaginal scan demonstrates a 4.2 cm simple cyst (c) in the right ovary. **B:** Follow-up study at 5 weeks shows spontaneous regression of the cyst, confirming its functional nature. u – uterus.

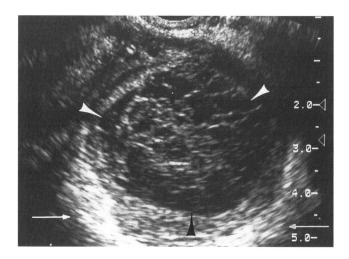

Fig. 3.13 Haemorrhagic cyst (arrowheads) of left ovary contains extensive internal echoes but maintains good through transmission (arrows), confirming the cystic nature of the mass.

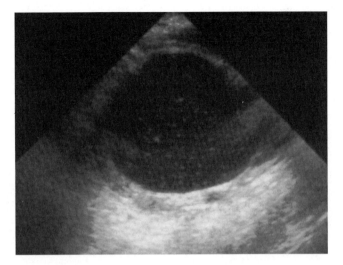

Fig. 3.14 Haemorrhagic functional cyst. A trans-vaginal view demonstrates the particulate matter representing clot breakdown products.

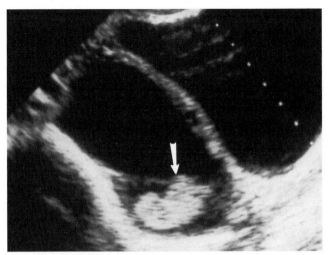

Fig. 3.15 Haemorrhagic cyst. Here the clot (arrow) lies in the most dependent position. On repositioning the patient the clot moved.

symptoms. Here too, haemorrhage may produce internal echoes in the form of debris or septations (Figs 3.16 and 3.17). Serial scans should document spontaneous regression of the cyst; this is of particular significance when the corpus luteum cyst coincides with pregnancy, as failure to regress by about 18–20 weeks gestation may be an indication for surgical intervention (Fig. 3.18). Torsion, spontaneous rupture and mechanical obstruction of delivery are problems associated with the persistence of a sizeable corpus luteum cyst. The functional role of the corpus luteum in early pregnancy is the production of progesterone, which supports the secretory endometrium.

Corpora lutea cysts may be seen in up to one third of normal pregnancies.

Congenital ovarian cyst

In the neonate congenital ovarian cysts can reach quite large sizes and occasionally contain internal septations or debris. There have been an increasing number of these detected during antenatal ultrasound examination. They are almost invariably benign but, when very large, can produce significant compression of the abdominal viscera (and even elevation of the diaphragm), requiring surgical

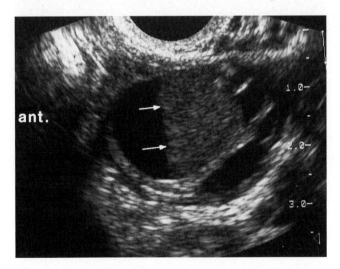

Fig. 3.16 Haemorrhagic cyst. Particulate matter forming a fluid–debris level (arrows) represents lysing clot in this haemorrhagic ovarian cyst. (ant. – anterior in this trans-vaginal scan, accounting for the orientation of the fluid level.)

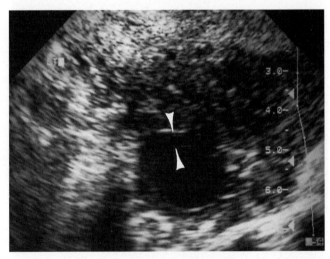

Fig. 3.17 Functional cyst. The relatively thick wall (arrowheads) of this functional cyst suggests a corpus luteum cyst rather than a follicular cyst, which characteristically has a thin wall. Distinction is frequently difficult and histological proof is often lacking, as both tend to regress spontaneously.

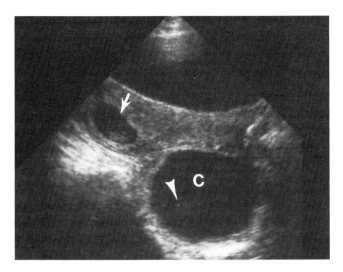

Fig. 3.18 Normal pregnancy and corpus luteum cyst. In association with a normal intra-uterine pregnancy of approximately 8 weeks gestation (arrow) there is a 7.5 cm corpus luteum cyst (C) with some low-level internal echoes (arrowhead). Usually these cysts can be followed to spontaneous resolution.

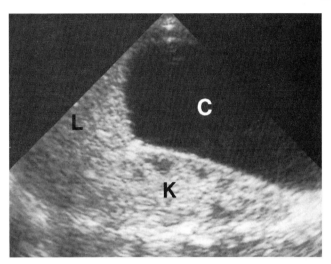

Fig. 3.19 Congenital ovarian cyst. A very large congenital ovarian cyst (C) rises out of the pelvis of this newborn infant; it lies immediately below the liver (L) and anterior to the right kidney (K). Note the high reflectivity of the normal neonatal kidney.

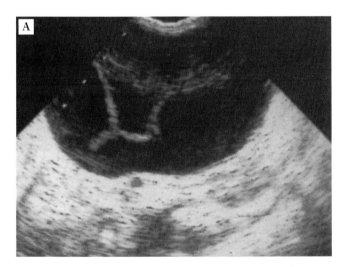

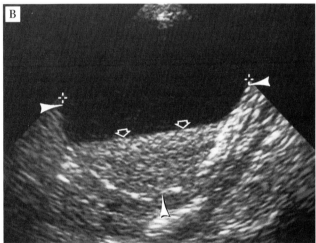

Fig. 3.20 Congenital ovarian cyst. A: Congenital ovarian cysts may display a variety of internal echo patterns beyond the simple fluid-filled cyst. Note the multiple internal septations in this congenital ovarian cyst. **B:** Congenital ovarian cyst (arrowheads) with fluid–debris level (open arrowheads) extended well up into the right upper quadrant. Percutaneous aspiration produced essentially complete resolution of the cyst.

intervention.[25,26] The growth of such cysts is presumed to result, at least in part, from the influence of maternal hormones (Figs 3.19 and 3.20).

Polycystic ovaries

The clinical triad of hirsutism, obesity and oligomenorrhoea constitutes the Stein–Leventhal syndrome.[27] The classic appearance is of enlarged, spherical ovaries (the ovary is normally ovoid) with multiple small peripheral cysts (Figs 3.21 and 3.22).[28] More than 10 cysts greater than 5 mm in diameter in an ovary whose volume exceeds the expected 14 ml is considered typical. As the patient is often obese, trans-vaginal scanning may be particularly useful for full evaluation. The characteristic morphology of polycystic ovaries is seen in less than half the patients with clinical and biochemical evidence of the syndrome.[29,30] Thirty percent have normal ovarian volumes at ultrasound and, in an additional 25%, echo-poor ovaries are seen without demonstrable follicles.[4,31]

Increased levels of luteinising hormone or elevated ratios of luteinising hormone to follicle-stimulating

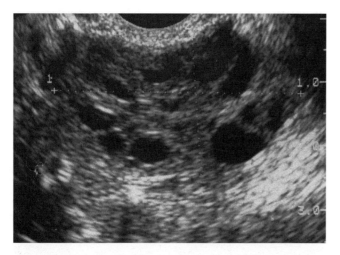

Fig. 3.21 Polycystic ovary. Trans-vaginal scan of a mildly enlarged ovary with multiple small, undeveloped follicles without a single dominant one.

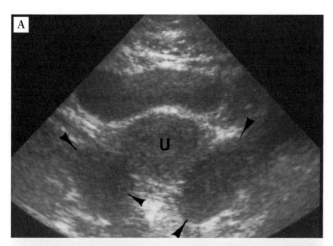

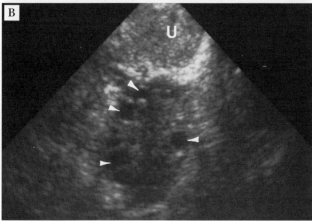

Fig. 3.22 Polycystic ovaries. A: Bilateral ovarian enlargement is seen in this transverse transabdominal scan of a patient with polycystic ovaries (arrowheads). The ovarian volumes were 15.4 and 21.4 ml. U – uterus. Visualisation is often compromised because of the patient's obesity. **B:** Trans-vaginal view of the ovary in the same patient demonstrates a number of follicles of different sizes (arrowheads). U – uterus.

hormone (LH/FSH) or direct pathological examination of the ovaries is definitive.[32] A decrease in the volume of the ovaries in response to LHRH analogue therapy for polycystic ovaries can be documented by ultrasound.[33]

The epidemiology of polycystic ovaries merits some consideration. The condition has been identified in 21% of all presentations to infertility clinics, as well as in 22% of the general population.[34,35] A strong familial tendency was documented in that same study in which polycystic ovaries were identified in 92% of pedigrees studied.[34] A significant association of polycystic ovaries has also been identified in patients with congenital adrenal hyperplasia: more than 80% of adults and 40% of post-pubertal girls with adrenal hyperplasia were found to have polycystic ovaries as well.[36,37]

Hyperstimulated ovaries

Increased circulating levels of human chorionic gonadotrophin (HCG) can produce cystic enlargement of both ovaries. Two situations are commonly responsible for this phenomenon: trophoblastic disease and exogenous administration in cases of infertility.

Trophoblastic disease produces extremely high levels of HCG irrespective of the histology of the disease (i.e. hydatidiform mole, chorioadenoma destruens or invasive mole, or choriocarcinoma). Large multiseptated ovaries are encountered in some 20–50% of cases, and in as many as 50% are bilateral (Fig. 3.23). These theca lutein cysts regress spontaneously following evacuation of the trophoblastic tissue from the uterus, but the ovaries may take several months to return to normal size and morphology.[8,38]

Therapeutic administration of HCG to stimulate ovulation in the infertile patient can produce similar multilocu-

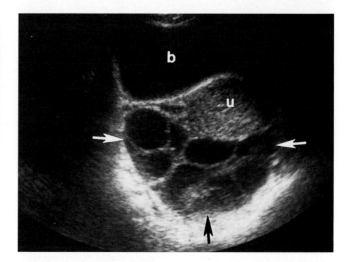

Fig. 3.23 Theca lutein cysts. Transverse transabdominal view of bilateral theca lutein cysts forming a confluent multilocular cystic mass (arrows) in the *cul de sac*. u – uterus; b – urinary bladder.

lated cystic enlargement of the ovaries (Fig. 3.24). A broad spectrum of hyperstimulated ovaries has been observed in this setting, ranging from several small cysts to ovaries that reach and exceed 10 cm in diameter (Figs 3.25 and 3.26). The presence of ascites and severe electrolyte imbalances which accompany the full-blown hyperstimulation syndrome may signal a life-threatening condition.[8,39] Even with simple bilateral cystic enlargement of the ovaries resulting from iatrogenic overstimulation, pursuit of pregnancy during that cycle is considered inadvisable because of the increased risk of multiple gestations.[40,41] A decrease in the fraction of mature follicles and an increase in the number of very small follicles correlates with the risk for development of the ovarian hyperstimulation syndrome.[42]

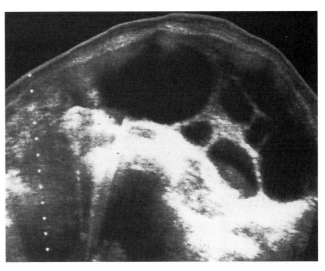

Fig. 3.25 Hyperstimulated ovaries. The static scan in this patient outlines a left ovary which measures more than 16 cm in diameter. No ascites is seen, however, and the patient did not display all the features of the hyperstimulation syndrome.

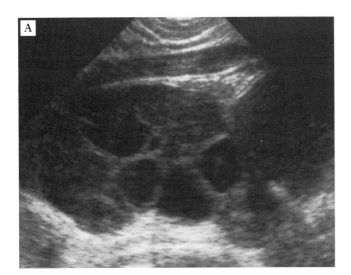

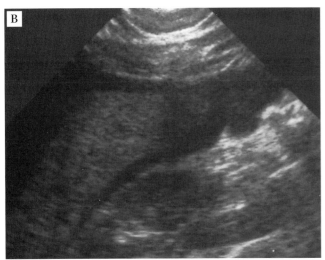

Fig. 3.24 Hyperstimulated ovaries. A: Longitudinal scan in the midline showing a massively enlarged ovary superior to the bladder. Under the influence of fertility drugs, such as clomiphene citrate, the ovaries may grow large with multiseptated cysts, as in this patient with hyperstimulated ovaries. **B:** A scan in the right upper quadrant showing ascites which is a complication of this condition.

The incidence of ovarian hyperstimulation syndrome in all degrees of severity has been reported as high as 23%, and varies from a mild, asymptomatic condition identifiable only by ultrasound to one in which massive shifts of fluid out of the vascular space produce ascites, hydrothorax and renal failure.[43,44] Classification of the severity of the syndrome is based on a combination of clinical, laboratory and ultrasound findings. In general, ovarian size is less than 5 cm in the mild form, 5–12 cm in the moderate, and more than 12 cm in severe cases. The syndrome is more common in patients with polycystic ovary disease who are treated with gonadotrophins (see Ch. 4).

Ovarian remnant syndrome

If even a small amount of functioning ovarian tissue is left behind at oophorectomy cyst formation may occur, producing confusion in the face of a history of prior surgical removal of both ovaries (Fig. 3.27). Both simple and haemorrhagic cysts have been reported in this context, and the possibility must be considered.[45]

Torsion

Torsion of the ovary is seen most commonly in teenagers and young adults; the presence of an ovarian mass, such as a functional cyst or dermoid, as well as inflammatory processes, is thought to predispose to this condition.[46] Such underlying pathology is reported to occur in as many as 70% of cases. Pain, fever, nausea and vomiting may constitute the presenting clinical picture; leukocytosis frequently accompanies torsion, which may therefore simulate

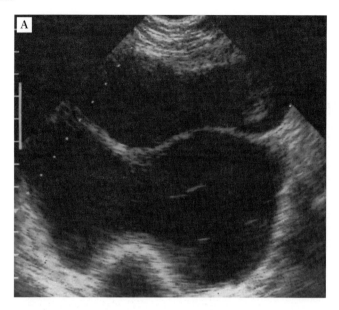

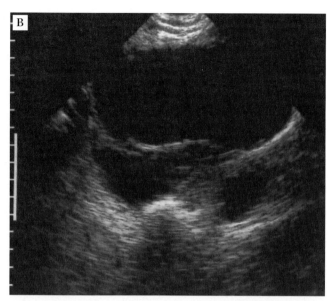

Fig. 3.26 Bilateral ovarian enlargement. A: Marked bilateral ovarian enlargement is seen in this patient on fertility drugs. **B:** Three weeks after cessation of therapy the ovaries have returned to near-normal size.

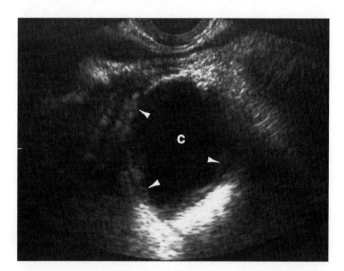

Fig. 3.27 Ovarian remnant. Trans-vaginal scan of patient who had previously undergone hysterectomy and bilateral oophorectomy demonstrates a 4.5 cm cystic mass (c) with a thin rim of solid tissue (arrowheads) representing an ovarian remnant.

a wide variety of clinical conditions, including gastro-enteritis, appendicitis and urinary tract infection.[47]

The ultrasound appearance of the torted ovary is highly variable. Enlargement to 4–10 cm in diameter is common; the texture varies from largely solid to nearly cystic, and good through-transmission of sound is generally preserved in either case (Fig. 3.28).[48] Free fluid is frequently found in the pelvis.

The position of the torted ovary is quite variable, with the midline being a common location; identification of the ovary superior to the uterus has also been reported.[49] The torsion may also involve portions of the tube, which becomes dilated.[50]

Both duplex and colour flow Doppler techniques may be helpful; some observers have noted a cluster of dilated vessels in the periphery of a torted ovary.

Epithelial neoplasms

Serous cystadenoma – cystadenocarcinoma

The most common neoplasms of the ovary are epithelial in origin. Serous cystadenoma, which constitutes approximately 20% of all benign neoplasms of the ovary, appears as a unilocular or multilocular cystic mass with thin septations, few or no internal echoes and sharply defined walls (Figs 3.29 and 3.30). The septa are sufficiently thin to undulate when gently palpated with the transducer. They are generally 2–3 mm thick, without nodularity or mural nodules of solid tissue. Although papillary projections may sometimes be encountered in the benign form, the greater the amount of solid tissue present the greater is the concern for borderline or malignant histology (Fig. 3.31).[51]

About 15% of epithelial malignancies of the ovary are of borderline histology: the ultrasound distinction between benign and malignant, always difficult, is nearly

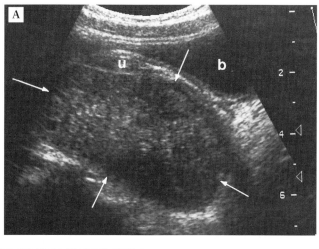

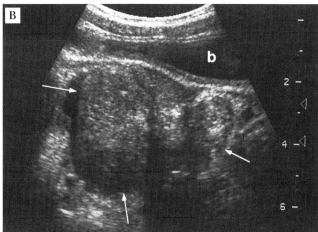

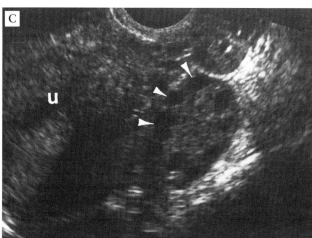

Fig. 3.28 Ovarian torsion. Heterogeneous soft tissue mass (arrows) in the right posterior adnexa seen on both **A:** sagittal and **B:** transverse views represents a torted ovary and tube. **C:** The peripheral arrangement of the follicles (arrowheads), although not specific, is said to be suggestive of ovarian torsion. b – bladder, u – uterus.

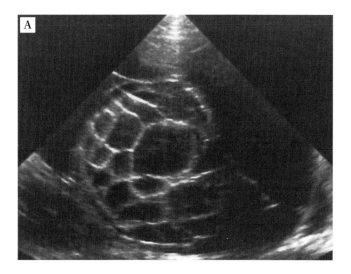

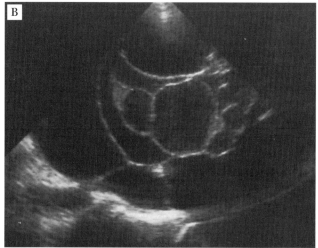

Fig. 3.29 Benign serous cystadenoma. **A:** Longitudinal and **B:** transverse scans. This very large benign serous cystadenoma has very thin septa, a characteristic finding in benign lesions. A few low-level echoes are present in some of the cysts.

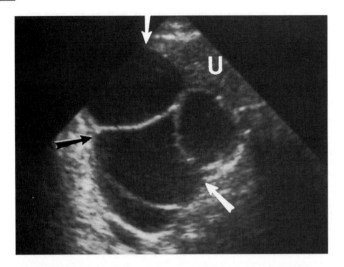

Fig. 3.30 Serous cystadenoma. A trans-vaginal scan demonstrates a small benign serous cystadenoma of the right ovary (arrows) with multiple thin septa. U – uterus.

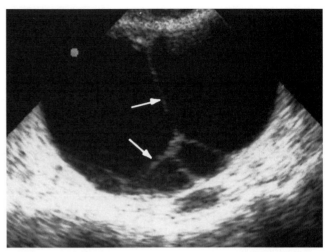

Fig. 3.31 This benign serous cystadenoma with few, thin septa (arrows) is otherwise purely cystic and without a wall of measurable thickness.

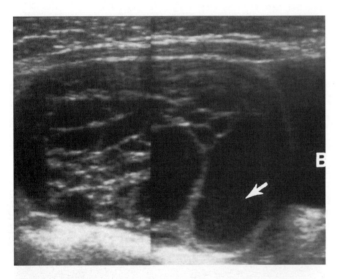

Fig. 3.32 Borderline mucinous cystadenoma. Increasing numbers of soft tissue septa are seen in this histologically borderline mucinous cystadenoma. The low-level echoes of contained mucin (arrow) are characteristic. B – bladder.

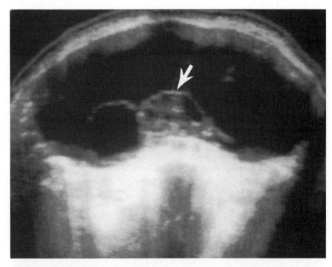

Fig. 3.33 This borderline mucinous cystadenoma displays more numerous and thicker septa (arrow) than the simple benign cystadenoma in Fig. 3.31.

impossible in this situation.[52] Serous cystadenocarcinoma accounts for approximately 40% of malignant tumours of the ovary. Features suggesting malignancy include thickening of the septa, increased numbers and size of mural nodules, foci of solid tissue and the presence of ascites (Figs 3.32 and 3.33). Ascites has been reported with a frequency of greater than 50% in ovarian cancer (and is always associated with peritoneal spread of the tumour), whereas it is said never to occur with benign disease.[53] Malignant tumours may be bilateral in as many as 62.5% of cases.[53,54] Ultrasound is relatively insensitive in the recognition of peritoneal spread of tumour (as is CT).

Mucinous cystadenoma – adenocarcinoma

Like their serous counterparts, mucinous tumours of the ovary display multiple septa dividing fluid-containing loculations. The septa in mucinous disease tend to be more numerous than in serous neoplasms and fine, low-level internal echoes are more common. These are thought to represent the viscid mucin and can often form fluid–debris levels (Fig. 3.34). Although most mucinous neoplasms are in the range of 15–30 cm in diameter, they can grow considerably larger and have been reported to reach 50 cm.[51]

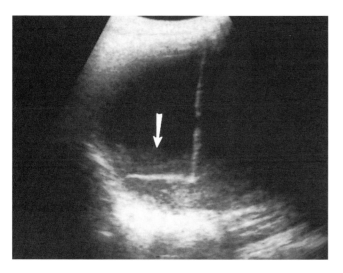

Fig. 3.34 **Benign mucinous cystadenoma.** Gravity-dependent low-level echoes (arrow) are seen in this benign mucinous cystadenoma. The septa are quite thin.

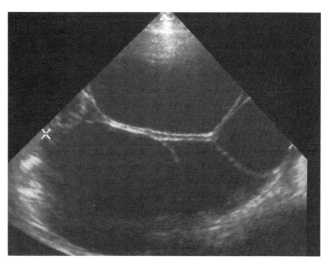

Fig. 3.35 **Mucinous cystadenocarcinoma.** With its thin septa and minimal soft tissue components, there is little to distinguish this well differentiated grade I mucinous cystadenocarcinoma from its benign counterpart.

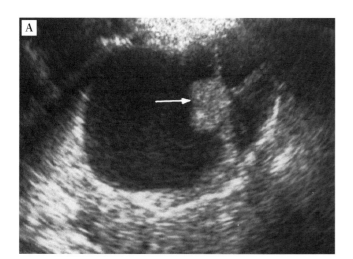

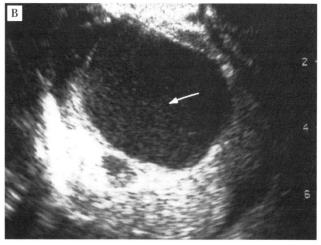

Fig. 3.36 **Mucinous cystadenocarcinoma** is characterised by **A:** the presence of soft tissue thickening of the septa (arrow) and **B:** low-level echoes within the cyst (arrow), representing mucin.

Mucinous neoplasms represent some 20% of ovarian masses and are more likely to be benign than malignant (Figs 3.35 to 3.38).

The larger a mass becomes the more difficult it is to identify its organ of origin with certainty. Large necrotic uterine leiomyomata, for example, can be difficult to distinguish from ovarian tumours. Identification of the ovary as separable from the mass is often extremely difficult but, if achieved, helps to make this distinction.

Germ cell tumours

Dermoid (teratoma)

Few other pathological processes or neoplasms display the broad spectrum of ultrasound appearances of which ovarian dermoid tumours are capable. Comprised of mixtures of fat, hair, sebum, calcium, epithelial tissue, neural elements and debris in varying proportions, dermoids may be cystic, complex or solid, and any combination of these, depending upon which component predominates.[47]

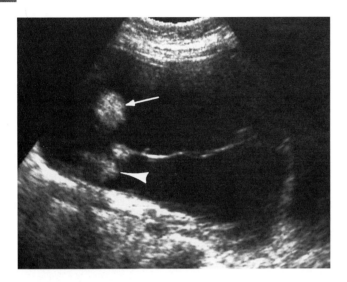

Fig. 3.37 Mucinous cystadenocarcinoma. Soft tissue nodule (arrow) and septal thickening (arrowhead) are seen in this stage I mucinous cystadenocarcinoma.

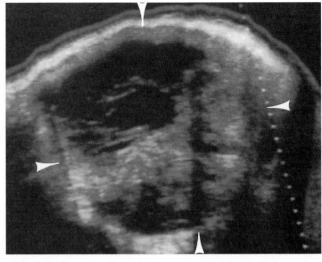

Fig. 3.38 Mucinous cystadenocarcinoma. A predominantly solid lesion with some areas of cyst formation is produced by this mucinous cystadenocarcinoma in combination with anaplastic carcinoid (arrowheads).

The classic and almost pathognomonic appearance of an ovarian dermoid is a well circumscribed mass containing a fluid–debris level with an internal focus of highly reflective material, which may produce an acoustic shadow. The fluid–debris level represents the interface between hair and sebum or sebum and cellular debris, and the reflective focus either fat (no acoustic shadow) or calcification (shadowing) (Fig. 3.39). A mural nodule of solid tissue, the 'dermoid plug', has also been described as strongly suggestive of the diagnosis (Fig. 3.40);[55] it may

also produce an acoustic shadow. Identification of a mural nodule or shadowing component in these tumours is much more common after puberty.[56]

Hair floating on sebum is strongly reflective and may produce shadowing distally, which obscures the tissues deep to it. In this case only the anterior margin of the dermoid will be visualised, giving rise to the 'tip of the iceberg' sign in which most of the volume of the mass is not seen.[57] It should be noted here that the stool-filled rectosigmoid colon can produce a similar appearance, at

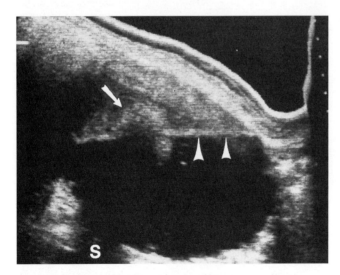

Fig. 3.39 Dermoid. This classic dermoid displays a fluid–debris level (arrowheads), probably representing hair floating on sebum, with a highly reflective focus of calcium (arrow) which produces an acoustic shadow (S).

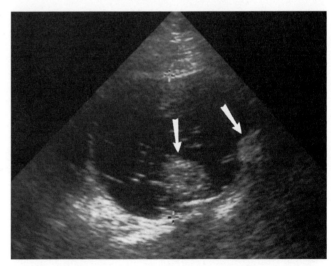

Fig. 3.40 Cystic dermoid. Two foci of solid tissue (arrows) are seen in the periphery of this largely cystic dermoid. These represent the so-called 'dermoid plug'.

least in the transverse plane. Sagittal views should demonstrate the linear pattern of the colon, thus distinguishing it from a dermoid.

By virtue of the broad range of appearances of ovarian dermoids the differential diagnosis includes haemorrhagic ovarian cyst, epithelial neoplasm, tubo-ovarian abscess, pedunculated leiomyoma, ectopic gestation and endometrioma, to list only the more common conditions (Figs 3.41 to 3.43).[58] Sacrococcygeal teratoma is a mass of equally heterogeneous composition and, particularly when large, can simulate an ovarian dermoid.

Malignant changes in ovarian dermoids are not common and tend to occur mainly in post-menopausal patients, with a reported frequency of 2–4%. Unfortunately there are no specific ultrasound signs that allow differentiation between benign and malignant teratomas (Fig. 3.44), unless liver metastases and ascites can be demonstrated (Figs 3.45 to 3.47).[51]

Sex cord – stromal tumours

The hormonally active tumours constitute approximately 10% of all ovarian tumours and 2% of malignant neoplasms.[59] Generally they show no distinguishing ultrasound features to allow definitive identification.

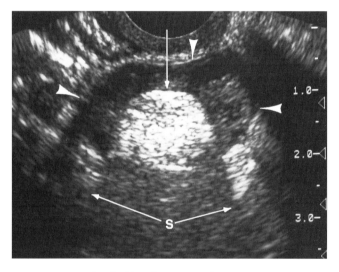

Fig. 3.41 Dermoid. A highly reflective mass (long arrow) with partial acoustic shadowing (s) represents hair in a dermoid within the ovary (arrowheads).

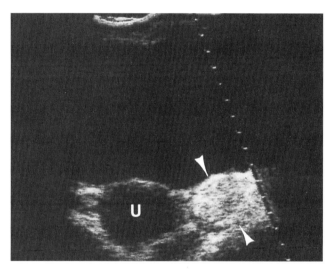

Fig. 3.42 Dermoid. A markedly reflective pattern without acoustic shadowing is produced by a dermoid which is mostly composed of fat (arrowheads). Compare the echoes to those of the muscle of the uterus (u).

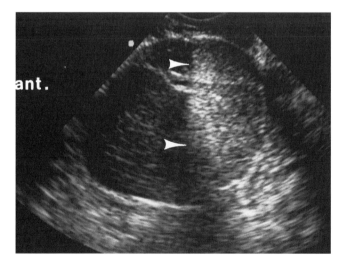

Fig. 3.43 Dermoid. Trans-vaginal view of a dermoid with a fluid–debris level (arrowheads), presumably produced by sebum, which is liquid at body temperature, with hair, debris etc.

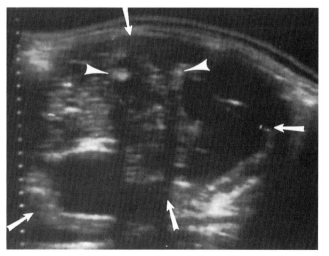

Fig. 3.44 Teratoma. This large teratoma (arrows) in a 13-year-old was a teratocarcinoma grade I. It contains a mixture of heterogeneous cystic and solid elements, including foci of calcification (arrowheads).

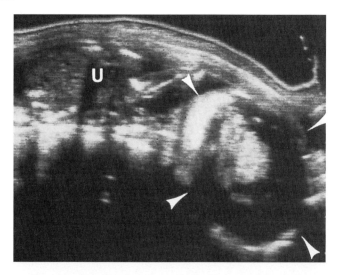

Fig. 3.45 Complex dermoid. This large complex dermoid (arrowheads) was initially thought to represent a bulging amniotic sac with fetal small parts in this patient who was 23 weeks pregnant. Gentle pressure demonstrated that the dermoid moved independently of the uterus (U).

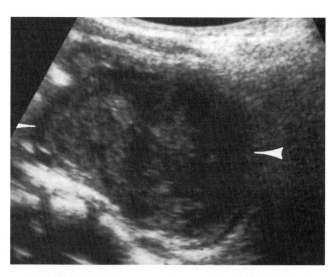

Fig. 3.46 Embryonal cell sarcoma. Other pelvic tumours may be indistinguishable from those arising from the ovary. This embryonal cell sarcoma (arrowheads) was of indeterminate origin; the mixed texture is similar to that of many ovarian tumours.

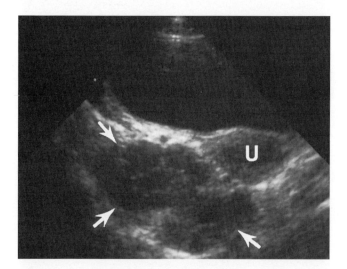

Fig. 3.47 Neurofibromas. Underscoring the wide variety of tumorous conditions that may present as adnexal masses are these lobular, echo-poor mass in the right adnexal region (arrows), which are neurofibromas. U – uterus.

Thecomas, which occur in the post-menopausal age group, are reported to produce extensive acoustic shadowing involving the entire extent of the tumour. No obvious explanation has been offered for this phenomenon. Thecomas are unilateral and are histologically benign.[60,61]

Granulosa cell tumours produce oestrogen in post-menopausal patients; although solid when small, when larger they may become cystic and septated and be difficult to distinguish by ultrasound from epithelial neo-plasms of the ovary, or even pedunculated fibroids of the uterus.[62]

Masculinisation is produced by Sertoli–Leydig cell tumours of the ovary; these account for less than 0.5% of ovarian neoplasms and display a non-specific ultrasound appearance.

Fibromas of the ovary may occur in both pre- and post-menopausal patients: they constitute about 5% of ovarian neoplasms. Although they are generally echo-poor, fibromas attenuate the sound beam quite markedly (Fig. 3.48). Enlarging to 5–10 cm and beyond, they can be associated with ascites and pleural effusion (Meig's syndrome) in a small percentage of cases (1–3%).[63,64] Although Brenner tumours are histologically classified as epithelial neoplasms they are ultrasonically indistinguishable from fibromas, being solid, echo-poor and with good transmission. They occasionally contain peripheral calcification (Fig. 3.49).[65]

Endometrioid carcinoma

Accounting for approximately 20% of ovarian malignancies, endometrioid carcinoma usually shows a solid appearance with areas of necrosis and/or haemorrhage in a significant number of cases (Fig. 3.50). This pattern is unlike that of the epithelial tumours of the ovary and should raise the possibility of endometrioid histology. It has been suggested that long-standing endometriosis predisposes to this malignancy, but this concept is not universally accepted.[66,67] It is true, however, that the histology of endometrioid carcinoma is quite similar to that of endometrial carcinoma of the uterus.[68]

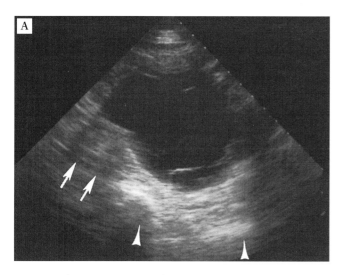

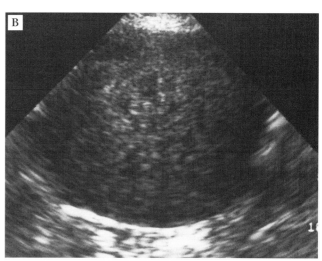

Fig. 3.48 Fibroma. A: Cystadenofibroma. On histological examination this mass proved to be a serous cystadenofibroma. Note that some areas demonstrate good through transmission (arrowheads), whereas others, despite an echo-poor texture, attenuate most of the beam (arrows). **B:** Ovarian fibroma with low-level echoes and characteristic moderate sound attenuation.

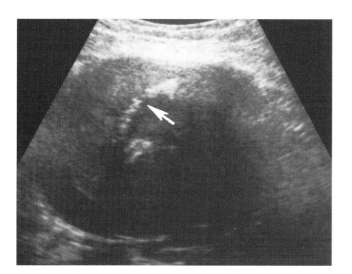

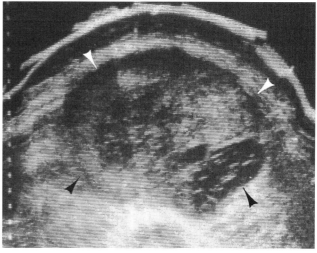

Fig. 3.49 Brenner tumour. The solid, echo-poor but attenuating character of this large Brenner tumour is indistinguishable from that of an ovarian fibroma. Brenner tumours occasionally contain peripheral calcification, as in this case (arrow).

Fig. 3.50 Endometrioid carcinoma. Although they may have large areas of cyst formation, endometrioid carcinomas are characteristically solid, as in this case (arrowheads).

Secondary ovarian neoplasms

The original description of the Krukenberg tumour was of metastases to the ovary from signet-ring cell mucin-producing malignancies of the gastrointestinal tract, chiefly the stomach. Over the years the term 'Krukenberg tumour' has come to be applied to a variety of malignancies that metastasise to the ovary, notably breast, lung, endometrium and the gastrointestinal tract. They account for approximately 10% of ovarian malignancies.[69,70] The ultrasound appearance is variable, but a predominant solid component is generally sufficient to direct the diagnosis away from the more common cystadenomatous disease, with its predominantly fluid structure and multiple septations (Fig. 3.51). No specific appearance of the ovaries at ultrasound enables identification of the primary malignancy.

The lymphoproliferative disorders, lymphoma and leukaemia, can also involve the ovary. Echo-poor enlargement of one or both ovaries is occasionally seen in leukaemia, but more often in lymphoma, chiefly non-Hodgkin's and Burkitt's, as opposed to Hodgkin's disease (Fig. 3.52).[71,72] Lymphadenopathy elsewhere, such as the

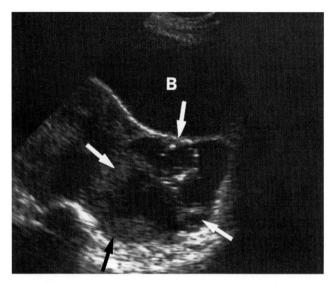

Fig. 3.51 **Krukenberg tumour.** Irregular, heterogenous enlargement of the ovary (arrows) by metastatic adenocarcinoma. B – bladder.

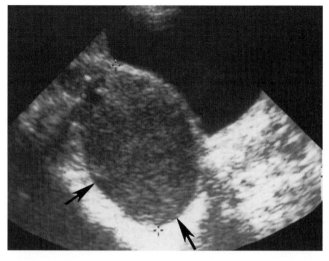

Fig. 3.52 **Ovarian lymphoma.** Homogeneous echo-poor enlargement of the ovary (arrows) is a typical pattern of involvement by leukaemia and lymphoma. This 8-year-old girl was found to have non-Hodgkin's lymphoma.

retroperitoneum, may serve to suggest this possibility. Involvement of the uterus may blend together with enlarged ovaries to form a lobular echo-poor mass with indistinct borders between the individual organs. CT is the method most often employed for monitoring disease regression with chemotherapy, but ultrasound can also be used to monitor tumour shrinkage.

Adnexal pathology

Pelvic inflammatory disease

A number of factors predispose to the development of pelvic inflammatory disease. Sexually transmitted infections, foreign bodies (e.g. intra-uterine contraceptive devices), and non-sterile instrumentation (e.g. septic abortion) are among the most common. *Neisseria*, chlamydial and streptococcal infections are frequently implicated, and clinical findings include pelvic pain, vaginal discharge, pyrexia, gastrointestinal symptoms and leukocytosis.

The ultrasound findings of early pelvic inflammatory disease (PID) may be minimal. Beginning as an endometritis from an ascending infection, PID may be manifest as mild uterine enlargement, sometimes with a small fluid collection within the endometrial canal.[73] However, as a small amount of free fluid is a frequent normal finding in the pelvis of a female of childbearing age this observation is of little diagnostic significance. Enlargement of the ovaries and thickening of the adnexal tissues has been described in PID but is difficult to identify with confidence.

With a clinical picture of PID but without demonstrable findings at ultrasound, antibiotic treatment should not

be delayed. The role of ultrasound will have been of value in excluding a frank abscess.[74]

With progression of the disease ultrasound demonstrates irregularly marginated fluid collections or complex masses in the adnexae and/or *cul de sac* representing abscess formation (Fig. 3.53). The fluid frequently contains echoes as a result of highly proteinaceous material or cellular debris (Fig. 3.54). It is often difficult or impossible to identify the ovaries separately from the inflammatory mass as they, along with the fallopian tubes, have been engulfed in the formation of what is now a tubo-ovarian abscess. The outlines of the uterus are commonly also obscured (Figs 3.55 and 3.56).

The occluded tube may produce a characteristic picture of a figure of eight-shaped fluid collection, often with internal echoes which may be gravity dependent (Figs 3.57 and 3.58). This represents a pyosalpinx and requires drainage, as does any other definable adnexal fluid collection. Some investigators have reported good results with percutaneous drainage of such pelvic abscesses.[74-77] In its chronic form the pyosalpinx may evolve into a hydrosalpinx, which often contains a fluid–debris level comprised of material that is now culture negative.

The ultrasound finding of a complex pelvic mass most often defies interpretation in the absence of clinical information, as such a picture can be produced by a wide variety of markedly different pathological processes. Epithelial neoplasms of the ovary (benign or malignant), haemorrhagic ovarian cysts, necrotic uterine leiomyomata, endometriomas, haematomata and ovarian dermoids represent some of the more common differential diagnostic considerations (Fig. 3.59).

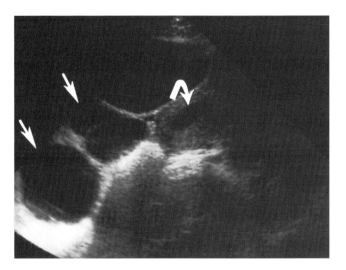

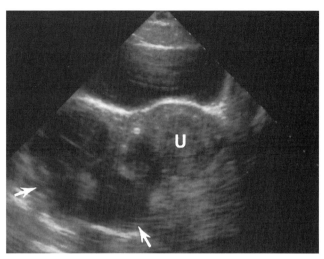

Fig. 3.53 **Tubo-ovarian abscesses.** Multilocular fluid collections (arrows) are seen in the right adnexa, representing tubo-ovarian abscesses. The uterus contains an empty fluid-filled sac (curved arrow) due to a missed abortion secondary to the inflammatory process.

Fig. 3.54 **Inflammatory mass.** A large complex mass occupies the right adnexa (arrows), with the inflammatory process engulfing the tube, ovary and broad ligament. U – uterus.

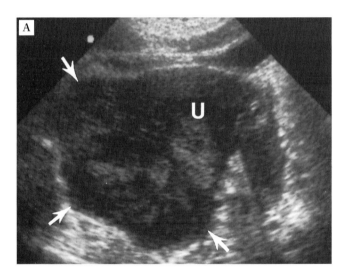

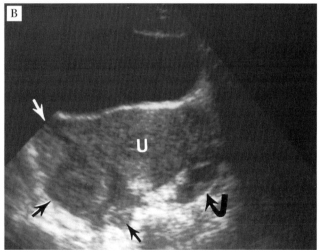

Fig. 3.55 **Tubo-ovarian abscess. A:** A large, poorly marginated complex mass in the right adnexa (arrows) represents a tubo-ovarian abscess obscuring the border of the uterus (U). **B:** After 5 days of intensive intravenous antibiotic therapy the inflammatory mass (arrows) is much smaller. Curved arrow – left ovary, U – uterus.

Chronic PID may cause a loss of the normal mobility of bowel and other pelvic structures because of peritoneal and mesenteric adhesions (Fig. 3.60). Gentle compression with the transducer may prove useful in demonstrating the lack of normal motion. A major contributing factor to infertility, PID is apparently on the increase. Its effects upon tubal patency and motility are significant and difficult to overcome.

It must also be remembered that not all inflammatory processes found in the pelvis are gynaecological in origin:

inflammatory bowel disease such as Crohn's disease, ruptured appendicitis and diverticulitis may all produce complex pelvic masses indistinguishable from those found in PID.

Endometriosis

Endometriosis is primarily a condition of young caucasian women and is estimated to occur in 5–20% of those of childbearing age. It is implicated as a major causative

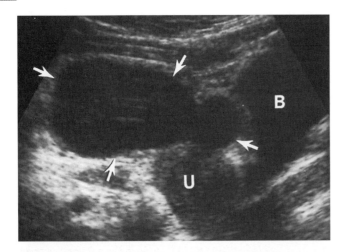

Fig. 3.56 Multilocular tubo-ovarian abscess. After several days of antibiotic therapy this multilocular tubo-ovarian abscess (arrows) became more sharply marginated. U – uterus, B – bladder.

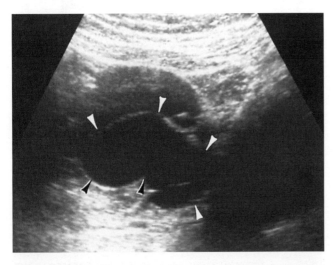

Fig. 3.58 Hydrosalpinx. Hydrosalpinx, particularly when chronic, may assume a figure-of-eight configuration, as in this patient (arrowheads).

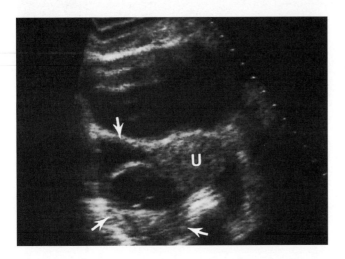

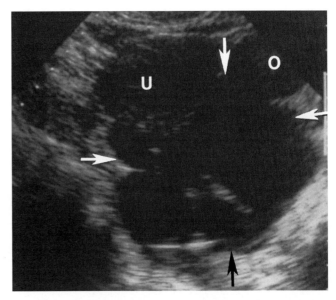

Fig. 3.57 Hydrosalpinx. The multilocular cystic mass (arrows) in the left adnexa and *cul de sac* represents a hydrosalpinx, the ultrasound appearance being produced by multiple folds of the distended fallopian tube. U – uterus, O – left ovary.

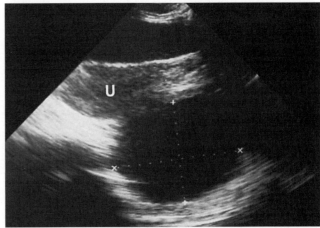

Fig. 3.59 Haematoma. This largely cystic haematoma (cursors) resulted from continued bleeding following caesarean section. Haematomas must be included in the differential diagnosis of cystic or complex pelvic masses. U – uterus.

Fig. 3.60 Multiple adherent bowel loops. Occasionally the appearance of a complex pelvic mass may be produced by postinflammatory or post-surgical adhesions of multiple bowel loops, as in this case. The apparent right adnexal mass (arrows) was produced by adherent bowel loops; the appearance persisted unchanged over 3 days. At operation no focal mass was identified. U – uterus.

factor in 40% of women presenting with infertility. Endometriosis has been reported in 10–25% of laparotomies in patients of menstrual age.[78–80] The presenting clinical picture includes infertility (defined as failure to conceive after 1 year of unprotected intercourse), dysmenorrhoea, abdominal pain and an abdominal mass. As implants of endometrial tissue can be found in a wide range of locations, reports of dysuria, bowel symptoms and even haemoptysis and pneumothorax are extant, indicating involvement of these organ systems.[81–83] Endometriosis, focal or diffuse, can also occur in the patient who has undergone hysterectomy.

Two general morphological types of endometriosis are recognised: a diffuse form and a tumefactive pattern. By far the more common is the diffuse variety, which consists of small, discrete implants of endometrial tissue on the serosal surfaces of abdominal and pelvic viscera and peritoneum. These foci are described at laparoscopy as 'powder burns' on the normally smooth and glistening surfaces; they are readily identified under laparoscopy but are too small to be detected by ultrasound. Reports of a diffuse increase in the reflectivity of the pelvis and increased arterial pulsations in the region as indicators of the diffuse form of endometriosis have not been widely reproducible, and it is generally considered that ultrasound is of minimal value in this context for diagnosis screening.[66,73]

Endometriotic cysts, or endometriomas, result from cyclical haemorrhage of functioning endometrial tissue into a confined space. Varying in size from 1 cm to large, relatively well circumscribed masses of 10–15 cm diameter, endometriomas are most often complex with low-level internal echoes, sometimes gravity dependent, but occasionally in the form of internal septations (Fig. 3.61).

The proportion of internal echoes tends to decrease over time. Throughout their course endometriomas display good through transmission of sound, despite the extensive internal echoes (Fig. 3.62).[84–86]

Because of the cyclical nature of the process multiple endometriomas may exhibit differing ultrasonic characteristics, as they are at different stages of resolution of the contained fluid (Figs 3.63 and 3.64). This variegated appearance places endometriomas in the rather lengthy differential diagnosis of complex pelvic masses, which includes epithelial ovarian neoplasms, tubo-ovarian abscesses, dermoids and necrotic uterine leiomyomata among the more common pathologies.

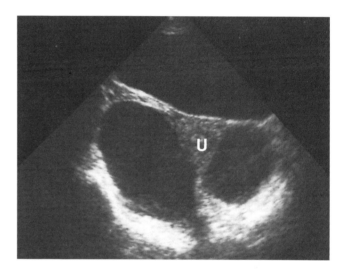

Fig. 3.62 Bilateral endometriomas. This transverse scan demonstrates bilateral endometriomas, both with low-level internal echoes. U – uterus.

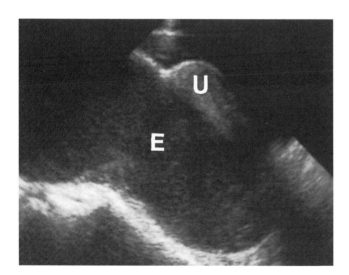

Fig. 3.61 Bilocular endometrioma. This large bilocular endometrioma (E) is filled with low-level echoes representing small fragments of clot breakdown. Note the excellent through transmission of sound, characteristic of any blood-filled structure. U – uterus.

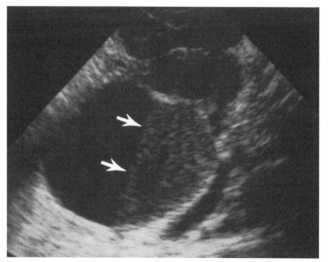

Fig. 3.63 Endometrioma. On this trans-vaginal view the particulate portions of the clot have settled out to form a fluid–debris level (arrows).

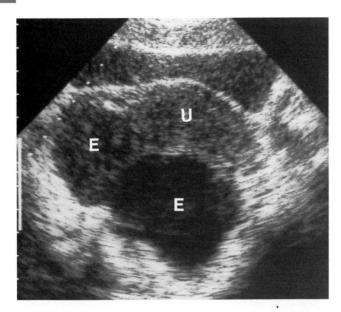

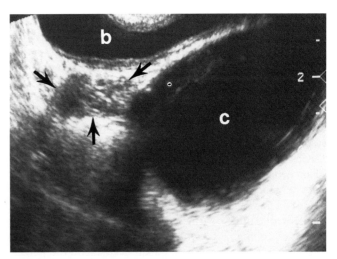

Fig. 3.65 **Para-ovarian cyst** (c) is adjacent to but separable from the normal ovary (arrows). b – urinary bladder.

Fig. 3.64 **Endometriomas.** The endometriomas in this patient (E) are at different stages in their natural history, with considerably more echoes still remaining in the mass on the right compared to that occupying the *cul de sac*. Through transmission of sound is excellent for both. U – uterus.

Para-ovarian cyst

The para-ovarian cyst represents a remnant of Gartner's duct and appears in the adnexa as a simple, smooth-walled cyst which may be indistinguishable from a functional cyst of the ovary (Fig. 3.65), though the better resolution of trans-vaginal probes and the ability to apply direct pressure to demonstrate movement of structures may allow them to be separated. Haemorrhage produces low-level internal echoes. Para-ovarian cysts are most commonly 3–5 cm in diameter and do not change with the menstrual cycle, as do functional cysts.[87,88] Failure of such a cyst to regress spontaneously will most often lead to surgical removal to ensure that it is not an epithelial neoplasm, particularly in the older premenopausal patient. In the post-menopausal age group, in which functional cysts should not occur, adnexal masses, cystic or solid, should be investigated further.

Ectopic pregnancy

The incidence of ectopic pregnancy continues to rise in developed countries secondary to the use of intra-uterine contraceptive devices (IUCD), the increased incidence of pelvic inflammatory disease and the more common use of tubal surgery for infertility or reversal of sterilisation.[89,90] Paradoxically, it is the successful treatment of pelvic infections with the newer antibiotic regimens that contributes to the frequency of ectopic pregnancies, by preserving tubal patency in the presence of adhesions that render

tubal mobility abnormal. Endometriosis, with the induction of fibrosis and adhesions, is also thought to be a predisposing factor for ectopic pregnancy.

The current incidence is reported to be 1.4% of all pregnancies; of the women who conceive following treatment for an ectopic pregnancy (60%), 10% will have another ectopic gestation, so that early ultrasound confirmation of the intra-uterine location of a subsequent pregnancy in such patients is important.

Confirmation of the presence of an intra-uterine gestation with a trans-vaginal probe should be possible at about 32 days menstrual age (i.e. from the first day of the last menstrual period) or with a serum β-HCG of 1000 mIU (Second International Standard).[91] Visualisation of either an embryo or a yolk sac (which is of fetal origin) is proof of an intra-uterine pregnancy; the so-called 'double decidual sac sign' is also excellent, if not absolute, evidence for an intra-uterine location of the pregnancy (see Ch. 7). Identification of an intra-uterine pregnancy is the most useful function of ultrasound, as for all practical purposes it rules out the presence of an ectopic gestation. The incidence of an intra-uterine pregnancy with an extra-uterine twin is now estimated to be 1 in 7000 at most, this occurring largely in the population under treatment for infertility; it would therefore be impractical and unrealistic to manage every possible ectopic pregnancy on the expectation of such a scenario.

The ultrasound findings in ectopic pregnancy are widely variable and, unless an intra-uterine gestation is identified, cannot be excluded by ultrasound. The differential diagnosis, without consideration of the clinical setting, includes endometriosis, tubo-ovarian abscess, haemorrhagic ovarian cyst and ovarian torsion.[92] Some 20% of ectopic gestations present with no ultrasound findings whatever, that is, the images are those of a normal, non-pregnant pelvis with no evidence of masses, fluid collections or other adnexal abnormalities.

Correlation with the serum β-HCG is of particular importance in such a situation, as a pregnancy, normal or ectopic, at less than 4 weeks menstrual age may not be visualised. If, then, the HCG level is commensurate with a 3-week gestation, observation may be the appropriate course of action.[93]

The trans-vaginal transducer has made it possible to detect a living embryo in 17% of ectopic pregnancies (Fig. 3.66).[94] A 'tubal ring', representing the reflective chorion, can be identified on trans-vaginal scanning in as many as 68% of patients.[95] It has been further observed that identification of this sac-like adnexal ring indicates functioning trophoblasts and an intact fallopian tube (Fig. 3.67). The finding of an adnexal mass of complex texture raises the suspicion of tubal haematoma or frank rupture.[96] Free fluid is also more easily detected. A small amount of fluid confined to the *cul de sac* or adnexae may be a normal finding in the non-pregnant pelvis; however, moderate to large amounts of fluid are abnormal.[97,98] Echoes within the fluid suggest a haemoperitoneum, with a high risk for ectopic gestation. Echogenic fluid was identified in 56% of patients with proved ectopic pregnancies in a recent study.[99]

Leakage of blood from the fimbriated end of the fallopian tube is thought to account for the haemoperitoneum in most women, though frank tubal rupture occurs in only 10–15% of cases (Figs 3.68 and 3.69).[100,101]

In some 20% of patients with ectopic gestations a ring-like structure is identified within the endometrial cavity (Fig. 3.70).[102] Mimicking a true gestation sac in some respects, this 'pseudosac' is thought to represent the hyperplastic endometrium responding to the increased hormone levels produced by the ectopic pregnancy. Lack of a double decidual reaction will generally distinguish the pseudosac from a true gestation sac.[103] It has been suggested that a pseudogestation sac is identified less frequently by the trans-vaginal route than by abdominal scanning, reaching only 8.8% in one study.[104] Doppler evaluation of the intra-uterine sac has shown some promise in the differentiation between true and pseudosacs.[105]

The vast majority of ectopic pregnancies occur in the ampullary portion of the tube. Approximately 1% may be situated in the interstitial segment of the tube (i.e. the intramural portion) and the cervical canal (Fig. 3.71). In both of these sites growth can persist for longer, so that when the ectopic ruptures haemorrhage is more catastrophic. Abdominal ectopics are quite rare (and unsuspected in 60% of cases) and can grow surprisingly large.[106–109] They are characterised by the absence of amniotic fluid, extension of fetal parts that often lie close to the maternal abdominal wall, an extra-uterine placenta and an empty uterus.

Infertility

Infertility is estimated to affect one in six couples, with ovarian dysfunction accounting for some 20% of female infertility.[110] Ultrasound and, in particular, trans-vaginal scanning, has become a cornerstone in the approach to infertility, with its ability to identify hydrosalpinges, endometriomas and other mechanical impediments to conception. Ultrasound salpinography is used to assess tubal patency by monitoring intra-uterine fluid injection, with documentation of peritoneal spillage.[111]

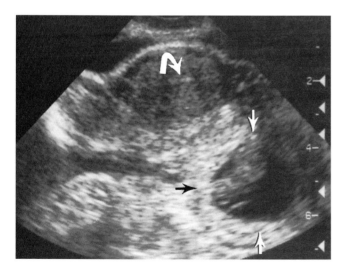

Fig. 3.66 Unruptured ectopic gestation. A living, unruptured ectopic gestation is identified in the left posterior adnexa (arrows). The endometrial echo (curved arrow) is seen, confirming an empty uterus.

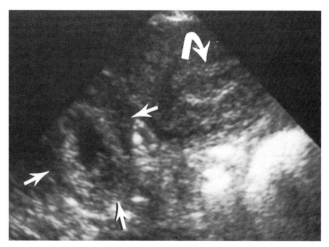

Fig. 3.67 Ectopic gestation. Curved arrow indicates a poorly formed intra-uterine sac-like structure representing a reactive endometrium felt to result from sloughing of hypertrophied endometrium. The unruptured ectopic gestation (arrows) is seen in the right posterior adnexa.

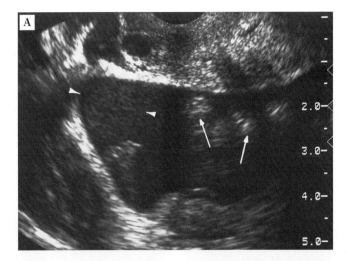

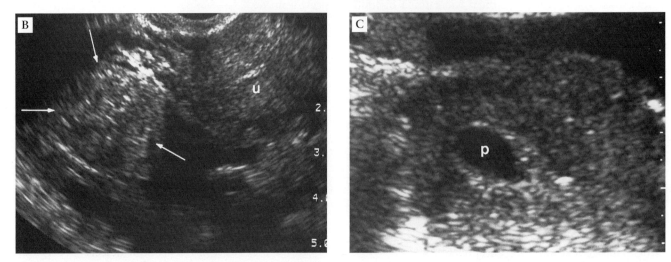

Fig. 3.68 Ectopic gestations. A: Ruptured ectopic gestation. Considerable free fluid containing low-level echoes from haemorrhage (arrowheads) and bowel loops (arrows). **B:** Semisolid right adnexal mass (arrows) represents clot from ruptured ectopic. u – uterus. **C:** Uterus containing pseudogestational sac (p).

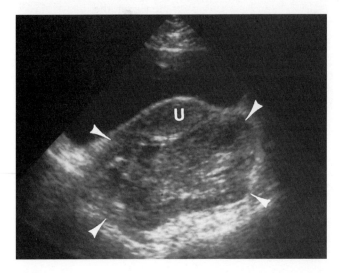

Fig. 3.69 Complex mass. A ruptured interstitial pregnancy has resulted in a complex mass (arrowheads) filling the *cul de sac*. The small empty uterus (U) is identified.

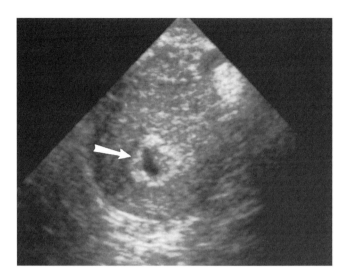

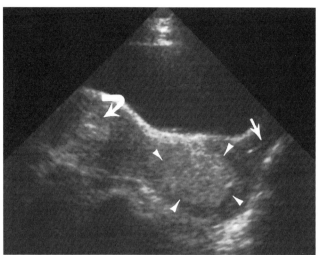

Fig. 3.70 **Intra-uterine pseudosac.** The intra-uterine pseudosac (arrow) accompanying an ectopic pregnancy can be quite confusing in its appearance, as in this case. However, the double decidual sign is absent.

Fig. 3.71 **Haemorrhage in a cervical ectopic gestation.** A reflective mass (arrowheads) occupies the region of the endocervical canal and represents haemorrhage in a cervical ectopic gestation lying between the vagina (arrow) and the empty endometrial canal (curved arrow).

Monitoring follicular development for timed insemination or oocyte retrieval in an *in vitro* fertilisation programme is easily and precisely accomplished with ultrasound.[112] Trans-vaginal ultrasound-guided oocyte retrieval has been shown to be as effective as its laparoscopic counterpart, with less discomfort, expense and time.[113,114] Maximum efficiency with minimum interobserver error is achieved by having the same sonographer scan the patient on each visit. In general, daily monitoring is begun on or about the 9th day of the cycle and carried through until ovulation has occurred. Sudden shrinkage or disappearance of the follicle, sometimes accompanied by the appearance of internal echoes representing haemorrhage, marks ovulation.

The follicle grows at about 2–3 mm per day from the 9th day of the menstrual cycle to reach a mature diameter of 17–24 mm at ovulation.[115,116] Identification of the precise time of ovulation is somewhat difficult, even with current techniques.[117] Oocyte retrieval, via either transvesical or trans-vaginal routes, is best accomplished under ultrasound guidance (see Ch. 4).[10]

Family history of ovarian cancer

Introduction

By 1994 the National Institutes of Health had determined ovarian cancer to be the leading cause of death from gynaecological malignancies in the United States, with an anticipated 24 000 new cases and 13 600 deaths from the disease annually. This translates to a prevalence of 30–50 cases per 100 000 women, with a lifetime incidence of 1 in 70 women. In 95% of cases ovarian carcinoma is sporadic, with no discernible pattern of inheritance. The 5-year survival has increased only slightly in the period from 1973 to 1990, from 36% to 40%.[118] The 5-year survival of patients with FIGO stage III or IV disease (approximately 70% of cases) is in the range of 15–20%; those presenting with stage I disease, however (some 30%), will have a 5-year survival of 80–90%. The impetus for early detection is obvious.[119–121]

Certain factors are associated with an increased risk of developing ovarian carcinoma: increasing age, nulliparity, North American or north European descent, a personal history of endometrial, colon or breast cancer and a family history of ovarian carcinoma. In one large study 13% of masses resected prior to menopause proved to be malignant, as opposed to 45% of those removed in postmenopausal patients.[122] Viewed another way, 85% of ovarian cancers occur in women over the age of 45.[121] Protective factors include more than one full-term pregnancy, oral contraceptive use and breastfeeding (the common denominator being the interruption of incessant ovulation). A very small percentage of women (less than 0.05%) are at significantly increased risk by virtue of three hereditary syndromes: breast–ovarian cancer syndrome, site-specific ovarian cancer syndrome, and hereditary nonpolyposis colorectal cancer, or Lynch II syndrome. For these women the lifetime risk of developing ovarian carcinoma approaches 40%, which is sufficient to recommend prophylactic oophorectomy at age 35, or when childbearing is complete. This recommendation does not extend to the woman with a single first-degree relative with ovarian cancer, despite the lifetime risk of 5% for developing the disease (increased over the 1 in 70 incidence in the general population) and 7% with two affected relatives.[123] It is to women presumed to have one of the heritable syndromes and, therefore, a significantly increased risk of developing ovarian cancer, that efforts at regular and methodical screening are directed.[124]

Familial ovarian cancer

Three heritable syndromes have been shown to be associated with a significantly increased incidence of malignant ovarian neoplasms. Although they constitute only a small percentage of women who develop ovarian cancer, they are at such an increased risk of the disease that they constitute a proper target population for screening. In all three conditions ovarian carcinoma develops at a significantly earlier age (40, 49 and 52 years) than those occurring sporadically in the general population (mean age 59 years).

Hereditary non-polyposis colorectal carcinoma syndrome (Lynch syndrome) is an autosomal dominant gene with a high degree of penetrance, manifesting as early colorectal cancer in women under 45 years of age. It is also associated with an increased incidence of endometrial carcinoma, and those affected show a 3.5-fold likelihood of developing ovarian cancer compared to the general population. Most are serous cystadenocarcinomas.[125]

Hereditary breast and ovarian cancer syndrome carries with it a 50% lifetime risk of ovarian cancer in first-degree relatives. The *BRCA1* gene on the long arm of chromosome 17 has recently been identified as the marker for this syndrome.[126,127] It is thought to be a tumour suppressor gene and its malfunction appears responsible for disease in 45% of families with multiple cases of breast carcinoma only, and most, but not all, families which have both breast and ovarian carcinoma.[128]

Hereditary site-specific ovarian cancer is considerably less common than the Lynch syndromes and carries with it only an increased incidence of ovarian neoplasia without the involvement of breast, colon or other organ systems.[127]

Screening

Current consensus holds that screening the general population for ovarian cancer is not warranted by virtue of its relatively low prevalence (in comparison, for example, with that of breast cancer, where mammographic screening is effective and worthwhile). In the subset of women at increased risk for the development of ovarian carcinoma (i.e. those with a family history of the disease, or heritable syndromes with an increased incidence of this neoplasm), annual screening is accepted and recommended, albeit without conclusive objective data currently available to confirm its value with respect to improved morbidity and mortality figures. It has been proposed that screening begin at age 25–30 years.[128,129] The three approaches in use are annual bimanual rectovaginal physical examination, serum CA125 levels and trans-vaginal ultrasound.

Physical examination

A key element of initial screening is the targeted family history, by which those at increased risk for ovarian cancer can be identified. Admittedly, physical examination has been found to be relatively insensitive as well as non-specific in the detection and evaluation of ovarian cancer, particularly in its early stages. In one study only 30% of ovarian masses identified at ultrasound were detected by physical examination.[129] However, physical examination, by its universal availability, non-invasive nature and low cost, would intuitively seem an appropriate starting point.[130]

CA125

CA125, a high molecular weight cell surface glycoprotein, is an antigenic determinant detected by radioimmunoassay; its serum level is elevated in 80% of epithelial ovarian cancers, but in fewer than 50% of those patients with stage I disease.[131] It has also been observed that mucinous neoplasms of the ovary generally do not elaborate CA125.[132,133] A significant number of healthy women and women with benign disease also demonstrate elevated levels of CA125, making the specificity of this determination unacceptably low. Generally, a level of greater than 30–35 U/ml is considered abnormal.[130,134,135] Most authors agree that CA125 determinations are, by themselves, insufficiently sensitive as a screening test for ovarian cancer. One investigator, Woolas, using three serum markers (CA125, M-CSF and OVX1) found at least one marker elevated in 98% of patients with stage I disease; CA125 was elevated in 67%.[136] However, at least one marker was also elevated in 11% of healthy individuals and 51% of patients with benign disease, rendering the specificity of this multiple-marker approach only moderate. Used in conjunction with trans-vaginal ultrasound, the CA125 was found by DePriest *et al.* to yield a specificity of 0.995.[129]

Ultrasound

Early work in the use of ultrasound as a method for screening for ovarian cancer used the technology available at the time, i.e. transabdominal instruments with frequencies generally in the range of 3.5 MHz. It is recognised that, although these efforts were the basis of present approaches, the transabdominal scan does not have a place in screening for ovarian malignancy.[137–140] Instead, attention is focused on trans-vaginal ultrasound as a means of identifying and characterising ovarian masses in an at-risk population. Three sonographic parameters have been extensively studied for their sensitivity, specificity, accuracy and predictive value in the assessment of ovarian masses: grey scale morphology, spectral Doppler and colour flow Doppler.

Morphology

With some degree of variation, all the investigators classifying ovarian masses as to the likelihood of malignancy or benignity examine the same features and characteristics of the mass. Size, wall thickness, number and thickness of septa, presence or absence of papillary excrescences (from the wall or septa) and reflectivity are evaluated and, in most series, assigned a numerical value (Fig. 3.72). The sum of the assigned values is then used to predict the likelihood of an individual mass being benign or malignant.[131,141,142]

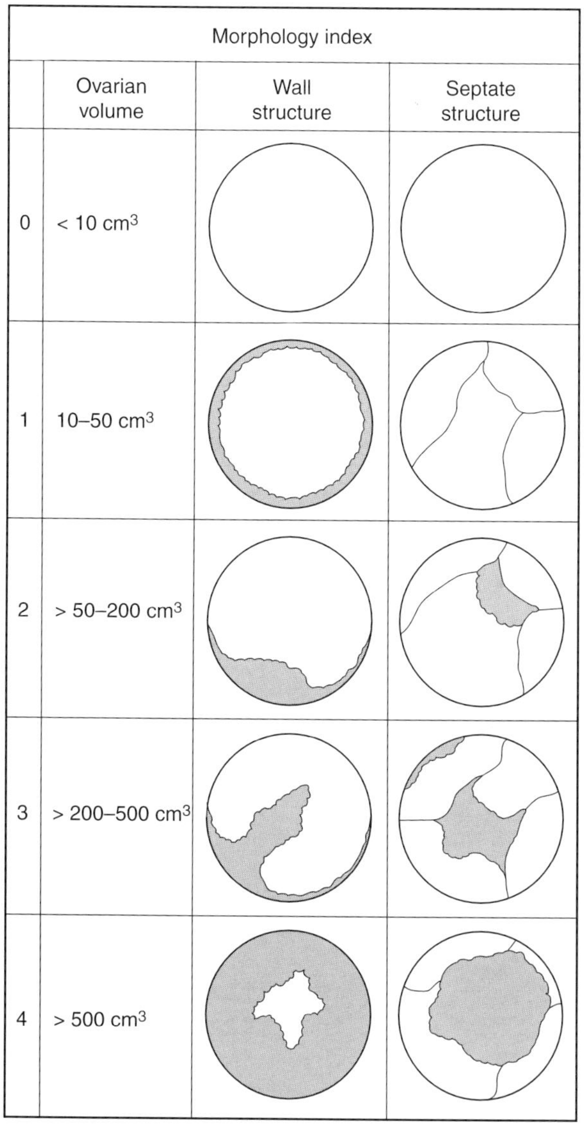

Size

The size of the ovary is determined by the standard formula for the volume of an ellipsoid: length (L) × width (W) × height (H) × 0.5233 (or, by rough estimation, one half of the product of the three dimensions in cm) (Fig. 3.73). Observers vary in the volume they consider to be the upper limit of normal, but the ranges are 5–8 ml in the postmenopausal woman and 15–18 ml in the premenopausal woman. Some allow for masses up to 9–10 cm as possibly still benign.[143] In one series the risk of malignancy was determined to be 3% for masses less than 5 cm, 10% for masses between 5 and 10 cm, and 65% for those larger than 10 cm.[144] DePriest *et al.* found no malignant tumour with a volume less than 10 ml.[141] Jain[145] reported the mean size of benign masses at 3.6 ± 1.9 cm and malignant at 8.0 ± 3.8 cm. Sassone *et al.*[142] found that ovaries larger than 5 cm on trans-vaginal sonography had a 2.5 times greater risk of malignancy than smaller ovaries, but admit that the inclusion of tumour size in their scoring system did not improve sensitivity. Others have found no correlation between size and likelihood of malignancy.[146]

Wall characteristics

The thickness and contour of the wall of a cystic ovarian mass are considered by all investigators to be important indicators of potential malignancy (Fig. 3.74).[143,147] Papillary projections from the inner surface of the wall of a cystic mass are worrisome for malignancy, as is irregular thickening of more than 3 mm.[142,145,148–150] DePriest *et al.*[151] found wall structure to be the most reliable morphological characteristic in distinguishing between benign and malignant masses. Several classifications distinguish between

Morphology index		
	Ovarian volume	Wall structure	Septate structure
0	< 10 cm³		
1	10–50 cm³		
2	> 50–200 cm³		
3	> 200–500 cm³		
4	> 500 cm³		

Fig. 3.72 Representative morphological classification (with numerical scoring system) considering size, wall structure with excrescences and thickness, and septal thickness. (Reproduced with permission from DePriest et al.[151]).

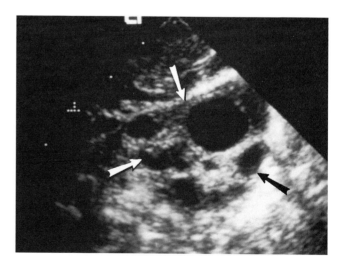

Fig. 3.73 Normal ovary. The normal ovary is outlined by arrows. Note several small echo-free follicles with a single dominant developing follicle. The volume may be calculated by the formula L × W × H × 0.5233.

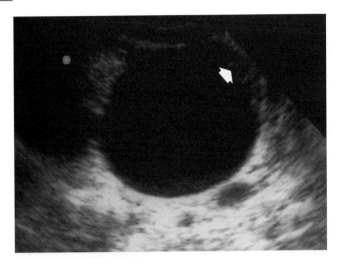

Fig. 3.74 **Simple functional cyst** with a rim of ovarian tissue (arrow) visible. No internal architecture or wall thickness is identifiable. Spontaneous resolution was confirmed on a follow-up study several weeks later.

papillary excrescences of less than or greater than 3 mm, for example, whereas some cite such features qualitatively. Nonetheless, an increasing number and/or size of solid tissue projections from the walls of a mass are taken to raise the level of suspicion of malignancy. Diagrammatic representation of these morphological characteristics, including septa and debris, is provided with a number of the studies to allow for numerical indices to be calculated. There are, expectedly, some variations in number assignment and detail of criteria – some are more specific (e.g. excrescences greater than 3 mm) and some less, but all take into account the same basic observations.

Septa

The presence, number and characteristics of septations within a complex mass are important and generally accepted factors (Figs 3.75 and 3.76). The more numerous, thicker and irregular the internal septations, the more suggestive of malignancy and the higher the score assigned by the various morphological classification systems; 3 mm in thickness is generally regarded as the threshold above which suspicion of malignancy rises (Fig. 3.77).[142,145,148,151,152] Although an increasing number of septations tends to raise the subjective concern about malignancy, no investigators have offered a number (or number per volume of tumour ratio) in an attempt to quantify this impression. The number of internal septations is said to be higher for mucinous than serous neoplasms, whether benign or malignant.

Echo pattern

Epithelial neoplasms of the ovary, which constitute the majority of true neoplasms, are cystic to a greater or lesser degree. The amount of solid tissue within the cystic mass and the echo pattern of the material within the mass vary considerably. In general, masses with a higher component of solid tissue admixed with the cystic areas (Fig. 3.78) (apart from the mural nodules and septal thickenings already described) and/or reflective internal debris tend to have a higher likelihood of malignancy than those without a significant solid component. Quantification of the percentage of solid tissue in a given mass would be difficult at best, and most observers have avoided such attempts.[142,148,153]

A significant exception to this tendency is seen in the case of ovarian teratomas (Fig. 3.79), which commonly have either a highly reflective nodule in the wall of a cystic

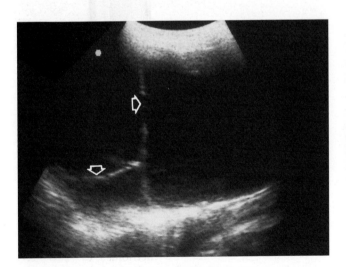

Fig. 3.75 **Benign mucinous cystadenoma.** Despite its considerable size (>15 cm) this cystic mass has few internal septations (arrows), all of which are thin (<3 mm) and without excrescences.

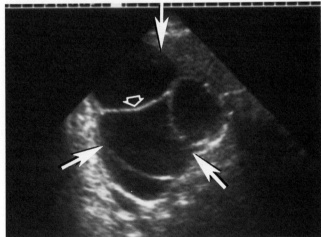

Fig. 3.76 **Benign serous cystadenoma.** Thin septations (open arrow) are seen in this well circumscribed cystic mass (outlined by arrows) adjacent to the uterus.

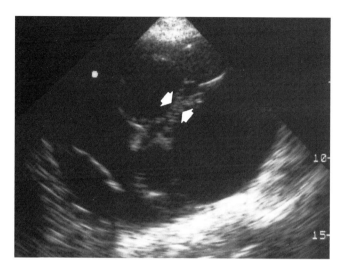

Fig. 3.77 Mucinous cystadenoma of low malignant potential. This cystic mass, which is histologically considered borderline in nature between benign and low-grade malignancy, demonstrates some thickening of its central septa (arrows). Septa greater than 3 mm in thickness begin to raise suspicion for malignancy.

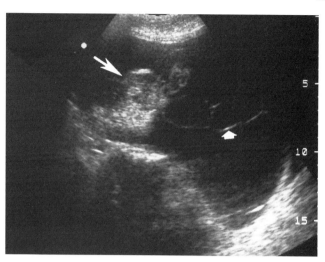

Fig. 3.78 Mucinous cystadenocarcinoma. Although several septa in this large cystic mass are quite thin (short arrow), significant solid components (long arrow) between them increase the likelihood of malignancy.

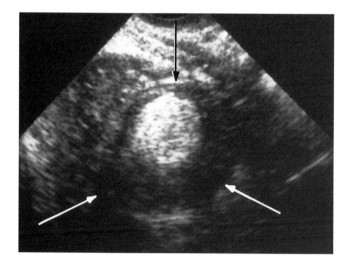

Fig. 3.79 Dermoid. Contained within the ovary (outlined by long arrows) is a well circumscribed, highly reflective mass representing fat within a dermoid. Such highly reflective material is characteristic of teratomas.

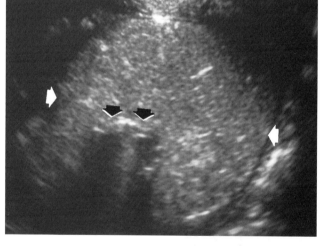

Fig. 3.80 Dermoid. A mass of uniformly moderate reflectivity (white arrows) contains a highly reflective focus (black arrows), which produces a distinct shadow. This represents calcification within a benign mature cystic teratoma.

structure (the so-called 'dermoid plug' or 'Rokitansky nodule') or a substantial amount of markedly reflective material layering in a fluid–debris or debris–fluid level, representing fat or hair. In addition, the presence of a shadowing focus within a cystic mass would suggest calcification and raise the consideration of an ovarian teratoma (Fig. 3.80). These characteristic compositions strongly favour ovarian teratomas and suggest a benign process, as only a very small percentage of dermoids are malignant (though it should be admitted here that there are no

specific sonographic signs that separate benign from malignant teratomas).[154–157]

In one recent series the grey scale morphological characteristics considered benign (completely cystic with no internal echoes; cystic with thin, smooth septations less than 3 mm; or complex cysts with internal echoes suggesting haemorrhagic cysts, endometriomas or cystic teratomas) resulted in a negative predictive value of 99%.[152] However, the positive predictive value of morphology for malignancy was only 50%.

Filly considers a simple unilocular cyst less than 6 cm in a premenopausal woman benign and appropriately followed at 1–2 months for spontaneous resolution;[90] similarly a unilocular thin-walled cystic lesion less than 5 cm in a post-menopausal patient may be followed.

High proportions of solid tissue are also seen in endometrioid carcinomas of the ovary, metastatic tumours from a variety of sources (lung, breast, gastrointestinal tract) now all grouped under the umbrella of Krukenberg tumours, germ cell tumours and lymphomas.[158–163] In general they do not resemble epithelial neoplasms and do not figure in the consideration of tumours with significant familial involvement.

Spectral Doppler

Malignant neoplasms produce neovascularity that is devoid of muscular walls and vasomotor control. Hence, the vascular bed in a malignant tumour characteristically produces a high-flow low-resistance perfusion pattern, resulting in a large passive diastolic forward flow component. Measurements of proportion of such diastolic flow to the systolic component should, therefore, reflect the altered perfusion pattern. A resistance index (RI) less than 0.4 and pulsatility index (PI) less than 1.0 have been cited by a number of investigators as suggestive of malignancy, as they reflect increased diastolic flow compared to benign neoplasms which demonstrate a high resistance vascular bed (and hence a high RI and PI).[143,148,149,164–170] Although the general tendency is for malignant processes to have low-resistance flow and benign masses higher resistance, the majority of recent papers indicate that the overlap between the distributions is sufficiently broad to render the discriminatory value of these determinations very low (Fig. 3.81).[145,146,150,152,153,171–173] In none of the recent studies could an acceptable sensitivity be coupled with an acceptable specificity for the spectral Doppler findings which, therefore, is not considered to be of value by itself in discriminating between benign and malignant ovarian masses.

Colour flow Doppler

Various investigators have focused on the presence or absence of colour flow signals within an ovarian mass and/or the distribution of such signals (i.e. peripheral versus central) in attempts to distinguish benign from malignant processes.[152,164,173] Although some have held that the absence of peripheral or internal flow carries a negative predictive value of 94%,[148,152] or that peripheral colour may be seen in benign masses but that central flow indicates malignancy,[174] others have concluded that even a complete lack of demonstrable colour flow does not exclude malignancy.[171] Complete absence of flow was documented in only 10% of proven benign masses in Stein's series, rendering the finding relatively insensitive.[152] She found demonstrable vascularity in all malignant vegetations greater than 1 cm and Buy *et al.* reported colour flow in all malignant tumours in their series.[148]

In short, although it is widely recognised that malignant tumours of the ovary have more flow signals on colour Doppler and lower-resistance vascular beds on spectral Doppler than benign processes, neither provides sufficient specificity and sensitivity to allow consistent distinction

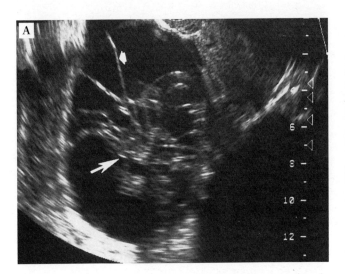 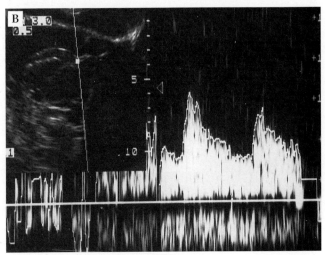

Fig. 3.81 Mucinous tumour of low malignant potential. A: Classified histologically as a mucinous tumour of low malignant potential (i.e. a borderline neoplasm), this cystic mass contains both thin (short arrow) and thick (long arrow) septa. **B:** Spectral Doppler tracing demonstrates a substantial passive diastolic forward flow component, which would be compatible with malignant neovascularity. The resistance index (RI) of 0.57 falls within the benign range (greater than 0.4), but the pulsatility index (PI) of 0.8 is below the normal value (greater than 1.0). Overlap of these indices between benign and malignant neoplasms has been found to be too broad to allow histological prediction on this basis.

between benign and malignant masses. They continue to be studied and are, in fact, used clinically to provide at least a subjective sense of the vascularity of a given mass. More flow signals and lower resistance at least raise the level of suspicion for malignancy.

Conclusion

The role of ultrasound in screening for ovarian malignancy is still evolving.[175] Certain tenets are currently established and are guiding its application today. Screening of the general population with trans-vaginal ultrasound does not appear to be warranted or cost-effective by virtue of the relatively low prevalence of the disease. Large-scale experimental screening programmes are now in progress to test that tenet; over the next several years results will be analysed to support or refute that belief.

Screening an at-risk population is broadly accepted more on a commonsense basis than because objective data are available to support it. Women with at least one first-degree relative with ovarian cancer and women with a family history of the heritable conditions that carry an increased risk of ovarian malignancy may properly undergo trans-vaginal ultrasonography as part of a yearly-screening programme, beginning at 25–30 years of age.

The criteria by which an ovary is judged to be abnormal currently centre on its morphological characteristics. An ovarian mass which enlarges the ovary beyond 15–18 ml in the premenopausal or 5–8 ml in the post-menopausal patient is considered suspicious, as is any ovarian mass that exhibits an irregular or thickened wall (greater than 3 mm), mural excrescences, thickened septa (greater than 3 mm) or a focus of solid tissue greater than 1 cm in diameter. Several morphological classifications are available providing both diagrammatic and scan representations of the features to be considered; assigning numerical values to each characteristic produces a scoring system which at least establishes the level of suspicion for malignancy. Under certain circumstances close follow-up may be acceptable, with rescanning in 6–8 weeks, along with measurement of the CA125 levels and thorough physical examination. However, the overwhelming bias in such situations is in favour of surgical removal of a suspicious ovary; this is largely predicated on the excellent prognosis for stage I and II disease against the dismal outcome for stages III and IV. Several authors suggest strong consideration of prophylactic oophorectomy at age 35, or whenever childbearing is complete, for women with two first-degree relatives with ovarian cancer.

The adjunctive use of spectral and colour Doppler information may prove helpful, but neither has been shown to have sufficient discriminatory value to allow its application as a sole criterion.

REFERENCES

1 Ivarsson S A, Nilsson K O, Persson P H. Ultrasonography of the pelvic organs in prepubertal and postpubertal girls. Arch Dis Child 1983; 58: 352

2 Orsini L F, Salardi S, Pilu G et al. Pelvic organs in premenarcheal girls: real-time ultrasonography. Radiology 1984; 153: 113

3 Munn C S, Kiser L C, Wetzner S M, Baer J E. Ovary volume in young and premenopausal adults: US determination. Radiology 1986; 159: 731

4 Nicolini U, Ferrazzi E, Bellotti M et al. The contribution of sonographic evaluation of ovarian size in patients with polycystic ovarian disease. J Ultrasound Med 1985; 4: 347–351

5 Sample W F, Lippe B M, Gyepes M T. Gray-scale ultrasonography of the normal female pelvis. Radiology 1977; 125: 477

6 Cohen H L, Tice H M, Mandel F S. Ovarian volumes measured by US: bigger than we think. Radiology 1990; 177: 189–192

7 Hall D A, McCarthy K A, Kopans D B. Sonographic visualization of the normal postmenopausal ovary. J Ultrasound Med 1986; 5: 9

8 Rankin R N, Hutton L C. Ultrasound in the ovarian hyperstimulation syndrome. J Clin Ultrasound 1981; 9: 473

9 Hackeloer B. The role of ultrasound in female infertility management. Ultrasound Med Biol 1984; 10: 35

10 Bonilla-Musoles F, Pardo G, Perez-Gil M, Serra V, Pellicer A. Abdominal ultrasonography versus transvaginal scanning: accuracy in follicular development. Evaluation and prediction for oocyte retrieval in stimulated cycles. JCU 1989; 17: 469–473

11 Andreotti R F, Thompson G H, Janowitz W et al. Endovaginal and transabdominal sonography of ovarian follicles. J Ultrasound Med 1989; 8: 555–560

12 Hilgers T W, Dvorak A D, Tamisiea D F, Ellis R L, Yaksich P J. Sonographic definition of the empty follicle syndrome. J Ultrasound Med 1989; 8: 411–416

13 Ganong W F. The gonads: development and function of the reproductive system. Review of medical physiology, 7th edn. Los Altos, CA: Lange, 1975; 310–341

14 Levine D, Gosink B B, Wolf S I et al. Simple adnexal cysts: the natural history in postmenopausal women. Radiology 1992; 184: 653–659

15 Wolf S I, Gosink B B, Feldesman M R et al. Prevalence of simple adnexal cysts in postmenopausal women. Radiology 1991; 180: 65–71

16 Hall D A, McCarthy K A. The significance of the postmenopausal simple adnexal cyst. J Ultrasound Med 1986; 5: 503–505

17 Rulin M C, Preston A L. Adnexal masses in postmenopausal women. Obstet Gynecol 1987; 70: 578–581

18 Andolf E, Jorgensen C. Simple adnexal cysts diagnosed by ultrasound in postmenopausal women. JCU 1988; 16: 301–303

19 Goldstein S R, Subramanyam B, Snyder J R et al. The postmenopausal cystic adnexal mass: the potential role of ultrasound in conservative management. Obstet Gynecol 1989; 73: 8–10

20 Shawker T H, Garra B S, Loriaux D L, Cutler G B, Ross J L. Ultrasonography of Turner's syndrome. J Ultrasound Med 1986; 5: 125–129

21 Sohval A R. The syndrome of pure gonadal dysgenesis. Am J Med 1965; 38: 615

22 Lippe B M. Primary ovarian failure. In: Kaplan S A, ed. Clinical pediatric and adolescent endocrinology. Philadelphia: WB Saunders, 1982; 286–287

23 Reynolds T, Hill M C, Glassman L M. Sonography of hemorrhagic ovarian cysts. JCU 1986; 14: 449

24 Baltarowich O H, Kurtz A B, Pasto M E et al. The spectrum of sonographic findings in hemorrhagic ovarian cysts. AJR 1987; 148: 901–905

25 Suita S, Ikeda K, Koyamagi T et al. Neonatal ovarian cyst diagnosed antenatally: report of two patients. JCU 1984; 12: 517

26 Nussbaum A R, Sanders R C, Hartman D S et al. Neonatal ovarian cysts: sonographic–pathologic correlation. Radiology 1988; 168: 817–821

27 Stein I F, Leventhal M L. Amenorrhea associated with bilateral polycystic ovaries. Am J Obstet Gynecol 1935; 29: 181–191

28 Rottem S, Levit N, Thaler I et al. Classification of ovarian lesions by high-frequency transvaginal sonography. JCU 1990; 18: 359–363

29 Yeh H C, Futterweit W, Thornton J C. Polycystic ovarian disease: US features in 104 patients. Radiology 1987; 163: 111

30 Orsini L F, Venturoli S, Lorusso R et al. Ultrasonic findings in polycystic ovarian disease. Fertil Steril 1985; 43: 709

31 Hann L E, Hall D A, McArdle C R, Seibel M. Polycystic ovarian disease: sonographic spectrum. Radiology 1984; 150: 531

32 Hall D A. Sonographic appearance of the normal ovary, of polycystic ovary disease, and of functional ovarian cysts. Semin Ultrasound 1983; 4: 149–165

33 Jaffe R, Abramowicz J, Eckstein N et al. Sonographic monitoring of ovarian volume during LHRH analogue therapy in women with polycystic ovarian syndrome. J Ultrasound Med 1988; 7: 203–206

34 Hague W M, Adams J, Reeders S T, Peto T E A, Jacobs H S. Familial polycystic ovaries: a genetic disease? Clin Endocrinol 1988; 29: 593–605

35 Polson D W, Wadsworth J, Adams J, Franks S. Polycystic ovaries – a common finding in normal women. Lancet 1988; i: 870–872

36 Adams J, Polson D W, Franks S. Prevalence of polycystic ovaries in women with anovulation and idiopathic hirsutism. BMJ 1986; 293: 355–359

37 Hague W M, Adams J, Rodda C et al. The prevalence of polycystic ovaries in patients with congenital adrenal hyperplasia and their close relatives. Clin Endocrinol 1990; 33: 501–510

38 Goldstein D P, Berkowitz R J, Cohen S M. The current management of molar pregnancy. Curr Probl Obstet Gynecol 1979; 3: 1

39 Geishovel F, Skubsch U, Zabel G et al. Ultrasonographic and hormonal studies in physiologic and insufficient menstrual cycles. Fertil Steril 1983; 39: 277

40 Queenan J T, O'Brien J D, Bains L M et al. Ultrasound scanning of ovaries to detect ovulation in women. Fertil Steril 1980; 34: 99

41 Ritchie W G M. Sonographic evaluation of normal and induced ovulation. Radiology 1986; 161: 1

42 Blankstein J, Shalev J, Saadon T et al. Ovarian hyperstimulation syndrome: prediction by number and size of preovulatory follicles. Fertil Steril 1986; 47: 597–602

43 Polishuk W Z, Schenker J G. Ovarian hyperstimulation syndrome. Fertil Steril 1969; 20: 443

44 Golan A, Ron-El R, Herman A et al. Ovarian hyperstimulation syndrome: an update review. Obstet Gynecol Surv 198; 44: 430–440

45 Phillips H E, McGahan J P. Ovarian remnant syndrome. Radiology 1982; 142: 487

46 Warner M, Fleischer A, Edell S et al. Uterine adnexal torsion: sonographic findings. Radiology 1985; 154: 773–775

47 Haller J O, Friedman A P, Schaffer R, Lebensart D P. The normal and abnormal ovary in childhood and adolescence. Semin Ultrasound 1983; 4: 213

48 Graif M, Itzchak Y. Sonographic evaluation of ovarian torsion in childhood and adolescence. AJR 1988; 150: 647–649

49 Helvie M A, Silver T M. Ovarian torsion: sonographic evaluation. JCU 1989; 17: 327–332

50 Farrell T P, Boal D K, Teele R L et al. Acute torsion of the normal uterine adnexa in children: sonographic demonstration. AJR 1982; 139: 1223–1225

51 Williams A G, Mettler F A, Wicks J D. Cystic and solid ovarian neoplasms. Semin Ultrasound 1983; 4: 166

52 Kliman L, Rome R M, Fortune D W. Low malignant potential tumors of the ovary; a study of 76 cases. Obstet Gynecol 1986; 68: 338–344

53 Buy J-N, Ghossain M A, Sciot C et al. Epithelial tumors of the ovary: CT findings and correlation with US. Radiology 1991; 178: 811–818

54 Czernobilsky B. Common epithelial tumors of the ovary. In: Kurman R J, ed. Blaustein's pathology of the female genital tract, 3rd edn. New York: Springer-Verlag, 1987; 560–606

55 Quinn S F, Erickson S, Black W C. Cystic ovarian teratomas: the sonographic appearance of the dermoid plug. Radiology 1985; 155: 477

56 Sisler C L, Siegel M J. Ovarian teratomas: a comparison of the sonographic appearance in prepubertal and postpubertal girls. AJR 1990; 154: 139–141

57 Gutman P H Jnr. In search of the elusive benign cystic ovarian teratoma: application of the ultrasound 'tip of the iceberg' sign. JCU 1977; 5: 403

58 Sheth S, Fishman E K, Buck J L et al. The variable sonographic appearance of ovarian teratomas: correlation with CT. AJR 1988; 151: 331–334

59 Robbins S L, Cotran R S, Kumar V, eds. Female genital tract. In: Pathologic basis of disease, 3rd edn. Philadelphia: WB Saunders, 1984; 1151–1155

60 Diakoumakis E, Vieux U, Seife B. Sonographic demonstration of thecoma: report of two cases. Am J Obstet Gynecol 1984; 150: 787

61 Yaghoobian J, Pinck R L. Ultrasound findings in thecoma of the ovary. JCU 1983; 11: 91

62 Novak E R, Woodruff J D. Novak's gynecologic and obstetrical pathology, 8th edn. Philadelphia: WB Saunders, 1979

63 Stephenson W M, Laing F C. Sonography of ovarian fibromas. AJR 1985; 144: 1239

64 Athey P A, Malone R S. Sonography of ovarian fibromas/thecomas. J Ultrasound Med 1987; 6: 431–436

65 Athey P A, Siegel M F. Sonographic features of Brenner tumor of the ovary. J Ultrasound Med 1987; 6: 367–372

66 Birnholz J C. Endometriosis and inflammatory disease. Semin Ultrasound 1983; 4: 184–192

67 Scully R E, Richardson C S, Barlow J F. The development of malignancies in endometriosis. Clin Obstet Gynecol 1966; 9: 384

68 Robbins S L, Cotran R S, Kumar V, eds. Female genital tract. In: Pathologic basis of disease, 3rd edn. Philadelphia: WB Saunders, 1984; 1142–1145

69 Peel K R. Benign and malignant tumors of the ovary. In: Whitfield C R, ed. Dewhurst's textbook of obstetrics and gynecology for postgraduates. Oxford: Blackwell Scientific Publications, 1986; 733–754

70 Griffiths C T, Berkowitz R. The ovary. In: Kistner R W, ed. Gynecology: principles and practice. Chicago: Year Book Medical Publishers, 1986; 289–377

71 Talerman A. Mesenchymal tumors and malignant lymphoma of the ovary. In: Blaustein A, ed. Pathology of the female genital tract, 2nd edn. New York: Springer-Verlag, 1982; 705–715

72 Bickers G H, Siebert J J, Anderson J C. Sonography of ovarian involvement in childhood acute lymphocytic leukemia. AJR 1981; 137: 399–401

73 Swayne L C, Love M B, Karasich S R. Pelvic inflammatory disease: sonographic–pathologic correlation. Radiology 1984; 151: 751–755

74 Nosher J L, Winchman H K, Needell G S. Transvaginal pelvic abscess drainage with ultrasound guidance. Radiology 1987; 165: 872

75 Tyrrel R T, Murphy F B, Bernardino M E. Tubo-ovarian abscesses: CT-guided percutaneous drainage. Radiology 1990; 175: 87–89

76 Worthen N J, Gunning J E. Percutaneous drainage of pelvic abscesses: management of the tubo-ovarian abscess. J Ultrasound Med 1986; 5: 551–556

77 Nosher J L, Needell G S, Amorosa J K, Krasna I H. Transrectal pelvic abscess drainage with sonographic guidance. AJR 1986; 146: 1047–1048

78 Dawood M Y. Endometriosis. In: Gold J F, Josimovich J B, eds. Gynecologic endocrinology, 4th edn. New York: Plenum Press, 1987; 387

79 Friedman H, Vogelzang R L, Mendelson E B, Neiman H L, Cohen M. Endometriosis detection by ultrasound with laparoscopic correlation. Radiology 1985; 157: 217–220

80 Sample W F. Pelvic inflammatory disease and endometriosis. In: Sanders R C, James A E Jnr, eds. The principles and practice of ultrasonography in obstetrics and gynecology, 2nd edn. New York: Appleton-Century Crofts, 1979; 322–333

81 Gorell H A, Cyr D R, Wang K Y, Greer B E. Rectosigmoid endometriosis. Diagnosis using endovaginal sonography. J Ultrasound Med 1989; 8: 459–461

82 Kumar R, Haque A K, Cohen M S. Endometriosis of the urinary bladder: demonstration by sonography. JCU 1984; 12: 363–365

83 Im J-G, Kang H S, Choi B I et al. Pleural endometriosis: CT and sonographic findings. AJR 1987; 148: 523–524

84 Athey P A, Diment D D. The spectrum of sonographic findings in endometrioma. J Ultrasound Med 1989; 8: 487

85 Deutsch A L, Gosink B B. Nonneoplastic gynecologic disorders. Semin Roentgenol 1982; 14: 269

86 Goldman S M, Minkin S I. Diagnosing endometriosis with ultrasound. Accuracy and specificity. J Reprod Med 1980; 25: 178

87 Alpern M, Sandler M, Madrazo B. Sonographic features of parovarian cysts and their complications. AJR 1984; 143: 157

88 Athey P, Cooper N. Sonographic features of parovarian cysts. AJR 1985; 144: 83

89 Loffer F D. The increasing problem of ectopic pregnancies and its impact on patients and physicians. J Reprod Med 1986; 31: 74–77

90 Filly R A. Ectopic pregnancy: the role of sonography. Radiology 1987; 162: 661–668

91 Nyberg D A, Mack L A, Laing F C, Jeffrey R B. Early pregnancy complications: endovaginal sonographic findings correlated with human chorionic gonadotrophin levels. Radiology 1988; 167: 619–622

92 Manor W F, Zweibel W J, Hanning R V, Raymond H W. Ectopic pregnancy and other causes of acute pelvic pain. Semin Ultrasound CT MR 1985; 6: 181–206

93 Peisner D B, Timor-Tritsch I E. The discriminatory zone of beta-hCG for vaginal probes. JCU 1990; 18: 280–285

94 Dashefsky S M, Lyons E A, Levi C S, Lindsay D J. Suspected ectopic pregnancy: endovaginal and transvescical US. Radiology 1988; 169: 181–184

95 Fleischer A C, Pennell R G, McKee M S et al. Ectopic pregnancy: features at transvaginal sonography. Radiology 1990; 174: 375–378

96 Cacciatore B. Can the status of tubal pregnancy be predicted with transvaginal sonography? A prospective comparison of sonographic, surgical, and serum hCG findings. Radiology 1990; 177: 481–484

97 Romero R, Kadar N, Castro D et al. The value of adnexal sonographic findings in the diagnosis of ectopic pregnancy. Am J Obstet Gynecol 1988; 158: 52–55

98 Mahony B S, Filly R A, Nyberg D A et al. Sonographic evaluation of ectopic pregnancy. J Ultrasound Med 1985; 4: 221–228

99 Nyberg D A, Hughes M P, Mack L A, Wang K Y. Extrauterine findings of ectopic pregnancy at transvaginal US: importance of echogenic fluid. Radiology 1991; 178: 823–826

100 Cacciatore B, Stenman U-H, Ylostalo P. Comparison of abdominal and vaginal sonography in suspected ectopic pregnancy. Obstet Gynecol 1989; 73: 770–774

101 Bateman B G, Nunley W C, Kolp L A, Kitchin J D III, Felder R. Vaginal sonography findings and hCG dynamics of early intrauterine and tubal pregnancies. Obstet Gynecol 1990; 75: 421–427

102 Marks W M, Filly R A, Callen P W, Laing F C. The decidual cast of ectopic pregnancy: a confusing ultrasonographic appearance. Radiology 1979; 133: 341–344

103 Nyberg D A, Laing F C, Filly R A et al. Ultrasonographic differentiation of the gestational sac of early intrauterine pregnancy from the pseudogestational sac of ectopic pregnancy. Radiology 1983; 146: 755–759

104 Hill L M, Kislak S, Martin J G. Transvaginal sonographic detection of the pseudogestational sac associated with ectopic pregnancy. Obstet Gynecol 1990; 75: 986–988

105 Dillon E H, Feyock A L, Taylor K J W. Pseudogestational sacs: Doppler US differentiation from normal or abnormal intrauterine pregnancies. Radiology 1990; 176: 359–364

106 Rahman M S, Al-Suleiman S A, Rahman J, Al-Sibai M H. Advanced abdominal pregnancy: observations in 10 cases. Obstet Gynecol 1981; 59(3): 366–372

107 Beacham W D, Hernquist W C, Beacham D W et al. Abdominal pregnancy at Charity Hospital in New Orleans. Am J Obstet Gynecol 1962; 84: 1257–1270

108 Strafford J C, Ragan W D. Abdominal pregnancy: review of current management. Obstet Gynecol 1977; 50(5): 548–552

109 Stanley J H, Horger E O III, Fagan C J, Andriole J G, Fleischer A C. Sonographic findings in abdominal pregnancy. AJR 1986; 147: 1043–1046

110 Fleischer A C, Pittaway D, Wentz A et al. The uses of sonography of monitoring ovarian follicular development. In: Ultrasound Annual 1983. New York: Raven Press, 1983; 163–705

111 Richman T S, Viscomi G N, deCherney A et al. Fallopian tubal patency assessed by ultrasound following fluid injection. Radiology 1984; 152: 507–510

112 Feldberg D, Goldman J A, Ashkenazi J et al. Transvaginal oocyte retrieval controlled by vaginal probe for in vitro fertilization: a comparative study. J Ultrasound Med 1988; 7: 339–343

113 Gonen Y, Blanker J, Casper R F. Transvaginal ultrasonically guided follicular aspiration: a comparative study with laparoscopically guided follicular aspiration. JCU 1990; 18: 257–261

114 Wiseman D A, Short W B, Pattinson H A et al. Oocyte retrieval in an in-vitro fertilization – embryo transfer program: comparison of four methods. Radiology 1989; 173: 99–102

115 Mendelson E B, Friedman J, Neiman H L et al. The role of imaging in infertility management. AJR 1985; 144: 415

116 Hull M E, Moghissi K S, Magyar D M et al. Correlation of serum estradiol levels and ultrasound monitoring to assess follicular maturation. Fertil Steril 1986; 46: 42

117 Zandt-Stastny D, Thorsen M K, Middleton W D et al. Inability of sonography to detect imminent ovulation. AJR 1989; 152: 91–95

118 Boring C C, Squires T S, Tong T. Cancer statistics. CA 1994; 43: 7–26

119 Ozols R F, Rubin S C, Dembo A J, Robboy S J. Epithelial ovarian cancer. In: Hoskins W J, Perez C A, Young R C, eds. Principles and practice of gynecologic oncology. Philadelphia: J B Lippincott, 1992; 731–781

120 Morrow C P. Malignant and borderline epithelial tumors of the ovary: clinical features, staging, diagnosis, intraoperative assessment and review of management. In: Coppleson M, ed. Gynecologic oncology. Edinburgh: Churchill Livingstone, 1992; 889–915

121 Westoff C, Randall M C. Ovarian cancer screening: potential effect on mortality. Am J Obstet Gynecol 1991; 165: 502–505

122 Koonings P P, Campbell K, Mishell D R et al. Relative frequency of primary ovarian neoplasms: a ten year review. Obstet Gynecol 1989; 74: 921–925

123 Kerlikowske K, Brown J S, Grady D G. Should women with familial ovarian cancer undergo prophylactic oophorectomy? Obstet Gynecol 1992; 80: 700–707

124 Ovarian cancer: screening, treatment and follow up. Consensus Development Conference Statement. National Institute of Health, 1994; 1–29

125 Lynch H T, Kimberling W J, Albano W A et al. Hereditary non-polyposis colorectal cancer: Lynch syndrome I + II. Cancer 1985; 56: 939–951

126 Lynch H T, Harris R E, Guirgis H A et al. Familial association of breast/ovarian carcinoma. Cancer 1978; 41: 1543–1548

127 Lynch H T, Albano W A, Black L et al. Familial excess of cancer of the ovary and anatomic sites. J Am Med Assoc 1981; 245: 261–264

128 Gallion H H, Smith S A. Hereditary ovarian carcinoma. Semin Surg Oncol 1994; 10: 249–254

129 DePriest P D, van Nagell J R Jr. Transvaginal ultrasound screening for ovarian cancer. Clin Obstet Gynecol 1992; 35(1): 40–44

130 Jacobs I, Bridges J, Reynolds C et al. Multimodal approach to screening for ovarian cancer. Lancet 1988; i: 268–271

131 van Nagell J R Jr, Higgins R V, Donaldson E S et al. Transvaginal sonography as a screening method for ovarian cancer: a report of the first 1000 cases screened. Cancer 1990; 65: 573–577

132 Jacobs I, Bast R C. The CA 125 tumour associated antigen: a review of the literature. Hum Reprod 1989; 4: 1–12

133 Bast R C, Klug T L, St John E et al. A radioimmunoassay using a monoclonal antibody to monitor the course of epithelial ovarian cancer. N Engl J Med 1983; 309: 883–887

134 Helzlsouer K J, Bush T L, Alberg A J et al. Prospective study of serum CA-125 levels as markers of ovarian cancers. J Am Med Assoc 1993; 269: 1123–1126

135 Zurawski V R Jr, Orjaseter H, Andersen A, Jellum E. Elevated serum CA 125 levels prior to diagnosis of ovarian neoplasia: relevance for early detection of ovarian cancer. Int J Cancer 1988; 42: 677–680

136 Woolas R P, Xu F-J, Jacobs I J et al. Elevation of multiple serum markers in patients with stage I ovarian cancer. J Natl Cancer Inst 1993; 85: 1748–1751

137 Campbell S, Bhan V, Royston P et al. Transabdominal ultrasound screening for early ovarian cancer. BMJ 1989; 299: 1363–1367

138 Davies A P, Jacobs I, Woolas R, Fish A, Oram D. The adnexal mass: benign or malignant? Evaluation of a risk of malignancy index. Br J Obstet Gynaecol 1993; 100: 927–931

139 DeLand M, Fried A, van Nagell J R, Donaldson E S. Ultrasonography in the diagnosis of tumors of the ovary. Surg Gynecol Obstet 1979; 148: 346–348

140 Goswamy R K, Campbell S, Whitehead M I. Screening for ovarian cancer. Clin Obstet Gynecol 1983; 10(3): 621–643

141 DePriest P D, van Nagell J R, Gallion H H et al. Ovarian cancer screening in asymptomatic postmenopausal women. Gynecol Oncol 1993; 51: 205–209

142 Sassone A M, Timor-Tritsch I E, Artner A et al. Transvaginal sonographic characterisation of ovarian disease: evaluation of a new scoring system to predict ovarian malignancy. Obstet Gynecol 1991; 78: 70–76

143 Kurjak A, Zalud I. Transvaginal colour Doppler in the differentiation between benign and malignant ovarian masses. In: Sharp F, Mason W P, Creasman W, eds. Ovarian cancer. London: Chapman & Hall, 1992; 249–264

144 Rulin M C, Preston A L. Adnexal masses in postmenopausal women. Obstet Gynecol 1987; 70: 578–581

145 Jain K A. Prospective evaluation of adnexal masses with endovaginal gray-scale and duplex and color Doppler US: correlation with pathologic findings. Radiology 1994; 191: 63–67

146 Levine D, Feldstein V A, Babcock C J, Filly R A. Sonography of ovarian masses: poor sensitivity of resistive index for identifying malignant lesions. AJR 1994; 162: 1355–1359

147 Rottem S, Levit N, Thaler I et al. Classification of ovarian lesions by high-frequency transvaginal sonography. JCU 1990; 18: 359–363

148 Buy J-N, Ghossain M A, Hugol D et al. Characterisation of adnexal masses: combination of colour Doppler and conventional sonography compared with spectral Doppler analysis alone and conventional sonography alone. AJR 1996; 166: 385–393

149 Bourne T H, Campbell S, Reynolds K M et al. Screening for early familial ovarian cancer with transvaginal ultrasonography and colour blood flow imaging. BMJ 1993; 306: 1025–1029

150 Bromley B, Goodman H, Benacerraf B R. Comparison between sonographic morphology and Doppler waveform for the diagnosis of ovarian malignancy. Obstet Gynecol 1994; 83: 434–437

151 DePriest P D, Shenson D, Fried A et al. A morphology index based on sonographic findings in ovarian cancer. Gynecol Oncol 1993; 51: 7–11

152 Stein S M, Laifer-Narin S, Johnson M B et al. Differentiation of benign and malignant adnexal masses: relative value of gray-scale, color Doppler and spectral Doppler sonography. AJR 1995; 164: 381–386

153 Taylor K J W, Schwartz P E. Screening for early ovarian cancer. Radiology 1994; 192: 1–10

154 Quinn S F, Erickson S, Black W C. Cystic ovarian teratomas: the sonographic appearance of the dermoid plug. Radiology 1985; 155: 477

155 Sisler C L, Siegel M J. Ovarian teratomas: a comparison of the sonographic appearance in prepubertal and postpubertal girls. AJR 1990; 154: 139–141

156 Gutman P H Jr. In search of the elusive benign cystic ovarian teratoma: application of the ultrasound 'tip of the iceberg' sign. JCU 1997; 5: 403

157 Sheth S, Fishman E K, Buck J L et al. The variable sonographic appearance of ovarian teratomas: correlation with CT. AJR 1988; 151: 331–334

158 Diakoumakis E, Vieux U, Seife B. Sonographic demonstration of thecoma: report of two cases. Am J Obstet Gynecol 1984; 150: 787

159 Yaghoobian J, Pinck R L. Ultrasound findings in thecoma of the ovary. JCU 1983; 11: 91

160 Talerman A. Mesenchymal tumors and malignant lymphoma of the ovary. In: Blaustein A, ed. Pathology of the female genital tract, 2nd edn., New York: Springer-Verlag, 1982; 705–715

161 Athey P, Malone R S. Sonography of ovarian fibromas/thecomas. J Ultrasound Med 1987; 6: 431–436

162 Athey P A, Siegel M F. Sonographic features of Brenner tumor of the ovary. J Ultrasound Med 1987; 6: 367–372

163 Young R H, Scully R E. Metastatic Tumours of the Ovary. In: Kurman R J, ed. Blaustein's pathology of the female genital tract, 3rd edn. New York: Springer-Verlag, 1987; 742–768

164 Kurjak A, Shalan H, Kupesic S et al. An attempt to screen asymptomatic women for ovarian and endometrial cancer with transvaginal color and pulsed Doppler sonography. J Ultrasound Med 1994; 13: 295–301

165 Hata T, Hata K, Senoh D et al. Doppler ultrasound assessment of tumor vascularity in gynecologic disorders. J Ultrasound Med 1989; 8: 309–314

166 Bourne T, Campbell S, Steer C et al. Transvaginal colour flow imaging: a possible new screening technique for ovarian cancer. BMJ 1989; 299: 1367–1370

167 Fleischer A C, Rodgers W H, Kepple D M et al. Color Doppler sonography of benign and malignant ovarian masses. Radiographics 1992; 12: 879–885

168 Hamper U M, Seth S, Abbas F M et al. Transvaginal Doppler sonography of adnexal masses: differences in blood flow impedance in benign and malignant lesions. AJR 1993; 160: 1225–1228

169 Weiner Z, Thaler I, Beck D et al. Differentiating malignant from benign ovarian tumors with transvaginal color flow imaging. Obstet Gynecol 1992; 79: 159–162

170 Bonilla-Musoles F, Ballester M J, Simon C et al. Is avoidance of surgery possible in patients with perimenopausal ovarian tumors using transvaginal ultrasound and duplex color Doppler sonography? J Ultrasound Med 1993; 12: 33–39

171 Brown D L, Frates M C, Laing F C et al. Ovarian masses: can benign and malignant lesions be differentiated with color and pulsed Doppler US? Radiology 1994; 190: 333–336

172 Hata K, Hata T, Manabe A et al. A critical evaluation of transvaginal Doppler studies, transvaginal sonography, magnetic resonance imaging and CA 125 in detecting ovarian cancer. Obstet Gynecol 1992; 80: 922–926

173 Carter J, Saltzman A, Hartenbach E et al. Flow characteristics in benign and malignant gynecologic tumors using transvaginal color flow Doppler. Obstet Gynecol 1994; 83: 125–130

174 Tekay A, Jouppila P. Validity of pulsatility and resistance indices in classification of adnexal tumors with transvaginal color Doppler ultrasound. Ultrasound Obstet Gynaecol 1992; 2: 338–344

175 Jacobs I J, Skates S J, MacDonald N et al. Screening for ovarian cancer: a pilot randomised controlled trial. Lancet 1999; 353: 1207–1210

4

Infertility

John H Parsons and Christopher V Steer

Introduction

Ultrasound was first used to demonstrate the pelvic organs in 1966.[1] In 1972 Kratochwil[2] demonstrated that follicles may be seen in the preovulatory stage of the cycle. The early work[3–9] was laborious as it was done using static scanners and a full bladder. The development of real-time equipment in the late 1970s[10] and the vaginal probe in the early 1980s[11] transformed pelvic ultrasonography into a technique that is simple to learn and use.

The incorporation of spectral Doppler, and more recently colour flow mapping, into ultrasound equipment has allowed changes in the uterine and ovarian blood supply to be studied during health and disease. The full potential of this is still being explored and looks likely to enhance the diagnostic yield significantly.

The importance of pelvic ultrasound in the investigation and treatment of infertility is demonstrated by the wide range of applications described in this chapter.

Technique and equipment

The pelvic organs may be scanned either transabdominally or trans-vaginally. The former requires a full bladder to displace the gas-containing bowel and to provide an 'acoustic window' through to the pelvic organs.

In most infertility units trans-vaginal ultrasound has become the routine method. However, when the ovaries are high in the abdomen, or when the uterus is enlarged, abdominal ultrasonography may be necessary for adequate visualisation.

During trans-vaginal ultrasound with the probe in the lateral and anterior fornices of the vagina only a few centimetres separate it from the uterus and ovaries, with no intervening bowel gas. The elasticity of the vaginal vault allows these structures to be approached individually. Because there is no need for a full bladder the patient is comfortable and appointment times may be fixed. The proximity of the probe to the structures being examined allows the use of high-frequency probes with a short focal length, giving enhanced resolution compared to transabdominal scanning.

The size of the trans-vaginal probe varies between manufacturers, the slimmer, round-ended probes being the least uncomfortable. Patients who have not had intercourse but who have used tampons will tolerate such a probe. Cooperative patients who are virgo intacta may, if the probe is slim, be scanned rectally with minimal discomfort. Patients bleeding heavily at the time of the examination are best advised to leave a tampon in the vagina; the probe may be positioned beside it. Great care must be taken while performing vaginal ultrasonography to minimise the patients' natural embarrassment at being exposed in the lithotomy position.

Whichever gynaecological organ is being examined it is good practice to review the whole pelvis routinely using a standard sequence. To obtain the maximum amount of information it is preferable to carry out serial examinations. This is particularly important when assessing ovarian morphology and function.

Potential dangers of ultrasonography

There is no evidence that diagnostic ultrasound by either the transabdominal or the trans-vaginal route has any adverse effect on either the oocyte, the pre-embryo or the early developing pregnancy.[12]

It is not practical to sterilise the trans-vaginal probe between procedures, so it is covered either by a specially designed sheath or by an ordinary contraceptive condom, although in infertility studies condoms lubricated with spermicidal gel must be avoided. Cross-infection remains a cause for concern as occasionally the protective sheaths break. Furthermore, the British Standard to which condoms should conform in the UK (BS 3704/1989; British Standards Institution, London) means only that there are holes in fewer than four condoms per 1000.

Ovarian ultrasound

Identification

The ovaries are usually identified lying lateral to the uterus, adjacent to the side wall of the pelvis. A useful landmark is their close relationship to the internal iliac vessels, which are usually easily identified (Figs 4.1 and 4.2).

The stroma has a characteristic appearance and is outlined by loops of bowel, in which peristalsis may be seen.

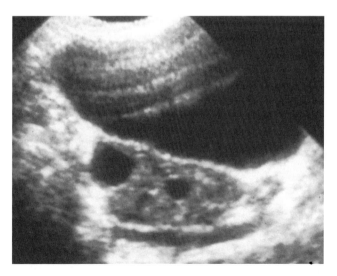

Fig. 4.1 Normal ovary. A transabdominal ultrasound scan of an unstimulated ovary. The internal iliac vein is seen immediately beneath the ovary.

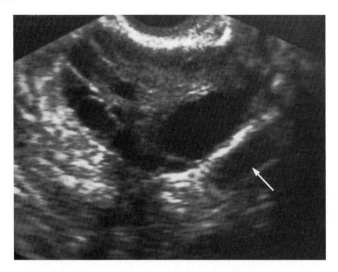

Fig. 4.2 Normal ovary. A trans-vaginal ultrasound scan of an ovary showing the close proximity to the internal iliac vein (arrow).

Identification is made easier by the presence of follicles or cysts. It is occasionally necessary to search more widely for the ovary: it may be found behind or above the uterus, or under the anterior abdominal wall. These unusual sites may be caused by excessive mobility, but are often attributable to adhesions (see Ch. 9).

A high ovary may sometimes be brought into the field of view of a trans-vaginal probe by pressing firmly on the lower abdomen. When the ovary will not descend in this manner a clear picture may sometimes be obtained by either a high-frequency (5–7.5 MHz) abdominal or trans-vaginal probe scanning transabdominally, without a full bladder (Fig. 4.3).

The normal ovary is ellipsoid in shape. Its volume (in ml when measuring in cm) may be estimated using the approximate formula for an ellipsoid: length × breadth × depth × 0.5.[5]

Ovarian morphology

The unstimulated ovary in women with regular cycles contains a small number of cystic structures (Fig. 4.1) and has a mean volume of 5.4 ml.[13] However, 23% of women have ovaries that contain 10 or more such structures (2–8 mm in diameter), often distributed peripherally round a central core of stroma (Fig. 4.4). Such ovaries have been termed polycystic and are associated with menstrual irregularity, raised luteinising hormone concentrations, hirsutism, anovulation and an increased incidence of miscarriage; 87% of women with oligomenorrhoea and anovulation have polycystic ovaries.[14,15]

Ovaries with a polycystic morphology have a mean volume greater than the non-polycystic ovary (11.1 ml), but there is a considerable overlap in size between the two types. The presence of polycystic ovaries is more likely to be associated with infertility if the woman has a raised body mass index (BMI).[16]

The ovaries of woman with a low BMI, those approaching the menarche and those suffering from anorexia nervosa pass through characteristic changes as their BMI increases. Initially the ovaries are small and featureless but, as the woman's weight rises, the ovarian volume increases and small cysts appear. Unlike the cysts in polycystic ovaries, these are associated with a normal amount of ovarian stroma, low or normal gonadotrophins and a small uterine volume. With further weight gain one of the cysts becomes dominant and the rest regress, so that the morphology returns to normal. This type of cystic ovary has been termed multifollicular[17] (Fig. 4.5) and its presence is suggestive of less than optimum weight in

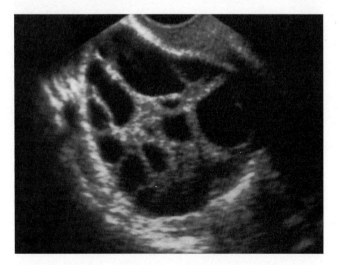

Fig. 4.3 A stimulated ovary seen immediately beneath the anterior abdominal wall with a 7 MHz probe.

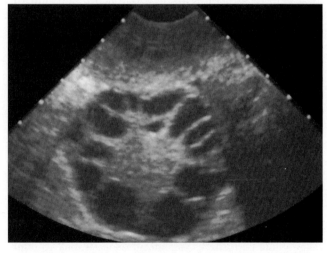

Fig. 4.4 A polycystic ovary showing the peripheral distribution of follicles and a central core of stroma (trans-vaginal).

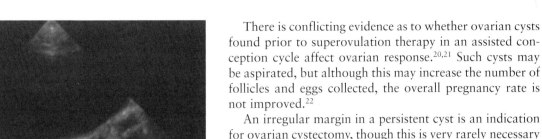

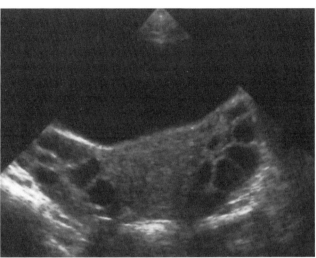

Fig. 4.5 Prepubertal ovary. Transabdominal ultrasound of an ovary 3 months before the menarche, showing the multifollicular appearance.

patients recovering from anorexia nervosa. If the patent conceives, the fetus has an increased risk of intra-uterine growth retardation.[18]

Functional ovarian cysts

Ovaries commonly contain follicular or luteal cysts (Fig. 4.6). These are characterised by their echo-free contents, failure to grow and disappear over the normal 2-week timespan of a follicle, and a tendency to resolve spontaneously. They are usually less than 5 cm in diameter but may reach 10 cm as long as their outline is sharp and smooth, the woman may be reassured.[19]

There is conflicting evidence as to whether ovarian cysts found prior to superovulation therapy in an assisted conception cycle affect ovarian response.[20,21] Such cysts may be aspirated, but although this may increase the number of follicles and eggs collected, the overall pregnancy rate is not improved.[22]

An irregular margin in a persistent cyst is an indication for ovarian cystectomy, though this is very rarely necessary in women seeking treatment for infertility. The blood flow to such cysts may be assessed with colour flow Doppler. In a study of 50 women, Bourne *et al*[23] found that the seven patients with primary ovarian cancer (two at stage 1a) had low pulsatility indices (0.3–1.0) which clearly differentiated them from those with normal ovaries (3.2–7.0).

Blood-filled ovarian cysts may be identified by their reflective contents.

Endometriosis

Endometriomas contain thick syrupy altered blood which typically generates numerous low-level echoes filling the space (Fig. 4.7). Endometriomas not adjacent to clear fluid-containing cystic structures may be difficult to differentiate from ovarian stroma. The presence of ovarian endometriomas indicates a significant degree of endometriosis, which may have an important bearing on the patient's response to treatment.[24]

Other benign ovarian cysts and tumours

Dermoid cysts and fibromata may occasionally be identified in the ovaries of women of reproductive age. These

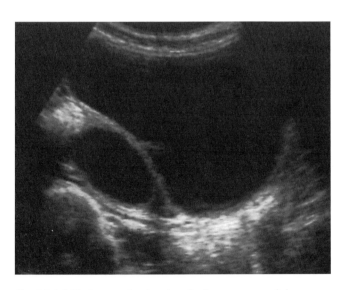

Fig. 4.6 A follicular cyst showing the echo-free contents and sharp outline.

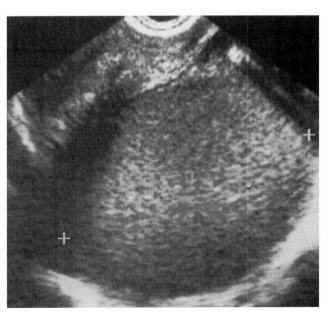

Fig. 4.7 Endometrioma. The characteristic ground-glass appearance of an endometrioma (trans-vaginal).

tumours may interfere with normal ovarian function, particularly if they are large.

Ovarian follicular monitoring

Serial monitoring of follicular development may be useful in both natural and stimulated ovarian cycles. Observation of a developing follicle, the prediction of impending ovulation and the detection of ovulation allow procedures such as post-coital testing, hCG administration, intercourse, donor and husband insemination and egg collection to be timed optimally. Patients shown not to be ovulating may be treated with ovulation induction agents.

A baseline scan early in the menstrual cycle should always be done to identify and record cystic structures which could later be misinterpreted as developing follicles. A luteal cyst (from the previous cycle) is commonly seen and may decrease in size during the follicular phase. A coiled hydrosalpinx may be mistaken as a group of follicles if care is not taken to identify continuity of the tubal lumen (Fig. 4.8).

Natural cycles

In the natural unstimulated ovarian cycle precursor follicles (2–4 mm) grow in each ovary in response to the intercycle FSH rise. There are usually about 20 such follicles, their number decreasing with age.[25] Under optimal conditions they may be identified on ultrasound. At a mean diameter of 10 mm (range 7–14) 7 days (range 9–6)

before the LH surge a dominant follicle takes over and there is very little further growth of other follicles. Non-dominant follicles within the ovary containing the dominant one tend to decrease in size during the late follicular and luteal phases of the cycle.[26] Occasionally (5% of cycles) two dominant follicles develop.[27,28]

Stimulated and superovulation cycles

Anovulation is treated by artificially raising the woman's serum follicle-stimulating hormone level to initiate the growth of follicles. This may be done with oral anti-oestrogens (e.g. clomiphene or cyclofenil), which bind to cytoplasmic oestrogen receptors in the pituitary causing a secondary rise in endogenous follicle-stimulating hormone (FSH), or parenterally with human menopausal gonadotrophin (hMG) or pure FSH. Preferably this should stimulate the development and ovulation of one, but no more than three follicles. If more are allowed to develop and ovulate, a high multiple pregnancy can result and there is a risk of the ovarian hyperstimulation syndrome (see below). Clomiphene (25–200 mg given for 5 days early in the follicular phase) rarely causes such problems; 10% of pregnancies are twin, but triplets are very unusual (Fig. 4.9). Parenteral ovulation induction was previously monitored by measuring serum or urinary levels of oestrogen. When the levels rose excessively the treatment had to be abandoned and a lower dose of gonadotrophin used in subsequent cycles. This technique does not differentiate one follicle from many follicles producing the same total amount of oestrogen. Ultrasound allows accurate monitoring of the numbers of follicles developing, but it may still be difficult to predict how many will ovulate (Fig. 4.8) because of the wide range of sizes at which follicles

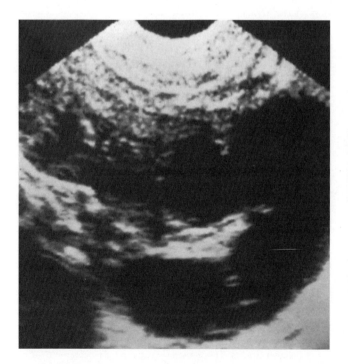

Fig. 4.8 A hydrosalpinx showing coiled shape and septa (trans-vaginal).

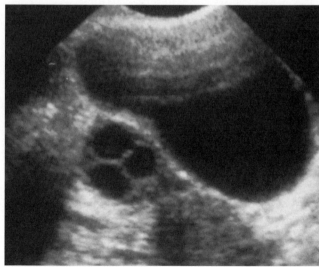

Fig. 4.9 Stimulated ovary. An ovary stimulated with clomiphene citrate (transabdominal).

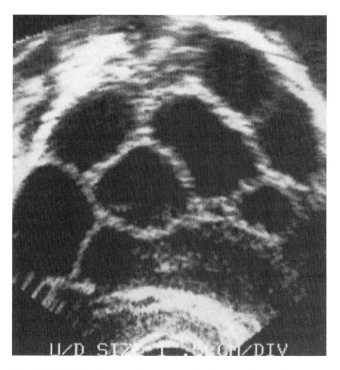

Fig. 4.10 Stimulated ovary. A trans-vaginal ultrasound scan of an ovary stimulated with hMG.

rupture. Patients with polycystic ovaries are particularly difficult to manage.

Superovulation therapy is used prior to assisted conception techniques such as gamete intrafallopian transfer (GIFT) or *in vitro* fertilisation (IVF). HMG or pure FSH, or a combination of both, with or without an anti-oestrogen, are used. The objective is to stimulate the synchronous development of many follicles, from which eggs are collected prior to ovulation (Fig. 4.10). Follicles which would have become suppressed by the dominant follicle are 'rescued' by the higher than physiological levels of FSH.[29] In some patients this strategy fails and one follicle remains dominant. Aspiration of this leading follicle may prevent it from triggering an endogenous luteinising hormone (LH) surge[30,31] and allow the treatment cycle to continue. Patients concerned that their increased production of eggs will mean an early menopause will usually be reassured when a simple explanation of the mechanism of superovulation is given. The risk of high multiple pregnancies is obviated by limiting the number of eggs or embryos replaced, but the risks of the ovarian hyperstimulation syndrome remain.

Ovarian blood supply before ovulation

Taylor, in 1985,[32] originally obtained Doppler signals from the ovarian arteries by scanning transabdominally through a full bladder. However, because of technical limitations

and patient obesity, it was not possible to obtain signals in 27% of the women studied. They found that the impedance of the ovarian artery decreased throughout the menstrual cycle, possibly before the dominant follicle could be recognised by its size or increased hormone production. This effect was noted to be more marked in clomiphene-stimulated cycles. Obtaining satisfactory ovarian artery Doppler signals trans-vaginally is difficult because from this direction the artery traverses the infundibulopelvic ligament at approximately 90° to the insonating ultrasound beam. A recent study using a trans-vaginal colour flow system has raised doubts as to whether intra-ovarian vessels can be identified during the follicular phase of the menstrual cycle.[33]

During gonadotrophin-stimulated cycles for IVF the ovarian artery impedance reduces during the follicular phase, in parallel to the increasing production of oestradiol. Furthermore, in an hMG-stimulated cycle the ovarian impedance is inversely proportional to the number of follicles larger than 15 mm which are present in the ovary, and to the number of oocytes subsequently harvested from the ovary.[34]

Follicle measurement

In the unstimulated ovary follicles are approximately spherical. They may, however, be flattened in one plane or have their shape altered by pressure from the ultrasound transducer or the bladder, so a mean of the maximum diameter in three planes is a better estimate of follicular size than measurements in only two planes (Figs 4.11 and 4.12).

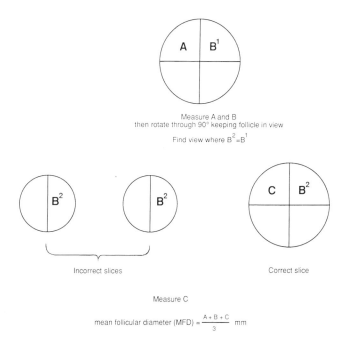

Measure A and B
then rotate through 90° keeping follicle in view
Find view where $B^2 = B^1$

Incorrect slices   Correct slice

Measure C

mean follicular diameter (MFD) = $\dfrac{A + B + C}{3}$ mm

Fig. 4.11 Technique for measuring the mean follicular diameter.

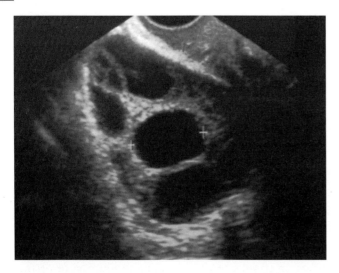

Fig. 4.12 **Follicle measurement:** the widest diameters should be selected.

Errors in measurement may arise as a result of difficulty in defining the follicle margin; this is more likely to occur when using transabdominal ultrasound.[35] A blind comparison between the two ultrasound approaches has shown that although the mean readings by a single observer of follicle size are likely to be similar whichever route is used, there is more scatter in the transabdominal readings and therefore more potential for inaccuracy.[36] The inter-observer variation of measurement is larger than the intra-observer measurement by either route, the least inter-observer variation being ±1.6 mm (95% confidence limit) for the trans-vaginal route. This suggests that serial follicular measurement is best done by the same observer using the trans-vaginal route.[37]

There is a significant correlation ($r = 0.64$) between the mean follicular diameter measured trans-vaginally and the follicular fluid volume aspirated laparoscopically.[38]

Follicular measurement is more difficult in stimulated and superovulation cycles as pressure from abutting follicles distorts the follicles, so that measurements often have to be a 'best estimate'. When there are many follicles, assessment may have to be limited to measurement of the two or three largest and a count of the total number. The count is performed by sweeping through the ovary from one edge to the other, in any plane.

Rate of follicular growth

During the 5 days prior to ovulation the dominant follicle in the natural cycle grows in a linear fashion at an average rate of 2–3 mm per day.[6,39] In clomiphene-stimulated cycles the growth rate during the 3 days preceding ovulation has been found to be greater than in the natural cycle.[40]

Subtle changes in the rate of follicular growth have been detected in patients with endometriosis.[41]

Prediction of ovulation

Follicular rupture occurs at a wide range of 13–30 mm, with a mean of 21 mm, and is unaffected by prior ovulation induction therapy.[28] There is a linear correlation between the mean level of serum oestradiol and the mean follicular diameter.[42] In stimulated cycles, where there are several follicles, this relationship holds good for total follicular volume.[43] The peak serum oestradiol (1500–1650 pmol/l per follicle) and the peak luteinising hormone levels occur in the majority of cases 2 days and 1 day, respectively, before ovulation.[39,44]

Because follicular size is no indication of imminent ovulation, other morphological features have been assessed in the hope that they will be a better guide. A poorly reflective halo around the follicle, thought to represent oedema in the theca cell layer, and a crenelated lining to the follicle, thought to indicate separation of the granulosa cell layer from the basement membrane, have been described as occurring within 24 and 6–10 hours, respectively, prior to ovulation.[45] A number of authors have identified echoes within the follicle which they ascribe to the presence of an expanded cumulus oophorus, either attached to the follicular wall or free floating (Fig. 4.13).[46] Unfortunately, none of these ultrasound signs has proved to be of practical value in the investigation or management of infertility.

Preceding ovulation, associated with the LH rise, perifollicular ovarian blood flow can be identified using transvaginal colour Doppler. In the few hours preceding ovulation there is a rapid increase both in the number of blood vessels that can be identified supplying the follicle and in the blood velocity within them.[33]

Ovulation pain (mittelschmerz) occurs in a minority of menstrual cycles,[28,47] it may occur either before or after ovulation[48] (usually before[49]) and does not necessarily correspond to the side on which ovulation occurs.[47]

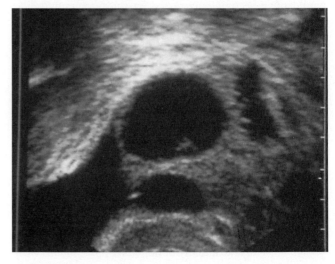

Fig. 4.13 **Cumulus oophorus.** Cone-shaped cumulus mass clearly visible within preovulatory follicle.

Timing of investigations and procedures

Because of the wide range of follicular size prior to ovulation, follicular monitoring can only form a guide to when ovulation might occur. During the 1980s follicle monitoring was used extensively but it has now been largely superseded by urinary LH dipsticks, which give 12–36 hours warning of ovulation; they may be purchased by the patient and used at home, which is convenient. Follicle monitoring may identify a growing follicle to enable the most appropriate moment to being testing the urine for LH to be chosen. This is particularly useful when the menstrual cycles are irregular or long.

Post-coital testing

Cervical mucus varies in consistency during the menstrual cycle in response to the changes in ovarian oestrogen production. Sperm can only swim well in the clear viscid mucus produced during the peri-ovulatory period. A positive post-coital test (many sperm swimming progressively through copious clear mucus) confirms that ejaculation of motile sperm has occurred into the vagina of an ovulatory woman, and carries a good prognosis.

A poor or negative post-coital test (no sperm, or few immotile or non-progressively motile sperm in low-volume cellular mucus) may indicate either a significant problem (apareunia, poor sperm quality, an immunological disorder, anovulation) or a mistimed test. Assessment with ovarian ultrasound, with or without urinary LH testing, improves the likelihood that post-coital tests are timed appropriately, sparing couples the unnecessary anxiety caused by a false negative test.

Sexual intercourse and artificial insemination

Serial ovarian ultrasonography may help women with irregular cycles identify their peri-ovulatory period and thus increase their chance of conception. Accurate identification of the fertile period is particularly important when artificial insemination is being used, as such treatment is demanding of both staff and patient time.

Donor semen is in short supply and it is therefore important to ensure that it is used efficiently. Insemination timed using ultrasound has been shown to be more successful than insemination timed using only a knowledge of previous menstrual cycle lengths and basal body temperature recording.[28]

Administration of human chorionic gonadotrophin

Oocyte maturation and ovulation may be induced with human chorionic gonadotrophin (hCG) when the follicle has reached a size at which it is likely to contain a suitably responsive egg. This approach is used during ovulation induction or superovulation with gonadotrophins, as therapy with these drugs may reduce or completely suppress the endogenous LH surge. Ovulation occurs 32–40 hours after the administration of hCG. If hCG is administered late at night, procedures such as insemination and egg collection may be performed at convenient times during the working day.

The actual follicular size at which hCG should be administered varies. Premature administration will damage the developing oocytes. When using clomiphene or hMG and sexual intercourse, good results may be achieved when hCG is administered at 17 mm. When using these drugs for superovulation prior to an egg collection, the hCG must be given before the endogenous LH surge to maintain control of the cycle. If serum or urinary LH measurements detect a premature surge, or there is a fall in the serum oestradiol level, there is a risk that the oocytes will be aged when collected 36 hours later and the treatment cycle should therefore be abandoned. When the endogenous gonadotrophins have been suppressed with a luteinising hormone-releasing hormone (LHRH) analogue (such as buserelin) there is no danger of being pre-empted by the endogenous LH surge and the hCG may then be delayed until the follicles are very much larger, without detrimental effect.[50] Delaying hCG administration allows smaller follicles to grow, thereby increasing the subsequent yield of oocytes and making the timing of the egg collection more flexible.

Ovulation

Usually the follicle simply disappears at ovulation.[28] However, an increase or decrease in size of the follicle, a change in shape or the development of irregular margins or internal echoes (Fig. 4.14) may all indicate that ovulation has occurred. During the peri-ovulatory period it is always possible to detect fluid in the pouch of Douglas. Only a relatively small percentage of women have a detectable increase in the volume of this fluid at ovulation.[28]

Contrary to popular belief, ovulation need not alternate between the two ovaries: there is a 75% chance of ovulation from the same ovary as the preceding cycle, and this may continue for several consecutive cycles.[51]

Ovarian blood flow after ovulation

The impedance in the artery supplying the ovary containing the corpus luteum falls in comparison to the contralateral ovary.[52] Presumably this signifies an increased blood supply, and the vessels within the ovarian substance may be seen relatively easily with colour flow imaging during the luteal phase. Immediately following ovulation there is a dramatic increase in blood velocity within the vessels

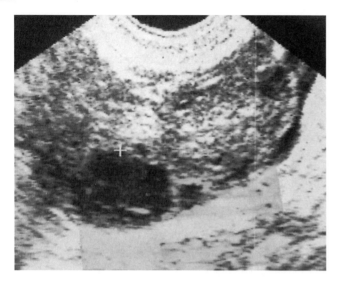

Fig. 4.14 Corpus luteum. A scan on the preceding day showed a 21 mm follicle. This has now developed an irregular outline and internal echoes following ovulation.

supplying the newly formed corpus luteum. This is due to the rapid formation of new blood vessels (neovascularisation). In the adult these blood vessels only develop in the corpus luteum and during wound healing and malignancy. They are unique in that they produce very low-impedance Doppler waveforms because the resistance vessels (arterioles) lack muscle lining in the media (Fig. 4.15).

In a group of women having IVF treatment, intra-ovarian flow velocity waveforms analysed 3 days following embryo transfer showed that those who became pregnant had a lower impedance compared to those who did not conceive.[53]

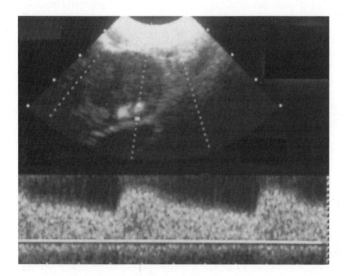

Fig. 4.15 Corpus luteum Doppler. Low-impedance vessels near a corpus luteum (trans-vaginal Doppler).

Corpus luteum

The corpus luteum may have a variety of ultrasound appearances. After ovulation the collapsed 'follicle' may fill in almost completely and be difficult to differentiate from the surrounding ovarian stroma. There is, however, usually a cystic component, which aids identification. It often increases in size and fills with echoes of varying amplitude. A haemorrhagic corpus luteum or luteal cyst (Fig. 4.14) may exceed 40 mm in diameter. As the ultrasound appearance of the corpus luteum is so varied, serial examinations may be required to document its resolution at the end of the secretory phase of the cycle.

Ultrasound assessment of non-conception cycles

Serial ovarian ultrasound can detect anovulation in both natural and stimulated cycles. Lower conception rates than expected after ovulation have led to attempts to define the characteristics of unsuccessful ovulation. Asynchrony between oestrogen and luteinising hormone levels and follicular rupture has been documented,[54] and some patients appear to undergo premature rupture of follicles.[55] Failure to detect follicular collapse but with infilling of the follicle suggests luteinisation without ovulation. The luteinised unruptured follicle (LUF) syndrome occurs more often in infertile than fertile patients and may be a cause of unexplained infertility.[56] The absence of an ovulatory stigma in such patients has been confirmed laparoscopically,[57] but the ultrasonic diagnosis was found to have a 15% false-positive rate. The LUF syndrome may be more common with endometriosis. Great care should be taken in diagnosing this syndrome, as ovulation may be associated with an increase in the size of apparent 'follicles' and these cystic corpora lutea may even indicate a conception cycle.[58]

Ovarian hyperstimulation syndrome

The ovarian hyperstimulation syndrome is potentially the most serious complication of ovulation induction with gonadotrophins. The syndrome occurs after hCG administration to patients with a large number of follicles and high serum oestradiol levels, and is particularly likely to occur in those with a polycystic ovarian morphology. HCG administration is less likely to be followed by clinically significant hyperstimulation syndrome if the follicles are subsequently aspirated at egg collection, probably because a substantial proportion of the oestrogen-secreting granulosa cells are removed with the follicular fluid. In principle, if the ovarian response is monitored with oestrogens or ultrasound, and cycles causing concern abandoned before hCG administration, hyperstimulation is avoidable. In practice, however, even in the most careful

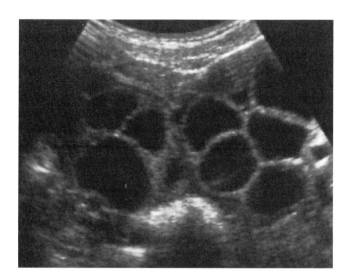

Fig. 4.16 Ovarian hyperstimulation. There is bilateral ovarian enlargement with multiple follicles.

hands, cases occur, particularly following superovulation therapy prior to assisted conception techniques. The syndrome may be divided into mild, moderate and severe depending on the degree of ovarian enlargement, symptoms and signs.

Mild hyperstimulation (lower abdominal discomfort, ovaries enlarged up to 5 × 5 cm) occurs in most patients who successfully superovulate prior to egg collection. Such patients may be observed and managed symptomatically. They do not require admission to hospital.

Patients with more serious hyperstimulation may be divided on ultrasound criteria into moderate (ovaries measuring more than 5 × 5 cm) (Fig. 4.16) and severe (ovaries measuring more more than 12 × 12 cm).[59] The clinical features that cause concern are nausea, vomiting, ascites, and pleural and pericardial effusions. These all compound to worsen the haemoconcentration, causing hyperviscosity and hypercoaguability which predispose to thrombosis, embolism and renal failure. Gross ascites may aggravate the discomfort, nausea and vomiting. Previously paracentesis was prescribed[59] because of the risk of damage to the fragile luteal cysts but, when performed under ultrasound control,[60] it has been found to be a safe and useful procedure.

Uterine ultrasound

Identification

The uterus is usually easily identifiable in the midline, its uniformly reflective myometrium contrasting with the varying reflectivity of the adjacent bowel. The opposing surfaces of the endometrium produce a characteristic midline echo, usually of high reflectivity. In patients with the pelvic anatomy distorted by an adnexal mass or fibroids it may be helpful to identify the external os and follow the endometrial cavity to the fundus. There is no relationship between uterine position (anteversion or retroversion) and infertility.

Congenital abnormalities

Trans-vaginal ultrasonography can be used to identify congenital uterine malformations,[61] the most common of which is the partially septate uterus, which is a leading cause of repeated first-trimester miscarriage.[62] However, major malformations such as uterus didelphys (Fig. 4.17) are not usually associated with infertility.[63] Visualisation of uterine malformations can be improved by filling the uterine cavity with saline.[64]

Cervix

Mucus retention cysts are commonly seen within the substance of the cervix (Fig. 4.18) (see Ch. 3). During the peri-ovulatory period a column of mucus may be seen extending from the external os to the uterine cavity.

Myometrium

Changes during the menstrual cycle

The uterus enlarges in response to the rising oestradiol levels during the follicular phase of the cycle.[65]

Rhythmic contractions of the subendometrial myometrium causing fluid within the uterine cavity to move may be observed with the trans-vaginal probe (Fig. 4.19). The amplitude and frequency of these contractions peak during the peri-ovulatory period.[66]

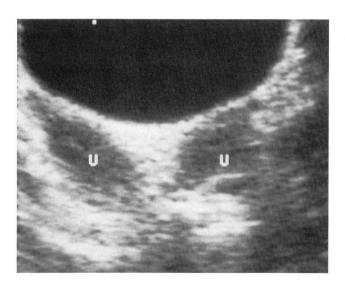

Fig. 4.17 Transabdominal scan of uterus didelphys; the separate uteri (U) may be seen.

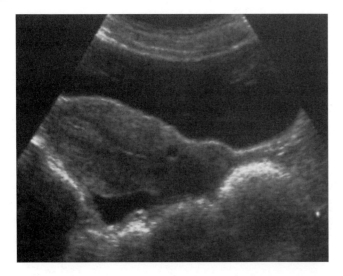

Fig. 4.18 Nabothian cyst. Endocervical mucus retention cyst. Note a little fluid in the pouch of Douglas.

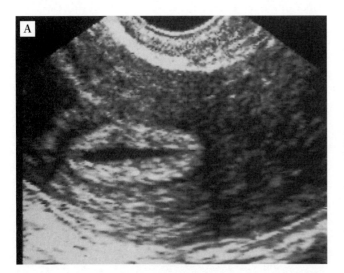
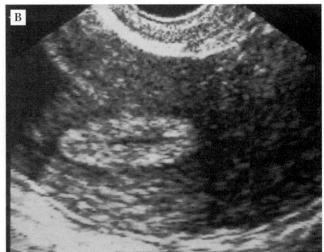

Fig. 4.19 Subendometrial contractions (every 18 seconds) moving fluid in endometrial cavity; 1 day post-ovulation in conception cycle.

Leiomyoma

Fibroids may be identified by their disruption of either the uniform myometrial reflectivity or the smooth uterine outline (Fig. 4.20). They often contain highly reflective regions which may cast acoustic shadows. Large fibroids are best seen with transabdominal ultrasound, as they often extend beyond the effective range of the trans-vaginal probe. The relationship of fibroids to the uterine cavity may be examined closely with trans-vaginal ultrasound. The effect of fibroids on fertility probably depends on their site: large fibroids may anatomically disturb oocyte pick-up by the fimbrial end of the tube, whereas those near the cornua may obstruct the fallopian tube. Submucous fibroids may interfere with implantation, particularly if they are pedunculated.

Endometrium

Changes during the menstrual cycle

During the menses the endometrium may be identified as a narrow strip of variable reflectivity on either side of the midline echo (Fig. 4.21).

The endometrium thickens as the serum oestrogen level rises. It is initially seen as a poorly reflective zone on either side of the midline echo (Fig. 4.22). Its outer margin, where it meets the myometrium, is defined by a band of increased reflectivity. Immediately outside this band is a 'halo' of reduced reflectivity thought to represent the inner layers of compact and vascular myometrium.[67] The reflectivity of the endometrium increases so that by mid-cycle it is iso-echoic with the myometrium (Fig. 4.23), but by the mid-

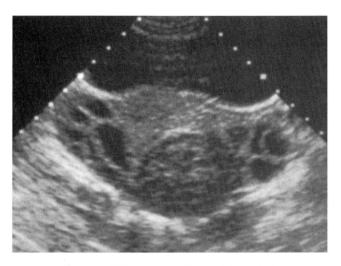

Fig. 4.20 Posterior wall fibroid seen with transabdominal ultrasound. The ovaries have been superovulated. (Figure courtesy of Ms V Sharma, St James' Hospital, Leeds.)

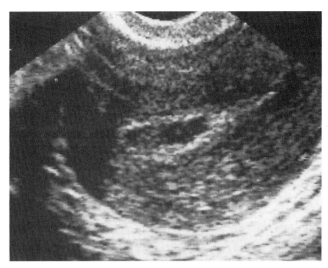

Fig. 4.21 Day 2 of menses; blood in endometrial cavity, thin endometrium.

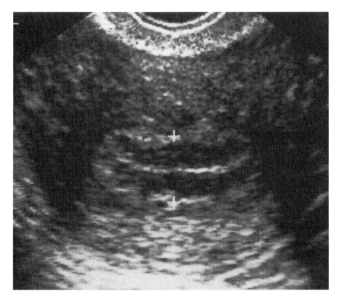

Fig. 4.22 Poorly reflective mid-follicular endometrium.

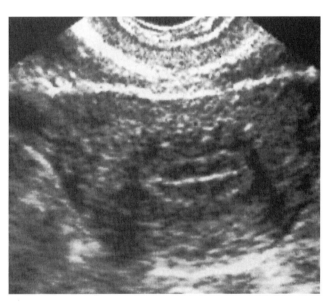

Fig. 4.23 Isoechoic late follicular endometrium.

luteal phase it is more reflective (Fig. 4.24).[68] Enlargement and tortuosity of the glands, along with an increase in glycogen and mucus content, are presumed to cause the increasing reflectivity.

The endometrial thickness increases through to the mid-luteal phase, then reaches a plateau before falling prior to the next menses.[69] If conception occurs the thickness increases further.

Endometrial indices and fertility

Endometrial growth in a stimulated cycle is very similar to that in the normal cycle, in spite of much higher oestrogen levels suggesting that the uterine response in the natural cycle is virtually maximal. There is a tendency for the endometrium to be thinner when clomiphene is used.[69,70] A positive correlation between endometrial thickness in the follicular phase and subsequent conception has been reported.[71,72] but the majority of authors have failed to confirm such a relationship.[67,69,73,74] Endometrial reflectivity may be used as a guide to variations in the end-organ response to oestrogen, thus allowing earlier administration of hCG than adherence to a fixed minimum mean follicular diameter would allow.[75]

Both in the late follicular phase and after egg collection in superovulated IVF cycles an endometrium of low

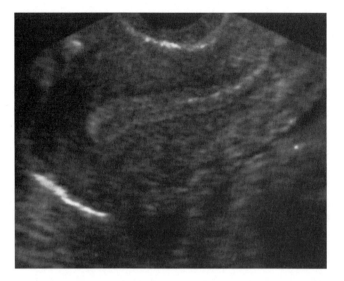

Fig. 4.24 Moderately reflective mid-luteal endometrium.

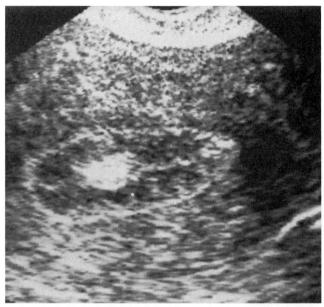

Fig. 4.25 Polyp. Small, clearly defined highly reflective ellipsoid polyp within the upper endometrial cavity.

reflectivity is associated with higher pregnancy rates than when the endometrium is more reflective.[74,76] This ultrasonic 'advancement' may be indicative of premature luteinisation, which would be expected to have an adverse effect on the cycle outcome.

Suboptimal levels of mid-luteal serum progesterone correlated with an endometrial thickness below 10 mm.[77] An attempt has been made to use endometrial thickness in the luteal phase to predict conception. A minimum thickness 11 days after hCG has been defined, but increased growth does not occur early enough to be useful.[73] In practice, assessment of the endometrium is of little use in the management of the infertile couple.

Adhesions

Intra-uterine adhesions may form following surgical trauma or infection. If these occur in the cervical canal or lower uterine segment, amenorrhoea will ensue (Asherman's syndrome) and a haematometra may be demonstrable. It may be possible to relieve the obstruction with a uterine sound under ultrasound guidance.[78]

Benign polyps

Endometrial polyps may be identified by ultrasound. Their relevance to fertility is unknown. The ultrasound appearances are variable, and range from apparent endometrial thickening to clearly defined lesions which may be either poorly or highly reflective (Fig. 4.25).

Endometrial ossification

The aetiology of this rare condition is unknown. Pieces of cartilage or bone are found at hysteroscopy or dilatation and curettage. They may act like an intra-uterine contraceptive device and inhibit implantation.[79] The highly reflective bone has a striking appearance (Fig. 4.26).

Intra-uterine contraceptive device

Very occasionally, examination of the uterine cavity reveals an intra-uterine contraceptive device, the removal

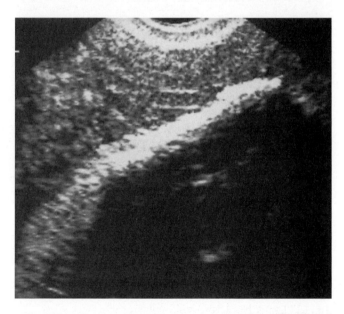

Fig. 4.26 Endometrial ossification – intensely reflective endometrium with acoustic shadow.

of which should rapidly resolve the patient's infertility problem!

Uterine artery blood flow

Trans-vaginal colour Doppler allows the ascending branch of the uterine artery to be identified and insonated at an optimal angle to obtain a spectral tracing. Changes in the uterine blood supply during the menstrual cycles of normal women,[80] subfertile women and in stimulated cycles have been investigated using this technique. Normally the rise in oestrogens in the follicular phase is associated with decreasing uterine artery impedance (Figs 4.27 and 4.28). At mid-cycle there is a transitory rise in resistance, followed by a further fall to the lowest value 7 days after ovulation. Prior to menstruation the impedance rises as the ovarian hormone levels fall.

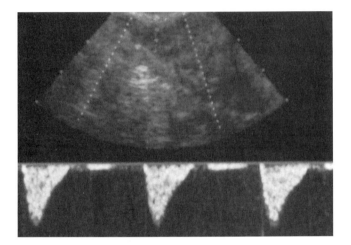

Fig. 4.27 Uterine blood flow – early follicular phase. No end-diastolic flow.

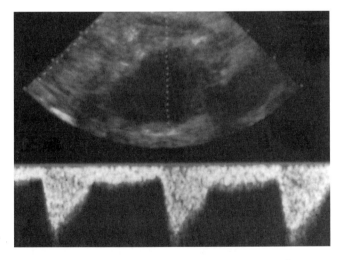

Fig. 4.28 Uterine blood flow – mid-luteal phase. Continuous flow through systole and diastole. (Figure courtesy of R. Schlief, Clinical Research Diagnostics, Schering AG, PO Box 65 03, 11, Berlin.)

Patients with a high uterine artery impedance immediately prior to embryo transfer during treatment with *in vitro* fertilisation, fail to conceive.[81] Attempts to improve results with oestrogen therapy and by cryopreserving the embryos for replacement in an artificial cycle have met with some success.[82,83]

Tubal ultrasound

The normal tube

The fallopian tube is not usually seen with ultrasound, though it is sometimes possible to visualise the reflective fimbrial end within fluid in the pouch of Douglas.[84] Fimbrial cysts are commonly seen as echo-free structures separate from the ovary.

The abnormal tube and pelvic inflammatory disease

Blockage of the fallopian tube with fluid accumulation (hydrosalpinx) may be demonstrated with ultrasound. Typically the distended tube is coiled around the ovary and the folds produce septa which do not completely cross the lumen (see Fig. 4.8). Conception rates following salpingostomy are less than 25% if the hydrosalpinx has a thick wall or a diameter greater than 15 mm.[85] Other damage from pelvic infection may be detectable with ultrasound. A tubo-ovarian abscess may be differentiated from an ovarian cyst by its thick wall and reflective contents. Pelvic adhesions may be seen as loculated fluid collections.

Tubal patency testing

Tubal patency is usually assessed either by hysterosalpingography or at laparoscopy. Following injection of saline through the cervix, ultrasound may be used to detect fluid in the pouch of Douglas.[64] It is as sensitive as hysterosalpingography at demonstrating the patency of at least one tube, but is less good at establishing the side that is patent. An ultrasound contrast medium (Echovist: Schering, Berlin) consisting of a suspension of galactose monosaccharide microparticles in an aqueous (20%) solution has been used to assess tubal patency (see Vol., Ch. 5). Unfortunately this technique overestimates the incidence of tubal blockage.[86] Ultrasound is unlikely to replace conventional techniques for the assessment of tubal patency.

Ultrasound-directed procedures

Introduction

Transabdominal oocyte harvesting was the first ultrasound-directed procedure used in the treatment of infertility.[87]

Since that time ultrasound has played an increasingly important role in the treatment of infertility.

Follicle aspiration

Historical review

In the first successful *in vitro* fertilisation attempts oocytes were collected during laparoscopy. This is an expensive procedure, requiring inpatient care and general anaesthesia; it fails when there are peri-ovarian adhesions and it has a significant serious complication rate,[88] including haemorrhage and infection. Demand for *in vitro* fertilisation and other assisted conception techniques requiring egg collection has increased as results have improved. Cost considerations have provided pressure to simplify the procedures. Ultrasound-directed follicle aspiration (UDFA) has reduced costs considerably because egg collection becomes an outpatient technique that requires minimal analgesia.

UDFA was initially guided by transabdominal ultrasound developed from experience with ultrasound-directed amniocentesis.[89] The ovary was approached either through the full bladder (transabdominal, through the bladder),[90] or directly, through the anterior abdominal wall (direct transabdominal). Subsequently trans-vaginal,[91] trans-vaginal/trans-vesical[92] and per-urethral approaches were developed.[93] However, these techniques, despite being as effective as laparoscopy,[94] were not easy to learn and so were not widely adopted. Oocyte collection using a trans-vaginal ultrasound transducer, first described by Wikland in 1985,[95] has become the technique of choice. Table 4.1 shows how the preferred route for egg collection at King's College Hospital has moved from transabdominal trans-vesical in 1983/84 to per-urethral in 1985/86, and finally to trans-vaginal with the trans-vaginal probe since 1987.

Patient preparation and analgesia

Most patients require some form of analgesia, such as pethidine, and a tranquilliser such as diazepam; the risk of vomiting necessitates starving for 6 hours and careful titration of the drugs against the patient's level of consciousness, and an oxygen supply should respiratory support become necessary. A benzodiazepine tranquilliser may be used as premedication pre-operatively to reduce anxiety. UDFA may be performed with no analgesia if there are few follicles or if the patient is particularly stoical, and some patients may find hypnotherapy adequate. Good rapport between patient and operator is crucial: excessive intravenous sedation may make the patient confused and uncooperative.

A paracervical block with lignocaine may be used prior to trans-vaginal egg collection: although this local anaesthetic is a known parthenogenetic activator and appears in the follicular fluid, it has not been found to have an adverse effect on oocyte quality.[96] Epidural anaesthesia renders the patient pain-free but the subsequent recovery time precludes its routine use.

Vaginal route

The patient is placed in the lithotomy position; preparation varies from simply cleansing the vagina with saline and culture medium[96] to preparation with povidone-iodine on both the day before and that of the procedure.[97] Antibiotics, both oral and intravenous, have been used.[98]

The trans-vaginal transducer is covered with a sterile spermicide-free condom. A biopsy guide is attached and the assembly is inserted into the vagina. The end of the transducer rests in the lateral fornix of the vagina on the side of the ovary to be punctured (Fig. 4.29). The follicles are identified and the electronic biopsy guides lined up with a follicle in the middle of the ovary. The distance

Table 4.1 Ultrasound-directed follicle aspiration. King's College Hospital, London, 1983–1990

Year	TA/TV	PU/TV	Direct TA	TV (abd. probe)	TV (vag. probe)	Mixed routes	Total
1983	45						45
1984	145	6		6			157
1985	48	188	1	1		55	293
1986	2	291	2	0	60	30	385
1987	0	57	0	0	338	23	418
1988	1	14	0	0	515	9	539
1989	4	4	0	0	648	3	659
1990	0	0	0	0	813	5	818
Total	245	560	3	7	2374	125	3314

TA/TV – transabdominal trans-vesical
TA – transabdominal
PU/TV – per-urethral trans-vesical
TV – trans-vaginal

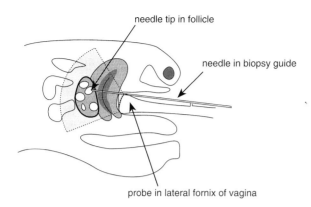

needle tip in follicle

needle in biopsy guide

probe in lateral fornix of vagina

Fig. 4.29 Diagram of trans-vaginal ultrasound-directed follicle aspiration.

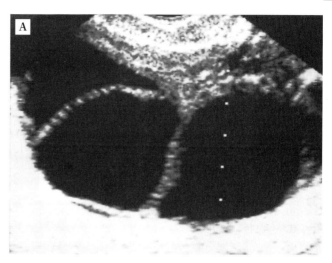

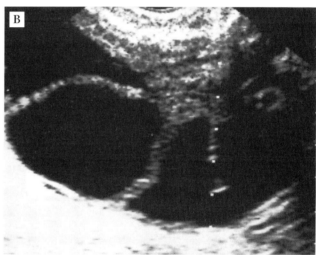

Fig. 4.30 Ultrasound-guided oocyte recovery. **A:** Ovary before and **B:** after needle passed into follicle under trans-vaginal ultrasound guidance.

from the end of the probe to the centre of the follicle is measured and, after warning the patient to expect a sharp stabbing sensation, the needle is passed rapidly into the ovary (Fig. 4.30). A single-channel needle is preferred,[99] although a double-channel needle that allows aspiration and flushing through separate channels has been used,[100] but this is slower and no more productive.

The follicular fluid is aspirated by applying suction from a pump at approximately 100 mmHg. It is important to ensure that the follicle is entirely empty before realigning the needle or moving on to the next follicle. It is usually possible to empty all the follicles in each ovary with one puncture on each side.

Alternative routes

Occasionally some or all the follicles are not accessible by the trans-vaginal approach. If an ovary is fixed on the posterior aspect of the uterus the operator has a choice between needling the follicles through the myometrium (Fig. 4.31) (avoiding the endometrium[101]) or filling the bladder and reaching them over the fundus of the uterus (Fig. 4.32; needle A). If an ovary is out of the range of the trans-vaginal transducer and does not descend with pressure on the lower abdominal wall, it may be approached using the direct transabdominal route (Fig. 4.32; needle B) or the per-urethral route (Fig. 4.32; needle C).

Transabdominal trans-vesical follicle aspiration. The patient is placed in the lithotomy position and a 12 Fr Foley catheter inserted. Throughout the procedure the bladder volume is adjusted with Hartmann's solution to optimise viewing of the follicles to be aspirated, with as little discomfort to the patient as possible.

After anaesthetising a small area of the skin on the anterior abdominal wall with 10 ml 1% lignocaine, a needle is passed under freehand ultrasound guidance into the bladder. The needle is then manipulated within the bladder to a suitable angle (Fig. 4.33) before passing it

through the posterior bladder wall into the ovary. It is often possible to aspirate all the follicles in each ovary through a single posterior bladder wall puncture, but withdrawal into the bladder and realignment may be necessary. The contralateral ovary is approached through a second anterior abdominal wall puncture.

Direct transabdominal follicle aspiration. The patient is placed supine: a full bladder may help by steadying the ovary but it is not always necessary. An ultrasound transducer with a short focal length and high frequency, such as a trans-vaginal probe, gives good images of the ovaries (see Fig. 4.3).

After anaesthetising the skin and abdominal wall a needle is passed directly into a target follicle either freehand or using a biopsy guide.

Withdrawal of the needle to the ovarian surface enables the operator to realign the needle for subsequent follicles.

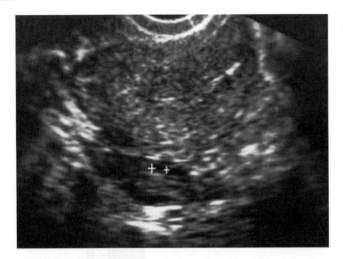

Fig. 4.31 Posteriorly sited ovary. Oocyte recovery from an ovary in this position is not practicable via the trans-vaginal route.

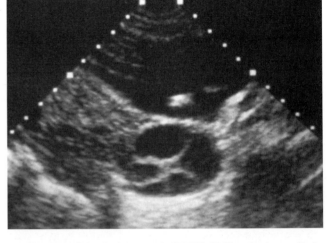

Fig. 4.33 Transabdominal trans-vesical UDFA; highly reflective needle tip seen immediately prior to posterior bladder wall and follicle puncture.

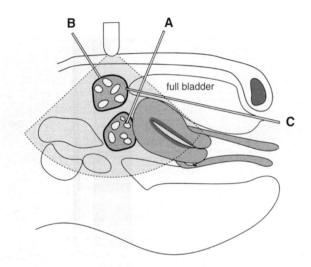

Fig. 4.32 Alternative routes for ultrasound-directed follicle aspiration.

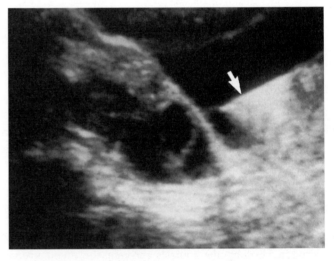

Fig. 4.34 Per-urethral UDFA; needle (arrow) poised to puncture posterior bladder wall and enter follicle. The entire length of the needle is visible.

This procedure is more difficult than either of the other techniques, particularly if the anterior abdominal wall is thick.

Per-urethral route. The patient is placed in the lithotomy position. A needle is introduced into the bladder with the tip sheathed in the side hole of a Foley catheter (14 Fr). Under transabdominal ultrasound control the bladder is filled with Hartmann's solution until the follicles are clearly seen. The needle is disengaged from the catheter and the follicles aspirated in a similar manner to that described for the transabdominal trans-vesical technique. As the needle is nearly at right-angles to the transducer, its entire length should be seen (Fig. 4.34).

Results

In 1990 in King's College Hospital, London a total of 818 cases of UDFA were performed, with a mean of 17 follicles aspirated (range 1–54). Each procedure took 35 minutes on average and 10 eggs were collected (range 1–37). During 1990 the follicles were aspirated and then routinely flushed. At the beginning of 1991 a policy of aspiration only was adopted, unless there were fewer than five follicles available, in which case we flushed as often as was necessary.

From 1 March to 28 May 1991 a total of 160 aspirations were performed with a mean of 18 follicles (range 3–55). The time for each procedure was shortened to

22 minutes (range 5–60), and on average 12 eggs were collected (range 1–36). The very significant reduction in procedure time with no reduction in the number of eggs collected per follicle is striking.

In 1990 it was necessary to resort to an alternative route in five cases. In one case an ovary was inaccessible on the posterior aspect of the uterus. In four cases an ovary was too high to be approached trans-vaginally.

Complications

All patients feel some pain as the needle is initially placed in the ovary. The amount of discomfort felt as the needle is moved within the ovary is variable, and much depends on the patient's personality and the theatre staff's ability to promote a relaxed atmosphere. The commonest complaint is of occasional sharp pain. Some patients feel virtually no pain, whereas a few find it very uncomfortable indeed.

Removal of the needle at the end of a trans-vaginal ultrasound-directed follicle aspiration procedure may be followed by haemorrhage. Inspection of the puncture site will reveal a spurting blood vessel, which invariably responds to direct pressure. One patient collapsed 18 hours after follicle harvest: laparotomy revealed significant bleeding from a large number of ruptured follicles without specific vascular damage.

It is common for the patient to complain of lower abdominal pain for a few days after the procedure. It may be difficult to determine whether this is due to a small intraperitoneal bleed, to infection, or to the hyperstimulation syndrome. Six cases of severe pelvic infection following trans-vaginal UDFA occurred in our series, but there were none when the transabdominal or per-urethral routes were used. In several of these cases large abscesses developed insidiously over a number of weeks.

Pelvic infections have occurred even after the administration of prophylactic antibiotics.[98] During UDFA using the transabdominal or per-urethral technique, if the bladder pressure becomes too high urine may extravasate into the tissues (Fig. 4.35). Postoperative clot retention (Fig. 4.36) or urinary tract infection may occur.

It is important that patients are warned of these complications before the procedure to ensure that significant symptoms are reported immediately.

Ultrasound-directed embryo transfer

Cervical embryo transfer

Routine blind trans-cervical transfer of embryos to the uterine cavity is followed by implantation in approximately 10% of procedures.[102] Many factors may explain this poor implantation rate, but mechanical failure may be contributory.

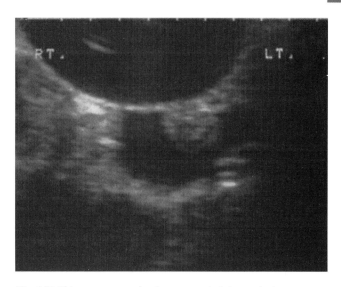

Fig. 4.35 **Urinary extravasation** into paravesical tissues during transabdominal trans-vesical UDFA.

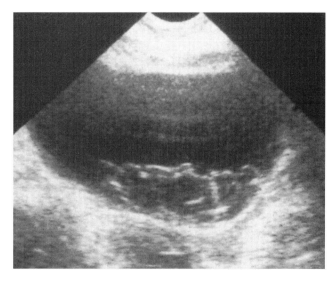

Fig. 4.36 **Blood clot within the bladder.** Clot causing retention after transabdominal trans-vesical UDFA.

Ultrasound may be used to measure the distance from the external os to the fundus before blind transfer to ensure that the embryos are placed in the uterine cavity rather than the cervical canal. This is particularly useful when the uterus is enlarged with fibroids. The most appropriate place to deposit embryos within the uterine cavity is not known. Embryo transfer may be observed ultrasonically, but in practice the catheters are not seen easily without moving them back and forth, which risks damage to the endometrium (Fig. 4.37). The only randomised controlled study comparing blind with ultrasound-guided embryo transfer failed to show a significant difference in pregnancy rate between the two groups.[103]

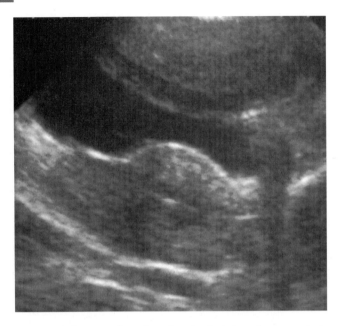

Fig. 4.37 Embryo transfer catheter. Longitudinal view of uterus pushed into an axial position by a full bladder. The embryo transfer catheter in the endometrial cavity is seen only with difficulty.

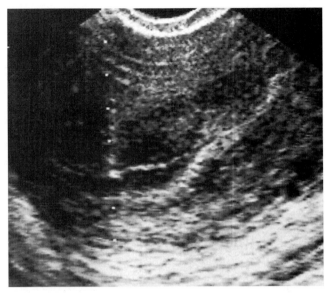

Fig. 4.38 Surgical embryo transfer; the needle may be seen passing through the myometrium, its tip in the endometrial cavity, the anterior and posterior surfaces of which are separated by injected fluid.

Some patients have a tortuous cervical canal which can only be negotiated under ultrasound control. Patients with a history of a difficult embryo transfer may benefit from a trial transfer between treatment cycles, during which ultrasound is used to assess the best way to manipulate the transfer catheter. The bladder volume may have a significant effect on the ease with which the catheter passes by altering the degree of uterine flexion.

Surgical embryo transfer

Very occasionally, when the cervix is severely stenosed or tortuous and both fallopian tubes are blocked, the only way to transfer embryos is surgically[104] through the myometrium.

The patient is placed in the lithotomy position, the vagina cleansed and a vaginal probe, mounted with a biopsy guide, inserted. The electronic guide line on the monitor is carefully lined up with the endometrial cavity just below the fundus. A 25 cm 19 gauge needle primed with culture medium is passed through the biopsy guide then, with a quick thrust, into the uterus. When the needle is correctly sited, injected culture medium will be seen transiently separating the reflective anterior and posterior surfaces of the endometrial cavity (Fig. 4.38). A long embryo transfer catheter with the embryos at its tip is then passed down the needle into the endometrial cavity. The embryos are injected and the catheter and needle withdrawn. Surgical embryo transfer may lead to pregnancy in up to 70% of cases in animals, but the success rate is very low in humans.

Direct intraperitoneal insemination (DIPI)

When this relatively simple assisted conception technique was introduced in 1986[105] it was hoped that it would prove to be an effective, low-cost treatment for patients with patent fallopian tubes. It has been used to treat couples with unexplained infertility, cervical mucus hostility, oligospermia, failed donor insemination, and women who have ovulated prior to egg collection.[106] The patient is gently superovulated with clomiphene and hMG or LHRH analogue and hMG. Care is taken to avoid stimulating the development of more than three follicles greater than 14 mm. If more do develop the cycle may either be abandoned or the follicles aspirated and the patient treated with either GIFT, peritoneal oocyte sperm transfer, or IVF and embryo transfer.

The procedure is performed 36 hours after administration of hCG. The patient is placed in the lithotomy position with a head-up tilt so that the peritoneal fluid gravitates to the pouch of Douglas. The vagina is cleansed with an antiseptic solution and a vaginal probe with a biopsy guide attached inserted. A pool of peritoneal fluid is identified (Fig. 4.39). After warning the patient that she will feel a sharp pain, a 19 gauge needle is passed along the guide and into the pool with a single rapid movement. Aspiration of peritoneal fluid confirms that the needle tip is correctly sited before the injection of a prepared sperm sample. The pregnancy rate after peritoneal implantation is 10%[107] or less.[108] This is better than after superovulation alone, but not better than after controlled superovulation and the intra-uterine insemination of prepared sperm[108] which probably achieves intraperitoneal insemination

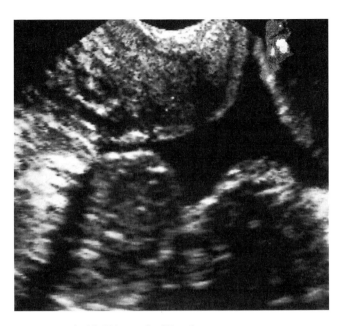

Fig. 4.39 Pool of fluid in pouch of Douglas.

without the need for a surgical procedure. DIPI is unlikely to find a role in the routine treatment of infertility.

Peritoneal oocyte sperm transfer (POST)

The establishment of ultrasound-directed follicle aspiration for oocyte collection removed the need for laparoscopy during treatment with IVF and embryo transfer. To units promoting the use of ultrasound techniques the introduction of GIFT in 1984 seemed like a retrograde step as it requires tubal catheterisation under laparoscopic control.

Reasoning that most patients with unexplained infertility will have gamete abnormalities rather than a problem with ovum pick-up by the fallopian tube, Mason and colleagues[109] placed both sperm and oocytes in the pouch of Douglas in the hope that they would achieve results comparable to GIFT.

The patients are first superovulated as if for *in vitro* fertilisation, with a view to collecting a minimum of three oocytes. Initially the follicles were aspirated by the trans-abdominal trans-vaginal route, but more recently the trans-vaginal approach has been used.[110] When all the follicles have been emptied, the needle is introduced under ultrasound guidance into the pouch of Douglas, which is repeatedly rinsed with culture medium until the aspirated fluid is clear. A long embryo transfer catheter, loaded with three eggs and 4 000 000 prepared sperm, is then passed down the needle and its contents injected into the pouch of Douglas.

Sharma *et al*[110] have reported a pregnancy rate of 24% for each procedure. This technique is simpler to perform than either GIFT or IVF and embryo transfer. It has two advantages over DIPI: first, egg release from the follicle is guaranteed; secondly, spare eggs not transferred may be inseminated to confirm the fertilising capability of the gametes.

This is an underrated procedure and its role has yet to be fully evaluated.

Transuterine intrafallopian transfer (TIFT)

Fertilisation and early embryo development to the morula stage normally occur in the fallopian tube. *In vitro* fertilisation is performed in culture medium, designed for rodents, in the artificial environment of the laboratory. The resultant embryos are transferred to the uterus at the two to six cell stage. The culture conditions may not be optimal and the uterine environment may not suit the embryo at this early stage of development. There are therefore good reasons to believe that results will be improved by the transfer of either gametes or embryos to the fallopian tube.

This hypothesis is supported by the higher implantation rates achieved after zygote intrafallopian transfer and tubal embryo stage transfer, compared to IVF and ET[111] and the good results achieved with zygote transfer.[112]

No prospective randomised trial to compare intrafallopian transfer techniques with conventional methods has been performed, so the relative success rates are not known. Intrafallopian tube methods require general anaesthesia and laparoscopy with their associated risks. The transuterine technique is being developed to overcome these major disadvantages. The technique was first used to transfer sperm,[113] but has since been used to transfer egg and sperm together,[114] zygotes[115] and cleavage-stage embryos.[116]

The transfer device most commonly used was developed in Australia (William Cook; Jansen Anderson Intratubal Transfer Set). It consists of a flexible Teflon 5.5 Fr outer cannula with a lateral curve designed to fit into the uterine angles, a metal obturator and a soft 3 Fr Teflon inner cannula which tapers to 2 Fr at its distal 5 cm.

The patient is placed in the lithotomy position and the cervix cleansed with antiseptic solution. The metal obturator is bent to the shape of the uterine cavity and placed inside the 5.5 Fr cannula, overriding its lateral curve. The two are then inserted into the uterus. A recent design change has been the addition of an olive tip to the end of the outer cannula, which allows it to be slid more smoothly into position.

The obturator is then removed, allowing the outer cannula's memory to carry the cannula tip into one or other of the uterine angles. The inner 3 Fr cannula, containing the sperm, eggs or embryos, is then passed through the outer cannula. The position of the cannulae may be confirmed with either trans-vaginal[113] or abdominal ultrasound.[115] Using a combination of operator 'feel' and ultrasound the cornual orifice is found and the tube catheterised. When this is successful the patient typically complains of lateralised discomfort. The flow of fluid as the contents of the inner cannula are injected may be seen on ultrasound.

Seven of 28 patients having eggs and sperm transferred and 18 of 76 having zygotes transferred conceived using this technique in Sydney, Australia, between 1989 and 1990.[116] Transuterine intrafallopian transfer certainly has the potential to replace laparoscopic techniques, but ultrasonic screening may prove unnecessary as operator skills and confidence improve. (Jansen 1991, personal communication).

Conclusion

The modern investigation of infertility would be incomplete without pelvic ultrasound. A very significant proportion of patients requiring treatment for infertility will need monitoring with ultrasound or an ultrasound-guided procedure, or both.

Colour flow Doppler equipment is generating more information on reproductive events during health and disease, from which we can expect the development of improved methods of treatment for infertile women.

REFERENCES

1   von Micsky L I. Ultrasonic tomography in obstetrics and gynaecology. In: Grossman C C, Holmer J H, Joyner C, Purnell E, eds. Diagnostic ultrasound. New York: Plenum Press, 1966; 348–368

2   Kratochwil A, Urban G, Friedrich F. Ultrasonic tomography of the ovaries. Ann Chir Gynae Fenniae 1972; 61: 211–214

3   Hackelöer B J, Hansmann M. Ultraschalldiagnostik in der fruhschwangerschaft. Gynäkologe 1976; 9: 108–122

4   Hackelöer B J, Nitschte S, Daume E, Sturm G, Buchholz R. Ultraschalldarstellung von ovarveranderungen bei gonadotropinstimulierung. Geburtsh u Frauenhheilk 1977; 37: 185–190

5   Sample W F, Lippe B M, Gyepes M T. Grey-scale ultrasonography of the normal female pelvis. Radiology 1977; 125: 477–483

6   Hackelöer B J, Robinson H P. Ultraschalldarstellung des wachsenden follikels und corpus luteum in normalen physiologisschen zyklus. Geburtsh u Frauenheilk 1978; 38: 163–168

7   Macler J, Jacquetin B, Ehret C, Dervain I, Plas-Roger S, Aron R, Renaud C. La surveillance échographique de l'induction de l'ovulation. J Gynecol Obstet Biol Reprod 1978; 7: 746–748

8   Robertson R D, Picker R H, Wilson P C, Saunders D M. Assessment of ovulation by ultrasound and plasma estradiol determinations. Obstet Gynecol 1979; 54: 686–691

9   Hackelöer B J, Fleming R, Robinson H P, Adam D H, Coutts J R T. Correlation of ultrasonic and endocrinologic assessment of human follicular development. Am J Obstet Gynecol 1979; 135: 122–128.

10 Queenan J T, O'Brien G D, Bains L M, Simpson J, Collins W P, Campbell S. Ultrasound scanning of ovaries to detect ovulation in women. Fertil Steril 1980; 34: 99–105

11 Morimoto N, Noda Y, Takai I, Yamada I, Tojo S. Ultrasonographic observation of ovarian follicular development via vaginal route. Acta Obstet Gynaecol Jpn 1983; 35: 151–158

12 Williams S R, Rothchild I, Wesolowski D, Austin C, Speroff L. Does exposure of preovulatory oocytes to ultrasonic radiation affect reproductive performance. In Vitro Fertil Embryo Transfer 1988; 5(1): 18–21

13 Polson D W, Wadsworth J, Adams J, Franks S. Polycystic ovaries – a common finding in normal women. Lancet 1988; i: 870–872

14 Adams J, Polson D W, Franks S. Prevalence of polycystic ovaries in women with anovulation and idiopathic ligutism. BMJ 1986; 293: 355–359

15 Homburg R, Armar N A, Eshel A, Adams J, Jacobs H S. Influence of serum luteinizing hormone concentrations on ovulation, conception and early pregnancy loss in polycystic ovary syndrome. BMJ 1988; 297: 1024–1026

16 Eshel A, Abdulwahid N A, Armar N A, Adams J M, Jacobs H S. Pusatile luteinizing hormone-releasing hormone therapy in women with polycystic ovary syndrome. Fertil Steril 1988; 49: 956–960

17 Adams J, Polson D W, Abdulwahid N et al. Multifollicular ovaries: clinical and endocrine features and response to pulsatile gonadotrophin releasing hormone. Lancet 1985; ii: 1375–1379

18 Editorial. Follicular multiplicity. Lancet 1985; ii: 1404

19 Granberg S, Wikland M. Ultrasound in the diagnosis and treatment of ovarian cystic tumours. Hum Reprod 1991; 6: 177–185

20 Hornstein M D, Barbieri R L, Ravnikar V A, McShane P M. The effects of baseline ovarian cysts on the clinical response to controlled ovarian hyperstimulation in an in vitro fertilisation program. Fertil Steril 1989; 52: 437–440

21 Thatcher S S, Jones E, Decherney A H. Ovarian cysts decrease the success of controlled ovarian stimulation and in vitro fertilization. Fertil Steril 1989; 52: 812–816

22 Rizk B, Tan S L, Kingsland C, Steer C, Mason B A, Campbell S. Ovarian cyst aspiration and the outcome of in vitro fertilisation. Fertil Steril 1990; 54: 661–664

23 Bourne T, Campbell S, Steer C, Whitehead M, Collins W. Transvaginal colour flow imaging: a possible new screening technique for ovarian cancer. BMJ 1989; 299: 1367–1370

24 Dlugi A M, Coy R A, Dieterle S, Bayer S R, Seibel M M. The effect of endometriomas on in vitro fertilisation outcome. In Vitro Fertil and Embryo Transfer 1989; 6: 338–341

25 Glasier A F, Baird D T, Hillier S G. FSH and the control of follicular growth. J Steroid Biochem 1989; 32: 167–170

26 Packe T D, Wladimiroff J W, DeJon F H, Hop W C, Fauser B C. Growth patterns of non-dominant ovarian follicles during the normal menstrual cycle. Fertil Steril 1990; 54: 638–642

27 O'Herlihy C, DeCrespigny L, Lopata A, Johnston I, Hoult I, Robinson H. Preovulatory follicular size: a comparison of ultrasound and laparoscopic measurements. Fertil Steril 1990; 34: 24–26

28 Marinho A O, Sallam H N, Goessens L K V, Collins W P, Rodeck C H, Campbell S. Real time pelvic ultrasonography during the periovulatory period of patients attending an artificial insemination clinic. Fertil Steril 1982; 37: 633–638

29 Hillier S G, Afrian A M M, Margara R A, Winston R M L. Superovulation strategy before in vitro fertilisation. Clin Obstet Gynecol 1985; 12: 687–723

30 Barash A, Shoham Z, Lunenfeld B, Segal I, Insler V, Borenstein R. Can premature luteinization in superovulation protocols be prevented by aspiration of an ill-timed leading follicle? Fertil Steril 1990; 53: 865–869

31 Pampiglione J S, Tan S L, Steer C V, Wren M, Parsons J H, Campbell S. Drainage of the dominant follicle in in-vitro fertilisation. Assisted Reproduction, Technology and Andrology 1991; 1: 76–80

32 Taylor K J W, Burns P N, Woodcock J P, Wells P N T. Blood flow in deep abdominal and pelvic vessels: ultrasonic pulsed Doppler analysis. Radiology 1985; 54: 487–493

33 Bourne T, Jurkovic D, Waterstone J, Campbell S, Collins W. Intrafollicular blood flow during human ovulation. Ultrasound Obstet Gynecol 1991; 1: 53–59

34 Dentinger J, Reinthaller A, Bernaschek G. Transvaginal pulsed Doppler measurement of blood flow velocity in the ovarian arteries during cycle stimulation and after follicle puncture. Fertil Steril 1989; 51: 466–470

35 Andreotti R F, Thompson G H, Janowitz W, Shapiro A, Zusmer N R. Endovaginal and transabdominal sonography of ovarian follicles. J Ultrasound Med 1989; 8: 555–560

36 Gonzalez C J, Curson R, Parsons J. Transabdominal versus transvaginal ultrasound scanning of ovarian follicles: are they comparable? Fertil Steril 1988; 50: 657–659

37 Eissa M K, Hudson K, Docker M F, Sawers R S, Newton J R. Ultrasound follicle diameter measurement: an assessment of inter observer and intra observer variation. Fertil Steril 1985; 44: 751–754

38 Yee B, Barnes R B, Vargyas J M, Marrs R P. Correlation of transabdominal and transvaginal ultrasound measurements of follicle size and number with laparoscopic findings for in vitro fertilisation. Fertil Steril 1987; 47: 828–832

39 Renaud R L, Macler J, Dervain I, et al. Echographic study of follicular maturation and ovulation during the normal menstrual cycle. Fertil Steril 1980; 33: 272–276

40 Leerentveld R A, Gent I, Stoep M, Wladimiroff J W. Ultrasonographic assessment of follicle growth under monofollicular and multifollicular conditions in clomiphene citrate-stimulated cycles. Fertil Steril 1985; 43: 565–569

41 Doody M C, Gibbons W E, Zamah N M. Linear regression analysis of ultrasound follicular growth series: statistical relationship of growth rate and calculated date of growth onset to total growth period. Fertil Steril 1987; 47: 436–440

42 Hackelöer B J, Sallam H N. Ultrasound scanning of ovarian follicles. Clin Obstet Gynecol 1983; 10: 603–620

43 Hillier S G, Parsons J H, Morgara R A, Winston R M L, Crofton M E. Serum oestradiol and preovulatory follicular development before in-vitro fertilisation. Endocrinology 1984; 101: 113–118

44 Smith D H, Picker R H, Sinosich M, Saunders D M. Assessment of ovulation by ultrasound and oestradiol levels during spontaneous and induced cycles. Fertil Steril 1980; 33: 387–390

45 Picker R H, Smith D H, Tucker M H, Saunders D M. Ultrasonic signs of imminent ovulation. JCU 1983; 11: 1–2

46 Kerin J F, Edmonds D K, Warners G M, et al. Morphological and functional relations of Graafian follicle growth to ovulation in women using ultrasonic, laparoscopic and biochemical measurements. Br J Obstet Gynaecol 1981; 88: 81–90

47 Marinho A O, Sallam H N, Goessens L, Collins W P, Campbell S. Ovulation side and occurrence of mittleschmerz in spontaneous and induced ovarian cycles. BMJ 1982; 284: 632

48 Depares J, Ryder R E J, Walker S M, Scanlon M F, Norman C M. Ovarian ultrasonography highlights precision of symptoms of ovulation as markers of ovulation. BMJ 1986; 292: 1562

49 O'Herlihy C, Robinson H P, Crespigny L J. Miteslchmerz is a preovulatory symptom. BMJ 1980; 986

50 Rutherford A J, Subak-Sharpe R J, Dawson K J, Margara R A, Frank S, Winston R M. Improvement of in vitro fertilisation after treatment with buserelin an agonist of luteinising hormone releasing hormone. BMJ 1988; 296: 1765–1768

51 Werlin L B, Weckstein L, Weathersbee P S, Parenicta K, White D, Stone S C. Ultrasound: a technique useful in determining the side of ovulation. Fertil Steril 1986; 46: 814–817

52 Scholtes M C W, Wladimiroff J W, Van Rijen H J M, Hop W C J. Uterine and ovarian flow velocity waveforms in the normal menstrual cycle: a transvaginal Doppler study. Fertil Steril 1989; 52: 981–985

53 Baber R J, McSweeney M B, Gill R W, et al. Transvaginal pulsed Doppler ultrasound assessment of blood flow to the corpus luteum in IVF patients following embryo transfer. Br J Obstet Gynaecol 1988; 95: 1226–1230

54 Polan M L, Totora M, Caldwell B V, Decherney A H, Haseltine F P, Kase N. Abnormal ovarian cycles as diagnosed by ultrasound and serum estrodiol levels. Fertil Steril 1982; 37: 342–347

55 Ying Y K, Daly D C, Randolph J F, et al. Ultrasonographic monitoring of follicular growth for luteal phase defects. Fertil Steril 1987; 48: 433–436

56 Bateman B G, Kolp L A, Nunley W C, Thomas T S, Mills S E. Oocyte retention after follicle luteinization. Fertil Steril 1990; 54: 793–798

57 Liukkonen S, Koskimies A I, Tenhunen A, Ylostalo P. Diagnosis of luteinized unruptured follicle (LUF) syndrome by ultrasound. Fertil Steril 1984; 41: 26–30

58 Hackelöer B J. Ultrasound scanning of the ovarian cycle. In Vitro Fertil Embryo Transfer 1984; 1: 217–220

59 Schenker J G, Weinstein D. Ovarian hyperstimulation syndrome: a current survey. Fertil Steril 1978; 30: 255–268

60 Borenstein R, Elhalah U, Lunenfeld B, Schwartz Z S. Severe ovarian hyperstimulation syndrome: a reevaluated therapeutic approach. Fertil Steril 1989; 51: 791–795

61 Nasri M N, Setchell M E, Chard T. Transvaginal ultrasound for diagnosis of uterine malformations. Br J Obstet Gynaecol 1990; 97: 1043–1045

62 Rrock J A, Schlaff W D. The obstetric consequences of uterovaginal anomalies. Fertil Steril 1985; 43: 681–692

63 Jones H W. Reproductive impairment and the malformed uterus. Fertil Steril 1981; 36: 137–148

64 Randolph J R, Ying Y K, Maier D B, Schmidt C L, Riddick D H. Comparison of real-time ultrasonography, hysterosalpingography and laparoscopy/hysteroscopy in the evaluation of uterine abnormalities and tubal patency. Fertil Steril 1986; 46: 828–832

65 Adams J M, Tan S L, Wheeler M J, Morris D V, Jacobs H S, Franks S. Uterine growth in the follicular phase of spontaneous ovulatory cycles and during luteinizing hormone-releasing hormone induced cycles in women with normal or polycystic ovaries. Fertil Steril 1988; 49: 52–55

66 Lyons E A, Taylor P J, Zheng X H, Ballard G, Levi C S, Kredenster J V. Characterisation of subendometrial myometrial contractions throughout the menstrual cycle in normal fertile women. Fertil Steril 1991; 55: 771–774

67 Fleischer A C, Herbert C M, Sacks G A, Wentz A C, Entiman S S, James A E. Sonography of the endometrium during conception and non-conception cycles of in vitro fertilisation and embryo transfer. Fertil Steril 1986; 46: 442–447

68 Randall J M, Fisk N M, McTavish A, Templeton A A. Transvaginal ultrasonic assessment of endometrial growth in spontaneous and hyperstimulated menstrual cycles. Br J Obstet Gynaecol 1989; 96: 954–959

69 Imoedemke D A G, Shaw R W, Kirkland A, Chan R. Ultrasound measurement of endometrial thickness on different ovarian stimulation regimens during in vitro fertilisation. Hum Reprod 1987; 2: 545–547

70 Leng S, Lindenberg S. Ultrasonic evaluation of endometrial growth in women with normal cycles during spontaneous and stimulated cycles. Hum Reprod 1990; 5: 377–381

71 Glissant A, Mouzon J, Frydman R. Ultrasound study of the endometrium during in vitro fertilisation cycles. Fertil Steril 1985; 44: 786–790

72 Gonen Y, Casper R, Jacobsen W, Blankier J. Endometrial thickness and growth during ovarian stimulation: a possible predictor of implantation in in vitro fertilisation. Fertil Steril 1989; 52: 446–450

73 Rabinowitz R, Laufer N, Lewin A et al. The value of ultrasonographic endometrial measurement in the prediction of pregnancy following in vitro fertilisation. Fertil Steril 1986; 45: 824–828

74 Walker B G, Gembruch U, Diedrich K, Al-Hasani S, Krebs D. Transvaginal sonography of the endometrium during ovum pick-up in stimulated cycles for in vitro fertilisation. J Ultrasound Med 1989; 8: 549–553

75 Smith B, Porter R, Ahuja K, Craft I. Ultrasonic assessment of endometrial changes in stimulated cycles in an in vitro fertilisation and embryo transfer program. In Vitro Fertil Embryo Transfer 1984; 1: 233–238

76 Sher G, Herbert C, Maassarani G, Jacobs M H. Assessment of the late proliferative phase endometrium by ultrasonography in patients undergoing in-vitro fertilisation and embryo transfer (IVF/ET). Hum Reprod 1991; 6: 232–237

77 Deichert I, Hackelöer B J, Dawne E. The sonographic and endocrinologic evaluation of the endometrium in the luteal phase. Hum Reprod 1986; 1: 219–222

78 Spitznagel E, Daly D. Sector ultrasound in the diagnosis and treatment of hematometra secondary to Asherman's syndrome. Fertil Steril 1988; 49: 370–372

79 Ombelet W. Endometrial ossification, an unusual finding in an infertility clinic. A case report. J Reprod Med 1989; 34: 303–306

80 Steer C, Campbell S, Pampiglione J, Kingsland C, Masson B, Collins W. Transvaginal colour flow imaging of the uterine arteries during the ovarian and menstrual cycles. Hum Reprod 1990; 5: 391–395

81 Steer C, Tan S L, Mills C, Rizk B, Mason B, Campbell S. Vaginal colour Doppler assessment of uterine artery impedance on the day of embryo transfer: a new screening technique for unsuccessful in vitro fertilisation. Lancet 1991; submitted

82 Goswany R K, Williams G, Steptoe P C. Decreased uterine perfusion – a cause of infertility. Hum Reprod 1988; 3: 955–959

83 Steer C, Mason B, Sathanandan M et al. Pituitary ovarian axis down regulation with LHRH agonist therapy increases frozen embryo

pregnancy rates abstract. In: Serono Symposia – Neuro Endocrinology of Reproduction, California, 4–9 Nov 1989

84 Rattern S, Thaler I, Goldstein S R, Timor-Tritsch I E, Brandes J M. Transvaginal sonographic technique: targeted organ scanning without resorting to 'planes'. JCU 1990; 18: 243–247

85 Donnez J, Casanas-Roux F. Prognostic factors of fimbrial microsurgery. Fertil Steril 1986; 46: 200–204

86 Schlief R, Deichert U. Hysterosalpingo–contrast sonography of the uterus and fallopian tubes: results of a clinical trial of a new contrast medium in 120 patients. Radiology 1991; 178: 213–215

87 Lenz S, Lauritsen J G, Kjellow M. Collection of human oocytes for in vitro fertilisation by ultrasonically guided follicular puncture. Lancet 1981; i: 1163–1164

88 Chamberlain G, Carron Brown J, eds. Gynaecological laparoscopy. In: Report on the confidential enquiry into gynaecological laparoscopy. London: Royal College of Obstetricians and Gynaecologists, 1978

89 Lenz S, Lauritsen J G. Ultrasonically guided perentaneous aspiration of human follicles under local anaesthesia: a new method of collecting oocytes for in vitro fertilisation. Fertil Steril 1982; 38: 673–677

90 Wickland M, Nilsson L, Hansson R, Hamberger L, Janson P O. Collection of human oocytes by the use of sonography. Fertil Steril 1983; 39: 603–608

91 Gleicher N, Friberg J, Fullan N, et al. Egg retrieval for in vitro fertilisation by sonographically controlled vaginal culdocentesis. Lancet 1983; i: 508–509

92 Dellenbach P, Nisand I, Moreau L, Feger B, Plumere C, Gerlinger P. Transvaginal sonographically controlled follicle puncture for oocyte retrieval. Fertil Steril 1985; 44: 656–662

93 Parsons J, Riddle A, Booker M et al. Oocyte retrieval for in vitro fertilisation by ultrasonically guided needle aspiration via the urethra. Lancet 1985; 1: 1076–1077

94 Lewin A, Laufer N, Rabinowitz R, Margalioth E J, Bar I, Schenker J G. Ultrasonically guided oocyte collection under local anaesthesia: the first choice method for in vitro fertilisation – a comparative study with laparoscopy. Fertil Steril 1986; 46: 257–261

95 Wikland M, Lennart E, Hamberger L. Transvesical and transvaginal approaches for the aspiration of follicles by the use of ultrasound. NY Sci 1985; 442: 182

96 Wikland M, Hamberger L, Enk L, Nilsson L. Sonographic techniques in human in vitro fertilisation programmes. Hum Reprod 1988; 3: 65–68

97 Itskovity J, Boldes R, Levron J, Thaler I. Transvaginal ultrasonography in the diagnosis and treatment of infertility. JCU 1990; 18: 248–256

98 Meldrum D R. Editorial. Antibiotics for vaginal oocyte aspiration. J In Vitro Fertil Embryo Transfer 1989; 6: 1–2

99 Scott R T, Hofmann G E, Muasher S J, Aeosta A A, Kreiner D K, Rosenwaks Z. A prospective randomized comparison of single- and double-lumen needles for transvaginal follicular aspiration. J In Vitro Fertil Embryo Transfer 1989; 6: 98–100

100 Parsons J, Pampiglione J S, Sadler A P, Booker M W, Campbell S. Ultrasound directed follicle aspiration for oocyte collection using the perurethral technique. Fertil Steril 1990; 53: 97–102

101 Wisanto A, Bollen N, Camus M, DeGrauwe E, Devroey P, Van Steirteghern A C. Effect of transuterine puncture during transvaginal occyte retrieval on the results of human in vitro fertilisation. Hum Reprod 1989; 4: 790–793

102 Waterstone J, Parsons J H, Bolton V. Elective transfer of two embryos. Lancet 1991; 337: 975–976

103 Hurley V A, Osborn J C, Leoni M A, Leeton J. Ultrasound-guided embryo transfer: a controlled trial. Fertil Steril 1991; 55: 559–562

104 Parsons J H, Bolton V N, Wilson L, Campbell S. Pregnancies following in vitro fertilisation and ultrasound-directed surgical embryo transfer by perurethral and transvaginal techniques. Fertil Steril 1987; 48: 691–693

105 Forrler A, Dellenback P, Nisand I, et al. Direct intraperitoneal insemination in unexplained and cervical infertility. Lancet 1986; i: 916–917

106 Pampiglione J S, Davies M C, Steer C, Kingsland C, Mason B A, Campbell S. Factors affecting direct intraperitoneal insemination. Lancet 1988; i: 1336

107 Curson R, Parsons J H. Disappointing results with direct intraperitoneal insemination. Lancet 1987; i: 112

108 Hovatta O, Kurunmaki H, Tutinen A, Lahteenmaki P, Kaskimies A I. Direct intraperitoneal or intrauterine insemination and superovulation in infertility treatment: a randomised study. Fertil Steril 1990; 54: 339–341

109 Mason B, Sharma V, Riddle A, Campbell S. Ultrasound-guided peritoneal oocyte and sperm transfer (POST). Lancet 1987; i: 386

110 Sharma V, Pampiglione J S, Mason B A, Campbell S, Riddle A. Experience with peritoneal oocyte and sperm transfer as an out-patient based treatment for infertility. Fertil Steril 1991; 55: 579–582

111 Yovich J L, Yovich J M, Edirisinghe W R. The relative chance of pregnancy following tubal or uterine transfer procedures. Fertil Steril 1988; 49: 858–864

112 Devroey P, Staessen C, Camus M, DeGrauwe E, Wisanto A, Van Steirteghem A C. Zygote intrafallopian transfer as a successful treatment for unexplained infertility. Fertil Steril 1989; 52: 246–249

113 Jansen R P S, Anderson J C, Radonic I, Smit J, Sutherland P. Pregnancies after ultrasound-guided fallopian insemination with cryostored donor semen. Fertil Steril 1988; 49: 920–922

114 Lucena E, Ruiz J A, Mendoza J C, et al. Vaginal intratubal insemination (VITI) and vaginal GIFT, endosonographic technique: early experience. Hum Reprod 1989; 4: 658–662

115 Scholtes M C W, Roozenburg B J, Alberda A, Zeilmaker G H. Transcervical intrafallopian transfer of zygotes. Fertil Steril 1990; 54: 283–286

116 Bauer O, Van der Ven H, Diedrich K, al Hasani S, Krebs D, Gembruch U. Preliminary results on transvaginal tubal embryo stage transfer (TV-TEST) without ultrasound guidance. Hum Reprod 1990; 5: 553–556

Fallopian tube patency

Josephine M McHugo

Introduction

Infertility is a common problem, with an incidence of between 1 in 10 to 1 in 7 couples. It is defined as a failure to conceive after regular sexual intercourse for 1 year. Tubal factors account for approximately 25% of the causes of the subfertility.[1]

There is a considerable investment of resources in the investigation and treatment of this problem. The assessment of tubal patency is an important part of the investigation of these couples. It is, however, important to remember that tubal function, and not just tubal patency, must be preserved for normal fertilisation and implantation. However, for the direct management of couples the demonstration of one patent tube is considered by many clinicians to be sufficient information to decide on a treatment strategy.[2] Primary or secondary infertility is therefore the clinical indication for the investigation of the fallopian tube in the majority of cases.[3]

Historically the fallopian tube has been investigated either by X-ray controlled hysterosalpingography (HSG) or by direct vision at laparoscopy. X-ray hysterosalpingography allows the internal anatomy of the uterine cavity and fallopian tube to be visualised (Fig. 5.1) by the instillation of contrast medium. This procedure was first described over 70 years ago. Initially oily contrast agents were used, but more recently non-ionic water-based media have been employed. Laparoscopy with instillation of dye into the uterine cavity allows direct vision of spillage of the dye from the tube into the peritoneal cavity (Fig. 5.2). The patency of the tube is assessed by spillage during fluoroscopic screening with HSG or by direct visualisation of spillage of dye at laparoscopy (hydrochromotubation). Laparoscopy gives additional information about the pelvis, in particular the presence of adhesions, but hysteroscopy must be used in addition to define the uterine cavity. The major disadvantage of laparoscopy is the operative intervention under general anaesthetic, with the increased

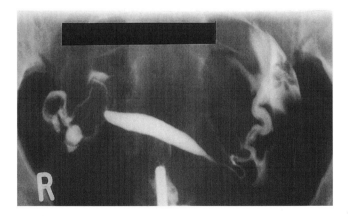

Fig. 5.1 X-ray hysterosalpingogram showing the normal anatomy of the uterine cavity and fallopian tube.

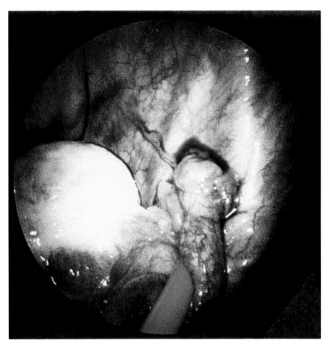

Fig. 5.2 Tubal patency, demonstrated by dye passing out of the fimbrial end at laparoscopy. (Image courtesy of Dr K Sharif.)

risks and cost compared to HSG. X-ray requires a small radiation dose, but this can be kept to a minimum if digital radiography is used.[4]

This chapter considers the ultrasound techniques available to assess tubal patency and the accuracy of this test compared to laparoscopy with hydrochromotubation and X-ray HSG.

Investigation of tubal pathology and patency

Transabdominal ultrasound was first used in assessment of tubal patency when a large volume of saline (approximately 500 ml) was instilled into the uterine cavity and spillage inferred when free fluid was detected within the pelvis on repeat scanning (Fig. 5.3). However, with the availability of trans-vaginal scanning and ultrasound echo-enhancing (contrast) agents the technique of hysterosonography has been developed.

Technique of hysterosonography

The basic technique consists of a routine trans-vaginal ultrasound examination followed by direct visualisation of the cervix with a speculum. Following cleansing of the cervix using a sterile agent under aseptic technique a soft flexible catheter (6–7 Fr) is inserted into the uterine cavity (Table 5.1). This technique is common to all procedures, regardless of the contrast agent chosen. A balloon catheter

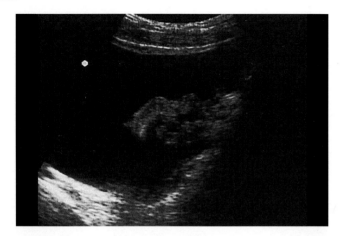

Fig. 5.3 **A transabdominal scan** demonstrated considerable free fluid in the pelvis.

Table 5.1 Technique for hysterosonography

Routine trans-vaginal ultrasound
Visualise and cleanse the cervix using a speculum
Introduce the balloon catheter (6–7 Fr) into the cervical canal
Remove the speculum
Reintroduce the trans-vaginal probe
Instil contrast under ultrasound control
Scan the length of each fallopian tube to the lateral pelvic wall.

is preferred as it is less likely to dislodge and creates a better seal at the internal cervical os. The tip of the catheter needs to be stiff enough to insert into the cervical canal, otherwise a catheter and stylet are required. The tip, however, must be atraumatic to avoid creating a false passage. The balloon needs to be positioned close to the tip, to allow the uterine cavity to be examined (Fig. 5.4). Various commercially available catheters are specifically designed for this investigation. In some instances it may be necessary to dilate the cervix prior to the insertion of the catheter; however, this is rarely necessary if the procedure is performed during the first half of the menstrual cycle. Following the insertion of the catheter the speculum is removed and the trans-vaginal ultrasound probe reinserted. Under ultrasound control the

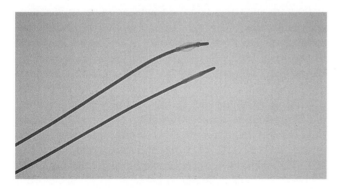

Fig. 5.4 **Balloon catheter used for hysterosalpingosonography.**

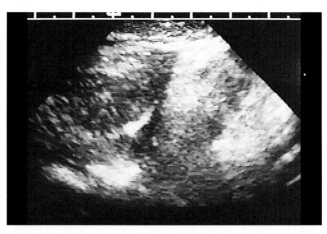

Fig. 5.5 **Cornual segment of the tube** demonstrated following instillation of Echovist into the uterine cavity.

echo-enhancing agent is instilled in small aliquots (1–2 ml). Tubal patency is assessed by direct imaging of flow within the segments of each tube. The operator should scan towards the fundus of the uterus in the transverse plane and identify the cornual segment of the tube following the instillation of a small volume of the agent. Once the origin of the tube has been identified (Fig. 5.5) further agent can be injected and sequential segments of the tube are examined by ultrasound, following its course out towards the lateral pelvic wall. Some operators instil only a small volume of agent (approximately 2 ml) and follow the spontaneous movement outwards without further instillation. This outward movement appears to occur only in a normal and patent tube.

Patency is confirmed by free spillage of the agent into the peritoneal cavity. The contralateral tube should then be examined in a similar way following the instillation of further agent if necessary. Some workers have inferred patency by observing continuous flow within the tube,[5] but this is less reliable than the visualisation of flow into the peritoneum. Spillage is assessed by imaging the flow of the agent around the ovary.

Colour Doppler imaging can be helpful but is not essential to assess the flow of the echo-enhancing agent in the tube and spillage into the peritoneal cavity.[6,7]

The indication for the investigation is screening for tubal patency as part of the preliminary work-up in infertility, either primary or secondary. Indications for investigation of the uterine cavity are not discussed further, as this is dealt with in Chapter 2; however, it is important that the cavity is examined as part of the standard work-up for infertility, and this may influence the choice of echo-enhancing agent used.

The contraindications (Table 5.2) are similar to those for X-ray HSG, i.e. current infection, menstruation and possible pregnancy. For this reason the author takes the precaution of performing this investigation prior to ovula-

Table 5.2 Contraindications for sonosalpingography

Contraindications for a trans-vaginal scan
Genital infection
Menstruation
Pregnancy
Hereditary galactosaemia (if using Echovist)

tion, with the couple abstaining from intercourse from the onset of menstruation until after the investigation.

If the chosen agent is Echovist (Schering Health Care) hereditary galactosaemia is a contraindication.

Echo-enhancing agents

Echo-enhancing agents that are available include saline, agitated saline, Echovist, and other microbubble-based agents. The majority of procedures to assess tubal patency using ultrasound in the UK are performed using a combination of saline for the assessment of the uterine cavity followed by Echovist for the assessment of patency of the fallopian tube. Patency is assessed by flow along the length of the tube (Fig. 5.6) or streaming of the contrast at the cornual segment for at least 10 seconds (Fig. 5.7), associated with spillage of contrast into the peritoneal cavity (Fig. 5.8).

Saline/agitated saline

Many commercial echo-enhancing agents are unsuitable for assessment of the uterine cavity because there is a marked increase in acoustic contrast within the cavity that masks any detail (Fig. 5.9). However, the less reflective saline is suitable. Tubal patency has also been assessed by a combination of 10 ml normal saline and 10 ml air agitated in a 20 ml syringe to create microbubbles.[8-10] With this technique there is a concordance of 88.7%, a sensitivity of

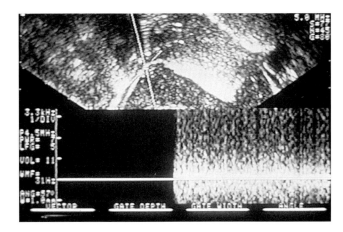

Fig. 5.7 Cornual segment flow with Doppler.

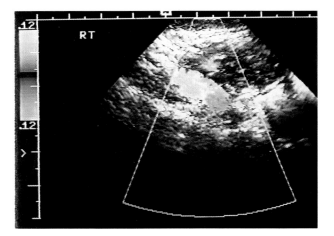

Fig. 5.8 Spillage of contrast into the peritoneal cavity around the ovary.

90% for tubal patency with a specificity of 83%, a positive predictive value of 94% and a negative predictive value of 71%. Therefore, as a screening test for tubal patency consideration should be given to the use of agitated saline, as the cost savings are great without a significant reduction in sensitivity. The criteria for patency are similar to those using commercial echo-enhancing agents, i.e. continuous flow in the cornual segment of the tube associated with spillage, as demonstrated by contrast flowing around the ovary. Chenia *et al*[8] reported a positive predicted value of tubal patency in 85%, compared to 81% when saline alone was used. However, in this study sonography was compared with X-ray HSG and no correlation with laparoscopy was given.

The majority of published data conclude that ultrasound assessment of tubal patency is suitable as a screening tool but not as a diagnostic test for pathology. Flow of contrast into an abnormally dilated distal tube can be demonstrated (Fig. 5.10). The accuracy of assessing patency in the abnormally distended tube is relatively low using ultrasound techniques.

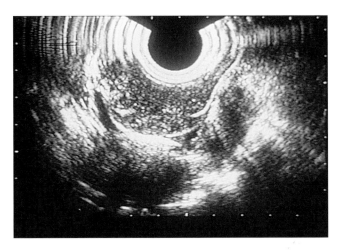

Fig. 5.6 Patency of the fallopian tube demonstrated following Echovist instillation.

5

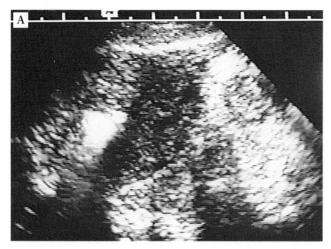
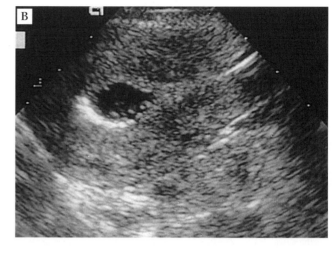

Fig. 5.9 Uterine cavity. A: Following instillation of Echovist and **B:** saline.

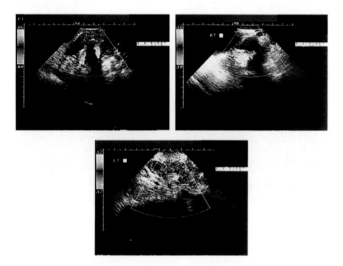

Fig. 5.10 Hydrosalpinx with ultrasound contrast.

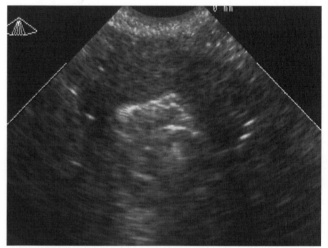

Fig. 5.11 Interrupted flow of contrast in the fallopian tube (string of pearls), suggesting tubal pathology. Courtesy of Mrs R Tetlow, Academic Department of Radiology. University of Hull.

Similarly, patent but damaged tubes, such as occur in salpingitis isthmica nodosa, may be inferred if there is abnormal streaming of the agent down the tube. This is seen when there is varying reflectivity resulting in an interrupted column of the agent (likened to a string of pearls) (Fig. 5.11). However, formal X-ray HSG is required to define this accurately (Fig. 5.12). This pathology is important to define as the ectopic pregnancy rate is high on assisted conception regimens.

Complications

The complications of ultrasound salpingography are procedure related and contrast related. In the first group the complications are directly related to the discomfort and pain of the instrumentation. This is similar to X-ray HSG and is quoted for the majority as discomfort experienced in 50% of cases.[11] However, there is a procedure failure due to the technical difficulties of either visualisation or canalisation of the cervix, which varies in the published literature between 2% and 8%.[12]

Contrast-related pain using Echovist is reported by many workers to be less than with HSG, although some have indicated a higher incidence of nausea and vasovagal reactions, which appears to be most common in those with patent tubes.[11,13] This may relate to the higher osmolarity of Echovist-200 compared to conventional X-ray contrast agents: 1699 mmol/kg H_2O compared to Iohexol 300 at 616 mmol/kg. Agitated saline appears less painful, probably again because of the low osmolarity of the injected solution.

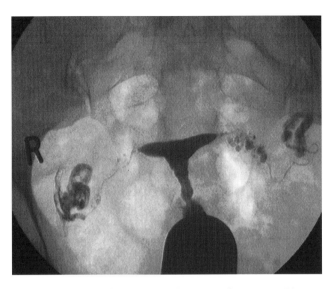

Fig. 5.12 **Salpingitis isthmica nodosa** demonstrated on X-ray HSG.

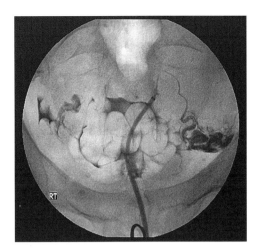

Fig. 5.13 **Selective catheterisation of the fallopian tube** under X-ray control.

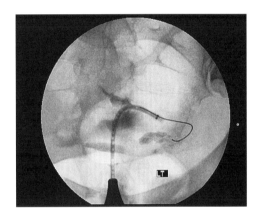

Fig. 5.14 **Tubal recanalisation** using a wire under fluoroscopic control.

The is a low reported post-procedural infection rate, but antibiotics should be prescribed for those with a dilated distal tube as this reduces the infection rate for X-ray HSG.

Correlation with HSG/laparoscopy and dye insufflation

The concordance for tubal patency between contrast sonography and laparoscopy and dye insufflation is 68–85%,[14] with a sensitivity of 85%, specificity of 85.6%, a positive predictive value of 71% and a negative predictive value of 92%.[13,15,16] Therefore, as a low-cost screening investigation for assessment of tubal patency ultrasound using contrast has an acceptable negative predictive value for occlusion. This is sufficient to allow management strategies to be planned in the apparently normal group. In view of the cost implications, with little loss of sensitivity or specificity, agitated saline should be considered as the agent of choice. However, it remains clear that further investigations for tubal abnormalities are appropriate for the abnormal group following this screening procedure. The type of investigation will depend on local working practice, but should include consideration of other diagnostic techniques such as X-ray HSG and selective catheterisation of the fallopian tube (Fig. 5.13). For some the consideration of recanalisation for proximal tubal occlusion is appropriate (Fig. 5.14). Other groups have suggested that a more rapid access to *in vitro* fertilisation is the most effective strategy to achieve a pregnancy, particularly when maternal age is more advanced. In those with distal disease further confirmation is appropriate.

Conclusion

Trans-vaginal ultrasound has revolutionised the practice of gynaecology and has a pivotal role in the assessment of the infertile couple, which is extended with the development of sonosalpingography for screening for tubal patency. The choice of contrast agent remains open, as both agitated saline and Echovist have been shown to be effective and safe. Saline remains the contrast of choice for assessment of the uterine cavity, an essential part of the investigation in infertility.

REFERENCES

1 Arronet G H, Eduljee S Y, O'Brien J R. A nine year survey of fallopian tube dysfunction in human infertility: diagnosis and therapy. Fertil Steril 1969; 10: 903–918

2 Gurriero S, Ajossa S, Mais V, Paoletti A M. The screening of tubal abnormalities in the infertile couple. J Assist Reprod Genet 1996; 13: 407–411

3 Pontifex G, Trichopoulos D, Karpathios S. Hysterosalpinography in the diagnosis of infertility (statistical analysis of 3437 cases). Fertil Steril 1972; 23(11): 829–833

4 Gregan A C M, Peach D, McHugo J M. Patient dosimetry in hysterosalpingography: a comparative study. Br J Radiol 1998; 71: 1058–1061

5 Dietrich M, Suren A, Hinney B, Osmers R, Kuhn W. Evaluation of tubal patency by hysterocontrast sonography (HyCoSy Echovist) and its correlation with laparoscopic findings. JCU 1996; 24: 523–527

6 Kalogriou D, Antoniou G, Botsis D, Kassanos D, Vitoratos N, Zioris C. Is colour Doppler necessary in the evaluation of tubal patency by hysterosalpingo-contrast sonography? Clin Exp Obstet Gynecol 1992; 79 (24): 101–103

7 Keinkauf-Houcken A, Huneke B, Lindner C, Braendle W. Combining ultrasound with pulsed wave Doppler for the assessment of tubal patency. Hum Reprod 1997; 12 (11): 247–260

8 Chenia F, Hofmeyer G J, Moolla S, Ratis P O. Sonographic hydrotubation using agitated saline: a new technique for improving fallopian tube visualisation. Br J Radiol 1997; 70: 833–836

9 Tekay A, Spalding H, Martikainen H, Joupilla P. Agreement between two successive transvaginal salpingosonography assessments of tubal patency. Acta Obstet Gynecol Scand 1997; 76 (6): 572–575

10 Inki P, Palo P, Anttila L. Vaginal sonosalpingography in the evaluation of tubal patency. Acta Obstet Gynecol Scand 1998; 77 (10): 978–829

11 Aidya G, Kennedy S, Barlow D, Chamberlain P. A comparison of patients' tolerance of hysterosalpingo-contrast sonography (HyCoSy) with Echovist-200 and X-ray hysterosalpingography for outpatient investigation of infertile women. Ultrasound Obstet Gynecol 1996; 7 (3): 201–204

12 Ayida G, Harris P, Kennedy S, Seif M, Barlow D, Chamberlain P. Hysterosalpingo-contrast sonography (HyCoSy) using Echovist-200 in the outpatient investigation of infertility patients. Br J Radiol 1996; 69: 910–913

13 Reis M M, Soares S R, Cancado M L, Camargs A F. Hysterosalpingo contrast sonography (HyCoSy) with SHU454 (Echovist) for the assessment of tubal patency. Hum Reprod 1998; 13 (11): 3049–3052

14 Splading H, Tekay A, Martikainen H, Joupilla P. Assessment of tubal patency with transvaginal salpingosonography after treatment for tubal pregnancy. Hum Reprod 1997; 12 (2): 306–309

15 Mitri F F, Andronikiou A D, Perinyal S, Hofmeyr G J, Sonnendecker E W W. A clinical comparison of sonographic hydrotubation and hysterosalpingography. Br J Obstet Gynaecol 1991; 98: 1031–1036

16 Heikkinen H, Tekay A, Volpie E et al. Transvaginal salpingosonography for the assessment of tubal patency in infertile women. Fertil Steril 1995; 64: 293–298

6

Embryology

Ian G Parkin

131

Introduction

This chapter summarises the development of the major organ systems. All timings are based on the time of fertilisation, about 2 weeks after the last menstrual period. Although the fetal period is not considered to start until the ninth week (and most fetal anomaly scanning is not done until about 16 weeks) the events of the previous 6 weeks (i.e. weeks 2–8) are crucial to the developing embryo and also to the understanding of organogenesis.

By the beginning of the third week (i.e. at the time of the first missed menstrual period) implantation has taken place, the chorion is forming and the embryo forms the bilaminar germ disc, with the prochordal plate (fused entoderm and ectoderm with no intervening mesoderm) visible at the cephalic end and the primitive streak at the caudal end.

The primitive streak becomes a groove, cells turn inwards and multiply in between the ectoderm and entoderm to form intra-embryonic mesoderm, which spreads in all directions to reach the extraembryonic mesoderm and create the trilaminar disc.

The cephalic end of the streak forms the primitive pit, which sinks inwards to create the notochord in the midline, pushing towards the prochordal plate. The neural plate, which then becomes the neural tube, forms from the ectoderm overlying the notochord.

The mesoderm forms somites (paired cubes) in the paraxial region, with intermediate mesoderm just adjacent and lateral mesoderm outside that. The intra-embryonic coelom forms as a horseshoe-shaped cavity in the lateral mesoderm, its posterior wall being somatic and its ventral wall (lining the entoderm) being splanchnic and forming the muscular wall of the developing gastrointestinal tract. Within the remainder of the mesoderm angiogenetic clusters coalesce to form the primordia of blood vessels, and the urogenital system will develop in the intermediate mesoderm.

During the fourth week these primordia fold in both cephalocaudal and lateral directions and the majority of organ systems commence their development. The prochordal plate becomes the buccopharyngeal membrane, while structures initially anterior to it rotate downwards to become the thorax, closed by lateral folding. Behind and above bulges the developing neural tube. The entoderm is pinched off to become the intestinal tract (epithelium). The intra-embryonic coelom becomes pericardial, pleural and peritoneal cavities. The mesoderm, which was originally at the anterior end of the horseshoe, swings inferiorly to become the septum transversum, and later the central tendon of the diaphragm.

The two-directional folds (cephalocaudal and lateral) ensure a pursestring closure of the anterior abdominal wall around the umbilicus, with ectoderm forming the epithelium. Failure of fusion of the lateral folds causes a defect in the body wall, allowing the intestine to lie in the extra-embryonic coelom. Such a defect may also cause failure of thoracic closure, resulting in ectopia cordis.

Central nervous system

The rapidly growing central nervous system is thought to control and induce much of the cephalocaudal embryonic folding, and consequently is the logical system to consider first. During the third week of embryonic life the cephalic end of the primitive streak forms the primitive knot (Hensen's node). From here cells move towards the prochordal plate and form the rod-like notochordal process between the entoderm and ectoderm (Fig. 6.1). The knot becomes pitted and the pit burrows along the notochordal process, converting it into a canal which fuses with the underlying entoderm and opens up to communicate with the yolk sac. (At this stage, through the original primitive pit, the yolk sac and amnion communicate via this neurenteric canal. As the surrounding ectoderm is induced to form the neural tube, and the entoderm the intestine, if this neurenteric canal remains open a connection between the intestine and the spinal cord central canal will exist.)

The notochordal canal effectively becomes a plate in the roof of the yolk sac; the plate folds inwards ventrally, to separate from the yolk sac again and become the notochord (Fig. 6.2). The overlying ectoderm thickens to become the neural plate (motor cells) and the immediately lateral cells become neural crest (sensory and autonomic cells).

Axially the plate grooves and cranially becomes broader, appearing almost bilobed. Caudally the plate envelops the primitive pit. As the embryonic disc grows so does the neural plate and its groove. By the seven-somite stage the edges of the groove meet dorsally in the midline and fuse, opposite the fourth to sixth somites. Cranial to this fusion the plate will become brain and caudally will be the upper cervical part of the cord. Continued caudal growth of the plate will form the remainder of the spinal cord (Fig. 6.3).

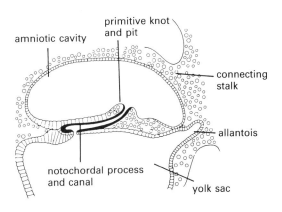

Fig. 6.1 Formation of notochordal process and its canal.

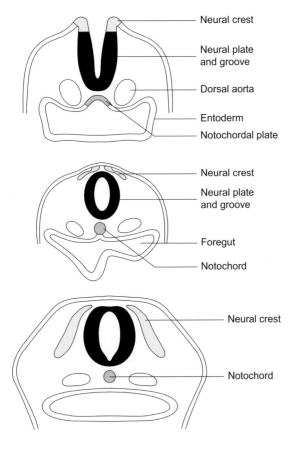

Fig. 6.2 Neural plate, groove and tube, with notochordal plate becoming notochord.

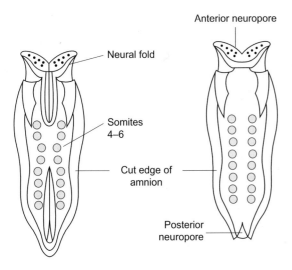

Fig. 6.3 Elongation and closure of the neural tube.

As fusion occurs anterior and posterior neuropores remain at either end, but the 'zip-up' extends in both directions, so that the anterior neuropore closes to become the

lamina terminalis by the 20-somite stage (3.5 weeks) and the posterior neuropore closes by the 25-somite stage (4 weeks). Consequently, by the late-somite stage the neural tube is present, with cranial swellings and a caudal part still forming to extend the full length of the embryo. As the disc folds the tube follows the concavity and the swollen cranial end is thrown forwards over the stomodeum, creating the cervical flexure at the junction of the cord and rhombencephalon. By 3 months the developing bone and cartilage of the vertebral column is growing more quickly than the spinal cord. Consequently, by birth the cord is 15–17 cm long and ends opposite L3.

Failure of closure of the neuropores causes neural tube defects as well as abnormalities in the overlying meningeal and skeletal elements. The various degrees of spina bifida are due to lack of closure of the posterior neuropore. Defects at the anterior neuropore are responsible for abnormalities of brain and cranium, including exencephaly and anencephaly.

Brain development

The somewhat bilobed cranial end of the neural tube becomes the familiar brain shape as a result of ventral cervical and mesencephalic flexures, dorsal pontine and telencephalic flexures and three primary dilatations, forebrain, midbrain and hindbrain (Fig. 6.4). Other secondary dilatations or vesicles are developed from the forebrain (prosencephalon) and hindbrain (rhombencephalon). The forebrain buds laterally on each side to become the lateral ventricles and overlying cerebral hemispheres, leaving the original dilatation as the third ventricle and its wall the diencephalon (thalamus). The pineal primordium separates forebrain and midbrain dilatations.

The midbrain shows the flexure but is largely unchanged, as is the cerebral aqueduct with tectum posteriorly, tegmentum and cerebral peduncles anteriorly.

The hindbrain thickens in its upper part, anteriorly to form the pons and posteriorly to form the cerebellum. The lower part remains as medulla oblongata. Between the two the dorsal concavity of the pontine flexure draws out the dorsal wall of the tube to create the thin roof of the fourth ventricle and the floor of the rhomboid fossa.

The telencephalic flexure throws the developing cerebral hemispheres dorsally over the diencephalon, which is consequently buried, and the hemispheres grow to overlap the midbrain and extend backwards to contact the cerebellum, as well as growing ventrally and rostrally to form the temporal lobes (Fig. 6.5).

As the lateral ventricles and fourth ventricle are formed the neural thinning allows ependyma and pia mater to come together, forming tela choroidea, and eventually the cerebrospinal fluid-producing choroid plexus. Defective circulation (aqueduct stenosis) or absorption of cerebrospinal fluid causes hydrocephaly.

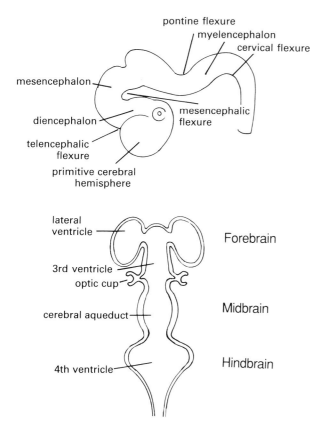

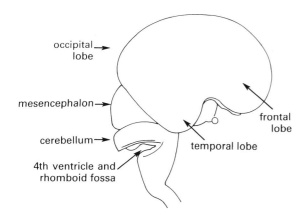

Fig. 6.4 Neural tube (brain) flexures and dilatations (early).

Fig. 6.5 Brain flexures (late).

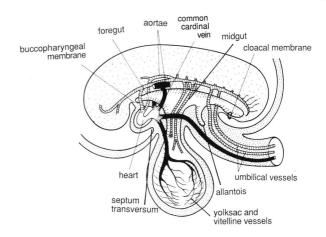

Fig. 6.6 Gastrointestinal tube and relations. (Reproduced with permission from Beck F, Moffat D B, Davies D P. Human embryology, 2nd edn. Oxford: Blackwell Scientific, 1985.)

Gastrointestinal tract

Following the cephalocaudal and lateral folding of the trilaminar disc the entoderm becomes converted into a tube, which will form the epithelium of the alimentary canal. This stretches from the buccopharyngeal to the cloacal membranes, where entoderm and ectoderm stick to each other. Elsewhere the tube has a covering of splanchnic mesoderm, which will differentiate to become the musculature and mesothelium (or surrounding fascia) of the tract. Mesoderm which remains and tethers the tract to either the dorsal or ventral body walls will become the corresponding mesentery. The entoderm maintains continuity with the yolk sac via the vitelline duct at what will become the umbilicus (Fig. 6.6).

Posterior to the tract lie the developing vertebral bodies and central nervous system. Anteriorly, throughout the length of the embryo, lie a number of structures: the septum transversum forms a division with the intra-embryonic coelom (peritoneal cavity) inferiorly, while the heart tube and pericardial and pleural cavities lie superiorly. The cephalic end of the heart tube (aortic sac) gives rise to the two dorsal aortae, which curve backwards to lie posterolateral to the canal. Further growth of the embryo and descent of the heart stretches the tube, creating a series of regions: oropharynx; oesophagus; foregut; midgut; hindgut and cloaca.

Oropharynx

Starting at the buccopharyngeal membrane this entodermal tube lies surrounded by mesoderm and ectoderm, which will become the body wall. At the start of the fourth week, sequentially with embryonic growth and not all clearly defined, a series of five pouches bulges outwards from the pharynx towards four ectodermal surface clefts, and create six intervening arches of mesoderm. Each arch receives: migrating neural crest cells, which surround the mesenchymal core and later become specific skeletal structures; an artery which runs from the aortic sac through the mesoderm to the dorsal aorta; and a nerve direct from the brain stem, which lies posteriorly.

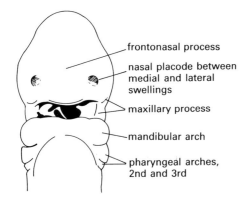

Fig. 6.7 Upper face development.

Between the fourth and eighth weeks the facial structure develops from five primordia. Cranial to the buccopharyngeal membrane (now broken down) a mesodermal thickening, the frontonasal process, grows towards the first arch thickenings (maxillary processes) at each side (upper cheek). Inferiorly lie the mandibular thickenings of first arch mesoderm, overlying Meckel's cartilages (derived from neural crest cells). Ectodermal thickenings, the nasal placodes, appear in the frontonasal process and the surrounding mesoderm thickens to form medial and lateral nasal swellings around the placodes, so that they become sunken and lie at the base of nasal pits (Fig. 6.7).

Each lateral swelling is initially separated from the maxillary arch by the nasolacrimal groove, but fusion occurs along these lines by the end of week 5. The medial prominences fuse with each other a week later to create the intermaxillary segment, which will form the philtrum of the lip, the premaxilla and associated gum, the primary palate and the nasal septum. At the same time maxillary prominences move medially, inferior to the lateral nasal swellings, to fuse with the medial swellings (intermaxillary segment). All the underlying mesenchyme is continuous, therefore there are no actual divisions underlying the grooves created externally by these prominences (Fig. 6.8).

The central part of the frontonasal process remains as the forehead, dorsum and apex of the nose. The alae curve from the lateral nasal swellings, which are now continuous with the cheeks. These early lips and cheeks, although structured originally from the first and second arch prominences, are invaded by second arch mesoderm, which differentiates to become the muscles of facial expression, carrying cranial nerve VII with it. The residual first arch mesoderm becomes the muscles of mastication, supplied by the mandibular nerve.

As the prominences above grow and develop around the nasal placode, the latter sinks more deeply so that the nasal pit becomes a nasal sac which grows backwards, in front of the overlying brain. The floor of this sac is the oronasal membrane, separating the nasal and oral cavities, but this soon disappears, leaving a single chamber. In the upper, nasal part, superior, middle and inferior conchae develop from the lateral wall.

While these developments have been continuing, the secondary palate has started its growth during the fifth week, to be completed by 12 weeks, with weeks 6–8 the most critical. The primary palate, from the intermaxillary segment, is already *in situ* but forms only the most anterior (incisive) part of the adult structure. Behind this two shelves (lateral palatine processes) push out horizontally from the internal aspect of the maxillary prominences and hang on each side of the tongue (Fig. 6.9).

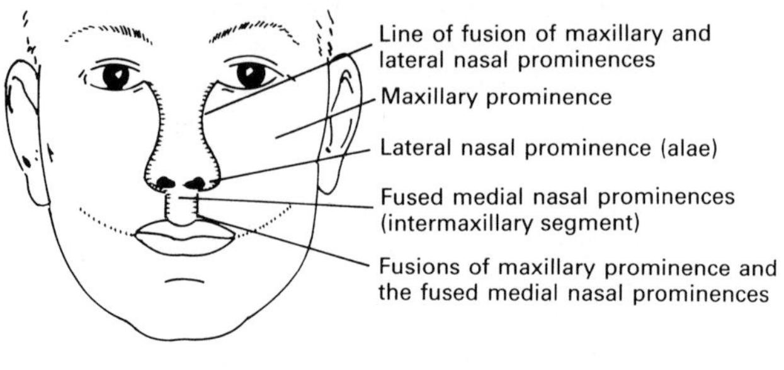

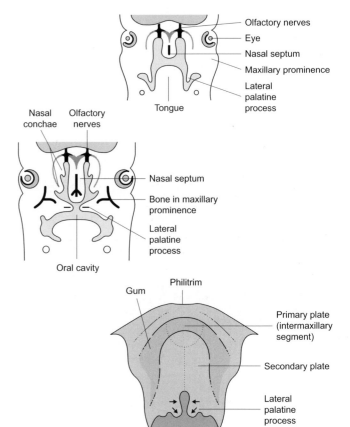

Fig. 6.9 **Palate formation.** (Reproduced with permission from Moore K L. The developing human, 4th edn. Philadelphia: W B Saunders, 1988.)

Fig. 6.8 **Facial lines of fusion.**

By the seventh week further growth makes the tongue relatively smaller and lie more inferiorly, allowing these palatal processes to elongate, swing upwards into a horizontal position and fuse with each other, to form the primary palate and the nasal septum (a downgrowth from the internal aspect of the intermaxillary segment). The fusion starts anteriorly during the eighth week and extends posteriorly until complete fusion occurs by the 12th week, at the uvula.

Clefts occur anteriorly following deficiencies in the intermaxillary segment (medial nasal prominences) and/or the maxillary prominences, so that they fail to fuse. Posterior clefts are due to faults in formation of the secondary palate, usually the lateral palatal processes.

Once into the fetal period (week 9) facial development is slow and depends on a reproportioning of the rather flat, underdeveloped but completed face, as described above. The growing brain forces a prominent forehead, the eyes move medially and the external ears grow from buds which appeared during week 5, from first and second arch components. By birth the lower face is still small and continues to grow, as dictated by the developing oronasal apparatus.

The primitive pharynx is wide behind the stomodeum and narrow towards the oesophagus. The laterally situated pouches give rise to many non-pharyngeal structures. The first pouch becomes the eustachian tube and middle ear. The second pouch forms the epithelium and crypts of the palatine tonsil (lymphoid tissue being derived from the underlying mesoderm). During weeks 6 and 7 buds of oral epithelium grow into the underlying mesoderm to become the salivary glands.

The floor of the pharynx, by the end of the fourth week, produces the midline tuberculum impar (median tongue bud) from first arch mesoderm. Beside this, also from first arch mesoderm, develop the lateral lingual swellings, which soon grow over, completely envelop and bury the tuberculum impar to form the connective tissue, lymphatic and blood vessels of the oral tongue, while overlying entoderm becomes the epithelium (Fig. 6.10).

A similar process exists for the pharyngeal tongue, which starts with a midline second arch swelling, the copula, which is soon overgrown and buried by the hypobranchial eminence of third, and far posteriorly, fourth arch origin. This accounts for the sensory innervation of the tongue being trigeminal (lingual) anteriorly and glossopharyngeal and vagus nerves posteriorly. The second arch is represented only by taste buds, supplied by the chorda tympani branch of the facial nerve.

Tongue musculature is derived from occipital somites, which bring the hypoglossal nerve with them.

During week 4 the laryngotracheal groove develops in the pharyngeal floor slightly further caudally, at the fourth/sixth arch level as the pharynx narrows to become the oesophagus. The groove enlarges to become the laryngotracheal diverticulum and its entodermal lining will become the epithelium and glands of the larynx, trachea and lungs.

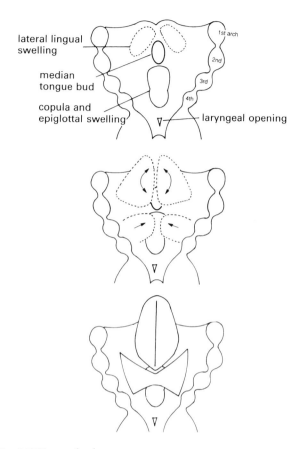

Fig. 6.10 Tongue development.

The diverticulum is separated from the pharynx and oesophagus by the tracheo-oesophageal septum, which leaves an opening (the laryngeal inlet) into the laryngotracheal tube at its cranial end. Consequently the developing larynx, trachea and lung bud now lie anterior to the oesophagus (Fig. 6.11).

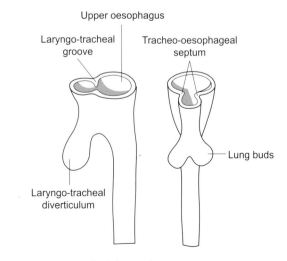

Fig. 6.11 Laryngotracheal diverticulum.

Should the tracheo-oesophageal septum deviate posteriorly the oesophagus narrows (atresia) and will not completely separate from the laryngotracheal tube (tracheo-oesophageal fistula).

Oesophagus

At the early stage (fourth week) the oesophagus is short, but heart descent and lung growth force it to elongate and reach its relative adult proportion by 7 weeks. During this time the epithelium (entoderm) proliferates to occlude the lumen. However, by the end of the eighth week the oesophagus usually reopens. Failure of this recanalisation causes oesophageal atresia and stenosis.

Epithelium and glands are derived from entoderm, whereas the surrounding musculature has two origins: in the cephalic portion, skeletal muscle comes from surrounding fourth and sixth arch mesoderm; in the caudal portion, smooth muscle from splanchnic mesoderm (both are supplied by branches of the vagus nerve). At this stage the oesophagus also has a flange of mesoderm behind it, forming a dorsal mesentery.

In front of the oesophagus and fused with its ventral mesoderm is the septum transversum, which now separates the pericardial cavity from the abdominal cavity and will become the central tendon of the diaphragm. Laterally the growing lungs and pleural cavities burrow into the body wall, creating medial pleuroperitoneal membranes which fuse with the septum transversum and the dorsal mesentery of the oesophagus to form a complete diaphragm separating the thoracic and abdominal cavities. Further body wall excavation forms costodiaphragmatic recesses, and myoblasts invade this thoraco-abdominal septum to create the musculotendinous sheet of the adult diaphragm.

Fusion of the various diaphragmatic elements (septum transversum, pleuroperitoneal membranes and dorsal mesentery of the oesophagus) occurs by 6 weeks and the sheet then 'descends' owing to relative body growth. Should this fusion fail or the pleuroperitoneal membranes be defective, the abdominal contents will herniate into the thorax when they return from the physiological hernia at 10 weeks.

Foregut

The foregut is the entodermal tube from the distal end of the oesophagus to the mid-duodenum, supplied by the coeliac axis. It also gives the epithelial primordia of liver, gallbladder, pancreas and associated ducts. Surrounding mesoderm forms the musculature and connective tissue of these structures, as well as the peritoneum and mesenteries. During the fifth week the stomach makes its first appearance as a dilatation of the tube. This portion then undergoes rotation around longitudinal and anteroposte-

rior axes (the adult position of the left and right vagus nerves providing good landmarks for following the former). The clockwise rotation in the longitudinal axis moves the left vagus to the anterior wall, the right vagus to the posterior wall, and swings the dorsal mesentery in a curve out to the left (Fig. 6.12).

The left (previously posterior) aspect grows more quickly than the right and forces the stomach to bend. Rotation of this curved tube around an anteroposterior axis throws the left side (greater curvature) to face inferiorly and slightly left, while the right side (lesser curvature) faces superiorly and slightly right.

The mesenteries are taken with these rotations, so that the dorsal mesentery, which grows considerably, appears to hang off the greater curvature (originally the posterior aspect of the dilatation) as the greater omentum, which maintains its connection to the posterior abdominal wall. The ventral mesentery connects the lesser curvature (originally anterior aspect) to the liver, developing in the septum transversum superiorly and to the right, then past the liver to the ventral wall as the falciform ligament (the umbilical vein lies in its free border). The repositioning pinches off a part of the peritoneal cavity to create the lesser sac posterior to the stomach and lesser omentum.

The caudal, pyloric, end of the stomach is also pushed to the right and takes the duodenum with it, so that the latter forms a C-shaped curve which rotates back on to the posterior abdominal wall, where its mesentery resorbs and it becomes mainly retroperitoneal.

As in the oesophagus epithelial proliferation causes duodenal obliteration (sixth week), which recanalizes after the eighth week. Failure to recanalise, which may have a number of causes (including Down's syndrome and vascular abnormalities), leads to duodenal atresia and stenosis.

During the fourth week the hepatic diverticulum arises from the lower end of the foregut ventrally. This bud of entoderm grows into the septum transversum (ventral mesentery) to become the cords of hepatocytes surrounded by mesodermally derived sinusoids, connective tissue, Kupffer cells and haemopoietic tissue. The embryonic liver is relatively large. Haemopoiesis commences by 6 weeks and bile production by 12 weeks.

The connection of the hepatic diverticulum to the duodenum sends another bud to become the cystic duct with the gallbladder, and the diverticulum itself remains as the bile duct (following obliteration and recanalisation).

In a similar way the pancreas springs from the entodermal tube, but as two buds. The ventral pancreas arises near the bile duct and the dorsal pancreas a little further cranially. The clockwise duodenal rotation forces the ventral bud to sweep all the way around to lie behind the dorsal bud. Both buds fuse and straddle the midline to nestle in the left aspect of the duodenal C-curve (Fig. 6.12).

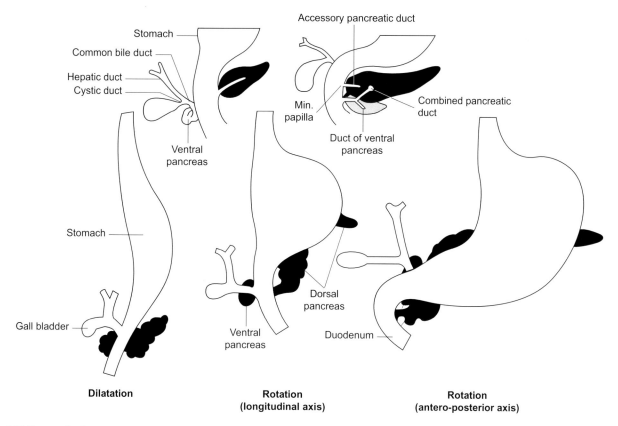

Fig. 6.12 Foregut development.

While rotating around the duodenum the pancreatic buds may form a ring around it (annular pancreas), which at birth may cause duodenal obstruction.

The main pancreatic duct is derived from the ventral pancreatic duct and the distal portion of the dorsal duct, opening with the bile duct into the duodenum. The proximal portion of the dorsal duct may remain as the accessory duct, opening into the minor papilla, cranial to the ampulla of Vater (major papilla).

Midgut and hindgut

Caudal to the bile duct opening the duodenum, jejunum, ileum, caecum, ascending colon and proximal two-thirds of the transverse colon are formed, as the midgut, from the entoderm of the yolk sac. This part of the tube communicates with the yolk sac via the vitelline duct (until 10 weeks), is supplied by the superior mesenteric artery and is suspended on a dorsal mesentery. Similarly, the hindgut continues to the rectum, supplied by the inferior mesenteric artery.

The midgut grows and outpaces the abdomen. Consequently, it forms the primary intestinal loop, pushing into the physiological umbilical hernia (6 weeks) with a much folded cranial limb and a straighter caudal limb con-

taining the caecal diverticulum. The loop rotates in an anti-clockwise direction around the superior mesenteric axis (viewed from the front), so that the cephalic limb (small intestine) moves downwards and to the right while the caudal limb (large intestine) moves up and left (Fig. 6.13).

As the hernia reduces (10 weeks) the small intestine returns first to lie centrally in the abdomen, posterior to the artery. (The vitello-intestinal duct should regress, but may remain as Meckel's ileal diverticulum.)

Failure of the lateral folds to fuse causes defects in the anterior abdominal wall (omphalocele), allowing the abdominal contents to lie externally, covered by the amnion. This problem often extends inferiorly to affect the cloaca, causing bladder exstrophy. Failure of the physiological hernia to reduce leaves loops of intestine in the umbilical cord. As this reduction should occur during the 10th week neither of these types of omphalocele can be diagnosed before that time.

As the large intestine returns to the abdomen, it rotates further anticlockwise so that the descending colon (part of the hindgut) falls into the left flank, with the transverse colon across the upper abdomen and the ascending colon to the right flank. The liver still takes up so much space that the caecum (last to return) has to lie tucked up close to its right lobe. Relative growth of body and decrease in

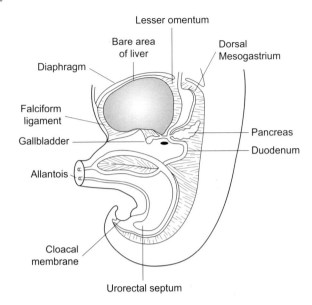

Fig. 6.13 **Midgut, physiological hernia and rotation.** (Reproduced with permission from Langman J. Medical embryology, 3rd edn. Baltimore: Williams & Wilkins.)

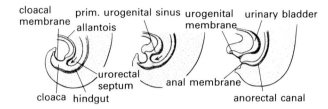

Fig. 6.14 **Division of cloaca.** (Reproduced with permission from Langman J. Medical embryology, 3rd edn. Baltimore: Williams & Wilkins.)

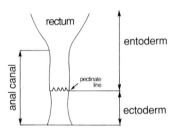

Fig. 6.15 **Anal canal.**

relative liver size then cause apparent descent of the caecum to the right iliac fossa.

The appendix is formed from the caecum owing to a slower rate of growth than that of the rest of the caecal diverticulum.

The dorsal mesentery for the full length of midgut and hindgut is forced away from its initial midline position. Where it is forced against the posterior abdominal wall it resorbs, and that part of the intestine becomes retroperitoneal and fixed. The small intestine, transverse and sigmoid colons keep their mesentery.

Cloaca

The distal end of the developing intestinal tract is sealed by the cloacal membrane, an apposition of ectoderm and entoderm with no intervening mesoderm. The allantois develops (second week) as a diverticulum of the yolk sac entoderm, but cephalocaudal folding moves its position so that it becomes a ventral bud of the entodermal tube, lying between the cloacal membrane and the vitelline duct/umbilicus.

The mesoderm between the duct and the allantois proliferates and pushes into the developing intestinal tube, behind the allantois, all the way to the cloacal membrane (Fig. 6.14). The mesoderm becomes the urorectal septum, which has the intestinal tube (lower end) posterior to it and the allantois in front. As the septum fuses with the cloacal membrane (7 weeks) it divides it into a dorsal anal membrane and a ventral urogenital membrane. Slight posterior deviation of the urorectal septum causes stenosis of the anorectal region.

Mesodermal proliferation around the anal membrane raises ectodermal swellings on either side and it comes to lie in the anal pit (proctodeum). Consequently, when at 8 weeks the anal membrane disappears, the lower third of the anal canal is formed from ectoderm and the upper two-thirds, joining the rectum, is entodermal hindgut (Fig. 6.15).

Failure of anal membrane breakdown causes imperforate anus; similar to the duodenum, failure of rectal recanalisation is another cause of stenosis.

Cardiovascular system

During week 3 (prior to folding) angiogenetic clusters form from proliferation in the intra- and extra-embryonic mesodermal cells. Clefts develop within the clusters and become confluent to form a lumen. The central cells detach into the lumen as primitive blood cells, while the peripheral ones flatten and form the endothelium of what are now called blood islands. These coalesce to form a vascular network, with circulation by the end of week 3. In this way a horseshoe forms in the mesoderm around the cephalic end of the notochord and prochordal plate (Fig. 6.16). This horseshoe will become the heart tube, and has vascular extensions: dorsal aortae and cardinal veins in the intra-embryonic mesoderm on each side of the notochord; vitelline vessels in the mesoderm around the yolk sac; and umbilical vessels in the mesoderm of the chorion and connecting stalk (Fig. 6.6).

Cephalocaudal folding throws the horseshoe, and the tube of the intra-embryonic coelom initially anterior to it, forward and downward to lie ventral to the developing

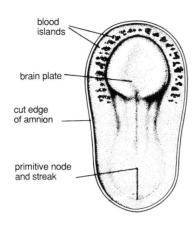

blood islands

brain plate

cut edge of amnion

primitive node and streak

Fig. 6.16 Blood islands forming a cephalic horseshoe. (Reproduced with permission from Langman J. Medical embryology, 3rd edn. Baltimore: Williams & Wilkins.)

pharynx (cervical region). Lateral folding ensures that the two limbs of the horseshoe move together and combine into a single tube, which lies dorsal to the single pericardial tube formed from similar fusion of the coelomic limbs. Growth of the heart and lungs later pushes both systems inferiorly into the definitive thoracic cavity. The heart tube invaginates into the pericardial cavity. Its superior end is arterial, receiving the two dorsal aortae into the aortic sac or truncus arteriosus. The inferior end is venous, receiving the cardinal, vitelline and umbilical veins into the sinus venosus.

Again as a result of folding, the dorsal aortae, which were continuations of the original horseshoe heart tube, curve bilaterally from the aortic sac past the pharynx to lie behind and parallel to the developing alimentary canal. This curve becomes incorporated into the first pharyngeal arch as the first aortic arch. As each pharyngeal arch develops an aortic arch grows into it, from the aortic sac dorsally to join the dorsal aorta (Fig. 6.6).

These events occurs sequentially between weeks 3 and 7. Heart descent and evolution of the pharyngeal derivatives forces the aortic arches to become (Fig. 6.17):

1. maxillary artery,
2. hyoid, stapedial arteries,
3. left common carotid, innominate arteries (the external carotid is a branch of the third arch),
4. left becomes arch of aorta, right becomes right subclavian artery,
5. disappears,
6. pulmonary arteries.

The aortic sac (truncus arteriosus) divides as the ascending aorta and pulmonary trunk. The initially paired dorsal aortae fuse to become a single aorta, which is continuous with the arch of the aorta derived from the left fourth aortic arch. The vitelline arteries become the coeliac axis, superior and inferior mesenteric arteries. The umbilical arteries originally carry deoxygenated blood to the placenta, but remain only as the internal iliac and superior vesical arteries.

The venous end of the heart remains for longer as a right and left horn of the sinus venosus. Each horn receives vitelline (yolk sac), umbilical (connecting stalk, oxygenated blood to embryo) and common cardinal veins (formed by the fusion of the anterior (head end) and posterior (rest of body) cardinal veins). Following left-sided venous obliteration, the left sinus horn regresses to remain as part of the coronary sinus and the right horn becomes incorporated into the atria.

The vitelline veins, on their way through the septum transversum to the sinus venosus, form a plexus around the duodenum and also link with the hepatic sinusoids of the developing liver. Consequently they become portal and hepatic veins, as well as contributing to the proximal inferior vena cava.

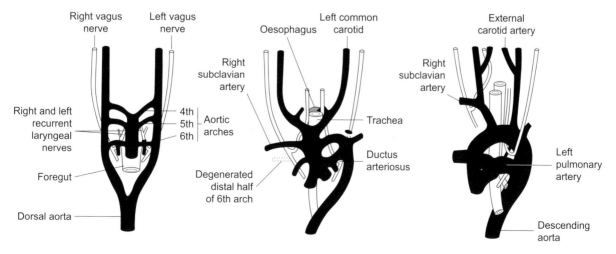

Fig. 6.17 Fate of aortic arches.

The umbilical veins run alongside the liver. The right degenerates and the left develops a large channel, the ductus venosus, sunk into the liver, to shunt deoxygenated blood directly to the inferior vena cava without circulating through the liver. After birth the left umbilical vein and ductus venosus become the ligamentum teres and ligamentum venosum.

Heart

The endothelium of the heart tube becomes surrounded by cardiac jelly and the mesodermal myoepicardial mantle. As the tube invaginates into the ventrally situated pericardial cavity these form the myocardium and epicardium. Each end of the tube is anchored, so that growth causes kinking and rotation to push the tube into the pericardium and place the atrium and sinus venosus dorsal to the truncus arteriosus and bulbus cordis end of the ventricle (Fig. 6.18). The partitions of the heart (concurrent, weeks 4–5) are created by: the constrictions formed at the sites of these flexures, dilatations on either side of these constrictions, and by the active growth of endocardial cushions (invaded by mesoderm) which push into the lumen and cause either narrowing or septum formation.

Flexural constriction narrows the junction between the bulbus cordis and the ventricle. The atrioventricular canal is divided into right and left openings by the growth and fusion of dorsal and ventral atrioventricular cushions. At the apex of the ventricle, opposite the bulboventricular constriction, a further endomyocardial ridge develops and pushes towards the fused atrioventricular cushions to become the inter-ventricular septum (Fig. 6.19). Initially this septum grows by the ventricles dilating and enlarging on either side of it, and consequently there is free communication between the ventricles over the upper edge of this ridge (the interventricular foramen).

In the meantime the fused atrioventricular cushions produce a thin extension which pushes into the interventricular foramen towards the upper edge of the muscular ridge. This will soon form the membranous part of the interventricular septum and, should it fail to develop, there would be a membranous ventricular septal defect.

Simultaneously truncal and bulbar ridges, continuous with each other, form in the truncus arteriosus and bulbus cordis. These ridges take a helical course as they grow and fuse to form a spiral aorticopulmonary septum, which divides the truncus arteriosus into aorta and pulmonary trunks which wind around each other. (Failure to form a helix causes transposition of the great vessels.)

The bulbus cordis becomes incorporated into the ventricles to form the right ventricular infundibulum and the left ventricular aortic vestibule. This incorporation, together with active growth of the septa, ensures that the bulbar ridges, the membranous extension of the atrioventricular cushions and the muscular inter-ventricular septum

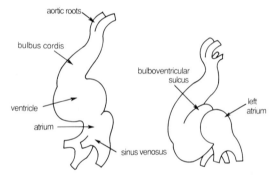

Fig. 6.18 Heart tube flexion and rotation to create septa.

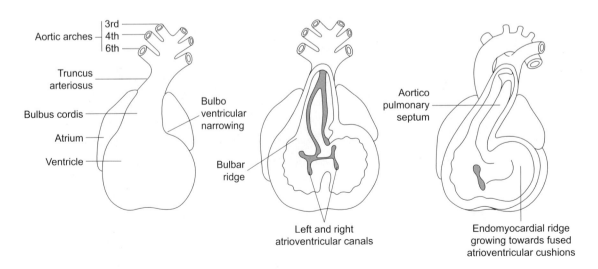

Fig. 6.19 Early positioning of atria and ventricles.

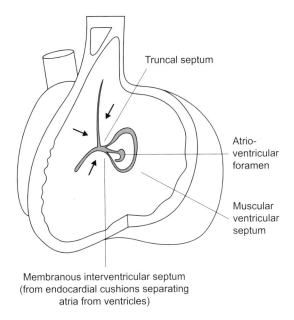

Fig. 6.20 Complete partitioning of heart chambers.

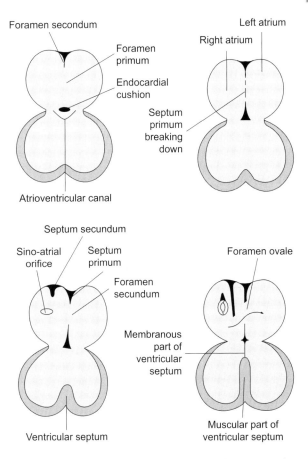

Fig. 6.21 **Formation of atrial septa.** (Reproduced with permission from Snell R S. *Clinical embryology for medical students*, 2nd edn. Boston: Little Brown.)

fuse to obliterate the inter-ventricular foramen (end of seventh week), producing separate right and left ventricles and outflows (Fig. 6.20). These divisions form the 'crux' seen on fetal cardiac ultrasound scans.

Cavitation of the ventricular wall undercuts the tissue to produce the trabeculae carneae, papillary muscles, chordae tendineae and atrioventricular valve cusps. The aortic and pulmonary valves are developed by the hollowing out and reshaping of three subendocardial valve swellings.

During weeks 4 and 5, as the ventricles and major arteries have been growing and partitioning, so has the primitive atrium. It divides by the active growth of septa, which meet and fuse with the endocardial cushion that divides the atrioventricular canal into right and left halves (the atrioventricular septum), but the septa develop in a way that ensures communication from left to right atrium.

The septum primum grows downwards from the atrial roof and creates the foramen primum, between its advancing inferior edge and the atrioventricular septum. As the septum primum fuses with the atrioventricular septum to obliterate the foramen primum, its upper aspect develops a series of perforations which coalesce and form the foramen secundum (Fig. 6.21).

Just to the right of the septum primum the thicker, stiffer septum secundum begins to grow inferiorly from the atrial roof. It advances to overlap the foramen secundum and form an incomplete partition with the foramen ovale in its inferior aspect. The lower part of the septum primum forms a flap valve, allowing the passage of blood from right to left atrium via the foramen ovale.

As mentioned above, many left-sided veins obliterate early, shunting blood to the right. Consequently, the right sinus horn increases in size and the sinoatrial orifice moves to the right. As the right atrium grows it incorporates the sinus venosus and right sinus horn, which now receives blood from the superior and inferior vena cavae. In the adult, the original fetal atrium is represented by the auricle and that part of the atrial wall with musculi pectinati. Posteriorly, demarcated by the crista terminalis, the atrium is smooth and developed from the sinus venosus.

On the left, initially a single pulmonary vein develops by budding from the atrium and branching to the lungs. Atrial growth incorporates the vein, so that only the left auricle is original atrium, the rest is vein derived and four pulmonary veins enter the chamber.

The ultimate division of the early heart tube into atrial and ventricular portions, each divided into separate left and right chambers, and each chamber connected to a specific vessel or vessels, is dependent upon the growth and fusion of many septa. Therefore, septal defects may have isolated consequences (probe patency of the foramen ovale, atrial septal defect, ventricular septal defect) or may lead to multiple abnormalities such as Fallot's tetralogy.

Urogenital system

The excretory and reproductive systems must be considered together as they develop adjacent to each other and utilise structures common to both. Growth tends to be sequential, as cranial sections regress, caudal sections proliferate. The primordia develop from intermediate mesoderm with its overlying coelomic epithelium, and from the allantois and cloaca lying anterior to the urorectal septum.

The embryo grows and creates new somites, with segments of intermediate mesoderm just laterally. These segments fuse and create a nephrogenic cord, which runs to the cloaca. As the lateral mesoderm splits to from somatic and splanchnic layers around the coelomic (peritoneal) cavity, folding then ensures that the intermediate mesoderm comes to lie on the posterior abdominal wall with a covering of coelomic epithelium (Fig. 6.22).

The first, and therefore most cranial, 'kidney' to develop in the nephrogenic cord is the non-functional pronephros. The remainder of the cord, caudal to the pronephros, forms the nephric duct to connect pronephros and cloaca.

As the pronephros regresses the mesonephros develops caudal to it (4–5 weeks), in the nephrogenic cord, and opens into the nephric duct. Consequently, the nephric duct is renamed the mesonephric or Wolffian duct. The mesonephros creates a ridge on the posterior abdominal wall. The coelomic epithelium on the medial aspect of the ridge proliferates to form the genital ridge, which grows inwards into the underlying mesoderm to form the gonadal primordium. Germ cells migrate into this primordium, so that the gonad is created from three tissue types: mesoderm, mesothelium and yolk sac (Fig. 6.23).

At this stage, there is a definite, joint urogenital ridge on the posterior wall, with the gonadal blastema medially and the mesonephros (nephrogenic cord) laterally. There is then an invagination of coelomic epithelium on the lateral aspect of the ridge (i.e. lateral to the mesonephros and its

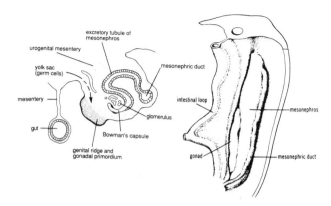

Fig. 6.23 **Urogenital ridge.** (Reproduced with permission from Langman J. Medical embryology, 3rd edn. Baltimore: Williams & Wilkins.)

duct) to form the paramesonephric duct (Müllerian), which maintains an opening into the coelom. Caudally the urogenital ridges swing medially to fuse in the midline, i.e. in the urorectal septum which divides the cloaca. As each ridge runs over the pelvic brim, it gains a mesodermal connection – the inguinal fold – to the anterior abdominal wall. The fate of structures within the urogenital ridge may be considered under the separate areas of urinary and reproductive development.

Kidney and ureter

As the mesonephros begins to regress cranially, the metanephros forms in the nephrogenic cord (5–6 weeks) in the sacral region, caudal to the mesonephros. Just above its point of entry into the cloaca, the mesonephric duct gives off the ureteric bud on its posteromedial aspect. The bud grows dorsally and migrates around the mesonephric duct to enter its posterolateral aspect. During its dorsal growth the ureteric bud expands and meets the metanephric blastema, which appears to ascend (because of

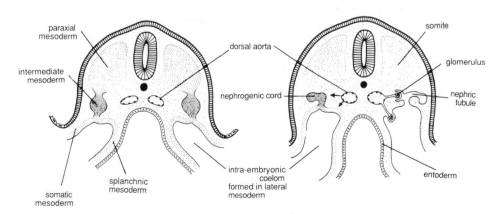

Fig. 6.22 **Folding to position the mesodermal regions and kidney development in the intermediate mesoderm.** (Reproduced with permission from Langman J. Medical embryology, 3rd edn. Baltimore: Williams & Wilkins.)

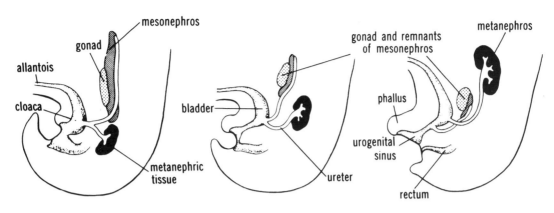

Fig. 6.24 Ureter and metanephric development. (Reproduced with permission from Langman J. Medical embryology, 3rd edn. Baltimore: Williams & Wilkins.)

embryo growth), reaching the adult position by week 9 (Fig. 6.24).

The ureteric bud may duplicate or divide abnormally, to create double ureters. The developing kidneys may fail to ascend and remain in the pelvis, or fusion may occur at their lower poles, resulting in horseshoe kidney.

The ureteric bud develops into major, then minor calyces, followed by further subdivision and a decrease in size to form collecting tubules (fifth month). Where the metanephros contacts a collecting tubule it forms a double-cell mass, the renal vesicle. Each vesicle becomes a nephron and differentiates to form a glomerulus, then proximal and distal convoluted tubules, with the loop of Henle between. The nephrons cluster around the collecting tubules as lobules and the lobules cluster around the major divisions of the ureteric bud as lobes. (The lobar nature of the kidney is visible into infancy, but usually is lost by adulthood.) The metanephros begins to function at about 11 weeks. Abnormal development of the collecting tubules allows the formation of blind renal vesicles, which become the cysts of congenital polycystic kidney diseases.

The ureter enters the mesonephric duct, the caudal part of which is now termed the common excretory duct. The latter joins the cloaca, which is divided by the urorectal septum so that the rectum lies posteriorly, with the allantois, urogenital ducts and primitive urogenital sinus anteriorly (6 weeks). The lower end of this urinary part of the cloaca is sealed by the urogenital membrane, around which mesoderm flows to create lateral genital swellings and an anterior midline genital tubercle (4 weeks), so that the membrane comes to lie in a depression, the external cloaca, which is forced to face inferiorly owing to formation of the anterior abdominal wall. The primitive urogenital sinus is considered in two parts. Cranial to the entry of the common excretory ducts is the vesico-urethral canal, continuous with the allantois, and caudal to their entry is the definitive urogenital sinus.

Bladder and urethra

The vesico-urethral canal will form the mucosa lining the bladder, whereas the muscle comes from the surrounding mesoderm. Most of the bladder remains abdominal and does not enter the true pelvis until after puberty.

The canal grows and incorporates the common excretory ducts, so that the mesonephric ducts and ureters now enter separately. (Failure to do so causes ectopic ureteric orifices.) The ureteric openings migrate cranially and laterally, leaving the trigone at what will be the base of the bladder (Fig. 6.25).

The vesico-urethral canal develops a dilated upper part, becoming the bladder, and remains narrow inferiorly to form the bladder neck and upper urethra, which in the male receive the mesonephric ducts. The allantois degenerates, with eventual obliteration of its lumen to leave the urachus (which later forms the median umbilical ligament) between bladder and umbilicus.

Below the entry of the mesonephric ducts, which either obliterate in the female or become the ejaculatory ducts/vas deferens, the definitive urogenital sinus forms the mucosa of the upper, pelvic portion of the urethra above the urogenital membrane. This pelvic portion in the female becomes the whole urethra, whereas in the male it will form the prostatic and membranous parts (the prostate gland being formed by buds from the urogenital sinus, with surrounding mesoderm forming the stroma) (Fig. 6.26).

Below the urogenital membrane the external cloaca is formed from the surface ectoderm in a depression between the genital tubercle (which will form penis or clitoris) anteriorly, and the genital swellings (scrotal wall or labia majora) laterally. Sandwiched just medial to each genital swelling, immediately below the urogenital membrane, are the bilateral, ectodermal urogenital folds. At about 7 weeks the urogenital membrane ruptures and sex differentiation and phallic development, starts at about 9 weeks.

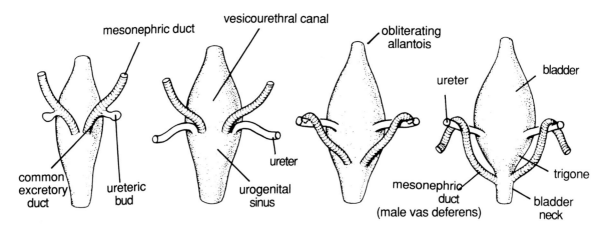

Fig. 6.25 Bladder, ureter and genital ducts. (Reproduced with permission from Langman J. Medical embryology, 3rd edn. Baltimore: Williams & Wilkins.)

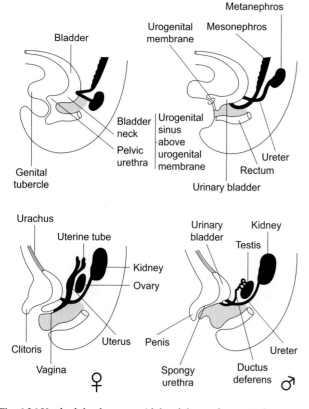

Fig. 6.26 Urethral development with breakdown of urogenital membrane and sex differentiation. (Reproduced with permission from Moore K L. The developing human, 4th edn. Philadelphia: W B Saunders, 1988.)

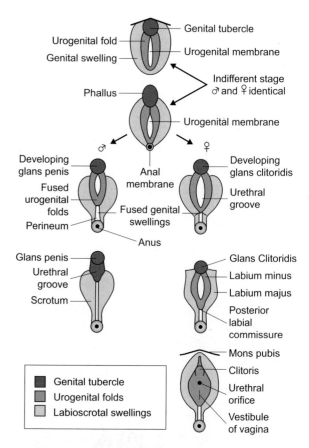

Fig. 6.27 Development of cloaca, below urogenital membrane. (Reproduced with permission from Moore K L. The developing human, 4th edn. Philadelphia: W B Saunders, 1988.)

In the male the genital tubercle grows and lengthens to form the penis, drawing the urogenital folds with it to form the lateral walls of the urethral groove on the ventral aspect of the penis. Meanwhile, entoderm from the membranous urethra (lower urogenital sinus) proliferates downwards as the urethral plate to line the walls of the urethral groove (Fig. 6.27).

The urethral folds begin to fuse in the ventral midline to form the penile raphe and enclose the entodermally lined spongy urethra. This 'zipping-up', which can be abnormally halted at any stage to produce hypospadias, ensures that the spongy urethra progresses down the length of the penis and meets the urethral canal of the glans, formed by ectodermal ingrowth.

In the female the genital tubercle, not stimulated by androgens, remains as the clitoris. The urogenital folds become the labia minora and the external cloaca the vestibule of the vagina, which receives the vagina and urethra between the labia majora (genital swellings).

Gonads and reproductive ducts

The gonadal ridge, described earlier, forms as an 'indifferent' stage at about 5 weeks, from mesodermal proliferation and the ingrowth of primary sex cords from the overlying coelomic epithelium (mesothelium). The primordial germ cells, from the yolk sac, are incorporated into the cords by week 6.

In the male, during week 7, and influenced by the Y-chromosome, the primary sex cords form the seminiferous tubules (also the sustentacular cells) and the blastema becomes surrounded by the characteristic tough fibrous tunica albuginea. The yolk sac germ cells give rise to spermatogonia, whereas the mesoderm provides the interstitial cells (Fig. 6.28).

In the female development occurs slightly later, as the primary sex cords degenerate and (at 10 weeks) are replaced by secondary sex cords, which break into primordial follicles, each containing an oogonium (16 weeks). The developing ovary is surrounded by a tunica albuginea, but it is rather thin (Fig. 6.29).

Within the ovary, during the fetal period only, the oogonia (from yolk sac germ cells) undergo active mitoses to form thousands of these primitive germ cells. Many of

these regress but, by birth, about 2 million are left as primordial follicles with oogonia which have entered the first meiotic division as primary oocytes. Further differentiation has been arrested by the follicle cells, and they remain quiescent until puberty.

Both male and female gonads become tethered to the anterior abdominal wall and genital swellings by a gubernaculum of mesonephric duct origin. Pelvic enlargement and abdominal elongation causes the apparent descent of the gonads, guided by the gubernaculum. The testis descends through the inguinal canal into the scrotum (formed from the genital swellings), whereas the ovary goes only as far as the pelvic brim.

The development of the reproductive duct system is controlled by the presence or absence of testicular androgens. Consequently, in the male, the paramesonephric ducts degenerate while the mesonephric duct joins to the testis to form the epididymis, then the vas deferens and ejaculatory duct entering the prostatic urethra.

In the female the mesonephric ducts regress while the paramesonephric ducts form the genital duct system. Cranially, fimbriae form where the ducts enter the coelomic (peritoneal) cavity, and this part becomes the uterine tube (Fig. 6.30). Further caudally the paramesonephric ducts fuse behind the bladder to form the uterovaginal canal. The cranial point of fusion forms the uterine fundus and the uterovaginal canal then grows caudally down the urorectal septum to meet and fuse with a pair of sinovaginal bulbs, which grow upwards from the entoderm of the urogenital sinus. These bulbs also fuse to create a solid plate of entoderm, the vaginal plate, which eventually canalises to receive the uterus (Fig. 6.31). The common sources of origin of the urinary and reproductive duct systems, the dependence of development upon local

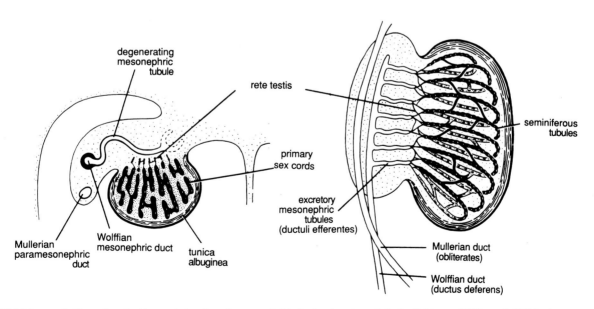

Fig. 6.28 Male gonad. (Reproduced with permission from Langman J. Medical embryology, 3rd edn. Baltimore: Williams & Wilkins.)

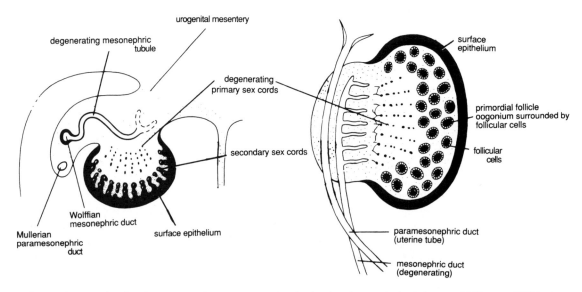

Fig. 6.29 Female gonad. (Reproduced with permission from Langman J. Medical embryology, 3rd edn. Baltimore: Williams & Wilkins.)

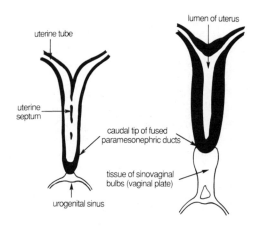

Fig. 6.30 Paramesonephric ducts fusing to form uterus.

hormone production, duct fusions, regressions and canalisations create many opportunities for congenital malformations to occur in this region.

Fetal period

As described above, by the start of the ninth week the major organ systems have largely developed. Between that time and birth (38 weeks post-fertilisation) there is rapid growth and reproportioning of these systems, but the fetus is less susceptible to teratogenic agents.

At the start of the fetal period the head is half the fetal length, male and female external genitalia are indistinguishable, coils of intestine protrude into the physiological hernia in the umbilical cord, the liver is the major site of erythropoiesis and the pronephros is non-functional.

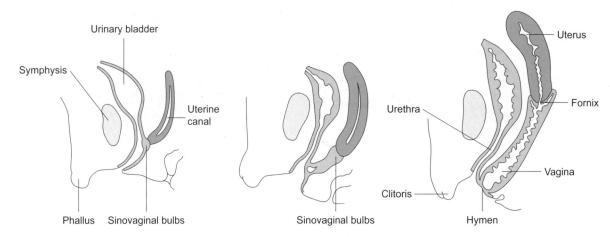

Fig. 6.31 Vaginal development. (Reproduced with permission from Langman J. Medical embryology, 3rd edn. Baltimore: Williams & Wilkins.)

By the 12th week the head is still relatively large but its growth has slowed in relation to the rest of the body; external genitalia show obvious sex differentiation; the intestine has returned to the abdomen; the spleen also commences erythropoiesis and urine is produced by the metanephros. Primary ossification centres appear, particularly in the skull and long bones, and the fetus will move in response to stimuli.

Over the following 4 weeks (to week 16) a more 'human' form is seen as the eyes face forward, ears are close to their final position and there is rapid growth. Skeletal ossification continues so that bones are visible on X-ray and both upper and lower limbs have almost reached normal relative proportions, although the lower ones are still rather small. Soon after this, limb movements may be felt by the mother.

By 20 weeks scalp hair, eyebrows, lanugo and vernix caseosa are well established. The ovary has had primordial follicles with oogonia for about 4 weeks, but now the uterus is formed and the vagina begins to canalise. The

			EMBRYOLOGICAL TIMING					
SOMITES	POST-FERTILISATION TIME	CROWN-RUMP LENGTH (APPROX.)	EVENTS					
			CVS		GIT	CNS		GUT
	6 days		Early implantation					
	8 days		Bilaminar disc					
	15 days		Trilaminar disc (mesoderm from primitive streak)					
Early presomite	16/17 days		Angiogenetic clusters (intra- and extra-embryonic) Development of allantois			Notochord		
Late presomite	18/19 days	1.4 mm				Neural plate Neural groove		
1–4	20		Folding of trilaminar disc		Formation of gut tube and pharyngeal system	Neural tube starts to form. Neural crest lies dorsolaterally		Pronephros – cells visible in intermed. mesoderm
10–12	23	2.2 cm	Formation of single heart tube Beating Folding of heart tube			'Zips up'. Ant., then Post. Neuropores close	Brain dilatations	Mesonephros developing/degenerating cranio-caudally
26–29	28 days	4 mm						
42–44	5 weeks	5–8 cm	Oblitn. of umb. and vit. vs. Formation of cardiac septa	Development and reformation of aortic arches SA Node	Liver forming Gut rotating Physiological hernia	Ant. spinal roots	Brain flexures Cerebral vesicles	Sex gland primordia Ureteric bud MN duct and ureter open separately into the VU canal
	6 wks	10–14 mm			Cloaca faces caudally Urorectal septum fuses			Paramesonephric ducts appear Renal vesicles in metanephros
	7 wks	17–22 cm	Complete ventricular septum		U.G. membrane disappears			Male gonadal blastema obvious
	9 wks	5 cm	Oblitn. L Cardinal V	Formation of main veins	Sex of ext. genit. Anal canal opens			Testicular tunica albuginea Prostatic buds appear.
	12 wks	8 cm			Gut returns to abdomen	Cord same length as whole embryo	Obvious adult brain architecture	
		9 cm						Rete canalises, joins to mesonephric tubules
	16 wks	10 cm						
	20 wks	15 cm						Distinction between uterus and vagina
	24 wks	20 cm						Processus vaginalis

testis has begun its descent but is still on the posterior abdominal wall.

The next 4 weeks see substantial weight gain, but weeks 26–29 are important as the lungs, pulmonary circulation and nervous system mature to sustain life. The eyes reopen, subcutaneous fat develops and bone marrow takes over erythropoiesis.

The last 9 weeks are for final maturation, so that the pupillary light reflex and the grasp reflex develop and the head circumference approaches that of the abdomen. Fetuses reach an average crown–rump length of 360 mm and a weight of 3400 g. In the male, by full term the testes have moved into the scrotum.

FURTHER READING

1 Moore K L. The developing human, 4th edn. Philadelphia: W B Saunders, 1988
2 Sadler T W. Langman's medical embryology, 7th edn. Baltimore: Williams & Wilkins, 1995
3 Hamilton W J, Boyd J D, Mossiman H W. Human embryology, 3rd edn. Cambridge: W Heffer, 1962
4 Snell R S. Clinical embryology for medical students, 2nd edn. Boston: Little, Brown, 1975
5 Williams P L, Warwick R, Dyson M, Bannister L M. Gray's anatomy, 37th edn. Edinburgh: Churchill Livingstone, 1989
6 Beck F, Moffat D B, Davies D P. Human embryology, 2nd edn. Oxford: Blackwell Scientific, 1985
7 Larsen W J. Human embryology. Edinburgh: Churchill Livingstone, 1993

The first trimester

Mike J Weston

Introduction

The major role of ultrasound in the first trimester of pregnancy is to establish the presence of a normal live intra-uterine pregnancy and to distinguish this from either pregnancy failure or ectopic pregnancy. There have been major developments in recent years both in the techniques and resolution of ultrasound and in hormonal assays that facilitate this diagnosis. It should be remembered that obstetric and radiology departments have had to respond to these advances in a relatively short time. Poor training, experience, equipment or departmental protocols can lead to erroneous diagnoses. A recent public inquiry highlighted the very strong emotions aroused by an incorrect diagnosis of pregnancy failure.[1] It was also apparent that in untrained hands ultrasound is a dangerous tool. If it were not for the protocols in place at the centre involved in the inquiry, then live pregnancies would have suffered unwanted evacuation. There are a number of reliable signs of a non-viable pregnancy that will be discussed below. These do, however, require good scanning technique, whether transabdominal or trans-vaginal. The inexperienced observer should be wary of applying signs that may be due more to their poor scanning technique than to reality. The added dimension of time with serial scans resolves many problems. Once the diagnosis of pregnancy failure has been made by experienced observers there is, of course, no worth in needlessly repeating scans.

Pregnancy failure in the first trimester is common – indeed, it is a physiological mechanism for removing maldeveloped or chromosomally abnormal embryos. The proportion that fails depends on what criteria have been used to define pregnancy initially. Not all ova exposed to fertilisation will become zygotes, and not all zygotes will implant. Of those that implant and produce detectable amounts of β-hCG (chemical pregnancy), some will abort at the time of the next menstruation before the woman knows she is pregnant. Only about half of the embryos will survive to become a recognised clinical pregnancy with a positive pregnancy test and a missed menstrual period.[2] In these clinical pregnancies about one-fifth will suffer bleeding before the 20th week, and over half of these will miscarry. This gives a miscarriage rate of about 12% of recognised clinical pregnancies.[3] Even this may be an underestimate, as these results do not take into account the estimated 10% of women who do not contact any health professional after a miscarriage.[4] First-trimester spontaneous abortions have a high rate of chromosomal abnormalities, ranging from 40% to 80%.[5-7] An underestimation of this rate may be caused by maternal contamination of the embryonic specimen, producing a false-normal 46XX karyotype.[7] It is an unavoidable conclusion that early pregnancy failure is both common and an essential physiological process.

Technique of transabdominal and trans-vaginal ultrasound scanning

Many hospitals have set up dedicated early pregnancy units (EPUs). These aim to deal efficiently and sensitively with the many women who present with bleeding or pain in early pregnancy, rather than subjecting them to long waits in unfriendly accident and emergency departments. Open access to these units has substantially relieved the pressure on out-of-hours services. Women who attend are seen by a clinician for history and examination and serum β-hCG measurement, as well as having an ultrasound scan. If there are pregnancy problems then counsellors and operating theatres are available. It is our practice to do a transabdominal scan first and then to decide whether a trans-vaginal scan is required.

Transabdominal ultrasound

The standard technique for pelvic ultrasound with a full urinary bladder is not always necessary, and may even be undesirable in early pregnancy. Useful information can be gained in women presenting with acute symptoms without having to wait for bladder filling.[8] In particular, slim women with an anteverted uterus can be imaged with an empty bladder by gentle pressure of the transducer on the abdominal wall. This can allow visualisation of the uterine contents in great detail (Fig. 7.1). A full bladder may be uncomfortable and can distort the appearance of the gestation sac, even preventing visualisation of an embryo by displacing the uterus away from the transducer into an area of poorer spatial resolution in the far field. This is not to say that a full bladder is not sometimes required. The full bladder displaces bowel filled with gas out of the pelvis and provides an acoustic window to the uterus and its adnexae. When an initial transabdominal scan has failed because the bladder is not sufficiently full, the decision can be made whether to proceed to fill the bladder or to use trans-vaginal ultrasound instead. The woman's own preferences will affect this decision. Filling the bladder needs a large fluid load of almost 1 litre in an hour. Once the bladder is full, longitudinal and transverse images through the pelvis can be obtained, with alteration of the scan plane to suit the orientation of the uterus. The adnexal structures are seen by moving the transducer to one side of the pelvis and angling it toward the contralateral side in order to maximise the advantage of the bladder's acoustic window. The retroverted uterus is usually best imaged by trans-vaginal ultrasound. The greater the gestational age of the pregnancy the more likely it is that transabdominal ultrasound will be able to answer the clinical question.

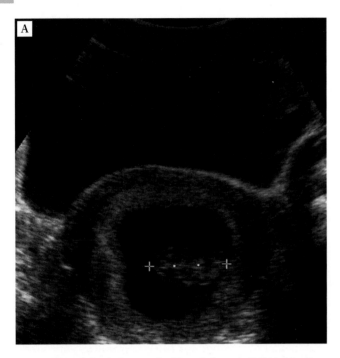
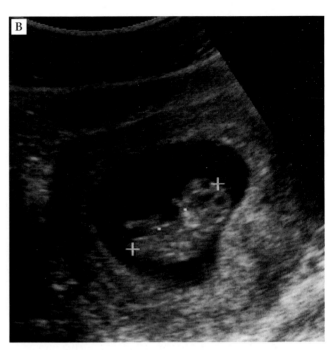

Fig. 7.1 Transabdominal scans of a 10-week fetus. A: Full bladder, **B:** empty bladder technique. Greater detail can be seen with the bladder empty as the fetus (between calipers) is within the near field of the transducer.

Trans-vaginal ultrasound

Nearly all ultrasound machines are now capable of supporting a trans-vaginal probe. The design of the probe has evolved from mechanical sector transducers to electronically focused multi-element ones. The shape has changed from an off-set bent handle with an out-of-line fan beam to a more versatile straight probe with an end-of-probe in-line beam. These newer probes are easier to manipulate and orientate, and the resolution of the electronically focused systems has surpassed that of the mechanical transducers. Assisted conception units may still prefer the offset probes, as these allow easier visualisation of lateral structures and easier placement of needle guides. Radiology departments usually find the end-fire probes better value as they can be used for trans-rectal scans and biopsies as well as trans-vaginal scans.

The choice of which frequency of probe to buy has been eased by the advent of multifrequency, broad-band probes which can be switched from their most efficient centre frequency to cover a range of frequencies, usually from 5 to 7.5 MHz. The higher frequency has a better resolution but poorer depth of penetration. The undoubted benefit of trans-vaginal ultrasound is the ability to place a higher-frequency probe adjacent to the organ of interest.

The procedure should be explained carefully to the patient. Most women are familiar with a speculum examination for cervical smear, and increasingly more women have had experience or have heard about trans-vaginal

scans. It has been shown that for many women trans-vaginal ultrasound is more comfortable than transabdominal ultrasound with a full bladder.[9,10] A study of acceptability in low-risk women in the normal first trimester showed that 88.1% agreed to undergo trans-vaginal scanning. Those who refused did so most commonly for fear of miscarriage or discomfort.[10] Those women who had had trans-vaginal scans before reported much less anxiety about the technique than those who had not.

An empty bladder is best for first-trimester trans-vaginal scans. A partially full bladder is only required if greater detail of cervical anatomy is needed. There is no need for the woman to be put into lithotomy stirrups: positioning her with her buttocks near the end of the couch and her feet supported on a ledge or chair just below the end of the couch allows good access. Raising the hips on a pillow may not give room to direct the probe anteriorly enough to view the fundus of an anteverted uterus, but is usually adequate. A head-down tilt is counter productive, as free fluid tends to run away from the pelvis.

The transducer should be covered with a protective sheath or condom. (This does not absolve the operator from having to clean the probe between patients, as contamination can still occur.) Gel is required to facilitate sound transmission and for lubrication. The labia should be parted to allow entry of the probe. Once in the vagina the probe can be manipulated by rotation, angling from side to side or up and down, and also by sliding the probe further in or out. A routine of examination should be developed. Most people start by examining the uterus and the endometrial cavity. This should include views of the cervix. The adnexae can then be searched for free fluid and any masses. The ovaries can be located either adjacent to the uterus, or in the pouch of Douglas, or lying anterior to the internal iliac vessels. Occasionally the ovaries lie above the uterus and transabdominal scanning may be needed to see them. The region of interest, once located, should be studied with optimum depth and focus settings. Extra information can be gained by using the free hand to press on the lower abdomen to bring structures into view. Moving the probe and pressing with the free hand can be used to test for adhesions by seeing if organs will slide freely, and can also help by localising a region of pain. Finally, on withdrawing the probe the bladder and urethra may be seen.[11]

Normal early pregnancy

There can be confusion when discussing early pregnancy, as embryologists describe embryonic age from the time of fertilisation, whereas clinicians use menstrual age measured from the first day of the last normal menstrual period. Consequently, blastocyst implantation into the endometrium occurs at the end of the first week of embryonic age, or 3 weeks menstrual age, assuming a 4-week menstrual cycle. It is at this stage that early chorionic villi develop and start to secrete hCG and the pregnancy test becomes positive, before the next menstruation is missed. A sign called the 'intradecidual' sign of a focus of high reflectivity with thickening of the adjacent endometrium is thought to represent the implantation site, and can be seen at 25 days menstrual age.[12] This is, however, an unreliable and difficult feature to detect and its appearances may be mimicked by secretory endometrium.

Gestation sac

The earliest that ultrasound is able to detect the gestation sac is debatable, and variously described as from 3.5 to 5 weeks menstrual age. However, most authors agree that a gestation sac of 2–3 mm mean sac diameter (MSD) is the smallest that can be seen (Fig. 7.2).[13] (MSD is calculated by averaging three orthogonal measurements of the sac, placing the cursors on the chorionic tissue–fluid interface.) Most machines are capable of identifying a 5 mm sac, either transabdominally or trans-vaginally, and there is agreement that this equates to a gestational age of 5 weeks (Fig. 7.3). For almost the next 3 weeks the sac grows at about 1 mm per day. At 5 weeks, when the sac can be consistently identified by sonography, the serum β-hCG levels lie between 500 and 1500 IU/l (second international standard).[14] Thereafter, in early pregnancy the β-hCG levels double approximately every 2 days.[15]

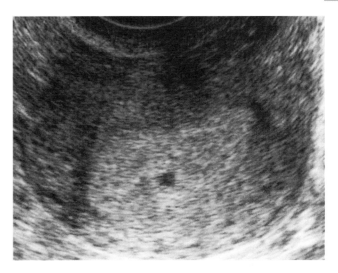

Fig. 7.2 Trans-vaginal scan. There is a 2 mm gestation sac seen within a thickened endometrium. This is the smallest size at which a sac can be seen.

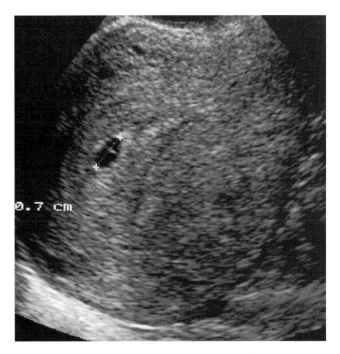

Fig. 7.3 Trans-vaginal scan of an early gestation sac. The longest diameter is measured at 7 mm (between calipers), but the MSD is 5 mm. The yolk sac is visible.

It is important to distinguish a gestation sac from other causes of intra-uterine fluid collections, such as bleeding, endometrial cysts, endometritis and, most importantly, the 'pseudosac' appearance associated with ectopic pregnancy. The most reliable indicators are the presence of a yolk sac or embryonic pole within the sac, but in early pregnancy these may not yet be present or visible and other ways of identifying a true sac are required. A gestation sac should lie within the endometrium and not within the cavity, where the other collections are seen. Collections in the endometrial cavity often have an elongated pointed configuration (Fig. 7.4). Gestation sacs are convex and appear rounded or ovoid, although care should be taken that the sac is not being distorted by an overfull bladder. A gestation sac characteristically has a rim of higher reflectivity around it, corresponding to a combination of chorion, trophoblast and decidua capsularis. This is called the 'chorionic rim' and is seen in 80% of gestational sacs (Fig. 7.5). It is open to misinterpretation and can be erroneously seen around 'pseudosacs', and so does not exclude ectopic pregnancy.[16] The 'double decidual sac' sign of two concentric reflective rings or a crescent around the sac is thought to be specific for an intra-uterine gestation sac.[17,18] The outer ring probably represents the deeper reflective layer of decidua vera beyond the gestation sac (Fig. 7.6). Unfortunately, in up to a third of normal gestation sacs this sign is not seen, and even when present it does not imply that the sac is viable, as it is also seen in blighted ova. Even so, when present it has value in confirming an intra-uterine pregnancy. Low-impedance endometrial arterial blood flow is another discriminator for an intra-uterine pregnancy.[16] The negative predictive value of endometrial blood flow for an ectopic pregnancy is of the order of 97% when cut-off values of peak systolic velocity and resistance index of over 15 cm/s and under 0.55 respectively are used.[16,19]

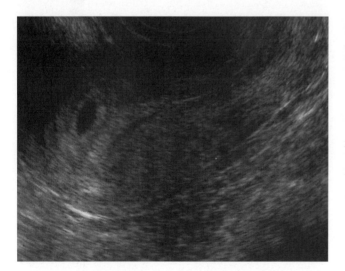

Fig. 7.4 Endometrial reaction. There is an elongated fluid collection (between calipers) within the endometrial cavity. This was an endometrial reaction (pseudosac) associated with an ectopic pregnancy. It can be confused with a gestation sac.

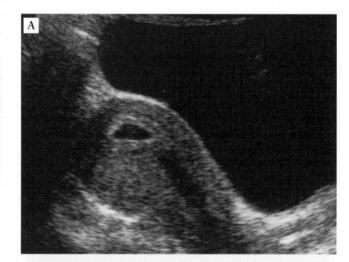

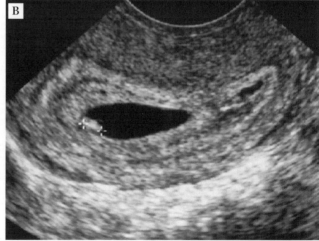

Fig. 7.6 The 'double decidual sac'. sign. A: Transabdominal and **B:** trans-vaginal images, demonstrating the two concentric rings or crescents around the sac that are thought specific but not sensitive for a gestation sac.

Fig. 7.5 The 'chorionic rim'. This is a ring of higher reflectivity seen around 80% of gestation sacs. It is a non-specific finding.

The yolk sac

The early gestation sac contains chorionic fluid. Within it develops the embryonic plate, with the yolk sac on one side and the developing amnion on the other. This produces the 'double bleb' sign that is described as occurring at about 5.5 weeks menstrual age, but which is rarely seen because it is such a transient feature as the amnion is growing rapidly (Fig. 7.7). The embryonic plate is not readily seen with transabdominal transducers at this stage, but the beat of the developing embryonic heart is often observed along the margin of the yolk sac. Trans-vaginal transducers may permit visualisation of the thickening along the yolk sac margin which is the embryo when it is less than 5 mm in length (Fig. 7.8).[20] The amnion grows and envelops the embryo. The yolk sac lies within the chorionic cavity, though this space is gradually obliterated by the growing amnion. The yolk sac remains close to the embryo and is joined to it by a stalk, the vitelline duct.

The yolk sac is seen by ultrasound from the 5th to the 12th weeks of menstrual age. At 5 weeks, when the yolk sac can be first seen on trans-vaginal scan, it occupies about half of the diameter of the gestation sac (Fig. 7.3). Transabdominal transducers do not consistently demonstrate the yolk sac until the MSD is over 15 mm (about 6.5 weeks menstrual age). Longitudinal studies of the yolk sac have shown that it grows in size from the 5th to the 10th week, when it reaches a diameter of 5–6 mm. Thereafter it shrinks until it is no longer seen, at around 12 weeks menstrual age.[21] Variations in the size of the yolk sac from normal, to small (less than 2 mm) or too large (greater than 6 mm), are an indicator of a poor prognosis.

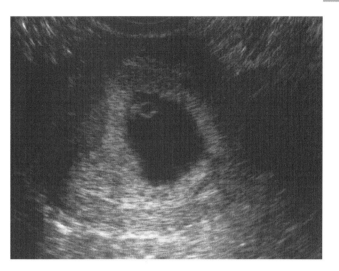

Fig. 7.8 An embryo with a CRL of less than 5 mm. The discoid thickening along the margin of the yolk sac represents the embryo. It measures less than 5 mm. A heartbeat may be visible but this is not always the case.

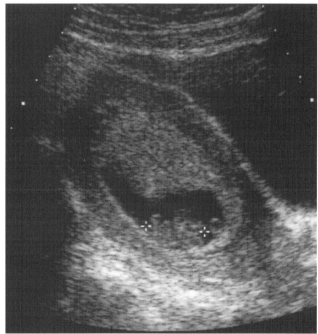

Fig. 7.9 An embryo with a CRL of 23 mm. Transabdominal scan showing an embryo (between calipers) with a CRL of 23 mm. There is a normal-sized yolk sac; however, sonographic interest is directed primarily at the embryo to look for a heartbeat.

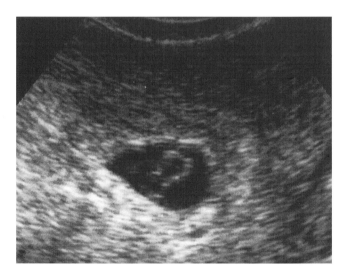

Fig. 7.7 The 'double bleb' sign. A transient early feature occurring at around 5.5 weeks menstrual age, when the two small rings within the gestation sac represent the yolk sac adjacent to the enlarging amniotic sac.

The main importance of the yolk sac in early pregnancy is to confirm that the collection of fluid seen does in fact represent a gestation sac. Once the embryo itself becomes visible it dominates the sonographic observations (Fig. 7.9).

The embryo

Trans-vaginal transducers are able to detect the thickening of the yolk sac margin that is the embryo when the crown–rump length is only 2–3 mm. This may be before cardiac activity is detectable, and has important implications when the diagnosis of pregnancy failure is considered. At 6 weeks menstrual age, when the crown–rump length of the embryo is 5 mm, it should be seen by trans-vaginal ultrasound as a separate structure from the yolk sac, and cardiac pulsation is usually visible. Mean gestational sac diameter at this stage is 18–20 mm.

Heart rate

The embryonic heartbeat is usually visible by trans-vaginal sonography from 6 weeks menstrual age. An M-mode trace taken through the cardiac pulsation is the best way of determining the heart rate (Fig. 7.10). There is a gradual increase in rate from 6 weeks until almost 9 weeks. A slow rate is a poor prognosis indicator for the pregnancy's survival. A study of 1185 early first-trimester ultrasound scans found that the mean heart rate increased from 110 beats per minute (bpm) at less than 6.2 weeks to 159 bpm at 7.6–8.0 weeks.[22] Another study found the peak mean heart rate of 175 bpm occurred at 9 weeks, and thereafter decreased to 166 bpm at 12 weeks.[23] Rates below 100 bpm before 6.2 weeks and below 120 bpm at 6.3–7 weeks are associated with a significantly increased incidence of first-trimester pregnancy failure, and rates below 80 bpm and 100 bpm at the same ages have a uniformly dismal prognosis. A slow rate should prompt appropriate counselling and early follow-up with a further scan.[24] Evacuation of the uterus should never be advocated on the basis of a slow heart rate alone.

Embryonic anatomy

Trans-vaginal ultrasound allows visualisation of embryonic structures at an earlier menstrual age than is generally possible with transabdominal transducers, usually by at least a week or two. Trans-vaginal ultrasound can just distinguish the head of the embryo during the 7th week of menstrual age, when the embryo has a crown–rump length (CRL) of about 12 mm, whereas transabdominal scans cannot usually make this distinction until 9–10 weeks. The early development of the brain is particularly interesting, as only a single large cerebral ventricle is seen on the scans, sometimes allowing the head of the embryo to appear very similar to the yolk sac. A knowledge of this early anatomy is important if errors in the diagnosis of malformations such as holoprosencephaly are not to be made (Fig. 7.11) (see also Ch. 14). Surprisingly detailed information on the embryonic hindbrain can be obtained using 7.5 MHz transducers. Blaas and colleagues[25] have shown that the

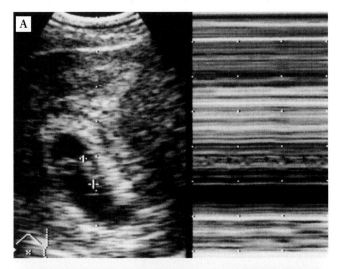

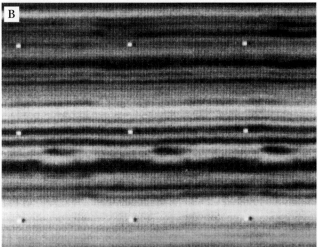

Fig. 7.10 Embryonic heartbeat. A: The heartbeat is demonstrated in M-mode. The cursor line on the image is placed through the cardiac pulsation. The M-mode trace shows the echoes received from this line mapped out against time. **B:** Magnified view of M-mode trace. The dotted vertical lines are half-second intervals. The heart rate is over 120 bpm.

single ventricle seen from 7 weeks onward represents the fourth ventricle within the rhombencephalon. The developing cerebellum could be seen in 80% of their population by 8 weeks, and the cerebellar hemispheres appeared to meet in the midline during weeks 11–12. These observations may in time allow the early diagnosis of Dandy–Walker and Arnold–Chiari malformations.[26] The trunk has relatively few recognisable structures in the first trimester, the heart, the stomach and the physiological midgut herniation predominating. Embryologically the lumen of the primitive gut is well defined after 6 weeks. Swallowing movements are thought to begin at 11 weeks, so before this time any fluid within the gut is probably epithelial secretions.[27] The stomach can be seen in most embryos by 10 weeks men-

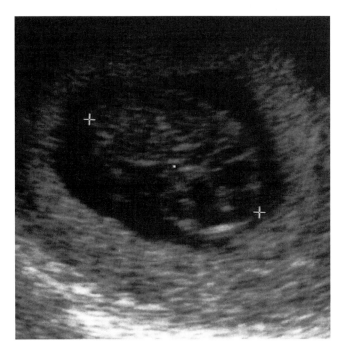

Fig. 7.11 Trans-vaginal image of a normal embryo at 8.5 weeks menstrual age. Note that at this stage of development, the cranium appears cystic.

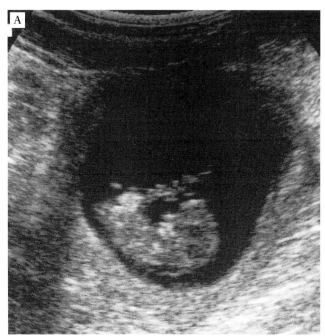

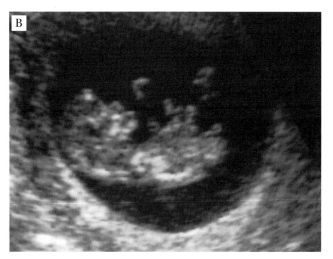

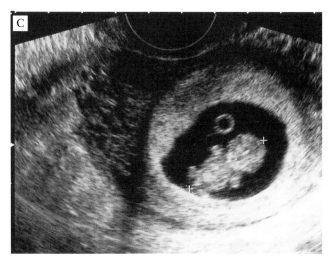

strual age, and in all by 11 weeks.[23] Physiological gut herniation, which leads to elongation and rotation of the bowel, can be identified as a swelling in the base of the cord in some embryos before 8 weeks, but can always be seen between 8.5 and 10.5 weeks (Fig. 7.12). The bowel should have returned to the abdomen in all fetuses by the 12th week, or 45 mm CRL. This has implications for the early diagnosis of exomphalos but does not exclude this diagnosis, as measurements of the size of the normal physiological herniation have been made.[23,28] If an exomphalos is large or contains the liver a presumptive diagnosis can be made in the 10th week.[29] Screening programmes for nuchal thickness at 11–14 weeks are able to detect exomphalos, and also show the strong association between exomphalos and trisomies 18 or 13.[30]

The limb buds can be seen trans-vaginally by 8 weeks menstrual age, and bones and joints become apparent by 9 weeks (Fig. 7.12C). Even transabdominal scans can identify digits by 12 weeks. Vermiform movements of the embryo can be seen from 7 weeks, and by the 8th week flexion and extension of the trunk may be seen. Movement becomes more coordinated during the 10th week and

Fig. 7.12 Normal embryonic development. A and B: Physiological gut herniation into the base of the umbilical cord can be seen in both these embryos (10 weeks). **C:** Limb buds are clearly visible in this 9-week menstrual age pregnancy.

by the 11th week there is an increase in limb movements, particularly the lower limbs, which produce sudden jumps of the embryo.

Three-dimensional (3D) ultrasound can elegantly demonstrate first-trimester anatomy, and may make it possible to appreciate some details earlier than by 2D trans-vaginal scans alone. Limb buds can be clearly seen at 7 weeks menstrual age. By 12 weeks the fetal face, orbits, nose, mouth and digits can be beautifully shown by 3D trans-vaginal scans.[31] The quality of the 3D image does depend on the quality of the source 2D images, and also on the embryo keeping still during the acquisition time. There are problems with the speed at which the 3D image can be produced, its resolution, and with making measurements on the produced image but, despite this, enthusiasts claim the technique has a valuable diagnostic role that can only increase as the technology evolves.

The embryo officially becomes the fetus at the end of the 10th menstrual week, when the period of organogenesis has finished. Thereafter the fetus shows maturation and growth of the tissues and organs.

It has been advocated that all pregnant women should be offered an anomaly scan at the end of the first trimester, not only to assign gestational age and assess the anatomy, but also to measure the nuchal thickness.[32] This latter has been shown to be a good screening test for chromosomal anomalies and heart defects. It should be remembered, though, that such a policy would not obviate the need for a further anatomy scan at 18–20 weeks menstrual age, or even a growth scan in the third trimester, as some anomalies, particularly those in the urinary tract, do not manifest themselves until later. A pilot screening study at 14 weeks gestation demonstrated that 53% of anomalies could be found, with another 32% being found at second-trimester rescreening and the remaining 15% later in pregnancy or after birth.[33] Inevitably, early trans-vaginal screening will be added to later screening, rather than as a replacement. This has obvious cost implications.

Placenta and membranes

The placenta and the chorionic membrane have the same origin. The early chorion surrounding the gestation sac has chorionic villi all around it. However, probably due to some nutritional disparity, there is more development near the deep endometrium (decidua basalis) and loss of villi elsewhere. This produces the differentiation into the chorion frondosum and the chorion laeve, the former becoming the placenta and the latter the chorionic membrane. Consequently these two structures are always joined, such that the chorionic membrane leads to the edge of the placenta and is inseparable from it. The chorionic membrane can easily be stripped from the underlying endometrium by any fluid accumulation. This is

usually blood, either occurring spontaneously or following needle placement for amniocentesis or other intervention. Such a collection is called a subchorionic haematoma (Fig. 7.13).

The amnion develops rapidly from the double bleb sign seen at 5.5 weeks, so that it surrounds the embryo but excludes the yolk sac. The amnion is often invisible at very early gestations, but once there is sufficient amniotic fluid to separate the amnion from the embryo it becomes visible. The amnion covers the umbilical cord also. The fluid within the gestation sac changes as the fluid-filled amnion grows to fill the chorionic space. The yolk sac lies within the diminishing chorionic fluid in the chorio-amniotic space. The amnion fuses with the chorion at around 12 weeks, though this fusion is not necessarily permanent and needle trauma can allow amniotic fluid into this space. Chorio-amniotic fluid can be distinguished from a subchorionic haematoma as the former can lie over the fetal surface of the placenta, whereas the latter cannot.

In summary, there are four regions where bleeding can occur:

1. behind the placenta – abruption, separating the placenta from the endometrium,
2. subchorionic – effectively in the endometrial cavity,
3. chorio-amniotic – in the chorionic cavity,
4. intra-amniotic.

The last two are not necessarily harmful to the fetus.

The site of placental formation can often be seen with trans-vaginal ultrasound at 8 weeks menstrual age, but more commonly it is only discernible after 9 weeks. The polarisation of the chorion into the placenta and chorionic membrane usually appears complete on ultrasound by 12 weeks, but may not be pathologically so until 17 weeks.[34] It is possible for trans-vaginal sonography to exclude a diagnosis of placenta praevia after 9 weeks.[35] However, the converse is not true, as 6% of patients at 9–13 weeks will appear to have a placenta praevia but, owing to subsequent villous atrophy and development of the lower uterine segment, the incidence of placenta praevia at term is only around 0.5%.

Colour Doppler can demonstrate the normal early placental circulation (Fig. 7.14). The earliest signals can be discerned in the retrochorionic space as soon as the gestation sac is seen. Venous Doppler signals can be obtained from the intervillous spaces as early as 5 weeks. Retrochorionic and umbilical peak systolic velocities increase, whereas their resistance and pulsatility indices decrease throughout the first trimester.[36] Some researchers have suggested that placental failure might be seen in early pregnancy using Doppler, enabling the prediction of those who will have growth restriction before growth actually slows down.[37] This concept has yet to be proven.

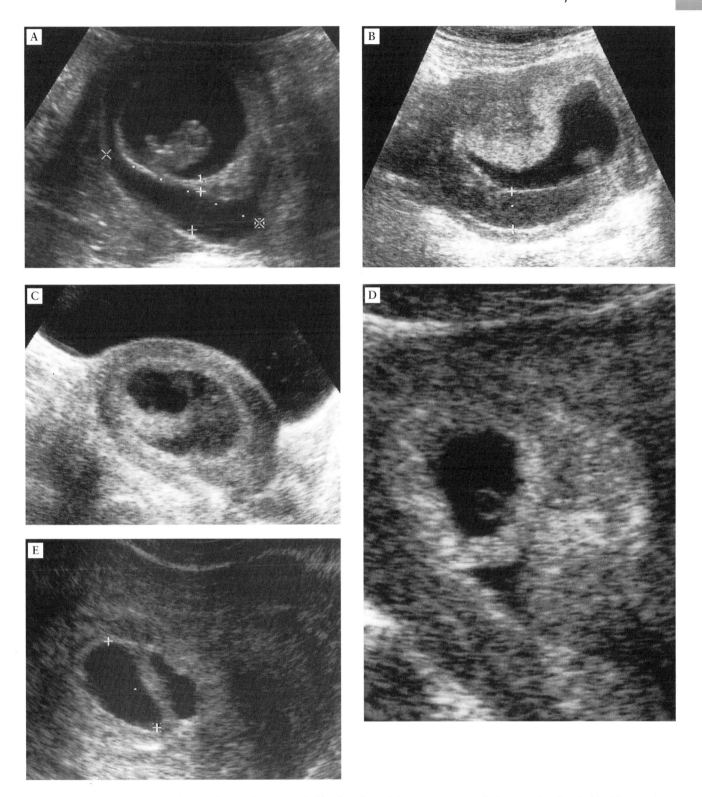

Fig. 7.13 Haemorrhage. A: A subchorionic haemorrhage is marked by the calipers. The contents are anechoic, suggesting that the bleed is not recent. **B:** This subchorionic haemorrhage (between calipers) contains echoes indicating fresh bleeding. Note how the chorionic membrane joins on to the edge of the placenta. **C:** This subchorionic haemorrhage is extending behind the placenta and separating the placenta from the endometrium. **D:** Six-week pregnancy. The small triangular area of fluid represents a small implantation bleed within the endometrial cavity and is of no consequence. **E:** This shows a failed pregnancy, diagnosed because of lack of growth. There is a haemorrhage adjacent to the sac that could at first sight mimic a twin pregnancy, a pitfall to be avoided.

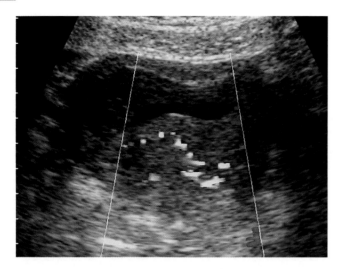

Fig. 7.14 Early placental blood flow. Colour flow Doppler showing early placental blood flow.

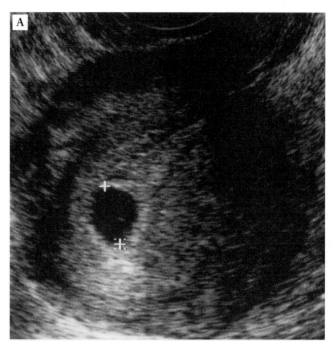

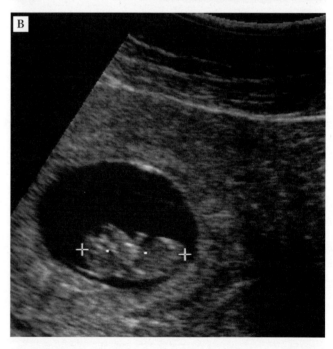

Fig. 7.15 Gestation sac diameter and crown–rump length measurements. A: Gestation sac diameter measurement (12 mm). The calipers are placed on the chorionic tissue–fluid interface. **B:** Crown–rump length measurement. There are no defined landmarks on which to place the calipers. The longest CRL obtained (26 mm) is assumed to be correct.

Measurements in the first trimester

Assignment of gestational age can be achieved from the woman's menstrual history or from measurements of gestation or embryonic size. If an ideal menstrual history can be obtained – that is, one in which the first day of the last period is known in a woman with regular periods, no unusual bleeding and no use of the contraceptive pill in the past 2 months – then it is as accurate at predicting the date of delivery as any measurement.[38] Unfortunately, such a history is only available for about a half of women and measurements are required.[39]

The measurements used to determine gestational age suffer inaccuracies because the positions of the measurement cursors may not be reproducible and because of biological variations in size. Furthermore, the charts against which the measurements are compared may not have been appropriately compiled.[40] The gestation sac dimensions and the crown–rump length of the embryo are commonly used in the first trimester (Fig. 7.15).

The gestation sac can be measured as a volume or as a mean sac diameter: both can acheive accuracies of ± 1 week, but only for a short period of time from 5 to 6.5 weeks.

Once the embryo is visible, measurement of the CRL supersedes gestation sac measurements.[41] There are potential sources of error in obtaining the CRL, not least that there are no defined anatomical markers from which to measure. The assumption is that the longest CRL obtained is the correct one. Pitfalls to be aware of are the inclusion of the yolk sac or other non-embryonic structure or artefact within the measurement (Fig. 7.16), and the curvature of the embryo. The embryo can flex and extend itself, altering the measurement, and later in the first trimester the fetus tends to lie with a flexed neck, causing under-

estimation of the CRL. Notwithstanding these comments, pregnancy is most accurately dated by measurements in the first trimester, even though a biparietal diameter measurement at 18 weeks is also reliable.[38] When ultrasound is used to date a pregnancy, the date should be determined at

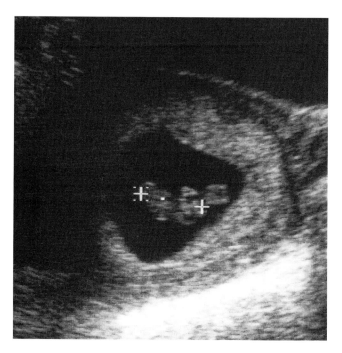

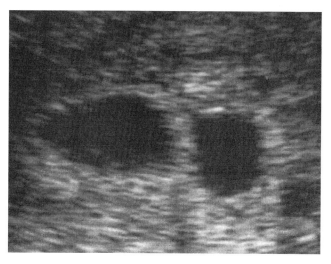

Fig. 7.17 **Twin gestation sacs.** There are two separate sacs with a thick dividing membrane, indicating a dichorionic pregnancy.

Fig. 7.16 **CRL measurement of 16 mm (8 weeks).** Care must be taken not to include the yolk sac in the measurement. The fetal head can mimic a yolk sac at this gestation.

the time of the first scan with acceptable measurements. Subsequent ultrasound measurements at later scans should not be used to adjust that date.[42]

Multiple pregnancy

It is possible to identify a multiple pregnancy as early as 5 weeks menstrual age, when more than one gestation sac is seen (Fig. 7.17). Caution should be exercised as there is a high rate of reduction – the so-called 'vanishing twin'. In one study of live twins detected by 7 weeks, only 71% went on to produce live twin neonates. Each twin, if live before 7 weeks, has a 19% risk of *in utero* death and, if alive between 7 and 10 weeks, an 11% risk of *in utero* death.[43] Another study gave a figure of 21% spontaneous reduction in twin pregnancy to singleton by the second trimester.[44] The possibility of impending death of one of the embryos is raised by seeing one sac smaller than the other, or the sac appearing too small for the embryo, and by one embryo being visibly smaller than the other (Fig. 7.18). The likelihood of reduction is unrelated to maternal age, method of conception or indication for the ultrasound scan, but is related to gestational age, chorionicity and the scan findings.[45] In summary, the earlier the

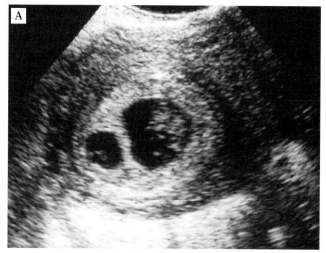

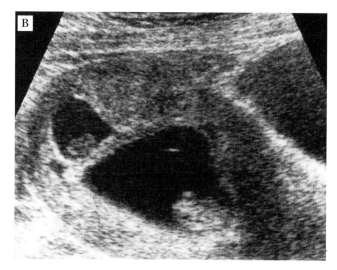

Fig. 7.18 **Failed twin. A:** The discrepancy in sac sizes indicates that the smaller sac has or will fail. **B:** The two embryos are different in size. The smaller one does not have a visible heartbeat and has died.

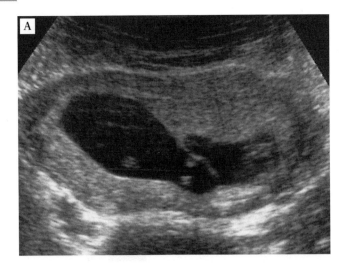

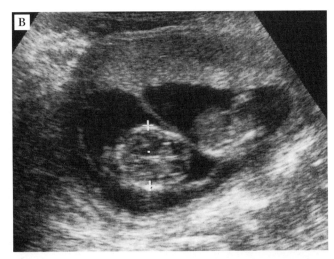

Fig. 7.19 The 'lambda' sign. A and **B:** Both these pregnancies show a triangular area of placenta extending into the inter-twin membrane base. This is a reliable sign of dichorionicity. There is also a subchorionic haemorrhage visible in **B**.

gestational age at which the twins are diagnosed, the greater the probability that spontaneous fetal loss will occur.

The first trimester is an ideal time during which to assess the chorionicity and amnionicity of a twin pregnancy. This information should always be recorded, as the chorionicity has significant implications for the prognosis of the pregnancy.[46] Monochorionic twins are at much higher risk of a poor perinatal outcome than dichorionic twins. A monochorionic pregnancy is at risk for twin–twin transfusion syndromes that can cause fetal death and neurological deficits in the survivor. If a co-twin dies in a dichorionic pregnancy there are no risks to its fellow, but in a monochorionic pregnancy the survivor may suffer hypotension and death or brain damage. Conjoint twins or entangled cords are rare complications occurring in monoamniotic twins. Chorionicity can be established in the second trimester by determining fetal sex, establishing that there are two separate placentae, and by assessing the thickness of the dividing membrane, but this assessment is time-consuming and not always achievable (see Ch. 12). Fortunately the 'lambda sign' in early pregnancy has been found to be highly reliable. This consists of the finding of chorionic tissue projecting into the base of the inter-twin membrane where it joins the placenta (Fig. 7.19). It is most reliable at 10 to 14 weeks gestation, when it is found in all dichorionic pregnancies and in no monochorionic ones. Later in pregnancy it becomes less useful because it is harder to see, and in 7% of dichorionic pregnancies may disappear by 20 weeks.[47] Before 10 weeks chorionicity and amnionicity can be determined very reliably by counting the number of gestation sacs (Fig. 7. 20) and by determining the presence or absence of an amnion around each embryo.[48–50] In addition, before 8 weeks menstrual age, when the amnion may be too thin

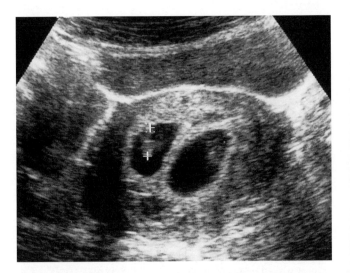

Fig. 7.20 Dichorionic twins. The two separate gestation sacs are clearly shown. CRL 8 mm. This is an ideal time at which to determine chorionicity.

to see, the amnionicity of a monochorionic pregnancy can be found by counting the number of yolk sacs. If there are two yolk sacs there must be two amnions, but if only one yolk sac can be found careful follow-up is required.[51]

Threatened abortion

Symptoms and signs

The commonest symptom in early pregnancy is vaginal bleeding, which occurs in about 25% of clinically apparent pregnancies. It is the main symptom of threatened abortion and identifies a group at increased risk of early pregnancy loss.[52] Pelvic and lower abdominal pain that is characteristically colicky or period-like may occur with or without bleeding. The symptoms of a normal pregnancy, such as nausea and vomiting or breast tenderness, may diminish, implying low hCG levels. Conversely hyper-emesis gravidarum may develop, suggesting molar change.

The physical signs include a uterus of inappropriate size for dates, i.e. either too small or too large. There may be focal or generalised tenderness, guarding, or occasionally cervical excitation. Vaginal examination may show an open cervix, which indicates that abortion is inevitable, particularly when in association with contraction-like pain and bleeding.

Expulsion of a non-viable gestation nearly always occurs spontaneously, but may be delayed for weeks after symptoms start; during that time the woman may suffer continued bleeding, infection and anxiety. There are hormonal assays (such as β-hCG and progesterone) that aid the diagnosis of pregnancy failure, but it is ultrasound that has become crucial in determining the prognosis and in facilitating the timely management of miscarriage.

Once trans-vaginal ultrasound has identified the successful development of each successive embryonic landmark the likelihood of pregnancy failure decreases. A study by Goldstein[53] showed that if a gestation sac developed there was a pregnancy loss rate of 11.5%; once a yolk sac was seen, the subsequent loss rate reduced to 8.5%. The loss rate was 7.2% with an embryo of up to 5 mm, reduced to 3.3% with an embryo of 6–10 mm, and further to 0.5% with an embryo larger than 10 mm. This study also suggested that there were two distinct periods of early pregnancy loss, the first in the embryonic period up to 10 weeks menstrual age, and the second, after a hiatus, in the fetal period from 14 to 20 weeks. In contrast, a screening study at 10–13 weeks menstrual age found a 3% prevalence of non-viable pregnancies, although some of these pregnancies will have failed prior to the 10th week and only been diagnosed as 'missed abortions' at the later menstrual age.[54] This background level of loss in apparently normal pregnancies should be borne in mind when calculating the loss rate from chorionic villous sampling in the first trimester.

Terms of pregnancy failure

Threatened abortion

This is a clinically descriptive term used for women in the first 20 weeks of pregnancy with vaginal spotting or bleeding, minor cramps and a closed cervical os.

Inevitable abortion

Inevitable abortion is a clinical diagnosis made with the finding of a dilated cervical canal and first-trimester uterine bleeding. There may be cramping pain approach-

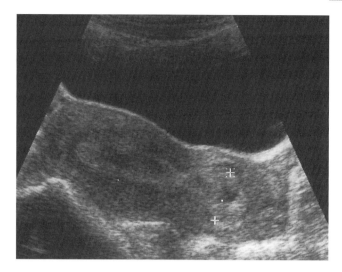

Fig. 7.21 Inevitable abortion. There is a separated gestation sac (between calipers) seen lying low within the uterus.

ing the severity of labour pains. 'Inevitable' implies that the abortion is in progress. Some prefer to subdivide this with a further diagnosis of imminent abortion, indicating that abortion is about to occur. Ultrasound is rarely required as the management is clinical. If an ultrasound is performed then the findings of a separated sac lying low in the uterus (Fig. 7.21) and a dilated cervical canal confirm the clinical impression, even though a heartbeat may still be detected. Rarely the sac will be seen to move position during the course of the scan (Fig. 7.22).

Missed abortion

The traditional definition of missed abortion is fetal death before 20 weeks menstrual age without expulsion of the fetus for at least 8 weeks afterwards.[55] This is obviously an inappropriate definition now that ultrasound is able to identify an embryo without a heartbeat from 6 weeks on, and the term is probably best not used.

Blighted ovum

When the gestational sac is at least 25 mm in diameter and no embryonic parts can be seen it is termed a blighted ovum (Fig. 7.23). This is synonymous with an 'anembryonic pregnancy'. The differentiation of an anembryonic pregnancy from an incomplete abortion on ultrasound criteria alone is not always possible, as a tiny non-viable embryo within the sac may be too small or too closely applied to the wall to find with ultrasound.

Incomplete abortion

This term is used if the embryo has died or failed to develop and the products of conception have not yet been

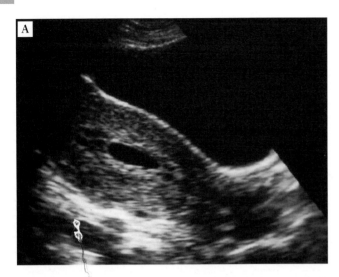

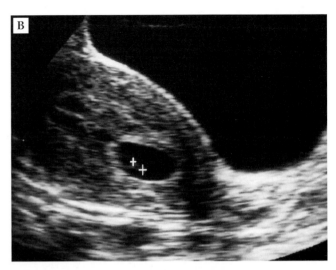

Fig. 7.22 Inevitable abortion. A and **B:** These images were obtained a few minutes apart. The sac can be seen to have migrated towards the cervix.

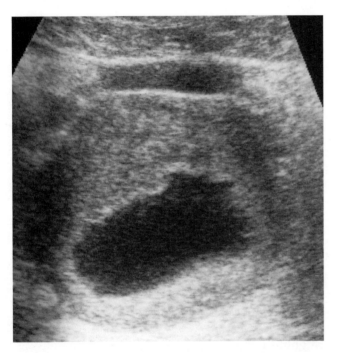

Fig. 7.23 Blighted ovum. This large irregular-shaped gestation sac with no visible embryonic parts is either a blighted ovum or an incomplete abortion. Ultrasound cannot make this distinction.

totally expelled from the uterus. This heading can include blighted ova and missed abortions under its rather large and non-specific umbrella. The differentiation between retained products of conception and simple retained blood clot can be difficult because the appearances of blood can be so variable. Some highly reflective clot may mimic the appearances of embryonic parts (Fig. 7.24). The clinical context should always be taken into account. Women in whom the vaginal bleeding is settling and only a little

reflective material is seen in the uterine cavity are best managed expectantly, with further ultrasound as required, rather than rushing to perform curettage with its risks of uterine perforation (Fig. 7.25).

Complete abortion

This is abortion in which all the products of conception have been expelled from the uterus (Fig. 7.26). The pitfall is to diagnose a normal-appearing uterus as complete abortion when in fact either the pregnancy is not as advanced as was thought and the gestation sac is not yet visible, or there is an ectopic pregnancy without a visible decidual reaction. Ideally the products of conception should be confirmed histologically to have been expelled before the diagnosis of complete abortion is made.

Ultrasound signs of pregnancy failure

'The primary objective is to formulate criteria for the ultrasound diagnosis of abnormal pregnancies that can be applied prospectively and with complete reliability in the active management of early pregnancy failures.' This statement is paraphrased from Robinson's early pioneering work on the subject and still holds true today.[56] One of the most important elements of any ultrasound examination is a judgement of its technical quality, as this will obviously influence the reliability of any sonographic sign sought. If an examination is thought to be of poor quality then any negative observation (such as an absent heartbeat) should be treated with caution and the scan repeated after an adequate interval to assess change. The signs of viability are often related to menstrual age. Certain features should always be present by a given age, such that their absence implies pregnancy failure. It is vitally important to under-

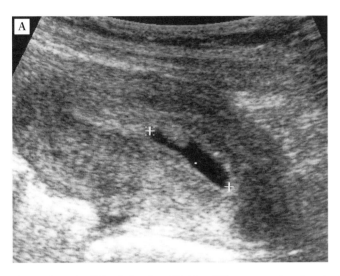

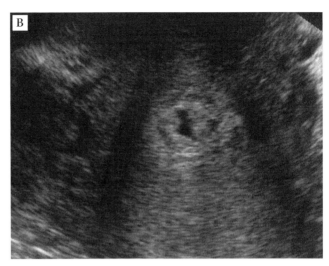

Fig. 7.24 Retained blood clot. A and **B:** Two different examples of retained blood clot following miscarriage. In both there is the potential for confusion with embryonic parts. No heartbeat is visible.

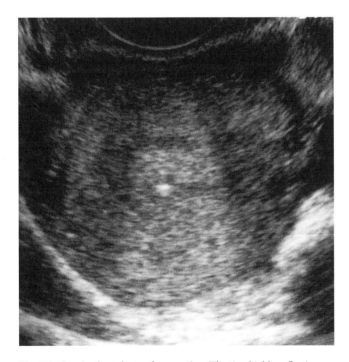

Fig. 7.25 Retained products of conception. The tiny highly reflective fleck within the endometrium represents retained products of conception following miscarriage. The management depends on the clinical context, but if bleeding is settling then expectant management is best.

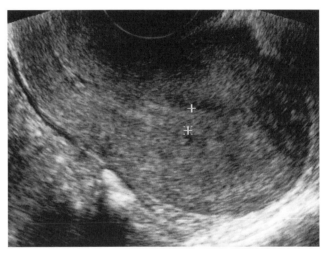

Fig. 7.26 Normal uterine appearances following a complete abortion.

stand the patient's reported dates may be unreliable, and that they should be excluded from any assessment of viability. Too often a pregnancy is thought non-viable when in fact it is merely less advanced than the patient thought. It was this error that led to the Cardiff inquiry.[1] The establishment of menstrual age should be based solely on measurable features on the scan. There is one exception to this rule: patients who have undergone assisted conception by methods such as artificial insemination or *in vitro* fertilisation know their date of conception, and it would be unwise to ignore this.

Heartbeat

The most reliable sign of a live embryo is the demonstration of a heartbeat. Unfortunately, the converse is no longer true now that trans-vaginal sonography can demonstrate very small embryonic poles of 2–4 mm, which can still be alive even though no heartbeat can be discerned: negative observations are much harder to make than positive ones. The first essential is to be sure that the structure being examined for a heartbeat is in fact the embryo. Once the CRL is larger than 10 mm this is easy, because there should be a definable head and body. Below this size only the presence of the heartbeat can confirm that the structure is an embryo; obviously this will not be present if the embryo is dead. The embryo should lie adjacent to the yolk sac and be surrounded by amnion. These features help differentiate it from a decidual reaction with a mimicking clot in the cavity. Once the embryo is identified enough time must be spent examining it for a heartbeat.

Transabdominal ultrasound cannot reliably find a heartbeat in a live embryo until the CRL is 10 mm; transvaginal scans cannot achieve this until the CRL is 6 mm. Consequently, if the embryo is smaller than this or the scan is technically poor, the absence of a visible heartbeat should not be used to diagnose pregnancy failure and a repeat scan should be done a week later. If the embryo is larger than these sizes and two independent trained observers agree that there is no heartbeat and the scan is of good quality, then pregnancy failure is diagnosed (Fig. 7.27).

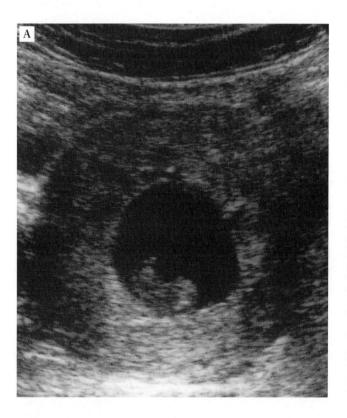

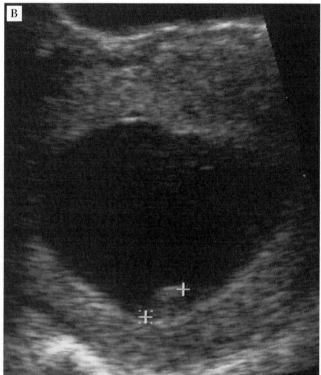

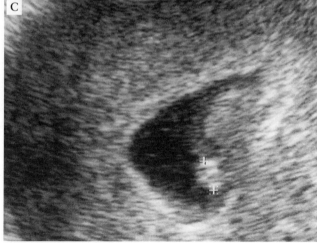

Fig. 7.27 Absent heartbeat. A: 16 mm CRL and **B:** 11 mm CRL embryos on transabdominal scans. No heartbeat was seen in either embryo and embryonic death was diagnosed once two trained observers agreed on the findings. The minor criterion of a poor decidual reaction around both sacs is shown. **B:** also demonstrates disproportion between the CRL and the gestation sac size. Notwithstanding these minor criteria, it is the absent heartbeat that is used to diagnose pregnancy failure. **C:** Trans-vaginal scan. 4 mm CRL. This is too small to diagnose pregnancy failure on the basis of an absent heartbeat. A repeat scan after an interval is required.

Gestation sac

The identification of a gestation sac over a certain size without identifiable embryonic parts is a major criterion of pregnancy failure. The debate lies in which sizes of sac are reliable. Criteria for transabdominal scans are relatively well accepted. A mean sac diameter of 20 mm or more without a visible yolk sac, or a size of 25 mm or more without a visible embryo, are major criteria for pregnancy failure with a 100% predictive value (Fig. 7.28).[57] Trans-vaginal ultrasound, with its greater resolution, has been thought able to make this diagnosis at smaller sac sizes. Caution should, however, be used in extrapolating results from expert centres looking at selected populations to less experienced staff looking at low-risk patients. Filly[2] advocated that gestation sac diameter values of 13 mm for visualisation of a yolk sac and 18 mm for visualisation of an embryo on trans-vaginal imaging were reliable. These are certainly more conservative than the 6 mm and 10 mm values suggested by Bree *et al*[58] but similar to the values of 13 mm and 17 mm found to be 100% specific by Tongsong *et al*[59] However, even Filly's recommendations may not be conservative enough. Another recent study on 2285 patients revealed 30 patients with gestation sacs of MSD 8–19 mm without visible yolk sacs who went on to develop normal pregnancies.[60] Likewise, there were five women with gestation sacs of 16–19 mm mean diameter without visible embryos who subsequently developed live embryos. These results suggest that pregnancy failure cannot be diagnosed with 100% confidence until the MSD is 20 mm and no embryo or yolk sac is seen. For simplicity, many centres will prefer to apply the same

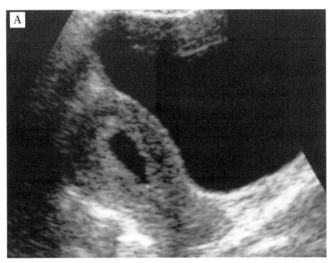

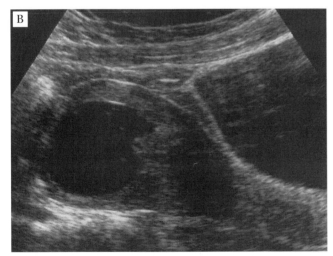

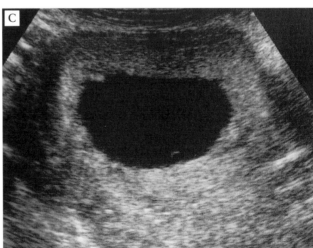

Fig. 7.28 Empty gestation sacs. A: Transabdominal scan showing an apparently empty gestation sac. MSD is, however, less than 20 mm, so no conclusion can be reached and a repeat scan in a week is required. **B:** Transabdominal scan of a 4 cm gestation sac. No embryo can be found and so the diagnosis of pregnancy failure can be made. **C:** Trans-vaginal scan showing a huge gestation sac containing a tiny yolk sac. No embryo is seen, so the pregnancy has failed.

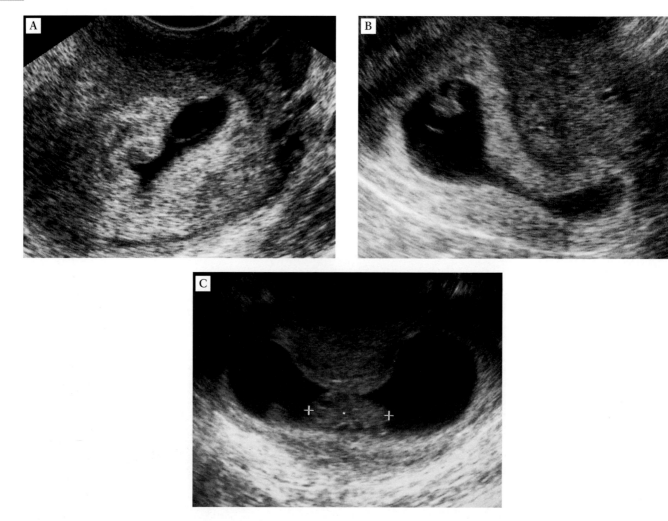

Fig. 7.29 Gestation sacs with unusual shapes. A: An irregular sac shape has been advocated as a minor criterion of pregnancy failure. This sac also shows the empty amnion sign. **B:** An unusual sac shape associated with a non-viable pregnancy. The absent heartbeat is the important sign. **C:** An unusual sac shape with a live pregnancy. This shape is due to a focal uterine contraction.

measurement criteria used for transabdominal scans to the trans-vaginal scans, even though this will increase the number of women who have to return for a rescan after an interval.[1]

The shape of the gestation sac, if very irregular, has been described as a further major criterion of pregnancy failure (Fig. 7.29).[57] Unfortunately this sign is only seen in about 10% of abnormal gestations, and is also rather subjective. The shape can be distorted by an overfull bladder, uterine contractions, fibroids and congenital anomalies of the uterus and not be used as the sole factor in making the diagnosis of a failed pregnancy.

In the first few weeks of pregnancy gestation sac growth is linear. A follow-up examination should show that its volume doubles every week between the fifth and eighth weeks. If it does not, this is suggestive of pregnancy failure. Even though this is interesting it is not clinically useful, because the repeat scan should be directed to determining whether a viable embryo or yolk sac appears. Furthermore, a gestation sac in a blighted ovum may continue to grow and produce β-hCG, though usually in reduced amounts.

The amnion

Between 6.5 and 10 weeks of gestation the length of the amniotic cavity is similar to that of the embryo. Consequently, if the amniotic sac can be seen then the embryo ought also to be visible (Fig. 7.30).[61] An empty amnion is a strong indicator that the pregnancy has failed, even though a yolk sac may also be visible (Fig. 7.31). The empty amnion sign is usually seen in conjunction with a gestation sac large enough that an embryo ought to be visible anyway, so it is useful corroboration of pregnancy

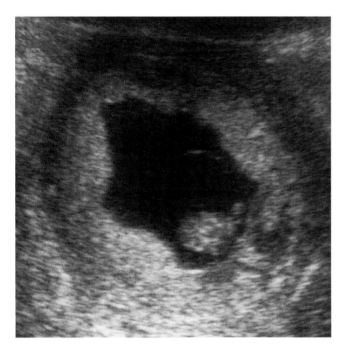

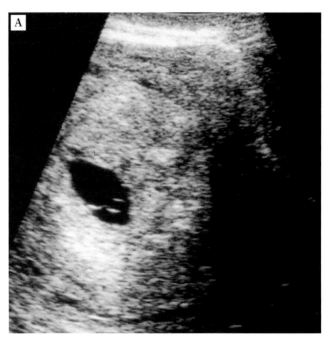

Fig. 7.30 The normal amnion is seen similar in size to the embryo. The two remain similar in length between 6.5 and 10 weeks.

failure rather than a sole diagnostic finding. Later in the first trimester it has also been noted that amniotic fluid volume tends to be excessive with failed pregnancies, and standards for amniotic fluid dynamics have been proposed.[62] Although interesting, this does not improve the diagnosis of a failed pregnancy over the major criteria discussed above.

Minor criteria

There are four minor criteria, all of which are subjective and non-specific and which may accompany a major criterion of failure. These are a thin decidual reaction, a poorly reflective decidual reaction, absence of the double decidual sac sign, and a low position of the sac in the uterus. Because they are non-specific and unreliable they should not be used alone to diagnose pregnancy failure.

Summary

The major criteria of pregnancy failure for reliable diagnosis are:

1. an embryo with a CRL of 6 mm or more on transvaginal ultrasound (10 mm transabdominal) without a heartbeat,
2. a gestation sac of mean diameter 20 mm or more without a yolk sac, or a sac greater than 25 mm MSD without a visible embryo,
3. the empty amnion sign,
4. the absence of growth after a 7–10-day interval.

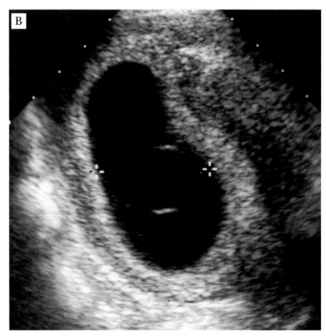

Fig. 7.31 Empty amnion sign. A: Although a yolk sac is seen, there is also a large amniotic cavity. An embryo of equivalent size should be seen and is not. The diagnosis of pregnancy failure can be made.
B: Huge gestation sac with an empty amnion sign. Both features can be used to diagnose pregnancy failure in the absence of an embryo.

Notwithstanding the above, it still remains imperative in desired pregnancies to establish the diagnosis of pregnancy failure properly before offering uterine evacuation. Serial scans or quantitative β-hCG assays, or both, may still be required.

Prognostic factors for pregnancy survival

Now that trans-vaginal ultrasound is able to identify very early live embryos which still have a substantial risk of failing later in the first trimester, there have been attempts to define signs other than the presence of a heartbeat on which to base a prognosis. The use of bradycardia was described earlier in this chapter, though heart rates of less than 85 can be seen in embryos that subsequently develop normally.

Oligohydramnios

Although this term is a misnomer in very early pregnancy, when the amnion is closely applied about the embryo and it is more likely the chorion that is small, it conveys the impression of a small gestation sac relative to the embryo. A difference of less than 5 mm between the MSD and the CRL in a pregnancy with a live embryo at 5.5–9 weeks menstrual age has been reported as predictive of miscarriage in 94% of cases.[63] Others have suggested that this sign is not as grave as originally predicted, and has a survival rate as high as 35%.[60]

Yolk sac

The yolk sac normally lies close to the wall of the gestation sac. Finding the yolk sac floating freely in the middle of the cavity implies that the pregnancy has failed. The size of the yolk sac has been related to prognosis (Fig. 7.32). A yolk sac with a diameter over 2 standard deviations above the mean has about a 60% positive predictive value for failure, and a yolk sac 2 standard deviations below the mean a positive predictive value of only 44%.[64] The same study also found six patients out of 486 who had a yolk sac diameter over 5.6 mm before 10 weeks menstrual age, and all of these had an abnormal outcome. Not everyone has found a large yolk sac size to be useful,[65] and this finding should not be relied on alone to predict failure (Fig. 7.33).

Bleeding

First-trimester pregnancies with vaginal bleeding and a live embryo have approximately twice the failure rate than those without bleeding.[66] Vaginal bleeding is also associated with other adverse pregnancy outcomes such as low birthweight, perinatal death and congenital malformation, but the magnitude of the risk has been found hard to quantify, probably because of lack of standardisation of the descriptions of timing and severity of the bleed.[67] Not

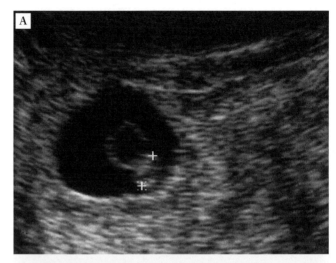

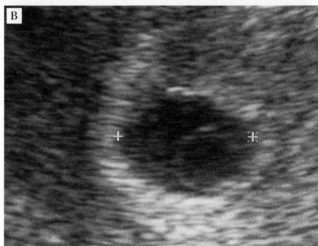

Fig. 7.32 Large yolk sacs. A: A large yolk sac associated with a 7 mm CRL embryo (between calipers). This pregnancy failed. **B:** 12.7 mm gestation sac (between calipers) containing a large yolk sac. This pregnancy also failed.

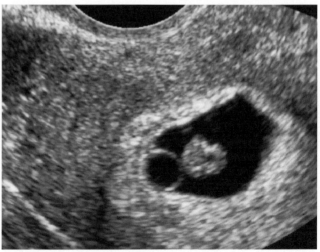

Fig. 7.33 A large yolk sac. A 6 mm yolk sac with a live embryo. Although this is a large sac size and a poor prognostic sign, the pregnancy continued uneventfully.

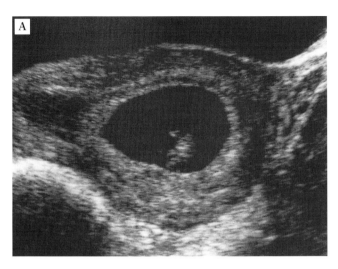

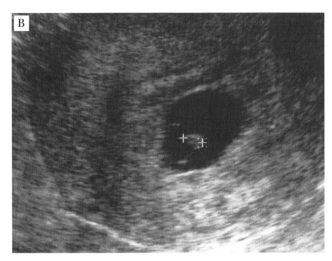

Fig. 7.34 Subchorionic haemorrhages. A: Subchorionic haemorrhage in a 7.5-week gestation. This pregnancy continued uneventfully. **B:** Subchorionic haemorrhage seen with a large yolk sac. This pregnancy failed.

all studies found such adverse outcomes, however. A series from India found that in continuing pregnancies, a history of threatened abortion between 6 and 12 weeks was not associated with any significant difference in preterm delivery, low birthweight or overall perinatal outcome.[68]

About a quarter of those who present with vaginal bleeding will have an intra-uterine haematoma demonstrated on ultrasound (Fig. 7.34). Again there is a discrepancy within the literature as to whether the presence of a haematoma increases the risk of failure. One early paper found no increase in loss,[69] and another found a subchorionic fluid collection to be associated with an increased loss only if there was clinical bleeding as well.[70] The weight of opinion, however, is that there is an increase in risk. The size of the haematoma relates to the subsequent risk of failure, with large subchorionic haematomas trebling the risk compared to those without a haematoma, and doubling it relative to those with only a small haematoma.[71]

Doppler

Doppler indices of the uterine and spiral arteries and the intervillous spaces may become abnormal in pregnancies complicated by embryonic death because of deficient placentation and disruption of the trophoblastic shell (Fig. 7.35).[72] There is as yet no consensus as to whether an abnormal Doppler finding can be used to predict which pregnancies will fail.

Kurjak *et al*[73] were able to show a statistical difference in the resistance index of the spiral arteries between normal pregnancy and threatened abortion, and also with molar pregnancies. Likewise, Jaffe *et al*[74] in a prospective study of 100 viable pregnancies, demonstrated that an abnormally high resistance to blood flow in the spiral

Fig. 7.35 Absence of blood flow in a failed pregnancy. Colour Doppler fails to show any trophoblastic blood flow in this failed pregnancy.

arteries and the presence of arterial blood flow in the intervillous spaces are associated with a high risk of early miscarriage. The cut-off used for resistance index was 0.55. It is of note that the miscarriage rate was relatively high in the study, which had a beneficial effect on the predictive value of the test.

In contradistinction, Lin *et al*[75] were unable to show any difference in the resistance index of the uterine arteries or the trophoblastic flow between normal and abnormal pregnancies. Another study of women with recurrent spontaneous abortion showed that although there was a difference in the subchorionic resistance index there was so much overlap between the failure group and the normal group that the measurement was not clinically useful.[76] In particular the resistance index value of 0.55 suggested

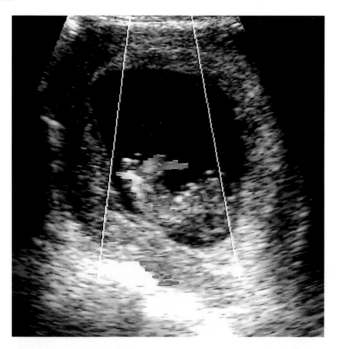

Fig. 7.36 **Normal flow to the embryo** shown on colour Doppler.

earlier was not discriminatory. A study of 38 first-trimester pregnancies complicated by retroplacental haematomas showed that Doppler studies of the fetal circulation were unable to predict which of the pregnancies would fail, and thus placental separation does not affect the fetal circulation prior to 14 weeks (Fig. 7.36).[77]

Pulsed (spectral) Doppler ultrasound can deposit high energy levels in the developing embryo, and that this is a time when the embryo might be most susceptible to any adverse effect. It is therefore inadvisable to use pulsed Doppler on the developing embryo outside a properly structured and ethically approved clinical trial (see Vol. 1 Ch. 3).[78]

Hormones

As pregnancy progresses the volume of trophoblastic tissue increases, leading to an increase in the production of β-hCG. There is a proportionate increase in the gestational sac size and the β-hCG levels until about 8 weeks, after which time the β-hCG levels plateau and then decline. It is therefore possible to construct a table of expected values against various measurements of early pregnancy size. If the β-hCG of a live embryo is below a certain level it could imply that there was inadequate trophoblastic activity to allow it to survive. One study of seven embryos with CRLs between 6 and 13 mm and heartbeats showed they all had an unfavourable outcome associated with low β-hCG levels for their gestational age (282–10 000 mIU/ml, mean 3033 mIU/ml Second International Standard).[79] The earlier use of β-hCG to try to diagnose a non-viable gestation sac before embryonic parts are visible is difficult

because of the differential diagnosis of ectopic pregnancy. A decidual reaction producing the appearance of a pseudosac may also have a low β-hCG.

Maternal serum progesterone has been measured and shown to be lower in pregnancies that failed or were ectopic than in normal pregnancies and threatened pregnancies that survived.[80] There is, however, overlap in the measurements between the two groups, so that the suggested discriminatory value of 45 nmol/ml is only 87% specific. This limits its usefulness in individual cases.

A disproportionally low maternal serum β-hCG or progesterone level is only supportive evidence of an abnormal pregnancy in the face of equivocal ultrasound findings, and repeat ultrasound and serum measurements are necessary after an interval.

First-trimester growth and chromosome anomaly

Fetuses with trisomy 18, trisomy 13 and triploidy have smaller than expected CRLs in the first trimester. Trisomy 21 does not demonstrate this shortening.[81] This is a difficult risk factor to apply prospectively because of the unreliability of menstrual dates. However, in precisely dated pregnancies, such as following *in vitro* fertilisation, using an observed minus expected CRL value can give a risk of aneuploidy that is useful in counselling regarding the need for karyotyping. The method can be refined by assessing growth rate over 2–3 weeks. This is also abnormal in trisomies 18 and 13, as well as triploidy, but not in trisomy 21 (Fig. 7.37). The advantage lies in its not being dependent on an accurate menstrual history.[82] Unfortunately there is still overlap with normal pregnancies, and as trisomies are relatively rare the clinical usefulness of first-trimester growth should only be used to corroborate other ultrasound findings, such as nuchal thickening.

Other factors

The identification of a heartbeat is normally a good prognostic sign as only 2–3% of these embryos will subsequently abort. This optimism may not be so justified in women with recurrent spontaneous abortion in whom a much higher proportion (22–55%) will go on to abort.[83,84] This is probably a reflection of the different mechanisms leading to abortion, notably that rates of chromosome anomalies are lower in the recurrent spontaneous abortion group.

Older mothers and those who undergo assisted conception are at a greater risk of spontaneous abortion.[85,86] However, it has also been shown that if the gestational age, indication for sonography and the scan findings are the same as those of a younger woman, or one who has conceived naturally, then the prognosis is the same. In other words, the prognostic validity of an ultrasound sign

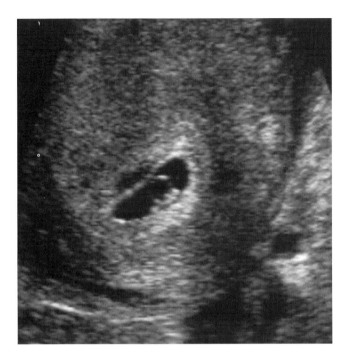

Fig. 7.37 Small subchorionic haemorrhage. This small subchorionic haemorrhage was seen early in pregnancy and was associated with an episode of vaginal bleeding. Later in pregnancy the embryo was found to have trisomy 21.

holds true even though older women and those with assisted conception are more likely to have bad prognostic ultrasound findings.[87]

Summary

The finding of a poor prognostic ultrasound feature in the presence of a live embryo with a heartbeat is used by some to prepare the parents for the worst. This is somewhat unfair on the parents, as it merely increases their anxiety without materially affecting management or eventual outcome. The finding of a heartbeat dominates any course of action, as the pregnancy must be managed expectantly. An embryo with poor prognostic features may nevertheless continue and confound predictions to produce a healthy neonate. Follow-up scans may be arranged if there are poor prognostic findings, but while there is a heartbeat the pregnancy must be allowed to continue.

Ectopic pregnancy

Incidence and risk factors

An ectopic pregnancy is defined as the implantation of a fertilised ovum outside the uterine cavity. It has been the leading cause of maternal mortality in the UK. The incidence is variously reported as between 0.3% and 1.6% of all pregnancies.[88,89] This has increased in the last two decades, and various theories have been put forward to account for this.[90] Women have a greater chance of carrying an ectopic pregnancy if they have previously had an ectopic, have undergone assisted conception, have an intra-uterine contraceptive device (Fig. 7.38), or have pre-existing tubal or pelvic inflammatory disease. There has been an increase in the use of assisted conception, but this probably accounts for only 5% of the ectopic pregnancies diagnosed. There has also been an increase in repeat ectopic pregnancies (recurrence risk is 10–20%[88]), but these two factors alone cannot account for the whole of the increased incidence.[90] The natural history of ectopic pregnancy almost certainly includes those that implant, die and resorb spontaneously. Some of the apparent increased incidence might be due to ectopic pregnancies that would formerly have remained undiagnosed but are now being diagnosed earlier, before they have resorbed spontaneously.[91] One modifiable behaviour that has been shown to be associated with an increased risk of ectopic pregnancy, probably via some effect on pelvic inflammatory disease, is vaginal douching. The risk increases with the increasing number of years of douching at least once per month.[92] It has been argued that symptom-free women known to fall into one of the high-risk categories for ectopic pregnancy should be screened early in the first trimester with ultrasound and serum β-hCG measurement. Such screening facilitates early diagnosis, reduces the risk of complications, and may make treatment easier.[93]

Symptoms

Ectopic pregnancy classically presents with the clinical triad of pain, vaginal bleeding and an adnexal mass. There may also be lower abdominal and pelvic peritonism. Unfortunately, these findings are not specific and may be absent. In one series of patients with ectopic pregnancy 9% reported no pain and 36% had no adnexal tenderness.[94] In another series only 41% had a definite palpable adnexal mass, with a further 23% possibly having a palpable mass.[95] In any woman of childbearing age presenting with pelvic or lower abdominal symptoms the first essential is to establish whether or not she is pregnant, by performing a pregnancy test.

Diagnosis of ectopic pregnancy

Blood markers

A great advance has been the development of highly sensitive radioimmunoassays to detect β-hCG. In the past, when the relatively insensitive haemagglutination studies were used, the relatively small amounts of β-hCG produced by an ectopic pregnancy might not be detected, so that a negative test did not exclude it. Nowadays, with the radioimmunoassays being approximately a thousandfold more

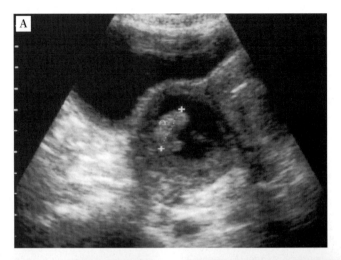

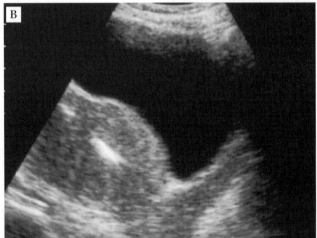

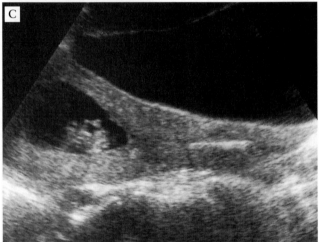

Fig. 7.38 **Intra-uterine contraceptive devices. A:** An ectopic pregnancy of CRL 21 mm associated with **B:** an intra-uterine contraceptive device (IUCD). **C:** Intra-uterine pregnancies can occur with an IUCD. In this case the IUCD is lying too low in the uterus and cervix to have been effective.

sensitive, this is no longer a limitation and has probably contributed the greatest impact of any new diagnostic tool.[96] There are different measurement standards available for calibrating β-hCG and it is important to know which is being used. The Second International Standard (2nd IS) is approximately half as sensitive as the purer standard of the International Reference Preparation (IRP, or 3rd IS), such that 500 mIU/ml 2nd IS is approximately equal to 1000 mIU/ml IRP. In a normal pregnancy an intra-uterine gestation sac should be visible on trans-vaginal sonography once the β-hCG level is above 1000 mIU/ml IRP.[97] If it is not, then the possibilities are either that products of conception have recently been passed or that there is an ectopic pregnancy.[98] If the initial β-hCG measurement is less than 1000 mIU/ml IRP then it is still possible that there is a normal intra-uterine pregnancy that is not yet visible on ultrasound. Serial measurements and ultrasound scans will be useful provided the clinical state is stable.

An ectopic pregnancy produces less β-hCG than a normally sited gestation of the same age. Unfortunately, because of the difficulty of establishing accurate dates, and because of overlap of the normal and abnormal ranges, it is not possible to establish an early cut-off concentration that predicts the presence of an ectopic pregnancy before the ultrasound signs become useful.[99]

Creatine kinase had been found to have a higher level in maternal plasma in ectopic pregnancy than in normal pregnancy. A cut-off level of 45 IU/l was suggested as a value over which ectopic pregnancy was more likely.[100] Unfortunately, others have shown that creatine kinase is valueless as a predictor of ectopic pregnancy.[101,102]

Ultrasound

The mainstay of ultrasound in suspected ectopic pregnancy is the demonstration of a normal intra-uterine pregnancy.

Well over half of those that are clinically thought at risk of an ectopic turn out to have an intra-uterine pregnancy. The identification of an intrauterine pregnancy virtually excludes the diagnosis of an ectopic, as the incidence of concurrent intra- and extra-uterine pregnancies is so low, nowadays thought to be about 1 in 7000.[103] However, there is the caveat that those undergoing assisted reproduction are at much greater risk, probably of the order of 1 in 100, and a thorough search of the adnexa must be made even in the presence of an intra-uterine pregnancy.[104-106] Even without assisted reproduction heterotopic pregnancies do occur, and considerable diagnostic difficulty can be encountered with an adnexal mass. Coexisting ectopic pregnancies have been thought to be ovarian carcinomas, and *vice versa*.[107,108]

Uterine appearances If there are no special risk factors then the exclusion of an ectopic pregnancy requires good sonographic demonstration of the uterine changes. There are statistical differences in the thickness of the endometrium between normal and ectopic pregnancy, even in the low non-discriminatory range of serum β-hCG. One study showed that if the endometrial width was 8 mm or less, then 97% had either an ectopic or a spontaneous abortion.[109] Another study found that a spheroidal 'endometrial three-layer' appearance (similar to the late proliferative phase endometrium) in patients with positive β-hCG and no visible gestation sac was specific for the presence of ectopic pregnancy, but was only seen in 62% of ectopic pregnancies.[110] These two studies appear contradictory, as the first suggests the endometrium is thin in ectopic pregnancy, whereas the second suggests it is thickened. The difference relates partly to different menstrual ages, but does serve to indicate that the main worth of the uterine appearances is to identify a correctly sited sac.

Once the serum β-hCG rises above 1000 mIU/ml IRP an intra-uterine sac should be visible on trans-vaginal scan. It must be distinguished from a decidual reaction forming a pseudosac (Fig. 7.39). Pseudosacs occur in 5–10% of ectopic pregnancies. They are usually elongated in shape in the centre of the endometrial cavity, and are surrounded by a ragged thickening of the endometrium. They can contain debris or blood clot that may mimic the appearances of embryonic structures, but do not exhibit the double decidual sac sign described earlier that is specific for a gestation sac. Trans-vaginal transducers have meant that there is really only a week-long period between the gestation sac becoming visible and the development of a visible yolk sac when the use of the double decidual sac sign remains useful.[111]

Free fluid Free fluid in the pelvis can be best seen with trans-vaginal ultrasound (Fig. 7.40), although the upper abdomen should also be checked with transabdominal ultrasound. It is a non-specific marker for the presence of an ectopic pregnancy if an intra-uterine sac cannot be seen. It usually accompanies other signs of ectopic pregnancy, but may be the only finding in 15% of proven ectopics.[112] Free fluid may occur in other conditions, such as a ruptured luteal cyst, and it may not be present in up to a third of ectopic pregnancies.[111] The more free fluid that is seen the more likely an ectopic becomes. Echogenic free fluid suggests a haemoperitoneum, and this is thought by some to greatly increase the likelihood of an ectopic being present. Culdocentesis to examine the *cul de sac* fluid for haematocrit is an old-fashioned diagnostic test: it has been refined by the use of trans-vaginal guidance to obtain the fluid[113]. Others have found that the level of β-hCG in *cul de sac* fluid is greater than the serum measurement in the presence of an ectopic pregnancy, and

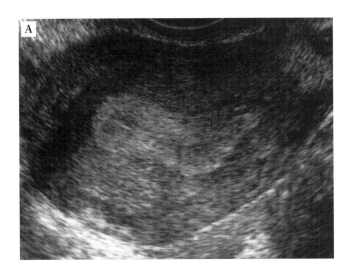
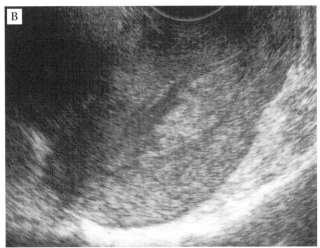

Fig. 7.39 Uterine appearances in ectopic pregnancies. A: Thickened endometrium with a spheroidal three-layer appearance seen in association with an ectopic pregnancy. **B:** Decidual reaction in an ectopic pregnancy mimicking the presence of retained products of conception.

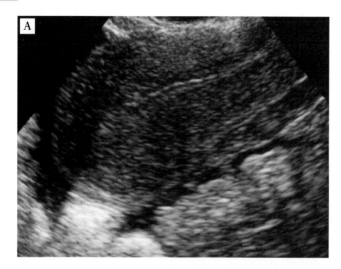
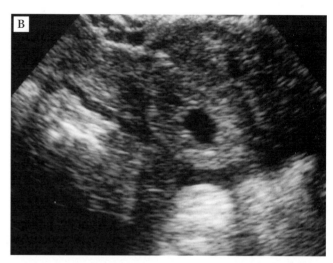

Fig. 7.40 Free fluid associated with an ectopic pregnancy. A: Trans-vaginal view of the uterus showing a small amount of surrounding free fluid containing low-level echoes. The echoes probably represent a haemoperitoneum. **B:** Reflective adnexal ring seen in the same patient that proved to be an ectopic pregnancy.

advocate trans-vaginal fluid aspiration when the pregnancy test is positive but there are no ultrasound signs other than free fluid. A fluid/serum β-hCG ratio over 1 has a high positive predictive value for ectopic pregnancy.[114,115]

Adnexal findings Of all ectopic pregnancies 95–97% occur in the fallopian tube, 2–5% occur in the cornual region of the uterus and only 0.5–1% occur in the ovary. Cervical ectopic pregnancy is extremely rare (0.1%). Some authors have noticed a small rise in the incidence of ovarian ectopic pregnancy.[116] Despite this, the finding of a cyst on the ovary should not be diagnosed as an ectopic as it is almost always just the corpus luteum. Furthermore, the side of the corpus luteum does not help in determining which side an ectopic will be, as up to a third implant contralaterally.

As most ectopic pregnancies are in the fallopian tubes, it is sensible when scanning to identify the ovary and then concentrate on the structures between the ovary and the uterus. If an abnormality is not found then the region of search can be widened. Pressure with the free hand on the lower abdomen when using a trans-vaginal probe may help to move bowel gas out of the way. The probe may identify a point of tenderness, which often indicates the site of the ectopic pregnancy.[98] Bowel should show peristalsis, which differentiates it from any suspected mass, though experience in interpretation is also important.[117]

The demonstration of an adnexal mass is the cornerstone of ectopic pregnancy diagnosis. These can be quite subtle, especially early in pregnancy at the 5–6-week stage, as any such mass is likely to be small. The most specific finding is that of an adnexal mass within which a yolk sac or embryo is demonstrated (Fig. 7.41). Unfortunately, this

will only be seen in 15–20% of ectopic pregnancies. It is more common to find complex adnexal masses with cystic and solid components likely to represent haematomas or ectopic trophoblastic tissue, and sometimes a ring-like structure with an echo-free centre and a reflective margin (tubal ring) (Fig. 7.42). A review of recently published studies has shown that, in the absence of an intra-uterine pregnancy, the identification of any non-simple, non-ovarian adnexal lesion can be used to diagnose ectopic pregnancy, with a sensitivity of 84.4% and specificity of 98.9%.[118] Trans-vaginal sonography performs better than transabdominal in the detection of ectopic pregnancy.[119]

There are, however, pitfalls in the detection of adnexal masses due to ectopic pregnancy. Adjacent structures may camouflage the mass in such a way that a predominantly solid ectopic merges with an adjacent structure, so that the only finding is asymmetrical enlargement of one ovary. An ectopic pregnancy may lie outside the range of a trans-vaginal transducer.[120] Overall, in up to 20% of ectopic pregnancies an adnexal lesion is not identified.[121] Likewise, the absence of free fluid does not exclude an ectopic pregnancy. A normal ultrasound, even though it has a negative predictive value of about 95%, should be viewed with some caution. A judgement has to be made on the technical adequacy of the examination, as the negative predictive value will be adversely affected in obese women and those with large fibroids. Likewise, the prior risk of an ectopic pregnancy has to be taken into account. Those who have undergone assisted conception, with their background high risk of ectopic, derive a much lower negative predictive value from a normal ultrasound examination. Some authors claim that 3D ultrasound will improve the accuracy,[122] though this has yet to be shown convincingly.

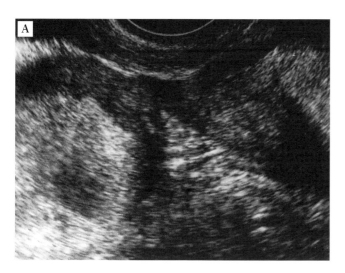
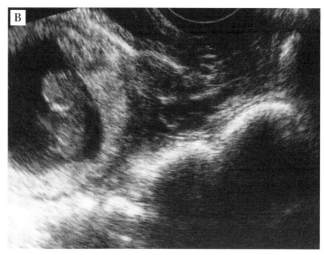

Fig. 7.41 Tubal ectopic pregnancy. Trans-vaginal images. **A:** The reflective gestation sac can be seen arising from the fallopian tube near to the cornual region of the uterus. **B:** A well formed living embryo is seen within the ectopic sac. Note that the sac is not surrounded by myometrium.

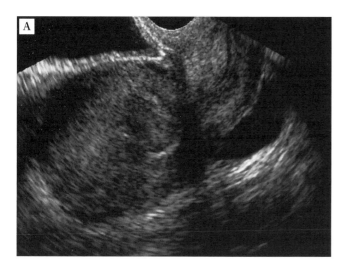
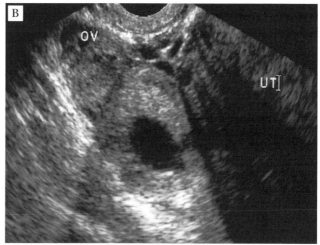

Fig. 7.42 Ectopic pregnancy. Trans-vaginal images. **A:** There is free fluid seen by the cervix and there is no visible intra-uterine sac. **B:** Lying between the uterus (UT) and ovary (OV) is a ring-like structure with a reflective margin. This is the ectopic pregnancy.

Doppler ultrasound in the diagnosis of ectopic pregnancy

Colour flow Doppler has the potential to improve the detection of ectopic pregnancy by being able to show peri-trophoblastic flow (Fig. 7.43). Adnexal areas of colour flow draw attention to small masses that might have been overlooked. Early studies suggested that colour Doppler did indeed perform better than grey scale ultrasound,[123,124] but the sensitivity of the grey scale findings in these studies was less than in other published work. More recent work, in which the grey scale ultrasound sensitivity was more in keeping with established rates, showed no benefit from using colour Doppler.[125] Another use of Doppler could be to define cut-off values for flow impedance on spectral pulsed Doppler that could differentiate between ectopic pregnancy and other adnexal masses. Unfortunately, although peritrophoblastic flow is of low impedance, it is not invariably so, and many other adnexal lesions also show low-impedance flow.

The finding of arterial flow in the endometrium has been suggested as a negative predictive index (97%) for an ectopic pregnancy.[19] Two-thirds of the patients in the study who did not have an ectopic pregnancy, and only three of the 55 patients with ectopic pregnancy, demonstrated arterial endometrial flow.

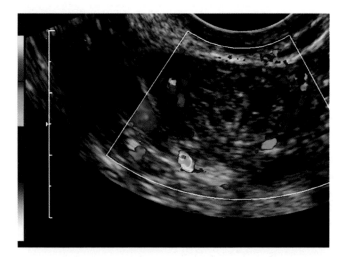

Fig. 7.43 Blood flow in an ectopic pregnancy. Colour Doppler showing trophoblastic blood flow around a mass from an ectopic pregnancy. The usefulness of this technique is still debated.

Uncommon forms of ectopic pregnancy

Chronic ectopic pregnancy

Chronic ectopic pregnancy is a form of tubal pregnancy in which slow disintegration of the tube, associated with small repeated bleeds rather than a single large episode of symptomatic bleeding, provokes an inflammatory response which leads to the formation of a mass, usually with numerous adhesions to adjacent structures. Clinically it presents as a long period of amenorrhoea, abdominal pain and a negative or very low serum β-hCG titre.[126] It has been thought to be rare, but one series of ectopic pregnancies classified 20% as being chronic.[127] In all their cases a complex adnexal mass was demonstrated and 8% had a negative β-hCG titre. There was also no evidence of increased vascularity, either within or around the mass. A single case report, however, has shown vascularity around a chronic ectopic pregnancy, though none within the mass.[128]

Delays in the diagnosis of an ectopic pregnancy or the diagnosis of a chronic ectopic pregnancy make it more likely that salpingectomy will be required. This reduces the woman's future fertility.[129]

Abdominal pregnancy

Abdominal pregnancies occur in up to 1% of all ectopic pregnancies. Diagnosis can be difficult, especially in later pregnancy, when less than 50% are correctly diagnosed before surgery.[130] In one case, of a woman who had three consecutive ectopic pregnancies, two progressed as undiagnosed abdominal pregnancies until the third trimester.[131]

Interstitial or cornual pregnancy

Interstitial pregnancies are those tubal pregnancies that implant in the intramural part of the tube, and the incidence is 2–5% of all ectopic pregnancies. Cornual pregnancy refers to an ectopic within a rudimentary uterine horn, but the term is often used interchangeably with an interstitial pregnancy.[98] An interstitial pregnancy is partly covered by myometrium and this enables the pregnancy to reach a later gestation than most ectopics before it causes symptoms. If it remains undetected and ruptures, profuse bleeding can occur. Ultrasound features of an interstitial pregnancy are its eccentric location and the absence or marked thinning of myometrium around it (Fig. 7.44). Diagnosis is difficult early in pregnancy as myometrium may still appear to surround the sac. The interstitial line sign of a thin reflective line extending from the uterine cavity to the margin of the sac has been suggested as an aid to diagnosis (Fig. 7.45).[132] Magnetic resonance imaging has also been used in conjunction with ultrasound to facilitate diagnosis, but this is still experimental.[133] Standard treatment is by surgical removal of the affected horn, but in up to 50% of cases hysterectomy becomes unavoidable. Alternative therapies include parenteral methotrexate or trans-vaginal ultrasound-guided puncture of the interstitial sac and the injection of methotrexate.[134] If such puncture is done, the sac should be approached with the needle from a medial trans-myometrial route, in order to reduce the chance of serious haemorrhage.

Cervical pregnancy

Cervical pregnancies are rare life-threatening forms of ectopic pregnancy, occurring in 1 of 8000 deliveries or

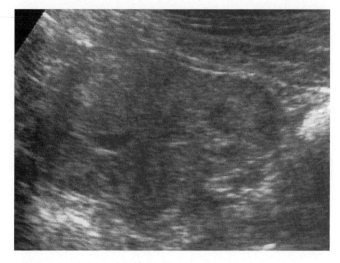

Fig. 7.44 Interstitial ectopic pregnancy. Fluid is present within the endometrial cavity on this transverse view through the fundus of the uterus. There is also a reflective ring representing a gestation sac in the interstitial region.

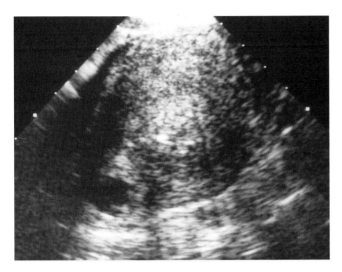

Fig. 7.45 Interstitial ectopic pregnancy. A reflective line is seen extending from the endometrium to the eccentric gestation sac. This is the 'interstitial line' sign.

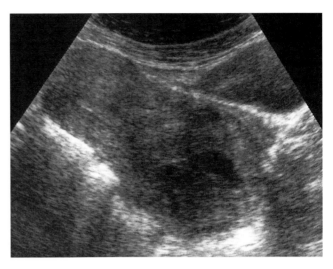

Fig. 7.46 Cervical ectopic pregnancy, seen on a longitudinal transabdominal view of the uterus.

about 0.15% of ectopic pregnancies.[135] Ultrasound shows an endocervical sac with trophoblastic invasion (Fig. 7.46), and Doppler may show peritrophoblastic flow indicating implantation. The main differential diagnoses are large nabothian cysts and inevitable abortion in progress.[98] Serial scans should show the sac of an inevitable abortion move and change shape, or alternatively the trans-vaginal transducer can be used to press gently and show sliding of the sac relative to the cervix. Nabothian cysts do not have embryonic parts or a reflective rim. About 60% of cervical ectopics have a live embryo.[135] Cervical pregnancies used to be managed by hysterectomy because of the risk of uncontrollable haemorrhage. Hysterectomy is still recommended for second- and third-trimester cervical pregnancy, but now that the diagnosis is made earlier with ultrasound, conservative management is possible. Control of bleeding can be achieved by Foley catheter balloon tamponade of the cervical canal. Systemic methotrexate causes the degeneration and resorption of the sac, with far less risk of haemorrhage than surgery.[136] Ultrasound-guided direct injection of methotrexate or potassium chloride has also been used, and in one case allowed the live birth of a concomitant intra-uterine twin.[137]

Treatment and monitoring of ectopic pregnancy

The standard treatment is by laparoscopy and removal of the ectopic pregnancy with the fallopian tube, or by removal of the ectopic on its own. This reduces the woman's chance of subsequent pregnancy. Reliable diagnosis with ultrasound is essential for non-surgical management, as surgery is the logical choice of treatment if laparoscopy is used for diagnosis.[138] Medical management involves either systemic methotrexate or local injection of methotrexate, or other agents such as potassium chloride or hyperosmolar glucose, into the sac. Expectant management with close monitoring has also been advocated.

Methotrexate, given either systemically or locally, has become most popular. It is considerably cheaper than surgical management.[139] The mass of ectopic pregnancy may transiently enlarge, have increased Doppler signals, and the serum β-hCG levels may also transiently increase.[140–142] A visible adnexal mass may persist for over 3 months, even after the hCG assay becomes negative. Local and systemic treatments are equally effective, but those who fail methotrexate management (8–20%) suffer greater morbidity than those who have primary surgical treatment.[143]

Asymptomatic women with an ectopic pregnancy can be offered expectant management. Excellent clinical, hormonal and ultrasound monitoring facilities are required. The criteria for expectant management are that the adnexal mass is less than 5 cm in size, the β-hCG levels are declining and the symptoms are minimal. Approximately 20% of women with ectopic pregnancy will fulfil these criteria.[144,145] Of these, between 48% and 69% have spontaneous resolution of the ectopic pregnancy. Features that predict a successful outcome are an initial β-hCG level below 2000 mIU/ml, and a decrease in size of the adnexal mass by day 7. An increasing volume of free fluid is a poor prognostic sign. Doppler flow patterns were not found helpful in one study,[145] but some have reported a useful difference in the resistance index of the corpus luteum and adnexal mass between developing and involuting ectopic pregnancies.[146] Involuting ectopic pregnancies demonstrate an increase in resistance index.

Molar pregnancy (see also Ch. 23)

Molar pregnancies comprise two distinct entities – partial and complete – which are distinct in epidemiology, genetics, clinical presentation, and the subsequent risk of persistent gestational trophoblastic disease.[147] It has an incidence of about 1 in 2000 pregnancies, but is far higher in the Far East. The classic presentation is with an enlarged uterus for menstrual age, elevated serum β-hCG levels and vaginal bleeding. The typical second-trimester appearance of a molar pregnancy is of a large soft tissue mass with numerous small cystic spaces filling the uterine cavity (Fig. 7.47). First-trimester molar appearances are much more varied, and can include features similar to a blighted ovum or a small reflective mass. Consequently they are much harder to diagnose.

The pathogenesis of a complete mole is thought to be due to the chorionic villi in a blighted ovum undergoing trophoblastic proliferation. An explanation for the falling incidence of molar pregnancy could be due in part to the earlier detection and evacuation of blighted ova than was previously the case.

A complete mole is characterised by diffuse trophoblastic proliferation in the absence of any embryonic parts. Its chromosomal material is entirely paternal in origin. Partial moles are characterised by focal trophoblastic proliferation and the presence of embryonic or fetal tissue. Partial moles are usually triploid, derived from fertilisation of an ovum by two sperms or by reduplication of a haploid sperm. Complete moles may coexist with a normal pregnancy and must have formed in a dizygotic twin pregnancy, tend to exhibit very high β-hCG levels and are more likely to be associated with theca lutein cysts, whereas partial moles are more likely to have a low β-hCG level.[147]

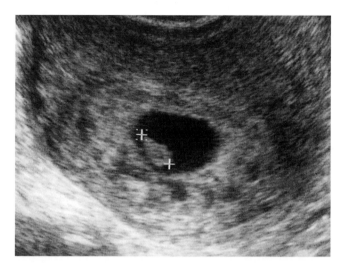

Fig. 7.48 Hydropic degeneration of the placenta. This failed first-trimester pregnancy demonstrates hydropic degeneration of the placenta. This should not be confused with molar change.

Serial scans in the first trimester have shown a living embryo becoming a molar pregnancy.[148] An abnormally large yolk sac at 8 weeks may be associated with a greater chance of molar pregnancy.[149] Trophoblastic disease is associated with a lower uterine artery impedance and a high-flow state on Doppler, but this may not be apparent in the early first trimester.[150] A prospective study in the late first trimester (11–15 weeks) has shown that the diagnosis of molar placental change is possible when ultrasound findings are taken in conjunction with the β-hCG levels and the uterine Doppler findings.[151] The β-hCG levels should help to distinguish a molar pregnancy from the differential diagnoses of hydropic degeneration of the placenta (Fig. 7.48) and degenerating fibroids, though histological examination may be required.

Uterine masses

Uterine fibroids (Fig. 7.49) may be confused with focal myometrial contractions. Focal contractions may be transitory or may persist for a considerable time and tend to occur under the placental implantation site.[152] Distinguishing features are that contractions are of the same reflectivity as the rest of the myometrium, whereas fibroids are not; a fibroid may attenuate the beam and have a heterogeneous pattern and may distort the serosal surface of the uterus. Contractions have a normal vascular pattern on Doppler, whereas most fibroids are avascular. These features are generalisations and some overlap in appearances does occur. Time should resolve the issue, but if a firm immediate diagnosis is required, ritodrine hydrochloride can be given orally to cause the contractions to relax.[152]

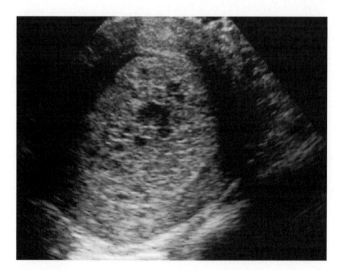

Fig. 7.47 Molar pregnancy. Classic appearance of a molar pregnancy with a large soft tissue mass with cystic spaces distending the uterine cavity.

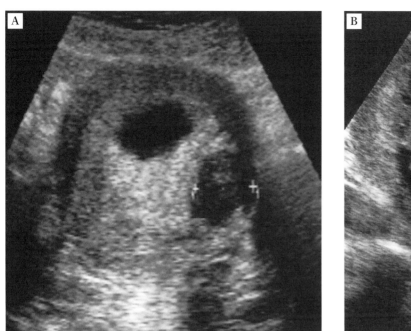

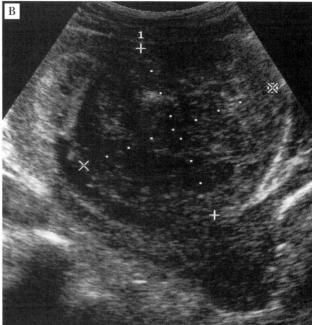

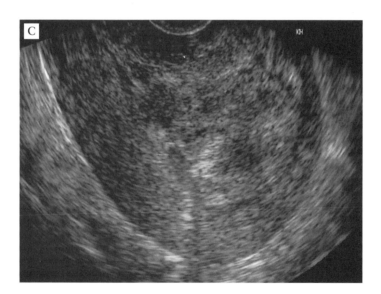

Fig. 7.49 Fibroids and pregnancy A: The calipers mark a small uterine fibroid associated with a first-trimester pregnancy. **B:** Huge anterior uterine wall fibroid (between calipers) associated with a failed first-trimester pregnancy. **C:** Same case as in B. The fibroid underwent degeneration such that at the time of uterine curettage for the failed pregnancy, large amounts of tissue were obtained. The surgeon thought he was obtaining molar tissue, but histology and this subsequent trans-vaginal scan proved otherwise.

There are other much rarer uterine masses. Adeno-myomas are benign tumours comprising smooth muscle and endometrial glands and are similar to adenomyosis. One has been reported complicating a first-trimester pregnancy and resulting in massive haemorrhage.[153]

Adnexal masses (Fig. 7.50) can be found coexisting with first-trimester pregnancies. Their diagnosis depends on the same ultrasound signs as in the non-pregnant patient.

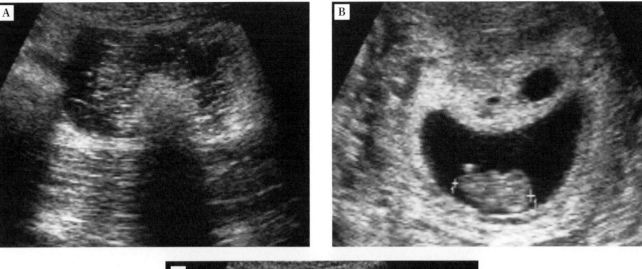

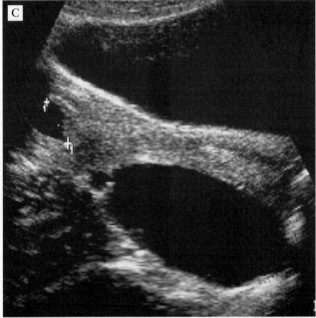

Fig. 7.50 Adnexal masses. A: Dermoid cyst exhibiting acoustic shadowing beyond a reflective mass seen in association with **B:** an early pregnancy.
C: Large simple cyst found in the pouch of Douglas in association with an intra-uterine gestation sac (between calipers).

REFERENCES

1 Hately W, Case J, Campbell S. Establishing the death of an embryo by ultrasound: report of a public inquiry with recommendations. Ultrasound Obstet Gynecol 1995; 5: 353–357

2 Filly R A. Ultrasound evaluation during the first trimester. In: Callen P W, ed. Ultrasonography in obstetrics and gynecology. Philadelphia: W B Saunders, 1994

3 Everett C. Incidence and outcome of bleeding before the 20th week of pregnancy: prospective study from general practice. BMJ 1997; 315: 32–34

4 Oakley A, McPherson A, Roberts H. Miscarriage. London: Fontana, 1984

5 Guerneri S R, Bettio D, Simoni G, Brambati B, Lanzani A, Fraccaro M. Prevalence and distribution of chromosome abnormalities in a sample of first trimester internal abortions. Hum Reprod 1987; 2: 735–739

6 Ohno M, Maeda T, Matsunobo A. A cytogenic study of spontaneous abortions with direct analysis of chorionic villi. Obstet Gynecol 1991; 77: 394–398

7 Goldstein S R, Kerenji T, Scher J, Papp C. Correlation between karyotype and ultrasound findings in patients with failed early pregnancy. Ultrasound Obstet Gynecol 1996; 8: 314–317

8 Wachsberg R H, Siegel J R. Ectopic pregnancy: value of transabdominal sonography without deliberate bladder distension. Emergency Radiology 1997; 4: 51–54

9 Guy R L, King E, Ayers A B. The role of transvaginal ultrasound in the assessment of the female pelvis. Clin Radiol 1988; 39: 669–672

10 Braithwaite J M, Economides D L. Acceptability by patients of transvaginal sonography in the elective assessment of the first trimester fetus. Ultrasound Obstet Gynecol 1997; 9: 91–93

11 Zimmer E Z, Timor-Tritsch I E, Rottem S. The technique of transvaginal sonography. In: Timor-Tritsch I E, Rottem S, eds. Transvaginal sonography, 2nd edn. New York: Elsevier, 1991

12 Yeh H C, Goodman J D, Carr L, Rabinowitz J G. Intradecidual sign: a US criterion of early intrauterine pregnancy. Radiology 1986; 161: 463–467

13 de Crispigny L C, Cooper D, McKenna M. Early detection of intrauterine pregnancy with ultrasound. J Ultrasound Med 1988; 7: 7–10

14 Nyberg D A, Filly R A, Mahony B S, Monroe S, Laing F C, Jeffrey R B Jr. Early gestation: correlation of hCG levels and sonographic identification. AJR 1985; 144: 951–954

15 Daya S, Woods S, Ward S, Lappalainen R, Caco C. Transvaginal ultrasound scanning in early pregnancy and correlation with human chorionic gonadotrophin levels. JCU 1991; 19: 139–142

16 Parvey H R, Dubinsky T J, Johnston D A, Maklad N F. The chorionic rim and low impedance intrauterine arterial flow in the diagnosis of early intrauterine pregnancy: evaluation of efficacy. AJR 1996; 167: 1479–1485

17 Bradley W G, Fiske C E, Filly R A. The double sac sign of early intrauterine pregnancy: use in exclusion of ectopic pregnancy. Radiology 1982; 143: 223–226

18 Nyberg D A, Laing F C, Filly R A, Uri-Simmons M, Jeffrey R B Jr. Ultrasonographic differentiation of the gestation sac of early intrauterine pregnancy from the pseudogestational sac of ectopic pregnancy. Radiology 1983; 146: 755–759

19 Dubinsky T J, Parvey H R, Maklad N. Endometrial color flow/image-directed Doppler imaging: negative predictive value for excluding ectopic pregnancy. JCU 1997; 25: 103–109

20 Levi C S, Lyons E A, Zheng X H, Lindsay D J, Holt S C. Endovaginal US: demonstration of cardiac activity in embryos of less than 5 mm in crown-rump length. Radiology 1990; 176: 71–74

21 Stampone C, Nicotra M, Muttinelli C, Cosmi E V. Transvaginal sonography of the yolk sac in normal and abnormal pregnancy. JCU 1996; 24: 3–9

22 Doubilet P M, Benson C B. Embryonic heart rate in the early first trimester: What rate is normal? J Ultrasound Med 1995; 14: 431–434

23 Blass H-G, Eik-Nes S H, Kiserud T, Hellevik L R. Early development of the abdominal wall, stomach and heart from 7 to 12 weeks of gestation: a longitudinal ultrasound study. Ultrasound Obstet Gynecol 1995; 6: 240–249

24 Stefos T I, Lolis D E, Sotiriadis A J, Ziakas G V. Embryonic heart rate in early pregnancy. JCU 1998; 26: 33–36

25 Blaas H-G, Eik-Nes S H, Kiserud T, Hellevik L R. Early development of the hindbrain: a longitudinal study from 7 to 12 weeks of gestation. Ultrasound Obstet Gynecol 1995; 5: 151–160

26 Achiron R, Achiron A, Yagel S. First trimester transvaginal sonographic diagnosis of Dandy–Walker malformation. JCU 1993; 21: 62–64

27 Diamant N E. Development of esophageal function. Am Rev Resp Dis 1985; 131: 29–32

28 Bowerman R A. Sonography of fetal midgut herniation: normal size criteria and correlation with crown-rump length. J Ultrasound Med 1993; 12: 251–254

29 Brown D L, Emerson D S, Shulman L P, Carson S A. Sonographic diagnosis of omphalocele during 10th week of gestation. AJR 1989; 153: 825–826

30 Snijders R J M, Brizot M L, Faria M, Nicolaides K H. Fetal exomphalos at 11 to 14 weeks of gestation. J Ultrasound Med 1995; 14: 569–574

31 Bonilla-Musoles F. Three-dimensional visualization of the human embryo: a potential revolution in prenatal diagnosis. Ultrasound Obstet Gynecol 1996; 7: 393–397

32 Bronshtein M, Zimmer E Z. Prenatal ultrasound examinations: for whom, by whom, what, when and how many? Ultrasound Obstet Gynecol 1997; 10: 1–4

33 D'Ottavio G, Meir Y J, Rustico M A, Conoscenti G, Maieron A, Fisher-Tamaro L, Mandruzzato G. Pilot screening for fetal malformations: possibilities and limits of transvaginal sonography. J Ultrasound Med 1995; 14: 575–580

34 Benischke K, Kaufmann P. Characterization of the developmental stages. In: Pathology of the human placenta, 2nd edn. New York: Springer-Verlag, 1990; 1–79

35 Hill L M, DiNofrio D M, Chenevey P. Transvaginal sonographic evaluation of first-trimester placenta previa. Ultrasound Obstet Gynecol 1995; 5: 301–303

36 Merce L T, Barco M J, Ban S. Color Doppler sonographic assessment of placental circulation in the first trimester of normal pregnancy. J Ultrasound Med 1996; 15: 135–142

37 Jauniaux E, Nicolaides K H. Placental lakes, absent umbilical artery diastolic flow and poor fetal growth in early pregnancy. Ultrasound Obstet Gynecol 1996; 7: 141–144

38 Campbell S, Warsof S L, Little D, Cooper D J. Routine ultrasound screening for the prediction of gestational age. Obstet Gynecol 1985; 65: 613–620

39 Geirsson R T. Ultrasound instead of last menstrual period as the basis of gestational age assignment. Ultrasound Obstet Gynecol 1991; 1: 212–219

40 British Medical Ultrasound Society Fetal Measurements Working Party report. Clinical applications of ultrasonic fetal measurements. London: British Institute of Radiology, 1990

41 Robinson H P, Fleming J E E. A critical evaluation of sonar crown–rump length measurements. Br J Obstet Gynaecol 1975; 82: 702–710

42 Altman D G, Chitty L S. New charts for ultrasound dating of pregnancy. Ultrasound Obstet Gynecol 1997; 10: 174–191

43 Sampson A, de Crespigny L C. Vanishing twins: the frequency of spontaneous fetal reduction of a twin pregnancy. Ultrasound Obstet Gynecol 1992; 2: 107–109

44 Landy H J, Weiner S, Corson S, Batzer F R, Bolognese R J. The 'vanishing twin': ultrasonographic assessment of fetal disappearance in the first trimester. Am J Obstet Gynecol 1986; 155: 14–19

45 Benson C B, Doubilet P M, David V. Prognosis of first trimester twin pregnancies: polychotomous logistic regression analysis. Radiology 1994; 192: 765–768

46 Sepulveda W. Chorionicity determination in twin pregnancies: double trouble? Ultrasound Obstet Gynecol 1997; 10: 79–81

47 Sepulveda W, Sebire N J, Hughes K, Kalogeropoulos A, Nicolaides K H. Evolution of the lambda or twin-chorionic peak sign in dichorionic twin pregnancies. Obstet Gynecol 1997; 89: 439–441

48 Monteagudo A, Timor-Tritsch I E, Sharma S. Early and simple determination of chorionic and amniotic type in multifetal gestations in the first fourteen weeks by high-frequency transvaginal ultrasonography. Am J Obstet Gynecol 1994; 170: 824–829

49 Copperman A B, Kaltenbacher L, Walker B, Sandler B, Bustillo M, Grunfeld L. Early first-trimester ultrasound provides a window through which the chorionicity of twins can be diagnosed in an in vitro fertilization (IVF) population. J Assist Reprod Genet 1995; 12: 693–697

50 Hill L M, Chenevey P, Hecker J, Martin J G. Sonographic determination of first trimester twin chorionicity and amnionicity. JCU 1996; 24: 305–308

51 Bromley B, Benacerraf B. Using the number of yolk sacs to determine amnionicity in early first trimester monochorionic twins. J Ultrasound Med 1995; 14: 415–419

52 Falco P, Milano V, Pilu G et al. Sonography of pregnancies with first trimester bleeding and a viable embryo: a study of prognostic indicators by logistic regression analysis. Ultrasound Obstet Gynecol 1996; 7: 165–169

53 Goldstein S R. Embryonic death in early pregnancy: a new look at the first trimester Obstet Gynecol 1994; 84: 294–297

54 Pandya P P, Snijders R J M, Psara N, Hilbert L, Nicolaides K H. The prevalence of non-viable pregnancy at 10–13 weeks of gestation. Ultrasound Obstet Gynecol 1996; 7: 170–173

55 Pridjan G, Moawad A H. Missed abortion: still appropriate terminology? Am J Obstet Gynecol 1989; 161: 261–262

56 Robinson H P. The diagnosis of early pregnancy failure by sonar. Br J Obstet Gynaecol 1975; 82: 849–857

57 Nyberg D A, Laing F C, Filly R A. Threatened abortion: sonographic distinction of normal and abnormal gestation sacs. Radiology 1986; 158: 397–400

58 Bree R L, Edwards M, Bohm-Velez M et al. Transvaginal sonography in the evaluation of normal early pregnancy: correlation with hCG level. AJR 1989; 153: 75–79

59 Tongsong T, Wanapirak C, Srisomboon J, Sirichotiyakul S, Polsrisuthikul T, Pongsatha S. Transvaginal ultrasound in threatened abortion with empty gestation sacs. Int J Gynecol Obstet 1994; 46: 297–301

60 Rowling S E, Coleman B G, Langer J E, Arger P H, Nisenbaum H L, Horii S C. First trimester US parameters of failed pregnancy. Radiology 1997; 203: 211–217

61 McKenna K M, Feldstein V A, Goldstein R B, Filly R A. The empty amnion: a sign of early pregnancy failure. J Ultrasound Med 1995; 14: 117–121

62 Birnholz J C, Madanes A E. Amniotic fluid accumulation in the first trimester. J Ultrasound Med 1995; 14: 597–602

63 Bromley B, Harlow B L, Laboda L A, Benacerraf B R. Small sac size in the first trimester: a predictor of poor fetal outcome. Radiology 1991; 178: 375–377

64 Lindsay D J, Lovett I S, Lyons E A et al. Yolk sac diameter and shape at endovaginal US: predictors of pregnancy outcome in the first trimester. Radiology 1992; 183: 115–118

65 Reece E A, Scioscia A L, Pinter E et al. Prognostic significance of the human yolk sac assessed by ultrasonography. Am J Obstet Gynecol 1988; 158: 1191–1194

66 Tongsong T, Srisomboon J, Wanapirak C, Sirichotiyakul S, Pongsatha S, Polsrisuthikul T. Pregnancy outcome of threatened abortion with demonstrable fetal cardiac activity: a cohort study. J Obstet Gynecol 1995; 21: 331–335

67 Ananth C V, Savitz D A. Vaginal bleeding and adverse reproductive outcomes: a meta-analysis. Paediatr Perinat Epidemiol 1994; 8: 62–78

68 Das A G, Gopalan S, Dhaliwal L K. Fetal growth and perinatal outcome of pregnancies continuing after threatened abortion. Aust N Z J Obstet Gynaecol 1996; 36: 135–139

69 Stabile I, Campbell S, Grudzinskas J G. Threatened miscarriage and intrauterine hematomas: sonographic and biochemical studies. J Ultrasound Med 1989; 8: 289–292

70 Dickey R P, Olar T T, Curole D N, Taylor S N, Matulich E M. Relationship of first trimester subchorionic bleeding detected by color Doppler ultrasound to subchorionic fluid, clinical bleeding and pregnancy outcome. Obstet Gynecol 1992; 80: 415–420

71 Bennet G L, Bromley B, Lieberman E, Benacerraf B R. Subchorionic hemorrhage in first trimester pregnancies: prediction of pregnancy outcome with sonography. Radiology 1996; 200: 803–806

72 Jauniaux E, Zaidi J, Jurkovic D, Campbell S, Hustin J. Comparison of colour Doppler features and pathological findings in complicated early pregnancy. Hum Reprod 1994; 9: 2432–2437

73 Kurjak A, Zalud I, Predanic M, Kupesic S. Transvaginal color and pulsed Doppler study of uterine blood flow in first and early second trimesters of pregnancy: normal versus abnormal. J Ultrasound Med 1994; 13: 43–47

74 Jaffe R, Dorgan A, Abramowicz J S. Color Doppler imaging of the uteroplacental circulation in the first trimester: value in predicting pregnancy failure or complication. AJR 1995; 164: 1255–1258

75 Lin S K, Ho E S, Lo F C, Peng S L, Lee Y H. Assessment of trophoblastic flow in abnormal first trimester intrauterine pregnancy. Chung Hua i Hsueh Tsa Chih – Chinese Med J 1997; 59: 1–6

76 Frates M C, Doubilet P M, Brown D L et al. Role of Doppler ultrasonography in the prediction of pregnancy outcome in women with recurrent spontaneous abortion. J Ultrasound Med 1996; 15: 557–562

77 Rizzo G, Capponi A, Soregaroli M, Arduini D, Romanini C. Early fetal circulation in pregnancies complicated by retroplacental hematoma. JCU 1995; 23: 525–529

78 European Federation of Societies for Ultrasound in Medicine and Biology (EFSUMB). Clinical safety statement for diagnostic ultrasound (October 1996). BMUS Bull 1997; 5(4): 9

79 Christodoulou C N, Zonas C, Loukaides T et al. Low hCG is associated with poor prognosis in association with an embryo with positive cardiac activity. Ultrasound Obstet Gynecol 1995; 5: 267–270

80 al-Sebai M A, Kingsland C R, Diver M, Hipkin L, McFadyen I R. The role of a single progesterone measurement in the diagnosis of early pregnancy failure and the prognosis of fetal viability. Br J Obstet Gynaecol 1995; 102: 364–369

81 Bahado-Singh R O, Lynch L, Deren O et al. First trimester growth restriction and fetal aneuploidy: the effect of type of aneuploidy and maternal age. Am J Obstet Gynecol 1997; 176: 976–980

82 Schemmer G, Wapner R J, Johnson A, Schemmer M, Norton H J, Anderson W E. First trimester growth patterns of aneuploid fetuses. Prenat Diagn 1997; 17: 155–159

83 Stern J J, Coulam C B. Mechanism of recurrent spontaneous abortion. I. Ultrasonographic findings. Am J Obstet Gynecol 1992; 166: 1844–1850

84 Opsahl M S, Pettit D C. First trimester sonographic characteristics of patients with recurrent spontaneous abortion. J Ultrasound Med 1993; 12: 507–510

85 Shoham Z, Zosmer A, Insler V. Early miscarriage and fetal malformations after induction of ovulation (by clomiphene citrate and/or human menotrophins), in vitro fertilization, and gamete intrafallopian transfer. Fertil Steril 1991; 55: 1–11

86 Smith K E, Buyalos R P. The profound impact of patient age on pregnancy outcome after early detection of fetal cardiac activity. Fertil Steril 1996; 65: 35–40

87 Benson C B, Doubilet P M, Cooney M J, Frates M C, David V, Hornstein M D. Early singleton pregnancy outcome: effects of maternal age and mode of conception. Radiology 1997; 203: 399–403

88 Chow W H, Daling J R, Cates W et al. Epidemiology of ectopic pregnancy. Epidemiol Rev 1987; 9: 71–94

89 Centers for disease control. Ectopic pregnancy – United States, 1988–1989. Morbid Mortal Weekly Rep 1992; 41: 591–594

90 Skjeldestad F E, Kendrick J S, Atrash H K, Daltveit A K. Increasing incidence of ectopic pregnancy in one Norwegian county – a population based study, 1970–1993. Acta Obstet Gynecol Scand 1997; 76: 159–165

91 El Farrar K, Grudzinskas J G. Ectopic pregnancy: what's new? Ultrasound Obstet Gynecol 1995; 5: 295–296

92 Kendrick J S, Atrash H K, Strauss L T, Gargiullo P M, Ahn Y W. Vaginal douching and the risk of ectopic pregnancy among black women. Am J Obstet Gynecol 1997; 176: 991–997

93 Cacciatore B, Stenman U H, Ylostalo P. Early screening for ectopic pregnancy in high-risk symptom-free women. Lancet 1994; 343: 517–518

94 Kaplan B C, Dart R G, Moskos M et al. Ectopic pregnancy: prospective study with improved diagnostic accuracy. Ann Emerg Med 1996; 28: 10–17

95 Weinstein L, Morris M B, Dotters D, Christian C D. Ectopic pregnancy: a new surgical epidemic. Obstet Gynecol 1983; 61: 698–701

96 Ankum W M, Hajenius P J, Schrevel L S, Van der Veen F. Management of suspected ectopic pregnancy. Impact of new diagnostic tools in 686 consecutive cases. J Reprod Med 1996; 41: 724–728

97 Cacciatore B, Stenman U H, Ylostalo P. Diagnosis of ectopic pregnancy by vaginal ultrasonography in combining with a discriminatory serum hCG level of 1000 IU/L (IRP). Br J Obstet Gynaecol 1990; 97: 904–908

98 Frates M C, Laing F C. Sonographic evaluation of ectopic pregnancy: an update. AJR 1995; 165: 251–259

99 Marcus S F, Macnamee M, Brinsden P. The prediction of ectopic pregnancy after in-vitro fertilization and embryo transfer. Hum Reprod 1995; 10: 2165–2168

100 Duncan W C, Sweeting V M, Cawood P, Illingworth P J. Measurement of creatine kinase activity and diagnosis of ectopic pregnancy. Br J Obstet Gynaecol 1995; 102: 233–237

101 Korhonen J, Alfthan H, Stenman U H, Ylostalo P. Failure of creatine kinase to predict ectopic pregnancy. Fertil Steril 1996; 65: 922–924

102 Darai E, Vlastos G, Benifla J L. Is maternal serum creatine kinase actually a marker for early diagnosis of ectopic pregnancy? Eur J Obstet Gynecol Reprod Biol 1996; 68: 25–27

103 Hann L E, Bachman D M, McArdle C R. Coexistent intrauterine and ectopic pregnancy: a reevaluation. Radiology 1984; 152: 151–154

104 Rizk B, Tan S L, Morcos S et al. Heterotopic pregnancies after in vitro fertilization and embryo transfer. Am J Obstet Gynecol 1991; 164: 161–164

105 Goldman G A, Fisch B, Ovadia J, Tadir Y. Heterotopic pregnancy after assisted reproductive technologies. Obstet Gynecol Surv 1992; 47: 217–221

106 Fisher A M, Goldberg B B. Unusual case of heterotopic pregnancies in an in vitro fertilization–embryo transfer patient. J Ultrasound Med 1997; 16: 703–706

107 Kuhl C K, Heuck A, Kreft B P, Luckhaus S, Reiser M, Schild H H. Combined intrauterine and ovarian pregnancy mimicking ovarian malignant tumor: imaging findings. AJR 1995; 165: 369–370

108 Riley G M, Babcook C, Jain K. Ruptured malignant ovarian tumor mimicking ruptured ectopic pregnancy. J Ultrasound Med 1996; 15: 871–873

109 Spandorfer S D, Barnhart K T. Endometrial stripe thickness as a predictor of ectopic pregnancy. Fertil Steril 1996; 66: 474–477

110 Lavie O, Boldes R, Neuman M, Rabinovitz R, Algur N, Beller U. Ultrasonographic 'endometrial three-layer' pattern: a unique finding in ectopic pregnancy. JCU 1996; 24: 179–183

111 Russell S A, Filly R A, Damato N. Sonographic diagnosis of ectopic pregnancy with endovaginal probes: what really has changed? J Ultrasound Med 1993; 3: 145–151

112 Nyberg D A, Hughes M P, Mack L A, Wang K Y. Extrauterine findings of ectopic pregnancy at transvaginal US: importance of echogenic fluid. Radiology 1991; 178: 823–826

113 Glezerman M, Press F, Carpman M. Culdocentesis is an obsolete tool in suspected ectopic pregnancy. Arch Gynecol Obstet 1992; 252: 5–9

114 Hinney B, Bertagnoli C, Tobler-Sommer M, Osmers R, Wuttke W, Kuhn W. Diagnosis of early ectopic pregnancy measurement of the maternal serum to cul-de-sac fluid hCG ratio. Ultrasound Obstet Gynecol 1995; 5: 260–266

115 Oettinger M, Odeh M, Tarazoua L, Snitkovsky T, Ophir E. Beta hCG concentration in peritoneal fluid and serum in ectopic and intrauterine pregnancy. Acta Obstet Gynecol Scand 1995; 74: 212–215

116 Gaudoin M R, Coulter K L, Robins A M, Verghese A, Hanretty K P. Is the incidence of ovarian ectopic pregnancy increasing? Eur J Obstet Gynecol Reprod Biol 1996; 70: 141–143

117 Wojak J C, Clayton M J, Nolan T E. Outcomes of ultrasound diagnosis of ectopic pregnancy. Dependence on observer experience. Invest Radiol 1995; 30: 115–117

118 Brown D L, Doubilet P M. Transvaginal sonography for diagnosing ectopic pregnancy: positivity criteria and performance characteristics. J Ultrasound Med 1994; 13: 259–266

119 Sadek A L, Schiotz H A. Transvaginal sonography in the management of ectopic pregnancy. Acta Obstet Gynecol Scand 1995; 74: 293–296

120 Zinn H L, Cohen H L, Zinn D L. Ultrasonographic diagnosis of ectopic pregnancy: importance of transabdominal imaging. J Ultrasound Med 1997; 16: 603–607

121 Parvey H R, Maklad N. Pitfalls in the transvaginal sonographic diagnosis of ectopic pregnancy. J Ultrasound Med 1993; 3: 139–144

122 Harika G, Gabriel R, Carre-Pigeon F, Alemany L, Quereux C, Wahl P. Primary application of three-dimensional ultrasonography to early diagnosis of ectopic pregnancy. Eur J Obstet Gynecol Reprod Biol 1995; 60: 117–120

123 Pellerito J S, Taylor K J W, Quedens-Case C et al. Ectopic pregnancy: evaluation with endovaginal color flow imaging. Radiology 1992; 183: 407–411

124 Emerson D S, Cartier M S, Altieri L A et al. Diagnostic efficacy of endovaginal color Doppler flow imaging in an ectopic pregnancy screening program. Radiology 1992; 183: 413–420

125 Chew S, Anandakumar C, Vanaja K, Wong Y C, Chia D, Ratnam S S. The role of transvaginal ultrasonography and colour Doppler imaging in the detection of ectopic pregnancy. J Obstet Gynaecol Res 1996; 22: 455–460

126 Cole T, Corlett R C Jr. Chronic ectopic pregnancy. Obstet Gynecol 1982; 59: 63–68

127 Ugur M, Turan C, Vicdan K, Ekici E, Oguz O, Gokmen O. Chronic ectopic pregnancy: a clinical analysis of 62 cases. Aust NZ J Obstet Gynaecol 1996; 36: 186–189

128 Abramov Y, Nadjari M, Shushan A, Prus D, Anteby S O. Doppler findings in chronic ectopic pregnancy: case report. Ultrasound Obstet Gynecol 1997; 9: 344–346

129 Robson S J, O'Shea R T. Undiagnosed ectopic pregnancy: a retrospective analysis of 31 'missed' ectopic pregnancies at a teaching hospital. Aust NZ J Obstet Gynaecol 1996; 36: 182–185

130 Alto W. Abdominal pregnancy. Am Fam Phys 1990; 41: 209–214

131 Moonen-Delarue M W G, Haest J W G. Ectopic pregnancy three times in line of which two advanced abdominal pregnancies. Eur J Obstet Gynecol Reprod Biol 1996; 66: 87–88

132 Ackerman T E, Levi C S, Dashefsky S M, Holt S C, Lindsay D J. Interstitial line: sonographic findings in interstitial (cornual) pregnancy. Radiology 1993; 189: 83–87

133 Bassil S, Gorolts S, Nisolle M, Van Beers B, Donnez J. A magnetic resonance imaging approach for the diagnosis of a triplet cornual pregnancy. Fertil Steril 1995; 64: 1029–1031

134 Timor-Tritsch I E, Monteagudo A, Lerner J P. A 'potentially safer' route for puncture and injection of cornual ectopic pregnancies. Ultrasound Obstet Gynecol 1996; 7: 353–355

135 Ushakov F B, Elchalal U, Aceman P J, Schenker J G. Cervical pregnancy: past and future. Obstet Gynecol Surv 1997; 52: 45–59

136 Jurkovic D, Hacket E, Campbell S. Diagnosis and treatment of early cervical pregnancy: a review and report of two cases treated conservatively. Ultrasound Obstet Gynecol 1996; 8: 373–380

137 Monteagudo A, Tarricone N J, Timor-Tritsch I E, Lerner J P. Successful transvaginal ultrasound guided puncture and injection of a cervical pregnancy in a patient with a simultaneous intrauterine pregnancy and a history of a previous cervical pregnancy. Ultrasound Obstet Gynecol 1996; 8: 381–386

138 Atri M, Leduc C, Gillett P et al. Role of endovaginal sonography in the diagnosis and management of ectopic pregnancy. Radiographics 1996; 16: 755–774

139 Yao M, Tulandi T, Kaplow M, Smith A P. A comparison of methotrexate versus laparoscopic surgery for the treatment of ectopic pregnancy: a cost analysis. Hum Reprod 1996; 11: 2762–2766

140 Brown D L, Felker R E, Stovall T G, Emerson D S, Ling F W. Serial endovaginal sonography of ectopic pregnancies treated with methotrexate. Obstet Gynecol 1991; 77: 406–409

141 Atri M, Bret B M, Tulandi T, Senterman M K. Ectopic pregnancy: evolution after treatment with transvaginal methotrexate. Radiology 1992; 185: 749–753

142 Schafer D, Kryss J, Pfuhl J, Baumann R. Systemic treatment of ectopic pregnancies with single-dose methotrexate. J Am Assoc Gynecol Laparosc 1994; 1: 213–218

143 Yao M, Tulandi T, Falcone T. Treatment of ectopic pregnancy by systemic methotrexate, transvaginal methotrexate and operative laparoscopy. Int J Fertil Menopaus Stud 1996; 41: 470–475

144 Shalev E, Peleg D, Tsabari A, Romano S, Bustan M. Spontaneous resolution of ectopic tubal pregnancy: natural history. Fertil Steril 1995; 63: 15–19

145 Cacciatore B, Korhonen J, Stenman U-H, Ylostalo P. Transvaginal sonography and serum hCG in monitoring of presumed ectopic pregnancies selected for expectant management. Ultrasound Obstet Gynecol 1995; 5: 297–300

146 Bonilla-Musoles F M, Ballester M J, Tarin J J, Raga F, Osborne N G, Pellicer A. Does transvaginal color Doppler sonography differentiate between developing and involuting ectopic pregnancies? J Ultrasound Med 1995; 14: 175–181

147 Goldstein D P, Berkowitz R S. Current management of complete and partial molar pregnancy. J Reprod Med 1994; 39: 139–146

148 Burmeister R, Tucker R. Ultrasonographic diagnosis of first trimester hydatidiform mole. JCU 1997; 25: 36–38

149 Zalel Y, Shalev E, Yanay N et al. A large yolk sac: a possible clue to early diagnosis of partial hydatidiform mole. JCU 1994; 22: 519–521

150 Chan F Y, Pun T C, Chau M T, Lam C, Ngan H Y, Wong R L. The role of Doppler sonography in assessment of malignant trophoblastic disease. Eur J Obstet Gynecol Reprod Biol 1996; 68: 123–128

151 Jauniaux E, Nicolaides K H. Early ultrasound diagnosis and follow-up of molar pregnancies. Ultrasound Obstet Gynecol 1997; 9: 17–21

152 Tadmoor O P, Rabinowitz R, Diamant Y Z. Ultrasonic demonstration of a local myometrial thickening in early intrauterine pregnancy. Ultrasound Obstet Gynecol 1995; 5: 44–46

153 Athas A M, Bluemke D A, Isacson C, Sheth S. Large cervical adenomyoma occurring in a first trimester gravid uterus: radiologic–pathologic correlation. AJR 1996; 167: 514–515

The normal fetus

David R Griffin

Introduction

In this chapter the normal fetal anatomical appearances are described from the time of a routine examination at approximately 18 post-menstrual weeks to term. The detailed embryology and developmental anatomy are described in Chapter 6. Recognition of abnormal fetal anatomy is founded upon a sound knowledge of normal appearances, which can only be attained through 'hands-on' experience.

A systematic approach to the examination of the fetus ensures that all regions are covered. Starting with the number of fetuses, the presentation, fetal activity, liquor volume, placental site and morphology and the number of cord vessels are assessed systematically. The fetal examination can conveniently begin with the head, so that gestational age can be confirmed by measurement of the biparietal diameter. The skull, brain and face are examined before progressing caudally to scan the thorax, heart, abdominal cavity and urogenital tract. The spine and limbs complete the picture. Fetal lie may make this order of examination impossible and, if it cannot be followd, a checklist will serve as a reminder so that no parts are missed. This approach is particularly important when the operator's attention is directed toward a particular fetal part or system because of suspected abnormality. It is all too easy to become so involved in abnormal features that other parts are forgotten. It is good practice to examine the whole fetus first, and to return to a detailed examination of abnormal features afterwards.

A three-dimensional image of the fetus is built up by scanning in three orthogonal planes (Fig. 8.1). Unfortunately there is no agreed terminology for these planes, and terms used in the head may differ from those in the trunk. The axial plane may also be known as horizontal or transverse, the coronal plane as the frontal plane, and the sagittal plane as the median plane. In this chapter the terminology in Figure 8.1 is used. An experienced operator frequently deviates from these standard views to obtain optimal imaging of a particular organ.

Head

Cranium and cranial contents

In examining the fetal head attention needs to be directed to the cranial vault, the intracranial contents and the soft tissue features of the face. These structures are examined in the three planes described above. Most routine measurements of the head and intracranial structures are performed in the axial plane, which should be orientated parallel to the fronto-occipital diameter (Fig. 8.2).

The skull

The skull is best examined in the axial plane.[1] Throughout pregnancy it should have an ovoid shape, the biparietal diameter (BPD) being 80–90% of the occipitofrontal diameter (OFD), and narrower in the frontal than in the occipital region (Fig. 8.3). If the fetus is presenting by the breech the head may be dolichocephalic, with an unusually low BPD/OFD ratio. Echoes from the vault should be very strong and an acoustic shadow should be evident across more distal structures in the ultrasound beam. These are more noticeable beyond the lateral extremities of the image, where the ultrasound beam is attenuated by a greater thickness of skull. This acoustic shadowing becomes more pronounced with increasing maturity, so that it becomes more difficult to examine intracranial structures at later stages without using the acoustic windows afforded by the sutures and fontanelles. Conversely, defective skull mineralisation may be suspected when there is enhanced imaging of intracranial detail. Breaks in the integrity of the skull outline will be evident at the sutures but, except in the mid-sagittal plane, where the anterior and posterior fontanelles are best seen, these gaps should be small.

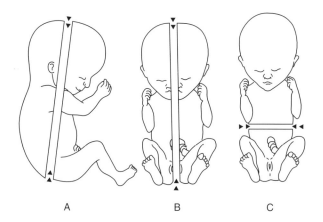

Fig. 8.1 Basic planes of ultrasound examination. A: Coronal plane. B: Sagittal plane. C: Axial plane.

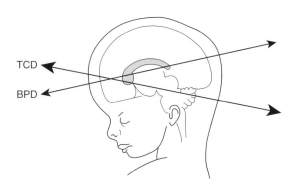

Fig. 8.2 Section for BPD measurement. Axial plane used for examination of the fetal head at the level used for measurement of the BPD, head circumference and ventricle–hemisphere ratios.

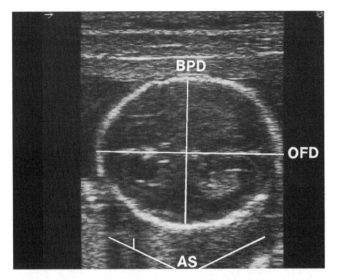

Fig. 8.3 Axial scan – 18 weeks. Axial scan of the fetal head at 18 weeks at approximately the level in Figure 8.2 to show BPD and OFD measurements. Note acoustic shadows (AS).

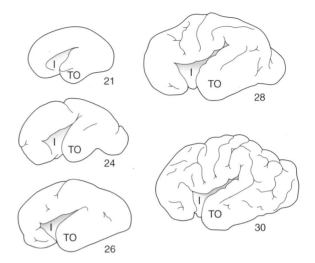

Fig. 8.4 Opercularisation of the brain. Diagrammatic representations of the fetal brain from 21 to 30 weeks showing opercularisation of the insula (I) and formation of gyri. TO – temporal operculum. (Drawn from *Gray's Anatomy*.)

Difficulty in obtaining a good axial view may occur in a cephalic presentation when the head is deep in the pelvis, when there is asynclitism, or when the spine lies perpendicular to the scanning plane, with the vertex immediately beneath the abdominal wall. This may be overcome by displacing the uterus upwards out of the pelvis and applying pressure to the anterior fetal shoulder. If this manoeuvre fails then tilting either the couch or the patient into a head-down position may be effective. Occasionally the patient may need to return for a further examination after an interval in the hope that the adverse position has changed.

The sagittal plane is mainly used in examining the fetal facial profile. Parasagittal sections clearly outline the full extent of the lateral ventricles, but they can be difficult to obtain except when the fetus lies in a direct occipito-anterior or occipitoposterior position.

In the coronal plane the skull should have a semi-circular outline. This view is used to examine soft tissue features of the face.

Abnormalities may occur in skull size (microcephaly, neural tube defects, macrocephaly), skull shape (brachy-cephaly, the 'lemon sign', scaphocephaly, clover-leaf skull, strawberry skull, microcephaly), skull integrity (anen-cephaly, encephalocele, exencephaly) or skull mineralisation (some skeletal dysplasias).

Intracranial structures

From the 16th week to term there is considerable growth of brain structures, both in size and in complexity. (Fig. 8.4). The lateral cerebral ventricles are a prominent feature of the brain in the early second trimester but they shrink relatively as the cerebral hemispheres grow. At 16 weeks the lateral ventricles consist of little more than an anterior horn, body and small inferior horn. The inferior and posterior horns become elongated with growth of the temporal and occipital lobes of the cerebrum (Figs 8.5 and 8.6). Until the 20th post-menstrual week the choroid plexus is a prominent, highly reflective feature on the inferolateral wall of the body of the lateral ventricle (almost filling it) and the roof of the inferior horn. Thereafter it becomes progressively less prominent, until in the third trimester it is barely visible.

Most of the essential structures of the fetal brain may be demonstrated in the axial plane at two positions (Figs 8.2 and 8.7). The first transects the anterior horns of the lateral ventricles, the cavity of the septum pellucidum, the thalamic nuclei and third ventricle, the body and posterior horns of the lateral ventricles and the insula and Sylvian fissure (lateral cerebral sulcus). The second is more caudal and angled to include the brain stem, cerebellum and cisterna magna.

As a consequence of disturbance of the ultrasound beam as it passes through the convex proximal skull table, detail of intracranial structures in the proximal hemisphere is frequently poor. The distal hemisphere is therefore chosen for measurements. This phenomenon should be borne in mind when intracranial pathology such as a choroid plexus cyst is detected unilaterally. Every effort should be made to view the brain from the other side, so that obscured contralateral pathology is not missed.

In the normal fetal brain the lateral wall of the body of the lateral ventricle runs parallel to the midline in the second trimester, so that measurement of the anterior horn is representative of the body. As the medial wall of the anterior horn is rarely seen, measurement is taken from the

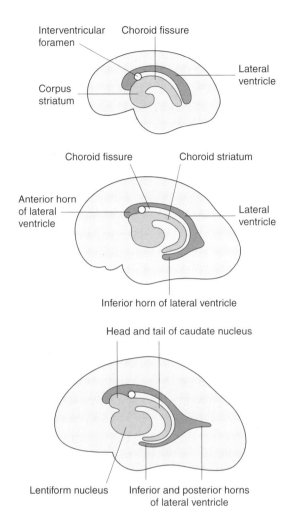

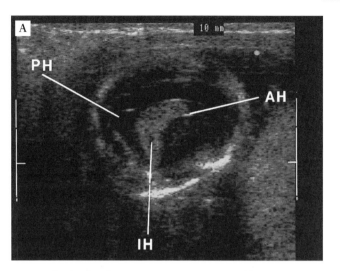

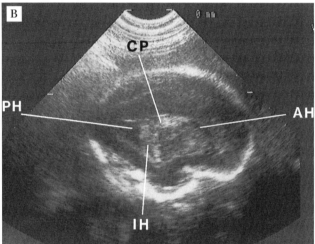

Fig. 8.5 Lateral ventricles. Diagram showing development of the lateral ventricular system. (From: Moore K L. The developing human. Philadelphia: WB Saunders, 1982; 400.)

Fig. 8.6 Developing ventricle. A: 18-week and **B:** 23-week parasagittal scans to demonstrate developing anterior (AH), posterior (PH) and inferior horns (IH) and the choroid plexus (CP), with the ventricular outlines highlighted.

midline echo. This measurement rarely exceeds 9 mm in the normal second-trimester brain. The body of the lateral ventricle has a measurable width posteriorly between its medial and lateral walls. The lateral wall is frequently obscured by the choroid plexus, and the lateral wall should then be taken to be the lateral border of the choroid plexus (Fig. 8.8). Later in the second trimester the posterior horns converge in the occipital poles, so that measurement of their maximum width will no longer be perpendicular to the midline but angled posteriorly (Fig. 8.9). Until about 20 weeks the width of the body of the lateral ventricle is similar to the anterior horn measurement, but as the medial wall of the body and posterior horn become indented by the calcar avis the width of the lateral ventricle decreases. Traditionally the anterior and posterior ventricle measurements have been compared as a ratio with the maximum width of the cerebral hemisphere. From the 16th week onwards this should be less than 0.5. Nomograms are available (see Appendix).[2]

Until the 20th week the brain has a smooth surface with few sulci or gyri (Fig. 8.4). The gyri and sulci extend and become more convoluted as the brain grows. Of particular clinical significance is the development of the lateral sulcus (Sylvian fissure) between the insula medially and the anteriorly migrating temporal operculum. From about the 22nd week this process, known as opercularisation, produces a linear echo in the same scanning plane as, but lateral to, the lateral ventricles. This may be mistaken for the lateral wall of the lateral ventricle and can lead to an erroneous diagnosis of ventriculomegaly (Fig. 8.10). If in doubt, identification of pulsations or the Doppler signals middle cerebral artery running in the lateral sulcus confirms the origin of the echo.

The medial walls of the lateral ventricle are formed anteriorly by the septum pellucidum, a double membrane

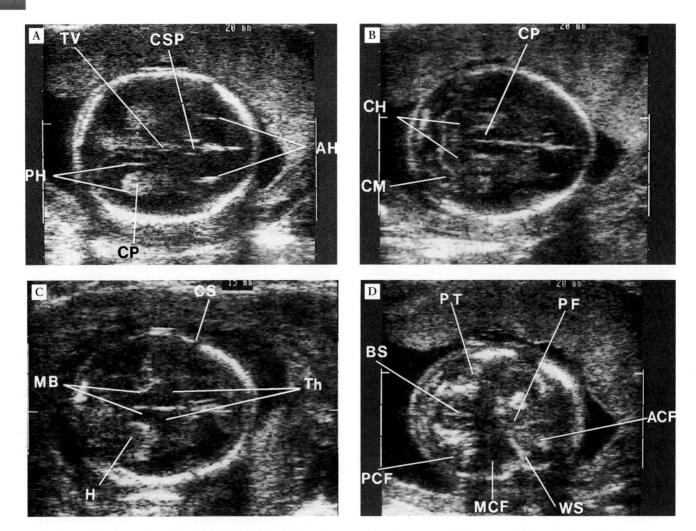

Fig. 8.7 Normal sections – 18 weeks. Axial sections of the fetal head at 18 weeks, each section slightly more caudal than the last. **A:** To show the lateral and third ventricles. AH – lateral wall of anterior horn of lateral ventricle, PH – posterior horn, CP – choroid plexus, CSP – cavity of the septum pellucidum, TV – third ventricle. **B:** Plane angulated about 15° to show the cerebellar hemispheres (CH), cisterna magna (CM), CP – cerebral peduncles. **C:** Section at the level of the thalamus (Th). H – hippocampus, MB – midbrain, CS – coronal suture. **D:** Section at the level of the base of the skull showing cranial fossae. ACF – anterior cranial fossa, MCF – middle cranial fossa, PCF – posterior cranial fossa, PF – pituitary fossa, WS – wing of the sphenoid bone, PT – petrous part of the temporal bone, BS – brain stem in the foramen magnum.

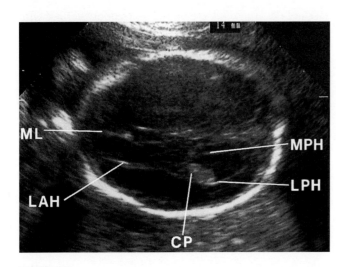

Fig. 8.8 Fetal head – 19 weeks. The anterior horn of the lateral ventricle is measured from the midline (ML) to the lateral wall (LAH). The posterior horn is measured from the medial wall (MPH) to the lateral wall (LPH) at its maximal width. The lateral wall of the posterior horn is frequently outlined by the choroid plexus (CP).

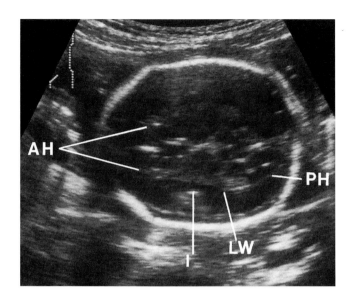

Fig. 8.9 Posterior horn – 25 weeks. Axial scan of the fetal head at 25 weeks to show narrowing and convergence of the posterior horn (PH). The lateral wall (LW) of the lateral ventricle can be followed to the anterior horn (AH) and should not be confused with the insula (I).

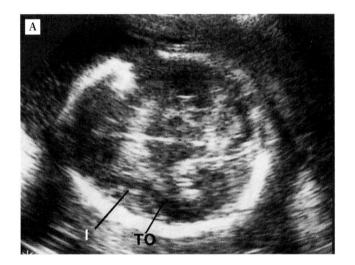

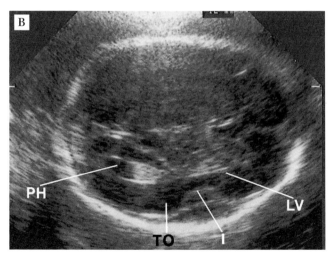

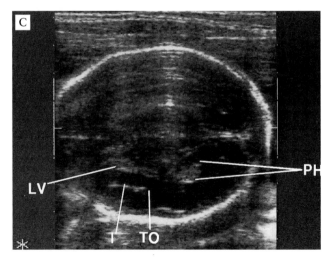

Fig. 8.10 Development of the insula. Axial scans at **A:** 18 weeks, **B:** 22 weeks and C: 25 weeks to demonstrate the insula. PH – posterior horn, LV – lateral wall of lateral ventricle, TO – temporal operculum, I – insula.

enclosing a narrow cavity (cavum septum pellucidum). This structure may be seen throughout gestation as a pair of parallel echoes close to the midline and just posterior to the echoes from the lateral walls of the anterior horns. The cavum septum pellucidum interrupts the midline (inter-hemispheric) echo about one-third of the distance from the frontal to the occipital calvarium. It should not be confused with the third ventricle, which lies postero-inferior to it between the thalamic nuclei (Fig. 8.7A) and is rarely visualised in the normal fetus. The bodies or antra of the lateral ventricles diverge and the medial wall can be identified. The choroid plexus is a highly reflective structure arising from the floor of the lateral ventricle (Figs 8.7A, 8.11 and 8.12). Usually it either fills the lateral ventricle from its medial to lateral wall, or a small anechoic rim

may be seen on its medial border. Under normal circumstances the lateral border of the choroid plexus may generally be taken to be that of the ventricle also.

The cerebellar hemispheres are seen at 18 weeks as bilaterally symmetrical, almost circular structures of low reflectivity but with a more reflective rim (Fig. 8.13). As pregnancy progresses the cerebellar hemispheres become more triangular in axial section and the more reflective vermis becomes prominent between the cerebellar hemispheres (Fig. 8.14). Anterior to the cerebellum the poorly reflective cerebral peduncles are evident. Posteriorly the cisterna magna is seen as an anechoic space between the posterior aspect of the cerebellum and the inner aspect of the occipital bone. The cerebellar hemispheres may also be well demonstrated in a posterior coronal plane (Fig. 8.15).

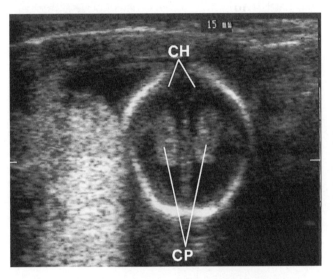

Fig. 8.11 Choroid plexus. Axial scan (17 weeks) from the occipital aspect showing the choroid plexus (CP) in each lateral ventricle. The occipital poles of the cerebral hemispheres (CH) are demonstrated.

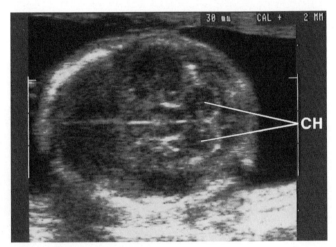

Fig. 8.13 Cerebellum – 21 weeks. Axial scan to show cerebellar hemispheres (CH) at 21 weeks.

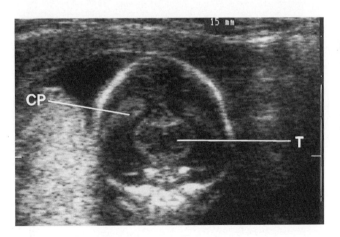

Fig. 8.12 Choroid plexus. Coronal scan angulated posteriorly to demonstrate the choroid plexus (CP) following the lateral ventricle into the inferior horn as it curves round the thalamus (T).

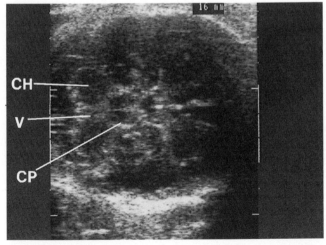

Fig. 8.14 Cerebellum – 30 weeks. Similar scan to Figure 8.13, showing cerebellar hemispheres (CH) and vermis (V) at 30 weeks. CP – cerebral peduncles.

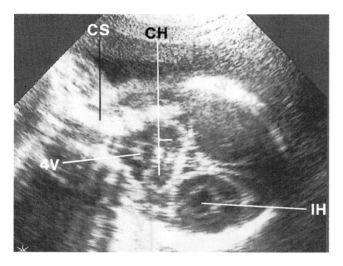

Fig. 8.15 Cerebellum – 19 weeks. Coronal scan to show cerebellar hemispheres (CH), fourth ventricle (4V) and inferior horn of the lateral ventricle (IH). CS – cervical spine.

The face

An examination of the face should be an essential part of any routine examination for fetal normality. It is not difficult or particularly time-consuming and may be rewarded by the discovery of a facial cleft, one of the more common congenital defects and a marker for some lethal or severely disabling genetic syndromes.

Coarse facial features start to be recognisable on ultrasound examination in the late first trimester. By the 14th post-menstrual week the nose, lips, ears etc. are evident, and by the time of a routine 18-week scan a detailed 3D image of the face may be constructed (Fig. 8.16). The added resolution of a higher-frequency transducer will often help in examining the finer details of the lips and ears.

Three views are employed: axial, coronal and sagittal (Fig. 8.17). In the coronal plane the chin, lips, external nares (Fig. 8.18), eyelids, lenses, cheeks and forehead may be demonstrated, as if in a direct frontal portrait. Slight adjustments of the plane are necessary to demonstrate all these features, but with a little perseverance the technique can be mastered. The axial plane demonstrates the orbits, lenses (Fig. 8.19), nasal bones (Fig. 8.20), palate, tongue, upper and lower lips and mandible (Fig. 8.21). The sagittal plane reveals the fetal profile (Fig. 8.22) and is useful when demonstrating the chin, tongue (with the mouth open), forehead, nasal bridge, philtrum etc.

The lips, nose and ears (Fig. 8.23) become increasingly clear as pregnancy advances, although they are more likely to be obscured by the upper limbs. It is unusual to be able to demonstrate both ears on a single occasion. The palate is most easily demonstrated in the axial plane at about 16–18 weeks, whereafter it becomes increasingly obscured by the maxilla.

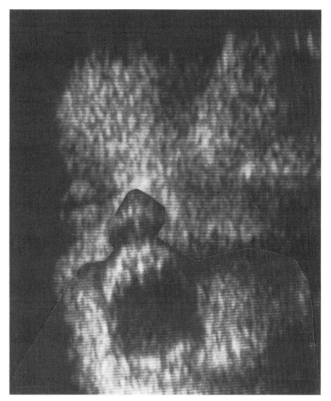

Fig. 8.16 Fetal face. Composite picture from two scans of the same fetal face at slightly different angles to give an indication of the three-dimensional mental image that can be built up during real-time scanning.

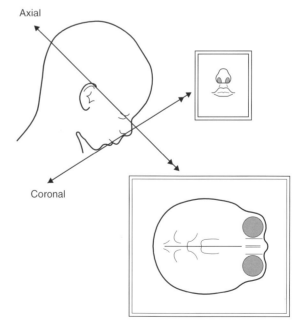

Fig. 8.17 Scan planes for the fetal face. Diagram of scanning planes for examination of the fetal face.

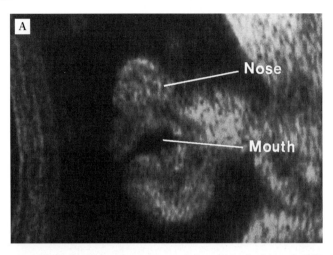

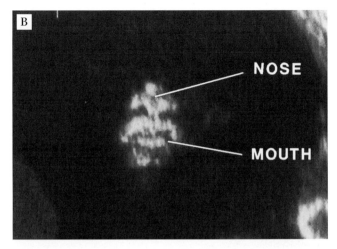

Fig. 8.18 Fetal mouth and nose. Coronal views of the fetal face. **A:** With the mouth open and **B:** mouth closed. The contours of the nostrils and lips are clearly demonstrated.

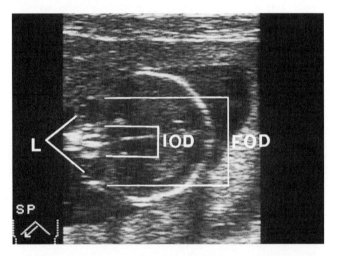

Fig. 8.19 Orbits. Axial scan of the fetal head to show measurement of the internal (IOD) and external orbital diameters (EOD) and the lenses (L).

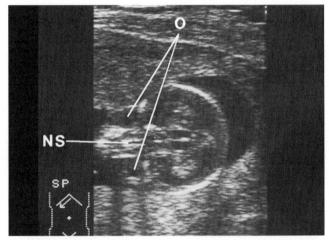

Fig. 8.20 Orbits and nasal bones. Axial scan to show the orbits (O) and nasal bones. Note that the nasal septum (NS) and turbinate bones normally give a double echo.

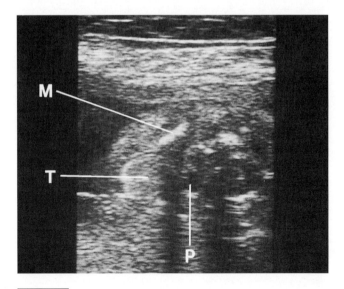

Fig. 8.21 Mouth. Axial scan demonstrating the tongue (T), ramus of the mandible (M) and pharynx (P).

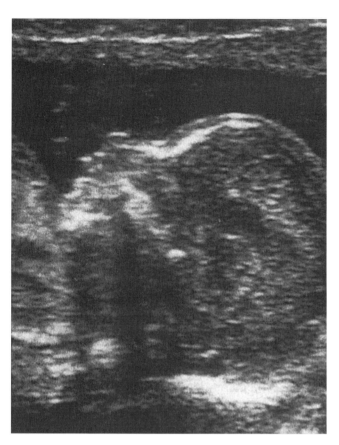

Fig. 8.22 Face – 19 weeks. Anterior sagittal scan of the fetal face demonstrating the profile.

The neck

The fetal neck may be examined for its external contours and its internal structure.

In axial section the neck should be circular with the cervical vertebrae centrally. Soft tissue or fluid-filled irregularities or swellings should suggest the possibility of neoplasms (haemangioma, teratoma) or cystic hygroma. Nuchal oedema posteriorly may be a marker for trisomy 21,[3] cardiac, musculoskeletal or other abnormalities.

The larynx is best demonstrated in the coronal plane. The epiglottis and the vestibular folds can usually be demonstrated (Fig. 8.24) and can be seen to move with fetal breathing and swallowing. Swallowing dysfunction from bulbar palsy is a rare cause of polyhydramnios.

Trunk

The fetal trunk comprises the axial skeleton (spine, shoulder and pelvic girdles and ribs) and the thorax and its contents divided from the abdominal cavity by the diaphragm.

Before attending to the detailed examination of the thoracic and abdominal contents an overall view of the whole trunk should be obtained to ensure that the relative proportions are correct. In sagittal and coronal planes the transition from the thoracic to abdominal wall should be a smooth curve (Fig. 8.25). Angulation between the base of the thorax and the abdominal wall (particularly in the sagittal plane) suggests the possibility of a reduced thorax (short ribs) or an abdominal mass (e.g. multicystic or polycystic kidney or enlarged viscus). Similarly, in transverse section the thoracic circumference at the level of the heart should be roughly similar to the abdominal circumference at the umbilical vein. In the same views the integrity of the

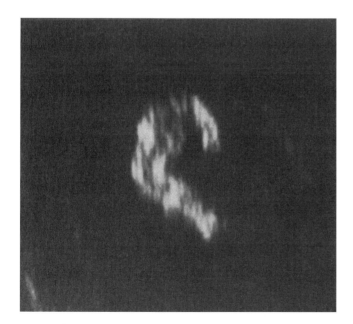

Fig. 8.23 Ear. Scan of the fetal ear in the mid-second trimester.

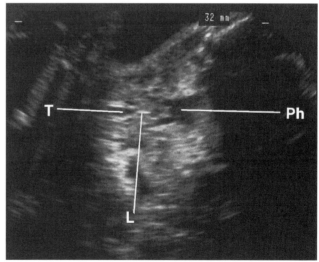

Fig. 8.24 Larynx. Sagittal scan of the fetal larynx (28 weeks). T – trachea, L – larynx, Ph – pharynx.

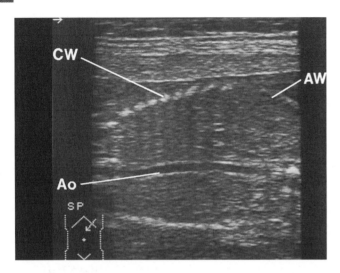

Fig. 8.25 Trunk – coronal. Longitudinal coronal section of the fetal trunk to show the smooth transition from the chest wall (CW) to the abdominal wall (AW). Ao – aorta.

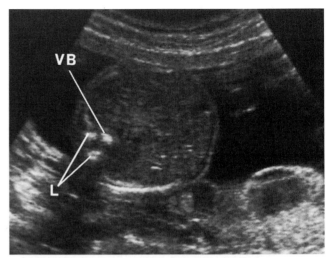

Fig. 8.27 Lumbar spine. Transverse section of the fetal lumbar spine (20 weeks) to show the three major ossification centres. Note the integrity of the skin overlying the spine. L – laminae, VB – vertebral body.

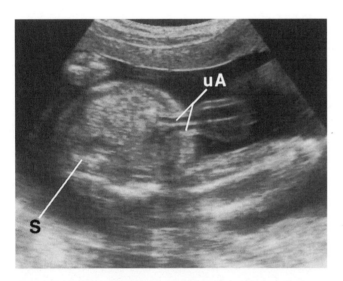

Fig. 8.26 Abdomen – transverse. Transverse scan of the fetal lower abdomen to show the insertion of the umbilical cord. uA – umbilical arteries, S – spine. Figure courtesy of the Portland Hospital.

skin coverings should be checked to exclude omphalocele, gastroschisis, bladder exstrophy, spina bifida, sacral teratoma or other surface tumours. Ensure that the umbilical cord contains one vein and two arteries, and that it has a normal insertion into the anterior abdominal wall (Fig. 8.26).

The spine

The vertebrae have three centres of ossification in fetal life: the vertebral body and each lamina of the neural arch (Fig. 8.27). The spinous process does not start to ossify

until after birth. Thus, ultrasonically in transverse section there are three reflective foci which represent these ossification centres surrounding the echo-free neural canal. In the cervical, thoracic and upper lumbar vertebrae they have an equilateral triangular orientation with its base posterior. Owing to the lumbar expansion of the neural canal the laminar echoes are more widely spaced in the lower lumbar vertebrae and may give a U-shaped appearance. The arms of the U should be parallel or convergent. Divergent arms raise suspicions of spina bifida and initiate a search for signs of a meningocele dorsally and Arnold–Chiari malformation in the fetal head (see Ch. 15). The normal lumbar and cervical expansions of the neural canal are best appreciated in the coronal plane. As part of a spinal examination, the integrity of the overlying skin should be noted.

The spinal curvatures are best examined in the sagittal plane (Fig. 8.28), where the posterior and anterior elements of vertebral bodies are recognised as a double row of strong echoes (the laminae posteriorly and the vertebral bodies anteriorly). The usual posture of the fetal spine is convex posteriorly (kyphotic). There may be a slight lordosis of the cervical spine when the head is extended, but the lumbar lordosis is variably evident depending upon fetal attitude. The spine approaches the skin surface in the sacral region. Spinal flexion may be very marked if there is limited amniotic fluid. The spine should be examined throughout its length for symmetry of both its curvature and its vertebral sequence. In low-risk cases this is first accomplished by a sagittal view, including the complete length of the spine if possible. The transducer is then rotated through 90° and the spine studied in transverse section, maintaining an orthogonal orientation to the ver-

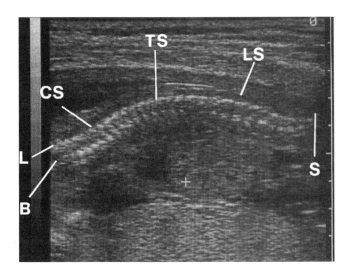

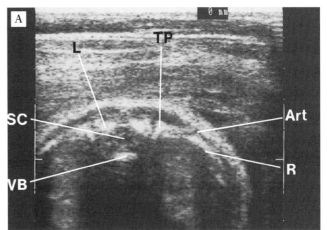

Fig. 8.28 Spine – sagittal. Sagittal section of the spine (18 weeks). The vertebrae are seen as paired reflective dots, the posterior representing the laminae (L) and the anterior representing the vertebral bodies (B). The spinal curvatures can be identified, convex in the thoracic (TS) and upper lumbar spine (LS) and concave in the cerevical (CS) and lumbosacral (S) spines. The skin can be seen overlying the cervical and thoracic spine.

tebrae by following the curvatures. A quick sweep along the spine will reveal gross defects. When an abnormality is suspected, such as spina bifida, Jarcho–Levin syndrome or hemivertebrae (see Ch. 16), more care is needed to examine each vertebra in succession. With good equipment and scanning conditions details of the vertebrae, spinal canal and spinal cord may be seen with increasing clarity as pregnancy advances (Fig. 8.29).

Ribs

The ribs are difficult to image in their full length. They should enclose about two-thirds of the thorax, which should be almost circular in transverse section. They should be evenly spaced and follow a smooth curve round the thorax. Where it is necessary to examine the ribs in detail the best views are:

1. tangential to the lateral thoracic wall to examine spacing and contour
2. longitudinal paramedian for counting
3. transverse for length and thoracic circumference.

Detailed examination of the ribcage tends to be time-consuming, frustrating, and hampered by fetal movement and shadowing by the shoulder girdle. 3D imaging could facilitate this examination.

Shoulder and pelvic girdles

The clavicles are S-shaped and easily identified and measured on a transverse scan in the upper thorax (Fig. 8.30).

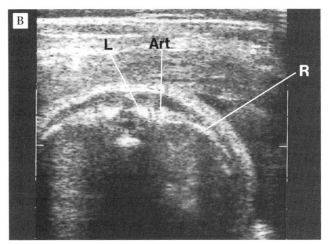

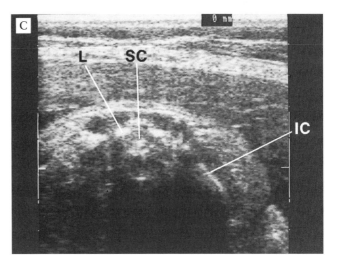

Fig. 8.29 Spine – third trimester. Transverse scans of the spine in the third trimester (33 weeks) to show detail. **A:** Mid-thoracic vertebra. The three major ossification centres in the vertebral body (VB) and the laminae (L) surround the spinal canal (SC). Detail of the transverse process (TP) and its articulations (Art) with the neck and head of the rib (R) are clear. **B:** The 12th rib (R) articulates with the lamina (L). **C:** Lumbar vertebra with lamina (L) spinal canal (SC) and iliac crest (IC).

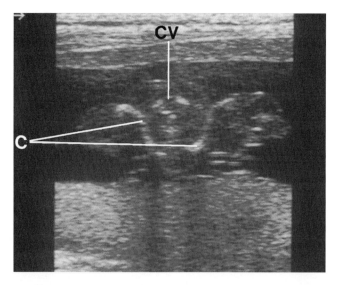

Fig. 8.30 Clavicles. Transverse scan to show the clavicles (18 weeks). CV – cervical vertebra, C – clavicles.

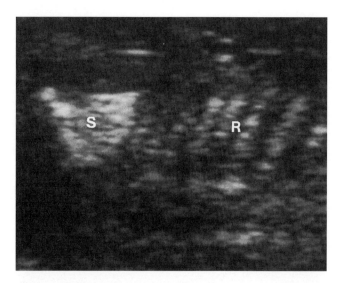

Fig. 8.31 Scapula. Scan tangential to the chest wall to demonstrate the scapula (S). R – ribs.

The triangular outline of the scapula and the spine of the scapula are seen in coronal section tangential to the ribcage (Fig. 8.31).

The iliac crest may be clearly seen in transverse and tangential scans (Figs 8.29C and 8.32). The pubis is usually obscured by the femora. In cloacal exstrophy it may show separation.

Thoracic contents

The major thoracic contents are the heart and great vessels and the lungs. The heart occupies about one-third of the chest and is situated with the apex towards the left side.

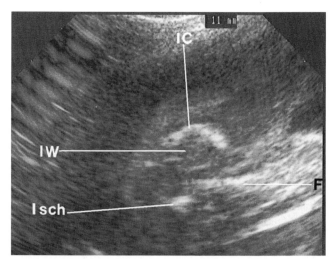

Fig. 8.32 Pelvis. Scan at 22 weeks to show the pelvic bones. IC – iliac crest, IW – wing of ilium, Isch – ischium, F – femur.

The left ventricle lies posterolaterally and the right ventricle anteromedially. Detailed normal anatomy of the heart is described in Chapter 18. The left lung lies behind the heart and is smaller than the right. The lobar divisions are not normally evident. The heart is normally in contact with the chest wall through most of its anterior border and at the apex. This relationship may be lost with a left-sided diaphragmatic hernia or in cystic adenomatoid malformation of the lung. The reflectivity of the lung at most gestational ages is greater than that of the liver, and often similar to the bowel (Fig. 8.33). As the bronchioles proliferate and the alveoli develop, lung reflectivity increases compared to the liver (Fig. 8.34).[4] Normally the pleural and pericardial cavities are not evident.

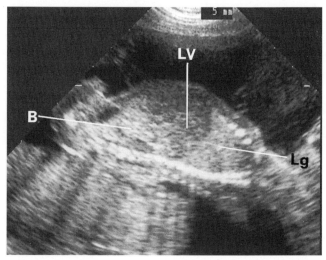

Fig. 8.33 Lung and liver. Right anterior parasagittal scan (19 weeks) to show relative intensity of lung (Lg), liver (LV) and bowel (B).

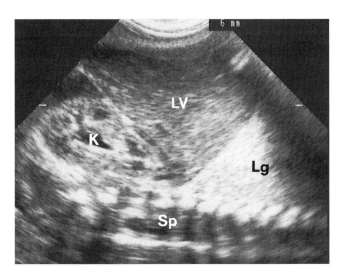

Fig. 8.34 Lung and liver. Sagittal scan at 34 weeks to demonstrate contrast between lung (Lg) and liver (LV) reflectivity (compare with Fig. 8.33). K – kidney, Sp – spine.

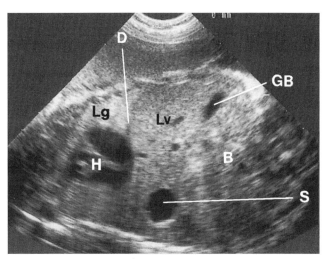

Fig. 8.35 Trunk. Coronal scan of the trunk. The heart (H) and lungs (Lg) are separated from the liver (Lv) by the diaphragm (D). The stomach (S) and gallbladder (GB) are seen at the lower border of the liver. Between them a faint line separates liver from bowel (B).

Breathing movements of the chest wall are evident from early in the second trimester. They can be recognised in either longitudinal or transverse section as rhythmic changes in thoracic diameter or excursions of the diaphragm or kidneys. Breathing is a useful indicator of fetal well-being[5] and is necessary for normal lung development.

The diaphragm

The diaphragm is a thin fibromuscular membrane that separates the thorax from the abdomen. Under good scanning conditions it is seen in sagittal and coronal views as a thin, upwardly convex, echo-poor line separating liver from lung and heart from stomach. In any routine examination it is important to confirm the normal relationships of these organs (Fig. 8.35). The chest should contain no echo-free structures apart from the heart and great vessels. The stomach should be beneath the left ventricle of the heart and separated from it by the diaphragm.

The abdomen

On general examination the abdominal portion of the trunk contains the liver, intestines, renal tract and great vessels. It should routinely contain three cystic structures – the stomach, the bladder and in later pregnancy the gallbladder – each of which should be identified.

The liver

The liver occupies the upper third of the abdominal cavity. Its right lobe is larger than the left, so that in coronal sections its outline approximates to a right-angled triangle, the

hypotenuse being the base of the liver facing caudally and to the left. It is of uniformly low reflectivity, lower than the lung or bowel which form its upper and lower borders, and similar to renal parenchyma. The umbilical vein enters the liver anteriorly and runs a 45° oblique course cephalad and posteriorly to join the portal veins and enter the inferior vena cava via the ductus venosus (Fig. 8.36). Just prior to its junction with the portal veins it takes a J-shaped turn, which is the level at which an abdominal circumference

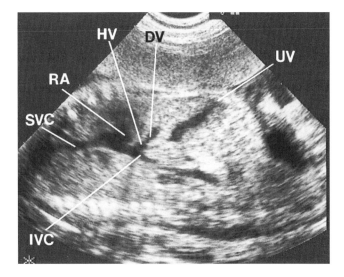

Fig. 8.36 Umbilical venous circulation. Longitudinal anteroposterior view of the fetal trunk to demonstrate the course of the umbilical venous circulation. The umbilical vein (UV) runs an oblique course through the liver from the cord insertion to the ductus venous (DV) and then into the right atrium (RA) via the hepatic vein (HV) and inferior vena cava (IVC). SVC – superior vena cava.

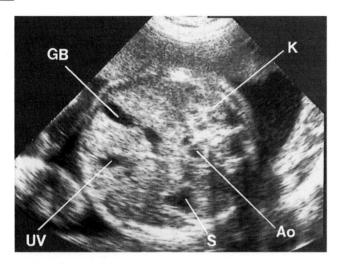

Fig. 8.37 Trunk. Transverse scan of the fetal abdomen showing stomach (S), umbilical vein (UV), gallbladder (GB) and kidney (K). The aorta (Ao) is anterior to the spine.

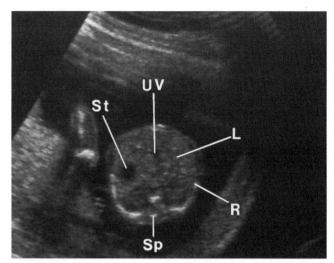

Fig. 8.38 Abdominal circumference. Typical transverse scan (17 weeks) at the level of the umbilical vein (UV) and stomach (St) suitable for abdominal circumference measurement. Sp – spine, L – liver, R – rib.

should be measured. At the right inferior border of the liver a further oblique anechoic structure, the gallbladder, is usually seen. This can be distinguished from the umbilical vein by its lateral position and lack of continuity with the umbilical insertion (Fig. 8.37).

The spleen

The left upper quadrant of the abdominal cavity is occupied by the spleen. Although its ultrasonic visualisation has been described and biometric tables have been published[6] (see Appendix), it may be difficult to identify routinely. It lies above the left kidney and behind the stomach. It has a uniform reflectivity, similar to the liver.

The stomach

The stomach should be identified in all routine scans, and if it is not the patient should be re-examined later the same day, or on another occasion. The stomach may be evident from the ninth to the tenth week onwards. In most cases it will be seen from the 14th week, and always by the time of a routine 18–20-week examination (Fig. 8.38). Its shape varies with fullness and gestation, the greater and lesser curvatures becoming more recognisable with increasing age. After the 16th week peristalsis may be seen on prolonged observation. Considering its dynamic state, the volume of the stomach has been found to be remarkably constant and biometric nomograms are available (see Appendix).[7] The stomach contents are echo-free.

The small intestine

In the second and early third trimesters the lumen of the small bowel is not usually obvious, but nearer term it can

be identified with occasional peristalsis. Widespread visualisation of the lumen and peristalsis should alert the sonographer to the possibility of bowel obstruction.

The colon

Like the small intestine, the lumen of the colon is not normally evident in the second trimester. However, in the third trimester colonic contents can be identified in the ascending colon at first, and progressively filling the transverse, descending and sigmoid colons by term. Haustrations are seen. Cellular debris produces low-level echoes in colonic contents which distinguish them from the echo-free fluid in the stomach or urinary tract, or other cystic abdominal or pelvic masses (Fig. 8.39).

The urinary tract

The ureters and urethra are not seen under normal circumstances, although the urethra may be evident in males during micturition.

The kidneys

The kidneys are situated on either side of the lumbar spine and may be consistently visualised from about the 14th week..At this stage they have a homogeneous appearance, with slightly lower reflectivity than the surrounding bowel and similar to the liver and are most readily demonstrated in a posterior transverse scan below the level of the liver. The renal pelvis may be seen as an echo-free slit-like space in the centre of the kidney (Fig. 8.40).

As pregnancy progresses, further details of the renal architecture appear. A thin reflective rim, representing the

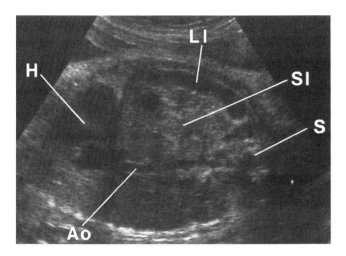

Fig. 8.39 Colon. Scan at 32 weeks showing large intestine (LI) containing meconium and enclosing the more reflective small intestine (SI). H – Heart, Ao – aorta, S – spine.

renal capsule, appears at about the 19th week. From about the 24th week fetal lobation becomes increasingly apparent, particularly in coronal and parasagittal sections. The medullary pyramids are arranged round the renal pelvis as a rosette of echo-poor foci with poorly defined margins (Figs 8.41 and 8.42). They should not be confused with cysts, which are echo-free and have well defined margins.

At all gestational ages the circumference of the kidney should be about one-third of the abdominal circumference.[8] The renal volume is calculated by multiplying the longitudinal, transverse and anteroposterior dimensions and dividing by two. Growth in all dimensions is roughly linear throughout pregnancy (see Appendix).[9]

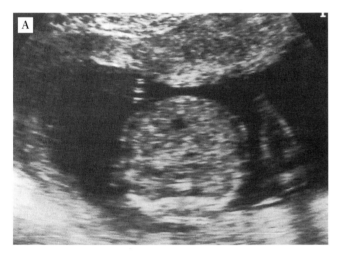

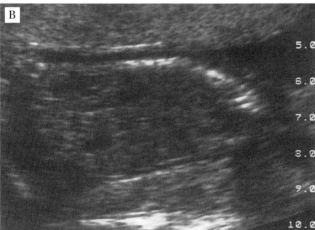

Fig. 8.40 Kidneys at 16 weeks. A: Transverse scan to show kidneys on either side of the lumbar spine. They have little architectural detail at this stage apart from the echo-free renal pelvis. **B:** Longitudinal scan of the same kidney.

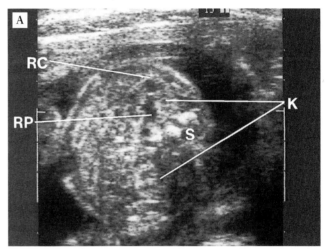

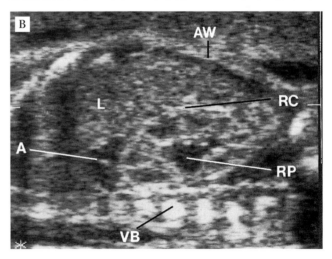

Fig. 8.41 Kidneys and adrenal at 24 weeks. A: The perimeter of the kidney (K) is more easily identified from the reflective renal capsule (RC). Renal architecture and the renal pelvis (RP) are evident. S – spine. **B:** Longitudinal scan clearly showing echo-poor pyramids and lobation of the kidney, the renal capsule (RC) and the intrarenal pelvis (RP). The adrenal gland is seen as a triangular structure above the upper pole of the kidney. VB – vertebral body, L – liver, AW – abdominal wall.

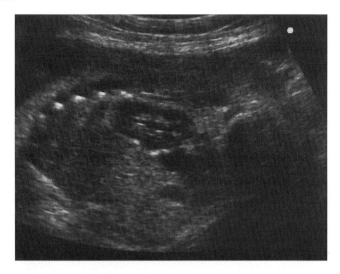

Fig. 8.42 Longitudinal scan of kidney at 36 weeks. The lobation is apparent and the renal capsule is highly reflective. Note shadowing of the adrenal by the 11th rib.

Comparisons of size and structure between the kidneys are best accomplished when they are simultaneously imaged in the prevertebral coronal plane. As in the adult, the left kidney lies slightly higher than the right and both should have an ovoid structure; the longitudinal axis is virtually parallel to the spine. In this view the renal pelves drain medially. In later pregnancy the renal vasculature may be seen at the hilum with colour Doppler.

In the early stages of pregnancy the kidneys may be quite difficult to image in obese patients, or if the fetus is lying with its spine either posteriorly or vertically in the scanning plane. Identification may be facilitated during fetal breathing, which causes longitudinal excursions of the kidneys against the spine. Visualisation is also often difficult in oligohydramnios, when the kidneys must be identified to exclude renal agenesis. A vaginal transducer may be helpful in these cases, as the fetus is often a breech presentation deep in the pelvis.

The renal pelvis

The prominence of the intrarenal pelvis is the subject of much debate. Studies are ongoing to ascertain the limits of normal size. For the present an arbitrary figure of 4 mm for the mean transverse and anteroposterior diameters has been chosen as the accepted upper limit in the mid-trimester.

Normally the extrarenal pelvis cannot be seen, but slight prominence may be a normal variant.

The bladder

The bladder is seen as an echo-free structure of variable size arising from the pelvis. Prior to the 14th week urine production is limited, so that the bladder may not be identified easily. Thereafter urine production increases progressively to a rate of approximately 50 ml per hour at term.[10] If the bladder cannot be identified, or if it seems excessively full, a repeat examination after about half an hour should show filling in the former case and emptying in the latter. Bladder volume is assessed by measuring the bladder outline in three dimensions and halving their product. The bladder should have no internal echoes.

The adrenal glands

The adrenal glands are situated between the upper pole of each kidney and the liver on the right and the spleen on the left (Figs 8.41B and 8.43). They may be difficult to identify owing to shadowing from the ribs. Nevertheless,

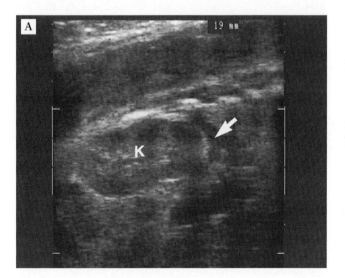

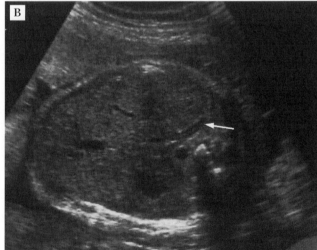

Fig. 8.43 Adrenal glands. A: Parasagittal and **B:** transverse scans at 36 weeks to show adrenal glands (arrow). K – kidney.

normal ranges for adrenal dimensions have been constructed (see Appendix).[11,12] Of importance in diagnostic ultrasonography is that in cases of renal agenesis the adrenal glands may take on an enlarged ovoid shape and be mistaken for kidneys.

Fetal genitalia

The male phallus may be demonstrated from quite early in the second trimester if the fetus is in a favourable supine position with its hips abducted (Fig. 8.44). However, sex assignation at this stage is imprudent as the clitoris may also be prominent. Later in pregnancy the scrotum is more evident and contains the testes (Fig. 8.45). These are best seen in a scan tangential to the upper thigh with the fetal legs flexed. In this plane the vulva may also be seen as fine

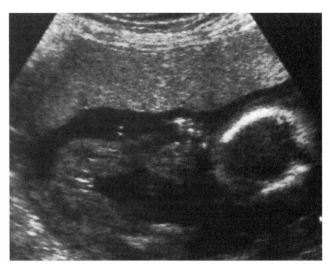

Fig. 8.46 **Female genitalia.** Scan of a female fetus at 22 weeks gestation.

lines (labia minora) between the mounds of the labia majora (Fig. 8.46).

Musculoskeletal system

Long bones (see Appendix)

It is important to measure femur length and to examine limb morphology in any routine 18–20-week scan, first because femur length has been shown to be as accurate an indicator of fetal gestational age as biparietal diameter,[13–15] and serves as a useful alternative in dating a pregnancy when the head is in a difficult position for measurement. Secondly, when checked against other fetal measurements pathologies such as limb reductions or microcephaly should be detected. Fetal limb reductions or deformities are a feature of many lethal or crippling congenital disorders (trisomy 18, the chondrodysplasias, arthrogryposis multiplex congenita, TAR syndrome etc.), most of which should be detected in the second trimester by careful ultrasound examination.

The femur is best located initially by scanning the fetus across the trunk in the axial plane and running down the fetal axis until the pelvic bones are identified. The proximal ends of one or both femora will then be seen. Keeping the femur in the image, the transducer is then rotated about the axis of the scanning plane until the whole of the ossified diaphysis (shaft) of the bone is in view (Fig. 8.47A). It is common practice to align the femur parallel to the transducer. However, this may give rise to an overestimate of the femoral length owing to beam spread effects. Alignment of the femur at about 45° to the transducer minimises this artefact, which can be further reduced by lowering the transmit power. A slight lateral shift of the scanning plane should cause the whole bone to disappear from view. If this manoeuvre causes apparent shortening or a lateral shift of the bone in the image, then the full length of the bone is not

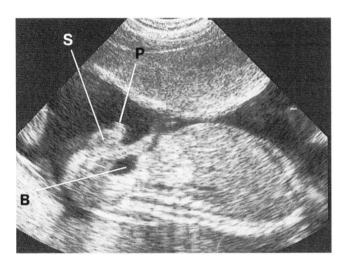

Fig. 8.44 **Male genitalia.** Sagittal scan of a 20-week fetus to show male genitalia. B – bladder, P – penis, S – scrotum.

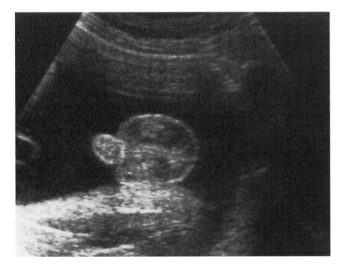

Fig. 8.45 Male genitalia at 36 weeks.

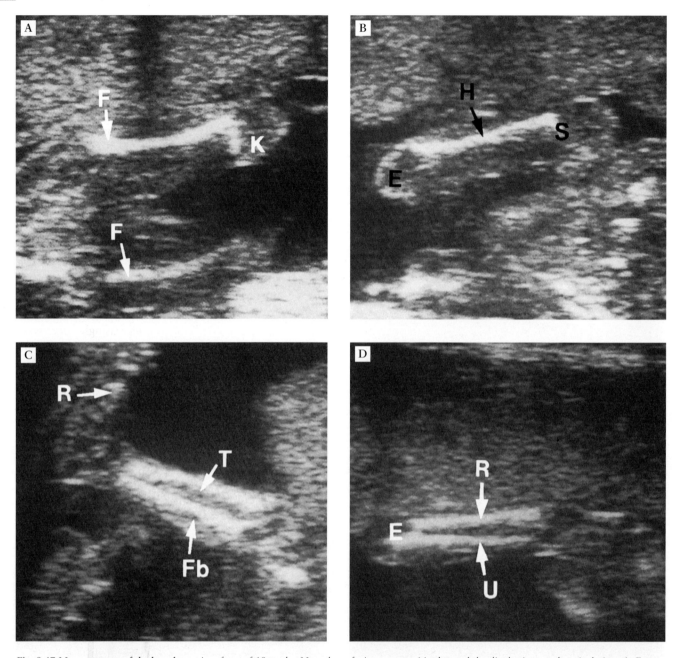

Fig. 8.47 Measurements of the long bones in a fetus of 18 weeks. Note the soft tissue extremities beyond the diaphysis at each articulation. **A:** Femur (F). Only the proximal femur is fully visualised. Note the expansion of the diaphysis at the femoral condyles and the knee (K) beyond. **B:** Humerus (H). S – shoulder, E – elbow. **C:** Tibia (T) and fibula (Fb). The heel and toes can be seen on the foot. **D:** Radius (R) and ulna (U). The ulna is longer because of the olecranon. E – elbow.

within the scanning plane and further rotational adjustment of the transducer is necessary. Inclusion of the limb extremities (knee and buttock, elbow and shoulder etc.) in the image will help in correct alignment. Finally, ensure that the diaphysis to be measured is not overshadowed by other bony structures and that adjacent bones are not included in the measurement. Accuracy may be improved if several measurements of the bone are taken until they are consistent.

The technique for humerus measurement is similar to that for the femur (Fig. 8.47B). With older machines it is sometimes difficult to differentiate the humeral extremities from their adjacent articulations (scapula/clavicle and olecranon process of the ulna), but with modern high-resolution equipment this should not be a problem. Humerus length is a useful alternative measure of fetal age if the femur is obscured, as may occur in a breech presentation.

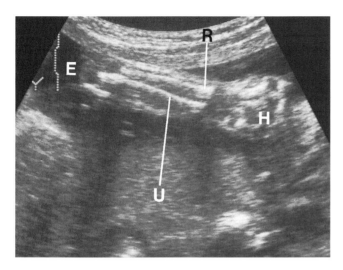

Fig. 8.48 Forearm. Radius (R) and ulna (U) at 28 weeks showing greater anatomical detail than in Figure 8.47D. E – elbow, H – hand.

The distal long bones are identified by following on from the proximal. One forearm is often obscured behind the fetal head or body, but will eventually move into view. Because radial hypoplasia or aplasia is a feature of many important syndromes the radius and ulna (Figs 8.47D and 8.48) should be visualised independently in all cases and measured separately in high-risk examinations. The tibia and fibula (Fig. 8.47C) are of such similar lengths that they need not be measured independently, but should be individually identified.

The upper tibial and lower femoral epiphyses will appear in the third trimester (Fig. 8.49). The exact timing of their appearance is variable and may be affected by growth impairment. The value of using them to date pregnancies in the third trimester is limited.

The feet may be viewed in three major planes (Figs 8.50 to 8.52) to identify deformities such as talipes, rocker-bottom feet, poly/syndactyly etc. Recently interest has been aroused in the ultrasonic recognition of clinodactyly of the fifth finger and the 'sandal gap' between the big and second toes, and its application to the diagnosis of Down's syndrome. Its application to clinical practice has yet to be evaluated. Foot length (heel to big toe) and femur length should be approximately equal in the second trimester, the foot usually being slightly larger. Hands should be examined so as to reveal four fingers and a normal thumb (Fig. 8.53). It may take a little time before the fetus opens the hand to reveal all digits.

Hip, knee, ankle, elbow, wrist and finger joints should be studied for normal position and movement.

Amniotic fluid

Prior to the 14th week of pregnancy the amniotic fluid is chiefly a transudate across the fetal skin and membranes. Thereafter, fetal urine production increasingly contributes to amniotic fluid, so that by the 20th week urine accounts for the majority. Amniotic fluid volume rises progressively from about 250 ml at 16 weeks to a fairly constant mean of 800 ml in the third trimester, with a slight reduction post-term.[16] Production is most rapid between 24 and 28 weeks. The constant volume is obtained by a balance of fetal swallowing and micturition. Any disturbance in this balance, such as reduced urine outflow (urinary tract obstruction, renal pathology or disturbed physiology), impaired intestinal absorption of fluid (duodenal atresia), or possibly excessive contribution of transudate from disrupted skin coverings (omphalocele, meningocele, teratoma), will cause the volume to rise or fall.

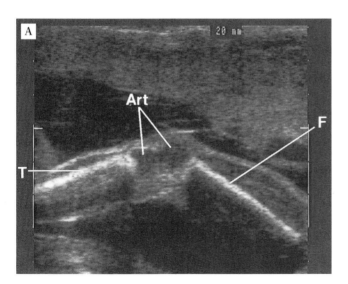

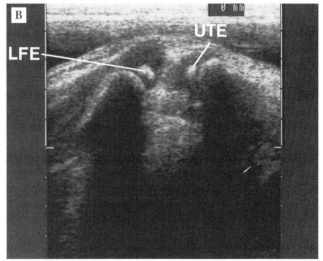

Fig. 8.49 Knee epiphyses. Scans to show development of the lower femoral and upper tibial epiphyses. **A:** At 29 weeks the unmineralised epiphyseal cartilages of the knee (Art). T – tibia, F – femur. **B:** At 38 weeks the lower femoral (LFE) and the upper tibial epiphyses (UTE) have begun to ossify.

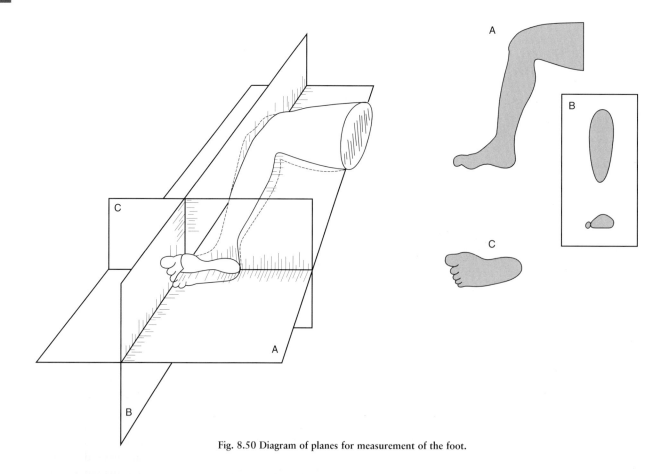

Fig. 8.50 Diagram of planes for measurement of the foot.

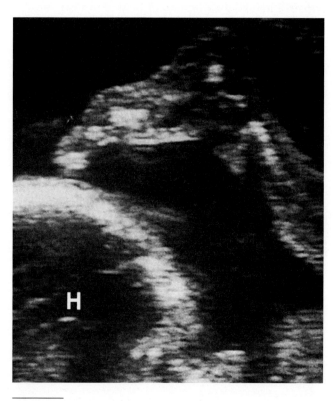

Fig. 8.51 Foot. Sagittal scan of the foot (22 weeks) – plane A. H – head.

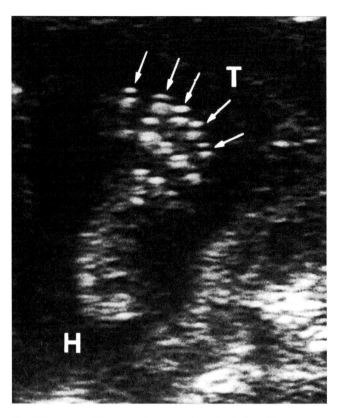

Fig. 8.52 Foot. Axial scan of the foot – plane C. H – heel, T – toes.

Accurate measurement of amniotic fluid is time-consuming. A simple estimate may be obtained by measuring the largest pool of amniotic fluid in two dimensions at right-angles. In the third trimester measurements between 2 and 8 cm are considered normal. Measurements below or above this range indicate oligohydramnios or polyhydramnios, respectively (see Ch. 11). The amniotic fluid index has been accepted as a more accurate assessment of volume when oligo or polyhydramnios is suspected.

Multiple pregnancy

The accepted incidence of twin pregnancies is 1 in 80. There are more dizygotic twins than monozygotic. The incidence of triplets is about 1 in 6000 pregnancies. These incidences are increasing with the more widespread use of ovulation stimulation and extracorporeal fertilisation.

Multiple pregnancies are at increased risk of fetal malformation, spontaneous abortion, growth retardation, placenta praevia, polyhydramnios and preterm labour. Routine ultrasound examination enables early detection of multiple pregnancy and timely institution of management regimes designed to reduce morbidity from these complications. All mothers of multiple pregnancies should be offered a full anomaly scan and serial scans for fetal growth. It is prudent to scan at 4-weekly intervals, with extra examinations according to clinical need.

Monochorionic twins are at considerably greater risk than dichoronic twins. Chorionicity should be carefully assessed as soon as twin pregnancy is diagnosed (see first-trimester scanning).

The only certain way to distinguish binovular from monovular twins is to identify different sexes. The thickness of the dividing membrane between the sacs (Fig. 8.54) or apparent placental unity are less reliable indications.

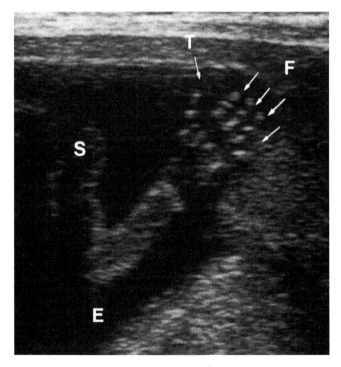

Fig. 8.53 Scan of the forearm and fanned hand (17 weeks). Contours of the shoulder (S), elbow (E), thumb (T) and fingers (F) can be seen. The fifth finger is partly obscured.

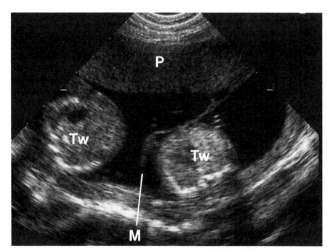

Fig. 8.54 Twin pregnancy. Showing the trunk of each twin (Tw) in transverse section and the membrane (M) dividing the two sacs. The attachment of the membrane to the placenta (P) can be seen on the left.

When no dividing membrane can be seen the differential diagnosis is between severe oligohydramnios in one sac and a monoamniotic pregnancy. Both situations carry a high risk and require skilled examination, as fetal abnormality or a shared circulation and twin–twin transfusion are distinct possibilities.

In examining fetuses in a multiple pregnancy a highly systematic approach should be adopted, starting with examination of the head and carefully following the continuity of the body through the trunk and on to the limbs. With mobile fetuses, and particularly with triplets, this is the only way to ensure full examination of each fetus. Ensuring that each fetus moves independently from the other excludes conjoint twins (Fig. 8.55). Shadowing of one fetus by the other is a frequent impediment to full examination, but patience will eventually be rewarded.

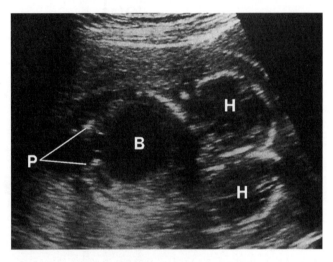

Fig. 8.55 Conjoint twins. Two heads (H) can be seen above a common trunk with fused pelvis (P) and a common, distended bladder (B). There were two complete spines, two legs and four arms.

REFERENCES

1　Shepard M, Filly R A. A standardized plane for biparietal diameter measurement. J Ultrasound Med 1982; 1(4): 145–150
2　Chudleigh P, Pearce J M. Obstetric ultrasound: how, why and when. Edinburgh: Churchill Livingstone, 1986; 65
3　Benaceraff B R, Chann A, Gelman R, Laboda L A, Frigoletto F D Jr. Can sonography reliably identify anatomic features associated with Down's syndrome in fetuses? Radiology 1989; 173: 377
4　Fried A M, Loh F K, Umer M A, Dillon K P, Kryscio R. Echogenicity of fetal lung: relation to fetal age and maturity. AJR 1985; 145(3): 591–594
5　Griffin D. Fetal activity. In: Studd J, ed. Progress in obstetrics and gynaecology, Vol 4. Edinburgh: Churchill Livingstone, 1984; 92–117
6　Schmidt W, Yarconi S, Jeanty P, Grannum P, Hobbins J C. Sonographic measurements of the fetal spleen: clinical implications. J Ultrasound Med 1985; 4: 667–672
7　Goldstein I, Reece E A, Yarkoni S, Wan M, Green J L, Hobbins J C. Growth of the fetal stomach in normal pregnancies. Obstet Gynecol 1987, 70(4): 641–644
8　Grannum P, Bracken M, Silverman R, Hobbins J C. Assessment of fetal kidney size in normal gestation by comparison of ratio of kidney circumference to abdominal circumference. Am J Obstet Gynecol 1980; 136(2): 249–254
9　Jeanty P, Dramaix-Wilmet M, Elkhazen N, Hubinont C, van Regemorter N. Measurements of fetal kidney growth on ultrasound. Radiology 1982; 144(1): 159–162
10　Nicolaides K H, Peters M T, Vyas S, Rabinowitz R, Rosen D J, Campbell S. Relation of rate of urine production to oxygen tension in small-for-gestational-age fetuses. Am J Obstet Gynecol 1990; 162(2): 387–391
11　Jeanty P, Chervenak F, Grannum P, Hobbins J C. Normal ultrasonic size and characteristics of the fetal adrenal glands. Prenat Diagn 1984; 4(1): 21–28
12　Lewis E, Kurtz A B, Dubbins P A, Wapner R J, Goldberg B B. Real-time ultrasonographic evaluation of normal fetal adrenal glands. J Ultrasound Med 1982; 1(7): 265–270
13　O'Brien G D, Queenan J T, Campbell S. Assessment of gestational age in the second trimester by real-time ultrasound measurement of the femur length. Am J Obstet Gynecol 1981; 139(5): 540–545
14　Hadlock F P, Harrist R B, Deter R L, Park S K. Fetal femur length as a predictor of menstrual age: sonographically measured. AJR 1982; 138(5): 875–878
15　Quinlan R W, Brumfield C, Martin M, Cruz A C. Ultrasonic measurement of femur length as a predictor of fetal gestational age. J Reprod Med 1982; 27(7): 392–394

Gestational age

Peter M Doubilet and Carol B Benson

Introduction

Accurate assessment of gestational age is critical for a variety of diagnostic and management considerations. A number of fetal abnormalities are diagnosed by comparing the size of the fetus and its component parts to norms for gestational age. These include skeletal dysplasias, microcephaly and pulmonary hypoplasia. In addition, diagnosis of intra-uterine growth restriction is made in part by estimating the fetal weight and assessing its percentile for gestational age. Interpretation of the maternal serum triple screen – human chorionic gonadotrophin, α-fetoprotein, and oestriol – also requires knowledge of the gestational age, because the normal levels of these substances vary with age.

Management decisions about the timing of delivery can best be made if gestational age is accurately known. The decision about when to deliver an abnormal pregnancy, such as one complicated by pre-eclampsia or intra-uterine growth retardation, should take gestational age into account. Knowledge of gestational age is essential to determine whether labour is premature, or to prompt the delivery of a post-dates fetus.

Definition of gestational age

Gestational age is important because fetal growth and development are assessed by comparing clinical and sonographic findings to expected milestones for gestational age. Ideally gestational age would be synonymous with conceptual age, the time elapsed since conception. Historically, however, the date of conception was unknown, whereas a related date – the first day of the last menstrual period (LMP) – was known in most cases. For this reason gestational age has long been used synonymously with menstrual age, the time elapsed since the first day of the LMP.

If all pregnant women knew their LMP and had regular 28-day cycles menstrual age would always be exactly 2 weeks more than conceptual age. Were this the case it would be reasonable to continue to use menstrual age to measure progression through pregnancy and ultrasound would play no role in dating pregnancies. In practice, however, dating via the LMP has a number of limitations.[1] Cycle lengths vary, so that the time interval between the LMP and conception may be greater or less than 2 weeks. Many women misremember their LMP, especially when questioned late in pregnancy. In addition, bleeding early in pregnancy, a fairly common occurrence, can be mistaken for a menstrual period. As a result the relationship between menstrual age based on reported LMP and conceptual age is inconstant.

The unreliability of the LMP to date a pregnancy led to on a new meaning for the term:

gestational age = conceptual age + 2 weeks.

With this definition a number of types of information can be used to assign age. When objective information is available to pinpoint the date of conception, as in cases of assisted conception, this should be used to assign gestational age. In women without objective data about the date of conception, LMP and ultrasound play complementary roles in establishing gestational age. The LMP provides a preliminary estimate. While the ultrasound findings are used to confirm or replace the gestational age based on the LMP. Ultrasound, especially when performed in the first half of pregnancy, is more accurate for assigning gestational age than even a well remembered LMP date in a woman with regular cycle lengths,[1,2] as ultrasound has been shown to be a better predictor of the date of delivery.[3–6]

It is important to note that the use of ultrasound to confirm or assign gestational age should be restricted to the first scan in a pregnancy.[7,8] From that point onward the gestational age (GA) should be calculated as:

GA = (GA at initial scan) + (time elapsed since initial scan).

Consider, for example, a woman who is assigned a gestational age of 10.0 weeks based on a scan in the first-trimaster. If she returns for another scan 15 weeks later, the gestational age at that time should be taken to be 25.0 weeks. The fetal measurements on this scan should not be used to redate the pregnancy, but rather should be compared to the norms for 25 weeks to assess whether the fetus is appropriate in size.

How ultrasound is used to date a pregnancy depends on the stage at which the first scan is performed. The various methods for ultrasound-based dating are discussed below.

Assignment of gestational age at initial ultrasound

First trimester

The development and growth of the gestational sac and its contents occur at a very predictable rate in the first trimester, with relatively little variation from pregnancy to pregnancy. When scanning trans-vaginally the gestational sac is first identifiable at, or very close to, 5.0 weeks gestational age.[9,10] At this age the sac appears as a small fluid collection with no discernable contents (Fig. 9.1). At 5.5 weeks the yolk sac can be seen as a round fluid-filled structure within the gestational sac (Fig. 9.2).[11] At 6.0 weeks the embryonic heartbeat is identifiable adjacent to the yolk sac (Fig. 9.3).[9,11] In some cases the heartbeat lies within a recognisable embryo, whereas in others it first appears as a flicker adjacent to the yolk sac.

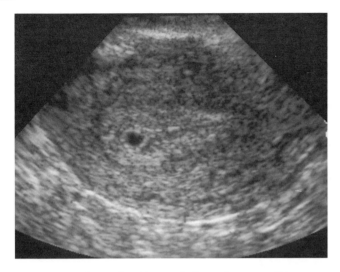

Fig. 9.1 5.0-week gestation. Trans-vaginal scan shows a small intra-uterine fluid collection with no visible contents (i.e. no yolk sac or embryo seen).

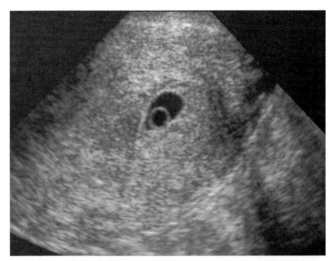

Fig. 9.2 5.5-week gestation. Trans-vaginal scan shows an intra-uterine gestational sac containing a yolk sac. No embryo is seen.

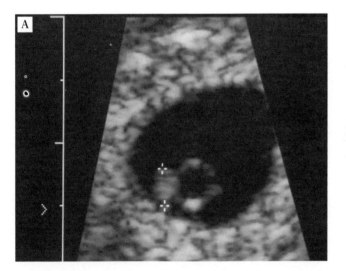

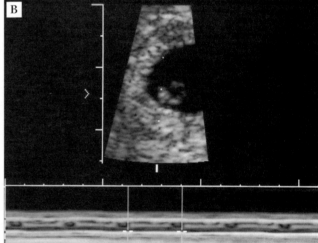

Fig. 9.3 6.0-week gestation. A: Trans-vaginal scan shows an intra-uterine gestational sac with a 2.9 mm embryo (delineated by calipers) adjacent to a yolk sac. B: M-mode demonstrates cardiac activity.

The mean sac diameter – average of the anteroposterior, transverse and sagittal diameters of the gestational sac – is typically 2 mm at 5.0 weeks. Over the next week it grows slightly more than 1 mm per day, reaching a mean of 10 mm at 6.0 weeks.[12]

The embryo is first visible at 6.0–6.3 weeks as an elongated structure without identifiable body parts. By the end of the first trimester the head, trunk and limbs can be identified. The length of the embryo or fetus, excluding the extremities when they are visible, is termed the crown–rump length (CRL). It is measureed by rotating the transducer until the full length of the embryo or fetus is imaged (Fig. 9.4). Care must be taken not to underestimate the CRL by scanning obliquely through a part of the embryo or fetus, and not to overestimate it by including the yolk sac in the measurement. The CRL is approximately 6 mm at 6.3 weeks, 9 mm at 7.0 weeks, and 64 mm at 13 weeks.[13]

These observations concerning the growth and development of the products of conception form the basis for the sonographic determination of gestational age in the first trimester (Tables 9.1 to 9.3). Between 5.0 and 6.0 weeks gestational age can be assigned using either the appearance (Table 9.1) or the size (Table 9.2) of the gestational sac.

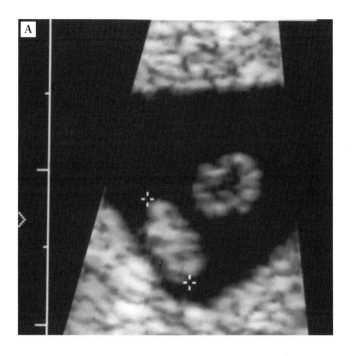

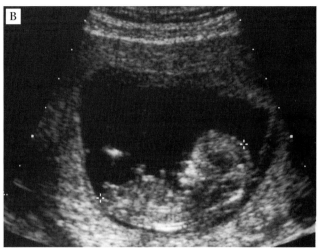

Fig. 9.4 Crown–rump length measurement. A: Cursors measure the length of an embryo with no identifiable body parts. The length is 6 mm, corresponding to a gestational age of 6.3 weeks. **B:** Cursors measure the length of a fetus with identifiable head and trunk. The length is 50 mm, corresponding to a gestational age of 11.9 weeks.

Table 9.1 Gestational age assignment based on trans-vaginal ultrasound findings in the early first trimester

Ultrasound finding	Gestational age (weeks)
Gestational sac, no yolk sac, embryo or heartbeat	5.0 weeks
Gestational sac and yolk sac, no embryo or heartbeat	5.5 weeks
Gestational sac, yolk sac and heartbeat; embryo not visible or ≤ 5 mm in length	6.0 weeks

Table 9.2 Gestational age assignment based on mean sac diameter in the early first trimester (Reprinted in part from (ref. 12) with permission)

Mean sac diameter (mm)*	Gestational age (weeks)
2	5.0
3	5.1
4	5.2
5	5.4
6	5.5
7	5.6
8	5.7
9	5.9
10	6.0
11	6.1
12	6.2
13	6.4
14	6.5

* Average of the anteroposterior, transverse and sagittal diameters of the gestational sac.

Using the former, an age of 5.0 weeks is assigned if sonography demonstrates a gestational sac with no identifiable internal structures, 5.5 weeks if the gestational sac contains a yolk sac but there is no visible embryonic heartbeat, and 6.0 weeks if there is a heartbeat but no embryo measuring greater than 5 mm in length (Table 9.1). Using the alternative approach of dating via the size of the gestational sac, the mean sac diameter is determined and the corresponding gestational age is assigned from a table (Table 9.2).[12] Either method is acceptable, although the latter may have greater variability owing both to interobserver differences in the selection of sonographic planes to measure sac diameter, and to distortions of the sac by uterine contractions.

When there is an embryo or fetus 6–75 mm in length gestational age is assigned via the CRL, using a table (Table 9.3), or calculated via a formula. In one of the early uses of medical ultrasound Robinson and Fleming[13] produced a table of gestational age versus CRL using measurements obtained by static B-mode ultrasound performed in women with regular 28-day menstrual cycles. Their work suggested that ultrasound dating using CRL is highly accurate, with an error range of only ±3–5 days. More recent studies involving women whose pregnancies were achieved via assisted conception[14] or with known ovulation dates[15] have confirmed the accuracy of the Robinson/Fleming data. In particular there are only minor discrepancies of 1–2 days between the Robinson/Fleming 'corrected regression analysis' table and a table generated from *in vitro* fertilisation patients.[14]

Table 9.3 Gestational age assignment based on crown–rump length (Based on ref 13 ('corrected regression analysis' data))

Crown–rump length (mm)	Gestational age (weeks)	Crown–rump length (mm)	Gestational age (weeks)
6	6.3	41	11.1
7	6.6	42	11.2
8	6.8	43	11.2
9	7.0	44	11.3
10	7.2	45	11.4
11	7.4	46	11.5
12	7.6	47	11.6
13	7.7	48	11.7
14	7.9	49	11.8
15	8.1	50	11.9
16	8.2	51	12.0
17	8.3	52	12.0
18	8.5	53	12.1
19	8.6	54	12.2
20	8.8	55	12.3
21	8.9	56	12.4
22	9.0	57	12.4
23	9.1	58	12.5
24	9.3	59	12.6
25	9.4	60	12.6
26	9.5	61	12.7
27	9.6	62	12.8
28	9.7	63	12.9
29	9.8	64	13.0
30	9.9	65	13.1
31	10.1	66	13.1
32	10.2	67	13.2
33	10.3	68	13.3
34	10.4	69	13.3
35	10.5	70	13.4
36	10.6	71	13.5
37	10.7	72	13.6
38	10.8	73	13.6
39	10.9	74	13.7
40	11.0	75	13.8

Second and third trimesters

After the first trimester, the CRL is not useful for determining gestational age. By the second trimester the measurement varies with fetal flexion and extension, and the fetal head and trunk do not easily fit on a single ultrasound scan image.

Measurements of one or more fetal body parts replace the CRL for gestational age determination in the second and third trimesters. In principle any body part can be used to determine gestational age, so long as norms have been established for the size of that body part in relation to gestational age. These have been published for a large number of body parts, including the head,[16–21] femur,[16,17,21–25] other long bones,[26,27] abdomen,[16,17,28] cerebellum,[29] spine,[30] foot,[31] binocular distance[32] and clavicle.[33] In practice, only the larger body parts merit serious consideration as bases for assigning gestational age, as

minor variations in caliper placement or scanning plane lead to lower relative errors in the measurement of large body parts than they do for small body parts. The parts most frequently used for pregnancy dating in the second and third trimester are the head and femur.

The fetal head is measured on an ultrasound image that displays the head in an axial plane at the level of the thalami and the cavum septum pellucidum (Fig. 9.5).[2,7,34–36] Gestational age can be determined by anumber of head measurements or derived values, including the biparietal diameter (BPD),[16,17,19,21] corrected BPD (cBPD)[37] and head circumference (HC).[16–18,20] The BPD is measured from the outer edge of the parietal bone nearer the transducer to the inner edge of the opposite parietal

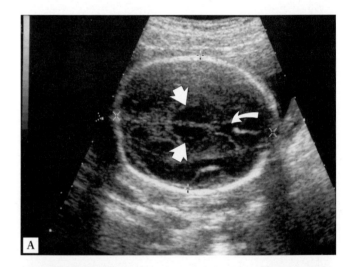

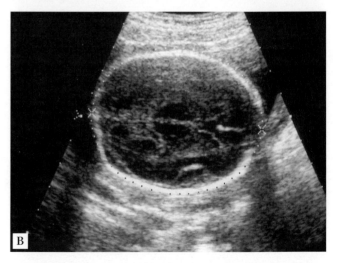

Fig. 9.5 Fetal head measurements. A: Axial plane through the fetal head at the level of the thalami (straight arrows) and cavum septum pellucidum (curved arrow). The biparietal diameter (+ ... + calipers, 54.1 mm) and the occipitofrontal diameter (× ... × calipers, 65.8 mm) are measured. **B:** On the same image the head circumference is measured by elliptical calipers to be 198.0 mm.

bone (i.e. from leading edge to leading edge). The occipitofrontal diameter (OFD) is measured from the middle of the occipital bone echo to the middle of the frontal bone echo.

The cBPD is a calculated value and is equal to the BPD of the standard-shaped head (i.e. one whose ratio of length to width is 1.265), whose cross-sectional area is the same as that of the fetus being measured.[37] It is calculated from the BPD and OFD using the equation:

$$cBPD = \sqrt{((BPD \times OFD)/1.265)}$$

The cBPD can be used in place of the BPD in any table or formula. Consider, for example, the fetal head in Figure 9.5, which has a BPD of 54.1 mm and an OFD of 65.8 mm. The cBPD is:

$$\sqrt{((54.1 \times 65.8)/1.265)} = 53.0 \text{ mm}.$$

To estimate gestational age the value of 53.0 mm is used as the BPD in any table or formula that relates BPD to gestational age.

The head circumference is the perimeter around the outer edge of the skull. It can be measured using electronic elliptical calipers, which are available on most ultrasound scanners. It can also be approximated from the BPD and the OFD using the formula:

$$HC \approx 3.14 \times ((BPD + OFD)/2).^{[38,39]}$$

The femur length (FL) is the measurement of the length of the femoral diaphysis, or shaft,[40] and is measured on an ultrasound image that displays the full length of the femoral shaft (Fig. 9.6). Occasionally the uncalcified epiphysis produces a thin line extending beyond the ossified diaphysis, and beam width or side lobe artefacts may also cause apparent echoes beyond the end of the diaphysis. These lines

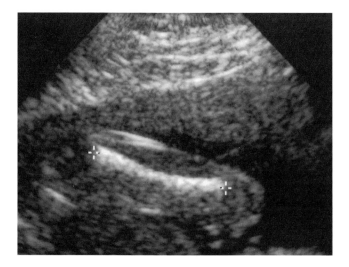

Fig. 9.6 Femur length. Cursors measure the length of the femoral diaphysis.

should not be included in the measurement.[40] Care must be taken to include the full length of the femoral shaft, as an oblique scan plane through a portion of the femur can lead to a falsely small measurement.

Tables and formulae have been published for gestational age assignment based on the BPD (or cBPD), HC and FL. Formulae have also been published for predicting gestational age from multiple indices, usually a combination of head measurements (BPD, HC or cBPD), FL and abdominal diameter or circumference.[16,17,21,41] Many of these however, systematically underestimate gestational age late in pregnancy. Formulae that avoid this bias provide a means for assigning gestational age that is largely free of systematic error throughout pregnancy.[21] These include:

GA from BPD (or cBPD):

$$GA = \begin{cases} \text{Exp } (2.27969 + & \text{if this value is} \\ \quad 0.015091 \text{ BPD}) & \text{equal to or less than 42} \\ 42 & \text{if above value is greater than 42} \end{cases}$$

GA from FL:

$$GA = \begin{cases} \text{Exp } (2.45132 + & \text{if this value is} \\ \quad 0.016590 \text{ FL}) & \text{equal to or less than 42} \\ 42 & \text{if above value is greater than 42.} \end{cases}$$

In the above formulae 'Exp' refers to the exponential function and BPD and FL are measured in millimetres. Tables based on these formulae (Tables 9.4 and 9.5) are presented here. (Although we have not developed a bias-free formula for predicting gestational age from HC, for completeness we have included a published table as Table 9.6.)

As there are a number of options for assigning gestational age in the second and third trimesters, including assignment via BPD, cBPD, HC, FL and multiple indices, the choice should be based on a comparison of their accuracies. The literature supports these conclusions:

1. Among the methods for assigning gestational age from head measurements, the HC and cBPD are equivalent in accuracy and both are more accurate than the BPD.[37,42] Their greater accuracy is because they take head shape into account, whereas the BPD alone does not.[37,43] To understand what this means, consider two fetuses whose heads are equal in width but different in length. Both have the same BPD, so that if age were assigned by the BPD alone, both would be estimated to have the same gestational age. The fetus with the longer head, on the other hand, has a greater cBPD and HC than the fetus with the shorter head, and so would be assigned a greater

Table 9.4 Gestational age assignment based on biparietal diameter or corrected biparietal diameter (Reprinted with permission from ref. 21)

BPD or cBPD (mm)	Gestational age (weeks)	BPD or cBPD (mm)	Gestational age (weeks)
20	13.2	59	23.8
21	13.4	60	24.2
22	13.6	61	24.5
23	13.8	62	24.9
24	14.0	63	25.3
25	14.3	64	25.7
26	14.5	65	26.1
27	14.7	66	26.5
28	14.9	67	26.9
29	15.1	68	27.3
30	15.4	69	27.7
31	15.6	70	28.1
32	15.8	71	28.5
33	16.1	72	29.0
34	16.3	73	29.4
35	16.6	74	29.9
36	16.8	75	30.3
37	17.1	76	30.8
38	17.3	77	31.2
39	17.6	78	31.7
40	17.9	79	32.2
41	18.1	80	32.7
42	18.4	81	33.2
43	18.7	82	33.7
44	19.0	83	34.2
45	19.3	84	34.7
46	19.6	85	35.2
47	19.9	86	35.8
48	20.2	87	36.3
49	20.5	88	36.9
50	20.8	89	37.4
51	21.1	90	38.0
52	21.4	91	38.6
53	21.7	92	39.2
54	22.1	93	39.8
55	22.4	94	40.4
56	22.8	95	41.0
57	23.1	96	41.6
58	23.5	97 or greater	42.0

BPD – biparietal diameter, cBPD – corrected biparietal diameter.

Table 9.5 Gestational age assignment based on femur length (Reprinted with permission from ref. 21)

Femur length (mm)	Gestational age (weeks)	Femur length (mm)	Gestational age (weeks)
10	13.7	45	24.5
11	13.9	46	24.9
12	14.2	47	25.3
13	14.4	48	25.7
14	14.6	49	26.2
15	14.9	50	26.6
16	15.1	51	27.0
17	15.4	52	27.5
18	15.6	53	28.0
19	15.9	54	28.4
20	16.2	55	28.9
21	16.4	56	29.4
22	16.7	57	29.9
23	17.0	58	30.4
24	17.3	59	30.9
25	17.6	60	31.4
26	17.9	61	31.9
27	18.2	62	32.5
28	18.5	63	33.0
29	18.8	64	33.6
30	19.1	65	34.1
31	19.4	66	34.7
32	19.7	67	35.3
33	20.1	68	35.9
34	20.4	69	36.5
35	20.7	70	37.1
36	21.1	71	37.7
37	21.4	72	38.3
38	21.8	73	39.0
39	22.2	74	39.6
40	22.5	75	40.3
41	22.9	76	40.9
42	23.3	77	41.6
43	23.7	78 or greater	42.0
44	24.1		

gestational age if dating were based on the cBPD or HC.

2. In the second trimester the cBPD and HC are more accurate that the FL.[42]
3. In the third trimester there is little difference in accuracy between HC, cBPD and FL.[42]
4. The abdominal circumference is less accurate than head or femur measurements through most of the second and third trimesters.[28,42]
5. Composite age prediction formulae are similar in accuracy to HC and cBPD in the second trimester, and slightly more accurate in the third trimester.[42] A potential disadvantage to the use of a composite formula is that, by pooling several measurements into one formula, the diagnosis of skeletal dysplasia or microcephaly might be obscured.
6. Using the best approach for assigning gestational age at each stage of pregnancy accuracy (measured as the width of the 95% confidence range) is ±1–2 weeks in the second trimester and ±3–4 weeks in the third trimester.[42]

Conclusion

Ultrasound is a reliable method for estimating gestational age throughout pregnancy and is the best method unless there is objective information about the date of conception. Its accuracy is greatest early in pregnancy and progressively declines as pregnancy advances, owing to the increasing biological variability in the size of the fetus and its parts. Because of this, only the initial ultrasound in a

Table 9.6 Gestational age assignment based on head circumference (Reprinted with permission from ref. 18)

Head circumference (mm)	Gestational age (weeks)	Head circumference (mm)	Gestational age (weeks)
80	13.4	225	24.4
85	13.7	230	24.9
90	14.0	235	25.4
95	14.3	240	25.9
100	14.6	245	26.4
105	15.0	250	26.9
110	15.3	255	27.5
115	15.6	260	28.0
120	15.9	265	28.1
125	16.3	270	29.2
130	16.6	275	29.8
135	17.0	280	30.3
140	17.3	285	31.0
145	17.7	290	31.6
150	18.1	295	32.2
155	18.4	300	32.8
160	18.8	305	33.5
165	19.2	310	34.2
170	19.6	315	34.9
175	20.0	320	35.5
180	20.4	325	36.3
185	20.8	330	37.0
190	21.2	335	37.7
195	21.6	340	38.5
200	22.1	345	39.2
205	22.5	350	40.0
210	23.0	355	40.8
215	23.4	360	41.6
220	23.9		

pregnancy should be used to assign gestational age. A pregnancy should not be redated based on measurements or findings on any subsequent scan.

The appropriate method for assigning gestational age on the initial scan depends on the stage of pregnancy at which it is performed (Table 9.7). For a singleton pregnancy the approach outlined in Table 9.7 is used directly. For a multiple pregnancy, gestation age assignment is a two-step process. First, each fetus is dated as if it were a singleton. If all of these ages are concordant (within ±0.5 weeks in the first trimester, within 1.5 weeks in the second trimester, and within 3 weeks in the third trimester), the ages are averaged to yield the best estimate of gestational age for the pregnancy. If one or more ages is lower than the others by more than 0.5 weeks in the first trimester, 1.5 weeks in the second trimester, and 3 weeks in the third trimester, these low values should be excluded from the average. For example, if a pair of twins have CRLs of 14 mm (corresponding to 7.9 weeks gestation) and 15 mm (corresponding to 8.1 weeks gestation) the pregnancy should be assigned a gestational age of 8.0 weeks. If, on the other hand, the CRLs are 9 mm (corrsponding to 7.0 weeks gestation) and 15 mm (corresponding to 8.1 weeks gestation), the smaller twin should be diagnosed as being abnormally small and the pregnancy should be assigned a gestational age of 8.1 weeks.

Table 9.7 Ultrasound approach to gestational age assignment on the initial scan in a pregnancy (Reprinted with permission from ref. 44)

Stage of pregnancy	Basis for GA	Accuracy (weeks)*
First trimester		
Early (5–6 wks)	Ultrasound findings (Table 9.1)	±0.5
	or	
	mean sac diameter (Table 9.2)	±0.7
Mid to late (6–13 wks)	Crown–rump length (Table 9.3)	
Second trimester		
If OFD measurable	cBPD (Table 9.4)	±1.2 (14–20)
	or	
	HC (Table 9.6)	±1.9 (20–26)
If OFD not measurable	BPD (Table 9.4)	±1.4 (13–20)
	or	
	FL (Table 9.5)	±2.1–2.5 (20–26)
Third trimester		
If OFD measurable	cBPD (Table 9.4),	±3.1–3.4 (26–32)
	HC (Table 9.6),	±3.5–3.8 (32–42)
	or	
	FL (Table 9.5)	
If OFD not measurable	BPD (Table 9.4)	±3.1 (26–32)
	or	
	FL (Table 9.5)	±3.5 (32–42)

* 2 standard deviations.

REFERENCES

1 Gardosi J. Dating of pregnancy: time to forget the last menstrual period. Ultrasound Obstet Gynecol 1997; 9: 367–368

2 Kurtz A B. Estimating gestational age. RSNA Special Course in Ultrasound 1996: 15–23

3 Tunon K, Eik-Nes S H, Grottum P. A comparison between ultrasound and a reliable last menstrual period as predictors of the day of delivery in 15,000 examinations. Ultrasound Obstet Gynecol 1996; 8: 178–185

4 Waldenstrom U, Axelsson O, Nilsson S. A comparison of the ability of a sonographically measured biparietal diameter and the last menstrual period to predict the spontaneous onset of labor. Obstet Gynecol 1990; 76: 336–338

5 Belfrage P, Fernstrom I, Hallenberg G. Routine or selective ultrasound examinations in early pregnancy. Obstet Gynecol 1987; 69: 747–750

6 Campbell S, Warsof S L, Little D, Cooper D J. Routine ultrasound screening for the prediction of gestational age. Obstet Gynecol 1985; 65: 613–620

7 American College of Radiology. Standards for antepartum obstetrical ultrasound. Reston, VA: 1995

8 American Institute of Ultrasound in Medicine. Standards for performance of the antepartum obstetrical ultrasound examination. 1994

9 Timor-Tritsch I E, Farine D, Rosen M G. A close look at early embryonic development with the high-frequency transvaginal transducer. Am J Obstet Gynecol 1988; 159: 676–681

10 Goldstein I, Zimmer E A, Tamir A, Peretz B A, Paldi E. Evaluation of normal gestational sac growth: appearance of embryonic heartbeat and embryo body movements using the transvaginal technique. Obstet Gynecol 1991; 77: 885–888

11 Bree R L, Edwards M, Bohm-Velez M, Beyler S, Roberts J, Mendelson E B. Transvaginal sonography in the evaluation of normal early pregnancy: correlation with HCG level. AJR 1989; 153: 75–79

12 Daya S, Woods S, Ward S, Lappalainen R, Caco C. Early pregnancy assessment with transvaginal ultrasound scanning. Can Med Assoc J 1991; 144: 441–446

13 Robinson H P, Fleming J E E. A critical evaluation of sonar crown–rump length measurements. Br J Obstet Gynaecol 1975; 82: 702–710

14 Daya S. Accuracy of gestational age estimation by means of fetal crown–rump length measurement. Am J Obstet Gynecol 1993; 168: 903–908

15 Chervenak F A, Brightman R C, Thornton J, Berkowitz G S, David S. Crown–rump length and serum human chorionic gonadotropin as predictor of gestational age. Obstet Gynecol 1986; 67: 210–213

16 Hadlock F P, Harrist R B, Shah Y P, King D E, Park S K, Sharman R S. Estimating fetal age using multiple parameters: a prospective evaluation in a racially mixed population. Am J Obstet Gynecol 1987; 156: 955–957

17 Hadlock F P, Deter R L, Harrist R B, Park S K. Estimating fetal age: computer-assisted analysis of multiple fetal growth parameters. Radiology 1984; 152: 497–501

18 Hadlock F P, Deter R L, Harrist R B, Park S K. Fetal head circumference: relation to menstrual age. AJR 1982; 138: 649–653

19 Kurtz A B, Wapner R J, Kurtz R J et al. Analysis of biparietal diameter as an accurate indicator of gestational age. JCU 1980; 8: 319–326

20 Ott W J. The use of ultrasonic fetal head circumference for predicting expected date of confinement. JCU 1984; 12: 411–415

21 Doubilet P M, Benson C B. Improved prediction of gestational age in the late third trimester. J Ultrasound Med 1993; 12: 647–653

22 Hadlock F P, Harrist R B, Deter R L, Park S K. Fetal femur length as a predictor of menstrual age: sonographically measured. AJR 1982; 138: 875–878

23 O'Brien G, Queenan J T, Campbell S. Assessment of gestational age in the second trimester by real-time ultrasound measurement of the femur length. Am J Obstet Gynecol 1980; 139: 540–545

24 Warda A H, Deter R L, Rossavik I K. Fetal femur length: a critical reevaluation of the relationship to menstrual age. Obstet Gynecol 1985; 66: 69–75

25 Hohler C W, Quetel T A. Fetal femur length: equations for computer calculation of gestational age from ultrasound measurements. Am J Obstet Gynecol 1982; 143: 479–481

26 Jeanty P, Rodesch F, Deibeke D, Dumont J E. Estimation of gestational age from measurements of fetal long bones. J Ultrasound Med 1984; 3: 75–79

27 Merz E, Kim-Kern M, Pehl S. Ultrasonic mensuration of fetal limb bones in the second and third trimesters. JCU 1987; 15: 175–183

28 Hadlock F P, Deter R L, Harrist R B, Park S K. Fetal abdominal circumference as a predictor of menstrual age. AJR 1982; 139: 367–370

29 Co E, Raju T N K, Aldana O. Cerebellar dimensions in assessment of gestational age in neonates. Radiology 1991; 181: 581–585

30 Birnholz J C. Fetal lumbar spine: measuring axial growth with ultrasound. Radiology 1986; 158: 805–807

31 Mercer B M, Sklar S, Shariatmadar A, Gillieson M S, D'Alton M E. Fetal foot length as a predictor of gestational age. Am J Obstet Gynecol 1987; 156: 350–355

32 Jeanty P, Cantraine F, Cousaert E, Romero R, Hobbins J C. The binocular distance: a new way to estimate fetal age. J Ultrasound Med 1984; 3: 241–243

33 Yarkoni S, Schmidt W, Jeanty P, Reece E A, Hobbins J C. Clavicular measurement: a new biometric parameter for fetal evaluation. J Ultrasound Med 1985; 4: 467–470

34 Campbell S, Thoms A. Ultrasound measurement of the fetal head to abdomen circumference ratio in the assessment of growth retardation. Br J Obstet Gynaecol 1977; 84: 165–174

35 Hadlock F P, Deter R L, Harrist R B, Park S K. Fetal biparietal diameter: rational choice of plane of section for sonographic measurement. AJR 1982; 138: 871–874

36 Shepard M, Filly R A. A standardized plane for biparietal diameter measurement. J Ultrasound Med 1982; 1: 145–150

37 Doubilet P M, Greenes R A. Improved prediction of gestational age from fetal head measurements. AJR 1984; 142: 797–800

38 Adler R S, Bowerman R A, Rubin J M. Circumference measurements in obstetrical ultrasound: ellipse vs. arithmetic mean. JCU 1988; 16: 361–363

39 Hadlock F P, Kent W R, Loyd J L, Harrist R B, Deter R L, Park S K. An evaluation of two methods for measuring fetal head and body circumferences. J Ultrasound Med 1982; 1: 359–360

40 Goldstein R B, Filly R A, Simpson G. Pitfalls in femur length measurements. J Ultrasound Med 1987; 6: 203–207

41 Hill L M, Guzick D, Hixson J, Peterson C S, Rivello D M. Composite assessment of gestational age: a comparison of institutionally derived and published regression equations. Am J Obstet Gynecol 1992; 166: 551–555

42 Benson C B, Doubilet P M. Sonographic prediction of gestational age: accuracy of second and third trimester fetal measurements. AJR 1991; 157: 1275–1277

43 Hadlock F P, Deter R L, Carpenter R J, Park S K. Estimating fetal age: effect of head shape on BPD. Am J Radiol 1981; 137: 83–85

44 Benson C B, Doubilet P M. Fetal measurements: normal and abnormal fetal growth. In: Rumack C, Charboneau W, Wilson S, eds. Diagnostic ultrasound. St. Louis: Mosby-Year Book, 1991; 723–728

Fetal growth

Martin J Whittle

Introduction

Although fetal growth problems are a serious cause of perinatal mortality and morbidity in current obstetric practice, understanding of the biology of intra-uterine growth remains incomplete. There are both growth-promoting and growth-restraining factors, most of which are under some form of genetic control. The issue is, however, complicated by extrinsic factors, which may include maternal nutrition, infection and habits such as smoking and alcohol abuse.

Fetal growth restriction remains an important problem and it seems likely that about 25% of babies who weigh less than 2.5 kg at birth and who contribute to the perinatal mortality are in fact growth restricted. In addition, babies who survive and who are severely growth restricted are over-represented among children who develop long-term handicap. For these reasons, reliable methods by which to detect intra-uterine growth restriction (IUGR) during pregnancy would seem desirable and a number of strategies have been developed, with varying degrees of success. In effect there are two approaches to the problem: the first is screening to identify the pregnancy at risk, and the second is to confirm a clinical suspicion. Unfortunately, fetal size alone may not be the most significant factor in the identification of true pathology. The use of other tests, such as the biophysical profile (see Ch. 11) and newer techniques such as Doppler, may have an important adjunctive role.

Normal intra-uterine growth

Intra-uterine growth is affected by both genetic factors and the supply to the fetus of essential nutrients.

Genetic control

Fetal growth and development goes through three phases:[1]

1. replication or proliferation, which may be called hyperplasia,
2. migration, during which cells move and aggregate to form tissue and organ rudiments,
3. hypertrophy, when the cells increase in size and become part of definitive functional structures.

These processes are under genomic control, but as all embryonic cells have the same 'blueprint', other influences must cause the differentiation of these early cells into structures with specific functions (see Ch. 6). This may be effected by alterations in the DNA or gene arrangement, which in turn influence the expression of one gene to alter the response of another. This cascade of genetic activity, which controls differentiation and growth, is influenced by macromolecules and growth factors, which also result from the expression of other genes. The biology of early growth is extremely complex: it forms one of the most challenging and exciting research areas in modern biology.

Growth problems that arise from disorders of the genome itself may be particularly severe. Thus aneuploidy, such as trisomy 18, is often associated with fetal growth disorders, and other more subtle abnormalities such as translocations and deletions are also important. There has been particular interest in the concept of genetic imprinting. In this process genes on the male-derived chromosome may produce phenotypic effects, of which differences in growth are just one, to those on the female-derived chromosome.[2] However, at present there is uncertainty as to the exact significance of imprinting as a cause of IUGR.[3]

Infection with certain viruses at a critical stage in embryonic development may interfere with the genomic message and cause either structural abnormalities or reduced growth potential. Rubella and cytomegalovirus are examples of viruses producing these effects; others such as varicella may also be significant.

The genome is also responsible for the production of growth-promoting factors such as insulin-like growth factor 1 (IGF-1). The stimulus for genetic expression may relate to nutritional status, so that if nutrient supply is diminished, IGF-1 manufacture may be reduced. Numerous other growth factors have been isolated and all provide a system which controls growth and differentiation, both from early embryonic existence and throughout life. Although current knowledge is limited, it is rapidly expanding to provide an important insight into the complexities of cellular control.

Nutrient supply

The fetus is uniquely vulnerable, as it must rely for its nutritional support on the vascular supply to the uterus[4] and on the function of the placenta.[5] Classic animal experiments indicated the importance of both of these factors in the restriction of fetal growth. Evidence from human pregnancies is also compelling.

The vascular supply is of particular importance; in a normal pregnancy the terminal branches of the uterine arteries, termed 'spiral arteries', become converted into flask-shaped vessels by the removal of the muscularis layer by trophoblasts.[6] This causes them to widen, allowing an unimpeded flow of maternal blood to the placental bed and thus maximising the exchange potential. Failure of this process seems to be associated with the development of serious complications such as pre-eclampsia and/or IUGR. It is also known that the mother with vascular disease (e.g. in long-standing diabetes or autoimmune diseases such as systemic lupus erythematosus) is much more likely to have a growth-restricted baby. Intravascular factors such as sickle cell disease and lupus inhibitor causing coagulopathy are also important.

Placental function is influenced by the maternal vascular supply but it is also possible that humoral factors from the mother control certain types of placental activity at a cellular level, including its own metabolism. The placental vascular space may well be sensitive to changes in the uterine circulation, and a clearer understanding of vascular control within the placenta is developing. Of particular interest are the ways in which the placenta may modulate fetal growth, not only by changes in nutrient supply but also through the secretion of growth-controlling substances.[7] It is possible that there is considerable metabolic 'cross-talk' between the fetus and the placenta.

Abnormal intra-uterine growth

Definition

Considerable confusion surrounds the terms 'small-for-dates' and 'intra-uterine growth restriction', such that they are often erroneously used interchangeably.

Small for dates

The term 'small-for-dates', is merely a statistical definition relating to a group of babies found at or below the tenth, fifth or third centiles for weight (depending on the chosen centile) of a normally distributed population (Fig. 10.1). Although the definition of a 'small-for-dates fetus' seems simple, difficulty is caused by the variation between birthweight charts: a baby defined as normal by one standard may be small by another. For many years the Lubchenko birthweight charts were used as the 'gold standard' but they were not always appropriate, as they were derived from a population in Denver, Colorado, some 5000 feet above sea level. It has become obvious that different populations show considerable variations in their birthweight characteristics. The Aberdeen birthweight data (the most commonly used in the UK), when applied to the Glasgow population for example, suggest that substantially more babies are small-for-dates than if local, Glasgow-derived figures are used.[8]

Whether standard deviation or centiles should be used on birthweight charts depends on the nature of the weight distributions around the mean. Standard deviations are more appropriate when the distribution is symmetrical. Early studies suggested a non-symmetrical distribution, hence the frequent use of centiles. In fact, adjustment of the data with accurate knowledge of the gestational age normalises the distribution, making standard deviation the more appropriate measure.[9] In practical terms it probably matters little, and other factors such as ethnic origin and the baby's sex may be much more important.

Intra-uterine growth restriction (IUGR)

This term is now used in preference to intra-uterine growth retardation. The definition of fetal growth restric-

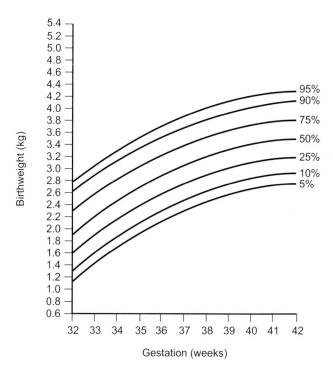

Fig. 10.1 Graph showing weight centiles for gestational age.

tion is inexact, but it may be diagnosed when the growth rate deviates significantly from an established norm. IUGR may be implied from the presence of other features, such as reduced amounts of amniotic fluid, diminished fetal activity and, more recently, abnormal Doppler waveforms in the umbilical artery. Alternatively, the diagnosis of growth restriction can be made retrospectively from the appearances and condition of the newborn, and measures such as the ponderal index or the baby's length related to its weight have their proponents. The rapid growth often observed in most of these babies once released from the *in utero* restraints, also suggests the diagnosis.

Clinical significance

The risk from being either small-for-dates or growth restricted is not easy to discern from the literature, which most often relates only to birthweight.

Perinatal loss in babies born weighing less than 2.5 kg represents just under 30% of the total perinatal mortality,[10] and probably about 20–25% of these babies are small-for-dates. How many of these are actually growth restricted is impossible to establish; this is also the case for babies weighing 2.5 kg and more. However, the importance of establishing the diagnosis in this group is underlined by the fact that when perinatal loss occurs it is much more likely to result in a stillbirth rather than a neonatal death.[11]

Small-for-dates fetuses who survive to the neonatal period may have problems, including the development of hypoglycaemia, hypothermia and birth asphyxia, whereas the preterm small-for-dates baby appears to have an excess mortality compared to one who is of an appropriate weight for dates.[12] In a Scottish study the small-for-dates babies born alive before 37 weeks had a mortality rate of 12.4%, in contrast to 5% in babies of appropriate weight.[13]

Long-term morbidity in the small-for-dates or IUGR baby is also difficult to assess, but there are indications of a statistically significant excess of learning and psycho-motor problems.[14,15] More recently evidence of long-term consequences of intra-uterine growth restriction have emerged with an apparent increase in the risk of developing hypertension and diabetes in later life.[16]

It would seem that the identification of the small-for-dates baby in the antenatal period should have an important impact on perinatal mortality and morbidity in current obstetric practice. Unfortunately the evidence that this is so is not convincing, possibly because of the diverse nature of the aetiological factors. The Growth Restriction Intervention Trial (GRIT),[17] currently running in the UK and Europe, is an attempt to establish the preferred intervention in these very difficult clinical circumstances. A recent study would suggest an advantage to early intervention, but larger numbers are required.[18]

Aetiology

Maternal factors

Numerous maternal factors may affect fetal growth.

1. Small for dates – constitutional maternal causes
   (a) maternal height/weight
   (b) ethnic group
   (c) socio-economic group/nutritional support
2. Toxins
   (a) smoking
   (b) alcohol abuse
   (c) drugs, both addictive and therapeutic
3. Illness
   (a) hypertensive disease: pre-eclampsia, renal disease etc.
   (b) autoimmune disorders: systemic lupus erythematosus
   (c) cyanotic heart and respiratory disease
   (d) haematological disease: sickle cell etc.
   (e) long-standing diabetes with microvascular involvement.

Apart from the problem of defining a normal population, important factors that influence birthweight include birth order, parental height (particularly the mother's) and ethnic group. This last has always been difficult to separate from economic and social factors, but studies in Singapore, which allow the comparison of three different ethnic groups living under similar circumstances, show clear differences in birthweight distributions.

Social and economic status remains an important influence on perinatal outcome, and fetal growth in particular; the reasons for this may be partly nutritional or related to habits such as smoking. The effect of diet is difficult to assess, but the starvation of women during the Dutch famine and the siege of Leningrad during the Second World War caused a significant increase in the number of small-for-dates babies. Nutritional supplementation may improve pregnancy outcome and have a small effect on birthweight.

Maternal disease, either pre-existing or coincidental with pregnancy, may interfere with fetal growth, and of particular importance are the vascular changes associated with hypertension and microvascular disease.

Fetal factors

The fetal causes for poor fetal growth include the following:

1. chromosome disorders, especially trisomies 13 and 18,
2. infections – viral, such as rubella, cytomegalovirus etc.,
3. non-chromosomal syndromes,
4. multiple pregnancy,
5. fetal sex,
6. birth order.

A variety of pathologies may be responsible which, as discussed above, usually relate to interference with the fetal genome. Severe damage usually results in spontaneous abortion, but occasionally the pregnancy survives to term, when the disturbance may manifest itself as growth restriction.

Fetal size is a particular problem in multiple pregnancy. In about two-thirds of twin pregnancies one of the babies is born weighing less than 2.5 kg.[19] This is partly because of preterm delivery, which occurs in almost half of twin pregnancies, compared to the singleton rate of about 5%.[19] Although perinatal loss in twins is often the result of immaturity, intra-uterine death occurs (with a frequency of two to three times the singleton rate) in pregnancies of 37 weeks or more in which the babies weigh less than 2.5 kg. Of particular importance is the situation in which there is discordant growth, when the smaller baby is at considerably greater risk.

Why babies from a multiple pregnancy should be smaller than singletons is unclear, but there may be good teleological reasons, including the biological advantage of keeping the intra-uterine contents to a minimum. However, it is also possible that there is a relative failure of nutrient supply, which may explain the higher incidence of intra-uterine death in the more mature babies.

Uteroplacental factors

Concepts of the role of the placenta in controlling fetal growth have already been discussed in some detail. This area of study may provide important information concerning the aetiology of currently 'unexplained' fetal growth restriction with or without maternal hypertension.

Methods of growth assessment

Biparietal diameter (BPD)

In early work using ultrasound to assess fetal growth the BPD was measured simply because it was the only measurement that could be made reliably. For it to have any value at all, the level in the head at which the measurement had to be taken needed to be carefully defined (Fig. 10.2), so that the section included the midline echo with the cavum septum pellucidum in the anterior third and the thalami on either side. With great care this is a reproducible measurement with an accuracy of about 1 mm.

Using this technique several workers observed that BPD increased steadily throughout gestation,[20,21] but that after about 32 weeks the rate of change decreased and the difficulty of accurate measurement increased. Nevertheless, it became obvious that up to about 20 weeks the BPD gives an accurate guide to gestational age, which in itself formed the basis upon which to judge whether growth restriction was a problem.

The use of BPD as a method of assessing growth has been largely abandoned because the concept that increases in BPD reflect overall fetal growth has been shown to be wrong. First, the increase in head size, which does reflect brain growth, may persist for some time in the face of quite severe growth restriction. Secondly, although an easy measurement to make, the BPD becomes increasingly inaccurate in the latter weeks of pregnancy, just when an assessment of growth may be most important. Finally, the spread of normal BPD size becomes very wide after 32 weeks, again reducing the value of the method as means of identifying a small fetus.

Head circumference (HC)

HC measurements are made at the same level as the BPD but involve a circumference rather than a diameter assessment, and this has led to the development of a number of measuring devices, including light-pen systems, joysticks and expanding ellipses.

A number of groups have produced charts of HC against gestational age: the two most often used are very similar.[22,23] Both show that changes in HC, like BPD, tend to tail off towards term (Fig. 10.3), but the standard deviations are much smaller, so the likelihood of identifying the growth-restricted fetus may be higher. In addition, HC is much less dependent on head shape, so that a dolichocephalic head, which is narrow but long, has an appropriate circumference for gestational age but a small BPD.

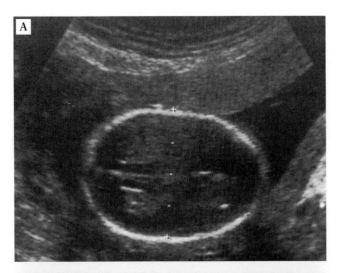

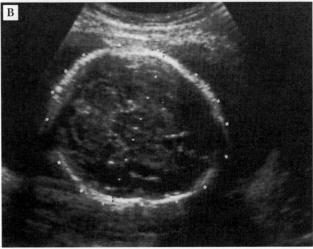

Fig. 10.2 Head measurements. A: Biparietal diameter and **B:** head circumference measurement.

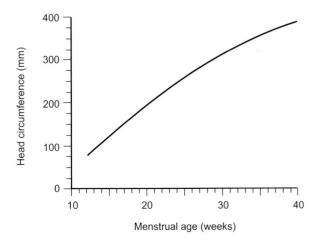

Fig. 10.3 Ultrasound measured head circumference chart (Deter[23]).

However, all head measurements become harder to perform in late pregnancy, and the brain-sparing effect in growth restriction affects both HC and BPD.

Cerebellar growth

Cerebellar growth has been shown to be reasonably linear from about 14 to 40 weeks,[24] with the transverse diameter in millimetres being roughly equivalent to the gestational age in weeks (Fig. 10.4). The measurement is more difficult to make in the latter weeks of pregnancy but the cerebellar diameter does offer an objective assessment of gestational age throughout pregnancy. Of particular importance is the fact that the cerebellum does not seem to be affected by intra-uterine growth restriction.

Femur length (FL)

FL is primarily a measurement for the estimation of gestational age, with good accuracy from around 15–25 weeks.[25] Its use in the estimation of fetal growth is limited, although it has been combined with other measurements to estimate fetal size (see below).

Abdominal circumference (AC)

The AC is undoubtedly the best index with which to assess both fetal size and growth because the measurement is taken at the level of the fetal liver, which constitutes about 4% of the total fetal weight and which steadily increases in size with gestational age.

Measurement of the AC must be at a carefully defined level in the fetal abdomen if consistency is to be achieved. A British Medical Ultrasound Society Bulletin[26] recommended the Deter tables[23] as the most appropriate. That recommendation has now been altered to the data of Jeanty *et al.*[27] Figure 10.5 shows a cross-sectional view of the fetal trunk with the intrahepatic portion of the umbilical vein situated in the anterior third of the abdominal

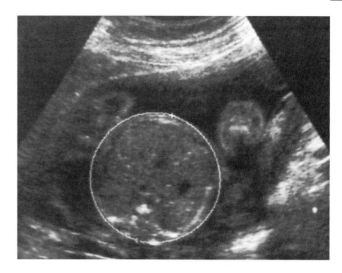

Fig. 10.5 Abdominal circumference measurement.

circumference. This view is best achieved by first aligning the ultrasound transducer with the fetal aorta and then turning it through a right-angle.

Tabular data for normal values of fetal growth and gestational age suggest a fairly linear growth throughout (Fig. 10.6), in contrast to head measurements, although the standard deviations widen towards term. Because of this linear relationship it has been proposed that a weight estimation taken at, say, 26 weeks may allow the prediction of weight at term.[28] The potential importance of this is embodied in the philosophy that each baby has its own growth profile which, if not followed, results in growth restriction regardless of absolute weight. A further modification of this principle has included other weighting factors, such as maternal size, which may allow a more accurate assignment of the fetal size to an appropriate centile.[29]

Complicated formulae have been devised for the estimation of fetal weight but none is very accurate and errors of between 10% and 15% are reported. Attempts to

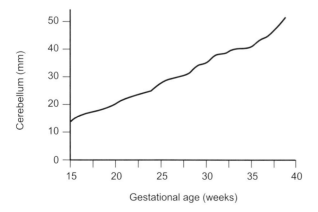

Fig. 10.4 Ultrasound-measured cerebellar diameter. Mean for gestational age (Goldstein[24]).

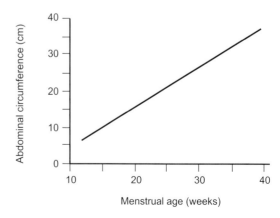

Fig. 10.6 Ultrasound-measured abdominal circumference chart (Jeanty[27]).

reduce these errors have been made by introducing other measurements, such as HC, FL and BPD,[30–34] but the best and probably the most accurate measurement sets include AC and FL, with an absolute error of 7.6%. Other measurements of the fetal abdomen have been used, including the area and transabdominal diameters. Although they have their proponents, their use seems to confer no additional value to the assessment of fetal growth or size.

Fetal growth dynamics

Normal growth

The original concepts about intra-uterine growth were extrapolated from birthweight data relying on two premises. The first was that the gestational age at the time of delivery was known accurately, and the second that those babies born prematurely were 'normal' and likely to be of an appropriate weight.

As previously mentioned, the sigmoid curve which is usually found for birthweight charts becomes more linear with adjustment of the gestational age, but nevertheless the distribution of weights is negatively skewed prior to 36 weeks,[9] implying that babies born prematurely tend to be smaller.

One of the advantages of ultrasound is that it allows repeated examinations of the fetus: both head and abdominal measurements have been used to plot fetal growth and normal patterns have been established for both these components, singly and in combination. Interestingly, estimations of weight using such measurements, especially prior to 36 weeks, tend to exceed the weight established from birthweight charts, which also suggests that babies born preterm are likely to be smaller than might be expected.

Asymmetrical and symmetrical growth patterns

Considerable debate surrounds the use of the terms 'asymmetrical' and 'symmetrical' to describe patterns of growth seen *in utero* in relation to head and abdominal circumferential measurements. Head size increases because of the progressive growth of the fetal brain and, as mentioned, this may be maintained for some time, despite intra-uterine starvation. Fetal liver size, which is the main contributor to the abdominal girth, normally increases steadily throughout pregnancy owing to the accumulation of glycogen and storage substances. However, in contrast to the brain, liver growth seems very sensitive to reductions in the supply of nutrients and so provides a potentially useful marker of intra-uterine starvation.

Thus an asymmetrical pattern of growth restriction develops because of continuing head growth with little or no increase in abdominal girth, leading to a high head/abdominal circumference ratio. These changes are prob-

ably most often observed when IUGR has a vascular or uteroplacental basis.

In contrast, symmetrical growth restriction, when both head and abdominal size are proportionally small, may be found either with a normal small-for-dates fetus or when there has been some serious early insult to the developing embryo, fetus, or even possibly the placenta.

From a clinical standpoint the symmetrically small baby has potentially more uncorrectable pathology than the asymmetrical type, as intrinsic problems are more likely. However, many of these babies are actually either just small but normal, or have incorrect dating. The latter group is now rare in the UK, although it remains a significant obstetric dilemma in countries where early ultrasound dating is not routinely available.

Identification of fetal growth restriction

Fetal growth is a dynamic process and yet often only a single measurement is available to evaluate fetal size at any time. Serial ultrasound measurements are required to measure a growth rate, but they are tedious and time-consuming and often not practical clinically. These concerns have led to a search for other methods to identify the pregnancy in which the fetus is IUGR, such as the biophysical profile, and Doppler studies of the umbilical and uterine arteries.

Abdominal measurements

It is apparent that unless serial measurements are taken of any of the indices discussed above it is unlikely that the slowing of growth in an individual fetus could be identified with any degree of certainty. Various strategies have been devised to overcome this difficulty, including the extrapolated growth curve discussed above.[28]

Most groups have used a two-stage system, with one early 'dating scan' and one later scan,[35] or just one late scan, in an attempt to identify the fetus at risk. Unfortunately none of the studies demonstrates that in low-risk groups screening in this way has any impact on pregnancy outcome,[36] in spite of the fact that the tests themselves have a reasonable positive predictive power of about 50–60%, which is well in excess of the 30–40% often quoted for most clinical methods.

The use of either a single abdominal circumference or, even better, a series of measures provides a better method of identifying the small-for-dates fetus than either umbilical or middle cerebral artery Doppler velocimetry, when compared using receiver operator characteristic curves.[37] This seems a logical conclusion, as the abdominal circumference measurements should correlate with birthweight. However, the Doppler results may be providing different information about the fetus than merely its size, under-lining the important distinction between the terms 'small for dates' and 'IUGR'.

Head circumference/abdominal circumference ratio

As alluded to above, one of the weaknesses of a single measurement of AC is that, even if it gives some indication of fetal size, it does not necessarily help in the identification of pathology. The measurement of both HC and AC allows the independent assessment of head and abdominal growth, which tends to differ under circumstances of vascular or placental failure such that head growth is maintained for some time while abdominal growth slows or even ceases. These changes cause the HC/AC ratio (Fig. 10.7) to rise, making it possible to identify the truly growth-restricted fetus from a single study. Unfortunately, the potential of the HC/AC ratio to assign fetal growth to either an asymmetrical or a symmetrical pattern does not run true in practice, although the sensitivity of the ratio for a small-for-dates baby is about 70%.[38]

Amniotic fluid volume (AFV)

The use of amniotic fluid volume in the evaluation of the fetal condition is well established and has been discussed at length in Chapter 11. A reduction in AFV is an important sign that the fetal condition may be impaired, and in these circumstances perinatal mortality rises sharply. From a strictly technical viewpoint accurate measures of AFV are impossible, and a number of strategies have been employed. The volume of single pockets of fluid rarely

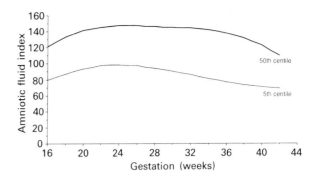

Fig. 10.8 Ultrasound-measured amniotic fluid index and gestational age (Moore and Cayle[39]).

gives a good overall impression and a subjective assessment is probably the most commonly used method. The amniotic fluid index (AFI) may prove to be useful, and involves the summing of amniotic fluid depth in the four quadrants of the uterus. Normal values have been produced (Fig. 10.8)[39] which suggest a minimum acceptable index of about 65 mm.

As for the HC/AC ratio, the AFV should provide direct evidence of pathological growth restriction, as the production of amniotic fluid is reduced in the presence of either vascular or placental deficiency. Most studies suggest that pregnancy outcome is impaired when the AFV is reduced.

Other methods

More recently alternative methods of fetal evaluation have been assessed, approaching the problem from a different direction. Often the identification of growth problems is 'retrospective' being noticed only when they are present. It is impossible to discuss IUGR without mentioning umbilical and uterine artery Doppler. Abnormalities in the flow velocity characteristics may predate the development of growth problems (see Ch. 13), and randomised studies involving the umbilical artery Doppler waveforms suggest a marginal benefit, but only in high-risk pregnancies.[40] However, what is generally unclear in the available studies is exactly how the technique is used, there being little standardisation. The situation is even less clear in uterine artery studies, some of which do suggest some relationship between abnormal results and the development of IUGR.[41]

Conclusion

Fetal growth restriction remains a serious obstetric problem, because of both the difficulties of identification and the associated perinatal mortality and morbidity. Unfortunately there is no clear definition of what is meant by growth restriction, and most statistics deal largely with babies that are small for dates, or perhaps even just small, rather than truly pathologically affected. However, ultrasound has given us the opportunity to classify a group of

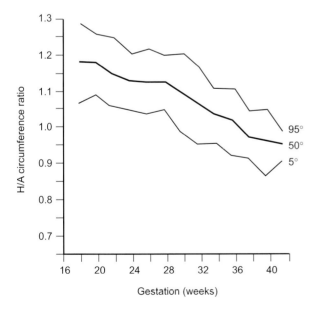

Fig. 10.7 Ultrasound-measured head/abdomen circumference ratio chart (Campbell and Thoms[38]).

truly IUGR fetuses on the basis of their size (less than the 5th centile), their poor growth in AC, reduced amniotic fluid volume, and the presence of abnormal umbilical (or uterine) Doppler waveforms.

It is clear that in the assessment of the baby suspected of growth problems a number of techniques need to be employed, of which ultrasound imaging is just one. Indicators that a pregnancy may be at risk of growth restriction, such as hypertension, renal disease or auto-immune problems, are important, together with the use of cardiotocography and possibly Doppler studies. The aim is to build an overall view of the fetal condition and what has led to it, and to develop a clinical strategy to ensure the optimal outcome.

REFERENCES

1 Han V K M. Genetic mechanisms of regulation of fetal growth. In: Sharp F, Milner R D G, Fraser R B, eds. Fetal growth. Ashton-on-Lyne: Peacock Press, 1989; 77–81

2 Hall J G. Genomic imprinting: review and relevances to human diseases. Am J Hum Gen 1990; 46: 857–873

3 Moore G E, Ali Z, Khan R U, Blunt S, Bennett P R, Vaughan J I. The incidence of uniparental disomy associated with IUGR in a cohort of 35 severely affected babies. Am J Obstet Gynecol 1997; 176: 294–299

4 Clapp J F, Szeto H H, Larrow R, Hewitt J, Mann L I. Umbilical blood flow response to embolization of the uterine circulation. Am J Obstet Gynecol 1980; 138: 60–67

5 Robinson J S, Kingstone J E, Jones C T, Thorburn G D. Studies on experimental growth retardation in sheep. The effect of removal of endometrial caruncles on fetal size and metabolism. J Devel Physiol 1979; 1(5): 379–398

6 Brosen I A, Dixon H G, Robertson W B. Fetal growth retardation and the vasculature of the placental bed. Br J Obstet Gynaecol 1977; 84: 656–664

7 Hay W W. Placental control of fetal metabolism. In: Sharp F, Milner R D G, Fraser R B, eds. Fetal growth. Ashton-on-Lyne: Peacock Press, 1989; 33–52

8 Forbes J F, Smalls M J. A comparative analysis of birthweight for gestational age standards. Br J Obstet Gynaecol 1983; 99: 297–303

9 Perrson P H. Fetal growth curves. In: Sharp F, Milner R D G, Fraser R B, eds. Fetal growth. Ashton-on-Lyne: Peacock Press, 1989; p 13–26

10 SHHD. Report on maternal and perinatal deaths in Scotland, 1981–1985. Edinburgh: HMSO, 1989

11 Whitfield C R, Smith N C, Cockburn F, Gibson A A M. Perinatally related wastage – a proposed clarification of primary obstetric factors. Br J Obstet Gynaecol 1986; 93: 694–703

12 Stewart A. Fetal growth: mortality and morbidity. In: Sharp F, Milner R D G, Fraser R B, eds. Fetal growth. Ashton-on-Lyne: Peacock Press, 1989; 403–412

13 Dickson D M, Forbes J F. Anthropometric standards and the risk of mortality in preterm infants. Social, paediatric and obstetric research unit, University of Glasgow, 1987

14 Neligan G A, Kolvin I, Scott D Mc I, Garside R F. Born too soon or born too small? A follow up study to seven years of age. Philadelphia: Spastic International Medical Publications, Heinemann Medical Books, 1976; 66

15 Fitzhardinge F M, Kalman E, Ashby S, Pape K. Present status of the infant of very low birthweight treated in a referral neonatal intensive care unit in 1974. In: Major mental handicap: methods and costs of prevention. Amsterdam: Elsevier Excerpta Medica, 1978; 139–150

16 Barker D J P, ed. Fetal and infant origins of adult disease. London: BMJ Publishing, 1992

17 The GRIT Study Group. When do obstetricians recommend delivery for a high risk preterm growth retarded fetus? Eur J Obstet Gynecol 1996; 67: 121–126

18 Schaap A H P, Wolf H, Bruinse H W et al. Influence of obstetric management on outcome of extremely preterm growth retarded infants. Arch Dis Child 1997; 77: 95–99

19 Scottish twin study. Social, paediatric and obstetric research unit, University of Glasgow, 1983

20 Willocks J, Donald I, Campbell S, Dunsmore I R. Intrauterine growth assessed by ultrasonic fetal cephalometry. J Obstet Gynaecol Br Common 1967; 74: 639–647

21 Campbell S, Dewhurst C J. Diagnosis of the small for dates fetus by serial ultrasonic cephalometry. Lancet 1971; ii: 1002–1006

22 Hadlock F P, Deter R L, Harrist R B, Park S K. Fetal head circumference: relation to menstrual age. AJR 1982; 138: 647–653

23 Deter R L, Harrist R B, Hadlock F P, Carpenter R J. Fetal head and abdominal circumference: II. A critical re-evaluation of the relationship to menstrual age. JCU 1982; 10: 365–372

24 Goldstein I, Reece A, Pilu G, Bovicelli L, Hobbins J C. Cerebellar measurements with ultrasonography in the evaluation of fetal growth and development. Am J Obstet Gynecol 1987; 156: 1065–1069

25 Hadlock F P, Harrist R B, Deter R L, Park S K. Fetal femur length as a predictor of gestational age: sonographically measured. AJR 1982; 138: 875–878

26 Evans J A, Farrant P, Gowland M, McNay M J. Clinical application of ultrasonic fetal measurement. Report of the Fetal Measurement Working Party. London: British Medical Ultrasound Society, 1990; 1–13

27 Jeanty P D, Cousaert M S, Cantraine F. Normal growth of the abdominal perimeter. Am J Perinatol 1984; 1: 129–135

28 Deter R L, Harrist R B, Hadlock F P, Poindexter A N. Longitudinal studies of fetal growth with the use of dynamic image ultrasonography. Am J Obstet Gynecol 1982; 143: 545–554

29 Gardosi J, Mongelli M, Wilcox M, Chang A. An adjustable fetal weight standard. Ultrasound Obstet Gynecol 1995; 6: 168–174

30 Campbell S, Wilkin D. Abdominal circumference in the estimation of fetal weight. Br J Obstet Gynaecol 1975; 82: 689–697

31 Warsof S L, Gohari P, Berkowitz R L, Hobbins J C. The estimation of fetal weight by computer-assisted analysis. Am J Obstet Gynecol 1977; 128: 881–892

32 Hill L M, Breckle R, Wolfram K R, O'Brien P C. Evaluation of three methods of estimating fetal weight. JCU 1986; 14: 171–178

33 Simon N V, Levisky J S, Shearer D M, O'Lear M S, Flood J T. Influence of fetal growth patterns as sonographic estimate of fetal weight. JCU 1987; 15: 376–386

34 Hadlock F P, Harrist R B, Sharman R S. Estimation of fetal weight by ultrasound. Am J Obstet Gynecol 1985; 151: 333–337

35 Neilson J P, Whitfield C R, Aitchison T C. Screening for the small for dates fetus: a two stage ultrasonic examination schedule. BMJ 1980; 280: 1203–1206

36 Thacker S B. Quality of controlled clinical trials. The case of imaging ultrasound in obstetrics: a review. Br J Obstet Gynaecol 1985; 92: 437–444

37 Chang T C, Robson S C, Spencer J A, Gallivan S. Prediction of perinatal morbidity at term in small fetuses; comparison of fetal growth and Doppler ultrasound. Br J Obstet Gynaecol 1994; 101: 422–427

38 Campbell S, Thoms A. Ultrasound measurement of the fetal head to abdomen circumference ratio in the assessment of growth retardation. Br J Obstet Gynaecol 1977; 84: 165–174

39 Moore T R, Cayle J E. The amniotic fluid index in normal human pregnancy. Am J Obstet Gynecol 1990; 162: 1168–1173

40 Neilson J P. Alfisevic. Doppler ultrasound in high risk pregnancies. In: Neilson J P, Crowther C A, Hodnett E D, Haffmeyr G J, Keirse M J N C, eds. Pregnancy and childbirth modules of the Cochrane Database of Systematic Reviews. (3.6.97) The Cochrane Collaboration Issue 3. Oxford: Update Software, 1997

41 Bower S, Harrington K F, Schuchter K, McGinn C, Campbell S. Prediction of pre-eclampsia by abnormal uterine Doppler ultrasound and modification by aspirin. Br J Obstet Gynaecol 1996; 103: 625–629

The biophysical profile

Martin J Whittle

Introduction

One of the major problems for the obstetrician in making an assessment of the fetus is its inaccessibility. In contrast, the physician can see his patient and determine, for example, his colour, activity and respiratory movements, information which until recent years has been denied to the fetal specialist. The development of ultrasound, however, has largely overcome these difficulties and allowed closer observation of the fetus and its activity, so that now considerable information concerning fetal condition can be obtained from a single examination.

Of course since ancient times the mother's appreciation of fetal life has been a traditional indication that the pregnancy is proceeding normally, although attempts to use the observation in a scientific way to identify a group of babies at risk of intra-uterine death has met with mixed success. Ultrasound has broadened the scope of the assessment of fetal activity as a means of determining fetal wellbeing, but nevertheless data on its value are conflicting.

This chapter explores the principles upon which the fetal biophysical profile is based, discusses the methods and indications, and considers the value of the test as a method of fetal assessment in current obstetric practice.

Physiological considerations

Fetal movement is the manifestation of central nervous system (CNS) activity, which may be influenced by a number of factors. Clearly, the progressive organisation of the fetal CNS will produce increasingly complex patterns of movement as the pregnancy advances.[1] In late pregnancy these patterns can be classified into defined behavioural groups which, although difficult to recognise in the fetus, undoubtedly exist and will be discussed later. CNS activity is also influenced by diurnal rhythm, maternal nutritional state, maternal drug therapy and hypoxia. In addition, however, it should be noted that activity may be altered when the brain has been damaged by intra-uterine infection, malformation or a non-hypoxic vascular catastrophe.

Behavioural states

Because the various forms of fetal activity appear to be influenced by the particular behavioural state of the fetus at that time, it is important to realise how these are deter-mined. Four states have been described,[2] corresponding to those seen in the neonate (Table 11.1). Only 1F and 2F persist for long enough to be identified with certainty in the fetus, and these are characterised as follows:

State 1F: quiescence which can be regularly interrupted by body movements, absent eye movements and a stable heart rate pattern with a small range of variation;

State 2F: frequent and periodic gross body movements, continuous eye movements and a heart rate with a wide range of variation and frequent accelerations;

State 3F and 4F occur infrequently in the fetus and do not show a developmental course and so are not considered further.

As gestational age advances the various activity patterns occur simultaneously with increasing frequency, so-called coincidence. Thus although at 32 weeks a recognisable state 1F exists only 29% of the time, by 38 weeks this rises to 67%.[2] These changes presumably relate to increasing maturation in the central nervous system.

The use of alterations in behavioural state as a method of fetal monitoring does not seem to have been considered practicable. Long periods of observation appear to be necessary, and in any case significant periods of coincidence do not develop until later in pregnancy, probably not until after 34 weeks. The problem of data handling is certainly surmountable with the use of suitable computer programs,[3] but even so the relevance of the data remains unclear.

Animal evidence

Evidence that specific types of fetal activity really existed in the normal fetus was disputed for some time. Chest wall movements had been seen in fetal lambs delivered into water baths, but in the more mature fetal lamb these were only seen when the cord was clamped and the fetus asphyxiated. The questionable validity of these early observations meant that fetal breathing came to be regarded as abnormal, and it was some years before new technology was available to show that in fact fetal breathing was not only normally present but could be observed throughout pregnancy.[4] Various factors were shown to influence the frequency of chest wall movements, including gestational age, diurnal rhythm, maternal nutritional

Table 11.1 Fetal behavioural activity

	1F	2F	3F	4F
Body movements	Incidental	Periodic	Absent	Continuous
Eye movements	Absent	Present	Present	Present
Heart rate patterns	Stable; few accelerations	Frequent accelerations	Stable; no accelerations	Large accelerations

state and, importantly, the blood gases. Thus, it was observed that chest wall movements increased when the fetus was hypercapnic but decreased or disappeared completely when there was hypoxia; in fact, in the very hypoxic fetus gasping movements were observed.

Other types of activity included forelimb movements, which were observed in the exteriorised fetal lamb.[5] This group also noted that the movements were influenced by a number of factors, including hypoxia, although they were unable to define a diurnal rhythm. These changes could be correlated with the pattern of eye movements and thus to the natural rest-activity cycles which become a feature of a normally functioning central nervous system, and increasingly prominent as the fetus develops.

Fetal activity

The clinical use of fetal movements as a method of evaluation was described by Sadovsky and Yaffe,[6] who used a series of case reports to demonstrate that fetal movements, as perceived by the mother, appeared to become markedly reduced or even cease days or occasionally only hours before fetal death. Pearson and Weaver[7] described the use of a fetal movement count chart, often called the 'kick chart', which allowed the mother to record the time at which she had felt 10 kicks over a 12-hour span. The results suggested that movements seemed to cease about 12–48 hours before death. In another fetal movement study[8] it was found that babies with reduced movements had a much poorer outcome and were more likely to be small for dates than those moving vigorously.

These observations led to the view that fetal activity indicated fetal health, and further, that a reduction in this activity preceded fetal death by a timespan of sufficient length to allow effective action to be taken to prevent an adverse outcome. Some support for this comes from a prospective randomised study involving 2250 patients[9] in which all the eight intra-uterine deaths occurred in the non-counting group, who were not monitoring fetal movements. In the counting group there were nine cases with reduced fetal movement and six of these babies were delivered by caesarean section; there were no deaths in this group, but two babies developed respiratory distress syndrome. The implication from this study is that these nine cases would have died if they had not been delivered at the appropriate time. However, later evidence derived from a large randomised study[10] comprising 68 000 patients showed that movement counting by the mother was unhelpful in reducing the risk of pregnancy loss, most babies being dead by the time of admission.

Although the maternal appreciation of fetal movement provides a simple method of assessing fetal condition on a day-to-day basis, it is relatively crude and gives no indication of the individual fetal activities. With the development of real-time ultrasound technology it became possible to observe these movements, and Manning[11] described a 'biophysical' assessment. Other methods of establishing the biophysical profile have been described,[12] and there are now innumerable modifications of the original Manning method.

The biophysical profile

Technique

The components of this score are shown in Table 11.2 and include fetal heart reactivity, fetal breathing movements, gross body movements, fetal tone and amniotic fluid pool depth. Each component is assigned an arbitrary value of 0 or 2, such that the minimum total score is 0 and the maximum 10.

Fetal heart rate activity

Antepartum heart rate testing has been used as a primary method of fetal assessment for a number of years, since the value of non-stressed testing was first discussed.[13] The concept depends on the inter-relationships between fetal movement and accelerations in fetal heart rate, which become disturbed in the presence of fetal hypoxia. Two movement-related accelerations in a 20-minute span are needed to deem the heart rate reactive (Fig. 11.1), although some groups use different criteria.

Table 11.2 Fetal biophysical score

Variable	Score 2	Score 0
Cardiotocography	At least 2 accelerations of 15 bpm, lasting 15 s in 20 min sessions	No accelerations
Fetal breathing	At least 30 s of sustained breathing in 30 min	<30 s breathing
Fetal movements	Three or more gross body movements in 30 min	<3 movements
Fetal tone	At least one motion of limb from flexion to extension and back	No movements
Amniotic fluid volume	A pocket of fluid at least 2 cm in depth	<1 cm^2 fluid

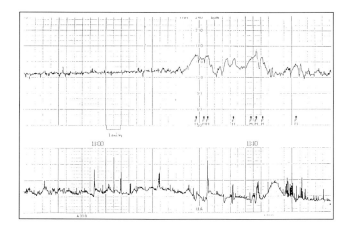

Fig. 11.1 A reactive fetal heart rate trace. FM indicates the time of fetal movement.

Fetal breathing

The observation of fetal breathing movements is not difficult but requires patience. At least 30 seconds of sustained breathing should be seen in a 30-minute span of observation. It is important to distinguish chest wall from trunk movement, and this is best achieved by scanning so that the fetal chest and abdominal walls appear on the screen together (Fig. 11.2). When the fetus breathes a see-saw apperance is seen, the chest moving in as the abdomen moves out. A further guide, which may be particularly helpful in cases with reduced amniotic fluid volume, is the movement of intra-abdominal structures such as the fetal kidney.

Fetal movements

Gross fetal activity is very easily observed using ultrasound and three or more movements should be seen in 30 minutes. Both limb and trunk movements are counted, but it is important to ensure that the limb movements are active and not merely occurring as the result of maternal activity. Trunk movements are usually of a rolling type.

Fetal tone

Although not self-evident it is possible to assess fetal tone most readily by observing the hands and feet, the clenched fist (Fig. 11.3) being obviously associated with normal tone, the same is true for feet undergoing dorsiflexion. In contrast, the fetus with absent tone lies with hands open and feet motionless.

Amniotic fluid volume

The measurement of amniotic fluid volume is very subjective but it is important that an empty pool is used, taking care that loops of cord are not mistakenly included in the measurement (Fig. 11.4). The original description of a significantly reduced volume as less than 1 cm is undoubtedly too rigorous. Indeed, this criterion probably originated from the use of amniotic fluid measurement in the evaluation of the post-dates pregnancy. Others[12] have considered 2 cm or less to be a more realistic amount (Table 11.3), although even this degree of oligohydramnios would be considered by many to be profound, and more recently the proposal is that the critical level should be defined as 2 cm in two perpendicular planes.[14]

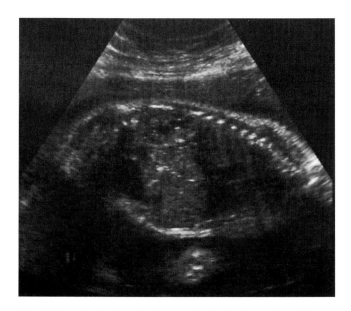

Fig. 11.2 **Longitudinal section through the fetal body** to show abdomen and thorax in the same plane.

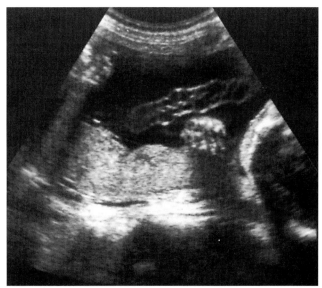

Fig. 11.3 **Fetal hand in clenched posture,** below the cord.

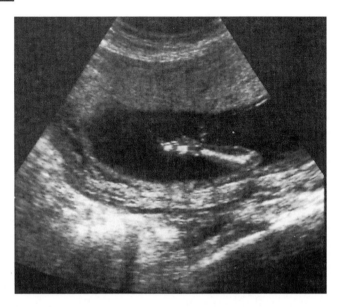

Fig. 11.4 Fetal forearm showing a clear pool of amniotic fluid.

One criticism of much that has been written concerning the biophysical profile relates to a lack of regard for the gestational age at the time of the assessment, and this applies particularly to amniotic fluid volume, which can change markedly with gestational age. Thus a 2 cm pool may be acceptable at term but almost certainly is not so at, say, 33 weeks. Unpublished data from our own department indicate that 90% of all pregnancies have a single depth of amniotic fluid of at least 3 cm, regardless of gestational age.

A better method of amniotic fluid assessment may be the use of the 'amniotic fluid index',[15] which is the sum of the vertical fluid depth in the four uterine quadrants. A total depth of 5 cm or more is considered normal. The amniotic fluid index has been stratified for gestational age[16] in a longitudinal study, but so far this approach has not been described as a feature of the biophysical profile technique.

Placental grading

Some systems include placental grading in the biophysical profile score (Table 11.3), but whether this is a helpful addition is uncertain. Vintzileos and colleagues suggest that a grade III placental score has a significant association with intrapartum distress and placental abruption.

Indications

In Manning's original description, common indications for study were the post-dates pregnancy and maternal diabetes. Since that time larger series have included pregnancies suspected to have a small-for-dates fetus and pregnancies complicated by hypertension.

Table 11.3 Criteria for scoring biophysical profiles

Non-stress test (NST)

Score 2 (NST 2):	>5 FHR accelerations of at least 15 bpm in amplitude and at least 15 s duration associated with fetal movements in a 20 min period.
Score 1 (NST 1):	2–4 accelerations of at least 15 bpm in amplitude and at least 15 s duration associated with fetal movements in a 20 min period.
Score 0 (NST 0):	<1 acceleration in a 20 min period.

Fetal movements (FM)

Score 2 (FM 2):	At least 3 gross (trunk and limbs) episodes of fetal movements within 30 min. Simultaneous limb and trunk movements were counted as a single movement.
Score 1 (FM 1):	1 or 2 fetal movements within 30 min.
Score 0 (FM 0):	Absence of fetal movements within 30 min.

Fetal breathing movements (FBM)

Score 2 (FBM 2):	At least 1 episode of fetal breathing of at least 60 s duration within a 30 min observation period.
Score 1 (FBM 1):	At least 1 episode of fetal breathing lasting 30–60 s within a 30 min observation period.
Score 0 (FBM 0):	Absence of fetal breathing or breathing lasting <30 s within a 30 min observation period.

Fetal tone (FT)

Score 2 (FT 2):	At least 1 episode of extension of extremities with return to position of flexion and also 1 episode of extension of spine with return to position of flexion.
Score 1 (FT 1):	At least 1 episode of extension of extremities with return to position of flexion, or 1 episode of extension of spine with return to position of flexion.
Score 0 (FT 0):	Extremities in extension. Fetal movements not followed by return. Open hand.

Amniotic fluid volume (AFV)

Score 2 (AFV 2):	Fluid evident throughout the uterine cavity. A pocket that measures >2 cm in vertical diameter.
Score 1 (AFV 1):	A pocket that measures <2 cm but >1 cm in vertical diameter.
Score 0 (AFV 0):	Crowding of fetal small parts. Largest pocket <1 cm in diameter.

Placental grading (PL)

Score 2 (PL 2):	Placental grading 0, I or II.
Score 1 (PL 1):	Placenta posterior, difficult to evaluate.
Score 0 (PL 0):	Placental grading III.

Other indications include circumstances in which the cardiotocograph (CTG) is equivocal, altered by drug treatment, e.g. β-blockers, complicated by the presence of variable decelerations or uninterpretable because of early gestational age. Alternatively, the profile may be indicated because the mother reports reduced fetal movements, or as a means of monitoring fetal condition during treatment, as in rhesus disease.

Method

Using real-time ultrasound the fetus may have to be observed for up to half an hour before the criteria are met for a normal result (Table 11.2). Although it has been proposed that the test interval of a week is adequate, this has been disputed,[17] the suggestion being that the test may need to be repeated sooner and should depend upon the underlying clinical problem. Indeed, in circumstances such as growth restriction daily assessment may be appropriate.

The order in which the tests are performed is not really important and, if all four ultrasound components of the profile are normal, fetal heart rate testing may not be necessary; indeed, in one series the CTG was always reactive.[18] It was found that when any one component was abnormal 64% of CTGs were normal, whereas if more than two were abnormal all the CTGs were non-reactive. The one single component most likely to be associated with an abnormal CTG was reduced amniotic fluid volume. The single component most likely to be absent was fetal breathing (72%), with a non-reactive CTG being found in 24% of cases. Very rarely was absent fetal tone or reduced amniotic fluid volume the single missing component.

Conversely, others[17] considered the CTG to be an integral part of the profile that needed to be retained. Although the observation of fetal activity, i.e. breathing, body and limb movement, may take some time, it is important that short-cuts are avoided.

The determination of fetal structural normality should be an integral part of the biophysical assessment, and this may be especially important either when the fetus appears small for dates or if oligohydramnios is noted.

Results

The results of biophysical testing appear to be remarkably impressive. Table 11.4 indicates the expected outcome in a large number of high-risk cases referred for evaluation by the profile.[19] When the score is 10 the outcome is excellent, and this also applies with a score of 8, so long as the

Table 11.4 Expected outcome following biophysical scoring

Score	PNM within a week
10/10	<1/1000
8/10	<1/1000
8/10 AFV = 0	89/1000
6/10 AFV = 2	Variable – retest within 24 h
6/10 AFV = 0	89/1000
4/10	91/1000
2/10	125/1000
0/10	600/1000

AFV = amniotic fluid volume
PNM = perinatal mortality

two points lost are not because the amniotic fluid is reduced, under which circumstances the perinatal loss rate rises dramatically. Scores less than 8 are associated with an increasingly high loss, scores 4–6 demand a repeat evaluation, and 2 or 0 indicate the need to deliver. One important point is the need to establish fetal normality when the profile score is abnormal and particularly if the amniotic fluid volume is reduced – renal agenesis features strongly in one series.[20]

The other approach to the biophysical profile has been the evaluation of each component. It was found[12] that although loss of fetal breathing occurred in many babies with impaired outcome (high sensitivity) it had a low positive predictive value. Conversely, loss of fetal tone was a very good predictor of a poor fetal outcome, usually with profound hypoxia, although by the time the fetus has reached this stage salvage may be impossible. Similar observations have been made by other groups,[21] who found absent fetal movements to be the most accurate predictor of perinatal death.

The association of the various components of the profile with hypoxia predicted the baby with marked acidosis.[22] In this study an abnormal profile score was predictive of a cord pH of less than 7.20 in 82% of cases. The fetal activity components of the score all provided a reasonable predictive value for acidosis, the weakest being absent fetal breathing and the strongest absent fetal tone.

The value of the biophysical profile in specific problems such as growth restriction has been addressed.[23] A false-negative result occurred more frequently when the baby was probably or definitely growth restricted. The implications of this are unclear and the reasons for the babies to be small for dates are not stated, although fetal abnormality had been excluded. It may be significant that in this report all of the losses followed the use of the modified profile (i.e. without CTG), although no comment is made concerning this. Further, in three of the cases the test interval was 7 days, and this may be inappropriately long when growth restriction is suspected. The same investigators, using a group of babies with neonatal evidence of growth restriction, found that the perinatal mortality rate was 27 per 1000 in babies suspected as small for dates and managed prospectively with the profile.[23]

The use of the biophysical profile in the evaluation of pregnancies with premature rupture of the membranes has been described[24] and the test appears to predict those babies in good condition. The specific use of the absence of fetal breathing movements as an indication of intrauterine infection has also been considered,[25] and certainly it appeared that infection was uncommon when breathing was seen. However, both these studies were retrospective and with few patients, making interpretation difficult. The technique does seem to show promise in this condition, but daily or alternate-day evaluation may be necessary.[26,27]

The use of the biophysical profile in multiple pregnancies has been described and recent evidence has suggested a predictive value for a poor outcome of about 50% and a sensitivity of 67%.[28] Interpretation of these data is difficult because of lack of information on chorionicity, but they suggest that the biophysical profile may have value in multiple pregnancies. Nevertheless, whether the full profile confers advantage over other methods of monitoring is unknown.

Diabetes mellitus represents a challenge in fetal assessment and in general the biophysical profile seems to have little to offer.[29] This may be because one component, amniotic fluid volume, may be artificially increased by the diabetic state of the mother and so be lost as a predictor of outcome.

Discussion

The biophysical profile as a method of fetal monitoring appears to be more firmly established in the USA than in Europe. A serious problem with the reported studies is that they use a variety of end-points with which to judge the test's value, making an objective evaluation difficult. Perinatal death, low cord blood pH values, poor Apgar scores and IUGR have all been used, and undoubtedly adverse outcome is associated with an abnormal profile. However, an association alone does not necessarily mean that the test will be an effective predictor of the adverse event, something which can only be assessed from a properly conducted randomised study of sufficient power to distinguish outcome variables between the groups chosen.

There are only four randomised studies evaluating the biophysical score.[30-33] Meta-analysis shows no particular advantage of biophysical profiles over other methods of monitoring. In fact, it would seem that biophysical profiles may increase the likelihood of induction of labour with no benefits from reduced morbidity or perinatal mortality.[34] The problem with interpreting these results comes from the variety of clinical problems encompassed and the relatively small size of the studies. In practice, the influence of prematurity and therapy such as betamethasone, and to a lesser extent, dexamethasone,[35] on fetal activity leads to difficulties in using the test clinically. However, in general the method appears to function well at the two extremes (very bad and very good), and so may provide helpful clinical information so long as caution is used.

To some extent the place of the biophysical profile, as well as the end-points, needs to be defined. Should the test be used primarily for screening, or as a method of evaluating a preselected group of at-risk pregnancies? Its use in screening would seem impracticable as it takes too long to

perform and can only be done effectively by staff with reasonable experience in ultrasound technique. Many modifications have been proposed, and a recent study has suggested that the use of non-stress testing together with an assessment of amniotic fluid volume is adequate, with a full biophysical profile being required in only 27% of cases.[36]

The advantage of biophysical profiling as a diagnostic test is that it does provide a semiquantitative assessment of fetal condition, which at least theoretically allows the progress of the pregnancy to be followed.[37]

If the profile has the ability to identify a deteriorating pregnancy it should provide some evidence about the degree of fetal hypoxia. The different components of the profile may relate to the functioning of various parts of the fetal central nervous system.[17] Thus, brain-stem function is considered most sensitive to hypoxia which, if present, would first produce changes in the CTG, followed by loss of breathing movements. As hypoxia deepens, the higher centres associated with movement and the maintenance of tone cease to function and the baby stops moving; the next stage is death. Although this hypothesis is attractive it does not fully explain observations in the hypoxic adult, in whom movement may cease early on but brain-stem function is maintained. It would seem likely that what is being observed in the fetus is the effect of progressive hypoxia on the central nervous system as a whole, and probably not in the selective way proposed.

If changing fetal activity represents the relatively acute response of the fetus to hypoxia the amniotic fluid volume reflects the effect of chronic hypoxia. Why amniotic fluid volume should decrease in IUGR is not clear, but it has been proposed that it is the result of reduced fetal urine output in the face of a redistributed fetal blood flow. Although this may be the case in some circumstances it cannot be the answer in all, as it is a common observation that perfectly adequate fetal activity is seen in oligohydramnios. Indeed, recent data suggest that in hypoxaemic sheep renal blood flow is maintained although amniotic fluid decreases.[38]

One serious criticism of the biophysical profile is that the various components are assigned the same value. This dates back to the origins of the test as an assessment based on the Apgar score, but with the evidence now available from a very large experience in its use perhaps the scoring system should be modified. Some groups have attempted this with the development of computerised analysis of variables, each of which are given different weightings.[39]

The advantages of the biophysical profile are that it provides a non-invasive method of fetal evaluation which can be performed daily, or more often if required. Further, it provides a biological assessment of fetal condition, in that it seems reasonable to assume that if the fetus is moving and breathing it will usually be healthy and not hypoxic.[17] In the growth restricted fetus invasive testing by fetal blood sampling has little to offer in the assessment of the blood gases, although it may provide useful information in terms of karyotype and infection.[40] A normal profile under these circumstances indicates the need to prolong the pregnancy, since functionally the baby's condition is satisfactory.

Conclusions

The biophysical profile has undergone major revisions since its use was first proposed. In addition, other methods of fetal evaluation have been developed to the extent that the original utility of the profile is largely no longer applicable. Further randomised studies have failed to show benefit. In spite of this, various components of the profile do have a use in clinical practice, but the results must be interpreted with caution. Studies are needed which define carefully not only outcome but also entry criteria, so that the use of the profile can be tested using discrete groups of problems.

REFERENCES

1 de Vries J I P, Visser G H A, Prechtl H F R. The emergence of fetal behavior. 1. Qualitative aspects. Early Hum Dev 1982; 7: 301–322

2 Nijuis J G, Prechtl H F R, Martin C B, Bots R S G M. Are there behavioral states in the human fetus? Early Hum Dev 1982; 6: 177–195

3 Rizzo G, Arduini D, Mancuso S, Romanini C. Computer-assisted analysis of fetal behavioural states. Prenat Diagn 1988; 8: 479–484

4 Boddy K. Fetal circulation and breathing movements. In: Beard R W, Nathanielsz P W, eds. Fetal physiology and medicine. London: W B Saunders, 1976; 302–328

5 Natale R, Clelow F, Dawes G S. Measurement of fetal forelimb movements in the lamb in utero. Am J Obstet Gynecol 1981; 140: 545–551

6 Sadovsky E, Yaffe H. Daily fetal movement recording and fetal progress. Obstet Gynecol 1973; 41: 845–850

7 Pearson J F, Weaver J B. Fetal activity and fetal wellbeing: an evaluation. BMJ 1976; 1: 1305–1307

8 Mathews D D. Maternal assessment of fetal activity in small-for-dates infants. Obstet Gynecol 1975; 45: 488–493

9 Neldum S. Fetal movements as an indicator of fetal wellbeing. Lancet 1980; i: 1222–1223

10 Grant A, Elbourne D, Valentin L, Alexander S. Routine formal fetal movement counting and risk of antepartum late death in normally formed singletons. Lancet 1989; ii: 345–349

11 Manning F A, Platt L D, Sipos L. Antepartum evaluation: development of a fetal biophysical profile. Am J Obstet Gynecol 1980; 136: 787–795

12 Vintzileos A M, Campbell W A, Ingardia C J, Nochimson D J. The fetal biophysical profile and its predictive value. Obstet Gynecol 1983; 62: 271–278

13 Keegan K A, Paul R H. Antepartum fetal heart rate testing. IV. The non-stress test as a primary approach. Am J Obstet Gynecol 1980; 136: 75–80

14 Manning F A. Dynamic ultrasound based fetal assessment; the fetal biophysical score. Clin Obstet Gynecol 1995; 38: 26–44

15 Phelan J P, Smith C V, Broussard P, Small M. Amniotic fluid assessment with the four quadrant technique at 36 to 42 weeks gestation. J Reprod Med 1987; 32: 540–542

16 Nwosu E C, Welch C R, Manasse P R, Walkinshaw S A. Longitudinal assessment of amniotic fluid index. Br J Obstet Gynaecol 1993; 100: 816–819

17 Vintzileos A M, Campbell W A, Nochimson D J, Weinbaum P J. The use and abuse of the fetal biophysical profile. Am J Obstet Gynecol 1987; 156: 527–533

18 Manning F A, Morrison I, Lange I R, Harman C R, Chamberlain P F C. Fetal biophysical scoring; selective use of the non-stress test. Am J Obstet Gynecol 1987; 156: 709–712

19 Manning F A, Morrison I, Harman C R, Lange I R, Menticoglou S. Fetal assessment based on fetal biophysical profile scoring: experience in 19 221 referred high risk pregnancies. Am J Obstet Gynecol 1987; 157: 880–884

20 Manning F A, Hill L M, Platt L D. Qualitative amniotic fluid volume determination by ultrasound. Antepartum detection of intra-uterine growth retardation. Am J Obstet Gynecol 1981; 139: 254–258

21 Baskett T F, Allen A C, Gray J H, Young D C, Young L M. Fetal biophysical profile and perinatal death. Obstet Gynecol 1987; 70: 357–360

22 Vintzileos A M, Gaffney S E, Salinger L M, Kontopoulos V G, Campbell W A, Nochimson D J. The relationships among the fetal biophysical profile, umbilical cord pH and Apgar score. Am J Obstet Gynecol 1987; 157: 627–631

23 Manning F A, Menticoglou S, Harman C R, Morrison I, Lange I R. Antepartum fetal risk assessment: the role of the biophysical profile score. In: Whittle M J, ed. Fetal monitoring. London: Baillière Tindall, 1987; 55–72

24 Vintzileos A M, Feinstein S J, Lodeiro J G, Campbell W A, Weinbaum P J, Nochimson D J. Fetal biophysical profile and the effect of premature rupture of the membranes. Obstet Gynecol 1986; 67: 818–823

25 Vintzileos A M, Campbell W A, Nochimson D J, Weinbaum P J. Fetal breathing as a predictor of infection in premature rupture of the membranes. Obstet Gynecol 1986; 67: 813–817

26 Gauthier D W, Meyer W J, Bieniarz A. Biophysical profile as a predictor of amniotic fluid culture results. Obstet Gynecol 1992; 80: 102–105

27 Vintzileos A M, Knuppel R A. Fetal biophysical assessment in preterm premature rupture of the membranes. Clin Obstet Gynecol 1995; 38: 45–58

28 Medina D, Vargas N, Bustos J C, Cadima R, Lavarello C. Biophysical profile in twin pregnancy: prospective study. Rev Chili Obstet Ginecol 1994; 59: 343–348

29 Bracero L A, Figueroa R, Byrne D W, Han H J. Comparison of umbilical Doppler velocimetry, non-stressed test and biophysical profile in pregnancies complicated by diabetes. J Ultrasound Med 1996; 1 5: 301–308

30 Platt L D, Walla C A, Paul R H et al. A prospective trial of the biophysical profile verses the non-stress test in the management of high-risk pregnancies. Am J Obstet Gynecol 1985; 153: 624–632

31 Manning F A, Morrison I, Lange I R, Harman C R. Fetal assessment based on fetal biophysical profile scoring: experience in 12 620 referred high risk pregnancies. Am J Obstet Gynecol 1985; 151: 342–350

32 Manning F A, Lange I R, Morrison I, Harman C R. Fetal biophysical profile score and the nonstress test: comparative trial. Obstet Gynecol 1984; 64: 326–331

33 Alfirevic Z, Walkinshaw S A. A randomised controlled trial of simple versus complex antenatal fetal monitoring after 42 weeks gestation. Br J Obstet Gynaecol 1995; 102: 638–643

34 Walkinshaw S A. Biophysical profiles. Curr Obstet Gynaecol 1997; 7: 1–8

35 Munder E J H, Derks J B, Visser G H A. Antenatal corticosteroid therapy and fetal behaviour; randomised study of the effects of betamethasone and dexamethasone. Br J Obstet Gynaecol 1997; 104: 1239–1247

36 Miller D A, Rabello Y A, Paul R H. The modified biophysical profile; antepartum testing in the 1990s. Am J Obstet Gynecol 1996; 174: 812–817

37 Druzin M L, Lockshin M, Edersheim T G, Hutson J M, Krauss A L, Kogut E. Second trimester fetal monitoring and preterm delivery in pregnancies with systemic lupus erythematosis and/or circulating anticoagulant. Am J Obstet Gynecol 1987; 157: 1503–1510

38 Cock M L, McCrabb G J, Wlodeck M E, Harding R. Effects of prolonged hypoxemia on fetal renal function and amniotic fluid volume in sheep. Am J Obstet Gynecol 1997; 176: 320–326

39 Devoe L D. Computerised fetal biophysical assessment. Clin Obstet Gynecol 1995; 38: 121–131

40 Morrison J J, Rodeck C H. Fetal blood sampling: does it have a place? Curr Obstet Gynaecol 1997; 7: 93–97

12

Twin pregnancy

Phillipa Kyle

Introduction

Multiple pregnancy carries a higher risk of morbidity and mortality than does singleton pregnancy. The risks become greater as the number of fetuses increase, when the placentation is monochorionic rather than dichorionic, and when there is only one amniotic sac. Ultrasound has become invaluable for the diagnosis, assessment and monitoring of multiple pregnancy, and this chapter focuses on some of the issues in which ultrasound is an integral component.

Incidence and outcome of twin pregnancy

The overall incidence of twin pregnancy has increased in recent years from 10 per 1000 pregnancies in 1982 to 13.6 per 1000 in 1995.[1] Most of the increase has been secondary to assisted conception techniques, such as ovulation induction and *in vitro* fertilisation. As a result the incidence is highest in older women (19.6 per 1000 in women aged 35 and over in 1995) and the greatest increase occurred in this group.[2] The increased number are mainly dizygotic twins, although this cannot be assumed as division of a fertilised ovum (i.e. monozygotic twinning) can occur in the course of infertility treatment. The incidence of monozygotic twin pregnancy is relatively constant at approximately 3–5 per 1000 twin pregnancies, and appears to be independent of genetics, age or environmental influences. Higher-order multiple pregnancies secondary to assisted reproduction have decreased since greater controls and surveillance have been introduced into reproductive medicine, although it remains to be seen whether these levels are maintained with time.

Embryology

All dizygotic twins commence as two fertilised ova, each developing into a blastocyst which has its own implantation site. All dizygotic twin pregnancies are dichorionic. In monozygotic twin pregnancy the pattern of chorionicity and amnionicity is dependent on the stage at which the single fertilised ovum splits. If the split occurs up to day 3 two blastocysts will develop, resulting in a dichorionic diamniotic pregnancy: this occurs in 25% of monozygotic twins. In the remainder cleavage occurs after day 3. If the split is between days 4 and 8 a monochorionic diamniotic pregnancy results; if between days 8 and 13 a monochorionic mono-amniotic twin pregnancy; and if after day 13 conjoined twins may result (Fig. 12.1).[3]

Morbidity and mortality in multiple pregnancy

All multiple pregnancies have higher rates of mortality than occur in singleton pregnancy, and the rate for triplets

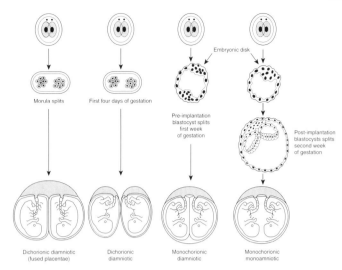

Fig. 12.1 The development and placentation of monozygotic twins (from Fox et al., 1978[3]).

is over twice as high as for twins. The factors responsible for the increased pregnancy loss in twins in general include an increased incidence of preterm delivery, intra-uterine growth retardation, intra-uterine twin–twin transfusion syndrome, malpresentation, and an increased incidence of congenital malformations.

The stillbirth rate is higher in multiple pregnancies: a rate of 19.6 per 1000, in contrast to 5.3 per 1000 in singletons, was recorded in 1994.[1] This trend also follows for early neonatal deaths (22.8 per 1000 for multiple versus 2.7 per 1000 singleton pregnancies) and for late neonatal, post-neonatal and infant death rates. This high loss rate in multiple pregnancy has gained increasing attention relative to a background of overall falling perinatal mortality.

The problems in multiple pregnancy are not just those of a high perinatal loss rate, but also those of a substantially increased handicap rate,[4] there being an eightfold increase in risk of cerebral palsy in twins and a 47-fold increase in triplets. There is also a strong suggestion that monozygosity confers an increased risk in pregnancy, as stillbirth and early neonatal death rates were highest in like-sex twin pregnancies.[2] Perinatal morbidity and mortality is three to five times higher in monochorionic than in dichorionic pregnancies.[5–7] The relative increase in risk of monochorionic compared to dichorionic twin pregnancies is therefore of similar magnitude to that of twins compared to singletons. Much of the increase is due to the presence of vascular anastomoses, which are implicated in twin–twin transfusion syndrome, co-twin death, and neurological sequelae in the surviving twin after the intra-uterine death of one fetus.

Preterm labour is the cause of substantial perinatal mortality and morbidity in multiple pregnancy: approximately 25–30% of twins and 80–95% of triplet pregnancies end spontaneously before 37 weeks gestation.[8] The major cause of neonatal death in multiple pregnancy is prematurity.

Zygosity and chorionicity

Figure 12.2 shows the relationship between zygosity and chorionicity. The most common misconception is that separate placentae denote dizygosity, but it must be remembered that if the fertilised ovum splits before day 3 separate placentae and membranes will form. Dichorionic placentae are separate, but in some cases are juxtaposed and therefore appear fused on ultrasound scans, which can make chorionicity determination more difficult.

Ultrasound determination of chorionicity

It has become increasingly possible over recent years to determine chorionicity *in utero* by ultrasound,[9,10] and routine prenatal determination of chorionicity has been widely recommended.[10–12] Appreciation of the importance of chorionicity has resulted in improved management of issues such as fetal reduction, prenatal diagnosis, twin–twin transfusion syndrome and intra-uterine growth retardation.

Chorionicity determination also pertains to higher-order pregnancies because, even with multiple pregnancies secondary to assisted reproduction techniques, splitting of one fertilised ovum can occur and thus cause monochorionic twins within a set of triplets.

Routine early assessment of chorionicity in multiple pregnancy is recommended because earlier in pregnancy its accuracy is higher, and by the time clinical indications for chorionicity determination present (growth retardation, stuck twin syndrome) it may be impossible to make an accurate assessment. These conditions are usually associated with oligohydramnios and fetal crowding, making it difficult to assess the fetal membranes and gender. Chorionicity determination needs to be routine if it is to be used in the prediction of risk in prenatal diagnosis, in ante-

natal care, fetal medicine, and in the management of twin complications in the second and third trimesters.

Chorionicity should be determined in the first trimester if possible, as the accuracy at this stage of pregnancy is 100%.[12] This is relatively easy in pregnancies resulting from assisted conception, as they are usually scanned in the first trimester, but in those resulting from spontaneous conception twins may not be diagnosed until the routine anomaly scan at 18–20 weeks. This may change if early pregnancy anomaly scans and nuchal thickness screening at 11–14 weeks gestation are introduced more widely.[13] Until that time chorionicity determination should be undertaken at the time the multiple pregnancy is diagnosed, although it must be recognised that mid-trimester assessment of chorionicity is inaccurate in at least 10% of cases.[14]

The determination of chorionicity is based on ultrasound to identify fetal gender, the number of placental masses, the dividing membrane thickness, and the characteristics of the dividing membrane's origin from the placenta.[9,10,15–18] The following steps should be taken in the mid-trimester:

1. Identify the external genitalia, which can be done relatively easily on the 18–20-week scan. Accuracy can be extremely high if positive visualisation of female external genitalia is used as the criterion for female gender, and technical difficulties with fetal position are acknowledged and the scan repeated if sex determination is suboptimal. Discordant external genitalia indicate dizygosity and dichorionicity.

2. Count the number of distinct placental masses. Separate placental masses indicate dichorionicity.

3. Assess the dividing membrane. Histologically the dividing membrane in dichorionic twins is formed by two layers of chorion and two of amnion, and in monochorionic twins there are only two layers of amnion. This means that monochorionic twins have a thinner membrane than dichorionic twins, and the difference can be seen on ultrasound (Fig. 12.3).[9,10] An accuracy of approximately 80% has been reported in several studies for the prediction of chorionicity using membrane thickness,[15,16] but these studies are limited by being retrospective, unblinded or qualitative. Furthermore, a subsequent study showed that quantitative measurements of membrane thickness have a high intra- and inter-observer variability,[19] making this sign on its own of limited use.

4. The final step for characterising chorionicity uses the appearance of the septum at its origin from the placenta. A tongue of placental tissue is seen ultrasonically within the base of dichorionic membranes and has been termed the 'twin peak'[18] or 'lambda' sign[20] (Fig. 12.4). This has a sound theoretical basis, presumably reflecting incomplete regression of the chorion laeve in the first trimester at its junction with the chorion frondosum, and appears to be accurate.[21] Absence of the lambda sign is found mainly in monochorionic placentation (Fig. 12.5).

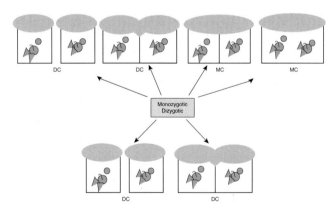

Fig. 12.2 The relationship between zygosity and chorionicity.
MC – monochorionic, DC – dichorionic

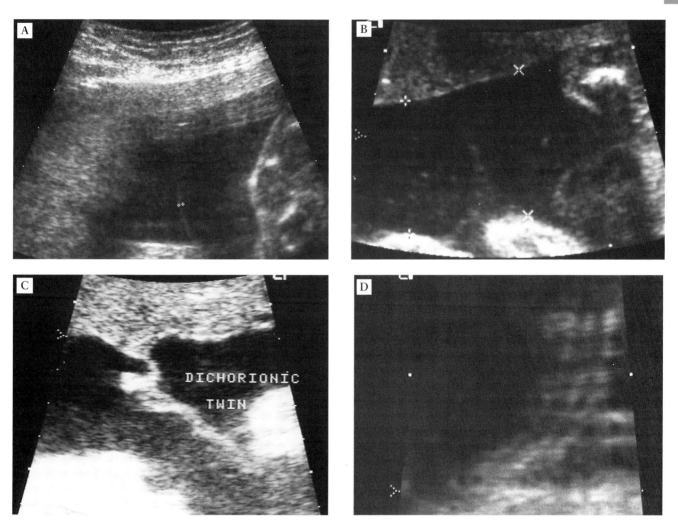

Fig. 12.3 The dividing membrane in twin gestations. A and **B**: Monochorionic gestations have a thin dividing membrane consisting of two layers of amnion only, whereas **C**: dichorionic twin gestations have a thick dividing membrane consisting of two layers of amnion and two layers of chorion, of which **D**: the individual layers may sometimes be apparent.

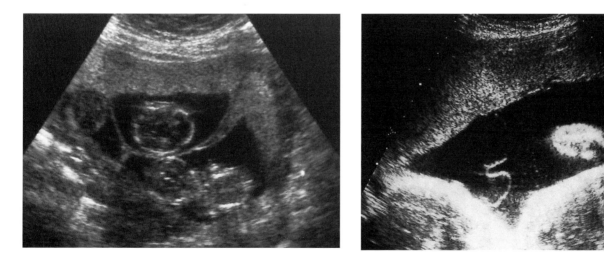

Fig. 12.4 The 'twin peak' or 'lambda sign' in dichorionic twin gestation.

Fig. 12.5 Absence of the lambda sign in monochorionic twin gestation.

247

A combination of all the signs should provide greater than 90% accuracy for chorionicity determination in the second trimester.[14] However, in the first trimester chorionicity determination has an accuracy of 100% and therefore this is the ideal time to perform the examination.[12] In the first trimester dichorionic twin pregnancies have a thick inter-twin septum, thicker than is seen in the mid-trimester (Fig. 12.6). Separate yolk sacs are seen within separate extraembryonic coeloms. In contrast, monochorionic twin pregnancy shows a tissue paper-thin midline septum (Fig. 12.7) and there is a single extraembryonic coelom containing both yolk sacs. Monteagudo *et al.*[12] reported a 100% accuracy in 43 twin and high-order multiple pregnancies using trans-vaginal ultrasound to look for the above features.

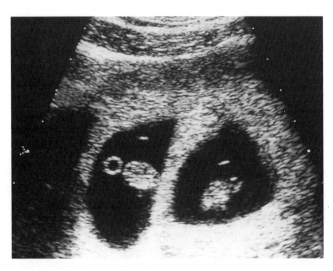

Fig. 12.6 The thick dividing septum found in the first trimester in dichorionic twin gestation.

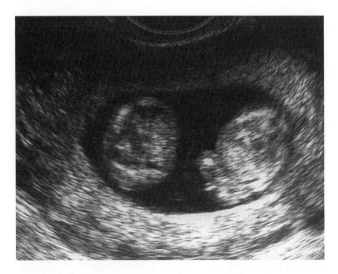

Fig. 12.7 The very thin dividing membrane in monochorionic twin gestation.

Zygosity can only be determined by ultrasound if the placentation is determined as monochorionic in the first trimester, or two fetuses of separate sex are identified in the mid-trimester. Otherwise zygosity can only be determined after birth from cord or infant blood samples.

Vascular anatomy of twin placentation

The presence of vascular anastomoses in dichorionic placentae is thought to be exceedingly rare,[22] although they may occasionally occur.[23] In monochorionic pregnancy there is a single placenta with one chorion and either two (diamniotic) or one (monoamniotic) sac(s). Almost 100% of these placentae will have communicating vascular anastomoses within them, and in up to 30–40% of these significant problems will occur as a result. The risk of problems related to anastomoses can generally be considered to be confined to monochorionic placentation.

The vascular anatomy of monochorionic placentae was first described over a century ago.[24] Subsequent studies have confirmed that the anastomoses are usually multiple, and may be superficial or deep.

Arterio-arterial and venovenous anastomoses are located on the surface of the chorionic plate, whereas arteriovenous anastomoses lie deep within the placental substance. The slow transfusion associated with chronic twin–twin transfusion syndrome is likely to be due to the deep arteriovenous anastomoses, which are unidirectional, whereas the superficial anastomoses may be implicated in the sequelae of co-twin intra-uterine death, where the cause of the transfusion is a sudden change in blood pressure leading to an acute large transfusion from the surviving twin into the dying twin.[25–27]

Twin–twin transfusion syndrome

Because of the vascular anastomoses that occur in monochorionic twin pregnancies a number of different forms of inter-twin transfusion can occur. Twin–twin transfusion syndrome (TTTS) is the most common form, and this term is used most frequently to refer to mid-trimester transfusion resulting in the oligohydramnios–polyhydramnios sequence. Although this represents a more chronic form of inter-twin transfusion there may be acute exacerbations of the underlying pathology. A more chronic form occurs as twin reversed arterial perfusion sequence in acardiac twin pregnancies, and the most acute form is that arising after the intra-uterine death of one of monochorionic twins.

TTTS complicates 4–35% of monochorionic diamniotic twin pregnancies[22,28] and accounts for 15–17% of perinatal mortality in twins.[29,30] The syndrome is attributed to the transfusion of blood via placental vascular anastomoses between the two fetal circulations, causing anaemia and growth retardation in the twin denoted the 'donor' and polycythaemia with circulatory overload in the 'recipient',[31] although recent data suggest that the mechanism is likely to be more complicated than this.

TTTS usually presents in the second trimester with maternal uterine over-distension, and is diagnosed by ultrasound. The most obvious finding is discordant amniotic fluid volume. The donor twin becomes oliguric and develops oligohydramnios, appearing enshrouded within its membrane and fixed to the uterine wall (Fig. 12.8). The recipient develops polyuria, with a persistently enlarged bladder, severe polyhydramnios, a hydropic cord, and ultimately hydrops fetalis (Fig. 12.9). The term 'stuck' twin syndrome, advocated by some authors,[32,33] refers to anhy-

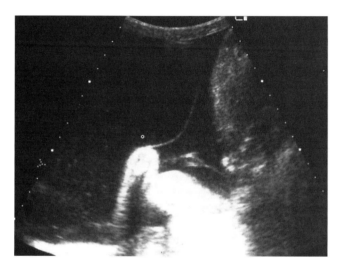

Fig. 12.8 The relative reduction in amniotic fluid causes the dividing membrane to enshroud the donor twin in twin–twin transfusion syndrome (TTTS).

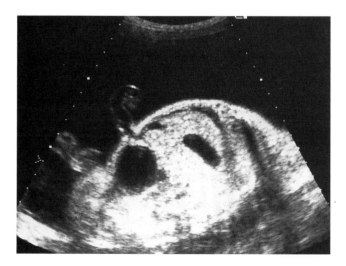

Fig. 12.9 The polyuric recipient twin in TTTS is at risk of becoming hydropic.

dramnios in the donor twin sac but does not refer to the polyhydramniotic recipient fetus. 'Stuck' twin may occur in some cases of dichorionic twin pregancies due to other causes,[33] and therefore the terminology is not recommended for TTTS. The diagnosis of mid-trimester TTTS should be restricted to monochorionic pregnancies with complete discordance of amniotic fluid volume. This is because there are no other known pathologies in monochorionic twins that result in severe oligohydramnios in one sac and severe polyhydramnios in the other.

Most cases of TTTS do have estimated fetal weight discordance *in utero*,[34] although as weight estimates are subject to error it is difficult to use this as an accurate diagnostic criterion. There is some evidence that pregnancies with a poor outcome have greater discrepancies in abdominal circumference than those with a good outcome.[35] At one time it was thought that all cases had a haemoglobin difference of more than 5 g/dl between donor (anaemic) and recipient (polycythaemic). However, such discordance has been shown to be present in approximately 20% of cases when sampled *in utero*. Therefore, the mainstay of diagnosis is discordant amniotic fluid volume in monochorionic diamniotic pregnancy (Fig. 12.10).

Presentation in the mid-trimester has, until recently, been associated with an 80–100% perinatal wastage rate, mainly from preterm delivery, secondary to polyhydramnios.[30,36] A large number of treatments have been tried, with no evidence of definite therapeutic effect. These range from trans-placental digoxin therapy,[37] intra-uterine venesection and exchange transfusion[38] to selective feticide.[39–41] More recently other therapeutic procedures have been introduced, with apparent improvement in survival to around 50%, although there is concern that neurological, cardiac and renal sequelae are common in some survivors. Serial amnioreduction is beneficial in prolonging gestation and improving survival, and until recently has been considered the treatment of choice. A randomised controlled trial would now be difficult to perform as the empirical evidence from the above series shows that amnioreduction is of major benefit, with an overall survival rate of 63% in recent series. Amnioreduction also improves uterine perfusion compared to control needling procedures,[42] and may improve fetal blood gas status.[43] Aggressive amnioreduction may therefore not only prevent complications such as preterm labour, but also improve fetal condition and possibly ameliorate the disease. In cases where amnioreduction fails more aggressive procedures may be required. Selective feticide of the donor has been used to allow survival of the recipient in seven cases, although this drastic procedure was performed primarily to prolong pregnancies threatened by gross polyhydramnios in the absence of hydrops or other fetal compromise.[40,41]

Fetoscopic laser ablation of placental vascular anastomoses has been performed in several centres worldwide. Theoretically this technique should be the ideal treatment

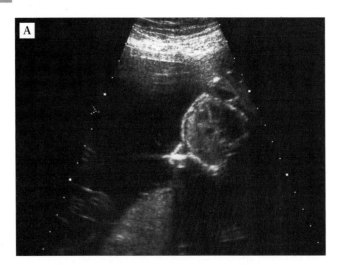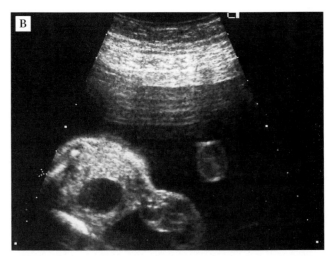

Fig. 12.10 A twin pregnancy with TTTS showing A: the donor twin trapped against the uterine side wall and B: the recipient twin in the polyhydramniotic sac.

for TTTS if the condition is due to the presence of anastomoses and they can be selectively ablated. However, the present technique relies on dividing all vessels at the membrane interface, which may not be identical to the vascular equator of the two circulations in which anastomoses are likely to occur. Indeed, this would explain why the survival rate is still just over 50%.[44,45] In one-third of cases both babies survive; in another third one baby survives, and in the remaining third both babies die. Nevertheless, initial data suggest that survivors may have less neurological damage than series reported from serial amniodrainage, but it does seem that further research to identify the type and location of the communicating channels needs to be performed, which will enhance the success of laser therapy.

We therefore feel that laser ablation of the placental vessels is suitable in cases of severe TTTS of early onset, around 18–24 weeks gestation, in which the prognosis is extremely poor. The ultrasound criteria used to diagnose severe TTTS include anhydramnios in the donor twin sac, empty 'donor' bladder, and polyhydramnios in the recipient twin sac. In such cases serial amnioreduction may result in survival but with a high incidence of neurological lesions.[46] In cases presenting with less severe TTTS, or after 24–26 weeks gestation, we would prefer to use serial amnioreduction to manage this condition.

Intra-uterine death in monochorionic pregnancies

The presence of fetal compromise, whether due to twin–twin transfusion or to intra-uterine growth retardation, raises particular difficulties in monochorionic twin pregnancies. Intra-uterine death in one twin is associated

with necrotic brain and renal lesions in 25% of co-twin survivors,[25] and there appears to be a similar risk of intra-uterine death in the healthy co-twin. The most likely mechanism of both these outcomes is ischaemia from severe hypotension, as the initially healthy twin transfuses blood into the dying twin's circulation.[26,27] There has been debate over the underlying cause for co-twin compromise. Previously it has been postulated that the death of a co-twin was due to the presence of DIC secondary to the dead twin, although this has never been found *in utero* or at birth. Okamura *et al.*[27] have examined the coagulation status of surviving twins following intra-uterine death and found no evidence to support DIC in the survivor. They did, however, demonstrate fetal anaemia, which was most marked the sooner the sampling procedure was performed after intra-uterine death, again suggesting that the surviving twin does transfuse a substantial proportion of its blood volume into the circulation of the dead twin.

Although knowledge of chorionicity influences prognosis and management after the intra-uterine death of one twin, its real value lies before such an event occurs, in that delivery may be expedited in monochorionic pregnancies with a potentially compromised fetus in order to avoid sequelae in the healthy co-twin. The decision to deliver is not difficult after 30 weeks gestation, but raises the greatest management problems at gestations of around 25–28 weeks. An option at such early gestations is to allow the death of the compromised twin and to arrange short- and long-term assessment of the survivor. It is not clear how one should respond to evidence of fetal distress in the surviving twin, should this manifest within 24–48 hours of the first twin's demise. There must be substantial concern that, were one to intervene in this situation, the surviving twin would be at risk of handicap, and yet it is difficult to monitor without considering delivery. Another option is to perform fetal blood sampling on the second twin and, if anaemic, to perform an intra-uterine red blood cell transfusion, although obviously this may only be available in a specialised centre. The least invasive policy is to wait and see if the second twin survives and, if so, arrange serial ultrasound assessment over the subsequent 2–4 weeks looking for evidence of cerebral ischaemic damage. If serious damage does become obvious then late termination should be considered. However, major problems occur with this approach, including the risk of preterm labour in the intervening period, difficulty in assessing intracranial structure in detail, and the fact that more subtle forms of cerebral compromise are undetectable using prenatal ultrasound. The parents need to be carefully counselled about the difficulties faced in such a situation.

In dichorionic pregnancies none of the above concerns apply, provided chorionicity has been accurately diagnosed and that another pathology was responsible for the twin death.

Twin reversed arterial perfusion sequence

Acardiac twinning is the most extreme presentation of the twin–twin transfusion syndrome, occurring in approximately 1% of monozygotic twin pregnancies. This disorder has also been called twin reversed arterial perfusion (TRAP) sequence because of the disruption in normal vascular perfusion, with the development of a recipient twin (acardiac) with an umbilical arterial-to-arterial anastomosis with the donor or pump twin.[47] Up until now at least 50% of donor twins die from congestive heart failure or preterm delivery, usually associated with polyhydramnios. All acardiac twins die from multiple malformations (Fig. 12.11). Prenatal treatment has been attempted,

including amniodrainage, administration of indomethacin to the mother, surgical removal of the acardiac twin, or occlusion of the umbilical cord.[48] Endoscopic laser coagulation of the umbilical vessels has been used with success, especially when performed in mid-trimester prior to the development of polyhydramnios and hydrops.[49] This appears to be the simplest method available. This twin abnormality should always be suspected when a 'nonviable' twin found on early scan continues to grow.

Conjoined twins

Conjoined twinning is an extremely rare sporadic event and rates of 1:33 000 to 1:165 000 have been quoted.[50] Such cases result from late and incomplete division of the monozygotic embryonic disc, sometime around days 13–15 post fertilisation. The mortality associated with conjoined twinning is high and only a few have sufficiently favourable anatomy to allow separation (Fig. 12.12). The degree of cardiovascular conjunction is usually the limiting factor to survival. Conjoined twins can be classified simply by describing where the fusion occurs, i.e. upper body, middle trunk or lower body. Central joining (thoraco-omphalopagus) represents around 80% of cases, cranial (syncephalus and craniopagus) 12% and caudal (pyopagus) 8%.[51]

Prenatal diagnosis

The prenatal diagnosis of structural, chromosomal and genetic abnormalities is an expanding field and, in cases of multiple pregnancy, many problems in this area are exacerbated owing to a conflict of loyalties to each fetus and heightened concern about pregnancy loss in what is often a very much wanted pregnancy. This means that very

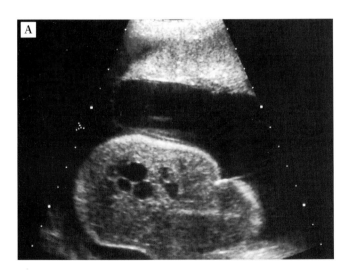
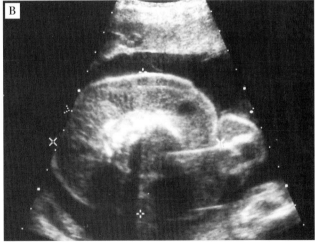

Fig. 12.11 An acardic twin at 22 weeks gestation which is **A:** hydropic and **B:** shows rudimentary tissue and bone formation.

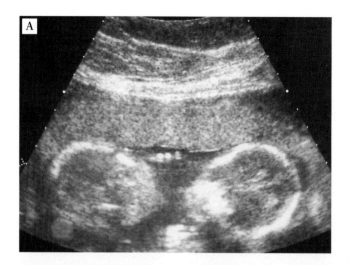

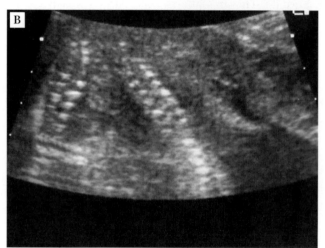

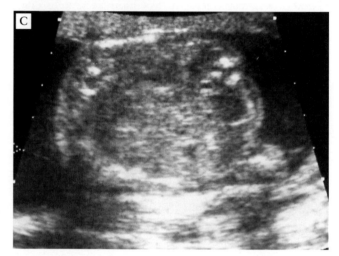

Fig. 12.12 A set of conjoined twins at 20 weeks gestation. A: The two separate heads, **B:** the two spines in longitudinal views descending into one common pelvis, and **C:** transverse section of the joined abdomens showing the two spines at 2 and 10 o'clock.

skilled management and counselling are required, providing a real challenge to the fetal medicine specialist.

Structural anomalies

There appears to be an increased risk of congenital malformation in twin pregnancies, particularly in monozygotic gestations. The defects may be concordant or discordant between twins, regardless of whether the pregnancy is mono- or dizygotic, and if it is in the former this must reflect an imbalance in the intra-uterine environment. Malformations seen in excess in monozygotic twins include neural tube defects (particularly anencephaly), holoprosencephaly, the sirenomyelia complex and cloacal exstrophy.[52] Monozygous twins have a higher risk of congenital heart disease, carrying a risk (32:1000) which is greater than that normally quoted to a couple who have already had a child with a heart defect (25:1000).

Therefore we recommend that a detailed evaluation of the fetal hearts is performed in monochorionic twin gestations, which are by default monozygotic pregnancies. Other structural abnormalities are secondary to a vascular disturbance related to vascular anastomoses and include microcephaly, hydranencephaly and porencephalic cysts.[53]

Screening for aneuploidy

In a dizygotic pregnancy each twin carries a maternal age-related risk of aneuploidy comparable to that of a singleton pregnancy, which means that a woman carrying dizygous twins should be counselled that the chance of either one of them having Down's syndrome is twice her age-related risk. In contrast, women with monozygous twins simply have their age-related risk that both twins will be aneuploid. Monozygotic twins may rarely be cytogenetically discordant, although this risk is unknown.

Biochemical screening for trisomy 21 in multiple pregnancies poses real difficulties as HCG and AFP are both increased in twin pregnancy, although some have advocated its use with adjusted ranges.[54] It is likely that fetal ultrasound in the first trimester (11–14 weeks gestation), with assessment of the nuchal thickness in each fetus, will become the optimal method for aneuploidy screening in multiple pregnancy.[55] Such an assessment also provides an opportunity to determine chorionicity, if this has not already been assessed. Preliminary information is available suggesting that increased nuchal thickness in a monochorionic twin gestation may be a marker for twin–twin transfusion syndrome in chromosomally normal fetuses.[55]

Invasive procedures

Prenatal diagnosis using invasive procedures involves testing of each fetus, although if monochorionic gestation is diagnosed in the first trimester some would advocate testing only one fetus, assuming that these twins are monozygotic and should therefore be chromosomally and genetically identical. Amniocentesis is the most common invasive procedure. Before commencing the procedure each amniotic sac must be mapped in detail and recorded, so that whether a two-needle procedure is performed (entry into each sac) or a single-needle technique (sampling one sac and then transversing the dividing membrane to then sample the second sac), there can be certainty as to the site of sampling and which result belongs to which fetus. The practice of injecting dye into the first sampling sac has been abandoned. Despite older studies suggesting a large increase in loss rate after amniocentesis, more recent studies suggest that the procedure-related loss rate may be no greater than with singletons.[56]

Chorion villous sampling (CVS) may be performed in twin pregnancy but problems may arise secondary to inter-twin contamination if there is one placental mass. Maternal contamination is unlikely using a transabdominal double-needle technique. Studies have estimated that contamination complicates 2–6% of CVS procedures in twins,[57–59] and therefore parents should be warned of this risk. Some have suggested zygosity testing in all cases of like-sexed dichorionic twins.[59] If they appear monozygous this could indicate either real monozygosity (20% chance) or contamination in dizygous twins – only subsequent amniocentesis could differentiate. Despite the concerns regarding contamination, CVS appears to be a safe procedure in twins, with few data to substantiate an increased procedure-related loss rate above that of singletons.

Fetal blood sampling can be performed in twin gestations. If the placental cord insertions are chosen as the sampling sites it is imperative that each is carefully identified, and in particular its relationship to which fetus. Some have advocated sampling from an intrahepatic vein in each fetus, to provide certainty that both twins have been sampled, but we have not found this to be necessary as long as the above precautions have been taken.

Selective feticide

In twin pregnancies discordant for fetal anomaly selective termination of the affected fetus is an option. A variety of fetoscopic and ultrasound-guided techniques to do this have been described, including fetal exsanguination and intracardiac injection of air or potassium chloride,[60,61] the latter now being the recommended technique.[62] Selective feticide is contraindicated in monochorionic pregnancies because of the risk of causing death of the normal twin, owing to the vascular communications within the shared placenta.[61] Therefore, as discussed previously, chorionicity determination is essential before contemplating such a procedure. The international experience in selective termination has been collected and shows that there is an overall pregnancy loss rate of 8.3%,[63] with procedures performed before 16 weeks gestation carrying a lower risk (5.4%) of subsequent loss. Furthermore, recent data have shown that reduction at 20 weeks gestation or later is associated with a worse perinatal outcome with earlier delivery and lower birthweight.[64]

Rarely, selective feticide has been intentionally performed in monochorionic twin pregnancies, not to terminate an abnormal fetus but to allow the survival of a fetus otherwise compromised by its co-twin. Robie *et al.*[48] delivered an acardiac monster by *sectio parva* with successful outcome for the pump twin left *in utero*, and intrapericardial injection has been used to tamponade the donor's heart in two fetuses with twin–twin transfusion syndrome, allowing prolongation of the pregnancy and survival of the recipient.[40,41] Recently cord ligation by endoscopic techniques has been reported,[65] and we have reported success with direct intravascular injection of pure alcohol.[66]

Multifetal pregnancy reduction

This procedure aims to reduce the markedly increased perinatal mortality in higher-order multiple pregnancies. The objective is to achieve either a twin or a triplet gestation. Initially trans-vaginal aspiration was performed, but this has been abandoned in view of the high loss rates[67] and now the majority are performed by transabdominal injection of potassium chloride into the fetal thorax.[68,69] As most of these pregnancies are the result of poorly controlled ovulation induction they are usually multizygotic and multichorionic. However, chorionicity must always be assessed.[70] Selective feticide is best delayed until 10–12 weeks, when the risks of abortion and spontaneous regression have subsided and the nuchal thickness can be measured. The optimal number of fetuses to be left remains controversial, but most centres reduce to twins. The risk of miscarrying the whole pregnancy is around 8%, although it is influenced by the starting and final number of embryos.[71,72] The outcome of twins and triplets delivered after 32 weeks gestation is similar to that of spontaneous multiple pregnancy.[72,73]

Routine surveillance of twins and higher-order pregnancies

It is recognised that it is difficult to monitor the growth and well-being of twins and higher-order pregnancies clinically (Fig. 12.13). In view of the growth disturbances that occur in multiple pregnancies, closer surveillance is required (Fig. 12.14). We follow a management protocol of scans every 4 weeks for growth and liquor volume in dichorionic twin gestations, and 2-weekly for monochorionic twin gestations, in view of their risk of developing twin–twin transfusion syndrome. The frequency is modified if an abnormality is detected. As in singleton pregnancies Doppler flow velocity of the umbilical artery is used to monitor and assess risk in the growth-restricted fetus(es), although in our experience abnormalites in the flow velocity pattern may persist longer than in singletons, and is not as useful for the timing of delivery.

Conclusion

Twin pregnancies are a challenge to the ultrasonographer and obstetrician in view of the large range of abnormalities that may develop. The aim in management is to assess the risk of complications by determining chorionicity in early pregnancy, to assess for congenital abnormalities and then to monitor for growth and fetal well-being. Monochorionic twin pregnancies have three to five times

the risk of perinatal mortality and morbidity as in dichorionic twin pregnancies, and therefore chorionicity should be determined as early as possible, ideally in the first trimester.

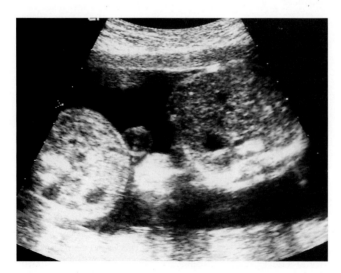

Fig. 12.13 A twin pair showing discordant sizes on ultrasound scan.

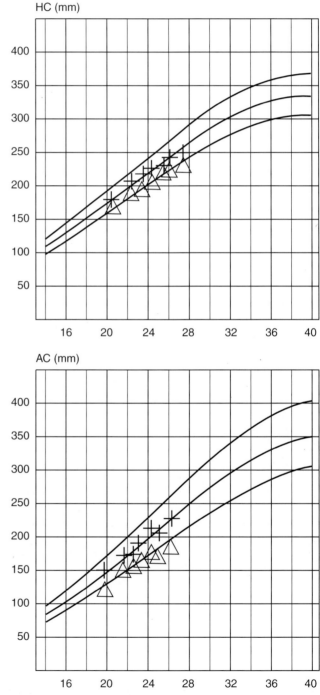

Fig. 12.14 A plot of serial growth scans in a set of discordant-sized monochorionic twins.

REFERENCES

1 Office of National Statistics. Series FM1, Birth statistics, 1990–1995. London: The Stationery Office, 1995

2 Office of National Statistics. Series DH3, Mortality statistics, 1990–1995. London: The Stationery Office, 1995

3 Fox H. Pathology of the placenta. London: WB Saunders, 1978

4 Petterson B, Nelson K B, Watson L et al. Twins, triplets, and cerebral palsy in births in Western Australia in the 1980s. Br J Obstet Gynaecol 1993; 307: 1239–1243

5 Benirschke K, Kim C K. Multiple pregnancy. N Engl J Med 1973; 288: 1276–1284

6 Neilson J P, Danskin F, Hastie S J. Monozygotic twin pregnancy: diagnostic and Doppler ultrasound studies. Br J Obstet Gynaecol 1989; 96: 1413–1418

7 Bejar R, Vigliocco G, Gramajo H et al. Antenatal origin of neurologic damage in newborn infants. II. Multiple gestations. Am J Obstet Gynecol 1990; 162: 1230–1236

8 Sassoon D A, Castro L C, Davis J L et al. Perinatal outcome in triplet versus twin gestations. Obstet Gynecol 1990; 75: 817–820

9 Mahony B S, Filly R A, Callen P W. Amnionicity and chorionicity in twin pregnancies: prediction using ultrasound. Radiology 1985; 155: 205–209

10 Barss V A, Benacerraf B R, Frigoletto F Jr. Ultrasonographic determination of chorion type in twin gestation. Obstet Gynecol 1985; 66: 779–783

11 Fisk N M, Bryan E. Routine prenatal determination of chorionicity in multiple gestation: a plea to the obstetrician. Br J Obstet Gynaecol 1993; 100: 975–977

12 Monteagudo A, Timor-Tritsch I, Sharma S. Early and simple determination of chorionic and amniotic type in multifetal gestations in the first fourteen weeks by high-frequency transvaginal ultrasonography. Am J Obstet Gynecol 1994; 170: 824–829

13 Sebire N J, Snijders R J, Hughes K, Sepulveda W, Nicolaides K H. Screening for trisomy 21 in twin pregnancy by maternal age and fetal nuchal translucency thickness at 10–14 weeks of gestation. Br J Obstet Gynaecol 1996; 103: 999–1003

14 Scardo J A, Ellings J M, Newman R B. Prospective determination of chorionity, amniocity and zygosity in twin gestations. Am J Obstet Gynecol 1995; 173: 1376–1380

15 Hertzberg B S, Kurtz A B, Choi H Y et al. Significance of membrane thickness in the sonographic evaluation of twin gestations. AJR 1987; 148: 151–153

16 Townsend R R, Simpson G F, Filly R A. Membrane thickness in ultrasound prediction of chorionicity of twin gestations. J Ultrasound Med 1988; 7: 327–332

17 Winn H N, Gabrielli S, Reece A, Roberts J A, Salafia C, Hobbins J C. Ultrasonographic criteria for the prenatal diagnosis of placental chorionicity in twin gestations. Am J Obstet Gynecol 1989; 161: 1540–1542

18 Finberg H J. The 'twin peak' sign: reliable evidence of dichorionic twinning. J Ultrasound Med 1992; 11: 571–577

19 Stagiannis K, Sepulveda W, Southwell D et al. Ultrasonographic measurement of the dividing membrane in twin pregnancy during the second and third trimester: a reproducibility study. Am J Obstet Gynecol 1995; 173: 1546–1550

20 Kurtz A B, Wapner R J, Mata J et al. Twin pregnancies: accuracy of first-trimester abdominal US in predicting chorionicity and amnionicity. Radiology 1992; 185: 759–762

21 Sepulveda W, Sebire N J, Hughes K, Kalogeropoulos A, Nicolaides K H. Evolution of the lambda or twin-chorionic peak sign in dichorionic twin pregnancies. Obstet Gynecol 1997; 89: 439–441

22 Robertson E G, Neer K J. Placental injection studies in twin gestation. Am J Obstet Gynecol 1983; 147: 170–174

23 King A D, Soothill P W, Montemagno R et al. Twin–twin blood transfusion in a dichorionic pregnancy without the oligohydramnios–polyhydramnios sequence. Br J Obstet Gynaecol 1995; 102: 334–335

24 Schatz F. Klinische Beiträge zur Physiologie des Fetus. Berlin: Hirschwald, 1990

25 Fusi L, Gordon H. Twin pregnancy complicated by single intrauterine death. Problems and outcome with conservative management. Br J Obstet Gynaecol 1990; 97: 511–516

26 Fusi L, McParland P, Fisk N et al. Acute twin–twin transfusion: a possible mechanism for brain-damaged survivors after intrauterine death of a monochorionic twin. Obstet Gynecol 1991; 78: 517–520

27 Okamura K, Murotsuki J, Tanigawara S et al. Funipuncture for evaluation of hematologic and coagulation indices in the surviving twin following co-twin's death. Obstet Gynecol 1994; 83: 975–978

28 Patten R M, Mack L A, Harvey D et al. Disparity of amniotic fluid volume and fetal size: problem of the stuck twin – US studies. Radiology 1989; 172: 153–157

29 Steinberg L H, Hurley V A, Desmedt E et al. Acute polyhydramnios in twin pregnancies. Aust NZJ Obstet Gynecol 1990; 30: 196–200

30 Weir P E, Ratten G J, Beischer N A. Acute polyhydramnios – a complication of monozygous twin pregnancy. Br J Obstet Gynaecol 1979; 86: 849–853

31 Tan K L, Tan R, Tan S H et al. The twin transfusion syndrome. Clinical observations on 35 affected pairs. Clin Pediatr Phila 1979; 18: 111–114

32 Bruner J P, Rosemond R L. Twin–twin transfusion syndrome: a subset of the twin oligohydramnios–polyhydramnios sequence. Am J Obstet Gynecol 1993; 169: 925–930

33 Reisner D P, Mahony B S, Petty C N et al. Stuck twin syndrome: outcome in thirty-seven consecutive cases. Am J Obstet Gynecol 1993; 169: 991–995

34 Fisk N M, Borrell A, Hubinont C et al. Fetofetal transfusion syndrome: do the neonatal criteria apply in utero? Arch Dis Child 1990; 65: 657–661

35 Saunders N J, Snijders R J, Nicolaides K H. Therapeutic amniocentesis in twin–twin transfusion syndrome appearing in the second trimester of pregnancy. Am J Obstet Gynecol 1992; 166: 820–824

36 Gonsoulin W, Moise K Jr, Kirshon B et al. Outcome of twin–twin transfusion diagnosed before 28 weeks of gestation. Obstet Gynecol 1990; 75: 214–216

37 De Lia J, Emery M G, Sheafor S A et al. Twin transfusion syndrome: successful in utero treatment with digoxin. Int J Gynecol Obstet 1985; 23: 197–201

38 Weiner C P, Ludomirski A. Diagnosis, pathophysiology, and treatment of chronic twin–twin transfusion syndrome. Fetal Diagn Ther 1994; 9: 283–290

39 Urig M A, Clewell W H, Elliott J P. Twin–twin transfusion syndrome. Am J Obstet Gynecol 1990; 163: 1522–1526

40 Weiner C P. Diagnosis and treatment of twin to twin transfusion in the mid-second trimester of pregnancy. Fetal Ther 1987; 2: 71–74

41 Wittmann B K, Farquharson D F, Thomas W D. The role of feticide in the management of severe twin transfusion syndrome. Am J Obstet Gynecol 1986; 155: 1023–1026

42 Bower S, Flack N, Sepulveda W et al. Uterine artery blood flow response to correction of amniotic fluid volume. Am J Obstet Gynecol 1995; 173: 502–507

43 Fisk N, Vaughan J, Talbert D. Impaired fetal blood gas status in polyhydramnios and its relation to raised amniotic pressure. Fetal Diagn Ther 1994; 9: 7–13

44 DeLia J, Kuhlmann R, Harstad T et al. Fetoscopic laser ablation of placental vessels in severe previable twin–twin transfusion syndrome. Am J Obstet Gynecol 1995; 172: 1202–1211

45 Ville Y, Hyett J, Hecher K et al. Preliminary experience with endoscopic laser surgery for severe twin–twin transfusion syndrome. N Engl J Med 1995; 332: 224–227

46 Denbow M, Nicholls M, Fisk N. Neurological lesions in neonates from pregnancies with twin–twin transfusion syndrome. Am J Obstet Gynecol 1998; 178: 479–483

47 Van Allen M I, Smith D W, Shepard T H. Twin reversed arterial perfusion (TRAP) sequence: study of 14 twin pregnancies with acardius. Semin Perinatol 1983; 7: 285–293

48 Robie G F, Payne G G, Morgan M A. Selective delivery of an acardiac twin. N Eng J Med 1989; 320: 512–513

49 Nicolaides K H, Hyett J, Ville Y, Hecher K. Management of severe twin–twin transfusion syndrome and twin reversed arterial perfusion sequence. In: Ward R H, Whittle M, eds. Multiple pregnancy. London: RCOG Press, 1995; pp 251–262

50 Baldwin V J. Pathology of multiple pregnancy. New York: Springer-Verlag, 1994

51 Edmunds L D, Layde P M. Conjoined twins in the United States, 1970–1977. Teratology 1982; 25: 301–308

52 Schinzel A A, Smith D W, Miller J R. Monozygotic twinning and structural defects. J Pediatr 1979; 95: 921–930

53 Anderson R L, Golbus M S, Curry C J R et al. Central nervous system damage and other anomalies in surviving fetus following second trimester antenatal death of co-twin. Prenat Diagn 1990; 10: 513–518

54 Spencer K, Salonen R, Muller F. Down's syndrome screening in multiple pregnancies using alpha-fetoprotein and free beta hCG. Prenat Diagn 1994; 14: 537–542

55 Sebire N J, D'Ercole C, Hughes K, Carvalho M, Nicolaides K H. Increased nuchal translucency thickness at 10–14 weeks of gestation as a predictor of severe twin–twin transfusion syndrome. Ultrasound Obstet Gynecol 1997; 10: 86–89

56 Ghidini A, Lynch L, Hicks C et al. The risk of second-trimester amniocentesis in twin gestations: a case-control study. Am J Obstet Gynecol 1993; 169: 1013–1016

57 Wapner R J, Johnson A, Davis G et al. Prenatal diagnosis in twin gestations: a comparison between second-trimester amniocentesis and first-trimester chorionic villus sampling. Obstet Gynecol 1993; 82: 49–56

58 Pergament E, Schulman J D, Copeland K. The risk and efficacy of chorionic villus sampling in multiple gestations. Prenat Diagn 1992; 12: 377–384

59 Brambati B, Tului L, Lanzani A et al. First-trimester genetic diagnosis in multiple pregnancy: principles and potential pitfalls. Prenat Diagn 1991; 11: 767–774

60 Rodeck C H, Mibashan R, Abramowitz J, Campbell S. Selective feticide of the affected twin by fetoscopic air embolization. Prenat Diagn 1982; 2: 189–194

61 Golbus M S, Cunningham N, Goldberg J D et al. Selective termination of multiple gestations. Am J Med Genet 1988; 31: 339–348

62 Isada N B, Pryde P G, Johnson M P, Hallak M, Blessed W B, Evans M I. Fetal intracardiac potassium chloride injection to avoid the hopeless resuscitation of an abnormal abortus: I. Clinical issues. Obstet Gynecol 1992; 80: 296–299

63 Evans M I, Goldberg J D, Dommergues M et al. Efficacy of second-trimester selective termination for fetal abnormalities: international collaborative experience among the world's largest centres. Am J Obstet Gynecol 1994; 171: 90–94

64 Lynch L, Berkowitz R L, Stone J, Alvarez M, Lapinski R. Preterm delivery after selective termination in twin pregnancies. Obstet Gynecol 1996; 87: 366–369

65 Quintero R, Reich H, Bardicef M, Evans M, Cotton D B, Romero R. Umbilical cord ligation of an acardiac twin by fetoscopy at 19 weeks' gestation. N Engl J Med 1994; 330: 469–471

66 Denbow M, Kyle P, Fogliani R, Johnson P, Fisk N. Selective termination by intrahepatic vein alcohol injection of a monochorionic twin pregnancy discordant for fetal abnormality. Br J Obstet Gynaecol 1997; 104: 626–627

67 Itskowitz J, Boldes R, Thaler I et al. Transvaginal ultrasonography-guided aspiration of gestational sacs for selective abortion in multiple pregnancy. Am J Obstet Gynecol 1989; 160: 215–217

68 Evans M, Fletcher J C, Zador I E, Newton B W, Quigg M H, Struyk C D. Selective first-trimester termination in octuplet and quadruplet pregnancies: clinical and ethical issues. Obstet Gynecol 1988; 71: 289–296

69 Berkowitz R L, Lynch L, Chitkara U, Wilkins I A, Mehalek K E, Alvarez E. Selective reduction of multifetal pregnancies in the first trimester. N Engl J Med 1988; 318: 1043–1047

70 Wenstrom K D, Syrop C H, Hammitt D G, Van Voorhis B J. Increased risk of monochorionic twinning associated with assisted reproduction. Fertil Steril 1993; 60: 510–514

71 Evans M I, Dommergues M, Wapner R, Lynch L, Dumez Y, Goldberg I D. Efficacy of transabdominal multifetal pregnancy reduction: collaborative experience amongst the world's largest centres. Obstet Gynecol 1993; 82: 61–66

72 Berkowitz R L, Lynch L, Stone J, Alvarez M. The current status of multifetal pregnancy reduction. Am J Obstet Gynecol 1966; 174: 1265–1272

73 Evans M I, Dommergues M, Timor-Tritsch I et al. Transabdominal versus transcervical and transvaginal multifetal pregnancy reduction: international collaborative experience of more than one thousand cases. Am J Obstet Gynecol 1994; 170: 902–909

13

Doppler in obstetrics

Sturla H Eik-Nes and Karel Marsál

Physics and technique

Basic Doppler ultrasound physics

The Doppler principle is named after Christian Doppler, who in 1842 described the relationship between the velocity of a moving reflector and the change in frequency of the transmitted wave – i.e. a sound wave. When the reflector is moving toward the source of sound, the reflected sound will be received at a frequency higher than that transmitted. Conversely, if the reflector is moving away from the source the frequency of the received sound will be lower than that transmitted. A similar effect also occurs when the source is moving in relation to a stationary reflector. The change in the frequency is called the Doppler shift and is described by the Doppler equation:

$$\Delta_f = \frac{(2 \times f_0 \times V \times \cos \Theta)}{c}$$

where

Δ_f = Doppler shift frequency,
f_0 = the frequency of the transmitted sound,
V = the velocity of the moving reflector,
Θ = the angle between the sound beam and the velocity vector of the moving reflector, and
c = the velocity of sound in tissue.

In blood flow velocity measurement ultrasound is transmitted by a piezoelectric crystal into the tissue at a given frequency, reflected by the moving red cells within the vessel and received at a different frequency. The velocity of the blood flow can be calculated when the angle of insonation is known. The ultrasound frequency is typically 1–10 MHz; the Doppler shift caused by the blood flow is then within the audible range. The detected Doppler shift is a spectrum of frequencies rather than a single frequency, as it originates from red cells moving at various velocities within the lumen of the vessel.

A loss of energy takes place as ultrasound passes through the tissue; the penetration of ultrasound is limited, the depth of penetration being inversely related to the ultrasound frequency. Accordingly, for measurements of blood flow in deep-lying vessels, low-frequency ultrasound must be used. For use on fetal and uteroplacental vessels an ultrasound frequency of 2–5 MHz is usually suitable.

Doppler ultrasound instruments

The continuous-wave Doppler technique

There are two piezoelectric crystals in a continuous-wave (CW) Doppler flowmeter, one continuously transmitting ultrasound signals, the other functioning as a receiver. The recorded spectrum of Doppler frequencies contains information on the movements of all interfaces traversed by the ultrasound beam, and the sampling is thus non-discriminative. As the construction of the CW Doppler instrument is technically quite simple, it is cheaper than the more complicated pulsed-wave variety. However, owing to the lack of range resolution the application of CW Doppler instruments is limited; in obstetrics their use is virtually confined to vessels where interference by signals from nearby vessels is not imminent, e.g. the umbilical artery and the uterine artery. An advantage of the CW Doppler technique is that there is no limitation to the highest blood velocity that can be measured.

The pulsed-wave Doppler technique

The sampling from a given depth range within the tissue is permitted with a pulsed wave (PW) Doppler instrument. In other words, using this technique blood velocity signals from a specific vessel can be recorded. The signal-to-noise ratio is usually better in the PW than in the CW Doppler mode. In the PW technique, a single piezoelectric crystal is used alternately as a transmitter and receiver. The ultrasound is transmitted in a short pulse; then the transducer gate is closed for a period corresponding to the time required for the pulse to travel to the vessel of interest and back. The gate then opens again to receive the ultrasound echoes returning from a defined region within the tissue, the so-called sample volume. The size of the sample volume is determined by the size of the emitting crystal, the shape of the ultrasound beam and the duration of the pulse. The positioning of the sample volume is governed by setting the interval between transmitting and receiving the ultrasound signals, i.e. between the opening and the closing of the transducer gate.

The PW Doppler technique is limited with regard to the maximum detectable velocity, owing to the fact that the maximum Doppler shift frequency that can be unambiguously detected is one-half of the pulse repetition frequency (the Nyquist limit). At high Doppler frequencies the aliasing phenomenon arises, i.e. the instrument cannot determine the true velocity direction. However, aliasing is seldom a problem in obstetrics, as the peak velocities in the fetoplacental and uteroplacental vessels do not usually exceed 1.5–2.0 m/s. It is important that the instrument allows optimisation of the depth–velocity product by adjustment of the pulse repetition frequency. Aliasing, when it occurs, can be avoided by changing the insonation angle, some of the instrument settings (scale, baseline position), or using a lower ultrasound frequency to produce lower-frequency echoes from moving structures.

Processing of Doppler signals

A relatively simple way of processing the Doppler signals is the determination of zero-crossing frequency, i.e. the number of zero crossing per unit time. However, this method is quite inaccurate and is dependent on the blood velocity profile. Therefore, the modern instruments are designed to be capable of more sophisticated analysis of the Doppler spectrum by digitising the signals, the most widely used way of spectral analysis being the fast Fourier transform. In this way almost all of the frequency information contained in the complex Doppler signal is retrieved.

From the Doppler spectrum both the maximum velocity (i.e. the envelope of the spectrum) and the mean velocity (i.e. the weighted average Doppler shift frequency) can be estimated. The waveform of the maximum velocity recorded from arteries can be further characterised by various indices (see below). A time-averaged mean velocity is used for the calculation of volume flow.

The received Doppler signals are usually passed through a high-pass filter to eliminate signals from any slow-moving interfaces in the path of the ultrasound beam. When a high-pass filter with a high cut-off level is used, a considerable part of the low-velocity flow signals will be eliminated. This results in overestimation of the mean velocity and sometimes in an erroneous diagnosis of absent end-diastolic flow. Therefore, it has been recommended that the use of high-pass filters with cut-off levels exceeding 100 Hz should be avoided. When examining fetal vessels very little disturbance is produced by the elastic vessel walls and little if any high-pass filtering is actually necessary.

Duplex systems

Both CW and PW Doppler instruments can be used as unassisted systems without imaging, the Doppler signals being monitored by ear. This approach is limited in application, however, and in obstetrics is virtually confined to recordings from the umbilical artery and uterine/uteroplacental vessels. In duplex ultrasound systems an imaging ultrasound scanner is combined with either a PW or a CW Doppler instrument. The vessel of interest is visualised and the Doppler ultrasound beam easily directed; in the PW mode the sample volume can be properly localised with the help of a cursor in the image. The two ultrasound systems are mutually exclusive and cannot be used simultaneously. During the Doppler recording the two-dimensional image is frozen; during updating of the image the recording of Doppler signals is interrupted. The use of electronic real-time scanners enables rapid switches to be made from one mode to the other.

Doppler instruments can be combined either with linear-array transducers or with sector transducers (phased-array or mechanical). The combination of an offset PW Doppler transducer and a linear-array transducer enables not only a longer section of the vessel to be visualised, but also a suitable angle of insonation to be selected. Both of these features are advantageous, for example when examining the fetal descending aorta. In a combination with a sector real-time scanner one of the image lines is usually used for Doppler recording. Particularly when examining such small vessels as fetal cerebral vessels, the latter duplex system is well suited.

Colour Doppler imaging

The first commercial colour Doppler imaging system was introduced in the early 1980s. Its primary application was thought to be in echocardiography to visualise intra-cardiac blood flow velocities, but the technique has proved its usefulness in almost all fields of medical ultrasound. The advent of the colour Doppler technique has also influenced ultrasound examination of the fetal and utero-placental circulation.

Colour Doppler imaging is a Doppler-based blood flow velocity mapping technique that superimposes colour-coded blood flow areas on the grey-scale anatomical two-dimensional image, producing a real-time representation of the spatial extent of blood flow. Colour Doppler images provide the opportunity to understand the haemodynamics and to point out the positions where more accurate and detailed assessment of velocity information is necessary. Colour velocity imaging might be seen as a complementary investigation tool to CW and PW Doppler.

The principles of colour Doppler mapping are similar to the pulsed-wave Doppler system. Both are based on transmitting short pulses and receiving echo information, with time delay proportional to depth. However, colour Doppler imaging is significantly different from PW Doppler in the way it gathers and processes echo information. PW Doppler displays the complete spectrum of blood velocities at one sample site on one scan line. In colour Doppler imaging each scan line is divided into a number of range gates (100–200). The mean velocity and direction of velocity for each range gate are estimated in real time. The velocity estimate has to be done on few transmitted lines (5–15) along a certain direction to maintain a frame rate high enough to visualise flow velocity changes satisfactorily in the interrogated organ. Echoes from the same location are compared for successively transmitted sound pulses, and phase differences are extracted and analysed. The phase difference is directly proportional to the Doppler shift. If 10 pulses are transmitted along one line, the average of nine phase differences will give the mean velocity in every location along the line. After interrogation of one line, the time delay for individual crystal elements will create a new direction for the second line. Because of the relatively slow process owing to multiple transmissions, a high frame rate is not easily accomplished. One way to handle this is to reduce the interrogated area and thereby decrease the number of lines included, or to reduce line density, i.e. to increase the distance between two neighbouring lines. In PW and CW Doppler, fast Fourier transformation (FFT) is the most common technique for calculating and displaying velocity information, but for colour Doppler FFT is too slow to calculate velocities in more than 15 000 locations within 10–30 ms time intervals. For two-dimensional flow display autocorrelation technique is the most commonly used technique, in which the echo is correlated to the corresponding one from the previous pulse.

When the frequency shift of blood flow exceeds the Nyquist limit, the display shows an aliased signal in PW Doppler. The same thing happens in colour Doppler: in areas where aliasing appears this will result in colour reversal. The maximum detectable velocity prior to the occurrence of aliasing depends on the pulse repetition frequency. A low pulse repetition frequency will give a low Nyquist limit. It can be a rather critical and difficult judgement to determine whether the cause for colour reversal is aliasing or true flow reversal.

The blood flow velocities are coded into colour maps which highlight differences in velocity. Blood flow moving toward the transducer is generally displayed with reds that gradually change to yellows as velocities increase. Blood flow moving away from the transducer is displayed with dark blues that gradually change to light blue as the velocities increase. To estimate the degree of turbulence the autocorrelation algorithm calculates the variance and the magnitude of variance is coded into a completely different colour – often green – to be overlaid across the standard red/blue map.

Power Doppler imaging

The development of power Doppler imaging represents a new approach to processing ultrasound Doppler signals returning from moving blood. This technique has many different names, e.g. colour Doppler energy, power angiography, Doppler angiography and colour power angiography. The echo signal returning from moving blood has two components, frequency and amplitude. The signal power calculated from the amplitude of Doppler shifts is a good estimate of the number of moving blood cells within a sample volume. In colour Doppler imaging the Doppler shift is coded into an appropriate colour scale, but the amplitude information is not used. Signal power from a sample volume can be calculated by squaring the Doppler shift amplitude. Energy estimation is accomplished by summation or integration of Doppler shifts returning from the individual sample volumes on the number of lines, corresponding to the summation/integration time. A single colour with gradually increasing intensity is used to visualise locations of blood flow in two dimensions and superimposed on a grey-scale two-dimensional B-mode image. Although the mean velocity of the Doppler signal has been an extremely valuable parameter in clinical practice, its usefulness can be extended even further by energy calculation and two-dimensional display. After summation, velocity and direction information will be lost as the intensity

of the signal depends on the number of moving scatters within a sample volume.

The power Doppler image will change very little with changing insonation angle as long as the velocities are higher than the vessel wall filter setting. This is because a changing angle just moves the power spectrum up and down along the velocity scale without influencing the integrated reflected power. As the power spectrum approaches zero velocity, the vessel wall filters might remove signals from the power spectrum and thereby reduce the integration value. Most algorithms used in power Doppler have low cut-off levels for suppression of vessel wall movement; this makes the method of imaging extremely sensitive to motion, sometimes giving massive colour artefacts.

One advantage of power Doppler imaging is that, as it does not utilise the velocity information, aliasing does not occur.

A most important advantage of using power Doppler imaging is its increased sensitivity to flow compared to colour Doppler imaging. Signal noise has a random frequency distribution and the autocorrelation algorithm very easily estimates noise as true velocities when the noise level becomes too high, e.g. by increasing the gain. The integrated amplitude of the noise is significantly smaller than the integrated amplitude of the power spectrum. The sensitivity of power Doppler imaging is 3–5 times higher than that of colour Doppler imaging. A power Doppler image is illustrated in Figure 13.1.

Safety aspects

Ultrasound with high intensity levels has known biological effects, e.g. thermal effects and cavitation.[1] Therefore, it is necessary that users are constantly alert to the possibility of adverse effects of diagnostic ultrasound. Hitherto, no harmful effects of ultrasound on mammalian tissues have

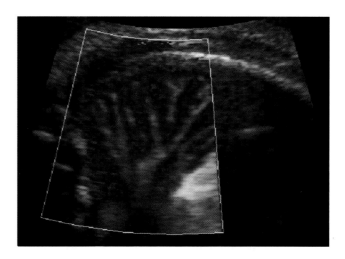

Fig. 13.1 Power Doppler image of the fetal lung showing the vessels branching.

been found at the intensities used for diagnostic purposes, and epidemiological follow-up studies have failed to elicit any evidence of adverse effects of exposure to diagnostic ultrasound *in utero*. Nevertheless, it is recommended that intensities exceeding 94 mW/cm^2 of the spatial-peak temporal-average *in situ* should be avoided, and that patients should be exposed to ultrasound only for valid clinical reasons.[2,3]

It is important that Doppler users are aware of the output ultrasound energy of the equipment they are using for examining pregnancies. Some of the PW Doppler devices can produce a considerable output energy, and it is therefore mandatory to use the mode with the lowest energy when applying it to a fetus. Owing to the specific physical conditions during the ultrasound examination of a fetus *in utero*, high-quality Doppler signals can usually be obtained even when using low-output energy.

Measurement techniques

Estimation of volume flow

Volume blood flow in a vessel – i.e. the amount of blood passing through the cross-section of the vessel per unit of time – can be estimated from the ultrasonically measured diameter of the vessel and the time-averaged mean blood velocity recorded with Doppler ultrasound. Vessel diameter is measured on the frozen images of the vessel. Usually an average value of several measurements is used to minimise the effect of pulsatile diameter changes in arteries. To enable comparison between intra-individual measurements at various stages of gestation and between fetuses, the flow is related to the ultrasonically estimated fetal weight and expressed in ml/min/kg.

The measurement of vessel diameter has been found to be the major source of error in estimating flow,[4] the risk of error being especially pronounced in vessels with diameters less than 6 mm. Therefore, the application of the method during pregnancy is limited to large fetal vessels, e.g. the descending aorta[5] and the intra-abdominal part of the umbilical vein.[6] Precision in measuring the diameter of pulsating vessels might be improved by using automatic phase-locked echo-tracking systems.[7]

The recording and estimation of the mean velocity is also susceptible to several sources of possible error. Uniform insonation of the whole cross-section of the vessel is a prerequisite, as is accurate positioning of the sample volume, which needs to be of suitable size. The recorded Doppler shift is corrected for the insonation angle. At large angles of insonation errors in the estimation of the true velocity might be considerable, and thus Doppler examinations should not be performed at insonation angles greater than 55°.[8]

The inherent sources of error outlined above have led to the abandonment of volume flow estimation in obstetrics.

During recent years the interest of researchers and clinicians has turned instead to velocity waveform analysis. However, as waveform analysis is not directly related to the blood flow, when the accuracy of estimating volume blood flow is improved in the future a renewal of interest in measuring flow in obstetrics is to be expected.

Velocity waveform analysis

The early reports on Doppler studies in fetuses showed an association between unfavourable fetal outcome and some typical changes of the velocity waveforms recorded from the fetal aorta[9,10] or umbilical artery.[11] Experience from the diagnostic use of Doppler ultrasound in peripheral vessels indicated that important information on circulation might be gained by analysing the maximum velocity waveforms.[12] In fetal arterial waveform analysis many of the possible errors involved in the volume flow estimation are avoided: there is no need to know the insonation angle to measure vessel diameter or to estimate fetal weight.

Many formulae and indices have been evolved to characterise the waveform mathematically. Most of the waveform indices express the degree of pulsatility of the velocity waveform. Some of them make use of only two points on the curve, e.g. the systolic-to-diastolic ratio (A/B ratio)[13] or the resistance index (RI) according to Pourcelot;[14] some include the average velocity over the heart cycle in the calculation, i.e. the pulsatility index (PI).[12] These indices eliminate the effect of the insonation angle by calculating a ratio (Fig. 13.2) (see Vol. 1, Ch. 6).

The shape of the velocity waveform recorded from the fetal arteries is dependent on several factors: heart action, blood velocity, vessel wall compliance and both proximal and distal resistance to flow. The vascular resistance peripheral to the site of measurement mainly affects the diastolic part of the velocity waveform, an increase in resistance causing a decrease in diastolic flow.

Owing to the presence of the placental vascular bed the fetal circulation as a whole is a low-resistance system. When resistance in the placenta increases, e.g. in pregnancies with hypertension or intra-uterine growth retardation, diastolic flow in the umbilical artery and the fetal descending aorta decreases and may even be absent.[9,10,15] With increasing peripheral resistance the values of the waveform indices increase. When the end-diastolic flow is absent the A/B ratio becomes infinite and thus not operational, and the RI is then equal to 1.0. The PI also reflects the area under the curve and is superior to the other two indices for practical purposes.[8] The disadvantage of the PI is that it entails more complex computation than does the A/B ratio or the RI.

In healthy fetuses during the second half of gestation, diastolic flow is always present in the descending aorta and umbilical artery during fetal apnoea.[16,17] Conversely, the absence of diastolic flow is often associated with an

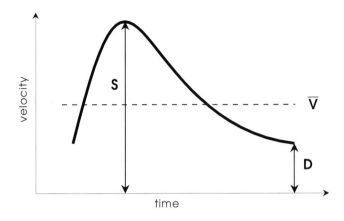

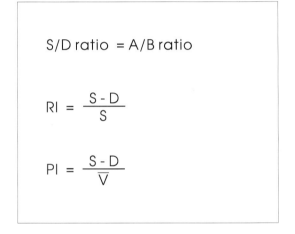

Fig. 13.2 **Resistance and pulsatility indices.** Waveform indices – S/D ratio, resistance index (RI), according to Pourcelot and pulsatility index (PI) according to Gosling. S – peak systolic velocity, D – minimum diastolic velocity, V – mean of the maximum velocity over the heart cycle.

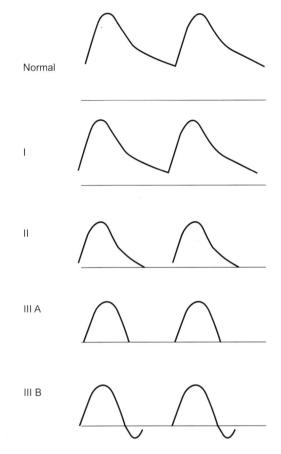

Fig. 13.3 **Blood flow classes (BFC) of the umbilical artery velocity waveform.** BFC normal, positive flow throughout the heart cycle, and a pulsatility index (PI) within the normal limits; BFC I, positive flow throughout the cycle, and a PI ≥ mean + 2 SD and < mean + 3 SD of the normals; BFC II, non-detectable end-diastolic velocity and/or PI ≥ mean + 3 SD of the normals; BFC III A, absence of flow throughout the major part of diastole; BFC III B, reversed flow in diastole.

adverse outcome of pregnancy, e.g. intra-uterine growth retardation and fetal hypoxia.[15,18,19] In extreme cases diastolic flow can even be reversed,[17] the extremely altered velocity waveform sometimes being referred to as ARED flow, i.e. absent or reversed end-diastolic flow.

The appearance of the diastolic part of the velocity waveform is a clinically important prognostic feature. On the basis of earlier findings that the degree of intra-uterine and neonatal morbidity is reflected in the degree of pathological changes of the fetal aortic velocity waveform, a semiquantitative method of assessing the waveform was designed (Fig. 13.3).[19] Four blood flow classes (BFC) were defined as follows:

1. BFC normal: positive flow throughout the heart cycle and a normal PI;
2. BFC I: positive flow throughout the cycle and a PI ≥ mean + 2 SD and < mean + 3 SD of the normal;
3. BFC II: PI ≥ mean + 3 SD of the normals and/or non-detectable end-diastolic velocity;

4. BFC III: absence of positive flow throughout diastole (BFC III A) or reversed flow in diastole (BFC III B).

This simple system of pattern recognition has been further refined and computerised using a classification based on 10 types of curves.[20]

Validation of the blood velocity waveform analysis
Waveform analysis has been evaluated from several points of view: the various waveform indices have been compared and the reproducibility of estimating maximum velocity from the Doppler spectrum and from calculating the indices has been studied, as has the dependence of the waveform shape and waveform indices on various flow factors. Recordings performed using CW versus PW Doppler ultrasound have been found to be fully comparable.[21,22]

Many reproducibility studies of various waveform indices and various vessels have been published. Very good reproducibility of the indices in the umbilical artery, regarding both the intra- and the interobserver variability, was found,[21,23] the coefficients of variation being reported to be below 10%.

The number of waveforms included to obtain the index value differs from one research group to another, often depending on the equipment used. Without doubt a large number of cycles improves the accuracy, the use of 10 consecutive cycles being probably the best but quite laborious approach. Provided the Doppler velocity recording is stable and the waveforms uniform, five cycles have been found to be as representative as 10 or more.[24] In one study a sequence of six heart cycles was found to be acceptably reproducible, even during periods of fetal breathing and movement.[25] It is important, however, to bear in mind that a Doppler recording made during a period of fetal breathing is not representative, as the breathing movements have a marked effect on blood flow.[26]

The fetal breathing movements profoundly modulate the blood velocities, not only in the venous circulation – in the umbilical vein and inferior vena cava – but also in the descending aorta, umbilical artery and other fetal arteries.[26] The increase in time-averaged mean blood velocity in the fetal aorta during breathing is dependent on the amplitude of breathing. As the vessel diameter cannot be measured simultaneously with the blood velocity, it is not possible to draw any conclusions regarding the effect of breathing on the venous return to the fetal heart and on fetal cardiac output. As the velocity waveforms in the fetal vessels are modulated during breathing, measurements taken during breathing are unacceptable for the purpose of waveform analysis. While recording signals from the umbilical cord it is easy to recognise the presence of fetal breathing as it causes modulation of the umbilical venous blood velocity.

Fetal blood velocity waveforms have been examined during different fetal behavioural states,[27,28] identified from the recordings of fetal heart rate (FHR) variability, fetal breathing, fetal movements and fetal eye movements. In the internal carotid artery and descending aorta of the fetuses, the PI levels changed with fetal behavioural state, being higher during quiet sleep (state F1) than during active sleep (state F2). In the umbilical artery no such difference was found. For strictly controlled physiological studies it might be of interest to record the behavioural states. However, in a clinical context the changes in the waveform indices due to pathological processes will exceed the changes due to fetal behaviour. It might therefore be sufficient to ensure that recordings are made during fetal quiescence, i.e. during periods of fetal apnoea and no general movement.

In maternal and fetal vessels waveform indices (A/B ratio, RI and PI) have been found to be inversely correlated to the heart rate. With increasing heart rate, the beat-to-beat interval shortens and the diastolic flow velocity

increases relative to the peak velocity. An opposite effect is seen in bradycardia. For both the fetal descending aorta and the umbilical artery this effect has been found to be not too pronounced provided the fetal heart rate (FHR) is within normal limits (120–160 beats/min).[10,16,29] Although some other investigators have reported a finding of a strong negative correlation,[30,31] their data included cases of FHR outside the normal limits as well.

Reference values of waveform indices have been published for various fetal vessels and all three indices (A/B ratio, RI and PI) have been found to be dependent on gestational age. Indeed, a variance analysis of data has shown gestational age and FHR to be the predominant determinants of the variance of umbilical artery waveform indices.[23] In the umbilical artery,[16,32] the fetal renal artery,[33] the common and internal carotid artery[34] and cerebral arteries[35,36] the indices have been found to decrease steadily with gestational age throughout the second half of pregnancy. Thus, when relating results of Doppler waveform analysis to reference values, curves corrected for gestational age should always be used.

As discussed, waveform analysis is much less prone to error than is the estimation of fetal blood flow. None the less, there are some pitfalls to be borne in mind. The importance of fetal apnoea and quiescence for recording reproducible Doppler signals has already been stressed. The small sample volume of some duplex scanners needs careful positioning in the axis of the vessel for proper detection of the maximum velocity; for this purpose, online control of the Doppler spectrum is invaluable.

The most important possible error in clinical application is obtaining false positive findings of missing end-diastolic velocities (see Vol. 1, Ch. 6). When the diastolic velocity is low it may fall below the cut-off level of the high-pass filter, and a waveform with erroneously missing end-diastolic flow will appear. The risk of this error increases with the increase of the insonation angle, as the shift frequency of the recorded velocities decreases proportionally to the increase of the angle. The risk of falsely missing diastolic velocities is most pronounced in situations where the insonation angle is unknown, e.g. in recordings of signals from the umbilical artery. Therefore, a finding of missing diastolic flow should be verified from at least two and preferably three different insonation angles.

The efficacy of the velocity waveform indices as indicators of the peripheral vascular resistance – in the case of the umbilical artery, of the resistance in the placental circulation – has been tested in a number of studies. Both with *in vitro*[37] and computer models[38,39] an increase in the resistance peripheral to the site of measurement has been shown to result in a decrease in the diastolic flow and an increase in the value of waveform indices (PI, RI, systolic/diastolic (S/D) ratio), when the pulse rate or pressure remained constant. Similar findings have also been reported from animal models, where placental resistance was increased either by embolising the fetal side of the placenta with microspheres[40,41] or by constricting the umbilical vein.[42,43] It may thus be concluded that the changes in the waveform indices are mainly, though not solely, determined by the peripheral vascular resistance.

Doppler measurement of fetal and maternal vessels

Umbilical artery In the early first trimester diastolic blood velocity in the umbilical artery is normally absent.[44] After 15 weeks of pregnancy umbilical blood flow is maintained throughout diastole, reflecting the low resistance in the fetoplacental circulation (Fig. 13.4). With increasing gestational age the PI and S/D ratio values fall as a sign of decreasing resistance to blood flow in the placenta.[16,45] The slight variation between published reference values is probably due to differences in processing flow signals in various commercially available Doppler instruments. For the above-mentioned reasons, gestational age-related reference curves of waveform indices specific for various Doppler instruments should be used. Recordings obtained by continuous or pulsed-wave Doppler instruments have been compared without any differences in velocity waveforms having been observed.[21]

The blood velocity signals recorded in the umbilical artery near the fetal abdomen show higher PI, RI or S/D ratio values than those recorded from the placental end of the umbilical cord.[46] The published reference curves are usually based on signals recorded from the free-floating mid-part of the cord.

Fetal descending aorta Non-invasive measurement in the human fetal aorta was first made by Eik-Nes *et al.* using a manually switched duplex scanning system.[5] The velocity waveforms recorded from the fetal thoracic descending aorta do not change significantly during the last trimester of pregnancy.[17] As in the umbilical artery, the aortic waveform is influenced mainly by the placental circulation and normally shows positive diastolic velocity. The aorta supplies some other vascular areas in addition to the placenta, e.g. kidneys, splanchnic area and fetal body wall and limbs, with vascular resistances higher than that of the placenta. Therefore, the aortic PI is usually higher than the umbilical artery PI, being typically within the range of 1.83–2.49.[47]

In complicated pregnancies the changes in the aortic waveform parallel those of the umbilical artery. For clinical use no significant difference has been found between the two vessels.[48] However, as it is much easier to examine in clinical contexts the umbilical artery is usually preferred.

Fetal middle cerebral artery Several of the fetal cerebral arteries can be identified using colour Doppler systems and the signals detected using PW Doppler. Among cerebral arteries the middle cerebral is the one most often examined, as its anatomy makes the examination easy. The insonation angle can be easily kept to zero, thus offering an optimal signal. In normal pregnancies the waveform of middle cerebral artery velocities has a positive, but relatively low, diastolic component. The PI increases from week 20 until 28–30 weeks of gestation; this increase is then followed by a continuous decrease towards term.[49]

From experimental studies on fetal lambs it is known that hypoxic fetuses redistribute their blood flow and give preferential supply to the brain.[50–52] This was named the brain-sparing phenomenon. It has been shown that the increase in cerebral flow in fetal lambs can be detected using Doppler ultrasound.[53] During experimental hypoxia there was both an increase in the mean velocity and dilation of the examined vessel (common carotid artery).

In the human fetus a number of reports have demonstrated a decrease in the middle cerebral artery PI and RI in pregnancies with intra-uterine growth retardation (IUGR).[54–57] A significant correlation between fetal hypoxaemia and the degree of reduction in the PI was shown in a study analysing fetal blood gases in samples taken via cordocentesis.[58] The abnormally low PI could be transiently normalised by giving oxygen to the mother.[54,59] In severely growth-retarded fetuses an increase in the PI was observed before intra-uterine demise, possibly due to preterminal cerebral oedema.[49,60]

For practical use a ratio between the waveform indices in the middle cerebral artery and the umbilical artery – so-called cerebral–placental ratio – has been proposed.[61] This approach has improved the diagnostic accuracy of Doppler velocimetry in predicting adverse perinatal outcome.[55]

Fetal renal artery Normally there is a positive diastolic flow in the fetal renal artery and the PI declines towards the end of pregnancy.[62] Abnormal renal artery velocity waveforms have been reported in IUGR, but the predictive value of this vessel seems low.[33]

Uteroplacental circulation The uteroplacental vascular tree branches from the main uterine arteries on each

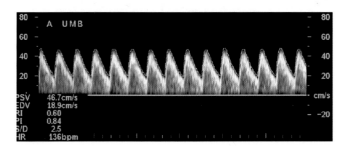

Fig. 13.4 Normal umbilical artery waveform. Normal flow velocity in the umbilical artery.

side of the uterus to end finally in the arcuate, radial and spiral arteries. Major morphological changes occur in the uteroplacental blood vessels during early normal pregnancy, facilitating an increase in blood flow to the uterus from about 50 to 700 ml/min at term.[63,64] Normally the trophoblast tissue invades the spiral arteries under the placenta. The arterial vessel wall dissolves, leaving the subplacental arteries as wide channels without contractile potential.[65]

During early gestation the relatively high vascular resistance in the uteroplacental circulation is characterised by a 'notch' in the early diastolic component of the Doppler velocity waveform recorded from the uterine artery (Fig. 13.5). This notch can be seen in normal pregnancies up to 26 weeks gestation.[66] Later the velocity waveforms from the uteroplacental circulation have a characteristic pattern, with high blood velocity during diastole as a sign of low vascular resistance. Arabin *et al.*[67] recorded blood velocities from different parts of the uteroplacental circulation and found that waveforms recorded under the central part of the placenta showed the lowest resistance, followed by those recorded within the placenta. Velocities at the margin of the placenta showed a still lower resistance, followed by recordings from the uterine artery on the same side as the placenta. The highest vascular resistances were recorded in the uterine artery on the nonplacental side of the uterus. This emphasises that blood velocities should be recorded from a specific location in the uteroplacental circulation using a standard technique. For evaluation of the results, reference charts for each location should be used.

In normal pregnancy vascular resistance to blood flow in the arcuate arteries seems to fall with gestational age.[16]

The uterine artery PI or S/D ratio decreases up to 20–24 weeks of gestation.[68,69] After 24 weeks the decline in resistance is limited and can be disregarded.

The reproducibility of Doppler signals recorded from the uteroplacental circulation using the 'blind' technique was relatively low. A much better reproducibility can be achieved when colour Doppler imaging is used for localisation of the main uterine arteries.[70]

Clinical application

Absent or reversed end-diastolic flow

Many studies have shown the finding of absent or reversed end-diastolic (ARED) flow in the umbilical artery to be associated with a bad outcome of pregnancy, very high perinatal mortality and a high degree of neonatal morbidity (Fig. 13.6).[15,71,72] Bell[73] reported that in 11 out of 40 fetuses a reappearance of the missing diastolic blood velocity was associated with an improved outcome of pregnancy compared to 29 cases with sustained ARED flow. The analysis was performed retrospectively, which makes it difficult to exclude the possibility of false positive findings, i.e. erroneously missing diastolic velocities. This possibility should be considered, especially in view of the fact that the ultrasound instruments used included high-pass filters with relatively high cut-off levels of 125 and 200 Hz.

Arduini *et al.*[74] serially examined 37 fetuses with ARED flow and evaluated the time interval between the onset of ARED flow and the occurrence of abnormal heart rate patterns. They found the interval to vary greatly between 1 and 26 days, depending on the gestational age, the

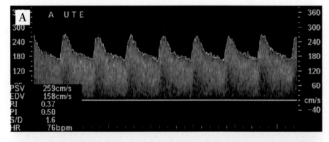

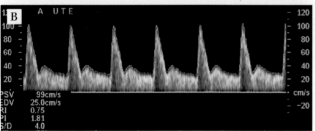

Fig. 13.5 Uterine artery waveforms. A: Normal flow velocity in the uterine artery. **B:** Uterine artery flow velocity with an early diastolic notch.

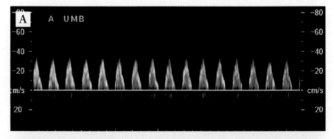

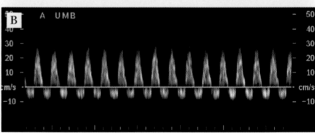

Fig. 13.6 Abnormal umbilical artery waveforms. ARED (absence of reversed end-diastolic flow velocity) in the umbilical artery. **A:** Blood flow class III A and **B:** blood flow class IIIB.

presence of maternal hypertension and pulsations in the umbilical vein. The occurrence of venous pulsations in the umbilical cord was a sign of impending fetal heart failure. The authors suggested that young fetuses (< 29 weeks gestational age) possibly have lower oxygen requirements and therefore develop a longer metabolic adaptation.

In an interesting study Farine *et al.*[75] examined the fate of subsequent pregnancies after the finding of ARED flow in the umbilical artery: 16 pregnancies with ARED flow were complicated with high perinatal mortality and severe IUGR. The outcome of 19 subsequent pregnancies in the 16 women was much better, 14 pregnancies being fully uncomplicated. The presence of autoantibodies was associated with complications of pregnancy. In only two pregnancies was there a recurrence of ARED flow.

Pre-eclampsia

The normal physiological trophoblast invasion in sub-placental spiral arteries with their subsequent dilatation is reduced in pre-eclampsia and IUGR.[65] As a consequence the uteroplacental blood flow is also reduced in pre-eclampsia, as has been shown also with radioisotope studies.[76]

The fetoplacental circulation in pre-eclampsia has been studied by several authors and the predictive value of the blood velocity waveform with regard to the perinatal outcome has been found to be similar to that described for IUGR pregnancies.[77–81] The uteroplacental circulation has also been examined in pre-eclampsia, using Doppler technique the results were inconsistent. The studies on arcuate artery blood velocity found no association between the blood velocity waveform and fetal outcome,[79] which might be due to the fact that one arcuate artery represents only about 10% of the uteroplacental circulation. The blood velocity waveform in the uterine artery seems to be more predictive of the outcome in pregnancies complicated by hypertension,[82] especially the presence of an early diastolic notch, which is associated with adverse perinatal outcome.[66]

As already mentioned, abnormal uterine blood velocity waveforms are associated with an increased risk of the subsequent development of pre-eclampsia and IUGR.[78] The uterine artery Doppler examination might therefore play an important role in targeting a subpopulation suitable for prophylactic treatment with low-dose aspirin. Recently, several publications[83,84] have confirmed the good experience of the first reports on Doppler screening of the total population.[78,85] In the early publications the sensitivity of uterine artery velocimetry was only 25%.[84] By adding colour Doppler technique for vessel localisation, the sensitivity for pregnancy-induced hypertension and IUGR has improved substantially, to 76%. Abnormal uterine artery blood velocities were recorded in 16% of all

pregnancies at 20 weeks of gestation, in 5.4% at 24 weeks and in 4.6% at 26 weeks. Thus, the selected group at risk is of reasonable size, allowing a more intense monitoring during the subsequent course of pregnancy. However, the optimal model of Doppler velocimetry screening, subsequent follow-up and prophylactic aspirin treatment does not yet seem to have been found.

Intra-uterine growth retardation

Uteroplacental blood flow is probably the single most effective determinant of fetal growth.[86] Restricted flow through the placental vascular bed can result in IUGR.[87] In the growth-retarded fetus the umbilical blood flow is reduced[88] and fetal blood flow redistributed to ensure preferential blood supply to vital organs such as the brain, myocardium and adrenals.[89] Before the ultrasound era the only possibility of finding a small fetus *in utero* was by manual palpation or by measuring the symphysis–fundus height. After the introduction of ultrasound imaging the abnormally small fetus could be detected, but the examination usually could not pinpoint which of the small fetuses were sick and needed special surveillance. All pregnancies suspected of IUGR were therefore usually monitored by tests that might give information on the availability of oxygen to the fetal brain, e.g. non-stress test of fetal heart rate or biophysical profile. Doppler velocimetry made it possible to evaluate the placental vascular resistance and to detect the signs of redistribution of blood flow within the fetus. Clinical Doppler velocimetry studies in pregnancies with small-for-gestational age (SGA) fetuses have improved our understanding of the pathophysiological processes leading to IUGR and our possibilities of monitoring fetal health.

In SGA fetuses with Doppler signs of increased vascular resistance in the placental circulation – elevated PI, RI or S/D ratio in the umbilical artery and/or uteroplacental vessels – morphological changes were found, indicating reduction of the fetal vessel bed in the placenta[90] and defective development of spiral arteries in the placental bed.[91] In severely growth-retarded fetuses developing signs of intra-uterine distress, the end-diastolic velocity of the aortic and umbilical artery waveform disappears or even becomes reversed (corresponding to BFC II and BFC III).[9,10,15,48,92–94]

In a prospective study of 159 fetuses where IUGR was suspected, the sensitivity of the method for predicting IUGR was 41% for aortic PI and 57% for aortic BFC; for the prediction of fetal distress the corresponding values were 63% and 87%.[19] In another study of 219 high-risk pregnancies, of which 141 fetuses were SGA and 37 of which suffered intra-uterine distress, receiver operating characteristic curves showed the mean velocity in the fetal descending aorta to be the single best parameter in the prediction of adverse fetal outcome.[95]

Gudmundsson and Marsal[48] compared Doppler velocimetry of the umbilical artery with that of the fetal aorta with regard to their clinical predictive capacity and found that there was only a marginal difference between the two vessels. The umbilical artery velocimetry was slightly more predictive of IUGR and the fetal aortic velocimetry was slightly better in identifying fetuses that subsequently developed intrauterine distress. As the Doppler signals of the umbilical artery are easier to record, this vessel seems preferable for clinical examinations.

Trudinger *et al.*[96] reported a highly significant association between increasing abnormality of umbilical artery velocity waveforms and fetal size at birth, as well as requirements for neonatal intensive care, in 2178 high-risk pregnancies. In a study by Maulik *et al.* the average sensitivity of umbilical artery Doppler velocimetry for the prediction of SGA neonates was 71% (range 45–91%).[97]

The sensitivity of umbilical artery Doppler velocimetry in predicting operative delivery for fetal distress (ODFD) in pregnancies where IUGR was suspected was 78% (range 62–95%). In our material,[48] when the blood flow velocity was normal in the umbilical artery (BFC 0) 10% underwent ODFD, which is about the same as for the general population. If the end-diastolic flow was absent (BFC II–III), nearly all fetuses (96%) showed signs of hypoxia/asphyxia at delivery. These results are clinically important, as they suggest that Doppler examination of the umbilical artery flow might find the pregnancies suspected of IUGR where the fetuses are truly at risk for asphyxia and therefore need special surveillance. Doppler findings seem to be better indicators of fetal health than of fetal size, which is not surprising in view of the multiplicity of determinants of fetal size. Probably only the IUGR cases of circulatory origin should be expected to be detected by umbilical artery velocimetry.

ARED flow in the umbilical artery or fetal aorta has been shown by many authors to be associated with severe IUGR and a high risk of perinatal death. The surviving neonates who had had ARED flow in utero had a significantly increased frequency of necrotising enterocolitis,[98,99] which might be secondary to a severe intestinal vasoconstriction as a part of fetal redistribution of blood flow during chronic hypoxaemia.

The time interval between the occurrence of ARED flow in the umbilical artery and cardiotocographic signs of fetal distress varies according to the severity of the blood velocity pattern and gestational age. The longer the period of absence of end-diastolic blood velocity in the umbilical artery, the closer the occurrence of pathological heart rate pattern. In our studies, the median time lag between the finding of BFC III in the umbilical artery and delivery due to signs of fetal asphyxia was 3 days (range 0–21 days).[19]

Analysis of blood gases in the umbilical cord blood, taken via cordocentesis or post-partum, have shown that the pathological umbilical artery blood velocity waveforms were associated with fetal hypoxaemia.[100–102]

Fetuses with ARED flow were more often hypoxaemic and acidaemic than those with positive end-diastolic flow.[103] However, the clinical value of cordocentesis for blood gas analysis in cases with ARED flow has been questioned, as it did not improve the outcome of the neonates.[104]

Abramowicz *et al.*[105] in their study on 250 high-risk pregnancies, concluded that Doppler umbilical artery velocimetry is as effective as the oxytocin challenge test when applied as a secondary diagnostic test in pregnancies with a non-reactive non-stress test. A comparison of several methods used for surveillance of SGA fetuses showed that Doppler velocimetry of the umbilical artery was a better predictor of perinatal morbidity than the ultrasonically measured fetal abdominal circumference, computerised fetal heart rate variability or biophysical profile score.[106] Similar results were reported by Arduini *et al.*[107] for low-risk pregnancies.

The results of the studies reviewed above indicate that Doppler velocimetry of the umbilical artery and fetal descending aorta is an excellent method for differentiating between healthy and truly growth-retarded SGA fetuses, and that it may help the clinician to identify pregnancies that need special surveillance. However, this is true only if Doppler velocimetry is applied as a secondary diagnostic test in preselected groups of high-risk pregnancies.[108–110] A recently published review of the few available prospective studies using umbilical artery velocimetry in low-risk populations could not show the umbilical Doppler to be of any value in the prediction of fetal compromise in unselected pregnancies.[111]

In a clinical context, as also demonstrated above, Doppler velocimetry of the placental and aortic circulation of growth-retarded fetuses gives reliable information on development of fetal distress, and the finding of ARED flow is accepted by many as an indication for intervention and delivery. This strategy seems to improve the outcome for the fetus when there is no risk of extreme prematurity. However, in pregnancies with a gestational age less than 30–31 weeks the clinical decision is often difficult, especially in view of cases with abnormal velocimetry findings reported to last for days or even weeks. Therefore, an additional parameter is needed to facilitate the clinical management. At present, the potentials of Doppler examination of fetal vessels other than the aorta and umbilical artery are being explored.

Abnormal umbilical venous pulsations have been described in third-trimester fetuses with imminent asphyxia (Fig. 13.7).[112] The venous pulsations might be a reflection of changes in fetal heart function or they might be due to dilatation of the ductus venosus during hypoxia, thereby allowing a transmission of pressure waves into the umbilical cord. In the inferior vena cava (IVC) an increased reversed blood velocity during atrial systole is probably a sign of heart failure or increased afterload. Recording venous blood velocities might be of value in deciding when to deliver the premature IUGR fetus.[113]

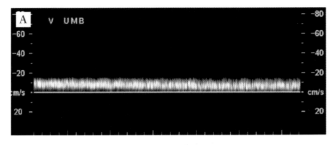

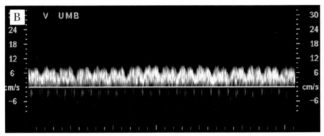

Fig. 13.7 Umbilical vein waveforms. A: Normal parabolic flow in the umbilical vein. **B:** Pulsations in the umbilical vein.

In a recent study on fetuses with ARED flow in the umbilical artery, an association was found between the finding of abnormal end-diastolic umbilical cord venous pulsations and perinatal mortality.[114] In a chronically instrumented fetal lamb model with experimental hypoxia maintained for 90 minutes, the preliminary results have shown that the end-diastolic blood velocity in the ductus venosus decreased at the onset of fetal hypoxia, and abnormal venous pulsations appeared in the intra-abdominal part of the umbilical vein before the changes in fetal blood pH occurred.[112] However, the venous and arterial blood velocities in the umbilical cord were unaffected during hypoxia. These results suggest that the brain-sparing effect and abnormal umbilical venous pulsations in the intra-abdominal part of the vein might be early signs of fetal hypoxia. On the contrary, abnormal umbilical cord venous pulsations are probably a late sign of hypoxia, indicating a poor prognosis.

Diabetes mellitus

In one of the very first reports on the use of Doppler studies in 40 diabetic pregnancies, it was not possible to demonstrate any velocity waveform changes in the umbilical artery and fetal descending aorta specific for fetuses of diabetic mothers.[115] Intra-uterine fetal distress and IUGR could be predicted from the Doppler signals in a similar way as in non-diabetic pregnancies. Bracero and Schulman[116] reported a significantly higher prevalence of abnormal uterine artery velocity waveforms in a consecutive series of 54 pregnancies complicated by diabetes mellitus than in a non-diabetic population. Among the diabetic women with abnormal uterine artery Doppler examination, a statistically higher incidence of poor glycaemic control, chronic hypertension, polyhydramnios, vasculopathy, pre-eclampsia, caesarean sections for fetal distress and neonatal respiratory distress syndrome was seen. However, there were no differences in the umbilical S/D ratio between the groups with normal and abnormal uterine artery velocity waveforms.

In another cross-sectional study of 65 well-controlled diabetic pregnancies, Doppler measurements from the uterine arteries, umbilical artery, fetal descending aorta and middle cerebral artery were performed.[117] No significant abnormalities of Doppler waveform indices could be demonstrated. It was suggested that the discrepancy between the results of the two studies might be explained by the fact that the former included patients with poor diabetic control. In accordance with the study by Salvesen *et al.*, no differences in RI in the umbilical artery were found between 128 diabetic and 170 non-diabetic pregnancies.[118]

Post-term pregnancy

A decrease in amniotic fluid in association with post-term pregnancy, with or without placental insufficiency, is an important risk factor for fetal morbidity and mortality.[119] The fetal renal system and renal haemodynamics play a major role in the regulation of the amniotic fluid volume. In a study of 50 normal human fetuses at or after 40 weeks gestation, Veille *et al.*[120] reported that the fetal renal artery S/D ratio was significantly higher in pregnancies with oligohydramnios than in those with normal amniotic fluid volume. Except for contributing to the development of oligohydramnios, the reason for and the importance of this increase in the renal vascular resistance in otherwise healthy and non-compromised fetuses is not clear.

In a prospective study on 102 pregnancies past 294 gestational days, with no other complication than prolongation of pregnancy, serial Doppler examinations were performed.[121] Velocity waveforms of the umbilical artery, the fetal descending aorta and common carotid artery, and the maternal uterine artery did not change. Abnormal waveforms had no significant relationship to fetal asphyxia. In another study[122] fetal heart rate monitoring, ultrasonic evaluation of the amniotic fluid volume and Doppler velocimetry of the umbilical and uterine arteries were used prospectively for surveillance of 140 post-term pregnancies. All methods were characterised by a low sensitivity and positive predictive value regarding fetal compromise; for the Doppler velocimetry the values were 17% and 29%, respectively. Used in combination, and considering any and at least one abnormal test as a positive result, the sensitivity increased to 67% and the positive predictive value to 33%. The limited value of the umbilical and uterine artery Doppler velocimetry for surveillance of prolonged pregnancies was also reported from another study, in which the possible role of the cerebral–placental RI ratio was evaluated.[123]

Pregnancy and autoimmune disease

Of the autoimmune diseases, systemic lupus erythematosus (SLE) holds an exceptional position because of its high rate of various fetal complications, e.g. pre-eclampsia, prematurity, IUGR and intra-uterine death. In a retrospective study of 27 pregnancies in 26 women with SLE, a pathological uteroplacental and umbilical Doppler velocimetry was reported to facilitate identification of the fetuses at risk of adverse perinatal outcome. Prediction of the perinatal outcome using velocimetry was better than using antiphospholipid antibodies.[124] In a study of 56 lupus anticoagulant pregnancies the finding of ARED flow accurately predicted fetal distress and delivery by caesarean section.[125] Pregnant women with SLE treated with aspirin and glucocorticosteroids were reported to have a normal Doppler velocimetry.[126]

Placental abruption

Placental abruption is not only a common cause of fetal morbidity and mortality but can also be life-threatening to the mother. Even though heavy smoking and pre-eclampsia are well known risk factors, the aetiology and the pathophysiological mechanisms are still incompletely understood.

Except for occasional case reports, few studies have been published using Doppler velocimetry in the surveillance of late pregnancies with clinical suspicion of placental abruption. In a prospective study of 67 third-trimester pregnancies complicated by vaginal bleeding and suspicion of placental abruption, weekly Doppler examinations of the umbilical artery and maternal arcuate artery were performed.[127] The odds ratio for placental abruption to occur was 2:1 in pregnancies with an abnormally elevated PI in the arcuate artery, compared to an odds ratio of 1:7 when the Doppler velocimetry was normal.

Premature rupture of membranes

Doppler velocimetry is being increasingly recognised as an excellent indicator of chronic impairment of uteroplacental and fetal circulation. However, in some more acute situations, e.g. in patients with premature rupture of the membranes, velocimetry does not seem sensitive enough to predict fetal distress or infection.[128] In another study, 10 out of 51 patients with premature rupture of membranes who developed chorioamnionitis did not show an abnormal systolic-to-diastolic ratio (S/D ratio).[129]

Twin pregnancies

The S/D ratio of the umbilical artery differs significantly between concordant and discordant twins, being higher in small discordant twins.[130,131] In 50 pairs of twins a significant association was found between the high umbilical

FVW indices and the occurrence of FHR abnormalities and IUGR.[132] Doppler velocimetry of the umbilical artery in twins predicted the SGA neonates earlier and with higher sensitivity than did real-time ultrasonography.[133] Nevertheless, Beattie et al.[134] recommend fetal biometry, biophysical profile score and Doppler velocimetry to be used as complementary methods in monitoring twin pregnancies.

Fetal cardiac arrhythmias

Doppler recording of fetal aortic velocities gives important information on the haemodynamic consequences of fetal cardiac arrhythmias. Simultaneous detection of Doppler signals from the fetal abdominal aorta, reflecting ventricular contractions, and the inferior vena cava, reflecting atrial contractions, can facilitate the classification of arrhythmias.[135-138] In most cases of fetal arrhythmias the estimated aortic volume flow remains within normal limits, indicating the ability of the fetal heart to maintain the cardiac output.[137,138] Abnormally low values of aortic flow were found in fetuses with severe arrhythmias causing heart failure.[139] In cases of brady- and tachyarrhythmias, a decrease in the aortic flow was observed when the fetal heart rate was outside the limits of 50 or 230 beats/min.[138]

In fetuses with premature heartbeats an increase of the peak aortic velocities was observed in the first post-extrasystolic beats.[140] Similarly, in fetuses with complete atrioventricular block the peak systolic velocities are higher than in fetuses with regular sinus rhythm.[139] This, together with the above-described compensation for negative effects of cardiac arrhythmias on fetal cardiac output, indicates that the Frank–Starling mechanism is also valid for fetal myocardium.

Fetuses with congestive heart failure caused by cardiac arrhythmia sometimes require transplacental treatment with digoxin or anti-arrhythmic drugs. Besides the effect of treatment on heart rhythm, the improved performance of the fetal heart can be followed by serial measurements of the fetal aortic volume blood flow.[137]

Fetal anaemia

In isoimmunised pregnancies the degree of fetal anaemia can be determined by analysing blood samples obtained by cordocentesis. However, it would facilitate the clinical management if the anaemic fetuses could be identified non-invasively. One of the early reports suggested that there was an inverse correlation between the cord haemoglobin at birth and the time-averaged mean velocity and volume blood flow recorded antenatally in the intra-abdominal part of the umbilical vein using Doppler ultrasound.[141] In the fetal descending aorta of previously untransfused isoimmunised fetuses, Rightmire et al.[142] reported an increased mean blood velocity and a negative correlation with the haematocrit of umbilical cord blood obtained by cord puncture under fetoscopic control. This was also confirmed by Nicolaides *et al.*,[143] who related the values of mean aortic velocity to the haemoglobin deficit in blood samples obtained by cordocentesis. The findings of increased fetal aortic velocities in anaemic fetuses are in accord with an increase in their cardiac output as a consequence of lowered blood viscosity, increased venous return and cardiac preload. Doppler cardiac studies of anaemic fetuses showed indications of increased cardiac output.[144,145] Contrary to the changes in the aortic time-averaged mean velocity in fetal anaemia, there were no changes in the waveform indices.

It can hardly be expected that Doppler ultrasound measurements would give an absolute measure of fetal anaemia. Nevertheless, a finding in pregnancy with iso-immunisation of fetal aortic velocity above the upper normal limit is suggestive of fetal anaemia. After intra-uterine transfusion, a decrease or even normalisation of the mean velocity in the fetal aorta has been observed.[146]

Recently Mari *et al.*[147] indicated that the blood flow velocity in the middle cerebral artery might provide the clinician with a non-invasive way of assessing the level of haemoglobin concentration in the anaemic fetus. In a series of 111 fetuses at risk for anaemia they obtained a sensitivity of 100% (confidence limit 86–100%) in detecting anaemia on the basis of an increase in the peak velocity. Their false positive rate was 12%. These results are promising but need to be verified by future studies.

Doppler velocimetry as a labour admission test

The revealed association between the abnormal Doppler velocity waveforms in the umbilical artery and fetal hypoxia initiated attempts to apply Doppler velocimetry in early labour as a test to predict subsequent development of fetal distress in labour.[148] Unfortunately, the initial expectations were not vindicated: Doppler velocimetry showed too low a sensitivity and positive predictive value to be of any use for this purpose. Both the amniotic fluid index and fetal heart rate monitoring proved superior in predicting the development of fetal asphyxia.[149] Arduini et al.[150] suggested a combined use of Doppler ultrasound and fetal heart rate monitoring to be of possible benefit if used in combination as a labour admission test. In the study by Malcus *et al.*[151] abnormal umbilical artery waveforms in early labour identified previously undetected small-for-gestational age fetuses, but were not predictive of fetal distress in labour. In one of the more recent papers Somerset *et al.*[152] considered Doppler velocimetry suitable for screening for fetal distress in labour. However, also in their study the overall sensitivity was lower than that of the heart rate monitoring used as a labour admission test.

Obviously, umbilical artery velocimetry has the capacity to reveal cases of fetal distress developing gradually on the basis of abnormal placental function with increased vascular resistance in the umbilical circulation, rather than identifying acute development of fetal distress. So far, no randomised controlled trial (RCT) has been published evaluating the possible clinical usefulness of Doppler velocimetry as a diagnostic test in labour.

Pharmacology

Antihypertensive drugs

The possible negative effect of drugs used for the treatment of pregnancy-induced hypertension (PIH) are of great concern to the clinician, as they readily cross the placenta and might directly influence the fetus or exert an influence on the fetus via the changed maternal haemodynamics. Therefore, it is important to test various treatment regimens for their possible haemodynamic effects.

Montan *et al.*[153] examined the fetal and uteroplacental flow velocity waveform before and after 1 week's treatment with methyldopa. The desired hypotensive effect was achieved without any significant influence on the utero-placental or fetal circulation. However, in the study by Rey,[154] methyldopa caused a decrease of PI in the umbilical and uteroplacental vessels of hypertensive women.

Walker *et al.*[155] followed the uteroplacental and umbilical artery waveforms in hypertensive pregnant women treated acutely with oral nicardipine and in women chronically treated with oral pindolol: 30 minutes after nicardipine there was a transient increase in the uteroplacental S/D ratio; 3 days after the commencement of the treatment with pindolol, the uteroplacental S/D ratio rose and then – at 7 days of treatment – it returned to the initial level. In the untreated control group a continuing rise in the S/D ratio was found. The umbilical FVW remained unchanged in all three groups. The finding of a transient PI increase after peroral pindolol is in disagreement with the randomised double-blind study of Montan *et al.*[156] which compared the effects of pindolol and atenolol. After pindolol there was no change in the uteroplacental or fetal FVW. Atenolol caused an increase in PI on both sides of the placenta, which confirmed the results from the previous open study.[157]

Oral treatment with labetalol, exerting both α- and β-blocking effects, had no adverse effects upon uteroplacental or umbilical blood flow.[158] However, fetal aortic mean velocity decreased and aortic PI increased, suggesting a direct effect on the fetus.

In a double-blind study the effects of placebo, peroral nifedipine and intravenous hydralazine were compared[159] and no differences were observed in the FVW of the uterine and umbilical arteries both within and between groups. In another study, dihydralazine given intravenously led to an increase in the PI of the uterine artery.[160]

The umbilical artery FVW remained unchanged. Recently, the role of nitric oxide was given special attention because of its role in maintaining low vascular tone in the fetal part of the placenta. Giles et al.[161] treated five pregnant women with abnormal umbilical FVW and PIH or IUGR with glyceryl trinitrate, which generates nitric oxide. The umbilical artery S/D ratio decreased significantly without any change in FHR, suggesting a vasodilatation in the fetal placental vessels.

Tocolytic drugs

Several papers have recently been published examining the effect of tocolytics on FVW in various uteroplacental and fetal vessels. Hallak et al.[162] followed the S/D ratio in the umbilical artery before and after the initiation of treatment, either with terbutaline, indomethacin or placebo, without being able to demonstrate any differences. Their findings are in agreement with a previous report on unchanged placental impedance after terbutaline.[163] In that study a positive chronotropic and inotropic effect on the fetal heart was reported, as reflected in blood flow changes in the fetal descending aorta. Faber et al.[164] found no changes in the PI of the uterine artery, umbilical artery, middle cerebral artery or descending aorta of fetuses following the administration of fenoterol. The effects of ritodrine have also been studied:[165] there was a decrease in umbilical PI after the infusion of ritodrine in a group of fetuses at 32–35 weeks gestation. Before that gestational age no PI change was observed.

During infusion of magnesium sulphate for tocolysis, the PI increased in the fetal middle cerebral artery and decreased in the maternal uterine artery.[166] This finding was explained by increased blood flow to the placenta and normalisation of the cerebral circulation in fetuses stressed by preterm labour.

Prostaglandins

Similar to the previous report on the vaginal application of prostaglandin E_2,[167] no effect on Doppler FVW indices was reported after the intracervical application of prostaglandin E_2 gel for ripening of the cervix.[168]

Glucose

Oral administration of 50 g glucose did not change the RI of FVWs recorded from the umbilical artery, fetal internal carotid or anterior cerebral artery, after correction for the effect of changed FHR.[169]

Application of Doppler in pregnancy: general evaluation

So far, four RCTs evaluating Doppler umbilical artery velocimetry in the late second and the third trimester of unselected pregnancies have been published.[170–173] Davies et al.[170] examined in a random fashion 2475 pregnant women at 19–22 gestational weeks and at 32 weeks. Both umbilical and uterine arteries were examined. The Doppler and control groups did not differ in the number of antenatal or neonatal admissions, number of cardiotocographic recordings, gestational age at delivery, rate of fetal distress or need for resuscitation. There were more perinatal deaths in the Doppler group (OR 2.29, 95% CI 1.02–5.11); however, only one of the fetuses that died during the perinatal period showed a previously abnormal blood flow pattern. The authors assumed that the difference in the perinatal deaths was most likely to be due to chance. They concluded that routine Doppler ultrasound screening of a general obstetric population did not improve the perinatal outcome. The finding of a possible increased rate of perinatal deaths in the study by Davies et al.[170] is in contrast to the findings in high-risk pregnancies,[174] and is also in disagreement with one of the prospective studies[175] and with two other RCTs[171,173] in unselected pregnancies. The two RCTs[171,173] found a tendency towards decreased perinatal mortality, OR being 0.79 (95% CI 0.21–2.92) and 0.34 (95% CI 0.10–1.07), respectively.

In the study by Mason et al.[171] 2025 low-risk primigravidae were allocated to either the Doppler or the control group. The Doppler examination was performed at 28 and 34 weeks gestation. There were no significant differences between the two groups with regard to the incidence of obstetric interventions and neonatal outcome. Thus, no benefit was shown from Doppler velocimetry used as a routine screening test in unselected pregnancies.

In 1993, Newnham and coworkers[172] published a randomised study comparing the effects of repeated Doppler umbilical artery examinations together with ultrasound biometry (at 18, 24, 28, 34 and 38 weeks of gestation) in 1415 pregnant women with a control group of 1419 women. There was no improvement of the outcome of pregnancy as measured by duration of neonatal stay, requirements for resuscitation and neonatal events. The only significant difference was in the rate of birthweight <10th centile and birthweight <3rd centile, the relative risk being 1.35 (95% CI 1.09–1.67) and 1.65 (95% CI 1.09–2.49), respectively. This finding might be a chance effect. However, to exclude the possibilities that repeated Doppler and imaging ultrasound examinations during low-risk pregnancies might influence fetal growth, larger randomised trials specifically addressing this question are required. In the study by Davies et al.[170] or in the RCTs in high-risk pregnancies, no negative effect on intra-uterine growth was observed.

Whittle et al.[173] included 2986 pregnant women in their RCT, scheduling Doppler velocimetry of the umbilical artery for 26–30 and 34–36 weeks of gestation. The knowledge of the Doppler results by the clinicians did not lead to any significant differences in the rates of antenatal or neonatal admissions, preterm deliveries, caesarean sections or need for assisted ventilation. As already mentioned, there was a trend toward fewer stillbirths in the Doppler group. Nevertheless, until the latter finding is confirmed in more studies, the authors do not consider screening with the Doppler method justified.

In a large Dutch study[176] 1598 unselected pregnancies were allocated to either a Doppler or a control group; however, the Doppler examination was performed only when clinical indications appeared subsequently. Thus, the velocimetry was done in a subpopulation (46% of the Doppler group) which was at a higher clinical risk than the original randomised population. The study used a predefined protocol for the management of abnormal Doppler findings, which might be the main reason for the prevention of intra-uterine deaths, and which resulted in a significant reduction of perinatal deaths of normally formed fetuses and infants with weight ≥500 g (risk ratio 0.33, 95% CI 0.13–0.82). Despite this important finding, because of the study design the Dutch trial cannot be included in the systematic RCT reviews of either high-risk or unselected pregnancies.

Conclusions

Doppler velocimetry is a rapid non-invasive test that provides valuable information about the haemodynamic situation of the fetus. The promising results from studies applying Doppler velocimetry of the uterine artery at midgestation as a screening for patients at risk for developing pre-eclampsia and/or IUGR still await final confirmation in randomised clinical trials. Abnormal velocimetry findings in the umbilical arteries and intrafetal arteries are associated with an adverse outcome of pregnancy and an increased risk of intrauterine death. Umbilical artery velocimetry has proved to be an efficient diagnostic test of fetal jeopardy and should be employed as a part of clinical management protocols in high-risk pregnancy. The available evidence does not support the use of Doppler velocimetry as a routine screening test of low-risk pregnancies.

The use of Doppler ultrasound has allowed extensive insight into physiological and pathophysiological fetal haemodynamics. After 20 years of Doppler ultrasound in fetal work, the technique is established as an invaluable tool for the assessment of the fetal status. The development of diagnostic applications has followed the technical evolution of the technique. The technical improvements and innovations are now taking place at an even greater pace than in the past, but the potential of the technique is by no means exhausted. On the contrary, combining 3D flow assessment and 3D imaging will most likely increase our diagnostic capability and help shed light on fetomaternal organs, such as the placenta, with complicated haemodynamics.

REFERENCES

1 (NCRP) NCoRPM. Biological effects of ultrasound: mechanisms and clinical implications. Bethesda: National Council on Radiation Protection & Measurements Report No. 74; 1983

2 AIUM. Bioeffects considerations for the safety of diagnostic ultrasound. J Ultrasound Med 1988; (Suppl 4)

3 Wells P. The safety of diagnostic ultrasound. Br J Radiol 1997; Suppl 20

4 Eik-Nes S H, Marsal K, Brubakk A, Kristoffersen K, Ulstein M. Ultrasonic measurement of human fetal blood flow. J Biomed Eng 1982; 4: 28–36

5 Eik-Nes S H, Brubakk A O, Ulstein M. Measurement of human fetal blood flow. BMJ 1980; 1: 283–284

6 Gill R W. Quantitative blood flow measurement in deep lying vessels using pulsed Doppler with the Octoson. Ultrasound Med Biol 1978; 4: 341–345

7 Stale H, Marsal K, Gennser G. Blood flow velocity and diameter changes in the fetal descending aorta: a longitudinal study. Am J Obstet Gynecol 1990; 163: 26–29

8 EAPM. Regulation for the use of Doppler technology in perinatal medicine. Barcelona; 1989

9 Jouppila P, Kirkinen P. Increased vascular resistance in the descending aorta of the human fetus in hypoxia. Br J Obstet Gynaecol 1984; 91: 853–856

10 Lingman G, Laurin J, Marsal K. Circulatory changes in fetuses with imminent asphyxia. Biol Neonate 1986; 49: 66–73

11 Trudinger B, Giles W, Cook C. Flow velocity waveforms in the maternal uteroplacental and fetal umbilical placental circulations. Am J Obstet Gynecol 1985; 152: 155–163

12 Gosling R, King D. Ultrasonic angiology. In: Harcus A, Adamson L, eds. Arteries and veins. Edinburgh: Churchill-Livingstone, 1975: 61–98

13 Stuart B, Drumm J, Fitzgerald D, Diugnan N. Fetal blood velocity waveforms in normal pregnancy. Br J Obstet Gynaecol 1980; 87: 780–785

14 Pourcelot L. Applications clinique de l'examen Doppler transcutane. In: Peronneau P, ed. Vélocimétrie ultrasonore Doppler. Paris: INSERM, 1974: 213–240

15 Rochelson B, Schulman H, Farmakides G et al. The significance of absent end-diastolic velocity in umbilical artery velocity waveforms. Am J Obstet Gynecol 1987; 156: 1213–1218

16 Gudmundsson S, Marsal K. Umbilical artery and uteroplacental circulation in normal pregnancy – a cross-sectional study. Acta Obstet Gynecol Scand 1988; 67: 347–354

17 Lingman G, Marsal K. Fetal central blood circulation in the third trimester of normal pregnancy. Longitudinal study. 2. Aortic blood velocity waveform. Early Hum Dev 1986; 13: 151–159

18 Gudmundsson S, Marsal K. Umbilical and uteroplacental blood flow velocity waveforms in pregnancies with fetal growth retardation. Eur J Obstet Gynecol Reprod Biol 1988; 27: 187–196

19 Laurin J, Lingman G, Marsal K, Persson P. Fetal blood flow in pregnancy complicated by intrauterine growth retardation. Obstet Gynecol 1987; 69: 895–902

20 Malcus P, Andersson J, Marsal K, Olofsson P-Å. Waveform pattern recognition – a new semiquantitative method for analysis of fetal aortic and umbilical artery blood flow velocity recorded by Doppler ultrasound. Ultrasound Med Biol 1991; 17: 453–460

21 Gudmundsson S, Fairlie F, Lingman G, Marsal K. Recording of blood flow velocity waveforms in the uteroplacental and umbilical circulation – reproducibility study and comparison of pulsed and continuous wave Doppler ultrasound. JCU 1990; 18: 97–101

22 Mehalek K, Berkowitz G, Chitkara U, Rosenberg J, Berkowitz R. Comparison of continuous-wave and pulsed Doppler S/D ratios of umbilical and uterine arteries. Obstet Gynecol 1988; 72: 603–606

23 Maulik D, Yarlagadda A, Youngblood J, Willoughby L. Components of variability of umbilical arterial Doppler velocimetry – a prospective analysis. Am J Obstet Gynecol 1989; 160: 1406–1412

24 Spencer J, Price J. Intraobserver variation in Doppler ultrasound indices of placental perfusion derived from different numbers of waveforms. J Ultrasound Med 1989; 8: 197–199

25 Spencer J, Price J, Lee A. Influence of fetal breathing and movements on variability of umbilical Doppler indices using different numbers of waveforms. J Ultrasound Med 1991; 10: 37–41

26 Marsal K, Lindblad A, Lingman G, Eik-Nes S H. Blood flow in the fetal descending aorta; intrinsic factors affecting fetal blood flow, i.e. fetal breathing movements and cardiac arrhythmia. Ultrasound Med Biol 1984; 10: 339–348

27 Eyck Jv, Wladimiroff J, Noordam M, Tonge H, Prechtl H. The blood flow velocity waveform in the fetal descending aorta: its relationship to fetal behavioural states in normal pregnancy at 37–38 weeks. Early Hum Dev 1985; 12: 137–143

28 Eyck Jv, Wladimiroff J, Wijngaard Jvd, Noordam M, Prechtl H. The blood flow velocity waveform in the fetal internal carotid and umbilical artery; its relation to fetal behavioural states in normal pregnancy at 37–38 weeks. Br J Obstet Gynaecol 1987; 94: 736–741

29 Thompson R, Trudinger B, Cook C. A comparison of Doppler ultrasound waveform indices in the umbilical artery. 1. Indices derived from the maximum velocity waveform. Ultrasound Med Biol 1986; 12: 835–844

30 Mires G, Dempster J, Patel N, Crawford J. The effect of fetal heart rate on umbilical artery flow velocity waveforms. Br J Obstet Gynaecol 1987; 94: 665–669

31 Mulders L, Muijers G, Jongsma H, Nijhuis J, Hein P. The umbilical artery blood flow velocity waveform in relation to fetal breathing movements, fetal heart rate and fetal behavioral states in normal pregnancy at 37–39 weeks. Early Hum Dev 1986; 14: 283–293

32 Thompson R, Trudinger B, Cook C, Giles W. Umbilical artery velocity waveforms: normal reference values for A/B ratio and Pourcelot ratio. Br J Obstet Gynaecol 1988; 95: 589–591

33 Vyas S, Nicolaides K, Campbell S. Renal artery flow-velocity waveforms in normal and hypoxemic fetuses. Am J Obstet Gynecol 1989; 161: 168–172

34 Wladimiroff J, Tonge H, Stewart P. Doppler ultrasound assessment of cerebral blood flow in the human fetus. Br J Obstet Gynaecol 1986; 93: 471–475

35 Kirkinen P, Müller R, Huch R, Huch A. Blood flow velocity waveforms in human fetal intracranial arteries. Obstet Gynecol 1987; 70: 617–621

36 Woo J, Liang S, Roxy L, Chan F. Middle cerebral artery Doppler flow velocity waveforms. Obstet Gynecol 1987; 70: 613–616

37 Legarth J, Thorup E. Characteristics of Doppler blood velocity waveforms in a cardiovascular in vitro model. 2. The influence of peripheral resistance, perfusion pressure and blood flow. Scand J Clin Lab Invest 1989; 49: 459–464

38 Adamson S, Morrow R, Bascom P, Mo L, Ritchie J. Effect of placental resistance, arterial diameter, and blood pressure on the uterine approach. Ultrasound Med Biol 1989; 15: 437–442

39 Thompson R, Stevens R. Mathematical model for interpretation of Doppler velocity waveform indices. Med Biol Eng Comput 1989; 27: 269–276

40 Morrow R, Adamson S, Bull S, Ritchie J. Effect of placental embolization on the umbilical arterial velocity waveform in fetal sheep. Am J Obstet Gynecol 1989; 161: 1055–1060

41 Trudinger B, Stevens R, Connelly A et al. Umbilical artery flow velocity waveforms and placental resistance: the effects of embolization of the umbilical circulation. Am J Obstet Gynecol 1987; 157: 1443–1448

42 Fouron J, Teyssiger G, Maroto E, Lessard M, Marquette G. Diastolic circulatory dynamics in the presence of elevated placental resistance and retrograde diastolic flow in the umbilical artery: a Doppler echographic study in lambs. Am J Obstet Gynecol 1991; 164: 195–203

43 Maulik D, Yarlagadda P, Nathanielsz P, Figueroa J. Hemodynamic validation of Doppler assessment of fetoplacental circulation in a sheep model system. J Ultrasound Med 1989; 8: 177–181

44 Wladimiroff J, Huisman T, Stewart P. Fetal and umbilical flow velocity waveforms between 10–16 weeks' gestation: a preliminary study. Obstet Gynecol 1991; 78: 812–814

45 Schulman H, Fleischer A, Stern W, Farmakides G, Jagani N, Blattner P. Umbilical velocity waveform ratios in human pregnancy. Am J Obstet Gynecol 1984; 148: 985–990

46 Sonesson S-E, Fouron J-C, Drblik S, Tawile C, Lessard M, Scott A. Reference values form Doppler velocimetric indices from the fetal and placental ends of the umbilical artery during normal pregnancy. JCU 1993; 21: 317–324

47 Marsal K, Gudmundsson S, Stale H. Doppler velocimetry in monitoring fetal heart during late pregnancy. In: Kurjak A, Chervenak F, eds. The fetus as a patient – advances in diagnosis and therapy. London: Parthenon Publishing, 1994: 455–476

48 Gudmundsson S, Marsal K. Fetal aortic and umbilical artery blood velocity waveforms in prediction of fetal outcome – a comparison. Am J Perinatol 1991; 8: 1–6

49 Mari G, Wasserstrum N. Flow velocity waveforms of the fetal circulation preceding fetal death in a case of lupus anticoagulant. Am J Obstet Gynecol 1991; 164: 776–778

50 Cohn H, Sacks E, Heymann M, Rudolph A. Cardiovascular response to hypoxemia and acidemia in fetal lambs. Am J Obstet Gynecol 1974; 120: 817–824

51 Kjellmer I, Karlsson K, Olsson T, Rosén K G. Cerebral reactions during intrauterine asphyxia in the sheep. I. Circulation and oxygen consumption in the fetal brain. Pediatr Res 1974; 8: 50–57

52 Peters L, Sheldon R, Jones M, Makowski E, Meschia G. Blood flow to fetal organs as a function of arterial oxygen content. Am J Obstet Gynecol 1979; 135: 637–646

53 Malcus P, Kjellmer I, Lingman G, Marsal K, Thiringer K, Rosén K-G. Diameters of the common carotid artery and aorta change in different directions during acute asphyxia in the fetal lamb. J Perinat Med 1991; 19: 259–267

54 Arduini D, Rizzo G, Romanini C, Mancuso S. Fetal hemodynamic response to acute maternal hyperoxygenation as predictor of fetal distress in intrauterine growth retardation. BMJ 1989; 298: 561–1562

55 Gramellini D, Folli M, Raboni S, Vadora E, Merialdi A. Cerebral–umbilical Doppler ratio as a predictor of adverse perinatal outcome. Obstet Gynecol 1992; 79: 416–420

56 Mari G, Deter R. Middle cerebral artery flow velocity waveforms in normal and small-for-gestational-age fetuses. Am J Obstet Gynecol 1992; 166: 1262–1270

57 Satoh S, Koyanagi T, Fukuhara M, Hara K, Nakano H. Changes in vascular resistance in the umbilical and middle cerebral arteries in the human intrauterine growth-retarded fetus, measured with pulsed Doppler ultrasound. Early Hum Dev 1989; 20: 213–220

58 Vyas S, Nicolaides K, Bower S, Campbell S. Middle cerebral artery flow velocity waveforms in fetal hypoxaemia. Br J Obstet Gynaecol 1990; 97: 797–803

59 Nicolaides K, Bradley R, Soothill P, Campbell S, Billardo C, Gibb D. Maternal oxygen therapy for intrauterine growth retardation. Lancet 1987; i: 942–945

60 Chandran R, Serra S, Sellers S, Redman C. Fetal middle cerebral artery flow velocity waveforms – a terminal pattern. Case report. Br J Obstet Gynaecol 1991; 98: 937–938

61 Arbeille P, Body G, Saliba E et al. Fetal cerebral circulation assessment by Doppler ultrasound in normal and pathological pregnancies. Eur J Obstet Gynecol Reprod Biol 1988; 29: 261–273

62 Mari G, Kirshon B, Abuhamad A. Fetal renal artery flow velocity waveforms in normal pregnancies and pregnancies complicated by polyhydramnios and oligohydramnios. Obstet Gynecol 1993; 81: 560–564

63 Assali N, Rauramo L, Peltonen T. Measurement of uterine blood flow and uterine metabolism. Am J Obstet Gynecol 1960; 79: 86–98

64 Metcalfe J, Romney S, Ramsey L, Reid D, Burvell C. Estimation of uterine blood flow in normal human pregnancy at term. J Clin Invest 1955; 34: 1632–1638

65 Sheppard B, Bonner J. The ultrastructure of the arterial supply of the human placenta in pregnancy complicated by fetal growth retardation. Br J Obstet Gynaecol 1976; 83: 948–959

66 Fleischer A, Schulman H, Farmakides G et al. Uterine artery Doppler velocimetry in pregnant women with hypertension. Am J Obstet Gynecol 1986; 154: 806–813

67 Arabin B, Bergmann P, Saling E. Quantitative Analyse von Blutflusspektren uteroplazentarer gefässe, der nabelarterie, der fetalen aorta und der fetalen arteria carotis communis innormaler schwangerschaft. Ultraschall Klin Prax 1987; 2: 114–119

68 Oosterhof H, Aarnoudse J. Ultrasound pulsed Doppler studies of the uteroplacental circulation: the influence of sampling site and placenta implantation. Gynecol Obstet Invest 1992; 33: 75–79

69 Schulman H, Fleisher A, Farmakides G, Bracero L, Rochelson B, Grunfeld L. Development of uterine artery compliance in pregnancy as detected by Doppler ultrasound. Am J Obstet Gynecol 1986; 155: 1031–1036

70 Arduini D, Rizzo G, Boccolini M, Romanini C, Mancuso S. Functional assessment of uteroplacental and fetal circulations by means of color Doppler ultrasonography. J Ultrasound Med 1990; 9: 249–253

71 Brar H, Platt L. Reverse end-diastolic flow velocity on umbilical artery velocimetry in high-risk pregnancies; an ominous finding with adverse pregnancy outcome. Am J Obstet Gynecol 1988; 159: 559–561

72 Mandruzzato P, Bogatti L, Fischer L, Gigli C. The clinical significance of absent or reverse end-diastolic flow in the fetal aorta and umbilical artery. Ultrasound Obstet Gynecol 1991; 1: 1926

73 Bell J, Ludomirsky A, Bottalico J, Weiner S. The effect of improvement of umbilical artery absent end-diastolic velocity on perinatal outcome. Am J Obstet Gynecol 1992; 167: 1015–1020

74 Arduini D, Rizzo G, Romanini C. The development of abnormal heart rate patterns after absent end-diastolic velocity in umbilical artery: analysis of risk factors. Am J Obstet Gynecol 1993; 168: 43–50

75 Farine D, Ryan G, Kelly E, Morrow R, Laskin C, Ritchie K. Absent end-diastolic flow velocity waveforms in the umbilical artery – the subsequent pregnancy. Am J Obstet Gynecol 1993; 168: 637–640

76 Nylund L, Lunell N-O, Lewander R, Sarby B. Uteroplacental blood flow index in intra-uterine growth retardation of fetal or maternal origin. Br J Obstet Gynaecol 1983; 90: 16–20

77 Jouppila P, Kirkinen P. Blood velocity waveforms of the fetal aorta in normal and hypertensive pregnancies. Obstet Gynecol 1986; 67: 856–60

78 Fairlie F, Moretti M, Walker J, Sibai B. Determinants of perinatal outcome in pregnancy-induced hypertension with absence of umbilical artery end-diastolic frequencies. Am J Obstet Gynecol 1991; 164: 1084–1089

79 Gudmundsson S, Marsal K. Ultrasound Doppler evaluation of uteroplacental and fetoplacental circulation in pre-eclampsia. Arch Gynecol Obstet 1988; 243: 199–206

80 Cameron A, Nicholson S, Nimrod C, Harder J, Davis D. Doppler waveforms in the fetal aorta and umbilical artery in patient with hypertension in pregnancy. Am J Obstet Gynecol 1988; 158: 339–345

81 Trudinger B, Cook C. Doppler umbilical and uterine waveforms in severe pregnancy hypertension. Br J Obstet Gynaecol 1990; 97: 142–148

82 Kofinas A, Penry M, Simon N, Swain M. Interrelationship and clinical significance of increased resistance in the uterine arteries in patients with hypertension or preeclampsia or both. Am J Obstet Gynecol 1992; 166: 601–606

83 Harrington K, Campbell S, Bewley S, Bower S. Doppler velocimetry studies of the uterine artery in the early prediction of the pre-eclampsia. Obstet Gynecol 1991; 42: 14–20

84 Campbell S, Pearce J, Hackett G, Cohen-Overbeek C, Hernandez C. Qualitative assessment of uteroplacental blood flow; early screening test for high-risk pregnancies. Obstet Gynecol 1986; 68: 649–653

85 Valensise H, Bezzeccheri V, Rizzo G, Tranquili A-L, Garzetti G. Doppler velocimetry of the uterine artery as a screening test for gestational hypertension. Ultrasound Obstet Gynecol 1993; 3: 18–22

86 Wootton R, Fayden IM, Cooper J. Measurement of placental blood flow in the pig and its relation to placental and fetal weight. Biol Neonate 1977; 31: 333–339

87 Brosens I, Dixon H, Robertson W. Fetal growth retardation and the arteries of the placental bed. Br J Obstet Gynaecol 1977; 84: 656–663

88 Clapp J, Szeto H, Larrow R, Hewitt J, Mann L. Umbilical blood flow response to embolization of the uterine circulation. Am J Obstet Gynecol 1980; 138: 60–67

89 Creasy R, Swiet MD, Kahanpää K, Young W, Rudolph A. Pathophysiological changes in the foetal lamb with growth retardation. In: Comline K, Cross G, Dawes G, Nathanielsz P, eds. Fetal and neonatal physiology. Cambridge: Sir Joseph Bacroft Centenary Symposium, 1973: 398–402

90 Giles W, Trudinger B, Baird P. Fetal umbilical artery flow velocity waveforms and placental resistance: pathological correlation. Br J Obstet Gynaecol 1985; 92: 31–38

91 Olofsson P, Laurini R, Marsal K. A high uterine artery pulsatility index reflects a defective development of placental bed spiral arteries in pregnancies complicated by hypertension and fetal growth retardation. Eur J Obstet Gynecol Reprod Biol 1993; 48: 161–168

92 Nicolaides K, Bilardo C, Soothill P, Campbell S. Absence of end diastolic frequencies in the umbilical artery: a sign of fetal hypoxia and acidosis. BMJ 1988; 297: 1026–1027

93 Arabin B, Siebert M, Jimenez E, Sailing E. Obstetrical characteristics of a loss of end-diastolic velocities in the fetal aorta and/or umbilical artery using Doppler ultrasound. Gynecol Obstet Invest 1988; 25: 173–180

94 Illyés M, Gati M. Reverse flow in the human fetal descending aorta as a sign of severe fetal asphyxia proceeding intrauterine death. JCU 1988; 16: 403–407

95 Arabin B, Mohnhaupt A, Becker R, Weitzel H. Comparison of the prognostic value of pulsed Doppler blood flow parameters to predict SGA and fetal distress. Ultrasound Obstet Gynecol 1992; 2: 272–278

96 Trudinger B, Cook C, Giles W et al. Fetal umbilical artery velocity waveforms and subsequent neonatal outcome. Br J Obstet Gynaecol 1991; 98: 378–384

97 Maulik D, Yarlagadda P, Youngblood J, Ciston P. The diagnostic efficacy of the umbilical arterial systolic/diastolic ratio as a screening tool: a prospective blind study. Am J Obstet Gynecol 1990; 162: 1518–1525

98 Hacket G, Campbell S, Gamsu H, Cohen-Overbeck T, Pearce J. Doppler studies in growth retarded fetuses predict neonatal death, necrotizing enterocolitis and haemorrhage. BMJ 1987; 294: 13–16

99 Malcolm G, Ellwood D, Devonald K, Beilby R, Henderson-Smart D. Absent or reversed end diastolic flow velocity in the umbilical artery and necrotising enterocolitis. Arch Dis Child 1991; 66: 805–807

100 Bilardo C, Nicolaides K, Campbell S. Doppler measurements of fetal and uteroplacental circulations: relationship with umbilical venous blood gases measured at cordocentesis. Am J Obstet Gynecol 1990; 162: 115–120

101 Gudmundsson S, Lindblad A, Marsal K. Cord blood gases and absence of end-diastolic blood velocities in the umbilical artery. Early Hum Dev 1990; 24: 231–237

102 Weiner C. The relationship between the umbilical artery systolic/diastolic ratio and umbilical blood gas measurements in specimens obtained by cordocentesis. Am J Obstet Gynecol 1990; 162: 1198–1202

103 Pardi G, Cetin I, Marxoni A et al. Diagnostic value of blood sampling in fetuses with growth retardation. N Engl J Med 1993; 328: 629–626

104 Nicolini U, Nicolaidis P, Fisk N et al. Limited role of fetal blood sampling in prediction of outcome in intrauterine growth retardation. Lancet 1990; ii: 768–772

105 Abramowicz J, Warsof S, Santolaya D, Nobles G, Levy D. Umbilical artery Doppler velocimetry and oxytocin challenge test in nonreactive nonstress tests. J Matern Fetal Invest 1992; 3: 41–45

106 Soothill P, Ajayi R, Campbell S, Nicolaides K. Prediction of morbidity in small and normally grown fetuses by fetal heart rate variability, biophysical profile score and umbilical artery Doppler studies. Br J Obstet Gynaecol 1993; 100: 742–745

107 Arduini D, Rizzo G, Soliani A, Romanini C. Doppler velocimetry versus nonstress test in the antepartum monitoring of low-risk pregnancies. J Ultrasound Med 1991; 10: 331–335

108 Berkowitz G, Mehalek K, Chitkara U, Rosenberg J, Cogswell C, Berkowitz R. Doppler umbilical velocimetry in the prediction of adverse outcome in pregnancies at risk for intrauterine growth retardation. Obstet Gynecol 1988; 71: 742–746

109 Gaziano E, Knox G, Wager G, Bendel R, Boyce D, Olson J. The predictability of the small-for-gestational-age infant by real-time ultrasound-derived measurements combined with pulsed Doppler umbilical artery velocimetry. Am J Obstet Gynecol 1988; 158: 1431–1439

110 Marsal K, Persson P. Ultrasonic measurement of the fetal blood velocity waveform as a second diagnostic test in screening for intrauterine growth retardation. JCU 1988; 16: 239–244

111 Beattie R, Hannah M, Dornan J. Compound analysis of umbilical artery velocimetry in low-risk pregnancy. J Matern Fetal Invest 1992; 2: 269–276

112 Gudmundsson S, Tulzer G, Huhta J, Marsal K. Venous Doppler velocimetry in fetuses with absent end-diastolic blood velocity in the umbilical artery. J Matern Fetal Invest 1993; 3: 196

113 Rizzo G, Arduini D, Romanini C. Inferior vena cava velocities in appropriate-and small for gestational age fetuses. Am J Obstet Gynecol 1992; 166: 1271–1280

114 Veille J, Kanaan C. Duplex Doppler ultrasonographic evaluation of the fetal renal artery in normal and abnormal fetuses. Am J Obstet Gynecol 1989; 161: 1502–1507

115 Olofsson P, Lingman G, Sjöberg N-O, Marsal K. Ultrasonic measurement of fetal blood flow in diabetic pregnancy. J Perinat Med 1987; 15: 545–553

116 Bracero L, Schulman H. Doppler studies of the uteroplacental circulation in pregnancies complicated by diabetes. Ultrasound Obstet Gynecol 1991; 1: 391–394

117 Salvesen D, Higueras M, Mansur C, Freeman J, Brudenell J, Nicolaides K. Placental and fetal Doppler velocimetry in pregnancies complicated by maternal diabetes mellitus. Am J Obstet Gynecol 1993; 168: 645–652

118 Johnstone F, Steel J, Haddad N, Hoskins P, Greer I, Chambers S. Doppler umbilical artery flow velocity waveforms in diabetic pregnancy. Br J Obstet Gynaecol 1992; 99: 135–140

119 Leveno K, Quirk J, Cunningham F. Postterm pregnancy. I. Observations concerning the cause of distress. Am J Obstet Gynecol 1984; 150: 465–473

120 Veille J-C, Penry M, Mueller-Heubach E. Fetal renal pulsed Doppler waveform in prolonged pregnancies. Am J Obstet Gynecol 1993; 169: 882–884

121 Malcus P, Marsal K, Persson P. Fetal and uteroplacental blood flow in prolonged pregnancies. Ultrasound Obstet Gynecol 1991; 1: 40–45

122 Weiner Z, Reichler A, Zlozover M, Mendelson A, Thaler I. The value of Doppler ultrasonongraphy in prolonged pregnancies. Eur J Obstet Gynecol Reprod Biol 1993; 48: 93–97

123 Brar H, Horenstein J, Medearis A, Platt L, Phelan J, Paul R. Cerebral, umbilical and uterine resistance using Doppler velocimety in postterm pregnancy. J Ultrasound Med 1989; 8: 187–191

124 Guzman E, Schulman H, Bracero L, Rochelson B, Farmakides G, Coury A. Uterine-umbilical artery Doppler velocimetry in pregnant women with systemic lupus erythematosus. J Ultrasound Med 1992; 11: 275–281

125 Kerslake S, Morton K, Versi E et al. Early Doppler studies in lupus pregnancy. Am J Reprod Immunol 1992; 28: 172–175

126 Weiner Z, Lorber M, Blumenfeld Z. Umbilical and uterine artery flow velocity waveforms in pregnant women with systemic lupus erythematosus treated with aspirin and glucocorticosteroids. Am J Reprod Immunol 1992; 28: 168–171

127 Malcus P, Laurini R, Marsal K. Doppler blood flow changes and placental morphology in pregnancies with third trimester hemorrhage. Acta Obstet Gynecol Scand 1992; 71: 39–45

128 Abramowicz J, Sherer D, Warsof S, Levy D. Feto-placental and uteroplacental Doppler blood flow velocity analysis in premature rupture of membranes. Am J Perinatol 1992; 9: 353–356

129 Leo M, Skurnick J, Ganesh V, Adhate A, Apuzzio J. Clinical chorioamnionitis is not predicted by umbilical artery Doppler velocimetry in patients with premature rupture of membranes. Obstet Gynecol 1992; 79: 916–918

130 Grab D, Hütter T, Sterzik K, Terinde R. Diskordantes wachstum bei geminigravidität stellenwert der Dopplersonographic. Geburtshilfe Frauenheilkd 1993; 53: 42–48

131 Shah Y, Gragg L, Moodley S, Williams G. Doppler velocimetry in concordant and discordant twin gestations. Obstet Gynecol 1992; 80: 272–276

132 Jensen R. Doppler velocimetry in twin pregnancy. Eur J Obstet Gynecol Reprod Biol 1992; 45: 9–12

133 Degani S, Shapiro RGI, Paltiely Y, Sharf M. Doppler flow velocity waveforms in fetal surveillance of twins. A prospective longitudinal study. J Ultrasound Med 1992; 11: 537–541

134 Beattie R, Dowell MM, Ritchie J. Optimizing fetal surveillance in twin pregnancy. J Matern Fetal Invest 1993; 3: 53–57

135 Chan F, Woo S, Ghosh A, Tang M, Lam C. Prenatal diagnosis of congenital fetal arrhythmias by simultaneous pulsed Doppler velocimetry of the fetal abdominal aorta and inferior vena cava. Obstet Gynecol 1990; 76: 200–204

136 Lingman G, Dahlström J, Eik-Nes S H. Hemodynamic evaluation of fetal heart arrhythmias. Br J Obstet Gynaecol 1984; 91: 647–652

137 Lingman G, Lundström N-R, Marsal K. Clinical outcome and circulatory effects of fetal cardiac arrhythmias. Acta Paediatr Scand 1986; Suppl 329: 120–126

138 Tonge H, Wladimiroff J, Noordam M, Stewart P. Fetal cardiac arrhythmias and their effect on volume blood flow in descending aorta of human fetus. J Clin Ultrasound 1986; 14: 607–612

139 Lingman G, Marsal K. Circulatory effects of fetal heart arrhythmias. J Pediatr Cardiol 1986; 7: 67–74

140 Marsal K, Eik-Nes S H, Persson P-H, Ulstein M. Blood flow in human fetal aorta in normal pregnancy and in fetal cardiac arrhytmia. Acta Obstet Gynecol Scand 1980; 93: 39

141 Kirkinen P, Jouppila P, Eik-Nes S. Umbilical venous flow as indicator of fetal anaemia. Lancet 1981; i: 1004–1005

142 Rightmire D, Nicolaides K, Rodeck C, Campbell S. Fetal blood velocities in Rh isoimmunization: relationship to gestational age and to fetal hematocrit. Obstet Gynecol 1986; 68: 233–236

143 Nicolaides K, Bilardo C, Campbell S. Prediction of fetal anemia by measurement of the mean blood velocity in the fetal aorta. Am J Obstet Gynecol 1990; 162: 209–212

144 Copel J, Grannum P, Green J. Fetal cardiac output in the isoimmunized pregnancy: a pulsed Doppler-echocardiographic study of patients undergoing intravascular intrauterine transfusion. Am J Obstet Gynecol 1989; 161: 361–365

145 Rizzo G, Nicolaides K, Arduini D, Campbell S. Effects of intravascular fetal blood transfusion on fetal intracardiac Doppler velocity waveforms. Am J Obstet Gynecol 1990; 163: 1231–1238

146 Bilardo C, Nicolaides K, Campbell S. Doppler studies in red cell isoimmunization. Clin Obstet Gynecol 1989; 32: 719–727

147 Mari G. Noninvasive diagnosis by Doppler ultrasonography of fetal anemia due to maternal red-cell alloimmunization. New Engl J Med 2000; 342: 9–14

148 Feinkind L, Abulafia O, Delke I. Screening with Doppler velocimetry in labor. Am J Obstet Gynecol 1989; 161: 765–770

149 Sarno A, Ahn M, Brar H. Intrapartum Doppler velocimetry, amniotic fluid volume, and fetal heart rate as predictors of subsequent fetal distress. I. An initial report. Am J Obstet Gynecol 1989; 161: 1508–1514

150 Arduini D, Rizzo G, Caforio L, Romanini C. Umbilical artery velocimetry versus fetal heart rate monitoring as labor admission tests. J Matern Fetal Invest 1992; 2: 37–39

151 Malcus P, Gudmundsson S, Marsal K. Umbilical artery Doppler velocimetry as a labor admission test. Obstet Gynecol 1991; 77: 10–16

152 Somerset D, Murrills A, Wheeler T. Screening for fetal distress in labour using the umbilical artery blood velocity waveform. Br J Obstet Gynaecol 1993; 100: 55–59

153 Montan S, Anandakumar C, Arulkumaran S, Ingemarsson I, Ratnam S. Effects of methyldopa on uteroplacental and fetal hemodynamics in pregnancy-induced hypertension. Am J Obstet Gynecol 1993; 168: 152–156

154 Rey E. Effects of methyldopa on umbilical and placental artery blood flow velocity waveforms. Obstet Gynecol 1992; 80: 783–787

155 Walker J, Mathers A, Bjornsson S, Cameron A, Fairlie F. The effect of acute and chronic antihypertensive therapy on maternal and fetoplacental Doppler velocimetry. Eur J Obstet Gynecol Reprod Biol 1992; 43: 193–199

156 Montan S, Ingemarsson I, Marsal K, Sjøberg N-O. Randomised controlled trial of atenolol and pindolol in human pregnancy: effects on fetal haemodynamics. BM J 1992; 304: 946–949

157 Montan S, Liedholm H, Lingman G, Marsal K, Sjøberg N-O, Solum T. Fetal and uterine haemodynamics during treatment of hypertension in pregnancy with the selective beta-1-blocker atenolol. Br J Obstet Gynaecol 1987; 94: 312–317

158 Olofsson P, Marsal K. Effects of labetalol antihypertensive treatment on uteroplacental and fetal blood circulation. J Matern Fetal Invest 1993; 3: 131–136

159 Duggan P, Cowan L M, Stewart A. Antihypertensive drug effects on placental flow velocity waveforms in pregnant women with severe hypertension. Aust NZ J Obstet Gynaecol 1992; 32: 335–338

160 Grunewald C, Carlström K, Lunell N-O, Nisell H, Nylund L. Dihydralazine in preeclampsia: acute effects on atrial natriuretic peptide concentration and feto-maternal hemodynamics. J Matern Fetal Invest 1993; 3: 21–24

161 Giles W, O'Callaghan S, Boura A, Walters W. Reduction in human fetal umbilical–placental vascular resistance by glyceryl trinitrate. Lancet 1992; 340: 856

162 Hallak M, Moise K, Smith E, Cotton D. The effects of indomethacin and terbutaline on human fetal umbilical artery velocimetry: a randomized, double-blind study. Am J Obstet Gynecol 1993; 168: 865–868

163 Lindblad A, Marsal K. Effects of maternal infusion of terbutaline on fetal blood flow. Int J Feto-Maternal Med 1990; 3: 98–102

164 Faber R, Ruckhäberle K-E, Robel R. Vergleich Dopplersonographisch gemessener utero-plazentofetaler perfusion zwischen normalen schwangerschaften und solchen mit drohender frühgeburt. Zentralbl Gynäkol 1993; 115: 27–32

165 Cosmi E, Luzi G, Fusaro P, Caserta G, Renzo GD. Short-term effects of ritodrine, aminophylline and atropine on umbilical artery blood flow velocity waveform. Eur J Obstet Gynecol Reprod Biol 1992; 46: 7–10

166 Keeley M, Wade R, Laurent S, Hamann V. Alterations in maternal–fetal Doppler flow velocity waveforms in preterm labor patients undergoing magnesium sulfate tocolysis. Obstet Gynecol 1993; 81: 191–194

167 Lindblad A, Ekman G, Marsal K, Ulmsten U. Fetal circulation 60 to 80 minutes after vaginal prostaglandin E$_2$ in pregnant women at term. Arch Gynecol 1985; 237: 31–36

168 Largier D, Rosselli A, Lindow S. Effect of intracervical dinoprostone (prostaglandin E$_2$) gel administration on fetal umbilical artery Doppler waveforms. J Obstet Gynecol 1992; 12: 390–393

169 Gillis S, Connors G, Potts P, Hunse C, Richardson B. The effect of glucose on Doppler flow velocity waveforms and heart rate pattern in the human fetus. Early Hum Dev 1992; 30: 1–10

170 Davies J, Gallivan S, Spencer J. Randomised controlled trial of Doppler ultrasound screening of placental perfusion during pregnancy. Lancet 1992; 340: 1299–1303

171 Mason G, Lilford R, Porter J. Randomised comparison of routine versus highly selective use of Doppler ultrasound in low risk pregnancies. Br J Obstet Gynaecol 1993; 100: 130–133

172 Newnham J, Evans S, Michale C. Effects of frequent ultrasound during pregnancy: a randomised controlled trial. Lancet 1993; 342: 887–891

173 Whittle M, Hanretty K, Primrose M, Neilson J. Screening for the compromised fetus: a randomized trial of umbilical artery velocimetry in unselected pregnancies. Am J Obstet Gynecol 1994; 170: 555–559

174 Neilson J, Alfirevic Z. Doppler ultrasound in high risk pregnancies. In: Neilson J, Crowther C, Hodnett E, Hofmeyr G, Keirse M, eds. Pregnancy and childbirth module of the Cochrane database of systematic reviews. Oxford: The Cochrane Collaboration, 1997

175 Beattie R, Dornan J. Antenatal screening for intrauterine growth retardation with umbilical artery Doppler ultrasonography. BMJ 1989; 298: 631–635

176 Omtzigt A, Reuwer P, Bruinse H. A randomized controlled trial on the clinical value of umbilical Doppler velocimetry in antenatal care. Am J Obstet Gynecol 1994; 170: 625–634

First trimester anomalies

Anna P Cockell and Lyn S Chitty

Introduction

First-trimester sonographic assessment of fetal anatomy has become an important component of prenatal diagnosis. With improved technology, particularly with the use of trans-vaginal probes,[1] it has become possible to assess fetal anatomy in detail within the first trimester.[2,3] Prenatal diagnosis early in pregnancy may be advantageous because it is said to lessen the morbidity of second-trimester diagnosis and abortion. Furthermore, the advent of maternal serum biochemistry testing, at 16 weeks gestation, has driven the need for a routine first-trimester scan to confirm gestational age for interpretation of these serological values. Early diagnosis of pregnancy failure, ectopic and multiple pregnancies has also stimulated this development.

Sonography in the first trimester requires a knowledge of embryological development, so that normal development is not misinterpreted as abnormal. The optimal gestational age for early fetal anomaly scanning will depend on when the majority of fetal structures can be reliably visualised. These are achieved at about 12 weeks, whether using the trans-vaginal (TV) or the transabdominal (TA) route (Table 14.1), although most authors report better overall visualisation using TV sonography.[1,4,5] The exception to this is a large study reporting the preferential use of the TA route to screen for anencephaly at 10–14 weeks.[6] The place of first-trimester sonography as the sole anomaly scan has yet to be proven, as not all anomalies are manifest so early in pregnancy, and standard transabdominal sonography in the second trimester is still recommended.

An increasing range of malformations of both the body wall and the truncal organs has been diagnosed within the first trimester. Diagnostic criteria, and limitations for specific anomalies, must be clearly established before ultrasound screening for anomalies can be introduced in the first trimester.[7] All of the abnormalities illustrated here are from transabdominal scans performed as first-trimester dating scans.

Table 14.1 Gestational age (weeks) at which fetal organs may be visualised in ≥70% of fetuses by transabdominal or trans-vaginal ultrasound (Derived from references 5,29,33,36,39,56)

Fetal structure	Transabdominal	Transvaginal
Cranium	11,12–13	11–12
Spine	12–13	11
Long bones	12–13	10–11
Feet	12	13
Four-chamber view of heart	12–13	12
Kidneys	12–13	11–12
Bladder	12–13	13
Anterior abdominal wall	12–13	12
Face	12–13	12
Stomach	13	11–12

System review

Head and neck

The finding of central nervous system (CNS) defects in the first trimester is relatively common, as the fetal head is the most prominent and easily recognised structure at early gestations. Moreover, CNS anomalies are more frequent at this gestation and comprise about 40% of all fetal malformations.[1] At 8 weeks gestation the intracranial anatomy appears as a single ventricle, the rhomboencephalic cavity and the Y-shape of the dividing telencephalon anteriorly. The large rhomboencephalon, in a posterior position, should not be confused with a Dandy–Walker malformation, which has been reported in the first trimester. An isolated large fourth ventricle in early pregnancy may be a benign transient phenomenon and a physiological variant in early fetal life.[8] Achiron and colleagues[9] described the early detection of a Dandy–Walker cyst at 11 weeks. The choroid plexus in the lateral ventricles becomes visible from 8 weeks, as reflective areas within the relatively poorly refuctive hemispheres. The division of the midline by the falx cerebri, the calcification of the calvarium and visualisation of the cerebellum are not apparent until the 10th week. The ventricles, with the prominent choroid plexuses, are seen filling the calvarium throughout the first trimester, within which choroid plexus cysts may be observed.[7] A small amount of cortex can be seen at the periphery by the end of the 12th week (Fig. 14.1). The corpus callosum does not develop fully until the second trimester, and so the third ventricle may appear both above the thalamus and higher than expected. The ratio of ventricular to biparietal diameter is greater in the first trimester than in the second. Hydrocephaly is

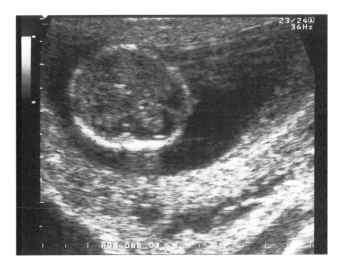

Fig. 14.1 Normal fetal head at 12 weeks: showing the relatively poorly reflective hemispheres with the bright choroid plexus filling the lateral cerebral ventricles.

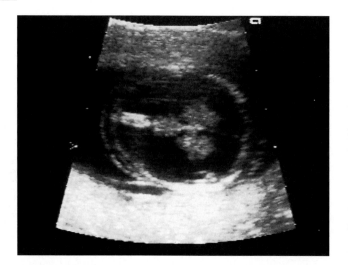

Fig. 14.2 Hydrocephalus at 12 weeks gestation: Note how the choroid plexus is compressed compared to Fig. 14.1. There is also a rim of scalp oedema present.

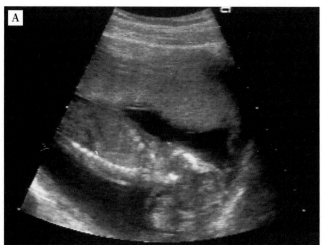

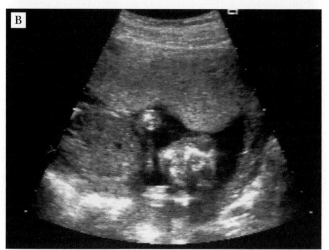

therefore a diagnosis which may be difficult to establish in the first trimester (Figs 14.2 and the Appendix).

Abnormalities of the cranial vault cannot be demonstrated until it becomes calcified. Exencephaly (acrania with preserved brain tissue) can be identified as a large irregular mass of disorganised cranial tissue without a normal cranium. Anencephaly (acrania without brain tissue) (Fig. 14.3), considered to be the natural progression of exencephaly, following abrasion of brain tissue can be seen from 11 weeks.[6,10] However, it is possible to miss the diagnosis of exencephaly owing to the appearance of preserved brain tissue – so-called angiomatous stroma – which may mimic normal neural tissue upon standard TA sonography.[11] Holoprosencephaly may be diagnosed from the end of the first trimester following the identification of the classic sign of lack of midline division anteriorly, together with the prominence of the thalami (Fig. 14.4).

Face

The midline structures are completely fused by the seventh week, but the mandible and maxilla are not clearly visualised until the 10th week. The use of 3D abdominal ultrasound has improved the detection rate of facial anomalies in the early second trimester[12] and may become a useful adjunct in the first trimester for the detection of these anomalies. There have been reports of prenatal diagnosis of midline clefting (Fig. 14.5) in the first trimester, in association with other anomalies such as holoprosencephaly and trisomy 13.[13] In the first trimester, the fetal ears are lower set than is observed in the second trimester, although low-set ears have been described as a sonographic feature in association with multiple anomalies.[4] Hypotelorism has been reported in

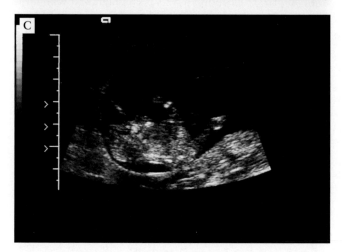

Fig. 14.3 Anencephaly at 12 weeks: with **A:** the parasagittal view showing lack of any ossification in the skull, and **B:** the coronal view demonstrating the typical facial appearance, with prominent eyes and lack of forehead, in this fetus, which also had cystic kidneys and Meckel's syndrome. **C:** shows a different fetus at 12 weeks; note how the fetus appears foreshortened because of the lack of cranial vault (Image courtesy of Sarah Russell.)

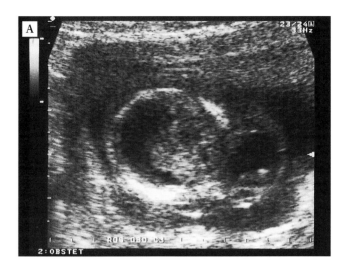

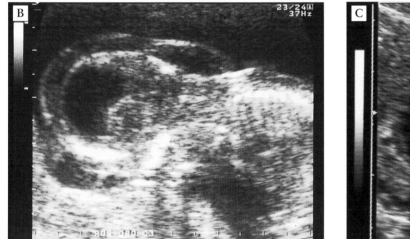

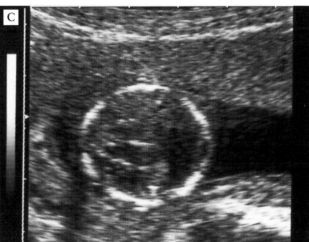

Fig. 14.4 Sonograph at 12+ weeks showing holoprosencephaly and increased nuchal fluid. A: Note the absence of midline anteriorly with prominent thalami. The nuchal fluid simulates an encephalocele in the axial plane, but the parasagittal view B: demonstrates that this echo-free area at the back of the skull is contiguous with the rim of fluid around the head. C: Holoprosencephaly at 13 weeks. Note how the thalami appear to occupy much of the brain.

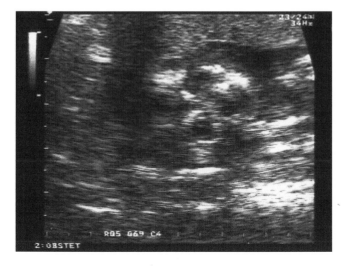

Fig. 14.5 Sonograph of a fetus at 12 weeks with holoprosencephaly and a large midline facial cleft.

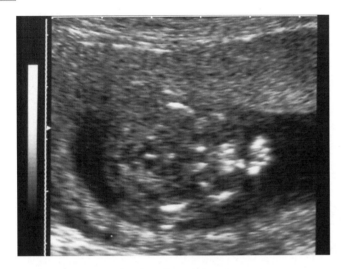

Fig. 14.6 Hypotelorism at 13 weeks gestation.

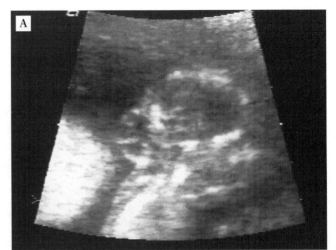

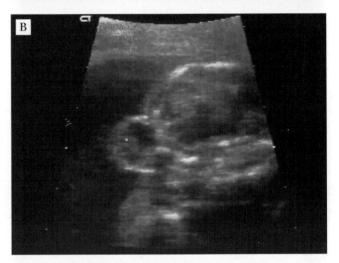

Fig. 14.8 Encephalocele at 13 weeks. A: Viewed in the parasagittal plane. B: Magnified view.

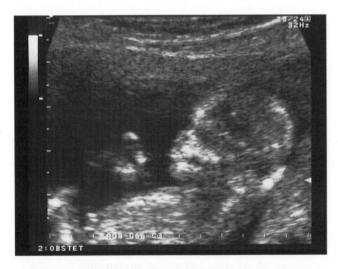

Fig. 14.7 Parasagittal view of the fetal face at 12 weeks gestation demonstrating a normal profile.

association with a neural tube defect (Fig. 14.6).[4] There are now sonographic reference charts available of mandibular and orbital measurements (see Appendix Tables 14, 16 and 17). However, micrognathia may either be too subtle to identify in the first trimester or only become evident in the second, although a normal profile may be discernible (Fig. 14.7).

Craniospinal abnormalities

The dorsal wall of the spine cannot be visualised until the sixth week. Closure of the neural pore and calcification of the lamina of the spine occurs at approximately 6 and 10 weeks, respectively. It is therefore possible to diagnose some neural tube defects (NTD) in the first trimester, e.g. encephalocele (Fig. 14.8) and myelomeningocele.[1] Screening for NTDs has been well established in the second trimester. Accuracy has been enhanced with the use of maternal serum biochemistry (α-fetoprotein) and by recognition of the cerebellar and cranial sonographic markers ('banana' and 'lemon' signs, respectively). First-trimester detection of neural tube defects is dependent on the identification of a spinal irregularity with an overlying skin defect (Fig. 14.9).[14] Detailed assessment requires obtaining both transverse and frontal plane views, which may be difficult to achieve at this early gestation. Indirect signs of NTDs, in the first trimester, such as microcephaly, dolichocephaly, or sharpening of the frontal carena with flattening of the skull at the level of the coronal sutures, is most likely to lead to successful diagnosis. It has been suggested that the fetal head appears acorn-shaped (Fig. 14.10) in association with NTDs in the first trimester, differing from the 'lemon shape' as reported in the second trimester.[14] In

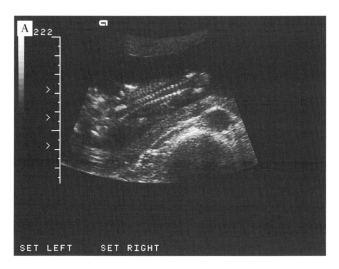

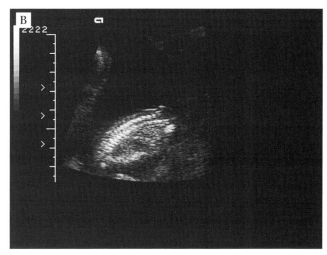

Fig. 14.9 Fetus with spina bifida at 14 weeks gestation. A: Splaying of the vertebral bodies seen in the coronal view; **B:** defect seen in the sacral region in the parasagittal view. (Image courtesy of Sarah Russell.)

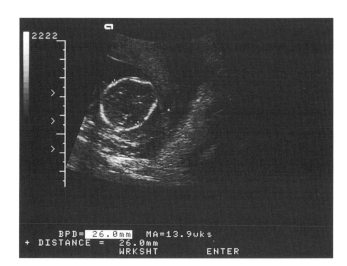

Fig. 14.10 Head of a fetus with spina bifida at 14 weeks. Note the 'acorn' shaped head. (Image courtesy of Sarah Russell.)

early pregnancy a prospective study of 8011 patients at low risk for open spina bifida identified six cases of lumbosacral open spina bifida by systematic screening by TV sonography at 12–17 weeks,[15] four of which were greater than 14 weeks. Other studies have reported false negatives for neural tube defects in the first trimester.[16]

The caudal regression syndrome is a sporadic event, with varying degrees of sacral agenesis to complete absence of the lumbosacral spine. It is more common in poorly controlled diabetics than in the general population.[17] Caudal regression syndrome has been reported in a pregnant woman who presented in diabetic ketoacidotic coma.[18] The diagnosis was suspected in the first trimester and confirmed in the second trimester. We have recently diagnosed sirenomelia (Fig. 14.11A) in a low-risk woman

undergoing a first-trimester scan for a nuchal thickness measurement. Marked cerebral ventriculomegaly was also present (Fig. 14.11B).

Nuchal thickness

An increased nuchal thickness (NT) measurement in the first trimester was reported by Bronshtein *et al.*[19] to have an association with aneuploidy. The NT is the maximum thickness of the subcutaneous translucency between the skin and the soft tissue overlying the cervical spine of the fetus (Fig. 14.12). NT can be conveniently assessed at the dating scan between the 11th and 12th weeks and is therefore a useful screening test for aneuploidy. A normal NT is described as less than 3 mm, but varies with gestational age. An accurate measurement depends on the distinction of both fetal skin and amnion, as at this gestation both structures appear as thin membranes.[20] The sensitivity of this test has been variously described from 0 to 88%, for a false positive rate of 2.7–9.9%, based initially on high-risk or selected populations. More recently Snijders et al.[21] in a multi-centre audit of 96 127 low-risk pregnancies, reported a sensitivity of 82% in the detection of aneuploidy.

Increased NT is also recognised to be associated with structural defects of the cardiovascular or skeletal systems, and also some genetic syndromes. However, not all of these are necessarily amenable to prenatal diagnosis in the first trimester (Tables 14.2 and 14.3). Brady *et al.*[22] reported abnormalities of the cardiovascular and skeletal systems in 10.1% (9 of 89 cases) of the group with increased NT (>3.5 mm), compared with 2% (5 of 302) in those with NT of less than 3.5 mm. This highlights the need to perform detailed second-trimester scanning following the identification of increased NT in a karyotypically normal fetus.

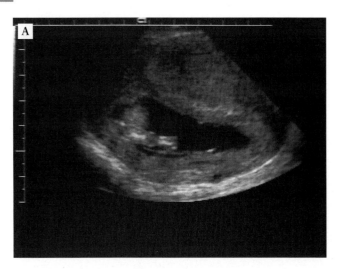

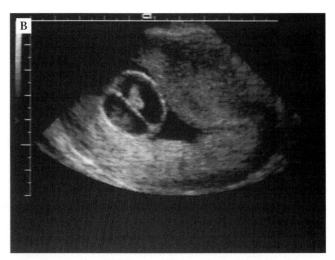

Fig. 14.11 Fetus with sirenomelia at 12 weeks gestation. A: A single femur was seen with two distal bones. **B:** Note the hydrocephalus, with the choroid plexus occupying relatively little space compared to normal (Fig. 14.1).

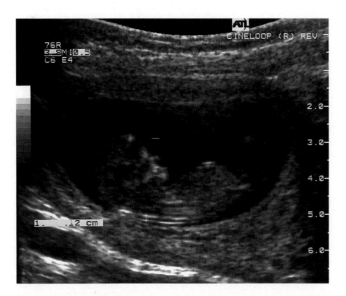

Fig. 14.12 Nuchal thickness measurement.

Table 14.2 Examples of structural abnormalities reported to be associated with an increased nuchal thickness measurement in the first trimester

Structural anomaly	Reference
Congenital diaphragmatic hernia	Sebire *et al.* 1997[38]
Body-stalk anomaly	Daskalis *et al.* 1997[52]
Lethal arthrogryposis	Hyett *et al.* 1997[57]
Heart and great arteries	Hyett *et al.* 1997[11];
	Brady *et al.* 1998[22]
Multicystic kidney	Brady *et al.* 1998[22]
Cystic hygromas	Trauffer *et al.* 1994[27]

Table 14.3 Examples of genetic syndromes reported to be associated with increased nuchal thickness measurement in the first trimester

Syndrome	Reference
Noonans	Trauffer *et al.* 1994[27]
Smith–Lemli–Optiz	Hobbins *et al.* 1994[25]
Pierre-Robin	Brady *et al.* 1998[22]
Roberts	Trauffer *et al.* 1994[27]
Meckel–Grüber	Sepulveda *et al.* 1997[59]

Hydrops and nuchal thickness

When the NT is greater than 4 mm it is often associated with more extensive skin oedema or hydrops (Fig. 14.13). In the first trimester fetal hydrops is unlikely to be due to the causes of hydrops that are common in the second trimester, such as blood group alloimmunisation.[23] It has been associated with haematological, cardiovascular, pulmonary, renal, gastrointestinal, hepatic, neoplastic, chromosomal, hereditary or infectious disorder of the fetus.[24] An increased NT may be a component of fetal hydrops and suggest cardiac or thoracic abnormalities affecting fetal venous and lymphatic return. Fetal hydrops in the first trimester has a high positive predictive value as a marker of aneuploidy in early pregnancy, particularly associated with Turner's syndrome and the more common trisomies (21, 18 and 13). The study by Iskaros *et al.*[24] described an incidence of chromosomal abnormalities of 77.8% in their series seen in a fetal medicine unit.

Genetic syndromes and nuchal thickness

A number of syndromes have been reported to be associated with increased NT, and therefore could be amenable to prenatal diagnosis in the first trimester (Table 14.3).

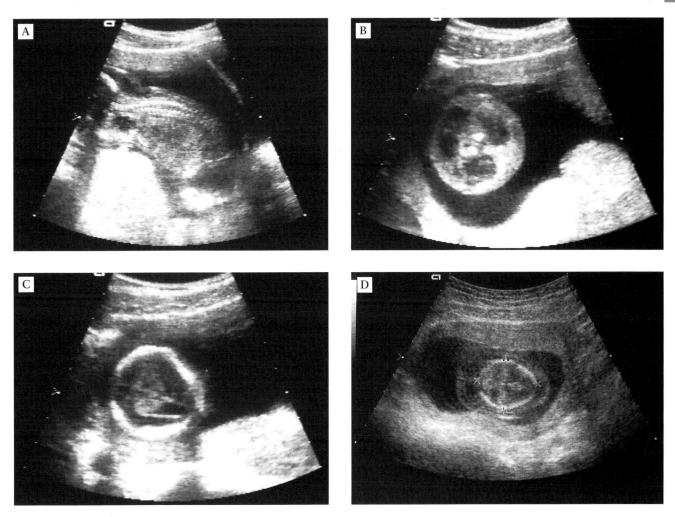

Fig. 14.13 Neck oedema in a fetus with trisomy 18 at 12 weeks. A: Parasagittal view. B: Transverse view through the fetal neck. C: View of the skull demonstrating the strawberry shape. D: Another case of hydrops the oedema spreads downwards over the trunk.

However, in most reports this has been a retrospective association with the syndrome, the diagnosis only becoming apparent post-natally. This association may be useful for early diagnosis of inherited syndromes where genetic diagnosis or linkage studies are not available but the parents are known to be at high risk. If the genetic syndrome has associated structural anomalies, diagnosis may be facilitated in the first trimester. For example, in Smith–Lemli–Opitz syndrome, an autosomal recessive syndrome of multiple congenital anomalies secondary to a defect in cholesterol synthesis, sonographic findings that may aid the diagnosis are cardiac, renal and skeletal malformations.[25]

Cystic hygromas

Cystic hygromas (Fig. 14.14) are fluid-filled sacculations of the lateral neck and nuchal region that probably result from lymphatic dysplasia.[4] They must be differentiated from the sonographic finding of an increased NT. In the first trimester cystic hygromas appear to be contained in the neck, whereas a comparable increased NT will extend to the chest, with more generalised skin oedema. Cystic hygromas tend to persist but may resolve without any adverse outcome,[26] the significance of which is not clear. Studies report high[4] and low[19] incidences of aneuploidy in association with this anomaly. Reports have associated cystic hygromas with Noonan's syndrome,[27] Turner's syndrome, Fryns' syndrome[28] and other genetic malformations. Bronshtein and colleagues[19] found that the septated cases have a poor outcome and are associated with chromosomal aberrations, whereas those with a non-septated appearance have a more favourable prognosis.

Skeletal abnormalities

The timing of the appearance of ossified regions of developing bone is important. TV sonography detects the mineralised regions of bones about a week earlier than does

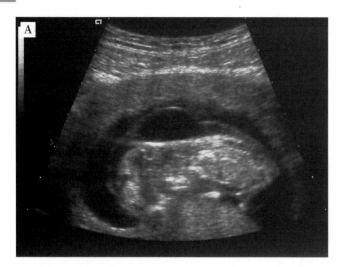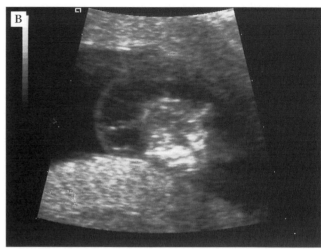

Fig. 14.14 Sonographs of a large cystic hygroma at 11 weeks gestation. A. Note the generalised skin oedema which can be seen in the parasagittal view. B: The septations are demonstrated in the transverse view.

the TA approach. Limb paddles can be seen at 6–7 weeks and ossification of the long bones appears at about the 10th week.[29] Distinct digits can readily be seen by this gestation, and by 12 weeks the limbs and digits can be seen using both TA and TV ultrasound. The sonographic diagnosis of radial club hand (Fig. 14.15) and postaxial polydactyly has been reported in the first trimester, as well as other skeletal anomalies such as talipes (Fig. 14.16); rib anomalies (Fig. 14.17) may also be amenable to prenatal diagnosis. For postural deformities the aetiology of the problem as well as the degree of deformity may well be a limiting factor in the timing of diagnosis. Where there is an absence or malformation of a bone(s) then the abnormality may be amenable to early diagnosis with ultrasound, as

the bony structure of the fetus is so readily examined, particularly between 13 and 14 weeks gestation. However, most anomalies of this type will arise in low-risk pregnancies, and diagnosis will depend on careful, systematic examination of many fetuses.

It is currently not known when many specific skeletal dysplasias will become manifest, but knowledge of the normal development of the ossification centres of the fetal skeleton remains the key to early prenatal diagnosis. However, short limb dysplasia,[30] mesomelic dysplasia[4] and achondrogenesis[31] have all been reported in the first trimester. Some conditions (e.g. achondroplasia, osteogenesis imperfecta types IIB, III) are not amenable to diagnosis until the second trimester, and others (e.g. spondyloepiphy-

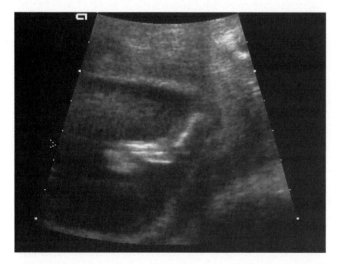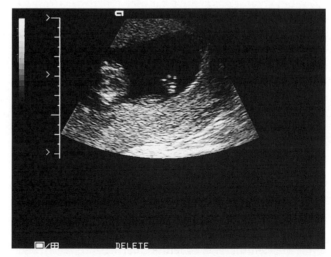

Fig. 14.15 Radial club hand in a 13-week fetus subsequently found to have trisomy 18.

Fig. 14.16 Talipes in a fetus at 13+ weeks gestation. (Image courtesy of Sarah Russell.)

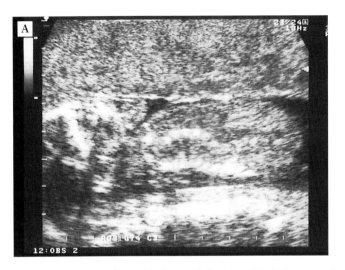 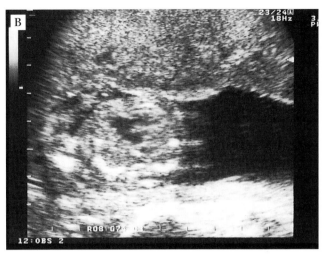

Fig. 14.17 A 13-week fetus with abnormal ribs. viewed in **A:** the parasagittal plane and **B:** transverse section. Note how the ribs appear short and irregular.

seal dysplasia congenita[32]), with even more severe degrees of short stature, have been shown to have normal limb lengths in the first trimester.

Cardiovascular system

The heart can easily be recognised by real-time ultrasound at 7 weeks[33] as a relatively large beating structure below the embryonic head. It is occasionally possible by TV sonography to identify the atrial and ventricular walls moving reciprocally as early as the end of the eighth week. By 10 weeks the moving valves and the inter-ventricular septum can be more readily identified. Detailed investigation of fetal cardiac anatomy performed in a segmental approach is feasible from 13 weeks gestation.[34] A four-chamber view of the heart can be obtained as early as 11 weeks, and evaluation of the cardiac chambers and atrioventricular valvular leaflets made from the 10th weeks.[33,35] However, chamber diameter discrepancies may not become apparent until later in pregnancy. Likewise, the great artery insertions may not be visualised. The use of colour Doppler complements classic 2D echocardiography in the first trimester, allowing visualisation of intracardiac blood flow and hence the detection of valvular insufficiencies and stenoses.[35]

First-trimester detected cardiac abnormalities are associated with a high incidence of karyotypic abnormalities: Gembruch and colleagues reported an incidence of 48.6%.[36] This may represent a high-risk population referred for early diagnosis of other structural anomalies, i.e. hydrops or extracardiac abnormalities, but also represents the identification of fetuses that will inevitably abort in the late first trimester.[37] Pericardial effusions may also be detected in the first trimester (Fig. 14.18).

Respiratory system

The fetal diaphragm is formed by 9 weeks gestation. To our knowledge there are no reports of the diagnosis of thoracic anomalies prior to 14 weeks, although diagnosis of some lesions is a possibility (Fig. 14.19). Although there have been no reported cases of diaphragmatic herniation in the first trimester, Sebire and colleagues[38] have reported increased NT in a series of cases that were later found to have diaphragmatic hernias in the second or third trimester. They suggested that up to 40% of fetuses with diaphragmatic hernia have an increased NT in the first trimester, suggesting that an increased NT is a marker of intrathoracic compression. The presence of intrathoracic herniation within the first trimester would increase the likelihood of pulmonary hypoplasia and significantly worsen the prognosis.

The identification of cystic adenomatous malformation in first-trimester fetuses has not been reported. This may indicate that this pulmonary disorder is gestation dependent and either evolve, or only be sonographically detectable, with the maturity of the pulmonary parenchyma.

Genitourinary system

Visualisation of the fetal urogenital tract has been greatly improved by TV sonography. Rosati and Guariglia[39] have compiled charts for kidney parameters at early stages of pregnancy, with growth patterns (transverse, longitudinal, anterior–posterior diameters and circumference) between 11 and 16 weeks' gestation (see also Appendix for charts derived for transabdominal measurements of the kidneys). This study reported smaller parameters than those obtained by TA sonography reported by other

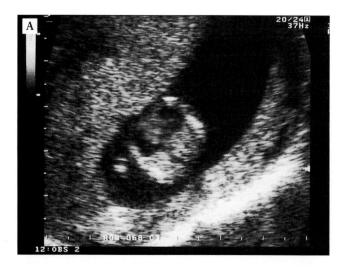 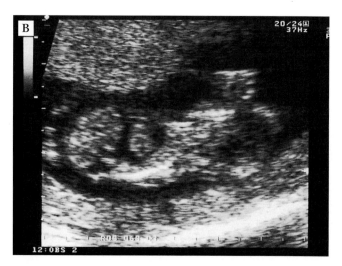

Fig. 14.18 Pericardial effusion at 11 weeks' gestation: The fluid collection surrounding the heart can be seen clearly in **A:** the transverse and **B:** longitudinal views. This resolved spontaneously over a period of several weeks and there were no obvious problems in the neonate.

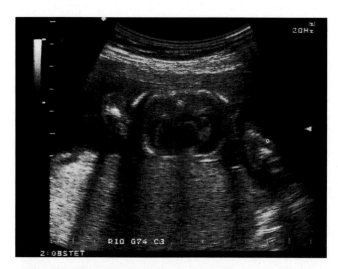

Fig. 14.19 Transverse view through the fetal chest at 13 weeks gestation showing bilateral pleural effusions.

authors,[40,41] as the cranial pole of the kidney is particularly difficult to define accurately by a TA scan in the longitudinal plane at this gestation. The fetal adrenal and renal parenchyma have very similar homogeneous patterns and are difficult to differentiate, resulting in an apparent increase in kidney length, but using the TV approach the disproportionately large fetal adrenals can be more easily identified.[39]

The normal sonographic parameters of the renal pelvis have not been established in the first trimester. In the study by Rosati and colleagues,[39] in accordance with the diameters proposed by Bronshtein et al.[42] 3 mm was chosen as the upper limit of normal of the fetal renal pelvis in the anterior–posterior diameter. Renal pyelectasis was diagnosed in 4.1% of fetuses in this study, 40.9% of which

were still present (>5 mm) at 18–26 weeks' gestation. There were no karyotypic abnormalities among these cases. In a screening study by Hernadi and colleagues[43] four cases of pyelectasis were identified in 3991 cases at 20 weeks, only one of which was diagnosed by TV scanning in the first trimester.

Bilateral renal agenesis has been reported in a few studies in the first trimester, suspected by an inability to demonstrate both the fetal bladder and the kidneys; however, classically this does not present until the second trimester, when fetal urine output is the predominant component in amniotic fluid production. Bronshtein et al.[44] reported five cases with renal agenesis where, at 14 weeks, large reflective masses were seen in the fetal abdomen which at post-mortem were later identified as enlarged adrenals.

Polycystic kidney disease may be difficult to diagnose in the first trimester and the sonographic appearances may not be detectable until the second trimester or later. In a report by Bronshtein et al.[44] a case of infantile polycystic kidney disease was detected at 26 weeks gestation; however, the retrospective review of the first-trimester videotape showed bilaterally large highly reflective kidneys. Multicystic kidney disease does not appear to be amenable to first trimester diagnosis. In the screening study by Hernadi et al.[43] three cases of unilateral multicystic dysplastic kidneys were identified at the second and third trimester scans, but had not been identified in the first trimester.

The bladder is visualised in 94% of cases by 12–13 weeks.[5] At 10–14 weeks a normal fetal bladder measures less than 6 mm and the bladder/crown–rump length (CRL) ratio is less than 10%.[45] Sebire et al.[45] reported megacystis in 10–14-week pregnancies, suggesting an incidence in a high-risk population of 1/1600 pregnancies. In seven of the 15 cases spontaneous resolution occured without obvious adverse consequences to the urinary system, whereas all those that had been shunted *in utero* miscarried. The aetiology of persistent megacystis is the same as later in pregnancy, with posterior urethral valves being the most common cause in males (Fig. 14.20); in females cloacal anomalies may predominate (Fig. 14.21).

The genital organs are often not completely formed until 11 weeks, although the male phallus can be seen at this time. However, gender assignment using ultrasound should be cautious until later in pregnancy.

Gastrointestinal system

In a longitudinal study Blaas *et al.*[33] reported the normal sonographic embryonic development of the truncal struc-tures (abdominal wall, stomach and heart) from 7 weeks gestation and established reproducible biometric para-meters. The initial sign of the physiological midgut herni-ation occurs during week 7, as a thickening of the cord containing a small refletive area at the abdominal inser-tion. Herniation of the fetal intestines into the coelom of the umbilical cord is present in all fetuses from 8 weeks 3 days to 10 weeks 4 days[33] (Fig. 14.22). The large reflective mass is most obvious between weeks 9 and 10, measuring maximally longitudinally at 10 weeks and 2–4 days (mean 4.1 mm, range 2.4–5.8 mm). The elongating and coiling intestine rotates through 90° in an anticlockwise direction and when returning to the abdomen rotates a further 180° during weeks 7–8.[46] The gut has always retracted into the abdominal cavity by 12 weeks gestation.[4,7,33,47] The bowel

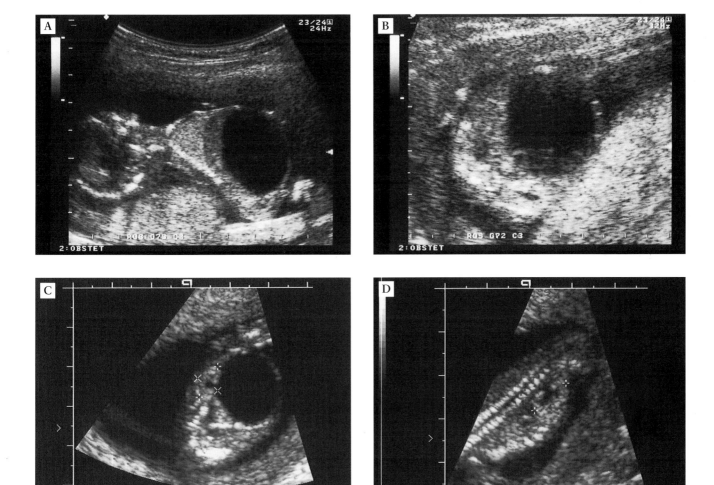

Fig. 14.20 Bladder outflow obstruction in a male fetus at 13 weeks gestation. Note the grossly dilated bladder seen in **A:** the parasagittal and **B:** transverse views. The reflective kidneys with minimal renal pelvic dilatation can be seen in the transverse section. The bladder was aspirated twice and then there was spontaneous resolution of the megacystis. The bladder remained thick walled throughout pregnancy, but kidneys and liquor volume appeared normal. A similar case is shown **C:** in transverse and **D:** longitudinal section, showing the reflective kidneys and pelvic dilatation, but in this case the megacystis persisted and the presence of posterior urethral valves was confirmed at post-mortem after termination of the pregnancy at 18 weeks.

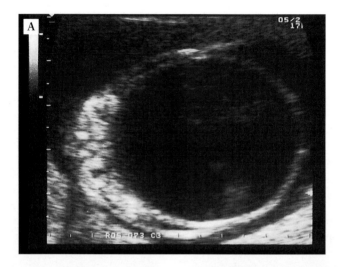

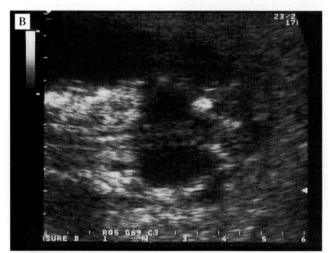
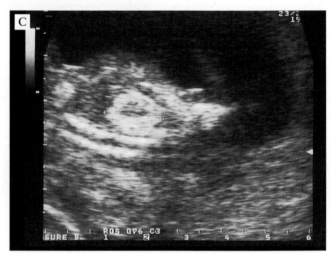

Fig. 14.21 Bladder outflow obstruction in a female fetus at 13 weeks gestation. A: The transverse view shows the hugely dilated bladder with highly reflective kidneys and prominent renal pelves. The kidneys appear very reflective both in transverse and **B:** longitudinal views, and **C:** remain so after aspiration of the bladder. The pregnancy was terminated at 17 weeks gestation and post-mortem examination revealed a complex cloacal anomaly.

may appear highly reflective as it returns to the fetal abdomen.

There are a number of reports of ventral wall defects at 11–12 weeks.[1,4,48] Exomphalos (Figs 14.23 and 14.24) is diagnosed after the expected time for the retraction of the physiological herniation, and in some cases the liver may be identified within the hernial sac[49] (Fig. 14.24). Gastroschisis is a paramedian anterior wall defect without a true peritoneal covering of the protruding bowel, and is identified at a small but detectable distance from the cord insertion (Fig. 14.25). Kushnir *et al.*[50] reported a fetus at 13 weeks with sonographic features of gastroschisis, a free-floating cauliflower-shaped mass protruding through the fetal abdomen. The diagnosis was confirmed later in gestation. Cullen *et al.*[4] have also reported gastroschisis at 11 weeks, but in association with both an encephalocele and kyphoscoliosis. The pregnancy was terminated.

Body-stalk anomaly is a lethal sporadic abnormality reported in about 1 in 14 000 births. It is characterised by a major abdominal wall defect, severe kyphoscoliosis and a rudimentary umbilical cord,[51] and may be diagnosed in the first trimester.[52,53] In a screening study of 3991 patients there were two cases of body-stalk anomaly diagnosed at the 11–14-week scan, and in one of these it was associated with increased NT thickness.[43]

The stomach is seen as a well delineated poorly reflective structure on the left side of the abdomen, inferior to the diaphragm, at 10–11 weeks. It can be identified as early as 8 weeks[33] and becomes more distinct with increasing gestation,[7] accumulating gastric and duodenal epithelial secretions. The finding of an empty stomach in the first trimester may be normal. Fetal swallowing movements are initiated at 11 weeks,[54] though amniotic fluid is not actually swallowed at this gestation. Abnormalities of the

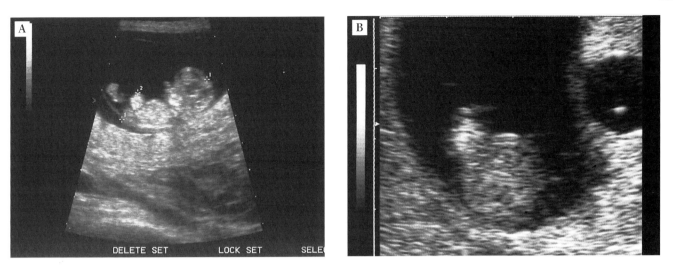

Fig. 14.22 A: **Longitudinal view of a fetus at 11 weeks gestation:** showing the physiological herniation of the gut (marked 2). **B:** A transverse view taken at 10 weeks and 4 days.

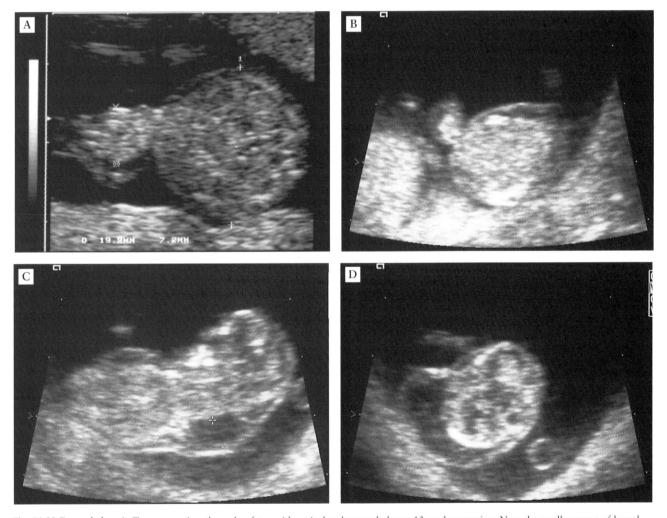

Fig. 14.23 **Exomphalos. A:** Transverse view through a fetus with an isolated examphalos at 13 weeks gestation. Note the small amount of bowel which has herniated into the base of the cord. **B:** The transverse view shows a small exomphalos in a 12-week fetus which **C:** also had an increased nuchal fold and **D:** generalised oedema, with underlying trisomy 18.

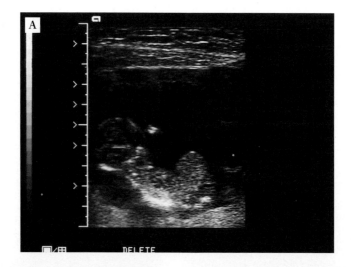

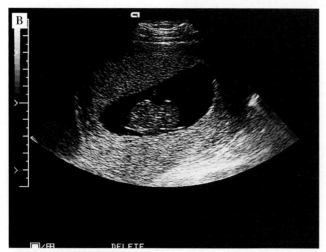
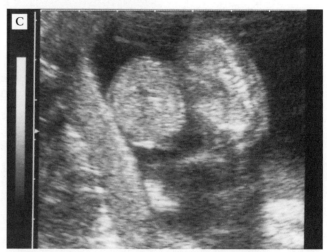

Fig. 14.24 Exomphalos. A: Longitudinal and **B:** transverse views, through a fetus with an exomphalos and trisomy 18 at 13 weeks gestation. Note the homogeneous nature of the contents and the larger sac in this fetus where the liver has herniated. (Image courtesy of Sarah Russell.) **C:** Similar appearances are seen in a fetus at 12 weeks, with virtually the entire liver herniated into the sac.

upper gastrointestinal tract have been reported in the first trimester. Tuskerman and colleagues[55] reported a 12-week fetus with a grossly dilated stomach and duodenum with oesophageal and duodenal atresia. However, gut anomalies often do not present until later in pregnancy, and the sensitivity of first-trimester ultrasound is poor in this area.

Other abnormalities

There are many other abnormalities that have not been covered in this brief description of first- and early second-trimester ultrasound. Some, such as tumours, may be detected, but early identification will depend on the rate of growth. Figure 14.26 shows a sacrococcygeal teratoma which was detected at 14 weeks gestation. However, such

abnormalities are more likely to be detected when a woman is scanned in the late second or third trimester because of a clinical finding such as polyhydramnios.

Early scanning can be useful for ascertaining the number of fetuses present and the zygosity of twins by looking for the twin peak sign (see Ch. 12). Structural abnormalities in twin pregnancies may be identified in the first trimester as for singletons, and other anomalies, such as conjoined twins (Fig. 14.27), may also be more readily identified in the first trimester.

Role of first trimester diagnosis

Screening for structural anomalies in the first trimester has some advantages over second-trimester screening. A

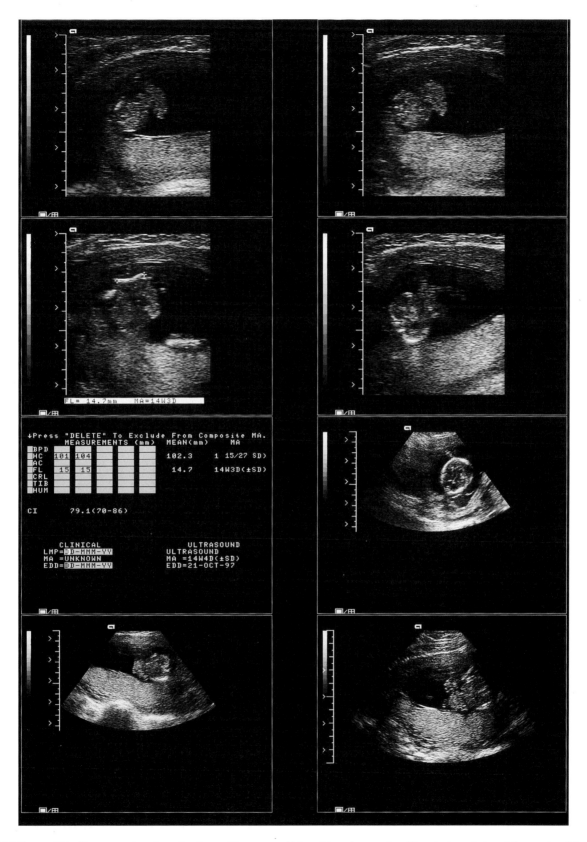

Fig. 14.25 Gastroschisis. Transverse view through a fetus with a gastroschisis at 14 weeks gestation. Note the irregularity of the margin of the herniated contents compared to the views of fetuses with an exomphalos (Figs 23 A and B and 24 B and C). Image courtesy of Sarah Russell.

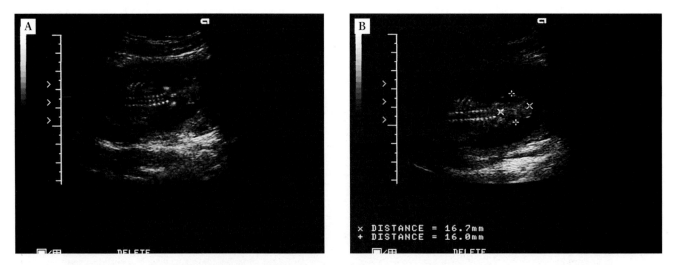

Fig. 14.26 Sacrococcygeal teratoma. Coronal views at 14 weeks showing a large tumour. protruding from the end of the spine in this fetus with a sacrococcygeal teratoma. Image courtesy of Sarah Russell.

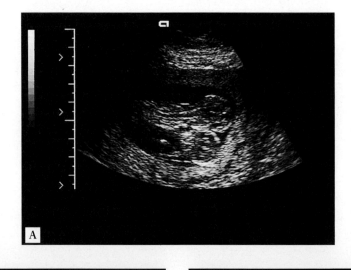

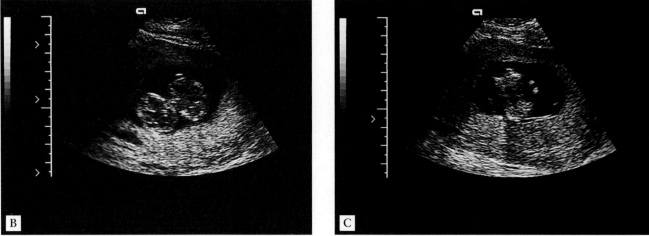

Fig. 14.27 Conjoined twins. A: Longitudinal and **B:** transverse view through the fetal heads and **C:** abdomens in conjoined twins at 11 weeks gestation, showing the extent of joining from head through to abdomen. Image courtesy of Sarah Russell.

normal sonographic assessment at 12 weeks can be reassuring, yet such reassurances must be guarded in view of the failure to detect some anomalies that are sonographically gestation dependent, e.g. duodenal atresia, hydrocephalus and many renal abnormalities. The natural history of some conditions detected in the first trimester remain unclear, e.g. bright reflective kidneys, choroid plexus cysts. Some findings resolve spontaneously with no long-term consequences, e.g. cystic hygroma. These sonographic findings may not have the same clinical significance as when detected in the second trimester, and may lead to considerable parental anxiety following identification.

When considering the implementation of first-trimester screening, whether for general structural or chromosomal abnormalities, it should be appreciated that many pregnancies complicated with serious abnormalities will spontaneously abort in the first or early second trimester. With inadequate data from longitudinal studies of sonographic findings in the first trimester and inadequate knowledge of the natural history, it is difficult to counsel parents appropriately. One of the potential advantages of a first-trimester diagnosis is the potential to offer surgical termination. This benefit must be carefully weighed against any potential harm that might result from making parents choose to terminate a wanted pregnancy that might have aborted spontaneously. Similarly, some karyotypically normal pregnancies and some that might abort spontaneously will be considered for invasive testing, with the inevitable risk of miscarriage. Furthermore, invasive testing for fetal karyotyping has a higher risk of miscarriage and other complications in the first trimester than in the second. The advantages of early fetal diagnosis is not supported at present by an early safe invasive test.

The future

With the rapid development of ultrasound technology, first-trimester ultrasound screening is becoming an important component of prenatal diagnosis. Many structural abnormalities have now been reported in the first trimester. However, the clinical cost–benefit ratio of this test needs to be fully evaluated before its true benefits and burdens become clear.

REFERENCES

1　Achiron R, Tadmor O. Screening for fetal anomalies during the first trimester of pregnancy: transvaginal versus transabdominal sonography. Ultrasound Obstet Gynecol 1991; 1: 186–191

2　Cullen M T, Green J J, Reece E A, Hobbins J C. Evaluation of the first trimester embryo. A comparison of transvaginal and abdominal sonography. J Ultrasound Med 1989; 8: 565–569

3　Timor-Tritsch I E, Farine D, Rosen M. A close look at early embryonic development with the high-frequency transvaginal transducer. Am J Obstet Gynecol 1988; 159: 676–681

4　Cullen M T, Green J, Whetham J, Salafia C, Gabrielli S, Hobbins J C. Transvaginal ultrasonographic detection of congenital anomalies in the first trimester. Am J Obstet Gynecol 1990; 163: 466–476

5　Braithwaite J M, Armstrong M A, Economides D L. Assessment of fetal anatomy at 12 to 13 weeks' of gestation by transabdominal and transvaginal sonography. Br J Obstet Gynaecol 1998; 103: 82–85

6　Johnson S P, Sebire N J, Snijders R J M, Trunkel S, Nicolaides K H. Ultrasound screening for anencephaly at 10–14 weeks of gestation. Ultrasound Obstet Gynecol 1997; 9: 10–14

7　Green J J, Hobbins J C. Abdominal ultrasound examination of the first-trimester fetus. Am J Obstet Gynecol 1988; 159: 165–175

8　Bronshtein M, Zimmer E Z, Blazer S. Isolated large fourth ventricle in early pregnancy – a possible benign transient phenomenon. Prenat Diagn 1998; 18: 997–1000

9　Achiron R, Achiron A, Yagel S. First trimester transvaginal sonographic diagnosis of Dandy–Walker malformation. JCU 1993; 21: 62–64

10　Johnson A, Losure T A, Weiner S. Early diagnosis of fetal anencephaly. JCU 1985; 13: 503–505

11　Goldstein R B, Filly R A, Callen N A. Sonography of anencephaly: pitfalls in early diagnosis. JCU 1989; 17: 397–402

12　Merz E, Weber G, Bahlmann F, Mirc-Tesanic D. Application of transvaginal and abdominal three-dimensional ultrasound for the detection or exclusion of malformations of the fetal face. Ultrasound Obstet Gynecol 1997; 9: 237–243

13　Parant O, Sarramon M F, Delisle M B, Toulouse-La Grave C H U. Prenatal diagnosis of holoprosencephaly. A series of 12 cases. J Gynécol Obstet Biol Reprod 1997; 26: 686–696

14　Bernard J P, Suarez B, Rambaud C, Muller F, Ville Y. Prenatal diagnosis of neural tube defect before 12 weeks' gestation: direct and indirect ultrasonographic semiology. Ultrasound Obstet Gynecol 1997; 10: 406–409

15　Blumenfeld Z, Siegler E, Bronshtein M. The early diagnosis of neural tube defects. Prenat Diagn 1993; 13: 1863–1871

16　Economides D L, Braithwaite J M, Armstrong M A. First trimester fetal abnormality screening in a low risk population. Proc Br Congress Obstet Gynaecol, Dublin, 1995; 455

17　Souka A P, Nicolaides K H. Diagnosis of fetal abnormalites at the 10–14-week scan. Ultrasound Obstet Gynecol 1997; 10: 429–442

18　Baxi L, Warren W, Collins M, Timor-Tritsch I E. Early detection of caudal regression syndrome with transvaginal scanning. Ultrasound Obstet Gynecol 1990; 10: 416–418

19　Bronshtein M, Rottem S, Yoffe N, Blumenfeld Z. First trimester diagnosis of nuchal cystic hygroma by transvaginal sonography: diverse prognosis of the septated and nonseptated lesion. Am J Obstet Gynecol 1989; 161: 78–82

20　Chitty L S, Pandya P P. Ultrasound screening for fetal abnormalities in the first trimester. Prenat Diagn 1995; 17: 1269–1281

21　Snijders R J M, Noble P, Souka A P. UK multicentre project on assessment of risk of trisomy 21 by maternal age and fetal nuchal-translucency thickness at 10–14 weeks of gestation. Lancet 1998; 351: 343–346

22　Brady A F, Pandya P P, Yuksel B, Greenough A, Patton M A, Nicolaides K H. Outcome of chromosomally normal livebirths with increased fetal nuchal translucency at 10–14 weeks' gestation. J Med Genet 1998; 35: 222–224

23　Jauniaux E, Van Maldergram L, De Munter C, Moscoco G, Gillerot Y. Non-immune hydrops fetalis associated with genetic abnormalities. Obstet Gynecol 1990; 75: 568–572

24　Iskaros J, Jauniaux E, Rodeck C H. Outcome of nonimmune hydrops fetalis diagnosed during the first half of pregnancy. Obstet Gynecol 1997; 90: 321–325

25　Hobbins J C, Jones O W, Gottesfeld S, Persutte W. Transvaginal sonography and transabdominal embryoscopy in the first trimester diagnosis of Smith–Lemli–Opitz syndrome type 2. Am J Obstet Gynecol 1994; 171: 546–549

26　Macken M B, Grantmyre E B, Vincer M J. Regression of nuchal cystic hygroma *in utero*. JCU 1989; 8: 101–103

27　Trauffer P M L, Anderson C E, Johnson A, Heeger S, Morgan P, Wapner R J. The natural history of euploid pregnancies with first trimester cystic hygromas. Am J Obstet Gynecol 1994; 170: 1279–1283

28　Hosli I M, Tercanli S, Rehder H, Holzgreve W. Cystic hygroma as an early first trimester ultrasound marker for recurrent Fryns' syndrome. Ultrasound Obstet Gynecol 1997; 10: 422–424

29 van Zalen-Sprock R M, Brons J T L, van Hugt J M G, van der Harten H J, van Geijn H P. Ultrasonographic and radiological visualization of the developing embryonic skeleton. Ultrasound Obstet Gynecol 1997; 9: 392–397

30 Benacerraf B R, Lister J E, DuPonte B L. First-trimester diagnosis of fetal abnormalities. A report of three cases. J Reprod Med 1988; 33: 777–780

31 Soothill P W, Vuthiwong C, Rees H. Achondrogenesis type 2 diagnosed by transvaginal ultrasound at 12 weeks' gestation. Prenat Diagn 1993; 13: 523–528

32 Nisbet D L, Heath V, Chitty L S, Sams V R, Hall C M, Rodeck C H. Prenatal ultrasound findings in compound heterozygote skeletal dysplasia – a report of two affected pregnancies. Prenat Diagn 2000; in press

33 Blaas H-G, Eik-Nes S H, Kiserud T, Hellvik L R. Early development of the abdominal wall, stomach and heart from 7 to 12 weeks of gestation: a longitudinal ultrasound study. Ultrasound Obstet Gynecol 1995; 6: 240–249

34 Gembruch U, Knopfle G, Chatterjee M, Bald R, Hansmann M. First-trimester diagnosis of fetal congenital heart disease by transvaginal two-dimensional and Doppler echocardiography. Obstet Gynecol 1990; 75: 496–498

35 Gembruch U, Knopfle G, Chatterjee M, Bald R, Hansmann M. Early diagnosis of fetal congenital heart disease by transvaginal echocardiography. Ultrasound Obstet Gynecol 1993; 3: 310–317

36 Gembruch U, Baschat A A, Knopfle G, Hansmann M. Results of chromosomal analysis in cardiac analysis in fetuses with cardiac anomalies as diagnosed by first and early second-trimester echocardiography. Ultrasound Obstet Gynecol 1997; 10: 391–396

37 Snijders R J M, Holzgreve W, Cuckle H, Nicolaides K H. Maternal age-specific risks for trisomies at 9–14 weeks' gestation. Prenat Diagn 1994; 14: 543–552

38 Sebire N J, Snijders R J M, Davenport M, Greenough A, Nicolaides K H. Fetal nuchal translucency thickness at 10–14 weeks' gestation and congenital diaphragmatic hernia. Obstet Gynecol 1997; 90: 943–946

39 Rosati P, Guariglia L. Transvaginal sonographic assessment of the fetal urinary tract in early pregnancy. Ultrasound Obstet Gynecol 1996; 7: 95–100

40 Bertagnoli L, Lalatta F, Gallicchio R et al. Quantative characterization of the growth of the fetal kidney. JCU 1983; 11: 349–356

41 Grannum P, Bracken M, Silverman R, Hobbins J C. Assessment of fetal kidney size in normal gestation by comparison of ratio of kidney circumference to abdominal circumference. Am J Obstet Gynecol 1980; 136: 249–254

42 Bronshtein M, Yoffe N, Brandes J M, Blumenfeld Z. First and early second trimester diagnosis of fetal urinary tract anomalies using transvaginal sonography. Prenat Diagn 1990; 10: 653–666

43 Hernadi L, Torcsik M. Screening for fetal anomalies in the 12th week of pregnancy by transvaginal sonography in an unselected population. Prenat Diagn 1997; 17: 753–759

44 Bronshtein M, Amit A, Achiron R, Noy I, Blumenfeld Z. The early prenatal diagnosis of renal agenesis: techniques and possible pitfalls. Prenat Diagn 1994; 4: 291–297

45 Sebire N J, Von Kaisenberg C, Rubio C, Snijders R J M, Nicolaides K H. Fetal megacystis at 10–14 weeks of gestation. Ultrasound Obstet Gynecol 1996; 8: 387–390

46 The digestive system, rotation of the midgut. In: Moore K. Moore K, eds. The developing human. Philadelphia: W B Saunders, 1988: 228–229

47 Timor-Tritsch I E, Warren W B, Peisner D, Pirrone E. First trimester midgut herniation: a high frequency transvaginal sonographic study. Am J Obstet Gynecol 1989; 161: 466–476

48 Rotten S, Bronshtein M. Transvaginal sonographic diagnosis of congenital anomalies between 9 weeks' and 16 weeks' menstrual age. JCU 1990; 18: 307–314

49 Gray D L, Martin C M, Crane J P. Differential diagnosis of first trimester ventral wall defects. J Ultrasound Med 1989; 8: 255–258

50 Kushnir O, Izquierdo L, Vigil L, Curet L B. Early transvaginal diagnosis of gastroschisis. JCU 1990; 18: 194–197

51 Mann L, Ferguson-Smith M A, Desai M, Gibson A A M, Raine P A M. Prenatal assessment of anterior abdominal wall defects and their prognosis. Prenat Diagn 1984; 4: 427–435

52 Daskalis G, Sebire N J, Jurkovic D, Snijders R J M, Nicolaides K H. Body stalk anomaly at 10–14 weeks of gestation. Ultrasound Obstet Gynecol 1997; 10: 416–418

53 Ginsberg N E, Cadkin A, Strom C. Prenatal diagnosis of body stalk anomaly in the first trimester. Ultrasound Obstet Gynecol 1997; 10: 419–421

54 Diamant N E. Development of esophageal function. Am Rev Respir Dis 1985; 131: 29–32

55 Tuskerman G L, Krapiva G A, Kirillova I A. First trimester diagnosis of duodenal stenosis associated with oesophageal atresia. Prenat Diagn 1993; 13: 371–376

56 Timor-Tritsch I E, Monteaguedo A, Peisner D B. High-frequency transvaginal sonographic examination of the potential malformation assessment of the 9-week to 14-week fetus. JCU 1992; 20: 231–238

57 Hyett J, Noble P, Sebire N J, Snijders R J M, Nicolaides K H. Lethal congenital arthrogryposis presents with increased nuchal translucency at 10–14 weeks of gestation. Ultrasound Obstet Gynecol 1997; 9: 310–313

58 Hyett J, Moscoso G, Nicolaides K H. Abnormalities of the heart and great arteries in first trimester chromosomally normal fetuses. Am J Med Genet 1997; 69: 207–216

59 Sepulveda W, Sebire N J, Souka A P, Snijders R J M, Nicolaides K H. Diagnosis of the Meckel–Grüber syndrome at eleven to fourteen weeks' gestation. Am J Obstet Gynecol 1997; 176: 316–319

15

CNS abnormalities

Alison Fowlie, Glyn Constantine and Olujimi Jibodu

Introduction

In the early days of obstetric ultrasound, in the era of the static B-scanner and before grey scale display, very little detail could be seen of the fetus, the part most easily visualized being the axial skeleton. This led initially to some chance diagnoses of hydrocephalus in the late part of pregnancy, when the fetal biparietal diameter was found to be abnormally large, and was followed by the first successful mid-trimester diagnosis of fetal abnormality when, in 1972, Campbell identified an anencephalic fetus of 19 weeks gestation.[1]

At about that time the incidence of anencephaly and spina bifida in England and Wales was particularly high. Considerable effort was put therefore into further development of ultrasonic antenatal diagnosis of neural tube defects. This led over the years, particularly with the increasing sophistication of ultrasound technology, to the ability to make many different diagnoses of abnormalities of the central nervous system.

Although neural tube defects themselves have declined in incidence, defects of the central nervous system (CNS) are among the commonest congenital abnormalities overall, occurring in one per 200 live births[2] and in 3–4% of spontaneous abortions.[3] Although α-fetoprotein (AFP) has had some part to play in identifying the neural tube defects, it has no part in the identification of the closed defects that make up the bulk of CNS abnormalities. Ultrasound remains the essential tool for the identification of these problems.

In assessing any structure with ultrasound it is important to have a thorough knowledge of the normal developmental anatomy and the appearance at different gestations. Prior to the development of ultrasound, knowledge of the development of the normal fetus was scanty and of course based on abortion specimens, in which normality could be questioned and trauma may have caused artefacts. This is particularly true for the fetal head. At about 12 weeks the fetal cerebral ventricles have a simple crescent-like shape and occupy the bulk of the cranium. By about 18 weeks, although the ventricles have not changed much in size, the cerebral cortex has grown considerably, and so the proportion of the cranium occupied by the ventricles is now much smaller (see Ch. 6). As pregnancy progresses the structure of the ventricles becomes more complex, with the development of the posterior and occipital horns. Initially the surface of the brain is very smooth, but late in the midtrimester gyri begin to develop. Thus care must be taken in conditions that rely on the size of the ventricles much before 18 weeks, and pure lissencephaly (agyri) cannot be diagnosed until the third trimester.

In several European countries, including Britain, the majority of pregnant women are scanned routinely. Most of these scans are in the second trimester, when the biparietal diameter (BPD), head circumference and cerebellum are measured. Central nervous system defects may be detected during the course of these routine antenatal measurements of the fetal head. In this way most CNS defects are potentially detectable, even in low-risk populations.[4–6]

The current practice is for this routine anomaly scan to be performed at about 19–20 weeks. Whilst the scan plane for the BPD is being aligned it should be possible to establish (a) the shape of the head in transverse section, noting whether there are any unusual contours or bulges; (b) the presence of a strong midline echo, the midline structures such as the cavity of the septum pellucidum, third ventricle and the bodies of the thalami; (c) the configuration of the lateral ventricles and (d) the configuration of the cerebellum and cisterna magna.

Examination of the spine in longitudinal and transverse sections reveals the typical appearance of the ossification centres and the parallel lines showing up the dorsal processes. The curvature of the spine must be taken into consideration, and optimum views obtained from the base of the skull to the sacrococcygeal region.

If any deviation from normal is noted, or the patient is at increased risk of fetal abnormality and on whom a detailed scan is being performed, further views should be sought. Most abnormalities to be discussed below can be detected and elucidated from these scan planes, but other views may be useful in specific cases, e.g. a sagittal section when assessing facial abnormalities such as in holoprosencephaly.

With technological advances, particularly the increasing usage of trans-vaginal scanning, interest has developed in first- and early second-trimester anomaly scanning. These high-frequency transducers produce higher-quality images and therefore better detail than is achieved with transabdominal transducers. Trans-vaginal scanning allows better visualisation of the fetus at a much earlier stage, and it is possible to detect a number of anomalies in the first trimester.[7–11] Because of the developmental changes occurring at this time, considerable care must be exercised in making early diagnoses.

Neural tube defects

These conditions have many features in common, the occurrence of one putting the woman at risk of the others in a future pregnancy.

Epidemiology

Neural tube defects (NTDs) have an incidence that varies over time and with geographical location.

Both long- and short-term temporal variations have been reported. A major confounding influence in determining the recent overall incidence, however, is the effect of prenatal diagnosis and termination of affected pregnancies. NTDs, in particular anencephaly, have in the past been noted to be more frequent in the winter months.[12] More recent reports have suggested that this seasonal variation has disappeared.[13] However, the experience from the West Midlands Region, England, during 1984–1990, was that of two peaks a year at approximately 6-monthly intervals, the larger peak of mid-trimester problems being apparent in August and September, implying conception in April and May. In addition to this seasonal variation a significant long-term variability in the incidence of neural tube defects has been found. Data from the eastern USA covering the years 1910–1970 show that in 1930 the rate was 2.5 times the levels in 1910 and 1970.[14] A similar variation in the incidence of anencephaly was reported in Birmingham, UK over the period 1936–1964. Here cyclical peaks occurred every 14 years, when the incidence was around 1.8 times the minimum.[2,15] Recently the incidence in the UK has fallen considerably:[16–19] between 1964 and 1986 the birth prevalence of NTDs declined from 31.5 to 6.2 per 10 000,[20] that of anencephaly declining by 94% and of spina bifida by 68%. When terminations for affected pregnancies were taken into account, however, the overall incidence of affected pregnancies fell by 50% and 32%, respectively.[16] In the light of previous experience it will be a long time before it is known whether this fall will be permanent.

Geographical variations are also important, with reported rates for NTDs ranging from 0.8 to 7.6 per 10 000, there being a tenfold difference between areas of highest and lowest incidence.[21] The highest recorded incidence was 10 per 1000 in some Welsh mining valleys.[22] Why the UK, and particularly the Celtic areas, has the world's highest incidence of NTDs, and the Japanese and the rest of Europe the lowest, is unclear.[23] It has been suggested that the variation within the UK is secondary to geological conditions, soft water areas having a higher prevalence of NTDs.[24] More intensive study, however, suggests this to be unlikely.[25,26]

As well as an apparent correlation with geographical area, a genetic predisposition among the inhabitants of those areas has been suggested. This is borne out by the studies of migrants from high- and low-risk areas. Thus those of Irish and Sikh descent tend to retain a higher rate of NTDs on emigration, whereas blacks and Jews retain a lower rate.[27–30]

The vast majority of NTDs therefore appear to be inherited in a multifactorial manner, with evidence of additional environmental factors. Other specific associations include the anticonvulsants sodium valproate and carbamazepine.[31–33]

Anencephaly and exencephaly

Anencephaly is a condition in which the cranial vault and much of the brain is absent, the residual brain being grossly malformed. In addition, the frontal, parietal and occipital bones are often malformed and deficient. The brain remnants are covered by a vascular membrane, the area cerebrovasculosa. It has for many years been thought that the defect resulted from failure of closure of the anterior neuropore at around 24 days gestation (see Ch. 6),[34] but a more recent theory suggests that an excess of CSF disrupts the normally formed cerebral hemispheres.[35,36]

Exencephaly is characterised by a partial absence of the cranial vault with a large amount of protruding brain tissue. This condition is considered to lie somewhere on the spectrum between anencephaly and encephalocele. It may be an embryological precursor of the more common anencephaly, the exposed brain slowly degenerating through trauma and exposure to amniotic fluid, finally reaching the anencephalic state.[37,38]

Incidence and aetiology

Anencephaly is the commonest of the open neural tube defects and is four times more frequent in females. As in the other neural tube defects geographical differences in incidence are marked, varying from 0.6 per 1000 in Japan to 3.5 per 1000 in parts of the UK. There is an increased familial incidence and these regional differences appear to be at least partly genetic in origin. Anencephaly has a multifactorial aetiology and genetic and geographical factors, specific teratogens have been implicated, including radiation, salicylates and sulphonamides.

Exencephaly is much less common than anencephaly, but it has the same aetiology and recurrence risk as the other neural tube defects.

Diagnosis

It was not uncommon for anencephaly to present clinically in the late second and third trimesters of pregnancy with polyhydramnios. Nowadays, most cases are detected earlier by a combination of ultrasound and maternal AFP screening.[1,39–43] The ultrasound diagnosis depends on visualising the cephalic pole of the fetus clearly, so that the absence of the cranial vault and fetal brain above the level of the orbits can be noted. The fetal face often has a 'frog-like' appearance, with prominent orbits, owing to the deficiency of the frontal bone. The neck is often short and this adds to the frog-like appearance (Fig. 15.1). The diagnosis is often considered when there is difficulty measuring the fetal biparietal diameter. The diagnosis can only be excluded by visualising a normal skull and made by having a good clear view of the cephalic pole (Fig. 15.2). Inattention to this may lead to both false positive and false diagnoses, although these are extremely rare. The calvarial bones are very small prior to 13 weeks and the angiomatous stroma above the orbits, which can occur in up to 45% of cases,[44,45] may be mistaken for a normal head by the unwary. A head low in the maternal pelvis, particularly in an obese patient, may be so poorly seen that it is mis-

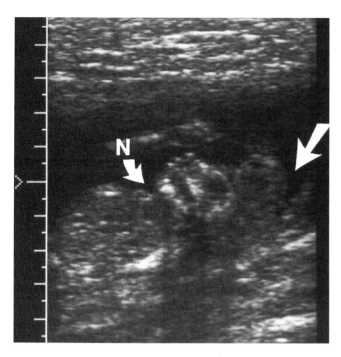

Fig. 15.1 Anencephaly. Longitudinal scan illustrating the absence of the cranial vault (arrowed), short neck (N) and frog-like face.

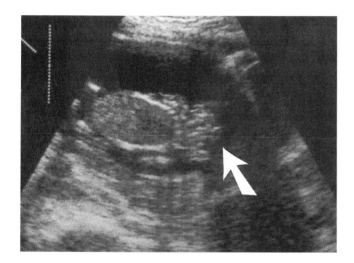

Fig. 15.2 Anencephaly. A view of the cephalic pole (arrowed) clearly illustrates absence of the cranial vault and disorganised brain tissue.

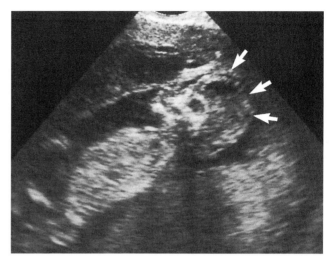

Fig. 15.3 Exencephaly. The calvarial bones are absent from the top of the skull (arrows) and the intracranial anatomy is abnormal.

early second trimester.[46–48] Because cranial ossification does not occur before 10 weeks gestation it may not be feasible to diagnose anencephaly by ultrasound at an earlier stage.[49]

For exencephaly, the diagnosis is much the same as for anencephaly, and in the majority of cases it would be unlikely to be recognised *in utero* as a different condition. The most striking feature is the large amount of disorganised cerebral tissue arising from the base of the cranium, as well as the non-visualisation of the calvarium (Fig. 15.3). The residual brain mass is bereft of normal features and there are convolutions on its surface. The facial structures and base of the cranium are always present.[50,51]

Differential diagnosis

In cases in which the fetal head appears small and difficult to visualise, the differential diagnosis lies between anencephaly, exencephaly, severe microcephaly, acrania and the amniotic band syndrome. It may be impossible to differentiate between anencephaly and exencephaly and even acrania antenatally, particularly if the diagnosis is being made very early in the second trimester. Acrania is a developmental abnormality with partial or complete absence of the cranium and nearly complete development of the brain tissue. In principle it should be possible to differentiate this from anencephaly by the presence of the cerebral cortex,[52] but in practice it may be difficult. In later pregnancy the differentiation from microcephaly may be made, not on the size of the head but on the presence of the skull vault, however small. Rarely amniotic bands may destroy most of the vault and brain.[53] When this occurs, however, the destruction is usually asymmetrical and, unlike anencephaly, is associated with oligohydramnios.[44] All these conditions have a very poor prognosis, but the risks of recurrence and therefore the implications for the future, differ.

taken for anencephaly. If the head is deep in the maternal pelvis and yet there is a strong suspicion that there is anencephaly, every attempt should be made to obtain a good view, including the use of head-down tilt, filling and emptying the bladder, and trans-vaginal scanning. If these fail amniocentesis and estimation of the liquor AFP and cholinesterase banding will produce a definitive diagnosis.

Although the diagnosis is usually made during a second-trimester anomaly scan, it is now feasible, particularly with trans-vaginal scans, to make the diagnosis in the first or

Associated malformations

Spina bifida is an associated finding in anencephaly. It may take the form of cranio-rrhachischisis, complete non-closure of the neural tube, or a coexistent sacral spina bifida. Exomphalos, cleft lip and palate and club foot have also been reported.[54] These findings are, however, of no practical significance as the condition is uniformly fatal. Exencephaly has been reported in association with exomphalos.[51]

Prognosis

Around 70% of fetuses with anencephaly will be still-born, the others surviving for only a matter of hours. Exencephaly is also incompatible with life.

Obstetric management

As these conditions are invariably lethal, termination of the pregnancy at any stage after the diagnosis is made is a reasonable option.[55]

Encephalocele

Encephalocele is a herniation of some of the cranial contents through a defect in the bony skull. Protrusion only of the meninges is strictly a meningocele; when brain tissue itself is extruding through the defect, this is an encephalocele. The lesion is thought to occur because of failed closure of the rostral end of the neural tube during the fourth week of fetal life. This may follow primary overgrowth of neural tissue in the line of closure, or failure of induction by adjacent neurodermal tissues interrupting this process (see Ch. 6).[56]

The majority of lesions occur in the midline and range in size from a few millimetres upwards; the protruded sac can be very small, or larger than the fetal skull. Although they usually protrude externally and are therefore visible, encephaloceles can occur through the base of the skull and protrude into the orbits, nose or mouth.[57] Sites of occurrence are occipital midline (75%), frontal midline (13%) and parietal (12%), most of the last resulting from the amniotic band syndrome, in which there is probably early disruption in the formation of the fetal skull. The resulting encephaloceles are atypical and the appearances very variable. Frontal encephaloceles almost always contain brain tissue and involve the bridge of the nose and nasal cavity in 60% and 30% of cases, respectively.[58] In some cases, the bulk of the brain is actually situated in the herniated sac.

Incidence and aetiology

Encephaloceles are uncommon. In 1984 the incidence in England and Wales was 0.8 per 10 000 births,[59] but it should be noted that the incidence of such disorders is much higher at stages of pregnancy.

Encephaloceles have a multifactorial aetiology; in common with most neural tube defects, genetic and geographical factors have been implicated and other defects occur with increased frequency in siblings.[58,60] Encephaloceles are commoner in females and have an increased incidence in certain races, e.g. Chinese. They are often found together with other abnormalities in a number of genetic syndromes (Meckel, von Voss, Chemke, Roberts, Knoblock) and non-genetic syndromes (cryptophthalmos, amniotic bands, warfarin, maternal rubella, diabetes).[61]

Diagnosis

The classic ultrasound picture is a mass arising from the occipital or frontal regions of the skull.[62–66] This may appear to be purely fluid filled (Fig. 15.4), or it can contain echoes from herniated brain tissue (Fig. 15.5). To make the diagnosis with certainty, the bony defect must be demonstrated. This may be difficult, because of its size or the presence of artefacts from shadowing mimicking a defect. In early pregnancy diagnosis is difficult because ossification of the calvarium is not completed before 12 weeks.[67] However, it has been reported that enlargement of the rhombencephalon cavity from 9 weeks may indicate the diagnosis.[67] Problems occur with meningoceles where a large lesion arises from a very small defect that is impossible to visualise.[66,68] It has been reported that, in the early first trimester, a meningocele may disappear by sliding in and out of the herniated sac.[69] The intracranial anatomy should therefore be assessed carefully as in the majority of cases it is abnormal. Once an encephalocele has been detected, a careful search must be made for associated anomalies.

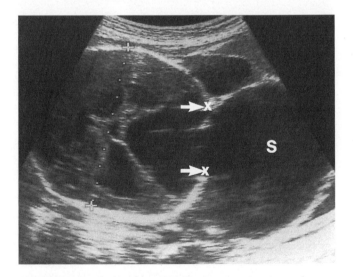

Fig. 15.4 Encephalocele. There is a large defect in the occipital bone (between arrows) through which protrudes a fluid-filled sac (S), a meningocele. The intracranial anatomy is grossly abnormal.

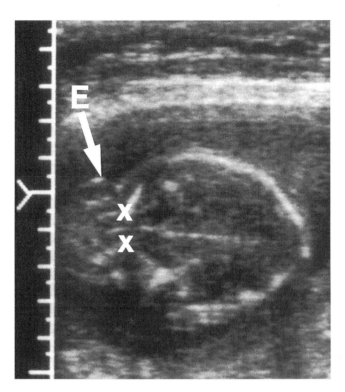

Fig. 15.5 **Encephalocele.** The defect is seen (between crosses) and, as the herniated sac (E) contains brain tissue, an encephalocele is diagnosed.

Differential diagnosis

The chief differential diagnoses lie between cystic hygroma, scalp oedema, branchial cleft cyst, nasal teratoma and clover-leaf skull deformity. Of these, encephaloceles are the only ones to be associated with a bony defect and, in the vast majority of cases there is some disorganisation or distortion of the intracranial anatomy, including hydrocephalus. Cystic hygromas are usually bilateral in origin and may contain septa; it should also be possible to see that scalp oedema affects the whole skull if scanning is carried out in different planes. Nasal teratomas are often irregular in outline. Haemangiomas can be distinguished by their vascular appearance and confirmed by the demonstration of blood flow on Doppler ultrasound. The clover-leaf skull is not a difficult diagnosis when it coexists with a skeletal dysplasia such as thanatophoric dwarfism because the associated abnormalities are obvious. When the head abnormality is isolated, careful evaluation of the skull shape is necessary (Fig. 15.6).

Associated malformations

Other malformations occur commonly. Some are parts of specific syndromes as previously mentioned, the common ones being polycystic kidneys in Meckel's syndrome or amputated limbs in the amniotic band syndrome. Other malformations, such as meningomyeloceles (7–33% of

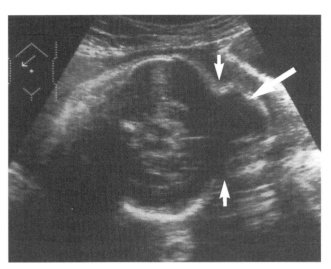

Fig. 15.6 **Craniosynostosis.** The frontal bulge (large arrow) caused by the premature fusion of the sutures (small arrows) may easily be mistaken for an encephalocele.

cases[62,70]), facial clefts, microcephaly (in 20% of cases[60]), hydrocephalus, Dandy–Walker syndrome and agenesis of the corpus callosum appear to be sporadic. Hydrocephalus occurs in up to 80% of occipital meningoceles and 65% of occipital encephaloceles (Fig. 15.7),[60] often being caused by herniation of the cerebellum into the encephalocele and/or aqueduct stenosis.[58] The rarer frontal encephalocele often occurs with the median cleft face syndrome[71] and, in 15% of cases, is associated with hydrocephalus.[63]

Prognosis

20% of fetuses with an encephalocele will be stillborn. The factors that result in this very poor prognosis, determined

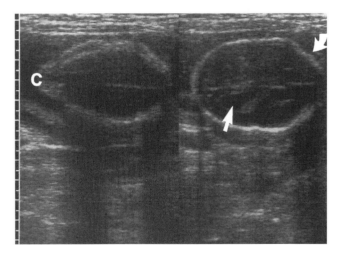

Fig. 15.7 **Encephalocele.** Small occipital encephalocele (C) but producing hydrocephalus (straight arrow – dilated posterior horn, curved arrow – 'lemon sign').

from groups of infants which were liveborn, are the coexistence of other abnormalities, the presence of brain in the herniated sac and microcephaly.[72,73] The impact of hydrocephalus is less certain. In general the mortality is lower if that is the only associated problem, but the intellectual impairment is very variable. Meningoceles have the lowest mortality, a 100% survival rate with 60% developing normally has been reported. This compares with a 56% survival rate with 9% normal development for cases where brain tissue is present in an encephalocele.[60] Frontal encephaloceles have a better prognosis than others.

Obstetric management

The prognosis for each encephalocele, based on its particular features, should be discussed with the parents: in the majority termination is chosen. If the abnormality is detected in later pregnancy, a caesarean section may be considered in cases where neonatal surgery is thought to be appropriate.

Spina bifida

Spina bifida is a midline bony defect of one or more vertebrae. Usually the defect is in the posterior arch and results in the absence of the arch, broadening of the vertebrae, lateral displacement of the pedicles and a widened spinal canal.[74] Occasionally the defect may be anterior, but this is very uncommon. Although the term refers only to the bony defect, the problems of the fetus are caused by maldevelopment of the spinal cord and the frequently associated hydrocephalus.

The suggestions concerning the origin of the condition are similar to those for anencephaly. The established theory has been that there is failure of closure of the caudal neuropore,[75] but more recently there has been a suggestion of overproduction or underabsorption of CSF in the embryonic period, the excess fluid causing a secondary rupture in the neural tube.[76] In 80–90% of cases the lesion affects the lumbar or lumbosacral regions; isolated sacral and cervical lesions account for most of the remainder. Spina bifida confined to the thoracolumbar, thoracic or cervicothoracic regions is rare.[77] Multiple defects are also unusual, being reported in only 1% of cases.[63]

At its most severe the lesion is overt and may present as a myeloschisis, in which the spinal cord is laid wide open, or as a meningomyelocele, a cystic protrusion of meninges containing central nervous system tissue. Meningomyeloceles are typically found in the lower thoracolumbar, lumbar and lumbosacral areas. Meningoceles are also cystic lesions that may contain peripheral nerves but no central nervous system tissue. These constitute only 5% of the total cases of spina bifida, and usually occur in the occipital, cervical or upper thoracic region or lower sacral region. Another form is spina bifida occulta. Here the lesion is usually small and completely covered by skin. There may be no abnormality on the overlying skin, but a tuft of hair or pigmentation is a clue in about 50% of cases. They are almost always found at the level of L5 or S1. In the majority of cases lesions such as these are asymptomatic, being picked up incidentally on X-ray examination. Some, however, do result in back pain and neurological disabilities, such as weakness in the lower limbs and poor sphincter control. Coexistent spinal cord abnormalities are common, hydromyelia and/or syringomyelia being present in around 43% of cases.[78]

The vast majority of cases of spina bifida also have the Arnold–Chiari type II malformation,[79] in which the cerebellar vermis herniates through the foramen magnum, leading to a displacement of the fourth ventricle, tentorium and medulla. The return flow of CSF to the intracranial arachnoid granulations is usually subsequently blocked, causing obstructive hydrocephalus (more than 90% of cases). The lesions without hydrocephalus tend to be meningoceles.

Incidence and aetiology

As discussed earlier, the incidence varies with season, geographical area and race. The UK, and especially Ireland, had a very high incidence of around three per 1000 births, but this has declined steadily over the past 15 years, Britain now having one of the lowest incidences in western Europe (0.6 per 1000 births).[80] The condition is commoner in caucasians than in orientals or blacks. Like the other neural tube defects, spina bifida appears to be most commonly inherited in a multifactorial manner. Other associations are with single mutant gene conditions (e.g. Jarco–Levin, Meckel, Robert and HARDE syndromes) and with teratogens such as sodium valproate and carbamazepine.

Diagnosis

The ultrasound appearances of spina bifida can be divided into those of the spinal lesion itself and those of associated findings in the fetal head. Often the latter are much more obvious than the lesion itself, and prompt a closer look at the spine.

The fetal vertebrae are composed of three ossification centres, which are present from the 10th week of gestation, giving rise to the typical view of the fetal spine seen in transverse section. The vertebral body arises from the anterior centre, whereas the laminae and neural arches arise from the two posterior centres, which develop an inward angulation. In longitudinal section the posterior ossification centres appear as two parallel dotted lines.[81] These normal relationships are the key to diagnosis of the spinal abnormality. Examination of the spine along its entire length should ideally be carried out in the transverse, sagittal and coronal planes. In transverse section the normal appearance of the spine in spina bifida is lost as the posterior ossification centres splay outwards, giving a U or V shape rather than the normal closed circle (Fig. 15.8). In addition the edges of the bones are rather sharp and highly reflective. In coronal section the parallel lines of the ossification centres splay out to give a characteristic bulge (Fig. 15.9), whereas in the sagittal midline section the posterior centres may not be visualised as the posterior arch is absent (Fig. 15.10). In addition, the normal curvature of the spine is often lost, particularly in the sacral region. Kyphoscoliosis may be present. The transverse and sagittal sections are preferable for identification of the characteristics of the soft tissue component.

It should be possible to distinguish between a myeloschisis (Fig. 15.8), when there is absence of skin or soft tissues over the spinal defect, and the cystic appearance of a meningocele or meningomyelocele (Fig. 15.11). It may not be easy to distinguish between a meningocele and a meningomyelocele on the ultrasound appearances, although the exact site of the lesion may help. Problems in scanning occur when the fetal back is pressed close to maternal tissue or placenta, or when the back is completely posterior and the fetus cannot be persuaded to move. If the spine lies directly at 3 or 9 o'clock in the field of view on a transverse scan, the beam spread artefact may cause difficulty in establishing the appearance of a closed

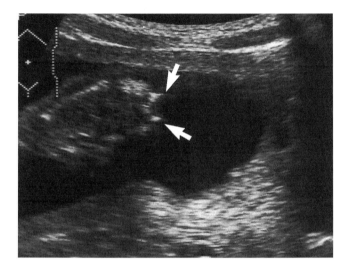

Fig. 15.8 Spina bifida. A transverse section of the sacral spine (arrowed) is shown. Note the sharpness of the bones, producing the typical U-shape and absence of any soft tissue covering, diagnostic of a myeloschisis.

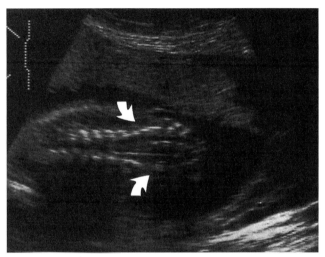

Fig. 15.9 Large lumbosacral spina bifida. The coronal section displays the characteristic bulge (arrowed) caused by the splaying out of the ossification centres.

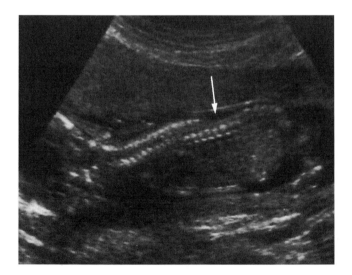

Fig. 15.10 Lumbosacral spina bifida displayed in sagittal section. The posterior arches are absent (arrowed).

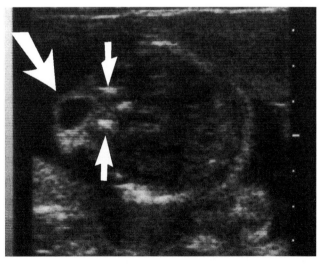

Fig. 15.11 Meningocele. Transverse scan of meningocele (large arrow) with widening of the posterior vertebral ossification centres (small arrows).

ring. In the future it may be possible to resolve diagnostic difficulties using MRI.[82–84]

It is very rare for spina bifida to be associated with an over-distended fetal bladder. Study of lower limb movement has not helped either with the diagnosis or the prognosis of the lesion, apparently normal movements occurring even with very severe lesions.

In the mid-trimester, hydrocephalus associated with the Arnold–Chiari malformation in fetuses with spina bifida is very characteristic and are different from those of isolated hydrocephalus. In transverse section, the head is irregular with a pointed frontal region,[85] described as the 'lemon' sign (Fig. 15.12). This is seen at the level used for measuring the biparietal diameter and was present in all 54 of the cases where such a view was available.[86,87] It has also been suggested that this sign is present by 12–14 weeks.[9] The anterior and the posterior horns of the lateral cerebral ventricles are large compared to the cerebral hemispheres. Ventricular to hemisphere width (V/H) ratios have been established for both horns (see Appendix).[88]

If these ratios are to be used, and particularly in the case of the anterior horn ratio, care must be taken in making a diagnosis before 18 weeks. When there is a wide normal range of ventricular size compared to the cerebral hemisphere is large (Fig. 15.13), so that follow-up studies are needed to demonstrate the normal growth of the cerebrum. These ratios were of considerable importance in the earlier days of antenatal diagnosis, when the amount of detail visible from the intracranial structures with ultrasound was minimal. With higher-resolution imaging,

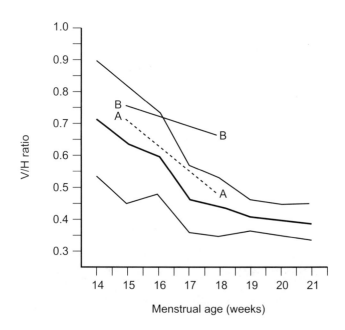

Fig. 15.13 Graph of the ventricular/hemisphere width ratio for the anterior horns of the lateral ventricles with the ratios of fetus A (normal) and fetus B (spina bifida with hydrocephalus) plotted at 15 and 18 weeks. This illustrates the pitfall of using the ratio before 18 weeks, when the normal range is wide.

however, their use is limited, though they are of particular help to the inexperienced scanner. The experienced sonographer with a thorough knowledge of the ultrasound anatomy of the fetal head can rely on qualitative assessment and readily identify abnormal cases.

Another important feature of the hydrocephalus associated with spina bifida is that of an apparently absent or bowed cerebellum.[86] Nicolaides *et al.* drew attention to abnormalities of the cerebellum in 21 cases.[86] They found it to be absent in eight, or with an anterior concavity (the 'banana' sign) in 12 (Fig. 15.14). These findings have been generally confirmed in other retrospective and prospective studies, although it seems more usual to have difficulty seeing the cerebellum because of its very low position or hypoplastic state.[89–91] It must be remembered that a normal cerebellum (see Appendix) does not exclude hydrocephalus or spina bifida (Fig. 15.15).

In addition, in contrast to the normal state, the medial borders of the anterior horns may be visible and prominent, deviating slightly away from the midline to give a feathered appearance (Fig. 15.16).

The BPD and head circumference may be small compared to dates or femur length. This applies even in late pregnancy. The abnormally large, fluid-filled hydrocephalic head is not found with spina bifida, but only with isolated hydrocephalus.

Abnormalities of the head are therefore found in the vast majority of cases of spina bifida. The presence of a normal head shape, normal cerebellum and cisterna magna, and

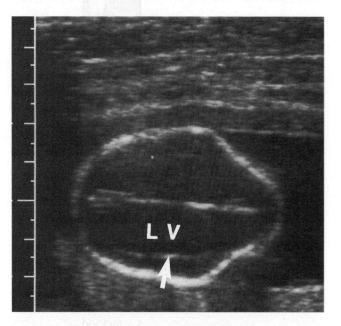

Fig. 15.12 Hydrocephaly. The characteristic appearances of hydrocephalus associated with spina bifida. Note the lemon-shaped head, the pointed end being anterior, and the enlarged lateral ventricles (LV). Arrow – lateral wall of ventricle.

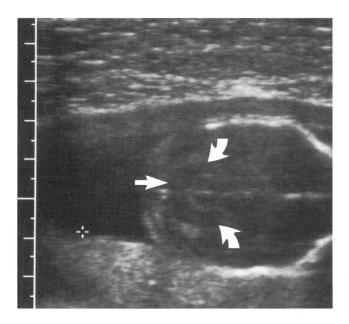

Fig. 15.14 'Banana sign'. Hydrocephalus associated with spina bifida displaying a bowed cerebellum – the 'banana' sign (curved arrows) – and obliterated cisterna magna (straight arrow).

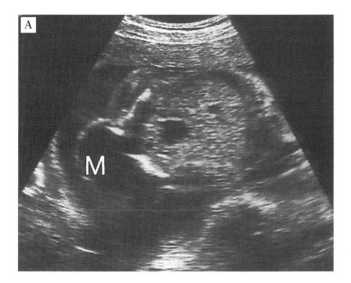

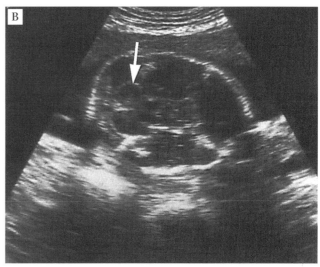

Fig. 15.15 Sacral meningocele. A: Large sacral meningocele (M) and **B:** normal appearance of the cerebellum. The pregnancy proceeded to term and the baby had no neurological deficit.

normal V/H ratios virtually rules out a serious neural tube defect. A normal appearance is found only in association with a spina bifida where there is a simple meningocele, which for the most part carries a good prognosis (Fig. 15.15). This has been borne out in the West Midlands series of 106 cases of spina bifida in which, in 102 (96%), there was obvious hydrocephalus. In one there was dilatation of the third ventricle only and in three there was no abnormality of the head. In these four cases the spinal lesions were very low and small, with no neurological deficit.

Amniocentesis with measurement of the amniotic fluid AFP and acetylcholinesterase has been used extensively in the diagnosis of neural tube defects. It is now rarely employed when there is a good ultrasound service, as ultrasound will not only detect the lesion, but indicate its extent and severity to give a guide to prognosis. In addition, amniocentesis is subject to errors (Fig. 15.17) and the incidence of abortion following amniocentesis is up to 1%.[92]

Effectiveness of ultrasound in diagnosing spina bifida

Ultrasound has been used both as a method of screening for neural tube defects and to investigate pregnancies singled out as being at high risk, either from the past history or because of raised serum AFP. These different

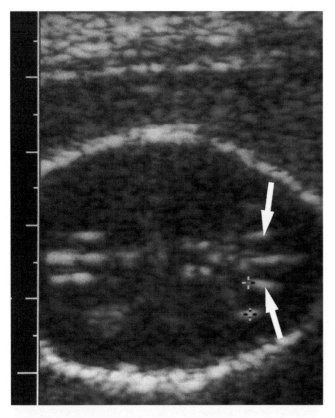

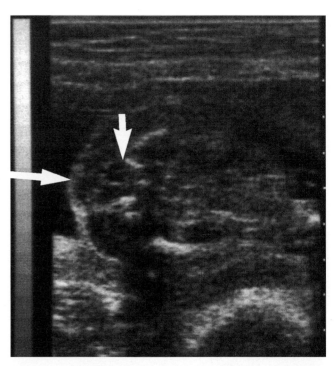

Fig. 15.17 **Closed spina bifida.** The skin covering (longer arrow) can be seen over the lesion (short arrow). The serum and liquor AFP were normal.

Fig. 15.16 **Hydrocephalus.** 15-week fetus with hydrocephalus associated with spina bifida in which the medial borders of the lateral ventricles are clearly seen (arrowed) and deviate away from the midline.

population groups must be borne in mind when evaluating reports, as well as the experience of the operators and the equipment employed. In addition, as knowledge of the appearance of the fetal head, equipment and expertise have all improved during the 1980s, earlier reports are unrepresentative. Taking the high-risk group, series dating from the early 1980s show sensitivities ranging from 30% to 87%, with specificities of 96% to 99%, positive predictive values of 80% to 92%, and negative predictive values of 99%.[42,93] More recent reports show a 91–100% sensitivity and 98% specificity in high-risk populations for open neural tube defects. The use of the 'lemon' sign and cerebellar abnormalities in the diagnosis of spina bifida has been reported.[9,11,89] The 'lemon' sign was shown to have a 100% sensitivity and 99% specificity, with a positive predictive value of 84% and negative predictive value of 100%, cerebellar signs showed figures of 96%, 100%, 100% and 100%, respectively. Small sacral lesions, usually particularly difficult to diagnose antenatally with ultrasound, were detected by use of these signs in four fetuses.

Ultrasound detection of NTDs without the benefit of maternal serum AFP results has improved remarkably over the years.[4,5] In a 1983 study by Persson *et al.*[98] ultrasound detected the only case of anencephaly and 2/3

encephaloceles, but missed 5/5 cases of open spina bifida. Rosendahl and Kivenen[99] reported in 1989 on an 8-year series of 9000 mid-trimester scans performed routinely at 18 weeks. During this time they detected 2/2 anencephalies, 3/4 meningoceles and 2/3 hydrocephalies, a very low instance of NTDs. Between 1984 and 1986, 1200 low-risk routine 18–20-week scans were performed at the Birmingham Maternity Hospital: 5/5 cases of spina bifida associated with hydrocephalus were detected. In this series all the abnormalities were noted in the first instance by recognition of changes in the fetal head. Chitty *et al.* diagnosed all the NTDs in their series of 8785 fetuses scanned in the mid-trimester in an unselected population.[4] In a similar study of 8849 women reported by Luck,[5] all the NTDs in a low-risk population were diagnosed by mid-trimester ultrasound. With improvements in technique, training and equipment, experience and knowledge of the important cranial signs, good results should be possible when a low-risk population is screened with ultrasound.

As with other aspects of ultrasound, first trimester diagnosis is increasingly feasible. Hernadi and Torocsik diagnosed 5/6 NTDs between 11 and 14 weeks in a series of 3991 women.[100]

Associated malformations

Other associated malformations are club and rocker-bottom feet, both occurring as a result of peripheral nerve damage,[101] and single gene disorders such as the Jarco–Levin and Kousseff syndromes.

Prognosis

Figures on prognosis are coloured by the effect of prenatal diagnosis and also by the preselection of those fetuses referred for treatment. However, before antenatal diagnosis up to 25% of fetuses with spina bifida were stillborn. Untreated, most of the remainder died in the first months of life, and even in the treated group 7-year survival was only 40%.[102] Of these children only 25% had no lower limb disability and only 17% normal continence. In a study of 213 children with spina bifida born between 1965 and 1972, before prenatal diagnosis was introduced, the 5-year survival was 36% for open lesions, 60% for closed lesions and 18% for unclassified lesions.[103] Among the survivors with open lesions 84% were severely handicapped, only 6% being normal. These children had spent an average of 6 months in hospital and had an average of six major surgical procedures during their first 5 years of life. In a second study between 1972 and 1979, 154 infants with spina bifida were followed up for 12 months.[104] Survival rates at 12 months were 64%, 73% and 45% for open, closed and unclassified lesions, respectively. A recent study of school-aged children in Western Australia confirmed the poorer prognosis of lesions containing neural tissue, with 76% having learning difficulties compared with 56% of those with meningoceles.[105] At birth, and even for months afterwards, the extent of neurological deficit may not be clear.[106]

Contemporary management ensures that a greater number of infants with this abnormality will survive and grow to be functional adults. Early closure of defects, ventriculoperitoneal shunting for hydrocephalus and management of urinary and faecal incontinence play a major role in their well-being.

It is not possible to predict with certainty which fetuses with spina bifida will die or have a major degree of disability, although certain features are known to be important, such as the level and the extent of the lesion, the presence of kyphoscoliosis and marked hydrocephalus. A large high lesion generally carries a poor prognosis, as do marked hydrocephalus and kyphoscoliosis. The presence of CNS tissue within a sac of meninges (Fig. 15.18) clearly affects the prognosis, although it may not be possible to distinguish a meningomyelocele from a meningocele with ultrasound. However, if a lesion is high but small and not causing hydrocephalus, this is likely to be a meningocele with a relatively good prognosis.

Obstetric management

Termination of pregnancy should be considered after appropriate counselling. With widespread adoption of either routine scanning or maternal serum AFP screening, late

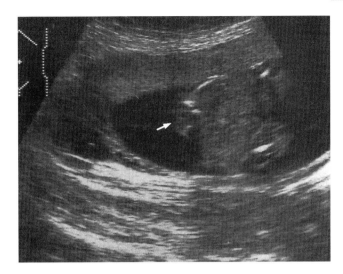

Fig. 15.18 Spina bifida. A transverse section of a spina bifida. The sac contains soft tissue (arrowed), suggesting that the lesion is a meningomyelocele.

diagnosis and the unexpected discovery of a neural tube defect at birth have become less common. Not all women wish for antenatal diagnosis however, and some women book late in pregnancy.[107] In these groups decisions have to be made about further management if a lesion is found at a late stage. A thorough evaluation of the fetus should be made in order to rule out additional abnormalities. Consultation should take place with the neonatal paediatricians and, if applicable, the neurosurgeons. If the decision is to continue with the pregnancy, all babies should be delivered in the best condition possible so that they may obtain maximum benefit from whatever post-natal treatment is available. It has been suggested that vaginal delivery could result in traumatising the defect or exposing it to infection,[108] and therefore caesarean section is advocated. *In utero* transfer to a tertiary centre is recommended.

Recurrence risks of neural tube defects

When a woman has had one pregnancy affected by a neural tube defect she should be carefully counselled about the chances of a recurrence in a subsequent pregnancy. The risk depends on the overall geographic incidence, which varies from 9% in Northern Ireland to 3% in southeast England.[109,110] In Britain overall recurrence risks are generally quoted as being 5% after one pregnancy with a neural tube defect, 12% after two and 20% after three. When one of the parents is affected the risk to any pregnancy is of the order of 3%.

Prevention of neural tube defects

Major advances have been made over the years in reducing the birth incidence of neural tube defects through antenatal screening and termination of affected fetuses. The risk may also be reduced in some specific cases, for example by altering the anticonvulsant therapy of epileptics who intend to become pregnant.[111] Dietary counselling and folic acid supplements at the time of conception and in early pregnancy have been shown to reduce the recurrence rate of NTDs in a high-risk area.[112,113] Similarly, a non-randomised multicentre study using a multivitamin preparation (Pregnavite Forte F) during the periconceptual period and the first trimester showed a marked decrease in the incidence of recurrent NTDs.[114] This has been confirmed[115,116] and by epidemiological data from the USA.[117] More recent studies have confirmed the benefit of folic acid supplements, and there are no apparent ill effects.[118,119] As the embryonic anterior and posterior neuropores close by 6 weeks, folic acid needs to be used before conception and in early pregnancy to be of benefit.[120] In cases of previous NTD the recommended daily dose is 4 mg. Such is the success of this supplementation that it has now been extended for prophylaxis in the general population, the dose here being 0.4 mg daily.[121]

Screening for NTDs with AFP

Because of the high incidence of NTDs and their devastating effects on the fetus (death or severe handicap) great efforts have been made to develop efficient screening techniques. The first practical technique was developed in the early 1970s, when Brock and Sutcliffe[122] measured AFP levels in amniotic fluid and found significantly higher levels in pregnancies complicated by an NTD. When expressed in multiples of the median for a specific gestation, there is a clear distinction between unaffected pregnancies and those with an open NTD. Around 20% of neural tube defects are, however, missed in cases where the lesion is closed, whereas other abnormalities, such as anterior wall defects and Finnish nephrosis, yield a positive result.

Between 1974 and 1977, a collaborative study using a system of rising cut-offs with increasing gestational age found a sensitivity of 98% for detection of open neural tube defects, with a false-positive rate of around 0.5%. Subsequently it was found that fetuses with open NTDs secreted acetylcholinesterase (AChE), which could be detected by electrophoresis into the amniotic fluid.[123] This was shown by the presence of a band which could be inhibited by the chemical BW284C51, in addition to the normally occurring pseudocholinesterase. Combining the two techniques eliminates most false positives.[70] Amniocentesis is not, however, a technique that can be employed for population screening.

α-fetoprotein is present in maternal serum during pregnancy at about 1/200th the concentration of that in amniotic fluid, and its measurement only became practical with improved assay techniques. Pregnancies affected with an open NTD have higher serum AFP levels than controls.[124,125] This finding was tested in a multicentre collaborative study which demonstrated that serum AFP varied with gestation, was best expressed in multiples of the median for gestation, and had a maximum sensitivity between 16 and 18 weeks gestation.[126] Most laboratories use a cut-off level of between 2.0 and 3.0 multiples of the median; this identifies NTDs with a sensitivity of 80–85% and a specificity of 96–98%.[98,127,128]

The group defined at high risk for NTDs also includes fetuses with other abnormalities, as well as those with incorrect dates, multiple pregnancies, previous threatened abortion and intra-uterine death. Once these diagnoses have been excluded, only about one in 20 actually has a fetal anomaly,[94] the remainder being at increased risk of abruption, growth retardation and pre-eclampsia. The raised maternal AFP thus designates these pregnancies as high risk. With high-resolution equipment and a skilled operator, ultrasound is now sensitive enough to make it the main tool in NTD screening.[4,5,129] The value of maternal AFP has diminished therefore but has been retained in many units because of its use in Down's syndrome screening.[130]

Diastematomyelia

This is characterised by the partial or complete clefting of a variable length of the spinal cord into two halves, usually by a midline bony spicule or fibrous band. It occurs most commonly in the lower thoracic and upper lumbar spine, and can be found with or without an associated meningomyelocele or neurocutaneous stigmata of spinal dysraphism. It is commoner in females.

Diagnosis and associated malformations

Prenatal diagnosis has been reported where a high-amplitude central echo was seen running through the spinal canal.[131] In addition there was widening of the posterior ossification centres of the spine. It is commonly associated with spina bifida (Fig. 15.19).

Prognosis

When diastematomyelia occurs in association with a spina bifida the prognosis is the same as for the spina bifida lesion. If it presents as a closed defect the prognosis is variable and may be good. The prognosis for neurological function is enhanced by early surgical removal of the septum dividing the spinal cord.

Hemivertebrae

Hemivertebrae develop when there is aplasia or hypoplasia of one of the two ossification centres that form the vertebral body.

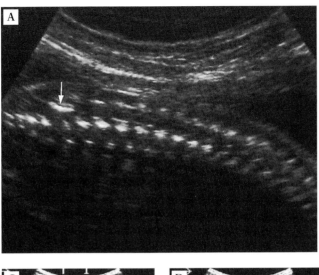

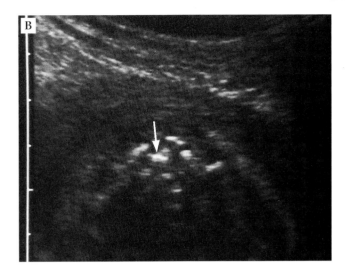

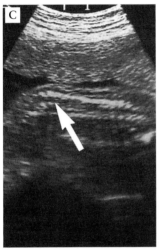

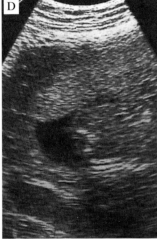

Fig. 15.19 Diastematomyelia. A and **B:** A case of lower lumbar diastematomyelia without spina bifida. Note the bony spur (arrow). **C:** Longitudinal and **D:** transverse scans of a spine with a large thoracolumbar spina bifida. At the lower end the bony spur is seen as a strong echo in the middle of the bulge (arrows).

Diagnosis

A single hemivertebra may be very difficult to identify. However, there is often more than one and they are frequently associated with rib abnormalities and scoliosis, which may be severe. The displacement of the anterior ossification centre from the straight line arrangement of the other centres is apparent on sagittal sections.[132] In coronal sections the normal tramline appearance is lost and there may be a bulge, which is easily mistaken for a spina bifida (Fig. 15.20). However, in transverse section, although there may be some distortion of the normal closed ring appearance of the spine, the distortion is anterior rather than posterior. Hemivertebrae may also be associated with neural tube defects.

Prognosis

If there is already marked scoliosis in early pregnancy the deformity of the child will be severe, albeit not life-threatening or associated with mental retardation. Multiple surgical procedures are likely to be needed and are seldom entirely successful. Fetuses without significant scoliosis *in utero* may develop severe problems after birth. These factors should be borne in mind when counselling the parents.

Caudal regression syndrome

An insult to the developing embryo during the third week of life may result in a wedge-shaped defect in the posterior axis caudal blastema. This may result in fusion of the early lower limb buds and the absence or incomplete development of intervening caudal structures. This results in the caudal regression syndrome, a disorder with a wide range of severity; the mildest form is represented by imperforate anus, and the most severe may result in lower limb fusion, sirenomelia, imperforate anus, urological deficits and lower vertebral and pelvic abnormalities, including agenesis (see Ch. 19).

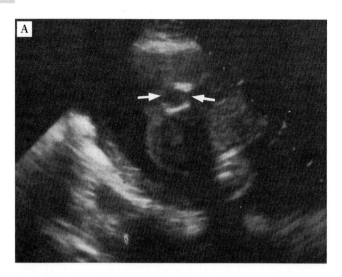

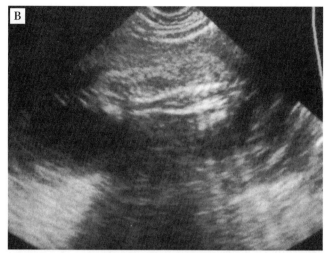

Fig. 15.20 Hemivertebrae. The fetus had three consecutive hemivertebrae. **A:** The lesion is seen in transverse section, the normal closed ring appears deficient both anteriorly and posteriorly (arrows) but the ossification centres do not diverge, nor are they sharp. **B:** In longitudinal section a bulge is noted which is indistinguishable from spina bifida.

Incidence and aetiology

Caudal regression syndrome occurs in about one in 60 000 neonates. It is strongly associated with diabetes mellitus and monozygotic twin pregnancies.[133,134]

Diagnosis

The mildest forms of caudal regression syndrome cannot be diagnosed antenatally. However, sacral agenesis may be recognised. When examining the spine in longitudinal section the normal sacral curve is lost, the spine being somewhat shortened (Fig. 15.21). The lower limbs may be hypoplastic and a large bladder may be present. In more severe cases the lower thoracic vertebrae may be malformed or absent. The pelvic bones may be absent or rudimentary and the legs may be asymmetrical, grossly

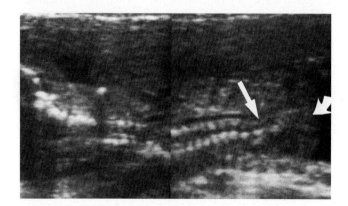

Fig. 15.21 Caudal regression syndrome. This fetus has sacral agenesis. The spine, shown in longitudinal section, appears to end in the lower lumbar region (straight arrow), stopping well short of the caudal pole (curved arrow).

shortened or fused. Ultrasound diagnosis between 11 and 14 weeks has been described.[135]

Associated abnormalities

Abdominal wall and genitourinary abnormalities may be present. The prognosis depends on the severity of the lesion: in its severest form it is incompatible with life. In cases with absent or deformed vertebrae there are likely to be neurological sequelae, such as limb weakness and loss of bladder and bowel sphincter control.

Obstetric management

This abnormality has a poor prognosis with major deformity and handicap, and termination of pregnancy should be offered.

Acardiac monster

This is a disorder occurring only in monozygotic twin pregnancies, when the head and upper part of the thorax of one twin, including the thoracic contents, are absent. Vascular anastomosis between the twins permits the acardiac fetus to survive and grow.

Incidence and aetiology

This rare disorder occurs in one in 35 000–48 000 births.[136]

Diagnosis

In addition to the absence of the fetal head no fetal heart movement can be detected in the abnormal fetus, but

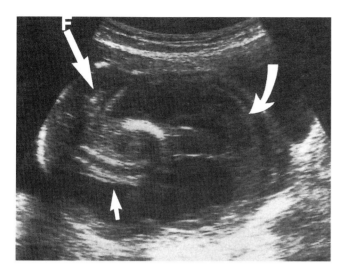

Fig. 15.22 Acardiac monster. In addition to a normal fetus, in the uterus was a bizarre mass that showed some movement. Part of a spine could be identified (small arrow). At one end legs could be seen (F). At the other end was a cystic and solid structure (curved arrow).

lower limb movements may be seen. The spine is short and is found to end abruptly. The lower part of the fetus may also exhibit abnormalities, but generally the femora and distal lower limb bones can be identified. The appearance is extremely bizarre (Fig. 15.22), so that the diagnosis will mostly be made by awareness of the possibility of the condition. Cardiac failure may occur in the normal fetus as it is providing the entire cardiac output for both fetuses; thus the normal fetus may become hydropic. Polyhydramnios may be present.

Obstetric management

The second fetus must be examined carefully for structural abnormalities. If normal, serial examinations are necessary to exclude cardiac failure. Early delivery or drug therapy through the maternal circulation, using digoxin or flecainide,[137,138] may be necessary if hydrops ensues. Platt *et al.*[139] advocated selective ligation of the umbilical artery of the abnormal fetus should hydrops occur. In two personal cases one abnormal fetus died *in utero* at 29 weeks and the other pregnancy developed severe polyhydramios, resulting in preterm labour at 31 weeks.

Iniencephaly

Iniencephaly is an uncommon anomaly first described in 1887,[140] in which a defect in the occiput resulting in exposure of the brain is combined with dysraphism of the cervical spine. This usually results in fusion of the occiput to the cervical spine and retroflexion of the head, with an exaggerated spinal lordosis. The condition is frequently associated with an encephalocele or spina bifida, the spine

appearing short and abnormal with pronounced kyphoscoliosis.

Embryologically iniencephaly is thought to be caused by an arrest of the embryo in physiological retroflexion in the third week of gestation, or by failure of normal forward bending in the fourth week.[141] Some authors consider that iniencephaly may belong to a group of disorders including Klippel–Feil, Dandy–Walker and Arnold–Chiari syndromes.[141–144]

Incidence and aetiology

Early reports of an incidence of 1 in 896 seem to be too high.[145] Other estimates in differing populations suggest a frequency varying from 1 in 1000 to fewer than 1 in 100 000.[142,146–148] It does not appear to be a familial condition. It is more common in females (male to female ratio 0.28) and in certain geographical areas. In humans it has been found in association with maternal syphilis[149,150] and sedative intake. In animal studies administration of vinblastine,[151] streptonigrin[152] and triparanol[153] have all resulted in iniencephaly.

Diagnosis

Hyperextension of the fetal head with fusion of the occiput to the dorsum of the spine, together with spinal deformities including shortening, lordosis, kyphoscoliosis (Figs 15.23 and 15.24) and myelomeningocele, are characteristic of iniencephaly.[154–159] Scanning longitudinally, it is difficult to locate the entire fetal spine in a single plane, but on transverse section the head is visualised at the same level as the thorax (Fig. 15.25).

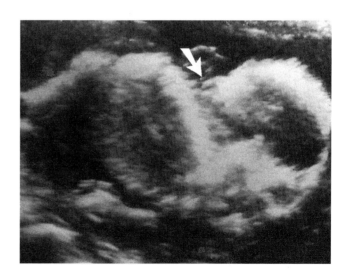

Fig. 15.23 Iniencephaly. The hyperextension of the fetal head and the fusion of the occiput to the dorsal spine (arrowed) is displayed in this longitudinal section.

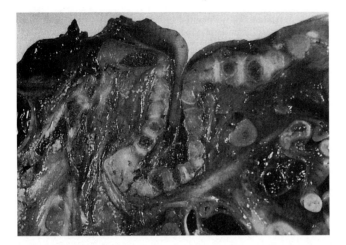

Fig. 15.24 Iniencephaly. Longitudinal section of an iniencephalic specimen at the level of the cervical spine, displaying its gross curvature. (With thanks to Dr Ian Rushton, Consultant Perinatal Pathologist, Birmingham Maternity Hospital.)

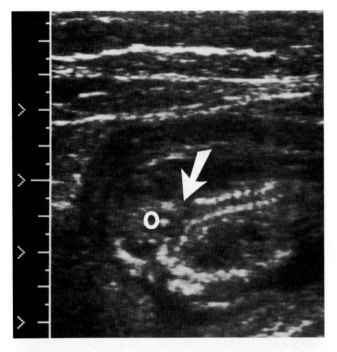

Fig. 15.25 Iniencephaly. In this scan the entire length of the spine cannot be located in a single plane and the occiput (O) is visualised adjacent to the thoracic spine (arrowed).

Associated malformations

Iniencephaly is associated with other abnormalities in around 84% of cases.[148,158,160,161] Morocz *et al.*[158] described 11 cases of iniencephaly diagnosed antenatally, five also having anencephaly, one an encephalocele, one a diaphragmatic hernia, and two lethal pulmonary hypoplasia. Other abnormalities reported were posterior fossa cysts, hydrocephalus, spina bifida, cyclopia, holoprosen-

cephaly, ventricular atresia, polymicrogyria, absence of mandible, facial clefts, cardiac anomalies, exomphalos, gastroschisis, situs inversus, polycystic kidneys, arthrogryposis, clubfoot, long upper limbs, thoracic cage deformities and talipes equinovarus.

Differential diagnosis

The main differential diagnosis is that of Klippel–Feil syndrome, where fusion of the cervical vertebrae leads to a short neck and deformed spine. It is in fact considered by some that Klippel–Feil syndrome is a mild form of iniencephaly.[158] Other abnormalities which may initially cause confusion include anencephaly and cervical meningomyelocele.

Prognosis

Severe iniencephaly is almost invariably fatal in the neonatal period. Out of over 250 cases in the literature very few are reported to have survived; these were cases with a mild abnormality and no associated problems.[144,157]

Obstetric management

When diagnosed early, termination should be offered. Later in pregnancy termination is still an option, but if it is decided to continue with the pregnancy it should be anticipated that hyperextension of the fetal head may cause obstruction of labour because of a face or brow presentation. Rarely neonatal surgery has been attempted.[157]

Hydrocephalus

Hydrocephalus is defined as an abnormal increase in the amount of cerebrospinal fluid within the cerebral ventricles. Cerebrospinal fluid (CSF) is formed by the choroid plexuses, which occupy much of the fetal ventricular system, flowing through the lateral and third ventricles before escaping into the subarachnoid space through the foramina of Luschka and Magendie in the fourth ventricle. After passing through the subarachnoid space and cisterna the fluid is reabsorbed by the arachnoid granulations lining the superior sagittal sinus. The system is normally in equilibrium, production being balanced by reabsorption. This increase in the amount of CSF distinguishes true hydrocephalus from conditions in which the ventricles appear large because of poor cerebral growth, e.g. colpocephaly or destruction/atrophy of the brain tissues, such as in hydranencephaly. Hydrocephalus does not necessarily imply a large head, this being a late and inconsistent sign.

Incidence and aetiology

Hydrocephalus has an incidence of between 0.1 and 2.5 per 1000 births in various series.[162–164] True hydrocephalus has many associations and causes, but is almost always caused by a relative or complete obstruction of CSF flow. Rarely, it is due to over-production.[165] If caused by obstruction it can be further subdivided into communicating and non-communicating varieties, the former being commonly associated with intracranial haemorrhage or meningitis in the neonatal period, and consequently rare in fetal life. Non-communicating hydrocephalus implies an obstruction within the ventricular system and is by far the commonest variety presenting in the antenatal period. The majority of cases of non-communicating or obstructive hydrocephalus are caused by stenosis of the aqueduct of Sylvius, which connects the third and fourth ventricles. This is a multifactorial condition in which genetic,[166] infective,[167] teratogenic and neoplastic aetiologies have been postulated. Antenatally, genetic and infective causes predominate, the stenosis being secondary to malformation or gliosis, respectively. Malformations include forking, narrowing and septation, narrowing being the most common finding in hereditary cases. In one neonatal autopsy series 50% of cases of aqueduct stenosis were due to gliosis, 46% to forking and 4% to simple narrowing of the canal.[168] Many studies have shown that aqueduct stenosis can be transmitted as an X-linked recessive trait.[169] However, it would appear to be inherited in this way in only about 25% of affected male fetuses, whereas in other families both sexes are affected.[170] Aqueduct stenosis is said to account for about 43% of all cases of congenital hydrocephalus. In other cases obstruction occurs at the foramen of Monro, caused by intracranial cysts, ventriculitis or neoplasms. When obstruction occurs at the foramina of Luschka and Magendie, the Dandy–Walker malformation and other brain cysts and neoplasms are implicated. Obstruction may also occur in the posterior fossa in achondroplasia or clover-leaf skull.

Diagnosis

Initial attempts at the antenatal ultrasound diagnosis of fetal hydrocephalus relied on measurements of the biparietal diameter. This is a late, crude and totally unreliable sign of hydrocephalus, and has long been superseded by more sophisticated techniques as technology has allowed increasingly detailed imaging. Unlike the hydrocephalus associated with spina bifida, the head is often rounded in transverse section (Fig. 15.26). Gross dilatation of the ventricles can easily be demonstrated, the third ventricle being evaluated in addition to the more obvious lateral ventricles (Fig. 15.27). More subtle degrees of ventricular dilatation, particularly in the second trimester, can be much more difficult to assess. This is partially due to the changing appearance of the ventricular system and choroid plexus during that time. It is also possible that mild and perhaps transient asymmetry of the lateral ventricles occurs without background pathology.[171]

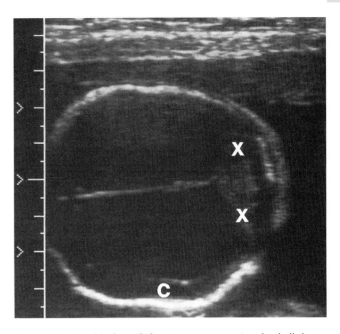

Fig. 15.26 Isolated hydrocephalus. In transverse section the skull shape is round. Gross dilatation of the lateral ventricle can be seen, the lateral wall being close to the skull, leaving only a rim of cortex (C). The cerebellum (crossed) is normal in shape and clearly seen.

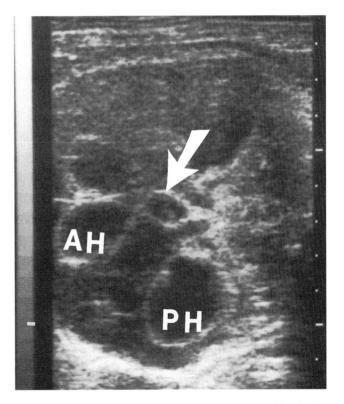

Fig. 15.27 Isolated hydrocephalus with marked dilatation of the third ventricle (arrowed) as well as the anterior (AH) and posterior (PH) horns of the lateral ventricles. This particular appearance, with a well-formed but ballooned ventricle, is consistent with a late pregnancy insult, rather than a genetic hydrocephalus.

Assessment of ventricular dilatation has traditionally been performed by measuring the width of either the anterior horns,[87,172] the posterior horns[88] or the body of the lateral ventricle[173] and comparing these measurements to the hemispheric width (see Appendix). The exact section as used by the authors must be reproduced. In many published graphs there is a large standard deviation, making detection of early changes difficult. This is borne out by reports of several false-negative diagnoses in early pregnancy.[174–176] Ventriculomegaly usually develops after 14 weeks. In a screening study using ultrasound at 11–14 weeks, with repeats at 18–20 weeks, only two out of eight were diagnosed at the early scan, the rest only being detectable at the later scan.[100] In addition, the lines initially thought to be the borders of the anterior horns of the lateral ventricles may actually represent reflections from vascular structures in the brain directly above the ventricle.[177] Some authors find the loss of concavity and 'ballooning' of the anterior horns of the lateral ventricles[178] and simultaneous visualisation of both walls of the lateral ventricles[63] useful signs.

A better assessment of ventricular size can be made by studying the choroid plexus and its relationship to the ventricular system.[178–182] At the start of the second trimester the choroid plexus has a prominent highly reflective 'bat's wing' appearance and proportionally occupies a large part of the cerebral hemispheres. As the head grows the choroid plexus becomes less prominent and on transverse section can be seen to occupy the atrial portion of the lateral ventricles. In the normal fetus the choroid plexus occupies the full width of the atrium. If the ventricular system is enlarged, the choroid plexus becomes compressed to a varying degree and settles to the lowest part of the atrium, leaving a fluid-filled gap between the medial walls of the ventricle and the choroid plexus (Fig. 15.28).[177–179] This has been quantified as a means of detecting mild hydrocephalus.[182] Mild ventricular dilatation is defined as a separation of 3–8 mm between the choroid plexus and the adjacent medial ventricular wall. The effect of gravity on the choroid plexus in cases of hydrocephalus also destroys its usual symmetry,[178] even causing the superior choroid to 'dangle' through an open septum into the inferior hemisphere.[181]

Measurement of the atria of the lateral ventricles themselves is also useful in the detection of hydrocephaly. In normal fetuses between 14 and 38 weeks gestation it has a constant mean width of 7.6 ± 0.6 mm.[88,183,184] If this exceeds 10 mm (more than 4 standard deviations) at any gestational age, ventriculomegaly can be diagnosed with a low false-positive rate (Fig. 15.29).[184] In a retrospective study of 112 fetuses with abnormalities of the CNS 99 (88%) had an atrial width greater than 10 mm, 81 (72%) exceeding 13 mm.[180] This suggests that measurement of the width of the atrium of the lateral ventricle is a sensitive and specific sign of fetal hydrocephalus with little intra- and inter-observer error.

Not uncommonly artefacts or structures other than the lateral ventricle wall give rise to the appearance of hydrocephalus, especially if insufficient gain has been applied to

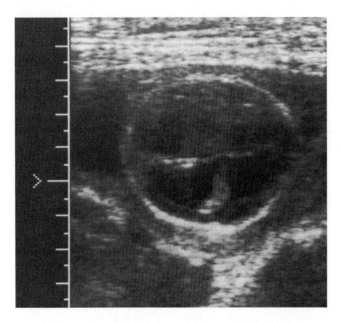

Fig. 15.28 Isolated hydrocephalus. Large lateral ventricles are displayed and the choroid plexus assumes a long thin appearance and hangs down vertically, leaving a gap between the medial wall of the atrium and its body.

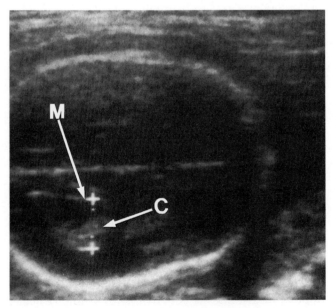

Fig. 15.29 Mild hydrocephalus. The atrial measurement (marked) is 11 mm, just above the upper limit of normal. The medial wall (M) is separated from the choroid plexus (C). The hydrocephalus was confirmed at autopsy.

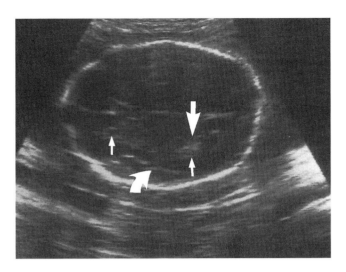

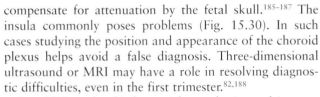

Fig. 15.30 **Normal insula.** In this transverse section of a fetal head the straight large arrow points to the medial border of the posterior horn and the curved arrow points to the insula, which is commonly mistaken for the lateral wall of the lateral ventricle, resulting in the mistaken diagnosis of hydrocephalus. The true lateral wall is indicated by the small arrows.

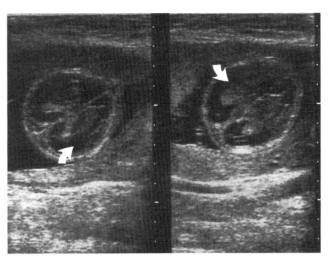

Fig. 15.31 **Osteogenesis imperfecta** in which lack of ossification of the bones of the skull results in reduced attenuation so that the cerebral structures (arrow to cortex) are more clearly seen, producing the impression of a fluid-filled structure and hence the false diagnosis of hydrocephalus.

compensate for attenuation by the fetal skull.[185–187] The insula commonly poses problems (Fig. 15.30). In such cases studying the position and appearance of the choroid plexus helps avoid a false diagnosis. Three-dimensional ultrasound or MRI may have a role in resolving diagnostic difficulties, even in the first trimester.[82,188]

In addition, the third ventricle can be imaged in most second- and third-trimester fetuses. Although there are changes in size and configuration as the gestation increases, a third ventricle greater than 3.5 mm in width should be viewed with concern at any gestation.[189]

It should be noted that in the vast majority of cases of isolated hydrocephalus the cerebellum is normal in size, in contrast to the hydrocephalus associated with the Arnold–Chiari malformation or neural tube defects (see Fig. 15.26).

Differential diagnosis

The main alternative diagnoses in cases of severe hydrocephalus are holoprosencephaly, hydranencephaly, Dandy–Walker syndrome and porencephalic cysts. In practice genuine hydrocephalus may coexist with, or be secondary to, these conditions. Pseudo-hydrocephalus and colpocephaly (apparent enlargement of the posterior horns secondary to poor development of the surrounding brain substance) may also cause confusion. Another anomaly which may be mistaken for hydrocephalus is osteogenesis imperfecta type II, where the normal brain structure is seen with remarkable clarity owing to the lack of ossification of the cranial vault (Fig. 15.31) (see Ch. 19).

Associated abnormalities

Around 85% of cases of fetal hydrocephalus are associated with other abnormalities, intracranial abnormalities occurring in 37% and extracranial in 63%.[190] Chromosomal abnormalities may be present in up to 12% of cases, including trisomy 21, balanced translocation and mosaicism.[154,191] Considering the cases of isolated hydrocephalus without spina bifida, 30% were associated with other abnormalities in one series, 3/30 having chromosomal abnormalities.[66] Other associated intracranial abnormalities include aqueduct stenosis, holoprosencephaly, hydranencephaly, Dandy–Walker malformation, absence of the corpus callosum, encephalocele and a clover-leaf skull deformity.

Extracranial anomalies range in frequency from 7% to 15% and include cardiac (VSD, Fallot's tetralogy), skeletal (sirenomelia, arthrogryposis, dysplastic phalanges), renal (agenesis, dysplasia), gastrointestinal (colonic and anal agenesis, duodenal atresia, malrotation of the bowel, anterior abdominal wall defects), Meckel's syndrome, gonadal dysgenesis and facial clefting, to name but a few.[66,192] Hydrocephalus can be found as part of many uncommon syndromes,[134] to which list may be added Walker–Warburg or HARD(E) syndromes.[193]

The success of ultrasonic diagnosis of hydrocephalus

This depends very much on the aetiology and time of onset and the degree of ventricular dilatation. Clearly if the hydrocephalus is caused by an insult such as infection occurring some time late in pregnancy, then the condition will not necessarily be detected by mid-trimester ultrasound scanning. If the condition is present at the time of scanning and is moderate to severe, then diagnosis should be reliable with no significant errors. The diagnosis of mild hydrocephalus is more difficult. Several authors have documented spontaneous resolution of ventriculomegaly in utero.[194,195] Although dilatation of the occipital or temporal horns may be an early sign,[176] the diagnosis of ventricular dilatation should not be based solely on these criteria as there is wide variation in this portion of the ventricular system in normal fetuses.[196] The finding of mild ventriculomegaly, defined as posterior horns between 10 and 15 mm diameter,[197] gives rise to problems. The predictive value of measurement is poor: some resolve or remain static, some progress, and some have chromosome abnormalities.[191] In our series, in 12 cases where the posterior horns were described as extremely prominent at 18–19 weeks, repeat examination 2–3 weeks later showed that seven had resolved spontaneously. Of the five that persisted, no other intracranial signs were found. One was shown to have multiple congenital abnormalities, one a chromosomal abnormality, and three had a normal outcome (Figs 15.32 and 15.33). Prominent posterior horns require further evaluation.

Prognosis

The prognosis of the hydrocephalic fetus depends on the exact type of concurrent anomalies. Several studies have reported the outcome in a series of hydrocephalic fetuses totalling in excess of 250 cases.[173,192,194,198,199] Although complicated by terminations of pregnancy and destructive

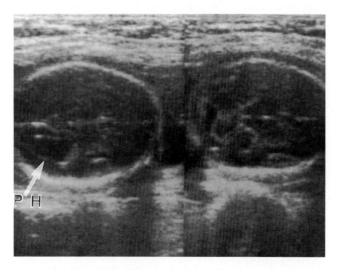

Fig. 15.32 **Prominent posterior horns** (PH) in a fetus with a chromosomal translocation. The rest of the intracranial anatomy is unremarkable. At autopsy multiple abnormalities were found, including mild hydrocephalus.

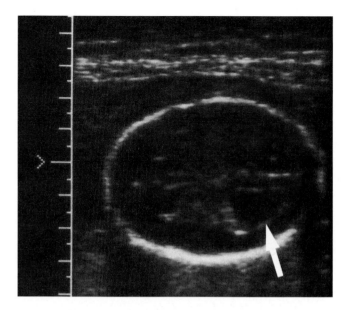

Fig. 15.33 **Prominent posterior horns** of the lateral ventricle in an otherwise normal head. The pregnancy proceeded to term and an apparently normal baby was delivered. If anything, the horns are more prominent in this normal case than in the abnormal one in Figure 15.32.

operations, quoted survival rates range from 15% to 34%. This leads to dilemmas in counselling and management, with outcome ranging from normal to mild developmental delay to serious handicap.[200] In one series only 4/41 were terminated, but only 34% survived.[194] Despite neonatal ventricular shunting, only 40–60% of those that survived were intellectually normal.[197] In another reported series of 47 cases 25 were associated with other abnormalities, of which none survived, 19 being terminated.[201] Of the 22 with isolated ventriculomegaly 14 were developmentally normal; nine required a shunting procedure, and of these nine, six were severely handicapped and two mildly delayed. Outcome is strongly affected by the presence of other abnormalities. In one series only 16% of patients with hydrocephalus had no associated abnormalities, whereas 56% had extra CNS abnormalities.[192] Some studies have suggested that a cortical thickness of less than 1 cm at birth predicts a poor outcome,[202] but this association has been questioned. Hydrocephalus present before 32 weeks appears to carry a worse prognosis.[203]

Recurrence risk

If associated with a chromosome abnormality or single gene defect the recurrence risk is that of the primary condition. Otherwise the empirical recurrence risk has been estimated at 1–2%.[170,204,205] If more than one male fetus with hydrocephalus has been born in a family, sex-linked recessive aqueduct stenosis is likely. If only one male infant has been affected with aqueduct stenosis, empirical recurrence risks of 4–7% are quoted.[169,170,206]

Obstetric management

Once a firm diagnosis of hydrocephalus has been made a very careful search for other abnormalities is mandatory, specific attention being paid to the fetal spine[201]. The detailed appearance of the hydrocephalus as previously described indicates whether a neural tube defect is likely or not. Termination may be offered, especially in the presence of other abnormalities. If the parents elect to continue with the pregnancy a karyotyping procedure and viral screen should be performed so that as much information as possible is available when the time comes for delivery. A dilemma is raised by the fetus which appears to have mild hydrocephalus and in which no other abnormality, including chromosomal, can be found.[182,191] Such cases should be carefully and thoroughly assessed and a guarded prognosis given.[178,182] If the parents elect to continue with the pregnancy serial assessments should be performed at regular intervals to detect any significant change. Prenatal paediatric neurosurgical consultation may improve management.[207]

If hydrocephalus is detected in later pregnancy a thorough search should still be made for other abnormalities, including performing a rapid karyotyping procedure. A decision must be made as to whether the pregnancy is terminated or whether intervention is justified, and the mode of delivery that should be attempted. Each case should be assessed on its merits, but most obstetricians adopt a conservative approach and aim for a vaginal delivery if the head size permits it. The fetus should be monitored serially to pick up progressive ventricular enlargement, this being an indication for early delivery.

If there is gross hydrocephalus together with macrocephaly, decompression of the fetal head may be performed abdominally or *per vaginam* during delivery. This procedure is destructive but it cannot be guaranteed to be lethal. A caesarean section should be considered if macrocephaly is present.[208]

Intra-uterine treatment with placement of a ventriculo-amniotic shunt has been attempted[201,209,210] but has not gained widespread acceptance. In one series of 39 treated fetuses the perinatal mortality was 18%, with 66% of the survivors having a moderate to severe handicap.[211] In a further series procedure mortality was 10% and only 33% of the survivors appeared to be developing normally.[212]

Holoprosencephaly

Holoprosencephaly is a spectrum of disorders resulting from absent or incomplete cleavage of the forebrain or prosencephalon during early embryonic development. It includes a range of disorders in which a single embryological defect affects the growth of both brain and face.[213] Depending on the degree of division, the condition is classified as alobar, semilobar or lobar.[214] If cleavage is absent alobar holoprosencephaly results, with a single ventricular cavity, fusion of the thalami and absence of the corpus callosum, falx cerebri, optic tracts and olfactory bulbs. The thin lining of the ventricular cavity may bulge out to occupy the space between the calvarium and cerebral cortex, forming a cyst filled with CSF known as the dorsal sac. In semilobar holoprosencephaly partial cleavage occurs, the cerebral hemispheres being separated posteriorly with variable degrees of fusion of the thalami and absent olfactory bulbs and corpus callosum. A single ventricle with rudimentary occipital horns is present.

Macrocephaly or microcephaly, together with facial defects, including cyclopia (fused or nearly fused orbits with a supraorbital proboscis), cebocephaly (hypotelorism, single nostril in nose), ethmocephaly (hypotelorism, high midline proboscis), median cleft and holotelencephaly, can occur with both these forms.[213,215]

In lobar holoprosencephaly the two hemispheres are separated anteriorly and posteriorly, with a certain degree of fusion of structures such as the lateral ventricles and cingulate gyrus, and absence of the cavum septum pellucidum.

Incidence and aetiology

The incidence of severe holoprosencephaly among live births has been variously reported to lie between one in 1660 and one in 16 000;[216,217] cyclopia and cebocephaly occur in one in 40 000 and one in 16 000 births, respectively.[214,216] The incidence among all pregnancies is considerably greater than this, as many abort spontaneously. In one series holoprosencephaly was reported to account for 16–19% of all cases of hydrocephalus detected prenatally,[218] but this has not been borne out in other series. Some cases of holoprosencephaly are associated with chromosomal abnormalities. In reported series the incidence of these has been around 55%, including trisomies 13, 13/15 and 18, ring chromosomes and deletions.[213,214,218,219] In these cases the recurrence risk is around 1% for a trisomy secondary to non-disjunction, and considerably more if related to the parents carrying a balanced translation. In other cases the condition appears familial, the mode of inheritance having been reported as both autosomal recessive and autosomal dominant with variable penetrance.[213,214,216,220] Other studies have implicated salicylates,[221] alkaloids and radiation in animals.[214] Insulin-dependent diabetes also appears to have a strong association.[222]

Diagnosis

Both alobar and semilobar holoprosencephaly are readily amenable to prenatal diagnosis,[218,219,223–228] and prenatal diagnosis of the lobar variety has been reported.[229,230] First and early second-trimester diagnosis has been reported by several authors.[7,231–234] The facial abnormalities associated with holoprosencephaly may be better demonstrated by

3D ultrasound,[235,236] which is useful when diagnostic difficulties occur.

In alobar and semilobar holoprosencephaly the midline echo of the fetal head, generated largely by echoes from the inter-hemispheric fissure, is either completely absent (in the former case) or incomplete (in the latter). The midline echo may also be deficient in hydranencephaly and where there is a large porencephalic cyst. However, in addition, in alobar holoprosencephaly a single sickle-shaped ventricle is found occupying the frontal portion of the cerebrum on axial scans. Anterior to this is a thin rim of cortex, shaped like a horseshoe or boomerang (Figs 15.34 and 15.35). Posteriorly the ventricle is bounded by the thalami, which appear fused: this is an important diagnostic feature. In alobar holoprosencephaly the dorsal sac, if present, can be seen on axial scans at a higher level, and by scanning in the coronal plane it may be possible to demonstrate a connection between the ventricle and the sac (Fig. 15.36).

Antenatally it may be impossible to distinguish between the alobar and the semilobar forms, but this is unimportant as the prognosis is similar (Fig. 15.37).

In addition to the cerebral features, associated facial abnormalities (Fig. 15.38), including cyclopia,[223,237] cebocephaly, ethmocephaly, hypotelorism,[219,238,239] median cleft and holotelencephaly, may aid diagnosis. If such abnormalities are found fortuitously, a more detailed examination of the fetal brain is indicated. Facial abnormalities

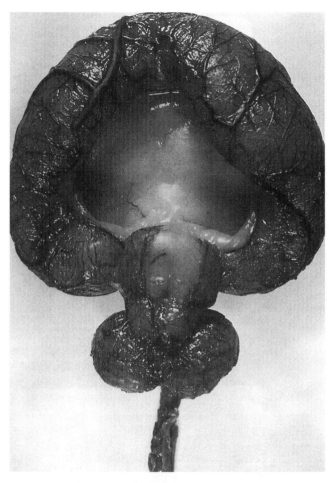

Fig. 15.35 Holoprosencephaly. Pathological specimen displaying the horseshoe-shaped cortex and fused thalami. (With thanks to Dr Ian Rushton, Consultant Perinatal Pathologist, Birmingham Maternity Hospital.)

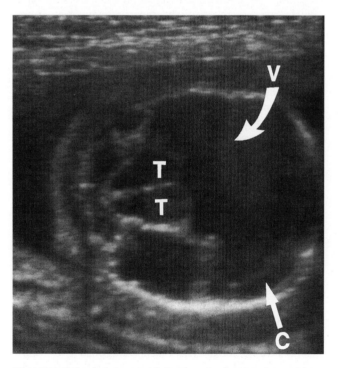

Fig. 15.34 Alobar holoprosencephaly. There is a large single ventricle (V) surrounded by a rim of cortex (C) anteriorly and the thalami (T) posteriorly. There is no midine echo.

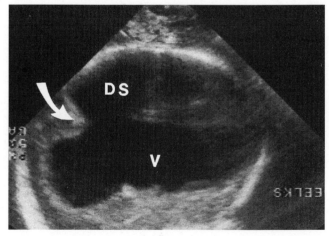

Fig. 15.36 Alobar holoprosencephaly. Vaginal scan of the head at the level of the dorsal sac (DS). The single ventricle (V) is seen inferiorly and the hippocampal ridge (arrowed) lies between the two. (With thanks to Charles Rodeck.)

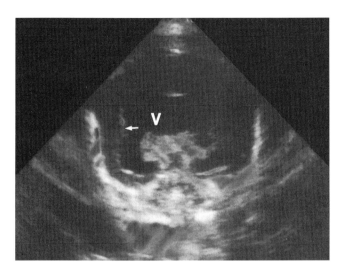

Fig. 15.37 Semilobar holoprosencephaly. Moderate hydrocephalus was initially diagnosed but the midline was partially deficient anteriorly, with no cavum septum pellucidum. In a coronal scan the single ventricle (V) could be identified surrounded by a thick rim of cortex (arrowed).

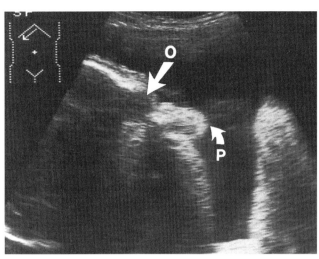

Fig. 15.38 Holoprosencephaly with anophthalmia and a proboscis. In a profile view of the fetal face the orbits (O) appear to be very shallow and no eye is visible. The nose is long and prominent (P).

usually but not inevitably predict an abnormal brain.[214] [215,218,240]

The lobar form is not so readily diagnosed because the inter-hemispheric fissure is well formed and the lateral ventricles are only fused anteriorly. The cavum septum pellucidum is absent, and this may alert the sonologist to this diagnosis in cases of apparent hydrocephalus. The antenatal ultrasound diagnosis of lobar holoprosencephaly has been reported;[229,230] the fusion of the anterior horns of the ventricular system and the central mass were identified.

Associated abnormalities

In addition to the facial features described above other abnormalities associated with holoprosencephaly include polydactyly, exomphalos, renal dysplasia and fetal hydrops.[218] This is to be suspected, as many cases have abnormal chromosomes.

Differential diagnosis

The major differential diagnoses of the more severe forms of holoprosencephaly are severe hydrocephalus and hydranencephaly. As the prognosis in all these conditions is uniformly poor, the exact prenatal diagnosis is unimportant. Particular features that point to severe forms of holoprosencephaly are facial abnormalities (including reduction in the interorbital distances, which can be measured and compared to established nomograms: see Appendix), a dorsal sac, fused thalami, an anterior boomerang cortical rim and the absence of a midline echo. In hydrocephalus the thalami may be seen to be separated by a dilated third

ventricle, whereas in hydranencephaly the anterior cortical rim is never seen. The presence of a cavum septum pellucidum effectively rules out any form of holoprosencephaly. Semilobar holoprosencephaly can present a similar appearance to complete absence of the corpus callosum, with a large inter-hemispheric cyst. Here the presence of a dilated third ventricle and frontal horns may point to the latter. The diagnosis of lobar holoprosencephaly relies mainly on the absence of the cavum septum pellucidum, together with variable enlargement of the lateral ventricles. These features are also seen in absence of the corpus callosum.

Prognosis

Alobar and semilobar holoprosencephaly have a very poor prognosis,[241] virtually all infants with the more severe form dying in the first year of life. Some with semilobar holoprosencephaly may survive into infancy with amentia.[214] Patients with lobar holoprosencephaly have some degree of mental impairment, but often a normal life expectancy.

Obstetric management

If the parents agree, termination of pregnancy is the best management in alobar and semilobar holoprosencephaly. In practice these are the varieties usually recognised prenatally. If termination is not an option, conservative management and delivery should be aimed for. Karyotyping should be performed in all cases to aid in management of this and future pregnancies. Lobar holoprosencephaly may pose a more difficult management problem, the degree of mental impairment being variable.

Risk of recurrence

An empirical risk of recurrence has been reported as 6% in the absence of chromosomal or genetic influences.[213,214,216] In cases with an autosomal dominant inheritance the penetrance is reduced such that the risk to first-degree relatives is 23–35%. If the fetus was chromosomally abnormal then the risk ranges from an assumed 1% if the parent's karyotypes are normal, to a much higher risk if one of the parents is a carrier for a balanced translocation.

Agenesis of the corpus callosum

The corpus callosum consists of bundles of white matter which connect the right and left cerebral hemispheres, forming a pathway via which information is exchanged and coordinated.[242] Development of the corpus callosum is later than the majority of the nervous system; it starts anteriorly at 8 weeks gestation and proceeds posteriorly, complete formation not occurring until after the fifth month.[243–245] Development may be arrested, leading to complete or partial agenesis. In the latter the posterior or caudal portion is absent. Post-natal diagnoses of agenesis of the corpus callosum (AGCC) have been made by pneumo-encephalography,[246] ultrasound[247–249] and CT scanning,[244,250] MRI may be useful where diagnosis is uncertain.

Incidence and aetiology

The true incidence of partial or complete agenesis of the corpus callosum in the general population remains unknown, figures ranging from one in 100 to one in 19 000 being suggested.[251] An autopsy study showed an incidence of 5.3%,[251] and a study of 6450 pneumo-encephalograms showed an incidence of 0.7%.[252] In mentally retarded persons a frequency of 2.3% has been quoted.[253] All of these series were of highly selected patients and are unlikely to be representative.

Absence of the corpus callosum may occur as an isolated entity.[254,255] In some cases familial transmission has been described following both autosomal dominant, recessive and sex-linked modes of inheritance.[251,254,256–258] Chromosomal abnormalities (trisomies 18, 13 and 8 and translocations)[253] have been found in association with AGCC. This condition can also occur in a variety of syndromes, examples being the median cleft face syndrome and Andermann's syndrome, and has been reported in association with maternal rubella and toxoplasmosis,[259,260] the fetal alcohol syndrome,[261] tuberous sclerosis,[262] mucopolysaccharidosis[243] and the basal cell naevus syndrome. In many cases, however, no obvious cause is found.

Diagnosis

When the corpus callosum is absent the fibres that were destined to develop into it run instead along the medial walls of the lateral ventricles in thick longitudinal bundles,[263] setting the ventricles further apart. In addition there is poor development of the white matter surrounding the occipital horns and atria, which consequently become enlarged, a condition known as colpocephaly (Fig. 15.39). As the corpus callosum normally forms the roof of the third ventricle, this is able to enlarge in a cranial direction, sometimes herniating upwards and forming a large interhemispheric cyst (Fig. 15.40). The development of the corpus callosum and septum pellucidum are closely related.[245,264] Absence of the latter is an easily noted ultrasound finding that should prompt careful evaluation of the corpus callosum. On routine transverse sections of the fetal head, appearances suggesting AGCC therefore include laterally displaced lateral ventricles, absence of the cavum septum pellucidum, disproportionate enlargement of the occipital horns and variable dilatation of the third ventricle.[265–267] If any of these findings is present, sagittal and coronal views should be obtained to assess the lateral ventricles and any upward extension of the third ventricle. A characteristic 'steerhorn' appearance is seen in frontal coronal sections.[240] A search should always be made for other associated abnormalities.

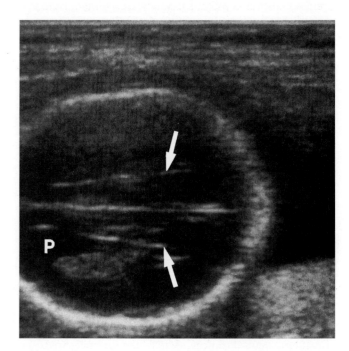

Fig. 15.39 Agenesis of the corpus callosum. A transverse scan of the head reveals the marked separation of the medial walls (arrows) of the anterior horns of the lateral ventricles, which normally nearly touch in the midline. The medial walls are also unusually obvious. Colpocephaly is illustrated by the marginal enlargement of the posterior horns (P).

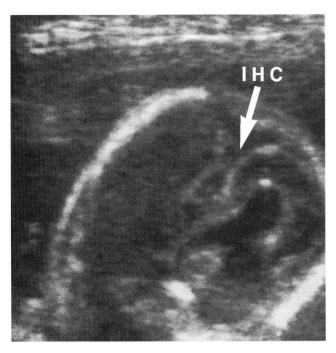

Fig. 15.40 Agenesis of the corpus callosum. A coronal view displays the inter-hemispheric cyst (IHC).

Associated malformations

The defects most commonly associated with this disorder are those of the holoprosencephaly series. Also occurring frequently are hydrocephalus, porencephaly and encephalocele.[253,264,268] In some series up to 88% of cases have other CNS abnormalities, and 65% have cardiovascular, gastrointestinal, genitourinary or other extra-CNS lesions.[267,268] When agenesis of the corpus callosum occurs as part of a syndrome it will have the specific abnormalities of that syndrome and condition.

Differential diagnosis

Lobar holoprosencephaly and mild hydrocephalus may be difficult to differentiate. In mild hydrocephalus the cavum septum pellucidum should always be present and only the lateral walls of the lateral ventricles are displaced outwards. This contrasts with AGCC, where both walls are displaced outwards. Holoprosencephaly and AGCC are frequently associated. Semilobar holoprosencephaly may be confused with AGCC and a large inter-hemispheric cyst. Determining whether the thalami are fused or separated by the third ventricle clarifies the situation, but this may not be possible.

Prognosis

Absence of the corpus callosum may have no or only subtle neurological sequelae,[251] and infants with complete AGCC are often mentally normal and asymptomatic. In one series, however, low intelligence occurred in 70% and fits in 60%.[264] Associated abnormalities may be the major determinant in prognosis in many cases.[269] Several series have reported follow-up following antenatal diagnosis in which[267,270] several fetuses had severe associated abnormalities and fits were common, although some children were developing normally.[267,270]

Obstetric management

Although AGCC as an isolated finding may not alter obstetric management, the frequency of other abnormalities should prompt a closer examination and karyotyping of the fetus. Each case should then be managed on its own merits and certainly, in view of the variable prognosis, termination should be considered as an option.

Recurrence risk

In most cases the recurrence risk is very low, the majority of cases being sporadic.[271] A small minority are part of a familial syndrome, chromosomal abnormality, or inherited in a Mendelian fashion.[258]

Lissencephaly

Lissencephaly is a brain malformation where there are essentially no sulci or gyri and a severe arrest of development of grey matter has occurred. The majority of cases are microcephalic. Other intracranial anomalies may be present, in particular hydrocephalus, agenesis of the corpus callosum and a Dandy–Walker type dilatation of the fourth ventricle, with hypoplasia of midline portions of the cerebellum.

Incidence and aetiology

This is an extremely rare condition thought to result from the homozygous state of an uncommon altered cerebral recessive gene.[272,273]

Diagnosis

In utero, there is commonly polyhydramnios in the second half of pregnancy. The associated microcephaly or hydrocephalus should easily be detected,[270,274,275] but definitive diagnosis by ultrasound is difficult. Definite prenatal diagnosis by MRI has been reported in two cases in which the features were barely detected by ultrasound.[276]

Associated abnormalities

In addition to the various intracerebral signs there are commonly other abnormalities, such as micromelia, polydactyly, congenital heart disease, renal abnormalities and duodenal atresia. Intra-uterine growth retardation is common.

Prognosis

This condition is invariably fatal in infancy or childhood.

Obstetric management

In a family at risk of lissencephaly, if there is an indication that the fetus has the condition termination of pregnancy may be offered.

Hydranencephaly

Hydranencephaly is a condition where the cerebral cortex and basal ganglia are destroyed, their place being occupied by CSF. The thalami and lower brain centres are usually preserved. The result is a fluid-filled skull lined by leptomeninges, into which these structures protrude.[66]

Incidence and aetiology

Hydranencephaly is a rare abnormality, said to be present in 0.2% of infant autopsies and approximately 1% of babies who are diagnosed clinically as having hydrocephalus.[277] It is thought to be the result of a destructive process involving the fetal brain early in gestation, and therefore could be considered as the extreme end of a spectrum which also includes porencephaly and schizencephaly. Support for the destructive aetiology, which may be secondary to vascular occlusion or a severe infective episode, comes from animal studies, fetal ultrasound changes seen *in utero* and post-mortem findings. Bilateral occlusion of the internal carotid arteries has been postulated as one mechanism for this destruction, but this does not account for the occurrence of the anomaly in dizygotic twins.[253] In studies in monkeys, partial placental abruptions have been shown to be precursors of hydranencephaly,[278] whereas changes leading to hydranencephaly have been documented in a fetus followed throughout pregnancy.[279] In post-mortem studies of affected fetuses, however, the vascular findings are variable. Absence,[280] thrombosis[278] and vasculitis of the cerebral vessels have been reported, but in many fetuses the internal carotid arteries are patent.[281] Hydranencephaly has also been reported to result from toxoplasmosis, probably secondary to vasculitis or local brain destruction.[282]

Diagnosis

An intracranial cavity filled with fluid is typical of hydranencephaly, the cerebral tissue and falx usually being totally absent (Fig. 15.41).[68,283–285] In less severe cases remnants of the cerebral tissue may remain, together with a midline

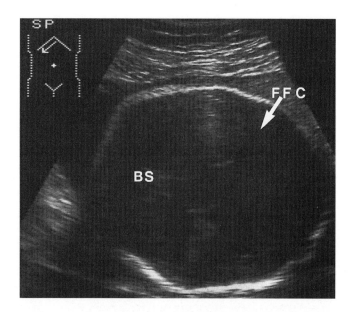

Fig. 15.41 Hydranencephaly. The cerebral hemispheres are entirely replaced by fluid and the brain stem (BS) protrudes into the fluid-filled cavity (FFC). No normal architecture is identified.

echo from the falx. Close examination shows that there is no rim of cortical tissue and that the brain stem typically bulges into the cavity, giving a characteristic appearance.[66] The head size may be normal or large.[286,287] First-trimester diagnosis of hydranencephaly has been reported.[288]

Differential diagnosis

Other causes of an apparently fluid-filled intracranial cavity include gross hydrocephalus and alobar holoprosencephaly. In both, cerebral tissue persists, either as a rim lining the vault, or surrounding the brain stem.

Prognosis

Not surprisingly, in view of the cerebral destruction the prognosis for infants with hydranencephaly is very poor. Some die at birth, whereas others initially appear normal, surviving for up to 3 years, but with no intellectual function.[286]

Obstetric management

Termination of the pregnancy is recommended once the diagnosis has been confirmed. As the prognosis is so poor cephalocentesis may be indicated if macrocrania develops when the condition is found in late pregnancy.

Recurrence risk

As expected, the vast majority of cases represent sporadic events. A handful of case reports have described familial hydranencephaly in association with other findings, such as talipes, absent kidneys and arthrogryposis.[286,289]

Porencephaly/schizencephaly

These terms refer to cystic intracerebral structures which, if communicating with the ventricular system or subarachnoid space, contain CSF. The nomenclature is confusing, some authorities using the term porencephaly to describe a lesion that follows local destruction of brain substance, and others referring to this as pseudoporencephaly. A similar appearance secondary to a developmental anomaly may be referred to as true porencephaly or schizencephaly when bilateral symmetrical clefts are present in the walls of the lateral ventricles. In the following description porencephaly is taken to refer to a destructive lesion, whereas schizencephaly denotes a developmental origin.

Incidence and aetiology

In an autopsy study of infantile brains schizencephaly was found to have an incidence of 2.5%.[290] The true incidence of porencephaly is unknown, although in one series of 112 CNS abnormalities one case of porencephaly was noted,[180] and in a series of 500 patients with epilepsy porencephaly was detected in 2%.[291]

Porencephaly follows destruction of cerebral tissue which is commonly a consequence of infarction or haemorrhage. Post-natally other recognised causes include trauma and infection.[290,292,293] The infarcted tissue becomes necrotic, forming a cystic space which may become confluent with the ventricular system but may occur in almost any position in the cerebrum, and may be single or multiple.

Schizencephaly is a developmental abnormality which arises from a failure of migration of cells destined to form the cerebral cortex. The result is a cleft-like deficiency in the cortex, commonly bilateral, which communicates with the subarachnoid space.[294–296] Such clefts usually occur around the Sylvian fissure in the region supplied by the middle cerebral arteries. Schizencephaly is a severe form of the migration anomaly, less severe forms being manifest as macrogyria or pachygyria (fewer larger cerebral gyri) and lissencephaly (absent gyri).[297]

Diagnosis

Both porencephaly and schizencephaly should be considered in the differential diagnosis of cystic lesions in the brain.[298]

Porencephalic cysts are usually unilateral and, because they are caused by destruction of normal tissue, do not create a mass effect.[240] Because there is often ischaemic damage and failure of growth of the surrounding brain tissue, the ipsilateral ventricle may enlarge and appear ragged owing to communication with the cyst. Neither of these causes of ventricular enlargement constitutes true hydrocephalus. The midline echo is present, but may be displaced. Some cortical substance should be recognised in each cerebral hemisphere (Fig. 15.42).

Schizencephaly is usually bilateral – although visualisation of the proximal ventricle may be difficult. The appearance is of fluid-filled spaces reaching from the skull inwards and communicating with the ventricles (Fig. 15.43).[296] In some cases shift of the midline may occur.[66] If apparent unilateral 'hydrocephalus' is seen schizencephaly and porencephaly should both be considered.

Differential diagnosis

This includes any cystic brain lesion, hydrocephalus, Dandy–Walker cyst, holoprosencephaly, arachnoid cyst, inter-hemispheric cysts in AGCC, etc. Each of these has characteristic features described in the appropriate sections.

Prognosis

Schizencephaly has a very poor prognosis. Mental retardation and neurological deficits are very common.

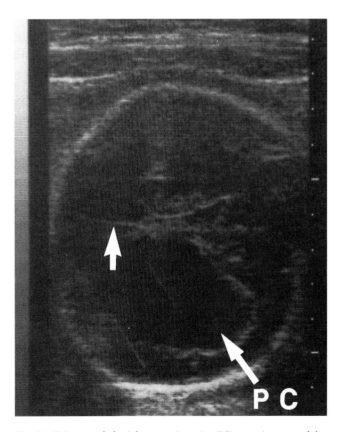

Fig. 15.42 Porencephaly. A large cystic cavity (PC) occupies most of the inferior hemisphere and the midline (short arrow) is shifted. There is no evidence of a cystic structure in the superior hemisphere.

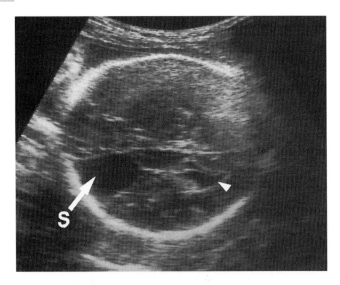

Fig. 15.43 Schizencephaly. A fluid-filled space (S) is seen anteriorly extending through the brain substance to the skull and communicating with the lateral ventricle (arrowhead).

Porencephaly also has a very poor outcome,[298] not least because ischaemic brain damage is likely to be more widespread than is visualised by antenatal ultrasound scan. Large lesions have a very poor prognosis, although smaller lesion may give rise to lesser degrees of disability.

Obstetric management

Because the prognosis of this condition is so poor, when diagnosed, termination of pregnancy should be discussed.

Recurrence risk

Both conditions appear to be sporadic, but autosomal dominant and recessive inheritance has been described in one and two families, respectively.[299,300]

Dandy–Walker malformation

The Dandy–Walker malformation (DWM) comprises a defect in the cerebellar vermis through which the fourth ventricle communicates with a posterior fossa cyst. Neonates usually have hydrocephalus of variable degree, although this may not be present antenatally. When first described it was thought to be secondary to atresia of the foramina of Luschka and Magendie,[301,302] although this appears unlikely as they are often patent at post-mortem. A more probable explanation is that the Dandy–Walker malformation is a complex abnormality of midline structures and should be classified together with holoprosencephaly, AGCC, etc.[303,304] In support of this an 18% incidence of other midline abnormalities has been reported in association with the Dandy–Walker malformation.[305]

Incidence and aetiology

The Dandy–Walker syndrome is reported to occur in approximately one in 25 000–35 000 pregnancies.[306] It is thought to represent a non-specific end-point resulting from a variety of diverse aetiologies,[305] including such inherited disorders as the Meckel–Gruber, Warburg and Aicardi syndromes and single gene disorders. Inheritance in the different syndromes ranges from dominant to sex-linked and recessive. In recent series three out of 40,[306] two out of seven[307] and four out of 12[308] cases had an abnormal karyotype, including trisomies 13, 18 and 21.

Diagnosis

The Dandy–Walker malformation is established early in fetal development and has been reported in a 14-week fetus.[309] It is therefore amenable to diagnosis at the mid-trimester scan. The finding of a posterior fossa cyst on ultrasound should suggest a Dandy–Walker malformation and initiate a detailed search for further confirmation.[307,308,310,311] The specific feature that differentiates this from other causes of a posterior fossa cyst is the cerebellar defect (Fig. 15.44) and so the cerebellum should be examined carefully. In some cases the cerebellar hemispheres are widely separated and compressed, whereas in others the connection may be small and difficult to visualise (Fig. 15.45). This is especially true where the superior vermis is intact, the defect occurring in the inferior vermis. In such cases the only finding may be an enlarged cisterna magna.[240] Although the cerebellum may appear small, its absence is not typical of the condition. Hydrocephalus is present antenatally in only 20% of cases.[306–308,312] If it occurs care should be taken to differentiate true hydro-

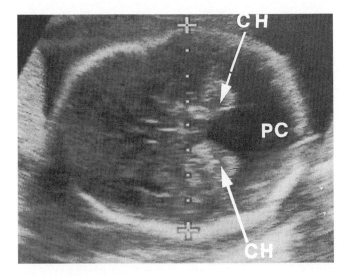

Fig. 15.44 Dandy–Walker malformation. A large posterior fossa cyst (PC) is seen. The cerebellar hemispheres (CH) are widely separated.

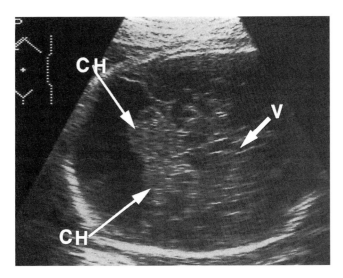

Fig. 15.45 Dandy–Walker malformation. In this case the cerebellar hemispheres (CH) are not obviously separated, the defect in the vermis being too small to image. Hydrocephalus was present and the dilated third ventricle (V) can be seen.

cephalus, with dilation of the third ventricle, from colpocephaly associated with agenesis of the corpus callosum, where this dilatation is absent. In fetuses with vertex presentation trans-vaginal scanning improves diagnostic accuracy.[313]

Differential diagnosis

Other causes of a cystic structure in the posterior fossa include a prominent cisterna magna, an arachnoid cyst and a dorsal cyst associated with holoprosencephaly. A prominent cisterna magna should never exceed 10 mm in depth,[311] and is associated with a cerebellum of normal size. An arachnoid cyst is often asymmetrical and again is not associated with cerebellar abnormalities.[314] A dorsal cyst is supratentorial, communicating directly with a single ventricle, and other features of holoprosencephaly are also present.

Associated malformations

Central nervous system abnormalities have been noted at autopsy in 68% of infants and adults with a Dandy–Walker malformation.[315] These include AGCC in 7–19% of cases,[306,307,315] lipomas, aqueduct stenosis and non-specific gyral abnormalities. Abnormalities outside the CNS occur in 25–60%, including polydactyly, cardiac defects, renal malformations and facial anomalies.[304–307,315] The latter includes an association noted with facial haemangiomas.[305,306] In cases where multiple abnormalities are present an underlying chromosomal problem should be sought.

Prognosis

Of cases not detected antenatally, 80% will present with symptoms of hydrocephalus before the age of 12 months,[306] overall mortality being reported as varying from 12% to 67%.[306,308] Many of these are attributable to associated congenital abnormalities. The functional outcome in survivors is variable. Subnormal intelligence (an IQ less than 83) has been reported in 41–71% of survivors.[306,316] Keogan *et al.* reported a good prognosis with isolated inferior vermian agenesis in a small series.[317]

Obstetric management

A careful examination for other anomalies should be undertaken, together with a karyotyping procedure. If the diagnosis is made in the mid-trimester, termination should be offered. At later gestations, full counselling with neurosurgical consultation is essential in deciding management.

Recurrence risk

Excluding certain autosomal recessive and X-linked dominant syndromes the recurrence risk for future pregnancies is between 1% and 5%.[305] There also appears to be a slightly increased risk of 7% that siblings may have other midline abnormalities.

Choroid plexus cysts

The choroid plexus occupies the lateral, the third and the fourth ventricles and is the major source of cerebrospinal fluid. Its size relative to the rest of the brain varies through embryonic life: it appears at around 7 weeks gestation, reaches the maximum proportions by the late first/early second trimester, and attains its adult appearance by 20 weeks.[318,319] During the early second trimester the size and the reflectivity of the choroid plexus make it one of the most easily recognised parts of the fetal brain. Cysts of the choroid plexus are common and have been reported in up to 50% of all autopsies, occurring in all age groups.[318]

Incidence and aetiology

Choroid plexus cysts (CPCs) are thought to represent neuroepithelial folds that subsequently fill with cerebrospinal fluid and cellular debris.[318,319] Their prevalence has been estimated at between 0.1% and 1%,[320–327] being noted to be highly dependent on the quality of both the ultrasound equipment and the operator.[325]

Diagnosis

Choroid plexus cysts are seen as discrete round or oval echo-free structures within the substance of the choroid

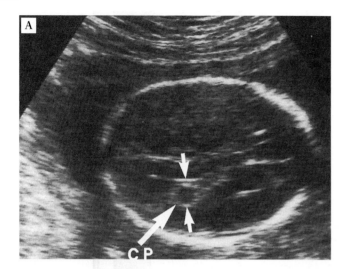

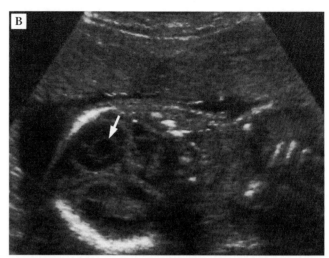

Fig. 15.46 Choroid plexus cyst. A: This small round cyst can be seen within the substance of the choroid plexus (CP) in the lateral ventricle (arrowed) in the inferior hemisphere. No cyst is seen in the superior hemisphere in the scan, but this is probably due to 'reverberation' artefact, when a change in position of the fetal head may reveal another cyst. **B:** When the placenta is anterior the proximal hemisphere may be better seen. Note the choroid plexus cyst (arrow).

plexus (Fig. 15.46), which must be identified as surrounding the cyst, most frequently at the level of the atrium of the lateral ventricle. They are usually detected between 16 and 20 weeks and are typically 3–14 mm in diameter. Larger cysts of up to 20 mm have, however, been reported. Unilateral and bilateral cysts have been said to occur with equal frequency, but in fact it is likely that bilateral cysts are the rule, the one present in the nearer hemisphere being difficult to see because of reverberation artefact.[320,325] Generally the cysts decrease in size as the gestation advances and the majority resolve by 26 weeks,[320,325,328] although some persist longer.

Associated malformations

There has been much discussion over the years on the association between choroid plexus cysts and chromosome abnormality, early studies suggesting links with trisomies 13, 18 and 21.[320,322,323,325,329–332] Overall, the risk of chromosomal abnormality in the presence of isolated CPCs has been estimated at 1 in 150 in an unselected population, the majority of these being trisomy 18. The risk of Down's syndrome in fetuses with isolated cysts has been estimated as 1 in 880,[333] or said to occur with similar frequency to the general population.[334] This significant association with trisomy 18 and negligible association with trisomy 21 has been confirmed by a number of authors.[328,330,335] Discussion has also taken place as to the relative importance of the size of the cysts, persistence beyond 22–24 weeks, and whether they are unilateral or bilateral.[320,325,336–338] Although there is some evidence that persistent and particularly large cysts have a greater association with trisomy 18,[335] this is not borne out by all authors.[326,339] Large choroid plexus cysts may cause obstructive hydrocephalus (Fig. 15.47).

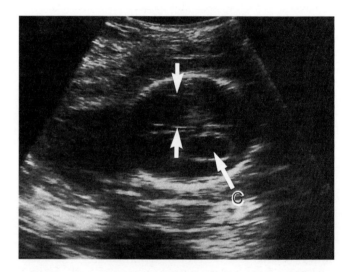

Fig. 15.47 Choroid plexus cyst causing hydrocephalus. In this case bilateral large cysts (C) caused obstructive hydrocephalus. The enlarged lateral ventricle can be seen between the small arrows.

Differential diagnosis

Porencephalic cysts and hydrocephalus may be confused with choroid plexus cysts at first glance. A closer inspection will always reveal that choroid plexus cysts arise within the choroid plexus, unlike the former.

Prognosis

Unless other abnormalities or a trisomy coexist, these lesions have an excellent prognosis.

Obstetric management

Choroid plexus cysts are common between 16 and 21 weeks gestation and normally resolve spontaneously. When found, a careful search must be made for any other fetal or pregnancy abnormality or soft marker. If any such problem is found the patient should be counselled as to the possibility of an underlying chromosomal abnormality, and a karyotyping procedure discussed.[340] Consideration should also be given to other risk factors, namely maternal age or biochemical screening results, and similar action taken.[341-343] Pregnancy termination may subsequently be indicated, either because of the particular nature of the other abnormalities or because of abnormal karyotype. If the cyst is truly isolated and there are no other risk factors then no further action need be taken at this stage.[328,335,343] It can be seen that the quality of the mid-trimester scan is extremely important: if there is any doubt as to its quality then a further detailed scan is advisable.[326] This may be best delayed 2–3 weeks so that the growth rate can be assessed and cardiac septal defects will be more amenable to detection. If at any time during the pregnancy a further risk factor becomes manifest, for example polyhydramnios, dilated fetal kidneys or early IUGR, then the situation should be reviewed.

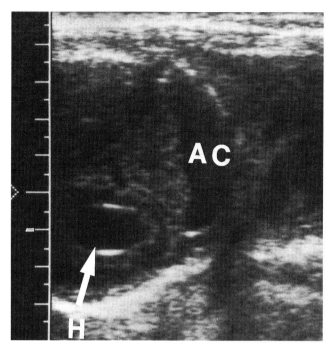

Fig. 15.48 Arachnoid cyst (AC) in the posterior fossa mimicking a Dandy–Walker malformation, although the cerebellar hemispheres are not separated. Hydrocephalus (H) is present. This fetus was affected with CMV and was severely growth retarded.

Arachnoid cysts

Arachnoid cysts are fluid-filled intracranial cavities lined wholly or partially by arachnoid. As such, they enter the differential diagnosis of any cystic intracranial structure, arising at any site within the CNS, including the spinal cord, the most frequent sites being the surface of the cerebral hemispheres in the region of the major fissures.[344] Other sites are the anterior and middle fossae[345,346] and the posterior fossa,[347] in the latter closely mimicking a Dandy–Walker malformation (Fig. 15.48).[314] The cysts may arise from either a localised enlargement of the subarachnoid space, a subarachnoid cyst, or between the inner and outer layers of arachnoid, an intra-arachnoid cyst.[348] They may grow either as a result of a valve-like effect, trapping CSF, or because of the presence of secreting tissue within the cyst itself.

Incidence and aetiology

Arachnoid cysts can be a congenital developmental abnormality or follow infection or haemorrhage.[344,349] The population incidence is unknown. In a series of 112 CNS abnormalities detected by ultrasound, two arachnoid cysts were found.[180] In our experience of over 300 cases of CNS abnormalities we have seen one case secondary to CMV infection.

Diagnosis

An arachnoid cyst always presents as a single cystic area within the brain or on its surface,[350] and can easily be confused with other anomalies, as described below. However, an arachnoid cyst does not communicate with the ventricular system and causes displacement of other structures, rather than being destructive. In the posterior fossa it thus displaces the cerebellum *en bloc*, rather than separating the hemispheres as in the Dandy–Walker malformation.[240] Compression of the ventricular system may lead to hydrocephalus.

Differential diagnosis

The differential diagnosis includes any discrete intracranial cystic structure, including choroid plexus cysts, porencephaly, schizencephaly, DWM, inter-hemispheric cysts, aneurysm of the vein of Galen, intracranial neoplasms, etc.[298] Often the diagnosis may be clarified by careful attention to detail, in other cases a precise diagnosis may be impossible.[66,351]

Prognosis

Antenatal diagnoses have been made and prognosis appears to be good.[298] In the infant period arachnoid cysts may be asymptomatic, or may cause hydrocephalus, epilepsy or mild neurological disturbances.[348,352] Some cysts have been successfully resected, and in general as they cause compression rather than destruction, the prospects for normal growth and development of the infant following treatment are good. However, if the aetiology of the cyst has been infection, such as CMV, this may prejudice the prognosis.

Obstetric management and recurrence risk

If such lesions are detected in the second trimester termination should be considered, as an accurate diagnosis may be impossible. In the third trimester, in the absence of hydrocephalus, a normal delivery should be anticipated. Where the diagnosis is moderately certain the labour and delivery should be managed in a normal fashion, but an infection screen for toxoplasmosis and cytomegalovirus, either on maternal, but preferably on fetal blood, should be performed, along with a rapid karyotyping procedure.

The recurrence risk is unknown but likely to be very low.

Posterior fossa abnormalities

Some abnormalities of the posterior fossa have been described under the appropriate headings. Some present as a cystic lesion, e.g. DWM and arachnoid cysts, whereas others are typified by an absent or abnormal cerebellum, e.g. Arnold–Chiari malformation. Any ultrasound examination of the fetal head should thus include an assessment of both the cerebellum and the posterior fossa. This can easily be done by measuring the cerebellum[353] and cisterna magna.[180,311,354] Nomograms for transverse cerebellar diameter can be used (see Appendix),[353] but a useful rule is that between 15 and 25 weeks the mean diameter in millimetres is within 1 mm of the gestational age in weeks. Measurement of the cisterna magna on the same section as that used for cerebellar measurements shows a mean depth of 5–7 mm, with an upper limit of 10 mm.[180,311,354] Care should be taken that the plane of measurement is not oblique.

Cerebellar abnormalities

The appearance of an absent cerebellum may be caused by the Arnold–Chiari type II malformation in association with spina bifida, when other features should clarify the diagnosis. True cerebellar hypoplasia may also occur, in some cases as an isolated finding in children with mental retardation;[355] experimentally it has been produced by parvovirus infection.[356] In other cases it occurs as part of a syndrome: in Joubert's syndrome it is in association with a unique respiratory abnormality, whereas in the Walker–Warburg or HARD(E) syndrome it is associated with hydrocephalus, agyria, retinal dysplasia and encephalocele.[357,358] These conditions may be inherited in an autosomal recessive manner. Other rare associations have also been noted.[359] If no definite entity can be found, a recurrence risk of 1 in 8 has been suggested.[360]

An abnormal cerebellar shape is associated with both the Arnold–Chiari malformation and the Dandy–Walker malformation, described elsewhere.

Enlarged cisterna magna

An enlarged cisterna magna may be obvious as a large cystic structure, or be detected only by careful measurement. Slight enlargement may be a benign variant of normal,[180] but other causes should be excluded, such as Dandy–Walker malformation, arachnoid cyst, communicating hydrocephalus, cerebellar hypoplasia and the dorsal cyst of holoprosencephaly.

Aneurysms of the internal cerebral veins

The cerebral veins may become enlarged as a result of direct arterial fistulae or secondary to adjacent arteriovenous malformations. The great vein of Galen, the major cerebral vein which runs over the thalami to join the inferior sagittal sinus as it runs along the lower edge of the falx, is one such vein which may be affected. In the 20–40 mm embryo fistulous connections may develop between the arterial and venous systems near the choroid plexus.[361] This results in a high-flow shunt between the cerebellar arteries and the vein of Galen, with progressive dilatation of the vein. The internal cerebral vein has also been reported as being affected by aneurysmal dilatation.

Incidence

Over 200 cases in total are recorded in the world literature.[362]

Diagnosis

The antenatal ultrasound diagnosis of an aneurysm of the vein of Galen has been reported on several occasions.[298,363–367] The salient features are an inter-hemispheric midline cyst of variable size that extends from the thalami to the straight sinus (Fig. 15.49), from which a characteristic high-frequency Doppler signal can be obtained. Aneurysms should be considered if any other unusual cystic structure is identified within the head, and Doppler ultrasound employed. MRI is a useful diagnostic adjunct.[367]

Associated abnormalities

Increased intracranial venous pressure or direct compression on the ventricular system, particularly the aqueduct

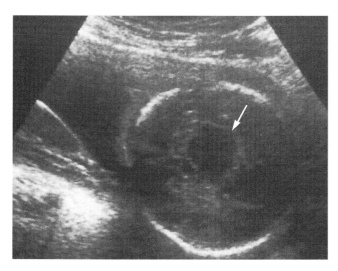

Fig. 15.49 Aneurysm of the internal cerebral vein displaying the large inter-hemispheric cyst (arrow).

of Sylvius, may give rise to hydrocephalus which, with macrocephaly, is frequently seen in the neonatal and infant periods. Ischaemic lesions such as porencephalic cysts may also be present owing to the decreased blood supply to the brain, most being shunted away. The size of the shunt may also lead to high-output cardiac failure and signs of hydrops fetalis.

Differential diagnosis

This is from other supratentorial cystic lesions, including choroid plexus cysts, porencephalic cysts, tumours, inter-hemispheric cysts in AGCC and dorsal cysts in holoprosencephaly. The differential diagnosis may be difficult to make, but a feature unique to an aneurysm is the high-frequency Doppler signal.[364]

Prognosis

In paediatric studies the prognosis appears to depend on the age at presentation. In the neonatal period severe high-output cardiac failure (non-immune hydrops) is the usual presentation.[298,368] In such cases the prognosis is very poor, the few survivors being grossly handicapped.[369] In another series only one out of nine survived, with severe handicap after treatment, results no better than without treatment.[370] In the infant and adult periods the results are much better, with a survival rate with no handicap of 20% after treatment.[370,371] It would seem likely that cases major enough to be noted and diagnosed in the antenatal period are likely to be at the severe end of the spectrum, with a poor prognosis.

Obstetric management

As the prognosis is generally poor, when the diagnosis is made early in the antenatal period termination should be

an option. If seen in later pregnancy associated hydrops and hydrocephalus should be sought. If either is present a poor prognosis is likely and termination should still be an option. If these signs are not present the parents should be given a guarded prognosis, especially if the precise diagnosis is in doubt.

Neoplasms

A wide variety of congenital intracranial tumours is recognised in the literature,[372] the vast majority being extremely rare. The most common is the benign or malignant teratoma, accounting for around 50% of cases,[373] glioblastomas being second in frequency. Even among these 'commoner' lesions only a handful have been diagnosed antenatally.[374,375] In addition to intracranial tumours teratomas of the sacrococcygeal region are found: these comprise over 50% of teratomas found at birth.

Incidence

Intracranial neoplasms account for 0.3% of all neonatal deaths before 28 days of life.[376] Some are asymptomatic and are therefore not detected until childhood or later. Sacrococcygeal tumours are the most common tumour encountered in the newborn, with an estimated incidence of one in 40 000 births and a high female to male ratio.

Diagnosis

The reported intracranial fetal neoplasms presented either with grossly disorganised intracranial contents owing to the bulk and mass effect of the tumour (Fig. 15.50), or

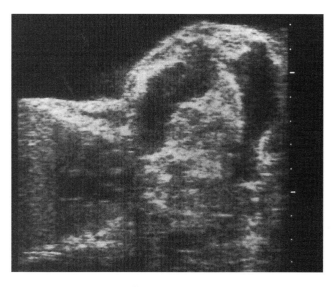

Fig. 15.50 Large intracranial teratoma expanding the fetal skull in this longitudinal section of a 26-week fetus. There is a complete loss of the normal anatomy, the greater part of the brain being replaced by a complex cystic/solid lesion.

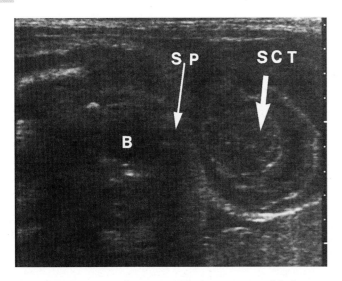

Fig. 15.51 Sacrococcygeal teratoma. This transverse scan of the lower pole of the fetus at the level of the bladder (B) shows a complex heterogeneous mass (SCT) behind the sacral spine (SP). The spine is intact and the mass does not communicate with the spinal canal.

distinct lesions which were of different reflectivity to the surrounding brain tissue. Such lesions may be solid or cystic, or contain elements of both.

Diagnosis of a sacrococcygeal tumour is made when a mass is seen to arise from the sacral area and extends around to the perineum. The mass may be cystic, solid or mixed. In cystic cases the initial appearance may be something like a meningomyelocele, but with sacrococcygeal tumours the spine is found to be intact (Fig. 15.51). The mass may be extremely large, as big as the fetal head or even bigger. One rare variety of this tumour does not present externally, occurring as an intra-abdominal mass. It is unlikely that it would be possible to determine the origin of such a mass antenatally. Although many teratomas contain neural tissue, MSAFP levels may be normal.[377]

Differential diagnosis

The main differential diagnosis is myelomeningocele or meningocele. Doppler imaging will help confirm the correct diagnosis.[378]

Associated abnormalities

In intracranial tumours hydrocephalus, from the compressive effect of the tumour on the ventricular system, is not uncommon.[374] In addition polyhydramnios is often present. The underlying mechanism is not clear, but it may be that fetal swallowing is affected by the intracranial mass.

Hydramnios may also be present with sacrococcygeal teratomas. Other associated anomalies may be of the muscular, skeletal, renal or nervous systems. Overall 18% of neonates with sacrococcygeal teratomas have been reported to have other abnormalities.[379]

Prognosis

Cerebral neonatal tumours, benign or malignant, have a poor prognosis, most babies being stillborn or dying in the neonatal period. The size and extent of the tumour and the histological type will have some effect on the outcome.

The prognosis for the sacrococcygeal teratomas is generally very good as the majority are benign. Early surgery is essential.

Obstetric management

Because of the poor prognosis of intracranial tumours, termination should be offered. If detected at a late stage, management depends very much on the size and extent of the tumour and the appearance of the rest of the brain.

Because of the good prognosis of the majority of sacrococcygeal teratomas, provided other significant abnormalities have been excluded, counselling should be towards continuation of the pregnancy. Serial scans are useful to detect polyhydramnios and also to measure the size of the tumour towards term to help decide the mode of delivery. With large tumours dystocia is a possibility and caesarean section should be carried out. Care must be taken at the delivery to ensure that the tumour is not damaged, as extensive haemorrhage may occur, compromising the fetus. Because of the malignant potential of some sacrococcygeal tumours early surgery is important.

Microcephaly

In paediatric terminology microcephaly is defined as a head which is two[380] or three[381] standard deviations below the mean for age, the quoted incidences varying with the cut-off employed. Three standard deviations below the mean for age is the better definition. If two standard deviations below the mean is used the condition is inconsistently associated with mental retardation, particularly as it includes 2.5% of the general population, as opposed to 0.3% when three standard deviations are used. Microcephaly results from a decrease in brain volume caused by a reduction in telencephalic neurons and, if severe, is associated with gross mental retardation.

Incidence and aetiology

The quoted incidence of microcephaly is extremely variable, ranging from 1.6 per 1000[163] to 1 in 25 000–50 000 births.[381] In one series of microcephalic infants diagnosed by the end of the first year of life, only 14% had been noted at birth.[163] Microcephaly is a heterogeneous entity with many different patterns and aetiologies. The causes can be divided into various non-genetic insults, such as infection, radiation, anoxia etc. and those where there appears to be a genetic component.[381]

Prenatal infections, including rubella, cytomegalovirus, herpes, toxoplasmosis and HIV, may all lead to microcephaly, as may maternal exposure to excess alcohol, radiation, phenytoin and aminopterin, and maternal phenylketonuria. Isolated microcephaly may have a genetic aetiology and be inherited as either an autosomal recessive or dominant condition. It may be found as part of some genetic syndromes, such as Fanconi pancytopenia, incontinentia pigmenti, Meckel–Grüber syndrome, Smith–Lemli–Opitz syndrome, or be one abnormality in trisomies 13, 18, 21 and 22.[382] In some forms of microcephaly it appears that the cerebellum has continued to develop while forebrain development has been impaired. As the growth spurt of the cerebellum is somewhat later than the forebrain, it is postulated that a teratogenic insult of short duration might inhibit the growth of one and not the other.[383]

Diagnosis

Antenatal diagnosis of microcephaly is for the most part based on the size of the head, its growth and its relative size compared to some other part of the fetal body. Rarely an intracranial abnormality may be detected, such as apparently enlarged ventricles due to cortical atrophy, or a brain thought to be featureless, but in the majority of cases the intracranial anatomy is unremarkable and the problem is solely the size of the brain. The diagnosis is made by using the head circumference measurement, the head-to-abdomen circumference ratio (Figs 15.52 and 15.53)[154,384,385] or the head perimeter-to-femur ratio (see Appendix).[96] The bipar-

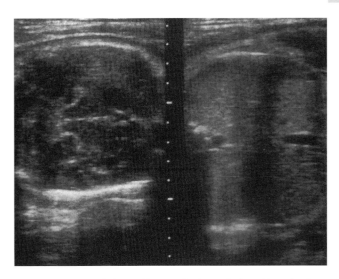

Fig. 15.53 Microcephaly. In this case of microcephaly at 31 weeks the head-to-abdomen circumference ratio is markedly abnormal but the intracranial anatomy is normal.

ietal diameter should never be used to make the diagnosis, as dolichocephaly and brachicephaly may lead to false-positive or false-negative diagnoses. Dolichocephalic heads are associated with breech presentations and reduced liquor, or occur for no apparent reason. Similarly, a rounded head shape may lead to false reassurance, and so the head circumference is a better measurement. The head/abdomen circumference ratio is the most reliable, but it must be remembered that the abdomen may be affected by intra-uterine growth retardation and this can conceal signs of disproportionate head growth. When using the head/abdomen circumference ratio it must also be remembered that on occasion the head will appear disproportionately small because the abdomen is disproportionately large, such as where there is hepatomegaly or macrosomia (which may occur with the Beckwith–Wiedemann syndrome, diabetes and early fetal hydrops), hence the need to use the absolute HC in these circumstances. Other fetal measurements will be of use in evaluating the situation, in particular the femur length. It is not safe to assume, when using a head circumference/femur chart, that skeletal growth has not been affected.

The diagnosis of microcephaly depends in part on the severity of the condition and in part upon the aetiology. In many cases the diagnosis cannot be made with confidence until after 25 weeks.[386] However, occasionally it is apparent at an earlier stage, whereas others remain undetected until the third trimester[154] and occasional cases go undetected through the antenatal period (Fig. 15.54); not all microcephalics can be diagnosed at birth.

If there is a family history of the condition it is advisable to date the fetus at an early stage, preferably by CRL in the first trimester, and then to begin making measurements of the head and abdomen circumference from about

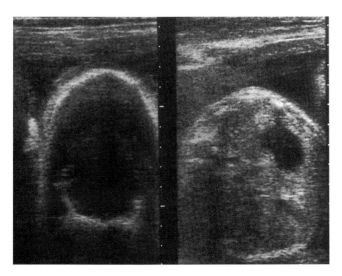

Fig. 15.52 Microcephaly. The head and abdomen of a severely microcephalic fetus at 26 weeks, showing the marked disproportion in size. No intracranial structures are seen.

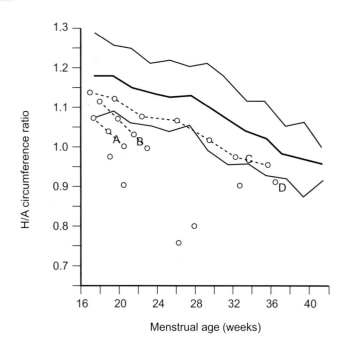

Fig. 15.54 Head circumference/abdomen circumference ratios. Serial and isolated HC/AC ratios in nine cases of microcephaly. **A** and **B**: show normal ratios, becoming frankly abnormal by 22–24 weeks. **C**: illustrates a case of microcephaly when the HC/AC ratio remained normal throughout pregnancy, the diagnosis not being made until 6 weeks post-partum. The HC/AC ratio **D** was suggestive but not diagnostic.

18 weeks. A disproportionate decrease in the head/abdomen (H/A) circumference ratio may alert one to the presence of the condition. The diagnosis should not be made on a single H/A ratio unless it is well below the lower limit of normal, or another abnormality of the brain is seen. However, when serial scans are available, a ratio that falls steadily to just below the normal limits is likely to be significant. Another useful aid to diagnosis is that these fetuses have a characteristic sloping forehead, which may be displayed on a profile scan.

Associated abnormalities

Because it is associated with a large number of chromosomal defects, gene disorders and syndromes, there are many associated abnormalities. Particular attention should be paid to the presence of neural tube defects, encephaloceles, alobar holoprosencephaly and Meckel's syndrome. A thorough examination of the fetus is mandatory.

Differential diagnosis

The major diagnostic difficulty is in the exclusion of normal fetuses. Other conditions may rarely be confused, including craniosynostosis and anencephaly or acrania.

Prognosis

Because of the diversity of the aetiologies and the poor correlation of brain size with the degree of mental retardation, deciding the prognosis of any particular microcephalic fetus poses problems. Clearly, if there are other associated abnormalities, and in particular if the microcephaly is part of a particular syndrome or abnormal karyotype, the prognosis will depend on this. Several series have examined the outcome in isolated microcephaly.[380,387,388] Taking a cut-off for head size of two standard deviations below the mean, normal intelligence has been variously reported in less than 1%,[380] 50%[387] and 82%.[388] Using the cut-off of three standard deviations below the mean, a normal intellect was found in 28%.[388] For those with smaller heads the prognosis became increasingly worse. If the head circumference was four to seven standard deviations below the mean the average IQ was 35.6, falling to 20 if the head size was less than seven standard deviations below the mean.[389]

Obstetric management

Sporadic cases of microcephaly often remain undetected until birth, a minority presenting as a chance finding at a routine ultrasound scan. If this diagnosis is suspected a thorough search should be made for other abnormalities and a karyotyping procedure performed. In cases with other associated abnormalities, a termination should be offered. Where the microcephaly appears to be isolated, if the head size is more than four standard deviations below the mean for gestation a termination can be offered, as there is an extremely high chance that the infant will be severely mentally retarded. When the head size is not as much reduced as this, the uncertainties regarding the prognosis should be discussed with the parents and termination may be considered as an option, particularly as brain size cannot be directly equated with IQ. In some cases a delay of 2 or 3 weeks to enable serial growth scans to be taken may aid the decision making if the head growth is seen to be falling off further. If there is a past history of microcephaly of genetic origin and if the head size is found to be small and the H/A ratio abnormal, counselling and management is somewhat easier as the previously affected children can be used as guides to the likely prognosis. The risk of shoulder dystocia should be borne in mind as the head may be delivered through a cervix that is not fully dilated.[390]

Recurrence risk

As microcephaly presents as part of such a large number of chromosomal abnormalities[253] and syndromes,[134] if the index case was associated with such abnormalities the recurrence risk will be that of the syndrome. Likewise, if an infectious aetiology was proven in a previous pregnancy, then the recurrence risk is very low indeed. However, most cases are isolated with no apparent chromosomal or infectious component, in which case both autosomal dominant[391] and recessive[392] inheritance patterns have been noted. Widely used recurrence risks for isolated microcephaly are 10–20%, increasing to 25% if the parents are consanguineous.[393,394]

Recent advances

First-trimester diagnosis

Using trans-vaginal ultrasonography it is now possible to diagnose a variety of fetal abnormalities, including those of the central nervous system, at earlier stages than was possible with conventional transabdominal scanning.[8,10,11,395] Scanning for intracranial structures requires vertex presentation of the fetus. The high-frequency transvaginal probe provides better-quality images than can be achieved through conventional transabdominal scanning. Blaas *et al.*[396] used this to study the early development of the hindbrain from 7 to 12 weeks of gestation, and Timor-Tritsch *et al.*[397] studied fetal CNS anatomy between 9 and 14 weeks. Definitive diagnosis of some conditions is feasible and diagnostic difficulties from transabdominal scanning may be resolved.[7]

Three-dimensional ultrasound imaging

Three-dimensional ultrasound produces images which give a far better assessment of the extent and size of fetal structures and abnormalities.[84,85,188] This is especially valuable when investigating abnormalities of the face and spine.[235,236] However, fetal movement produces artefacts and its use is limited in studying moving parts. Although useful, this is currently only available in a small number of centres in a research setting.

Conclusions

There is a wide variety of abnormalities of the CNS that can be detected antenatally by ultrasound. Initially only women at high risk of an abnormality were scanned. Contemporary practice, however, is for the majority of pregnant women to be scanned routinely between 19 and 20 weeks of gestation in an effort both to date the pregnancy accurately and to detect fetal anomalies. Indeed, the Royal College of Obstetricians and Gynaecologists of the UK has recommended that all pregnant women should normally be offered a detailed fetal anomaly scan between 18 and 20 weeks gestation.[398] The success of this approach depends on the quality of the equipment available and, much more importantly, on the training and quality of the sonographers who perform the routine scanning. They must be experts in the normal appearance of the fetus and

have a good knowledge of the possible abnormalities that may be encountered. The time required for a detailed scan in a high-risk patient is not usually available when performing a routine mid-trimester scan. Attention to key observations that may be made quickly and easily will rule out major CNS anomaly. These findings are summarised in two key papers[86,180] and are listed below:

1. shape of the fetal head: a normal shape virtually rules out spina bifida, anencephaly and encephalocele,
2. cerebellum and cisterna magna: a normal cerebellum rules out the majority of significant spina bifida lesions, Dandy–Walker malformation and cerebellar hypoplasia, whereas a cisterna magna of less than 10 mm will exclude Dandy–Walker malformation and infratentorial arachnoid cysts,
3. cavum septum pellucidum: the presence of a normal cavum rules out AGCC and major degrees of holoprosencephaly,
4. atria of the lateral ventricles: a width of less than 10 mm rules out hydrocephalus,
5. choroid plexus: inspection of the choroids and their positions relative to the atrium eliminates choroid plexus cysts and hydrocephalus.

All these observations can be made extremely quickly from the sections required to measure the biparietal diameter and head circumference. Thus the diagnosis of CNS abnormalities in the general population by antenatal ultrasound scanning is potentially extremely successful.

REFERENCES

1 Campbell S, Johnstone F D, Holt E M, May P. Anencephaly: early ultrasonic diagnosis and active management. Lancet 1972; ii: 1226–1227
2 Leck I. Changes in the incidence of neural tube defects. Lancet 1966; ii: 791–792
3 Creasy M R, Alberman E D. Congenital malformations of the central nervous system in spontaneous abortions. J Med Genet 1976; 13: 9–16
4 Chitty L S, Hunt G H, Moore J, Lobb M O. Effectiveness of routine ultrasonography in detecting fetal structural abnormalities in a low risk population. BMJ 1991; 303: 1165–1169
5 Luck C A. Value of routine ultrasound scanning at 19 weeks: a four year study of 8849 deliveries. BMJ 1992; 304: 1474–1478
6 Chan A, Robertson E F, Haan E A, Keane R J, Ranieri E, Carney A. Prevalence of neural tube defects in South Australia, 1966–91: effectiveness and impact of prenatal diagnosis. BMJ 1993; 307: 703–706
7 Stagianis K D, Sepulveda W, Bower S. Early prenatal diagnosis of holoprosencephaly: the value of transvaginal ultrasonography. Eur J Obs Gynecol Reprod Biol 1995; 61(2): 175–176
8 Van Zalen-Sprock R M, van Vugt J M, van Geijn H P. First and second trimester diagnosis of anomalies of the central nervous system. J Ultrasound Med 1995; 14(8): 603–610
9 Sebire N J, Noble P L, Thorpe-Beeston J G, Snijders R J, Nicolaides K H. Presence of 'lemon' sign in fetuses with spina bifida at the 10–14 week scan. Ultrasound Obstet Gynecol 1997; 10(6): 403–405
10 Gembruch U, Baschat A A, Reusche E, Wallner S J, Greiwe M. First trimester diagnosis of holoprosencephaly with a Dandy–Walker malformation by transvaginal ultrasonography. J Ultrasound Med 1995; 14: 619–622

11 Blumenfeld Z, Siegler E, Bronshtein M. The early diagnosis of neural tube defects. Prenat Diagn 1993; 13(9): 863–871

12 McKeown T, Record R G. Seasonal incidence of congenital malformations of the CNS. Lancet 1951; i: 192–196

13 Leck I, Record R G. Seasonal incidence of anencephalus. Br J Prev Soc Med 1966; 20: 67–75

14 MacMahon B, Yen S. Unrecognised epidemic of anencephaly and spina bifida. Lancet 1971; i: 31–33

15 MacMahon B, Record R G, McKeown T. Secular changes in the incidence of malformations of the central nervous system. Br J Prev Soc Med 1951; 5: 254–258

16 Cuckle H S, Wald N J, Cuckle P M. Prenatal screening and diagnosis of neural tube defects in England and Wales in 1985. Prenat Diagn 1989; 9: 393–400

17 Laurence K M. The apparently declining prevalence of neural tube defects in 2 counties in South Wales over 3 decades illustrating the need for continuing action and vigilance. Zeitschr Kinderchir Grenzgeb 1985; 40: 58–60

18 Northern Regional Health Authority. A regional fetal abnormality survey. First progress report. March 1988

19 Carstairs V, Cole S. Spina bifida and anencephaly in Scotland. BMJ 1984; 289: 1182–1184

20 Cuckle H S, Wald N J. The impact of screening for open neural tube defects in England and Wales. Prenat Diagn 1987; 7: 91–99

21 Stevenson A C, Johnson H A, Stewart M I P, Golding D R. Congenital malformations: a report of a series of consecutive births in 24 centres. Bulletin of the World Health Organization 1966; 34: 1–125

22 Laurence K M, Carter C O, David P A. Major central nervous system malformations in South Wales. 1. Incidence, local variations and geographical factors. Br J Prev Soc Med 1968; 22: 212–222

23 Anon. Prevalence of neural tube defects in 20 regions of Europe and the impact of prenatal diagnosis, 1980–1986. EUROCAT Working Group. J Epidemiol Commun Health 1991; 45(1): 52–58

24 Penrose L S. Genetics of anencephaly. J Mental Defic Res 1957; 1: 4–15

25 Fielding D W, Smithells R W. Anencephalus and water hardness in South West Lancashire. Br J Prev Soc Med 1971; 25: 217–219

26 Lowe C R, Roberts C L, Lloyd S. Malformations of the central nervous system and softness of local water supplies. BMJ 1971; 2: 357–361

27 Leck I. Ethnic differences in the incidence of malformations following migration. Br J Prev Soc Med 1969; 23: 166–173

28 Naggan L, MacMahon B. Ethnic differences in the prevalence of anencephaly and spina bifida in Boston. N Engl J Med 1967; 227: 1119–1123

29 Naggan L. Anencephaly and spina bifida in Israel. Pediatrics 1971; 47: 577–586

30 Searle A G. The incidence of anencephaly in a polytypic population. Ann Hum Genet (London) 1959; 23: 279–287

31 Main D M, Mennuti M T. Neural tube defects: issues in prenatal diagnosis and counselling. Obstet Gynecol 1986; 67: 1

32 Lammer E J, Sever L E, Oakley G P. Teratogen update: valproic acid. Teratology 1987; 35: 465–473

33 Anon. Epilepsy and pregnancy. Drug Therapeutics Bull 1994; 32(7): 49–51

34 Moore K L, Persaud T V N. The central nervous system. In: The developing human: clinically orientated embryology, 5th edn. Philadelphia: W B Saunders, 1993; 385–422

35 Gardner W J. The dysraphic states from syringomyelia to anencephaly. Amsterdam: Excerpta Medica, 1973

36 Giroud A. Anencephaly. In: Vinken P J, Bruyn G W, eds. Handbook of clinical neurology. Amsterdam: Elsevier/North Holland Biomedical Press, 1977; 30: 173–208

37 Ganchrow D, Ornoy A. Possible evidence for secondary degeneration of central nervous system in the pathogenesis of anencephaly and brain dysraphia: a study in young human fetuses. Virchows Arch (A) 1979; 384: 285–294

38 Papp Z, Csecsei K, Toth Z, Polgar K, Szeifert G T. Exencephaly in human fetuses. Clin Genet 1986; 30(5): 440–444

39 Skolnick N, Filly R A, Callen P W, Golbus M S. Sonography as a procedure complementary to alpha fetoprotein testing for neural tube defects. J Ultrasound Med 1982; 1: 319–322

40 Hashimoto B E, Mahony B S, Filly R A, Golbus M S, Anderson R L, Callen P W. Sonography: a complementary examination to alpha fetoprotein testing for neural tube defects. J Ultrasound Med 1985; 4: 307–310

41 Lindfors K K, McGahan J P, Tennant F P, Hanson F W, Walter J P. Midtrimester screening for open neural tube defects: Correlation of sonography with amniocentesis results. AJR 1987; 149: 141–145

42 Roberts C J, Hibbard B M, Roberts E E, Evans K T, Laurence K M, Robertson I B. Diagnostic effectiveness of ultrasound in detection of neural tube defect. The South Wales experience of 2509 scans (1977–1982) in high risk mothers. Lancet 1983; ii: 1068–1069

43 Hogge W A, Thiagarajah S, Ferguson J E, Schnatterly P T, Harbert G M. The role of ultrasonography and amniocentesis in the evaluation of pregnancies at risk for neural tube defects. Am J Obstet Gynecol 1989; 161: 520–524

44 Goldstein R B, Filly R A. Prenatal diagnosis of anencephaly: spectrum of sonographic appearances and distinction from the amniotic band syndrome. AJR 1988; 151: 547–550

45 Goldstein R B, Filly R A, Callen P W. Sonography of anencephaly: pitfalls in early diagnosis. JCU 1989; 17: 397–402

46 Rottem S, Bronshtein M, Thaler, Brandes J M. First trimester transvaginal sonographic diagnosis of fetal anomalies. Lancet 1989; i: 444–445

47 Kennedy K A, Flick K J, Thurmond A S. First trimester diagnosis of exencephaly. Am J Obstet Gynecol 1990; 162: 461–463

48 Bronshtein M, Ornoy A. Acrania: anencephaly resulting from secondary degeneration of a closed neural tube defect: two cases in the same family. JCU 1991; 19: 230–234

49 O'Rahilly R, Gardner E. The initial appearance of ossification in staged human embryos. Am J Anat 1974; 134: 291–308

50 Cox G C, Rosenthal S J, Holsapple J W. Exencephaly: sonographic findings and the radiologic–pathologic correlation. Radiology 1985; 155: 755–756

51 Hendricks S K, Cyr D R, Nyberg D A, Raabe R, Mack L A. Exencephaly–clinical and ultrasonic correlation to anencephaly. Obstet Gynecol 1988; 72: 898–900

52 Mannes E J, Crelin E S, Hobbins J S, Viscomi G N, Alcebo L. Sonographic demonstration of fetal acrania. AJR 1982; 139: 181–182

53 Mahoney B S, Filly R A, Callen P W, Golbus M S. The amniotic band syndrome: antenatal sonographic diagnosis and potential pitfalls. Am J Obstet Gynecol 1985; 152: 63–68

54 Frezal J, Kelley J, Guillemot M L, Lamy M. Anencephaly in France. Am J Hum Genet 1964; 16: 336–350

55 Chervenak F A, Farley M A, Walters L, Hobbins J C, Mahoney J. When is termination of pregnancy in the first trimester morally justifiable? N Engl J Med 1984; 310: 501–504

56 Leong A S, Shaw C M. The pathology of occipital encephalocele and a discussion of the pathogenesis. Pathology 1979; 11: 223–234

57 Carlan S J, Angel J L, Leo J, Feeney J. Cephalocele involving the oral cavity. Obstet Gynecol 1990; 75: 494–495

58 McLaurin R L. Encephalocele and cranium bifidum. In: Vinken P J, Bruyn G W, Klawans H L, eds. Handbook of clinical neurology. Amsterdam: Elsevier/North Holland Biomedical Press, 1987; 50: 97–111

59 International Clearing House for Birth Defects Monitoring Systems. Annual Report 15; 1983

60 Lorber J. The prognosis of occipital encephalocele. Dev Med Child Neurol 1966; 13 (Suppl): 75–86

61 Cohen M M, Lemire R J. Syndromes with cephaloceles. Teratology 1982; 25: 161–172

62 Chervenak F A, Isaacson G, Mahoney M J, Berkowitz R L, Tortora M, Hobbins J C. Diagnosis and management of fetal cephalocele. Obstet Gynecol 1984; 64: 86–91

63 Fiske C E, Filly R A. Ultrasound evaluation of the normal and abnormal fetal neural axis. Radiol Clin North Am 1982; 20: 285–296

64 Graham D, Johnson T R B, Winn K, Sanders R C. The role of sonography in the prenatal diagnosis and management of encephalocele. J Ultrasound Med 1982; 1: 111

65 Chatterjee M J, Bondoc B, Adhate A. Prenatal diagnosis of occipital encephalocele. Am J Obstet Gynecol 1985; 153: 646–647

66 Pilu G, Rizzo N, Orsini L F, Bovicelli L. Antenatal recognition of cerebral anomalies. Ultrasound Med Biol 1986; 12: 319–326

67 van Zalen-Sprock R M, van Vugt J M G, van Geijn H P. First trimester sonographic detection of neurodevelopmental abnormalities in some single-gene disorders. Prenat Diagn 1996; 16: 199–202

68 Nicolini U, Ferrazzi E, Massa E et al. Prenatal diagnosis of cranial masses by ultrasound: report of 5 cases. JCU 1983; 11: 170–174

69 Bronshtein M, Zimmer E Z. Transvaginal sonographic follow-up on the formation of fetal cephalocoele at 13–19 weeks' gestation. Obstet Gynecol 1991; 78: 528–530

70 Haddow J E. Prenatal diagnosis of neural tube defects. In: Levene M I, Bennett M J, Punt J, eds. Fetal neurology and neurosurgery. Edinburgh: Churchill Livingstone, 1988: 279–289

71 De Myer W. The median cleft face syndrome: differential diagnosis of cranium bifidum occultum, hypertelorism, and median cleft nose, lip and palate. Neurology 1967; 17: 961–971

72 Field B. The child with an encephalocele. Med J Aust 1974; 1: 700–703

73 Lorber J, Schofield J K. The prognosis of occipital encephalocele. Zeitschr Kinderchir Grenzgeb 1979; 28: 347–351

74 Friede R L. Developmental neuropathology. New York: Springer-Verlag, 1975

75 Patten B M. Embryological stages in myeloschisis with spina bifida. Am J Anat 1953; 93: 365–395

76 Gardner W J. Myelomeningocele, the result of rupture of the embryonic neural tube. Cleveland Clin Q 1960; 27: 88–100

77 Barson A J. Spina bifida: the significance of the level and extent of the defect to the morphogenesis. Dev Med Child Neurol 1970; 12: 129–144

78 Emery J L, Lendon R G. The local cord lesion in neurospinal dysraphism (meningomyelocele). J Pathol 1973; 110: 83–86

79 Lorber J. Systematic ventriculographic studies in infants born with meningomyelocele and encephalocele. The incidence and development of hydrocephalus. Arch Dis Child 1961; 36: 381–389

80 Smithells R W, Sheppard S, Wild J. Prevalence of neural tube defects in the Yorkshire region. Commun Med 1989; 11: 163–167

81 Campbell S. Early prenatal diagnosis of neural tube defects by ultrasound. Clin Obstet Gynecol 1977; 20: 351–359

82 D'Ercole C, Girard N, Boubli L et al. Prenatal diagnosis of fetal cerebral abnormalities by ultrasonography and magnetic resonance imaging. Eur J Obstet Gynecol Reprod Biol 1993; 50(3): 177–184

83 Mueller G M, Weiner C P, Yankowitz J. Three-dimensional ultrasound in the evaluation of fetal head and spine anomalies. Obstet Gynecol 1996; 88(3): 372–378

84 Merz E, Bahlmann F, Weber G, Macchiella D. Three-dimensional ultrasonography in prenatal diagnosis. J Perinat Med 1995; 23(3): 213–222

85 Fowlie A. An ultrasonic method of screening for the neural tube defects. Proceedings of the North of England Obstetrics and Gynaecological Society, 1982

86 Nicolaides K H, Gabbe S G, Campbell S, Guidetti R. Ultrasound screening for spina bifida: cranial and cerebellar signs. Lancet 1986; ii: 72–74

87 Thoms A, Campbell S. The diagnosis of spina bifida and intracranial abnormalities. In: Sanders R C, James A E, eds. Principles and practice of ultrasonography in obstetrics and gynaecology. Norwalk: Appleton Century Crofts, 1980: 179–190

88 Campbell S, Pearce J M. Ultrasound visualisation of congenital malformations. Br Med Bull 1983; 39: 322–331

89 Campbell J, Gilbert W M, Nicolaides K H, Campbell S. Ultrasound screening for spina bifida: cranial and cerebellar signs in a high risk population. Obstet Gynecol 1987; 70: 247–250

90 Pilu G, Romero R, Reece E A, Goldstein I, Hobbins J C, Bovicelli L. Subnormal cerebellum in fetuses with spina bifida. Am J Obstet Gynecol 1988; 158: 1052–1056

91 Nyberg D A, Mack L A, Hirsch J, Mahony B S. Abnormalities of the fetal cranial contour in sonographic detection of spina bifida – evaluation of the lemon sign. Radiology 1988; 167: 387–392

92 Tabor A, Madsen M, Obel E B, Philip J, Bang J, Pedersen B N. Randomised controlled trial of genetic amniocentesis in 4606 low risk women. Lancet 1986; i: 1287–1292

93 Allen L C, Doran T A, Miskin M, Rudd N L, Benzie R J, Sheffield L J. Ultrasound and amniotic fluid alpha-fetoprotein in the prenatal diagnosis of spina bifida. Obstet Gynecol 1982; 60: 169–173

94 Richards D S, Seeds J W, Katz V L, Lingley L H, Albright S G, Cefalo R C. Elevated maternal serum alphafetoprotein with normal ultrasound: is amniocentesis always appropriate? A review of 26 069 screened patients. Obstet Gynecol 1988; 71: 203–207

95 Hogge W A, Thiagarajah S, Ferguson J E, Schnatterly P T, Harbert G M. The role of ultrasonography and amniocentesis in the evaluation of pregnancies at risk for neural tube defects. Am J Obstet Gynecol 1989; 161: 520–524

96 Romero R, Pilu G, Jeanty P, Ghidini A, Hobbins J C. Prenatal diagnosis of congenital anomalies. Connecticut: Appleton and Lange, 1988

97 Gough J D. In: Wald N J, ed. Ultrasound, antenatal and neonatal screening. Oxford: Oxford University Press, 1984: 432–433

98 Persson P H, Cullander S, Gennser G, Grennert L, Laurell C B. Screening for fetal malformations using ultrasound and measurements of alpha fetoprotein in maternal serum. BMJ 1983; 286: 747–749

99 Rosendahl H, Kivinen S. Antenatal detection of congenital malformations by routine ultrasonography. Obstet Gynecol 1989; 73: 947–951

100 Hernadi L, Torocsik M. Screening for fetal anomalies in the 12th week of pregnancy by transvaginal sonography in an unselected population. Prenat Diagn 1997; 17: 753–759

101 Sharrard W J W. The mechanism of paralytic deformity in spina bifida. Dev Med Child Neurol 1962; 4: 310–313

102 Lorber J. Results of treatment of myelomeningocele. An analysis of 524 unselected cases, with special reference to possible selection for treatment. Dev Med Child Neurol 1971; 31: 279–303

103 Althouse R, Wald N J. Survival and handicap of infants with spina bifida. Arch Dis Child 1980; 55: 845–850

104 Adams M M, Greenberg F, Khoury M J, Marks J S, Oakley G P. Survival of infants with spina bifida: Atlanta 1972–1979. Am J Dis Child 1985; 139: 514–517

105 Kalucy M, Bower C, Stanley F. School-aged children with spina bifida in Western Australia – parental perspectives on functional outcome. Dev Med Child Neurol 1996; 38(4): 325–334

106 Steinbok P. Dysraphic lesions of the cervical spinal cord. Neurosurg Clin North Am 1995; 6(2): 367–376

107 Williamson P, Alberman E, Rodeck C, Fiddler M, Church S, Harris R. Antecedent circumstances surrounding neural tube defect births in 1990–1991. Br J Obstet Gynaecol 1997; 104: 51–56

108 Chervenak F A, Duncan C, Ment L R, Tortora M, McClure M, Hobbins J C. Perinatal management of meningomyelocele. Obstet Gynecol 1984; 63: 376–380

109 Nevin N C, Johnstone W P. A family study of spina bifida and anencephalus in Northern Ireland (1964–1968). J Med Genet 1980; 17: 203–211

110 Seller M J. Recurrence risks for neural tube defects in a genetic counselling clinic population. J Med Genet 1981; 18: 245–248

111 Anon. Epilepsy and pregnancy. Drug Therapeutics Bull 1994; 32(7): 49–51

112 Laurence K M, James N, Miller M, Campbell H. Increased risk of recurrence of pregnancies complicated by neural tube defects in mothers receiving poor diets, and possible effects of dietary counselling. BMJ 1980; 281: 1592–1594

113 Laurence K M, James N, Miller M, Tennant G B, Campbell H. Double blind randomised controlled trial of folate treatment before conception to prevent neural tube defects. BMJ 1981; 282: 1509–1511

114 Smithells R W, Nevin N C, Seller M J et al. Further experience of vitamin supplementation for prevention of neural tube defect recurrences. Lancet 1983; i: 1027–1031

115 Seller M J, Nevin N C. Periconceptual vitamin supplementation and the prevention of neural tube defects in South East England and Northern Ireland. J Med Genet 1984; 21: 325–330

116 Seller M J. Periconceptual vitamin supplementation to prevent recurrence of neural tube defects. Lancet 1985; i: 1392–1393

117 Mulinare J, Cordero J F, Erickson J D, Berry R J. Periconceptual use of multivitamins and the occurrence of neural tube defects. JAMA 1988; 260: 3141–3145

118 MRC Vitamin Study Research Group. Prevention of neural tube defects: Results of the Medical Research Council Vitamin Study. Lancet 1991; 338: 131–137

119 Czeizel A E, Dudas I. Prevention of first occurrence of neural tube defects by periconceptual vitamin supplementation. N Engl J Med 1992; 327: 1832–1835

120 Milunsky A, Jick H, Jick S S. Multivitamin/folic acid supplementation in early pregnancy reduces the prevalence of neural tube defects. JAMA 1989; 262: 2847–2852

121 Anon. Folic acid to prevent neural tube defects. Drug Therapeutics Bull Emp 1994; 32(4): 31–32

122 Brock D J H, Sutcliffe R G. Alpha fetoprotein in the antenatal diagnosis of spina bifida and anencephaly. Lancet 1972; ii: 197–199

123 Smith A D, Wald N J, Cuckle H S, Stirrat G M, Bobrow M, Lagercrantz H. Amniotic fluid acetylcholinesterase as a possible diagnostic test for neural tube defects in early pregnancy. Lancet 1979; i: 685–690

124 Wald N J, Brock D J H, Bonnar J. Prenatal diagnosis of spina bifida and anencephaly by maternal serum alpha fetoprotein measurement. Lancet 1974; i: 765–767

125 Brock D J H, Bolton A E, Scrimgeour J B. Prenatal diagnosis of spina bifida and anencephaly through maternal plasma alpha-fetoprotein measurement. Lancet 1974; i: 767–769

126 Wald N J, Cuckle H S. Collaborative study on alpha fetoprotein in relation to neural tube defects. Lancet 1977; i: 1323–1332

127 Burton B K, Sowers S G, Nelson L H. Maternal serum alpha fetoprotein screening in North Carolina: experience with more than 12 000 pregnancies. Am J Obstet Gynecol 1983; 146: 439

128 Wald N J, Cuckle H S, Boreham T, Turnbull A C. Effect of estimating gestational age by ultrasound cephalometry on the specificity of alpha fetoprotein screening for open neural tube defects. Br J Obstet Gynaecol 1982; 89: 1050–1053

129 RADIUS Study Group. A randomised trial of prenatal ultrasonic screening: impact on the selection, management and outcome of anomalous fetuses. Am J Obstet Gynecol 1994; 171: 392–399

130 Wald J N, Huttly W, Ward K, Kennard A. Down's syndrome screening in UK. Lancet 1996; 347: 330

131 Williams R A, Barth R A. In utero sonographic recognition of diastematomyelia. AJR 1985; 144: 87–88

132 Benacerraf B R, Greene M F, Barss V A. Prenatal diagnosis of congenital hemivertebra. J Ultrasound Med 1986; 5: 257–259

133 Harlow C L, Partington M D, Thieme G A. Lumbosacral agenesis: clinical characteristics, imaging and embryogenesis. Pediatr Neurosurg 1995; 23(3): 140–147

134 Smith D W. Recognisable patterns of human malformation, 3rd edn. Philadelphia: W B Saunders, 1982

135 Baxi L, Warren W, Collins M, Timor-Tritsch I E. Early detection of caudal regression syndrome with transvaginal scanning. Obstet Gynecol 1990; 75: 485–489

136 Napolitani F D, Schreiber I. The acardiac monster: a review of the world literature and presentation of 2 cases. Am J Obstet Gynecol 1960; 80: 582–589

137 Simpson P C, Trudinger B J, Walker A, Baird P J. The intrauterine treatment of fetal cardiac failure in a twin pregnancy with an acardiac, acephalic monster. Am J Obstet Gynecol 1983; 147: 842–844

138 Barjot P, Hamel P, Calmelet P, Maragnes P, Herlicoviez M. Flecainide against fetal supraventricular tachycardia complicated by hydrops fetalis. Acta Obstet Gynecol Scand 1998; 77(3): 353–358

139 Platt L D, Devore G R, Bieniary A, Benner P, Rao R. Antenatal diagnosis of acephalus acardia: a proposed management scheme. Am J Obstet Gynecol 1983; 146: 857–859

140 Lewis H F. Iniencephalus. Am J Obstet Gynecol 1887; 35: 11–53

141 Aleksic S, Budzilovich G, Greco M A, Feigin I, Epstein F, Pearson J. Iniencephaly: neuropathologic study. Clin Neuropathol 1983; 2: 55–61

142 Gunderson C H, Greenspan R H, Glaser G H, Lubs H A. The Klippel–Feil syndrome: genetic and clinical reevaluation of cervical fusion. Medicine 1967; 46: 491–512

143 Gardner W J. Klippel–Feil syndrome, iniencephalus, anencephalus, hindbrain hernia and mirror movements: overdistension of the neural tube. Child's Brain 1979; 5: 361–379

144 Sherk H H, Shut L, Chung S. Iniencephalic deformity of the cervical spine with Klippel–Feil anomalies and congenital elevation of the scapula. J Bone Joint Surg 1974; 1254–1259

145 Paterson S J. Iniencephalus. J Obstet Gynaecol Br Emp 1944; 51: 330

146 Jayant K, Mehta A, Sanghvi L D. A study of congenital malformations in Bombay. J Obstet Gynaecol India 1960; 11: 280

147 Bowden R A, Stephens T D, Le Mire R J. The association of spinal retroflexion with limb anomalies. Teratology 1980; 21: 53–59

148 Lemire R J, Beckwith B, Shepard T H. Iniencephaly and anencephaly with spinal retroflexion, a comparative study of eight human specimens. Teratology 1972; 6: 27–36

149 Abbott M E, Lockhart F A L. Iniencephalus. J Obstet Gynaecol Br Emp 1905; 8: 236

150 Howkins J, Lowrie R S. Iniencephalus. J Obstet Gynaecol Br Emp 1939; 46: 25

151 Cohlan S Q, Kitay D. The teratogenic effect of vincaleukoblastine in the pregnant rat. J Pediatr 1965; 66: 541–544

152 Warkany J, Takacs E. Congenital malformations in rats from streptonigrin. Arch Pathol 1965; 79: 65–79

153 Roux C. Action tératogèn du triparanol chez l'animal. Arch Franc Pediatr 1964; 21: 451

154 Campbell S, Allan L D, Griffin D, Little D, Pearce J M, Chudleigh P. The early diagnosis of fetal structural abnormalities. In: Lerski R A, Morley P, eds. Ultrasound '82. Oxford: Pergamon Press, 1983: 547–563

155 Drogan M M, Ekici E, Yapar E G, Soysal M E, Soysal S K, Gokmen O. Iniencephaly: Sonographic–pathologic correlation of 19 cases. J Perinat Med 1996; 24(5): 501–511

156 Santos-Ramos R, Duenhoelter J H. Diagnosis of congenital fetal abnormalities by sonography. Obstet Gynecol 1975; 45: 279–283

157 Katz V L, Aylsworth A S, Albright S G. Iniencephaly is not uniformly fatal. Prenat Diagn 1989; 9: 595–598

158 Morocz I, Szeifert G F, Molnar P, Toth Z, Csecsei K, Papp Z. Prenatal diagnosis and pathoanatomy of iniencephaly. Clin Genet 1986; 30: 81–86

159 Foderaro A E, Abu-Yousef M M, Benda J A, Williamson R A, Smith W L. Antenatal ultrasound diagnosis of iniencephaly. JCU 1987; 15: 550–554

160 David T J, Nixon A. Congenital malformations associated with anencephaly and iniencephaly. J Med Genet 1976; 13: 263–265

161 Meizner I, Levi A, Katz M, Maor E. Iniencephaly: a case report. J Reprod Med 1992; 37(10): 885–888

162 Myrianthopoulos N C, Kurland L T. Present concepts of the epidemiology and genetics of hydrocephalus. In: Fields W J, Desmond M M, eds. Disorders of the developing nervous system. Springfield, Illinois: Charles Thomas, 1961: 187–202

163 Myrianthopoulos N C. Epidemiology of central nervous system malformations. In: Vinken P J, Bruyn G W, Klawans H L, eds. Handbook of clinical neurology. Amsterdam: Elsevier/North Holland Biomedical Press, 1987; 50: 49–69

164 Habib Z. Genetics and genetic counselling in neonatal hydrocephalus. Obstet Gynecol Surv 1981; 36: 529–534

165 Chuang S. Perinatal and neonatal hydrocephalus. Perinatology 1986; Sept–Oct 8

166 Edwards J H. The syndrome of sex-linked hydrocephalus. Arch Dis Child 1961; 36: 486–493

167 Salam M Z. Stenosis of the aqueduct of Sylvius. In: Vinken P J, Bruyn G W, eds. Handbook of clinical neurology. Amsterdam: Elsevier/North Holland Biomedical Press, 1977; 30: 609–622

168 Milhorat T H. Hydrocephalus and the cerebrospinal fluid. Baltimore: Williams & Wilkins, 1972

169 Halliday J, Chow C W, Wallace D, Danks D M. X-linked hydrocephalus: a survey of a 20 year period in Victoria, Australia. J Med Genet 1986; 23: 23–31

170 Burton B K. Recurrence risks for congenital hydrocephalus. Clin Genet 1979; 16: 47–53

171 Achiron R, Yagel S, Rotstein Z, Inbar O, Mashiach S, Lipitz S. Cerebral lateral ventricular asymmetry: is this a normal ultrasonographic finding in the fetal brain? Obstet Gynecol 1997; 89(2): 233–237

172 Denkhaus H, Winsberg F. Ultrasonic measurement of the fetal ventricular system. Radiology 1979; 131: 781–787

173 Pretorious D H, Drose J A, Manco-Johnson M L. Fetal lateral ventricular determination during the second trimester. J Ultrasound Med 1986; 5: 121–124

174 Chervenak F A, Berkowitz R L, Tortora M, Chitkara U, Hobbins J C. Diagnosis of ventriculomegaly before fetal viability. Obstet Gynecol 1984; 64: 652–656

175 Fiske C E, Filly R A, Callen P W. Sonographic measurement of lateral ventricular width in early ventricular dilation. JCU 1981; 9: 303–307

176 Jeanty P, Dramaix-Wilmet M, Delbeke D, Rodesch F, Struyven J. Ultrasound evaluation of fetal ventricular growth. Neurology 1981; 21: 127–131

177 Hertzberg B S, Bowie J D, Burger P C, Marshburn P B, Djang W T. The three lines: origin of landmarks in the fetal head. AJR 1987; 149: 1009–1012

178 Benacerraf B R, Birnholz J C. The diagnosis of fetal hydrocephalus prior to 22 weeks. JCU 1987; 15: 531–536

179 Chinn D H, Callen P W, Filly R A. The lateral cerebral ventricle in early second trimester. Radiology 1983; 148: 529–531

180 Filly R A, Cardoza J D, Goldstein R B, Barkovich A J. Detection of fetal central nervous system anomalies: a practical level of effort for a routine sonogram. Radiology 1989; 172: 403–408

181 Cardoza J D, Filly R A, Podrasky A E. Exclusion of pseudohydrocephalus by a simple observation: the dangling choroid sign. AJR 1988; 151: 767–770

182 Mahoney B S, Nyberg D A, Hirsch J H, Petty C N, Hendricks S K, Mack L A. Mild idiopathic lateral cerebral ventricular dilatation in-utero: sonographic evaluation. Radiology 1988; 169: 715–721

183 Siedler D E, Filly R A. Relative growth of fetal higher brain structures. J Ultrasound Med 1987; 6: 573–576

184 Cardoza J D, Goldstein R B, Filly R A. Exclusion of ventriculomegaly with a single measurement: the width of the lateral ventricular atrium. Radiology 1988; 169: 711–714

185 Case K J, Hirsch J, Case M J. Simulation of significant pathology by normal hypoechoic white matter in cranial ultrasound. JCU 1983; 11: 281

186 Jeanty P, Chervenak F A, Romero R, Michiels M, Hobbins J C. The Sylvian fissure: a commonly mislabeled cranial landmark. J Ultrasound Med 1984; 3: 15–18

187 Schoenecker S A, Pretorious D H, Manco-Johnson M L. Artifacts seen commonly on ultrasonography of the fetal cranium. J Reprod Med 1985; 30: 541–544

188 Blaas H G, Eik-Nes S H, Kiserud T, Berg S, Angelsen B, Olstad B. Three-dimensional imaging of the brain cavities in human embryos. Ultrasound Obstet Gynecol 1995; 5(4): 228–232

189 Hertzberg B S, Kliewer M A, Freed K S et al. Third ventricle: size and appearance in normal fetuses through gestation. Radiology 1997; 203(3): 641–644

190 Chervenak F A, Berkowitz R L, Romero R et al. The diagnosis of fetal hydrocephalus. Am J Obstet Gynecol 1983; 147: 703–716

191 Tomlinson M W, Treadwell M C, Bottoms S F. Isolated mild ventriculomegaly: associated karyotypic abnormalities and in utero observations. J Maternal-Fetal Med 1997; 6(4): 241–244

192 Nyberg D A, Mack L A, Hirsch J, Pagon R O, Shepard T H. Fetal hydrocephalus: sonographic detection and clinical significance of associated anomalies. Radiology 1987; 163: 187–191

193 Pagon R A, Clarren S K, Milam D F, Hendrickson A E. Autosomal recessive eye and brain anomalies: Warburg syndrome. J Pediatr 1983; 102: 542–546

194 Cochrane D D, Myles S T, Nimrod C, Still D K, Sugarman R G, Wittman B K. Intrauterine hydrocephalus and ventriculomegaly: associated anomalies and fetal outcome. Can J Neurol Sci 1985; 12: 51–59

195 Glick P L, Harrison M R, Nakayama D K, et al. Management of ventriculomegaly in the fetus. J Pediatr 1984; 105: 97–105

196 Hyndman J, Johri A M, MacLean N E. Diagnosis of fetal hydrocephalus by ultrasound. NZ Med J 1980; 91: 385–386

197 Den Hollander N S, Vinkesteijn A, Schmitz-van Splunder P, Catsman-Berrevoets C E, Wladimiroff J W. Prenatally diagnosed fetal ventriculomegaly: prognosis and outcome. Prenat Diagn 1998; 18: 557–566

198 Chervenak F A, Duncan C, Ment L R et al. Outcome of fetal ventriculomegaly. Lancet 1984; ii: 179–181

199 Serlo W, Kirkinen P, Joupila P, Herva R. Prognostic signs in fetal hydrocephalus. Childs Nerv Syst 1986; 2: 93–97

200 Twining P, Jaspan T, Zuccollo J. The outcome of fetal ventriculomegaly. Br J Radiol 1994; 67: 26–31

201 Hudgins R J, Edwards M S B, Golbus M S. Management of fetal ventriculomegaly. In: Levene M I, Bennett M J, Punt J, eds. Fetal and neonatal neurology and neurosurgery. Edinburgh: Churchill Livingstone, 1988: 577–585

202 Vintzileos A M, Ingardia C J, Nochimson D J. Congenital hydrocephalus: a review and protocol for perinatal management. Obstet Gynecol 1983; 62: 539–549

203 Oi S, Honda Y, Hidaka M, Sato O, Matsumoto S. Intrauterine high resolution magnetic resonance imaging in fetal hydrocephalus and prenatal estimation of postnatal outcomes with 'perspective classification'. J Neurosurg 1998; 88(4): 685–694

204 Carter C O, David P A, Laurence K M. A family study of major central nervous system malformations in South Wales. J Med Genet 1968; 5: 81–106

205 Adams C, Johnston W P, Nevin N C. Family study of congenital hydrocephalus. Dev Med Child Neurol 1982; 24: 493–498

206 Howard F M, Till K, Carter C O. A family study of hydrocephalus resulting from aqueduct stenosis. J Med Genet 1981; 18: 252–255

207 Crombleholme T M, D'Alton M, Cendron M et al. Prenatal diagnosis and the paediatric surgeon: the impact of prenatal consultation on perinatal management. J Pediatr Surg 1996; 31(1): 156–162

208 Kuller J A, Katz V L, Wells S R, Wright L N, McMahon M J. Caesarean delivery for fetal malformations. Obstet Gynecol Surv 1996; 51(6): 371–375

209 Clewell W H, Johnson M L, Meier P R, et al. A surgical approach to the treatment of fetal hydrocephalus. N Engl J Med 1982; 306: 1320–1325

210 Chervenak F A, Berkowitz R L, Tortora M, Hobbins J C. The management of fetal hydrocephalus. Am J Obstet Gynecol 1985; 151: 933–942

211 International F A. International fetal surgery register: 1985 update. Clin Obstet Gynecol 1986; 29: 551–557

212 Manning F A, Harrison M R, Rodeck C. Catheter shunts for fetal hydronephrosis and hydrocephalus. N Engl J Med 1986; 315: 336–340

213 Cohen M M. An update on the holoprosencephalic disorders. J Pediatr 1982; 101: 865–869

214 DeMyer W. Holoprosencephaly (cyclopia–arhinencephaly). In: Vinken P J, Bruyn G W, Klawans H L, eds. Handbook of clinical neurology. Amsterdam: Elsevier/North Holland Biomedical Press, 1987: 225–244

215 DeMyer W, Zeman W, Palmer C. The face predicts the brain: diagnostic significance of median facial abnormalities for holoprosencephaly (arhinencephaly). Pediatrics 1964; 34: 256–263

216 Roach E, DeMyer W, Palmer K, Conneally M, Merritt A. Holoprosencephaly: birth data, genetic and demographic analysis of 30 families. Birth Defects 1975; 11: 294–313

217 Saunders E S, Shortland D, Dunn P M. What is the incidence of holoprosencephaly? J Med Genet 1984; 21: 21–26

218 Nyberg D A, Mack L A, Bronstein A, Hirsch J, Pagon R. Holoprosencephaly: prenatal sonographic diagnosis. AJR 1987; 149: 1051–1058

219 Chervenak F A, Isaacson G, Hobbins J C, Chithara U, Tortora M, Berhowitz R C. Diagnosis and management of fetal holoprosencephaly. Obstet Gynecol 1985; 66: 322–326

220 Dallaire L, Clarke Fraser F, Wigglesworth F W. Familial holoprosencephaly. Birth Defects Original Article, series VII, 1971; 7: 136–142

221 Benawra R, Mangurten H H, Duffell D R. Cyclopia and other anomalies following maternal ingestion of salicylates. J Pediatr 1980; 96: 1069–1071

222 Barr M Jr, Hanson J W, Currey K et al. Holoprosencephaly in infants of diabetic mothers. J Pediatr 1983; 102(4): 565–568

223 Blackwell D E, Spinnato J A, Hirsch G, Giles H R, Sackler J. Antenatal ultrasound diagnosis of holoprosencephaly: a case report. Am J Obstet Gynecol 1982; 143: 848–849

224 Hidalgo H, Bowie J, Rosenberg E R et al. In utero sonographic diagnosis of fetal cerebral anomalies. AJR 1982; 139: 143–148

225 Hill L M, Breckle R, Bonebrake C R. Ultrasonic findings with holoprosencephaly. J Reprod Med 1982; 27: 172–175

226 Filly R A, Chinn D H, Callen P W. Alobar holoprosencephaly: ultrasonographic prenatal diagnosis. Radiology 1984; 151: 455–459

227 Cayea P D, Balcar I, Alberti O, Jones T B. Prenatal diagnosis of semilobar holoprosencephaly. AJR 1984; 142: 401–402

228 Greene M F, Benacerraf B R, Frigoletto F D. Reliable criteria for the prenatal sonographic diagnosis of alobar holoprosencephaly. Am J Obstet Gynecol 1987; 156: 687–689

229 Hoffman-Tretin J C, Horoupian D S, Koenigsberg M, Schnur M J, Llena J F. Lobar holoprosencephaly with hydrocephalus: antenatal demonstration and differential diagnosis. J Ultrasound Med 1986; 5: 691–697

230 Young I D, Zuccollo J M, Barrow M, Fowlie A. Holoprosencephaly, telecanthus and ectrodactyly. Clin Dysmorphol 1992; 1: 47–51

231 Toth Z, Csecsei K, Szeifert G, Torok O, Papp Z. Early prenatal diagnosis of cyclopia associated with holoprosencephaly. JCU 1986; 14: 550–553

232 Van Zalen-Sprock R, van Vugt JMG, van der Harten H J, Nieuwint AWM, van Geijn HP. First trimester diagnosis of cyclopia and holoprosencephaly. J Ultrasound Med 1995; 14: 631–633

233 Gonzalez-Gomez F, Salamanca A, Padilla M C, Camara M, Sabatel R M. Alobar holoprosencephalic embryo detected via transvaginal sonography. Eur J Obstet Gynecol Reprod Biol 1992; 47: 266–270

234 Bronshtein M, Wiener Z. Early transvaginal sonographic diagnosis of alobar holoprosencephaly. Prenat Diagn 1991; 11(7): 459–462

235 Pretorius D H, Nelson T R. Face visualization using three-dimensional ultrasonography. J Ultrasound Med 1995; 14(5): 349–356

236 Merz E, Weber G, Bahlman F, Miric-Tesanic D. Application of transvaginal and abdominal three-dimensional ultrasound for the detection or exclusion of malformations of the fetal face. Ultrasound Obstet Gynecol 1997; 9(4): 237–243

237 Benacerraf B R, Frigoletto F D, Bieber F R. The fetal face. Ultrasound examination. Radiology 1984; 153: 495–497

238 Mayden K L, Tortora M, Berkowitz R L, Bracken M, Hobbins J C. Orbital diameters: a new parameter for prenatal diagnosis and dating. Am J Obstet Gynecol 1982; 144: 289–297

239 Pilu G, Romero R, Rizzo N, Jeanty P, Bovicelli L, Hobbins J C. Criteria for the prenatal diagnosis of holoprosencephaly. Am J Perinatol 1987; 4: 41–49

240 Filly R A. Ultrasound evaluation of the fetal neural axis. In: Callen P W, ed. Ultrasonography in obstetrics and gynaecology. Philadelphia: W B Saunders, 1988: 83–135

241 Whiteford M L, Tolmie J L Holoprosencephaly in the west of Scotland 1975–1994. J Med Genet 1996; 33(7): 578–584

242 Sperry R W. Hemispheric disconnection and unity in conscious awareness. Am J Psychol 1968; 23: 723–733

243 Loeser J D, Alvord E C. Agenesis of the corpus callosum. Brain 1968; 91: 553–570

244 Guibert-Tranier F, Piton J, Billerey J, Caille J M. Agenesis of the corpus callosum. J Neuroradiol 1982; 9: 135–160

245 Rakic P, Yakovlev P I. Development of the corpus callosum and cavum septi in man. J Comp Neurol 1968; 132: 45–72

246 Davidoff L M, Dyke C G. Agenesis of the corpus callosum: diagnosis by encephalography. AJR 1934; 32: 1–10

247 Babcock D S. The normal, absent, and abnormal corpus callosum: sonographic findings. Radiology 1984; 151: 449–453

248 Gebarski S S, Gebarski K S, Bowerman R A, Silver T M. Agenesis of the corpus callosum: sonographic features. Radiology 1984; 151: 443–448

249 Levine D, Barnes P D, Madsen J R, Li W, Edelman R R. Fetal central nervous system anomalies: MR imaging augments sonographic diagnosis. Radiology 1997; 204(3): 635–642

250 Byrd S E, Harwood-Nash D C, Fitz C R. Absence of the corpus callosum: computed tomographic evaluation in infants and children. Can Assoc Radiol J 1978; 29: 108–112

251 Ettlinger G, Blakemore C B, Milner A D, Wilson J. Agenesis of the corpus callosum: a further behavioural investigation. Brain 1974; 97: 225–234

252 Grogono J L. Children with agenesis of the corpus callosum. Dev Med Child Neurol 1968; 10: 613–616

253 Warkany J, Lemire R, Cohen M M. Mental retardation and congenital malformations of the nervous system. Chicago: Year Book Medical Publishers, 1981: 224–243

254 Vergani P, Ghidani A, Strobelt N et al. Prognostic indicators in the prenatal diagnosis of agenesis of corpus callosum. Am J Obstet Gynecol 1994; 170(3): 753–758

255 D'Ercole C, Girard N, Cravello L et al. Prenatal diagnosis of fetal corpus callosum agenesis by ultrasonography and magnetic resonance imaging. Prenat Diagn 1998; 18: 247–253

256 Fuchigami T, Mazaki R, Nishimura A et al. A mother and daughter with agenesis of the corpus callosum. Acta Pediatr Jpn 1996; 38(1): 52–56

257 Menkes J H, Philippart M, Clark D B. Hereditary partial agenesis of the corpus callosum. Arch Neurol 1964; 11: 198–208

258 Young I D, Trounce J Q, Levene M I, Fitzsimmons J S, Moore J R. Agenesis of the corpus callosum and macrocephaly in siblings. Clin Genet 1985; 28: 225–230

259 Friedman M, Cohen P. Agenesis of corpus callosum as a possible sequel to maternal rubella during pregnancy. Am J Dis Child 1947; 73: 178–185

260 Bartoleschi B, Cantore G P. Agenesia del corpus calloso in paziente affeto da toxoplasmasi. Riv Neurol 1962; 32: 79

261 Pfeiffer J, Majewski F, Fishback H, Bierich J R, Volk B. Alcohol embryo and fetopathy. J Neuro Sci 1979; 41: 125–137

262 Elliot G B, Wollin D W. Defect of the corpus callosum and congenital occlusion of the fourth ventricle with tuberous sclerosis. AJR 1966; 85: 701–705

263 Probst F P. Congenital defects of the corpus callosum: morphology and encephalographic appearances. Acta Radiol 1973; 331: 1–152

264 Kendall B E. Dysgenesis of the corpus callosum. Neuroradiology 1983; 25: 239–256

265 Comstock C H, Culp D, Gonzalez J, Boal D B. Agenesis of the corpus callosum in the fetus: its evolution and significance. J Ultrasound Med 1985; 4: 613–616

266 Meizner I, Barki Y, Hertzanu Y. Prenatal sonographic diagnosis of agenesis of corpus callosum. JCU 1987; 15: 262–264

267 Bertino R E, Nyberg D A, Cyr D R, Mack L A. Prenatal diagnosis of agenesis of the corpus callosum. J Ultrasound Med 1988; 7: 251–260

268 Parrish M L, Roessmann U, Levinsohn M W. Agenesis of the corpus callosum: a study of the frequency of associated malformations. Ann Neurol 1979; 6: 349–354

269 Gupta J K, Lilford R J. Assessment and management of fetal agenesis of the corpus callosum. Prenat Diagn 1995; 15(4): 301–312

270 Romero R, Pilu G, Jeanty P, Ghidini A, Hobbins J C. In: Prenatal diagnosis of congenital anomalies. Connecticut: Appleton and Lange, 1988

271 Baraitser M. The genetics of neurological disorders. Oxford: Oxford University Press, 1982

272 Dieker H, Edwards R H, Zurhein G, Chou S M, Hartman H A, Opitz J M. The lissencephaly syndrome. Birth Defects 1969; 5: 53–64

273 Garcia C A, Dunn D, Trevor R. The lissencephaly (agyria) syndrome in siblings. Computerized tomographic and neuropathologic findings. Arch Neurol 1978; 35: 608–611

274 Holzgreve W, Feil R, Louwen F, Miny P. Prenatal diagnosis and management of fetal hydrocephaly and lissencephaly. Childs Nerv Syst 1993; 9(7): 408–412

275 Van Zelderen-Bhola S L, Breslau-Siderius E J, Beverstock G C et al. Prenatal and postnatal investigation of a case with Miller-Dieker syndrome due to a familial cryptic translocation t(17;20) (p13.3;q13.3) detected by fluorescence in situ hybridisation. Prenat Diagn 1997; 17(2): 173–179

276 Okamura K, Murotsuki J, Sakai T, Matsumoto K, Shirane R, Yajima A. Prenatal diagnosis of lissencephaly by magnetic resonance image. Fetal Diagn Ther 1993; 8(1): 56–59

277 Halsey J H. Hydranencephaly. In: Vinken P J, Bruyn G W, Klawans H L, eds. Handbook of clinical neurology. Amsterdam: Elsevier/North Holland Biomedical Press, 1987; 50: 337–353

278 Myers R E. Brain pathology following fetal vascular occlusion: an experimental study. Invest Ophthalmol 1969; 8: 41–50

279 Green M F, Benacerraf B, Crawford J M. Hydranencephaly: US appearance during in-utero evolution. Radiology 1985; 156: 779–780

280 Johnson E E, Warner M, Simonds J P. Total absence of the cerebral hemispheres. J Pediatr 1951; 38: 69–79

281 Muir C S. Hydranencephaly and related disorders. Am J Dis Child 1959; 34: 231

282 Altshuler G. Toxoplasmosis as a cause of hydranencephaly. Am J Dis Child 1973; 125: 251–252

283 Carrasco C R, Stierman E D, Harnsberger H R, Lee T G. An algorithm for prenatal ultrasound diagnosis of congenital central nervous system abnormalities. J Ultrasound Med 1985; 4: 163–168

284 Lee T G, Warren B H. Antenatal diagnosis of hydranencephaly by ultrasound: correlation with ventriculography and computed tomography. JCU 1977; 5: 271–273

285 Strauss S, Bouzouki M, Goldfarb H, Uppal V, Costales F. Antenatal ultrasound diagnosis of an unusual case of hydranencephaly. JCU 1984; 12: 420–422

286 Hambey W B, Krauss R F, Beswick W F. Hydranencephaly: clinical diagnosis. Presentation of seven cases. Pediatrics 1950; 6: 371–383

287 Sutton L N, Bruce D A, Schut L. Hydranencephaly versus maximal hydrocephalus: an important clinical distinction. Neurosurgery 1980; 6: 34–38

288 Lin Y, Chang F, Liu C. Antenatal detection of hydranencephaly at 12 weeks' menstrual age. JCU 1992; 20: 62–64

289 Siber M. X linked recessive microencephaly, microphthalmia with corneal opacities, spastic quadriplegia, hypospadias and cryptorchidism. Clin Genet 1984; 26: 453–456

290 Gross H, Jellinger K. Morphologische aspekte cerebraler midbildungen. Wien Zeitscher Nervenheilk 1969; 27: 9–37

291 Gastaut H, Gastaut J L. Demonstration of a little known cause of infantile epilepsy, occipital porencephaly, by computerised tomography (CT). Comput Tomogr 1977; 1: 323–330

292 Benda C E. The late effects of cerebral birth injuries. Medicine 1945; 24: 71–110

293 Cantu R C, Le May M. Porencephaly caused by intracerebral haemorrhage. Radiology 1967; 88: 526–530

294 Page L K, Brown S B, Gargano F P, Shortz R W. Schizencephaly: a clinical study and review. Childs Brain 1975; 1: 348–358

295 Miller G M, Stears J C, Guggenheim M A, Wilkening G F. Schizencephaly: a clinical and CT study. Neurology 1984; 34: 997–1001

296 Klingensmith W C, Cioffi-Ragan D T. Schizencephaly: diagnosis and progression in utero. Radiology 1986; 159: 617–618

297 Larroche J C. Cytoarchitectonic abnormalities (abnormalities of cell migration). In: Vinken P J, Bruyn G W, eds: Handbook of clinical neurology. Amsterdam: Elsevier/North Holland Biomedical Press, 1977; 30: 479–506

298 Pilu G, Falco P, Perolo A et al. Differential diagnosis of fetal intracranial hypoechoic lesions: report of 21 cases. Ultrasound Obstet Gynecol 1997; 9(4): 229–236

299 Berg R A, Aleck K A, Kaplan A M. Familial porencephaly. Arch Neurol 1983; 40: 567–569

300 Airaksincn E M. Familial porencephaly. Clin Genet 1984; 26: 236–238

301 Dandy W E, Blackfan K D. Internal hydrocephalus. An experimental, clinical and pathological study. Am J Dis Child 1914; 8: 406–482

302 Taggart J K, Walker A E. Congenital atresia of the foramens of Luschka and Magendie. Arch Neurol Psychiatry 1942; 48: 583–612

303 Benda C E. The Dandy–Walker syndrome or so-called atresia of the foramen Magendie. J Neuropathol Exp Neurol 1954; 13: 14–29

304 Gardner E, O'Rahilly R, Prolo D. The Dandy–Walker and the Arnold–Chiari malformations. Clinical, developmental and teratological considerations. Arch Neurol 1975; 32: 393–407

305 Murray J C, Johnson J A, Bird T D. Dandy–Walker malformation: etiologic heterogeneity and empiric recurrence risks. Genetics 1985; 28: 272–283

306 Hirsch J F, Pierrekahn A, Renier D, Sainterose C, Hoppehirsch E. The Dandy–Walker malformation: a review of 40 cases. J Neurosurg 1984; 61: 515–522

307 Nyberg D A, Cyr D R, Mack L A, Fitzsimmons J, Hickok D, Mahony B S. The Dandy–Walker malformation: prenatal sonographic diagnosis and its clinical significance. J Ultrasound Med 1988; 7: 65–71

308 Russ P D, Pretorius D H, Johnson M J. Dandy–Walker syndrome: a review of 15 cases evaluated by prenatal sonography. Am J Obstet Gynecol 1989; 161: 401–406

309 Ulm B, Ulm M R, Deutinger J, Bernaschek G. Dandy–Walker malformation diagnosed before 21 weeks of gestation: associated malformations and chromosomal abnormalities. Ultrasound Obstet Gynecol 1997; 10: 167–170

310 Hatjis C G, Horbar J D, Anderson G G. The in utero diagnosis of a posterior fossa intracranial cyst (Dandy–Walker cyst). Am J Obstet Gynecol 1981; 140: 473–475

311 Mahony B S, Callen P W, Filly R A, Hoddick W K. The fetal cisterna magna. Radiology 1984; 153: 773–776

312 Pilu G, Romero R, DePalma L et al. Antenatal diagnosis and obstetrical management of Dandy–Walker syndrome. J Reprod Med 1986; 31: 1017–1022

313 Blazer S, Berant M, Sujov P O, Zimmer E Z, Bronshtein M. Prenatal sonographic diagnosis of vermal agenesis. Prenat Diagn 1997; 17: 907–911

314 Dempsey P J, Kock H J. In utero diagnosis of the Dandy–Walker syndrome: differentiation from extra-axial posterior fossa cyst. JCU 1981; 9: 403–405

315 Hart M N, Malamud N, Ellis W G. The Dandy–Walker syndrome: clinicopathological study based on 28 cases. Neurology 1972; 22: 771–780

316 Sawaya R, McLaurin A L. Dandy–Walker syndrome: clinical analysis of 23 cases. J Neurosurg 1981; 55: 89–98

317 Keogan M T, DeAtkin A B, Hertberg B S. Cerebellar vermian defects: antenatal sonographic appearance and clinical significance. J Ultrasound Med 1994; 13(8): 607–611

318 Shuangshoti S, Netsky M G. Neuroepithelial (colloid) cysts of the nervous system: further observations on pathogenesis, location, incidence and histochemistry. Neurology 1966; 16: 887–903

319 Shuangshoti S, Netsky M G. Histogenesis of choroid plexus in man. Am J Anat 1966; 118: 283–316

320 Chitkara U, Cogswell C, Norton K, Wilkins I A, Mehalek K, Berkowitz R L. Choroid plexus cysts in the fetus: a benign anatomic variant or pathological entity? Report of 41 cases and review of the literature. Obstet Gynecol 1988; 72: 185–189

321 Clark S L, DeVore G R, Sabey P L. Prenatal diagnosis of cysts of the fetal choroid plexus. Obstet Gynecol 1988; 72: 585–587

322 Twining P, Zuccollo J, Swallow J, Clewes J. Choroid plexus cysts – a marker for trisomy 18. A prospective study and review of the literature. Br J Radiol 1989; 63: 385

323 Furness M E. Choroid plexus cysts and trisomy 18. Lancet 1987; ii: 693

324 DeRoo T R, Harris R D, Sargent S K, Denholm T A, Crow H C. Fetal choroid plexus cysts: prevalence, clinical significance and sonographic appearance. AJR 1988; 151: 1179–1181

325 Ostelere S J, Irving H C, Lilford R J. Choroid plexus cysts in the fetus. Lancet 1987; i: 1491

326 Geary M, Patel S, Lamont R. Isolated choroid plexus cysts and association with fetal aneuploidy in an unselected population. Ultrasound Obstet Gynecol 1997; 10: 171–173

327 Walkinshaw S, Pilling D, Spriggs A. Isolated choroid plexus cysts – the need for routine offer of karyotyping. Prenat Diagn 1994; 14: 663–669

328 Kilby M, Whittle M, North L, McHugo J. Isolated choroid plexus cysts and aneuploidy. Prenat Diagn 1997; 17(8): 785

329 Bundy A L, Saltzman D H, Pober B, Fine C, Emerson D, Doubilet P M. Antenatal sonographic findings in trisomy 18. J Ultrasound Med 1986; 5: 361–364

330 Nicolaides K H, Rodeck C H, Gosden C M. Rapid karyotyping in non-lethal fetal malformations. Lancet 1986; i: 283–287

331 Benacerraf B R. Asymptomatic cysts of the fetal choroid plexus in the second trimester. J Ultrasound Med 1987; 6: 475–478

332 Thorpe-Beeston J G, Gosden C M, Nicolaides K H. Is karyotyping for choroid plexus cysts necessary? Br J Radiol 1990; 63: 385

333 Gupta J K, Cave M, Lilford R J, Farrell T A, Irving H C, Mason G, Hau C. Clinical significance of fetal choroid plexus cysts. Lancet 1995; 346: 724–729

334 Bromley B, Lieberman E, Benacerraf B R. Choroid plexus cysts: not associated with Down's syndrome. Ultrasound Obstet Gynecol 1996; (8): 232–235

335 Gray D L, Winborrn R C, Suessen T L, Crane J P. Is genetic amniocentesis warranted when isolated choroid plexus cysts are found? Prenat Diagn 1996; 16: 983–990

336 Ostler S J, Irvine N C, Lilford R J. Fetal choroid plexus cysts. A report of 100 cases. Radiology 1990; 175: 753–755

337 Platt L D, Carlson D E, Madearis A L. Fetal choroid plexus cysts in the second trimester of pregnancy: a cause for concern? Am J Obstet Gynecol 1991; 164: 1652–1656

338 Benacerraf B R, Harlow B, Frigoletto F D Jr. Are choroid plexus cysts an indication for second trimester amniocentesis? Am J Obstet Gynecol 1990; 162: 1001–1006

339 Montemagno R, Soothill P W, Scarcelli M, Rodeck C H. Disappearance of fetal choroid plexus cysts during the second trimester in cases of chromosomal abnormality. Br J Obstet Gynaecol 1995; 102: 752–753

340 Reinsch R C. Choroid plexus cysts – association with trisomy: prospective view of 16,059 patients. Am J Obstet Gynecol 1997; 176: 1381–1383

341 Cuckle H S, Thornton J G. Aneuploidy risk with isolated choroid plexus cysts. Prenat Diagn 1996; 16: 967–972

342 Gratton R J, Hogge W A, Aston C E. Choroid plexus cysts and trisomy 18: risk modification based on maternal age and multiple marker screening. Am J Obstet Gynecol 1996; 175: 1493–1497

343 Sharony R. Fetal choroid plexus cysts – is a genetic evaluation indicated? Prenat Diagn 1997; 17(6): 519–524

344 Starkman S P, Brown T C, Linell E A. Cerebral arachnoid cysts. J Neuropathol Exp Neurol 1958; 17: 484

345 Geissinger J D, Kohler W C, Robinson B W, Davis F M. Arachnoid cysts of the middle cranial fossa: surgical considerations. Surg Neurol 1978; 10: 27–33

346 Smith R A, Smith W A. Arachnoid cysts of the middle cranial fossa. Surg Neurol 1976; 5: 246–252

347 Roach E S, Laster D W, Sumner T E, Volberg F M. Posterior fossa arachnoid cyst demonstrated by ultrasound. JCU 1982; 10: 88–90

348 Shaw C M, Alvord E C. Congenital arachnoid cysts and their differential diagnosis. In: Vinken G W, Bruyn P W, eds. Handbook of clinical neurology. Amsterdam: Elsevier/North Holland Biomedical Press, 1977; 31: 75–135

349 Oliver L C. Primary arachnoid cysts. Br Med J 1958; 1: 1147

350 Diakoumakis E E, Weinberg B, Mollin J. Prenatal sonographic diagnosis of a suprasellar arachnoid cyst. J Ultrasound Med 1986; 5: 529

351 Sauerbrei E E, Cooperberg P L. Cystic tumours of the fetal and neonatal cerebrum: ultrasound and computed tomographic evaluation. Radiology 1983; 147: 689–692

352 Anderson F M, Landing B H. Cerebral arachnoid cysts in infants. J Pediatr 1966; 69: 88–96

353 Goldstein I, Reece E A, Pilu G, Bovicelli L, Hobbins J C. Cerebellar measurements with ultrasonography in the evaluation of fetal growth and development. Am J Obstet Gynecol 1987; 156: 1065–1069

354 Comstock C H, Boal D B. Enlarged fetal cisterna magna: appearance and significance. Obstet Gynecol 1985; 66: 25–27

355 Lyon G, Beaugerie A. Congenital developmental malformations. In: Levene M I, Bennett M J, Punt J, eds. Fetal and neonatal neurology and neurosurgery. Edinburgh: Churchill Livingstone, 1988: 231–248

356 Kilham L, Margolis G. Cerebellar ataxia in hamsters inoculated with rat virus. Science 1964; 143: 1047–1048

357 Walker A E. Lissencephaly. Arch Neurol Psychiatry 1942; 48: 13–29

358 Dobyns W B, Kirkpatrick J B, Hittner H M, Roberts R M, Kretzer F L. Walker–Warburg and cerebro-ocular-muscular syndromes and a new syndrome with type II lissencephaly. Am J Med Genet 1985; 22: 157–195

359 Young I D. Genetics of neurodevelopmental disorders. In: Levene M I, Bennett M J, Punt J, eds. Fetal and neonatal neurology and neurosurgery. Edinburgh: Churchill Livingstone, 1988: 249–257

360 Bundy S. Genetics and neurology. Edinburgh: Churchill Livingstone, 1985

361 Padget D H. The cranial venous system in man with reference to the development, adult configuration and relation to the arteries. Am J Anat 1956; 98: 307–355

362 Vintzileos A M, Eisenfeld L I, Campbell W A, Herson V C, DiLeo P E, Chameides L. Prenatal ultrasonic diagnosis of arteriovenous malformation of the vein of Galen. Am J Perinatol 1986; 3: 209–211

363 Reiter A A, Huhta J C, Carpenter R J, Segall G K, Hawkins E P. Prenatal diagnosis of arteriovenous malformation of the vein of Galen. JCU 1986; 14: 623–628

364 Hirsch J H, Cyr D, Eberhardt H, Zunkel D. Ultrasonographic diagnosis of an aneurysm of the vein of Galen in utero by duplex scanning. J Ultrasound Med 1983; 2: 231–233

365 Mao K, Adams J. Antenatal diagnosis of intracranial arteriovenous fistula by ultrasonography: case report. Br J Obstet Gynaecol 1983; 90: 872–873

366 Chisholm C A, Kuller J A, Katz V L, McCoy M C. Aneurysm of the vein of Galen: prenatal diagnosis and perinatal management. Am J Perinatol 1996; 13(8): 503–506

367 Campi A, Scotti G, Filippi M, Gerevini S, Strigimi F, Lasjaunias P. Antenatal diagnosis of vein of Galen aneurysmal malformation: MR study of fetal brain and postnatal follow-up. Neuroradiology 1996; 38(1): 87–90

368 Silverman B K, Brekzt T, Craig J, Nadas A S. Congestive failure in the newborn caused by cerebral arteriovenous fistula. Am J Dis Child 1959; 89: 539–543

369 Norman M G, Becker L E. Cerebral damage in neonates resulting from arteriovenous malformation of vein of Galen. J Neurol Neurosurg Psychiatry 1974; 37: 252–258

370 Hoffman H J, Chuang S, Hendrick E B, Humphreys R P. Aneurysms of the vein of Galen. Experience at the Hospital for Sick Children, Toronto. J Neurosurg 1982; 57: 316–322

371 Amacher A L, Shillito J. The syndromes and surgical treatment of aneurysms of the great vein of Galen. J Neurosurg 1973; 39: 88–98

372 Mori K. Anomalies of the central nervous system. Neuroradiology and neurosurgery. New York: Thieme-Stratton, 1985

373 Koos W, Miller M H. Intracranial tumours of infants and children. Stuttgart: G Thieme, 1971

374 Lipman S P, Pretorious D H, Rumack C M, Manco-Johnson M L. Fetal intracranial teratoma: US diagnosis of 3 cases and a review of the literature. Radiology 1985; 157: 491–494

375 Kirkinen P, Suramo I, Joupila P et al. Combined use of ultrasound and computed tomography in the evaluation of fetal intracranial abnormality. J Perinat Med 1982; 10: 257–265

376 Fraumeni J F, Miller R W. Cancer deaths in the newborn. Am J Dis Child 1969; 117: 186–189

377 Kirkinen P, Heinoven S, Vanamo K, Ryynanen M. Maternal serum alpha-fetoprotein and epithelial tumour marker concentrations are not increased by fetal sacrococcygeal teratoma. Prenat Diagn 1997; 17(1): 47–50

378 Sherer D M, Fromberg R A, Rindfusz D W, Harris B H, Sanz L E. Colour Doppler aided prenatal diagnosis of a type 1 cystic sacrococcygeal teratoma simulating a meningomyelocoele. Am J Perinat 1997; 14(1): 13–15

379 Altman R P, Randolph J G, Lilly J R. Sacrococcygeal teratoma: American Academy of Pediatrics Surgical Section Survey – 1973. J Pediatr Surg 1974; 9: 389–398

380 O'Connell E J, Feldt R H, Stickler G B. Head circumference, mental retardation and growth failure. Pediatrics 1965; 36: 62–66

381 Book J A, Schut J W, Reed S C. A clinical and genetical study of microcephaly. Am J Ment Def 1953; 57: 637–660

382 Haslam R H A. Microcephaly. In: Vinken P J, Bruyn G W, Klawans H L, eds. Handbook of clinical neurology. Amsterdam: Elsevier/North Holland Biomedical Press, 1987; 50: 267–284

383 Dobbing J, Sands J. Quantitative growth and development of human brain. Arch Dis Child 1973; 48: 757–767

384 Thoms A, Campbell S. Ultrasound measurement of the fetal head and abdomen circumference ratio in the assessment of growth retardation. Br J Obstet Gynaecol 1977; 84: 165–174

385 Kurtz A B, Wapner R J, Rubin C S, Cole-Beuglet C, Ross R D, Goldberg B B. Ultrasound criteria for in utero diagnosis of microcephaly. JCU 1980; 8: 11–16

386 Bromley B, Benacerraf B R. Difficulties in the prenatal diagnosis of microcephaly. J Ultrasound Med 1995; 14(4): 303–306

387 Avery G B, Meneses L, Lodge A. The clinical significance of 'measurement microcephaly'. Am J Dis Child 1972; 123: 214–217

388 Martin H P. Microcephaly and mental retardation. Am J Dis Child 1970; 119: 128–131

389 Pryor H B, Thelander H. Abnormally small head size and intellect in children. J Pediatr 1968; 73: 593–598

390 Chervenak F A, Isaacson G, Streltzoff J. Craniospinal and facial defects. In: James D K, Steer P J, Weiner C P, Gonik B, eds. High risk pregnancy; management options. London: WB Saunders, 1997; 871–899

391 Haslam R H A, Smith D W. Autosomal dominant microcephaly. J Pediatr 1979; 95: 701–705

392 Quazi Q H, Reed T E. A problem in diagnosis of primary versus secondary microcephaly. Clin Genet 1973; 4: 46–52

393 Bartley J A, Hall B D. Mental retardation and multiple congenital abnormalities of unknown etiology: frequency of occurrence in similarly affected sibs of the proband. Birth Defects Original Article Series XIV 1978; 6B: 127–137

394 Opitz J M, Kaveggia E G, Durkin-Stamm M V, Pendleton E. Diagnostic/genetic studies in severe mental retardation. Birth Defects Original Article Series XVI 1978; 6B: 1–38

395 Monteagudo A, Tharakan T, Timor-Tritsch I E. Sonographic neuroembryology of the central nervous system. J Assoc Acad Minority Phys 1995; 6(1): 34–37

396 Blaas H G, Eik-Nes S H, Kiserud T, Hellevik L R. Early development of the hindbrain: a longitudinal ultrasound study from 7 to 12 weeks of gestation. Ultrasound Obstet Gynecol 1995; 5(3): 151–160

397 Timor-Tritsch I E, Monteagudo A, Warren W B. Transvaginal ultrasonographic definition of the central nervous system in the first and early second trimesters. Am J Obstet Gynecol 1991; 164(2): 497–503

398 Report of the RCOG Working Party: Ultrasound screening for fetal abnormalities. London: RCOG Press, 1997

The urinary tract

*Alison Fowlie, Josephine M McHugo
and David Churchill*

Introduction

One of the earliest congenital abnormalities diagnosed *in utero* was that of polycystic kidneys, reported by Garrett in 1970.[1] Later, in 1975, obstructive nephropathy was recognised in a fetus.[2] These were both gross pathologies found in late pregnancies. Over the last 20–25 years improvements in ultrasound technology and techniques, and in the understanding of fetal anatomy and physiology as revealed by ultrasound, have led to increasingly early diagnoses of abnormalities of the urinary tract, even at 12–15 weeks,[3–8] and the recognition on ultrasound of virtually every possible pathology.

Congenital abnormalities of the urinary tract are common[9–11] but the true incidence is uncertain. Although exceeded only by malformations of the central nervous and cardiovascular systems as causes of death in infancy from congenital malformation, the majority (approximately 70%) are not lethal.[12] This makes assessment of the true incidence very difficult: it is approximately two or three per 1000 live births.[12,13]

As with other organs, the use of routine ultrasound scanning in low-risk pregnancies has resulted in early detection of many cases of urinary tract abnormalities. Lethal conditions may thus be terminated. Forewarning is given of moderate to severe pathologies, allowing planned delivery and post-natal treatment, counselling and preparation of the parents for the problems their baby will have, and opening up avenues for prenatal treatment.[14] Particularly importantly, clinicians are alerted to the presence of asymptomatic and clinically silent lesions (about 65% of abnormalities in live births[9]) which otherwise would be missed in the neonatal period, and perhaps remain unrecognised until late presentation with renal failure and chronic infection.

As with all developing fields, problems have occurred with the ultrasonic diagnosis and subsequent management of urinary tract problems. Its accuracy in prenatal diagnosis has been reported to be between 60 and 96%.[15,16] There have been errors, such as the large fetal adrenal mistaken for a fetal kidney[17] and confusion between pelvi-ureteric junction obstruction and duodenal atresia.[18,19] There may be difficulty in differentiating between multicystic dysplasia and an obstructed kidney,[18] but these problems are now well recognised and mistakes are few.

However, the differentiation of physiological dilatation of the urinary tract from minor degrees of obstructive pathology remains difficult[20] and this is an area that is still incompletely resolved. In addition, even when obstructive uropathy is present the degree of urinary tract dilation as visualised on ultrasound does not correlate well with the pathological state of the renal tissue or its function.

Attempts have been made to evaluate the presence or degree of dysplasia of the renal tissue and thus infer something about renal function. Increased renal reflectivity, together with cortical cysts in the presence of hydronephrosis, is strongly suggestive of renal dysplasia.[21] However, increased reflectivity has been found in 20% of normal fetal kidneys, and 25% of those with dysplasia were not detected,[21,22] casting doubts on the reliability of ultrasound for this.

One method of evaluating renal function is the assessment of amniotic fluid volume – a useful but fairly crude measure. Although severe oligohydramnios is associated with poor renal function, Glick *et al.* in 1984[22] found that one-third of pregnancies with only a mild reduction in amniotic fluid resulted in infants with severe reduction in renal function and one-third with moderately severe oligohydramnios actually had a reasonable outcome.

Attempts to correlate renal function with urine production are made difficult because of several factors:[22–24] polyuria, not oliguria, is the usual response to renal damage; reflux often coexists with obstruction, making accurate assessment of flow impossible; and maternal dehydration can severely affect the rate of fetal urine production.[25] More recently direct measurement of electrolytes, urea and creatinine in aspirated fetal urine has been used to evaluate renal function.[22,26,27] Although this correlates better with outcome, single or repeated aspiration of fetal urine is not always feasible or acceptable and procedure-related complications are not uncommon.

Despite these problems ultrasonic antenatal diagnosis of fetal urinary tract abnormalities has been useful in the prevention of serious renal damage in the child or young adult and its role here is likely to increase.

Normal urinary tract

Urine production begins at 11–13 weeks gestation.[28] Prior to this amniotic fluid is primarily a dialysate of fetal blood across the skin, which is permeable.[29] At about the time urine production begins the skin starts to keratinise, making it less permeable to water. Thus, between 13 and 20 weeks menstrual age there is a gradual change from fetal dialysate to urine as the main component of amniotic fluid.[30] Hence by 16–18 weeks absent or non-functioning kidneys are invariably associated with oligohydramnios.

The fetal kidneys may be imaged in the first trimester,[31] but with transabdominal ultrasound are more usually seen from 14 weeks onward[32] and reliably visualised in 90% of cases between 17 and 22 weeks.[33] With the advent of trans-vaginal ultrasonography the renal tract can now be visualised from 11 weeks onward in over 80% of individuals.[34] In the first part of the second trimester they are seen in transverse section, usually as areas of low reflectivity (Fig. 16.1) on either side of the spine, just inferior to the level where measurements for the abdominal circumference are made. In longitudinal section a bean-shaped structure is seen with very little internal architecture visible (Fig. 16.2). Later, as renal fat is laid down around

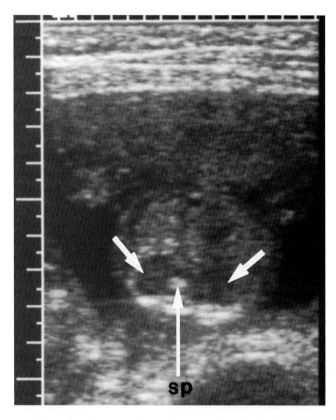

Fig. 16.1 Normal kidneys – 18 weeks. Transverse section of the fetal abdomen at 18 weeks. The kidneys (arrows) are seen as two echo-poor areas posteriorly within the fetal abdomen and touching the spine (sp) medially. The renal pelves are not visible.

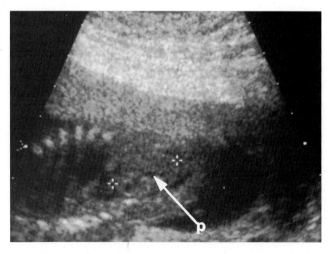

Fig. 16.2 Normal kidneys – 18 weeks. Longitudinal section of a fetal abdomen at 18 weeks. The kidney is seen in longitudinal section. The cortex and medulla cannot be differentiated. A normal 'slit-like' renal pelvis (p) is seen.

the renal fascia and in the central renal sinus, the fetal kidney is more easily seen and its appearance correlates well with that seen in the neonatal period (Fig. 16.3). The

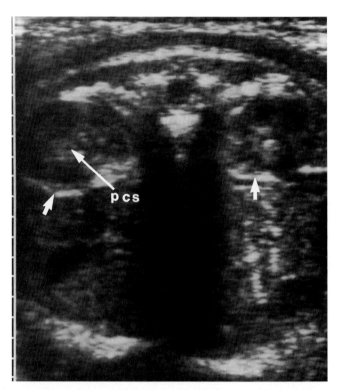

Fig. 16.3 Normal kidney – 22 weeks. Transverse section of the fetal abdomen at 22 weeks. The renal capsule (arrows) is well delineated and the pelvicalyceal system (pcs) can be seen.

marked corticomedullary differentiation and lobed outline that are normal for this age group may confuse the inexperienced operator into mistaking the pyramids for dilated calyces or renal cysts (Fig. 16.4). However, in hydronephrosis the dilated calyces communicate with the renal pelvis, and renal cysts do not surround the renal pelvis so uniformly.

The normal growth pattern of the fetal kidney has been well established in dead fetuses,[34–36] and *in utero* using ultrasound from the first trimester.[33,37–39] Standard measurements for renal circumference, volume, thickness, width and length related to menstrual age are available. Renal width, thickness (AP diameter) and circumference are measured in a transverse section of the fetal kidney. Length is measured from the upper to the lower pole on a longitudinal scan, care being taken to avoid including the adrenal gland in the measurement, particularly in early pregnancy. The ratio of the transverse renal circumference to the abdominal circumference is a simple screening measurement for conditions affecting renal size,[38] being fairly constant from 17 weeks to term at 0.27–0.30. These measurements, however, have limited value, as improved ultrasound equipment has allowed diagnoses of polycystic kidneys to be made on the appearances alone.

The normal fetal ureters are never visualised but the bladder can be seen as early as 11 weeks, and is consist-

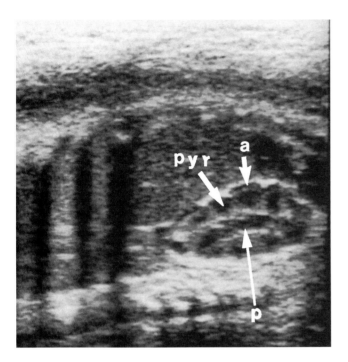

Fig. 16.4 Normal kidney – 22 weeks. Longitudinal section of the fetal abdomen at 22 weeks, displaying the kidney. The corticomedullary differentiation is well shown, with the arcuate vessels (a) seen at the base of the echo-poor medulla or pyramids (pyr). The renal pelvis (p) is seen centrally.

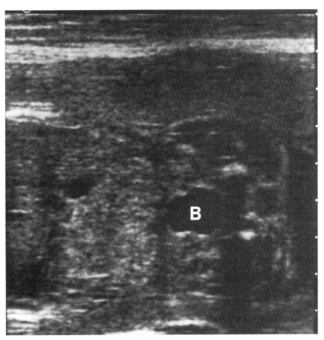

Fig. 16.5 Fetal bladder. Longitudinal section showing a normally filled fetal bladder (B).

ently identified from 16 weeks onward, when it may be observed to fill and empty regularly (Fig. 16.5). Failure to identify a fetal bladder in the course of an ultrasound examination may be because the fetus has just voided (voiding occurs at least once an hour).[23] In the routine situation, if the anomaly scan, including the urinary tract, is otherwise unremarkable and the liquor volume is normal, it is not essential to demonstrate the bladder. However, it should be noted that in some instances with severely abnormal kidneys, the volume of liquor may be relatively normal, causing diagnostic confusion. Urine production normally increases with menstrual age.[40] Calculating fetal urine production may be of help in such cases.[41]

Renal agenesis

Renal agenesis occurs because of failure of development of the ureteric buds of the mesonephros. It may be complete or partial, unilateral or bilateral. Ureteric remnants may be present.

Incidence and aetiology

Between 1974 and 1977 the birth frequency of bilateral renal agenesis was estimated to be 1.2 per 10 000 in England and Wales. Of these, 75% were isolated malformations in that only the kidney and embryologically related tissues were involved. The male:female ratio was 3:1.[42] Almost identical figures were obtained in British Columbia.[43] The incidence of unilateral renal agenesis is more difficult to establish as many cases are probably never identified. The British Columbia series identified an incidence of 0.15 per 1000 births, with a sex ratio of 1:1.[43]

Renal agenesis is an isolated anomaly in approximately 33–50% of cases. The aetiology is unclear. Families containing many members with renal agenesis or dysgenesis have been reported; postulated patterns of inheritance include autosomal recessive,[44,45] X-linked recessive,[46] autosomal dominant[47] and multifactorial.[47,48]

Chromosomal abnormalities have been described as producing bilateral renal agenesis as well as other abnormalities, but are rare. Trisomy 7 has been noted more than once.[49] Familial marker chromosome involving the presence of a small extra chromosome, possibly a segment of 22, has been reported,[50] as has renal agenesis in 4p syndrome.[51]

Bilateral renal agenesis may accompany cardiac and other abnormalities. A number of autosomal recessive syndromes include bilateral renal agenesis, namely cerebro-oculofacial skeletal syndrome, a syndrome with microcephaly, spinal and renal abnormalities,[52] and acrorenal mandibular syndrome comprising severe split extremity abnormalities and renal and genital malformations.[53] Renal agenesis is part of the autosomal dominant disorder of branchio-otorenal syndrome[54] and occurs with Müllerian duct abnormalities.[55]

Only insulin-dependent diabetes mellitus has been implicated as a teratogen in renal agenesis.[56]

Diagnosis

The most obvious ultrasound finding in bilateral renal agenesis in the second trimester is severe oligohydramnios, the fetus often being curled up and appearing squashed (Fig. 16.6). No fetal bladder is seen.[17] In the majority of cases the oligohydramnios results in such poor visualisation of the internal structure of the fetus that a definite diagnosis of absent kidneys is extremely difficult. Diagnosis may be easier in the first trimester, when the liquor volume is not reduced, as at this stage of pregnancy it is not dependent upon fetal urine production.[8]

This combination (severe oligohydramnios with no bladder) is not specific for bilateral renal agenesis: it may occur in many multiple abnormalities and in bilateral multicystic dysplastic kidneys. However, these also have a poor outcome and differentiation is therefore not essential. More importantly, these may be the findings in premature spontaneous rupture of membranes and early intrauterine growth retardation (IUGR). A very poor prognosis for all such cases of severe oligohydramnios[57–59] neglects the fact that the outcome in cases of IUGR and premature ruptured membranes may in fact be good in 20%. These cases consist entirely of early IUGR (62% good outcome) and premature spontaneous rupture of membranes (55% good outcome).[60]

Observations of urine production might be expected to prove the presence of functioning kidneys. Because in the normal situation voiding takes place at least once an hour,[23] failure to demonstrate the bladder in prolonged or serial examinations half hourly over 2–3 hours suggests renal agenesis. In order to speed up the process frusemide may be administered intravenously to the mother.[24] The fetus is then scanned at half-hourly intervals over a period of 2 hours, a filling bladder clearly ruling out bilateral renal agenesis. However, several authors have reported failure of diuresis even when renal tissue is present, particularly in early IUGR.[61,62] There is some controversy as to whether frusemide does in fact cross the placenta consistently, or in high enough doses to be effective, and, in fact, whether the kidneys of the early mid-trimester fetus will respond to it.[24,61,63,64] Urine production, assisted or unassisted, is less useful than might be expected in the diagnosis of bilateral renal agenesis.

Attempts to visualise the fetal kidneys directly are also fraught with difficulty. The fetal adrenal gland may be mistaken for the kidney, particularly in renal agenesis,[17,65] as it is a surprisingly large organ in the first and second trimesters of pregnancy and, in renal agenesis, does not conform to the usual shape, but forms an oval disc lying against the posterior abdominal wall, presumably owing to the absence of the compressive effect of the kidney (Fig. 16.7).[66] Positive identification of the kidneys therefore depends on defining the renal pelvis, capsule and early pyramid structure, which in many cases can be identified at 18–20 weeks. For more confident identification of the kidneys, instillation of normal saline into the amnion or fetal intraperitoneal space has been used. However, this may not be successful and causes uterine discomfort and contractions. The improved imaging of modern equipment usually enables a confident diagnosis of renal agenesis using either the abdominal or the transvaginal route (if the fetus is presenting by the breech low down in the pelvis). Colour flow Doppler may be of assistance when the diagnosis remains uncertain.

The diagnosis of isolated unilateral renal agenesis may well be missed unless the ultrasonographer painstakingly attempts to obtain ideal views of both kidneys in every case. Associated abnormalities may lead to the diagnosis. Aplastic

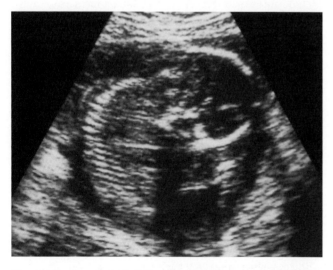

Fig. 16.6 Renal agenesis. Typical appearance of a pregnancy affected by renal agenesis. Anhydramnios with a curled up, poorly visualised fetus.

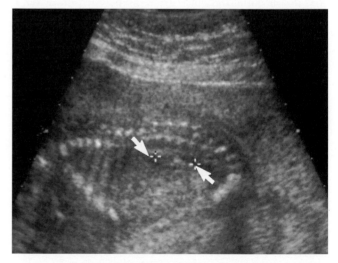

Fig. 16.7 Renal agenesis. In this longitudinal section of a fetus with renal agenesis the fetal adrenal (arrows) is seen. It was considered at the time to be either the adrenal gland or a hypoplastic kidney.

aplasia may be mistaken as unilateral renal agenesis, the aplastic kidney consisting of a nodule of tissue which microscopically represents dysplastic metanephric elements; however, renal agenesis and aplasia may represent a continuum and the differentiation between these two conditions on morphological and genetic grounds is probably not valid.[67]

Associated abnormalities

In 1946 Potter described infants with characteristic facial abnormalities, limb deformities and lethal pulmonary hypoplasia associated with bilateral renal agenesis.[68] This subsequently became known as the 'Potter syndrome'. It is now recognised that these appearances and the lung hypoplasia are a consequence of any condition leading to severe oligohydramnios[69,70] and that a better term to use is that of Potter sequence.[47] In this the lungs often weigh less than half that expected from the fetal weight, there being a reduction in the number of both alveoli and conducting airways. This suggests that the responsible insult occurs before the 16th conceptual week.[71] In Potter sequence the ears are low set, the skin is redundant, the nose is shaped like a parrot's beak and the chin recedes. There is abnormal hand and foot positioning, with bowed legs, clubbed feet and congenital dislocation of the hip.

The true associated abnormalities are divided into those involving the other genitourinary organs and those involving other systems. Abnormalities involving the genital organs are common (50–60% of cases[72,73]), including absence of the vas deferens and seminal vesicles, or absence of the uterus and upper vagina. Anomalies of other organ systems have been reported in 44% of patients.[72] Major deformities of the lower half of the body or limbs are common, occurring in about 40% of cases,[43] including lumbar hemivertebrae, sacral agenesis, caudal regression or absent radius and fibula, and digital abnormalities. Gastrointestinal abnormalities are common (19% of cases[43]), including anal atresia, absent sigmoid and rectum, and oesophageal and duodenal atresia. Cardiovascular malformations[43] occur in about 14% of cases, including septal defects, hypoplastic left heart, coarctation of the aorta, transposition of the great vessels, total anomalous pulmonary venous drainage and tetralogy of Fallot. Central nervous system malformations, including hydrocephaly, microcephaly, holoprosencephaly, spina bifida and iniencephaly, are found in some 10%.[43] Renal agenesis and cystic dysplasia have also been associated with the XYY chromosomal malformation when presenting with the Potter sequence of abnormalities. This emphasises the need to consider karyotyping in such cases.[74]

Prognosis

Bilateral renal agenesis is incompatible with life. About 40% of these infants are stillborn; the majority of those born alive die within 4 hours. Very rarely an infant will survive for more than 2 days. The cause of death *in utero* is not certain but other associated congenital abnormalities may be implicated.

Nearly 50% of infants with bilateral renal agenesis are growth retarded,[75] the incidence seeming to be higher in later pregnancy. Unilateral renal agenesis is no longer regarded as a relatively innocuous anomaly compensated for by enlargement of the contralateral kidney. Significantly higher frequencies of renal infection and calculus formation with resulting renal failure occur.[76] However, associated congenital abnormalities are similar to those found in bilateral renal agenesis and these therefore have a bearing on the prognosis.[43]

Obstetric management

If a positive diagnosis of renal agenesis has been made, termination should be offered. If the parents decline this option management should be conservative, with a non-interventional policy instituted if growth retardation or fetal distress ensues.

In many cases, however, for reasons already discussed, the diagnosis is in doubt. The conditions that may initially mimic renal agenesis, but which potentially carry a reasonable prognosis, are premature rupture of membranes and early intra-uterine growth retardation. A careful history to elicit any evidence of leaking liquor, speculum examination of the patient, the testing of any secretion found with nitrazine indicator sticks, and serial observations of the amniotic fluid volume over about 2 weeks, will in most cases indicate whether or not the membranes have ruptured. Either the fluid continues to leak, or serial scans show it to be reaccumulating. In early IUGR serial scans may be useful, looking for growth increments and any change in amniotic fluid volume, as this may well vary in IUGR. Doppler studies may be helpful.[77] Thus, study of the pregnancy over 2–3 weeks should rule out the more benign causes of severe oligohydramnios.

Recurrence risk

In bilateral renal agenesis there is an increased risk of a subsequent child being severely affected (3.5–4.4%[48,72]). In addition, the parents and their unaffected children are at increased risk of having silent genitourinary malformations: all first-degree relatives (the parents and siblings) of affected infants should be screened for asymptomatic malformations using ultrasound.[72] Part of the justification for this is the finding that unilateral renal agenesis has medical importance for the affected person, as it may be associated with abnormalities such as bicornuate uterus and absence of the vas deferens. Patients with unilateral renal agenesis should also be monitored more closely for infection and stone formation in the solitary kidney.

Renal cystic disease

Renal cystic disease encompasses a number of diverse hereditary and non-hereditary disorders. The original Potter classification[78–81] of type I infantile polycystic disease, type II multicystic dysplastic kidney, type III adult polycystic disease and type IV obstructive cystic dysplasia, although useful, is inadequate to cover the range of disorders and has largely fallen out of use. The main problems that concern the antenatal ultrasonographer are renal dysplasia and polycystic disease.

Renal dysplasia

Renal dysplasia is defined as the abnormal development of nephronic structures resulting in total or partial renal malformations.[82] Formation of the normal kidney is the result of interaction between the metanephric blastema, the metanephric diverticulum or ureteric bud, and the egress of urine from a non-obstructive collecting system.[83] The ureteric bud forms the collecting system, the stalk becoming the ureter and the expanded cranial end forming the renal pelvis[28] and the pelvicalyceal system. A crucial function of the cranial end is the induction of nephrons from the metanephric blastema. According to Potter[84] the pathogenesis of dysplasia is failure of this portion of the ureteric bud to divide, resulting in abnormal collecting tubules and nephrons. Dysplasia (excluding hereditary-cystic dysplasia) is frequently associated with lower urinary tract malformations, mainly obstructive. The severity of the obstruction, and also its site, corresponds well with the patterns of dysplasia.[82,85]

Multicystic dysplasia

Incidence and aetiology

Complete multicystic dysplasia is the most common form. Its precise incidence is unknown but is probably of the order of 1 in 10 000,[86] with a male to female ratio of 2:1.[87] It is usually sporadic but has been associated with maternal diabetes. Normal parenchyma cannot usually be identified on histological examination of the dysplastic kidney, only multiple cysts, varying from a few millimetres to 8 cm in diameter, being evident (Fig. 16.8). A unilateral severely dysplastic multicystic kidney is invariably associated with ureteric atresia and profound bilateral maldevelopment is accompanied by bilateral ureteric atresia or urethral atresia.[82,88]

Diagnosis

An affected kidney classically appears as a multilobulated mass of multiple thin-walled cysts containing clear fluid, surrounding a more or less centrally located solid core of

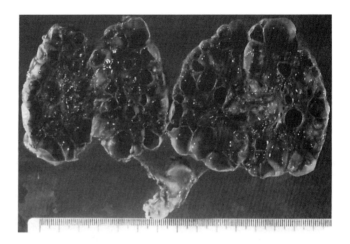

Fig. 16.8 Bilateral multicystic dysplastic kidney. Note that the substance of the kidneys is entirely replaced by cysts of varying sizes. (Courtesy of Dr Jane Zuccollo, Queens Medical Centre, Nottingham.)

fibrous tissue. The reniform shape is totally lost, so that the kidney resembles a bunch of grapes.[89] Thus the typical ultrasound appearance is a paraspinal mass with obvious cysts[86] which do not communicate and which are randomly distributed with variable sizes. It has an irregular shape and no renal pelvis can be demonstrated. Highly reflective islands of tissue may be seen between the cysts but there is no normal renal tissue (Fig. 16.9).

The appearances of the kidney may change throughout the course of the pregnancy, both enlargement and shrinking of the component cysts being reported.[90] Such changes in size may correlate with the degree of residual renal function. Although the multicystic dysplastic kidney is classically described as being functionless some nephrons may survive,

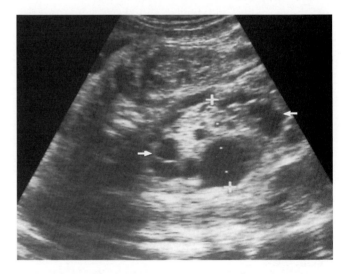

Fig. 16.9 Multicystic dysplastic kidney (marked). Longitudinal section showing the cysts of varying sizes and fibrous tissue replacing all normal renal substance.

giving partial residual function.[91] As long as the kidney can filter plasma, the overall renal size increases. As the nephrons become fibrotic, the amount of filtrate decreases and growth stops, leading eventually to involution.

Many reported cases were diagnosed during the late second and third trimesters.[92] In one series the earliest diagnosis made was at 21 weeks, despite earlier scans.[93] A further study involved scanning at 11–14 weeks and then 18–20 weeks. There were three cases of multicystic dysplastic kidney: none were detected at the early scan, two at the second and one at 31 weeks.[94] Such late detection may be because the cysts are only macroscopically evident after the completion of nephron induction (at around 20 weeks) with enough urine production to distend the dysplastic tubules; if so, multicystic dysplasia cannot be excluded by a routine mid-trimester scan performed before 20 weeks. Nevertheless, multicystic dysplastic kidney has been diagnosed earlier, at 15 weeks[7] and 12 weeks,[95] and all but one of our 47 cases were manifest by 19 weeks. In that case moderate oligohydramnios was present at 18 weeks but the kidneys were unremarkable. The patient defaulted until 24 weeks, by which time the renal abnormality was obvious.

In bilateral multicystic dysplastic kidney there is severe oligohydramnios and no fetal bladder is seen. If unilateral multicystic dysplastic kidney is diagnosed the rest of the urinary tract must be scanned carefully, as the prognosis depends on the state of the other kidney and the rest of the urinary tract. Contralateral renal abnormalities are present in up to 40% in this condition.[96] The abnormalities include pelvi-ureteric junction obstruction, renal agenesis and renal hypoplasia.

Differential diagnosis

The classic multicystic dysplastic kidney may be confused with hydronephrosis.[86] Here the normal reniform shape persists, renal parenchyma is present peripherally and the 'cysts' of calyceal dilatation are orderly and anatomically aligned around and communicate with the renal pelvis.[32] Despite careful attempts using these criteria, it may be impossible to distinguish between the two conditions (Fig. 16.10),[97] difficulty occurring even in the neonatal period. However, the situation may be changing. In a preliminary report, Doppler waveforms in the renal arteries were absent in multicystic kidneys, but present in normal and cystic nephrotic kidneys with normal function. Clearly much more work needs to be done to determine the value of this finding but it may offer hope in the future for differentiating between these two renal pathologies.[98] A necrotic Wilms' tumour or hamartoma producing a large cystic mass can also be confused with a multicystic dysplastic kidney. The former conditions are extremely rare and necrotic cystic spaces are unlikely to be as smooth walled as those of cystic dysplasia.

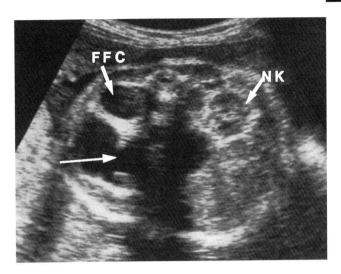

Fig. 16.10 Multicystic dysplastic kidney. Transverse section at 32 weeks showing one normal kidney (NK) and one fluid-filled kidney (FFC), with a dilated structure below. The appearance of communication (arrow) between the various parts of this led to the incorrect diagnosis of hydronephrosis and hydro-ureter.

Associated abnormalities

Bilateral multicystic dysplasia always leads to the Potter sequence. In addition it may be associated with other multiple abnormalities, such as cardiovascular malformations, CNS abnormalities, diaphragmatic hernia, cleft palate, duodenal stenosis and imperforate anus,[84] tracheo-oesophageal fistula and bilateral absence of the radius and thumb.[99] The XYY syndrome has also been associated with the Potter sequence.[74]

In unilateral multicystic dysplastic kidney other urinary tract abnormalities are common,[96] as previously discussed. Anomalies in other systems, similar to those with bilateral disease, are also found.[97,100] Recently cystic dysplasia of the testis has been associated with multicystic renal dysplasia: although it has been more commonly associated with renal agenesis, this finding may point to a common pathogenesis for all three abnormalities.[101]

Prognosis

Bilateral multicystic dysplastic kidney is a condition incompatible with life. All patients have Potter facies at birth and die within a few days. Isolated unilateral multicystic dysplastic kidney has a good outlook, although it is usual to follow up such infants at regular intervals. In the majority the kidney shrinks away; in a few cases the mass is large enough to necessitate nephrectomy. Complications resulting from the abnormal renal tissue, such as hypertension, may also necessitate its removal. When unilateral multicystic dysplastic kidney is not isolated, the prognosis depends on the type and severity of the associated conditions.

Obstetric management

When bilateral multicystic renal dysplasia is diagnosed, termination should be offered because of the poor outcome. If this is refused, conservative management should be adopted; growth retardation or fetal distress should not result in intervention. Careful examination for other abnormalities should be made, and ideally fetal karyotyping should be performed to provide information for counselling in future pregnancies.

In isolated unilateral multicystic disease normal obstetric management should be pursued. If other abnormalities have been detected as well, a full assessment of these should be made along with fetal karyotyping; the subsequent management is based on the likely prognosis.

Recurrence risk

As the condition is almost always sporadic there is usually no increased risk of recurrence. Rarely familial cases have been reported.[102]

Peripheral cortical cystic dysplasia

Aetiology and incidence

Peripheral cortical cystic dysplasia is associated with non-atretic urinary tract abnormalities, most commonly posterior urethral valves. It results from severe but incomplete obstruction of the lower urinary tract and development of the kidney is affected, possibly somewhat later in the embryological period (after the 10th week) than in multicystic dysplasia.[85,86] The later the obstruction the less severe the effect on development. In fetal lambs, obstruction late in gestation produces simple hydronephrosis with no dysplasia.[103] In humans less severe obstructions are rarely associated with dysplasia.[82] Baert[104] suggests that the structural abnormalities of multicystic dysplasia and of peripheral cortical cystic dysplasia are essentially identical, the severity of the changes being the only difference. The cysts are rarely visible macroscopically but histology reveals microscopic cysts, sometimes with cartilaginous and increased fibrous tissue intervening. The collecting tubes are dilated and the interstitial tissue is fibrotic and oedematous.

Diagnosis

In the presence of urinary tract obstruction (usually by posterior urethral valves or occasionally at the pelvi-ureteric junction level) the kidneys may appear abnormally reflective (Fig. 16.11); rarely the cortex may be seen to contain small cysts (Fig. 16.12)[105] The increased reflectivity is due to the multiple microscopic cysts, too small to be imaged clearly by ultrasound, and to the increased fibrous tissue within the dysplastic kidney. The normal

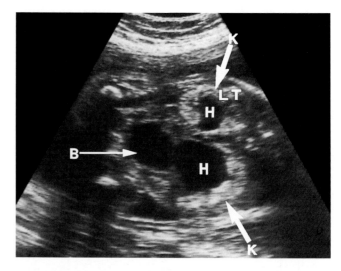

Fig. 16.11 Peripheral cortical dysplasia. The bladder (B) and both kidneys (K) are seen. There is hydronephrosis (H) and the renal substance (arrows) is extremely reflective.

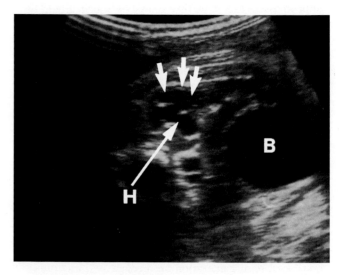

Fig. 16.12 Peripheral cortical dysplasia. The bladder (B) is dilated secondary to posterior urethral valves. There is hydronephrosis (H) and small cysts (arrows) were seen in the cortex.

reniform appearance of the kidney is usually undisturbed. As the majority of dysplastic kidneys do not contain macroscopic cysts and the microscopic cyst and fibrous tissue may not produce a marked increase in reflectivity (which is a subjective finding), the presence of renal cortical dysplasia cannot be predicted accurately.[21] Harrison[106] found that, although renal parenchymal reflectivity did correlate well with moderate to severe dysplasia, mild dysplasia was not easily detectable. Furthermore, not all kidneys that appear of increased reflectivity to the observer are dysplastic.[107]

Associated malformations

These are the associated malformations of obstruction of the urinary tract, namely other genitourinary abnormalities, tracheo-oesophageal fistula, imperforate anus and cardiovascular and skeletal abnormalities.[108,109]

Prognosis

The presence of renal dysplasia in urinary tract obstruction worsens the prognosis; however, if the obstruction is at the pelvi-ureteric junction and the dysplasia unilateral, with a normal contralateral kidney, the prognosis is better. If the dysplasia is bilateral (as occurs with posterior urethral valves) an accurate prognosis cannot be given as long-term follow-up in patients with biopsy-proven peripheral cystic dysplasia is not available.[110] Although generally the greater the increase in reflectivity the worse the dysplasia, we have followed at least one case with strikingly high reflectivity secondary to posterior urethral valves and reflux who post-natally had marked dysplasia on biopsy but retained near-normal renal function. In an attempt to assess each case the volume of liquor should be graded, oligohydramnios indicating failing renal function, particularly if the urinary tract is not grossly dilated. Aspiration of fetal urine, particularly from the pelves of both the affected kidneys, and catheter measurement of urine production may be useful.[106] A poor prognosis can be predicted for the fetus with bilateral obstructive uropathy and a decreased output of isotonic urine. Conversely, a fetus with an output of more than 2 ml/hour of normal hypotonic urine has a good prognosis. Normal hyptonic fetal urine implies intact glomeruli and continued tubular function.[108]

Obstetric management

If bilateral cortical dysplasia is suspected in a case of urinary tract obstruction, termination should be discussed. Aspiration of fetal urine from the renal pelves may aid in management. If termination is not required normal obstetric management should be given. Decompression of the urinary tract may be considered to prevent further damage to the renal tissue.[111]

Segmental dysplasia

Aetiology and incidence

Segmental dysplasia usually involves the upper pole of the kidney and is associated with renal or ureteric duplication, with an ectopic ureterocele and ureteric reflux.[112,113] Cysts, if present, are found in the cortical and medullary remnants and do not reach the dimensions of those of multicystic dysplasia.[110] This condition is also sporadic and the incidence is unknown.

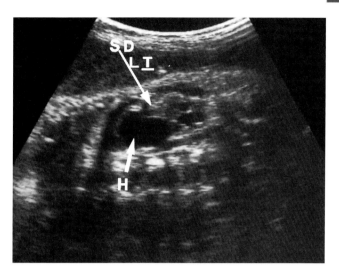

Fig. 16.13 Segmental dysplasia. In this case of a duplex collecting system and ureter, hydronephrosis (H) of the upper moiety is clearly seen. There appears to be some increased reflectivity (SD) around the dilated system which was more striking post-natally.

Diagnosis

The appearances are not unlike those of cortical dysplasia, but small cysts are more common along with increased reflectivity, and the changes usually involve the upper pole only (Fig. 16.13). The kidney retains its shape and dilated calyces and ureter can be identified.[108] The condition is usually unilateral.

Prognosis

If the contralateral kidney is normal the prognosis is good but hypertension may occur.[114] In the rare bilateral cases function is maintained by the lower moieties but hypertension may be a problem.

Obstetric management

After the exclusion of other abnormalities an expectant management policy can be pursued.

Heredofamilial cystic dysplasia

Aetiology and incidence

Cystic dysplasia occurs in a number of rare inherited syndromes, when it is non-obstructive in origin. In the Meckel–Grüber syndrome, which is autosomal recessive, there is bilateral non-obstructive multicystic dysplastic kidney, a craniospinal defect, usually occipital encephalocele, and postaxial polydactyly (Fig. 16.14). Cystic dysplasia may occur in Jeune syndrome (asphyxiating thoracic dystrophy) short-rib polydactyly syndrome and

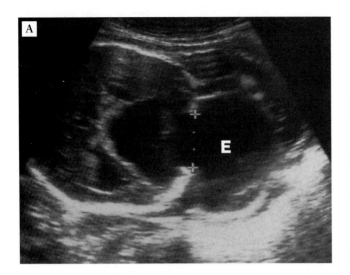

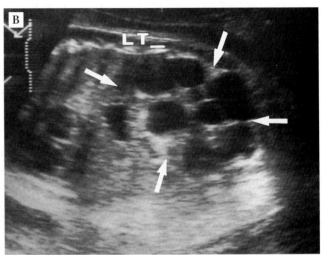

Fig. 16.14 Heredofamilial cystic dysplasia (Meckel's syndrome). A: There is a large occipital encephalocele (E). **B:** The kidney (arrows) is enlarged and cystic, the appearance being identical to multicystic dysplastic kidney.

trisomy 18.[115] It also occurs in Zellweger's syndrome (cerebrohepatorenal dysplasia), in which the appearance of the kidneys is identical to that in obstructive multicystic dysplasia.

Diagnosis

The renal abnormalities in these rare syndromes are not constant. The appearance of the kidneys may be identical to multicystic dysplastic kidneys, peripheral cortical dysplasia or the adult type of polycystic kidney disease. As the kidneys are not obstructed there is no dilatation of the upper or lower tracts. The ability of these kidneys to function is also variable, and therefore the amount of liquor present is variable. Diagnosis usually depends on the identification of the other abnormalities in the syndrome. The Meckel–Grüber syndrome has been confidently diagnosed in the first trimester. The ultrasound diagnosis may in fact be easier at this gestation, when the liquor volume is relatively normal, thus aiding visualisation of the fetus.[116]

Prognosis

These syndromes all comprise multiple abnormalities incompatible with sustained existence. The individual prognosis will be that of the particular syndrome.

Obstetric management

Parents should be given the option of termination, but if this option is refused a non-interventional management plan would seem to be prudent.

Recurrence risk

This is again the individual risk of the syndrome, these tending to be either autosomal recessive or autosomal dominant and carrying a recurrence risk of 25 or 50%, respectively. Polycystic kidney disease refers to two familial disorders, infantile polycystic kidney disease (IPCKD), which appears in the first two decades of life with an autosomal recessive inheritance, and adult polycystic kidney disease (APCKD), presenting in adulthood and rarely in children, with an autosomal dominant inheritance.

Polycystic disease

Infantile polycystic disease – congenital hepatic fibrosis complex (type I cystic disease of Potter)

In IPCKD there is bilateral and symmetrical enlargement of both kidneys, which retain their reniform appearance. Innumerable cortical and medullary cysts 1–3 mm in size are present throughout the kidney (Fig. 16.15).[108] Microscopically the cysts are radially arranged, fusiform structures located from the pelvis to the capsule in the orientation typical of the renal collecting tubules. Uninvolved nephrons are present in the intervening tissues. Infantile polycystic renal disease is actually a disease spectrum with a variable severity of renal and liver involvement.[117,118] The relative severity of the cystic change varies, with the most extensive cyst formation having the worst outcome.[109] Invariably associated with the renal cysts are liver changes, including bile duct proliferation with portal fibrosis. In cases demonstrating less severe cystic change of the renal

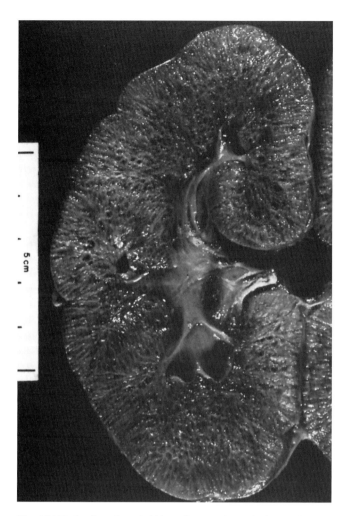

Fig. 16.15 Infantile polycystic kidney disease. The multiple tiny, fairly uniform cysts are seen, along with a normal pelvicalyceal system. (Courtesy of Dr Jane Zuccollo, Queens Medical Centre, Nottingham.)

tubules survival is prolonged, with the eventual development of more severe portal fibrosis.[89] There is no obstruction, the bladder, renal pelves and ureter being normal.

Aetiology and incidence

The disease is inherited as an autosomal recessive disorder which, in its most severe and typical form, manifests in the newborn or young infant with renal failure. The pathogenesis has not been fully established. Osathanondh and Potter[78] found fusiform sacculation and cystic diverticula of the collecting tubules that communicated freely with functioning nephrons. The most distal, earliest-forming tubules are the most severely affected. They suggested that the changes occurred after induction of the metanephric blastema and attachment of nephrons. Hyperplasia of the interstitial portions of the collecting tubules was the postulated cause, and that this hyperplasia began distally and progressed proximally. Thus milder forms of medullary

tubular ectasia when IPCKD presents at a later stage would reflect lesser degrees of collecting tubule hyperplasia.

Potter reported an incidence of two cases in 110 000 infants,[119] but rates of 1 in 6000 to 1 in 16 000 live births have been noted subsequently.[120,121]

Diagnosis

The typical ultrasound appearance includes bilaterally enlarged, highly reflective kidneys that retain their smooth shape.[122,123] The majority of the innumerable cysts are below the limit of ultrasound resolution and the multiple interfaces produced by them result in the characteristic increased reflectivity (Fig. 16.16).[107] Some cysts between 1 and 2 mm can be imaged with high-resolution scanners (Fig. 16.17). The enlargement may be assessed by measurement, but should not be used as a sole diagnostic criterion as isolated nephromegaly has been reported with no demonstrable pathological significance.[124] The degree of oligohydramnios is variable owing to the broad spectrum of renal compromise, and the liquor volume may remain within the normal range late into the second or even the third trimester.[125]

The presence of smoothly enlarged highly reflective kidneys, with some small cysts scattered throughout, seen in the fetus at risk for IPCKD, confirms the diagnosis. This condition has been diagnosed as early as 16 weeks.[107] There is a suggestion that diagnosis may be possible earlier, but this is yet to be confirmed.[126] However, the spectrum of disease is such that accurate diagnosis is not always possible, particularly not as early as the routine 18–20-week scan.[122,127] In the majority of cases there is evidence of the condition by 24 weeks, but occasionally the diagnosis cannot be made until the third trimester.[128,129]

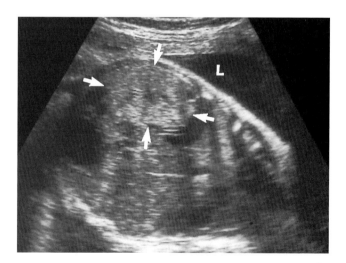

Fig. 16.16 Infantile polycystic kidney disease. The kidney (arrows) is large and highly reflective owing to the multiple tiny cysts. The other kidney was similar in appearance but not well displayed in this section. Note the normal amount of liquor (L) at 22 weeks.

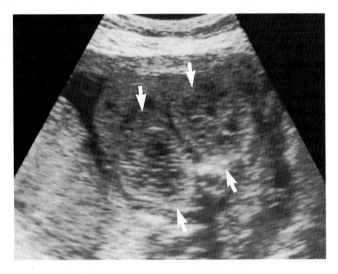

Fig. 16.17 **Infantile polycystic kidney disease.** Both kidneys (arrows) are seen to be enlarged and generally highly reflective, but with some small cysts visible.

IPCKD is associated with raised maternal serum α-fetoprotein levels, and must be considered along with many types of renal disease when this is evaluated.[130]

Differential diagnosis

The main differential diagnosis is from adult polycystic kidney disease, which can also produce large reflective kidneys.[131,132] It has been reported that with modern ultrasound equipment the two conditions – adult type and infantile polycystic kidneys – are amenable to differentiation in infancy and childhood. Whether in time this ability can be achieved *in utero* remains to be discovered.[133]

Associated abnormalities

Apart from the cystic changes in the liver, infants do not have increased risk of associated abnormalities.[87]

Prognosis

Blythe and Ockenden[118] suggested that IPCKD may represent a heterogeneous group of clinical and pathological disorders, and recognised four types:

1 a perinatal form, with nephromegaly at birth, absent hepatic symptomatology, probably Potter facies, and death in early infancy. The kidneys are massively enlarged, with 90% cystic change,
2 a neonatal form, with nephromegaly present at birth or noted between 1 week and 1 month of age. The kidneys are somewhat smaller than in the perinatal form, with about 60% of tissue involved. Death is in the first year of life,

3 an infantile form, with hepatomegaly with or without palpable kidneys, there being about 20% renal involvement, recognisable between 3 and 6 months of age, and with progressive portal hypertension and renal failure leading to death in the first or second decade of life,
4 a juvenile form, presenting between 1 and 5 years of age with hepatomegaly, portal hypertension and variable renal involvement.

The prognosis is therefore generally poor, but the exact nature will depend on the form of the disease. The larger the kidneys and the greater or earlier the onset of oligohydramnios, the more likely the disease will be at the severe end of the spectrum, resulting in neonatal death.

Obstetric management

In view of the poor prognosis termination should be offered if appropriate, or non-interventional management practised.

Recurrence risks

The recurrence risk is 25%.

Adult polycystic kidney disease (type III cystic disease of Potter)

APCKD is inherited as an autosomal dominant condition with variable expression and is usually asymptomatic until the fourth or fifth decade of life, when it presents with hypertension or renal failure. The kidneys are bilaterally enlarged with a bosselated outline produced by the innumerable cysts, which may be so numerous that normal renal parenchyma is apparent only microscopically in the intervening renal tissue. The cysts vary in size from a few millimetres to several centimetres (in the adult) and are thin walled. The calyceal system may be distended, but the pelvis and ureters show no abnormalities.[89]

Aetiology and incidence

The disorder is inherited as an autosomal dominant trait, the gene being located on chromosome 16.[134] The pathogenesis remains unknown. Milutinovic[135] examined renal biopsies from a group of patients between 11 and 26 years of age at risk for APCKD, and found that individuals who subsequently went on to develop the disease showed focal tubular dilatation and ultrastructural changes of the tubular lumen. (Other means of assessing the kidneys before the age of 20 years, including ultrasound, are not sensitive enough to pick up the preclinical states of the disease.[136])

One in 1000 people carry the gene for APCKD, it being one of the most common genetic disorders and the third most prevalent cause of chronic renal failure.[135] The expression of the gene is variable, ranging from severe forms which result in neonatal death to asymptomatic forms found only on autopsy.[137]

Diagnosis

Although autosomal dominant polycystic kidney disease is more common in the general population than is IPCKD, perinatal presentation is rare. There have, however, been several documented cases of prenatal diagnosis,[138–140] the time ranging from 14 weeks[6] to late in the third trimester.[140] In some cases serial examinations have shown normal appearances initially, abnormalities only developing at 30–36 weeks.[139] The ultrasound appearance may be similar to IPCKD, with enlarged highly reflective kidneys and multiple small cysts (Fig. 16.18), which tend to be larger than the adult form of the disease; they represent dilated nephrons. The corticomedullary junction may be accentuated in APCKD, and this forms a useful differentiating feature from other causes of an enlarged, not grossly cystic, kidney.[141] Initially the abnormality may appear to be unilateral, the lesions often being more prominent in one kidney.

The quantity of amniotic fluid ranges from normal to severely reduced. Examination of the parents may be helpful, one parent at least demonstrating innumerable renal cysts. However, if the parents are young ultrasound may be insufficiently sensitive to pick up the precystic form of the abnormal kidneys, as ultrasound is only diagnostic in 66% of cases before 20 years of age.[136] APCKD should be suspected when bilateral cystic enlargement of the kidneys is detected in association with a normal amount of amniotic fluid. Diagnosis of the condition has also been made using DNA markers on chromosome 16 after chorionic villus sampling.[142,143]

Differential diagnosis

The differential diagnosis when the kidneys are seen to be bilaterally enlarged is from the infantile form of the disease. Kidneys in the adult form rarely reach the very large size of the infantile form.[132] The accentuated cortico-medullary junction may be useful.[141] Examination of the parents may prove helpful but, as previously mentioned, ultrasound may not be sufficiently sensitive to pick up early forms if the full cystic form has not yet become manifest. However, with modern equipment this situation may well change. Correlations have been drawn between the two kinds of polycystic disease and different sonographic findings, but the preliminary study reporting these differences will need to be confirmed in much larger series.[133]

Associated abnormalities

APCKD is associated with cystic lesions in other organs, including the liver, pancreas, spleen and gonads,[137] but these are unlikely to be manifest prenatally. Cardiovascular abnormalities may be prominent in patients with this condition, including dilatation of the aortic root, bicuspid aortic valve and coarctation of the aorta.[144] This type of polycystic disease is also part of some syndromes, namely Meckel's and tuberous sclerosis.

Prognosis

APCKD usually becomes manifest in the fourth or fifth decade of life, with hypertension or gradual onset of renal failure; occasionally flank pain attributed to associated renal calculi, haemorrhage into a cyst or ureteric obstruction by a blood clot is reported as the initial presentation. However, it is becoming increasingly recognised in the newborn infant,[87] usually as an abdominal mass. Other signs or symptoms of renal disease are rare, although renal failure has been described[145] and hypertension has also been reported. Although it is reasonable to assume that cases detected clinically in early childhood are likely to be those detectable antenatally, it is not yet conclusively proven that, in the long-term, these cases carry a worse prognosis than those detected in adulthood. Therefore, the prognosis of antenatally detected cases is so far unknown, although it is certain that oligohydramnios carries a very poor prognosis.[146]

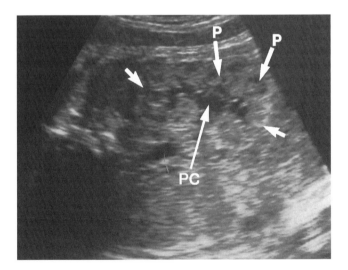

Fig. 16.18 Adult polycystic kidney disease. The kidney (small arrows) is enlarged and highly reflective, with well demarcated renal pyramids (P). The pelvicalyceal system (PC) (and distal urinary tract) are normal, ruling out cortical dysplasia.

Obstetric management

If the liquor volume is decreased in the presence of APCKD, termination should be offered. In the presence of normal liquor volume the parents should be advised that the fetus is suffering from a hereditary kidney disease, and that one of the parents must also have the disease. The usual course of the disease should be discussed so that the parents are aware of the likely prognosis. Termination should be considered.

Recurrence risk

The condition is autosomal dominant, therefore the recurrence risk is 50%.

Dilatation of the urinary tract

Dilatation of the urinary tract usually results from distal obstruction but may occur without obstruction.[147–149] Sites of obstruction are at the pelvi-ureteric junction, the ureterovesical junction and the urethra. Obstruction may be complete, partial, unilateral or bilateral. Non-obstructive causes of urinary tract dilatation are vesico-ureteric (VU) reflux, neurological lesions, primary (non-refluxing, non-obstructive) mega-ureter and part of the megacystis–microcolon syndrome.

Whereas moderate to severe examples of urinary tract dilatation are immediately obvious to the ultrasonographer and pose few problems in interpretation, minor changes which may nevertheless have important consequences on prognosis continue to present problems. To date the criteria developed for differentiating the normal from the dilated renal pelvis are not ideal.[150] Minimal pyelectasis in the fetus is common and can be seen from 13 weeks gestation; however, it is unlikely to be significant in every case (Fig. 16.19). In one study 59% of kidneys in fetuses between 24 and 33 weeks showed demonstrable

amounts of fluid in the renal pelves; in 41% the diameter of the renal pelvis measured 1–2 mm, and in 18% the measurement was 3 mm and over.[151] Although the pathogenesis remains unclear, it is possible that the fetal urinary tract is responding similarly to the maternal urinary tract to the circulating pregnancy hormones, maternal pelvicalyceal dilatation in pregnancy being well recognised.

In the second trimester it is firmly established that fetal renal pelves measuring less than 5 mm in the anteroposterior diameter are within the normal range.[147] Some researchers have suggested lower cut-off points. The problem with this is that the number of false-positive diagnoses rises considerably, causing more undue anxiety and unnecessary intervention to a larger number of parents and infants than those who would genuinely be identified with VU reflux.[149] However, fetal renal pelves measuring more than 10 mm in diameter,[147,148] although usually pathological, are not always so,[152] and the significance of anteroposterior measurements between 5 and 10 mm is problematical.[147,149,153]

It should be noted that in all series to date these cut-off points have been chosen on results obtained from groups of fetuses with widely varying gestational ages. A renal pelvis measuring, for example, 6 mm is of more concern at 18 weeks than at 38 weeks. There are as yet no data available relating renal pelvic size to fetal age.

The ratio of the anteroposterior diameter of the pelvis to the anteroposterior diameter of the kidney has been suggested as another means of differentiating pathological pyelectasis from normal.[147] Hydronephrosis is considered present if this ratio is greater than 0.5.

Calyceal dilatation is much more significant.[94] This indicates hydronephrosis even when the pelvis/kidney ratio is less than 0.5, and always persists into the post-

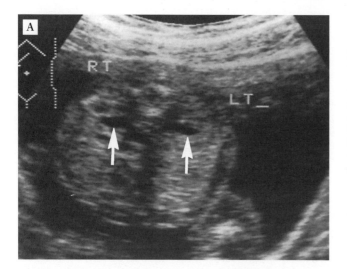
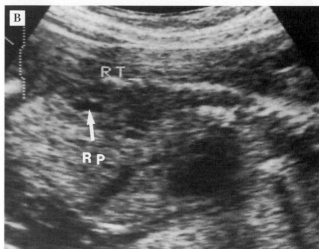

Fig. 16.19 Filled renal pelvis. A: Transverse section of a 19 week fetus showing prominent (full) renal pelves (arrows). No calyceal dilatation is apparent. **B:** Longitudinal section showing a prominent (full) renal pelvis (RP) but no calyceal dilatation is apparent.

natal period. If rounded calyces are present with a renal pelvic anteroposterior measurement of 10–15 mm there is significant hydronephrosis, which rarely regresses, often progresses, and frequently requires surgical treatment.[152] Grignon *et al.*[154] devised a classification of urinary tract dilatation according to the ultrasound appearances of the pelvicalyceal system and the renal pelvic size. Grades 2 and 3 were defined as renal pelvic measurements of 10–15 mm and more than 15 mm, respectively, along with normal to slight dilatation of the calyces, and resulted in 47% of infants with definite pathology. Grades 4 and 5 with renal pelves greater than 15 mm and moderate to severe dilatation of the calyces were always pathological.

When the pelvis appears prominent at the 18–20 week routine scan there is often uncertainty as to whether or not a mild degree of calyceal dilatation is present (Fig. 16.20). It is therefore useful to repeat the examination between 22 and 24 weeks, by which time considerable renal growth has occurred with deposition of fat. The improved renal images at this stage usually allow an accurate definition of calyceal dilatation. One possible source of error is compound upper pole calyces, which may simulate calyceal dilatation (Fig. 16.21).

In order not to miss significant changes, fetuses with more than 5 mm dilatation of the renal pelvis, as well as those with calyceal dilatation, should be followed up postnatally. Vesico-ureteric reflux is said to be present in 1%

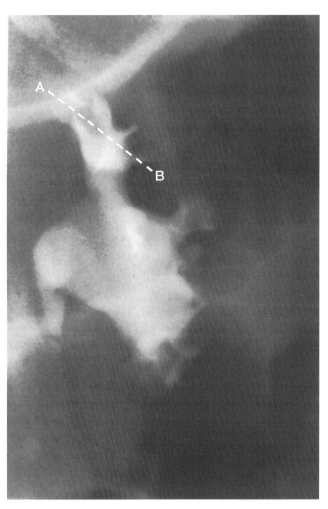

Fig. 16.21 Compound cystic calyces. Intravenous urogram showing compound cystic calyces. Ultrasound scanning in the A–B plane results in apparent calyceal dilatation.

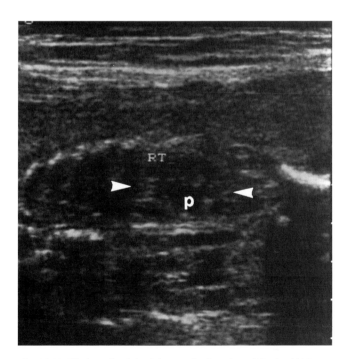

Fig. 16.20 Filled renal pelvis. A longitudinal section of the fetal kidney (arrowheads) is seen at 18 weeks gestation. A full renal pelvis (p) is seen but calyceal definition is such that it is uncertain whether or not they are dilated. A repeat examination at 22 weeks confirmed prominent renal pelves without calyceal dilatation.

of newborns and primary vesico-ureteric reflux, resulting from an anatomical defect at the ureter/bladder interface, in 1–2% of asymptomatic children. Clearly there is a large pool of infants and children who are at risk of suffering from significant renal damage caused by reflux. This in turn leads to significant long-term morbidity from recurrent renal infections, hypertension and renal failure.[155] The majority of affected newborns show *in utero* evidence of renal pelvis dilatation, with a small number of these fetuses going on to develop overt hydronephrosis during the course of the pregnancy. Closer examination of the family histories in these individuals has revealed that genuine reflux is often inherited in an autosomal dominant manner.[156] It is possible that it may turn out to be one of the most common inherited conditions. Once fetal renal pelvic dilatation is identified enquiries should be made to discover whenever any other family member suffers from renal disease. A positive family history may add further weight to the *in utero* finding, suggesting that it is truly representative of primary vesico-ureteric reflux in that fetus. However, only post-natal investigation can confirm the diagnosis with complete surety.

Dilatation of the ureter is always pathological. Gross dilatation of the fetal bladder is easily recognised, but lesser degrees are not as easily diagnosed. The fetal bladder fills and empties over the course of an hour,[23] so variations in size are normal. In doubtful cases prolonged observation and repeated scanning over 4–6 hours to see if the bladder changes in size or empties are useful. Hypertrophy of the bladder wall may also aid diagnosis, thickening greater than 2 mm being pathological.[107] Early post-natal diagnosis of urinary tract obstruction or reflux is seldom possible because the clinical signs of an abdominal mass, haematuria or recurrent urinary tract infections (UTIs) are often symptomless until irreversible renal damage has occurred. The timing of surgical correction is thought to be important in reducing chronic renal insufficiency, as the best results are achieved in infants operated on in the first year of life.[157] Therefore when pathological dilatation is diagnosed or suspected prenatally, post-natal follow-up is essential. Except in severe cases this is best performed at 5–7 days post-partum to avoid the false-negative finding of an empty renal pelvis caused by the dehydration that is common in the first 48–72 hours after birth.[25,158] Further assessment at 4–6 weeks is important even if the early neonatal scan is negative, as it can take that length of time before urine production in the infant has risen back to the levels of a term fetus. In cases of minimal dilatation of the pelvis it is common practice to leave the first post-natal examination until that time. Recently one follow-up study of 66 infants diagnosed antenatally with renal pelvis dilatation discovered that, if post-natal sonography at 72 hours was added to the assessment protocol, the positive predictive value of vesico-ureteric reflux for the two tests taken together is 17%. This, if replicated in further studies, is a considerable improvement upon screening with antenatally detected renal pelvis dilatation alone, which is a weak predictor of vesico-ureteric reflux. However, a negative scan at 72 hours is not completely reassuring, and further follow-up as stated above is still necessary for doubtful cases.[150] A full range of urinary tract investigations, including nuclear scintigraphy or voiding cystography may be needed to assess the problem, as ultrasound alone, even with prolonged follow-up, can lead to incomplete diagnoses.[159]

A team approach for the care of mothers with antenatally diagnosed fetal urinary tract abnormalities is best,[160] with the team ideally consisting of the ultrasonographer, obstetrician, neonatologist and paediatric nephrologist. This will ensure that parents are correctly and adequately counselled, and that the investigations in the post-natal period are planned in advance.

It has been suggested that screening for vesico-ureteric reflux (VUR) should begin antenatally. A study in the northeast of England showed that urinary tract disease in the mother herself, or a positive family history of urinary tract disease, identified a particularly high-risk group of infants. Of those so labelled, 31% of the resulting babies were confirmed as having VUR, which is many times higher than the background rate for VUR at 1–2%.[161] Therefore, the obstetrician counselling mothers whose fetuses have been found to have significant renal pelvic dilatation, should enquire if the mother or anyone in the immediate family (siblings in particular) does or did suffer from urinary tract disease. This information may be extremely helpful to the paediatrician when assessing the child post-natally and planning their further care. In addition, it is prudent to ensure that the kidneys of those fetuses in whom the antenatal family history is positive for VUR are properly assessed for renal pelvis dilatation by an experienced sonographer.

There is a definite association between renal tract dilatation and chromosomal abnormalities. Of 72 cases of obstructive uropathy reported in the Fetal Surgery Registry 1986[111] 8% had karyotypic abnormalities. Nicolaides *et al.*[162] reported an incidence of 24% abnormal karyotypes in a series of 38 cases of obstructive uropathy. However, in the majority of these cases many of the other multisystem abnormalities which are part of the expression of the abnormal gene are detectable on ultrasound examination, particularly as more subtle markers of chromosomal abnormality can be recognised and confirmed by a rapid karyotyping procedure. The situation in isolated hydronephrosis, and particularly in mild renal pelvic dilatation, is less clear. Nicolaides[163] reports an incidence of 3% abnormal karyotypes in these cases. In our series of 249 cases, where there was more than one structural abnormality a 3% incidence of karyotypic abnormalities was identified.

Thus although problems in the interpretation of urinary tract dilatation remain, there seems little doubt that prenatal diagnosis and subsequent follow-up improves the management of children with renal tract abnormalities.[10,158,164] It is also interesting to note that patients with renal scarring are more at risk of pre-eclampsia and premature birth. Therefore, for females who suffer from VUR their management as children could have a bearing upon their own wellbeing when they in turn become pregnant.[165]

Pelvi-ureteric junction obstruction

This is the most common cause of neonatal hydronephrosis,[109] being a stenosis at the junction of the renal pelvis and ureter. Unilateral obstruction is common,[154] more frequently affecting the left side.[166] The condition is bilateral in about 30% of cases, the degree of obstruction usually being different on the two sides. Thinning of the renal parenchyma and kidney enlargement are unusual in the fetus and are signs of severe obstruction.[167] Irreversible parenchymal damage is also unusual, as is a reduction in or absence of amniotic fluid. Occasionally polyhydramnios is reported, presumably the result of extrinsic compression of the retroperitoneal portion of the duodenum by an enlarged renal pelvis.[168]

Aetiology and incidence

The true incidence is unknown. There is an increased frequency in males, with a sex ratio of 5:1.[169] In the majority of cases the obstruction seems to be functional, as the pelvi-ureteric junction is anatomically patent, the abnormality being in the initiation or propagation of the peristaltic activity in the ureter that normally results in boluses of urine being passed from the pelvis down the ureter. Histologically the ureter shows signs of chronic inflammation, with disruption and disorganisation of the collagen fibres and muscle in the wall. Abnormality of the circular but not the longitudinal muscle layers has been demonstrated in approximately 70% of cases.[170] Anatomical causes found in a minority of cases are fibrous adhesions, bands, kinks, ureteral valves, aberrant lower pole vessels, abnormal ureteral insertion and odd shapes of the pelvi-ureteric outlet.[171]

Diagnosis

Diagnosis depends on the findings of a dilated renal pelvis with or without calyceal dilatation. The criteria for the diagnosis of pathological dilatation have already been discussed. Harrison *et al.*[14] have suggested a semiquantitative estimate, mild dilatation showing enlarged renal pelves, branching infundibula and calyces, and severe dilatation being characterised by a large unilocular fluid collection. We have found a classification of hydronephrosis into mild, moderate and severe more helpful, the appearances fitting fairly closely to Grignon's gradings.[148] Grade 2 approximates to our mild cases, except that we would classify renal dilatation as being 5 mm or greater (Fig. 16.22). Grades 3 and 4 are equivalent to moderate hydronephrosis (Figs 16.23 and 16.24) and grade 5 to severe (Fig 16.25).

The rest of the renal tract must be examined carefully looking particularly for evidence of peripheral cortical dysplasia and oligohydramnios. The latter is not usually a feature of this condition and implies a second disease process (e.g. IUGR) or a misdiagnosis (e.g. bilateral multicystic dysplastic kidney).[167] Transient hydronephrosis *in utero* has occasionally been noted;[31,149] its significance is unclear, but serial scans are necessary to pick up changes in the condition. If dilatation is identified on only one occasion and is mild, pathology is extremely unlikely. This form of transient dilatation may be due to the state of maternal hydration, but this has not been proved.[151] If the

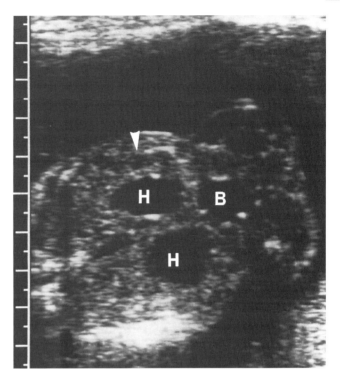

Fig. 16.22 Mild bilateral hydronephrosis. Oblique scan showing normal bladder (B) and two dilated renal pelves (H), with normal renal tissue (arrow) and no calyceal dilatation. This was a case of pelvi-ureteric junction obstruction.

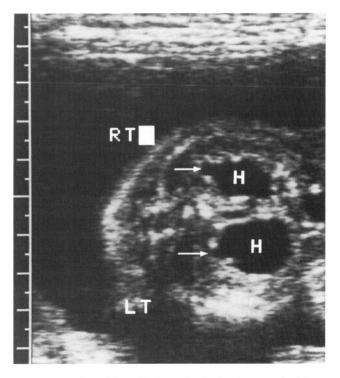

Fig. 16.23 Moderate bilateral hydronephrosis. Another case of pelvi-ureteric junction obstruction with dilated renal pelves (H) and mild calyceal dilatation (arrows).

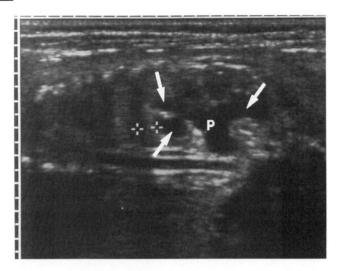

Fig. 16.24 Moderate bilateral hydronephrosis. This longitudinal scan of a hydronephrotic kidney shows an enlarged renal pelvis (P) and moderately dilated and rounded renal calyces (arrows). There is normal parenchymal thickness and reflectivity.

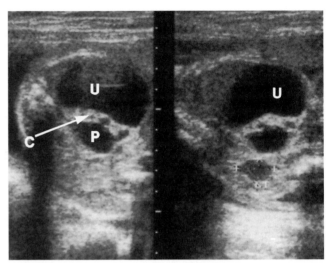

Fig. 16.26 Hydronephrosis with urinoma. Oblique sections displaying a hydronephrotic kidney with an enlarged pelvis (P), dysplastic cortex (C) and a retroperitoneal urinoma (U) following spontaneous decompression of pelvi-ureteric junction obstruction.

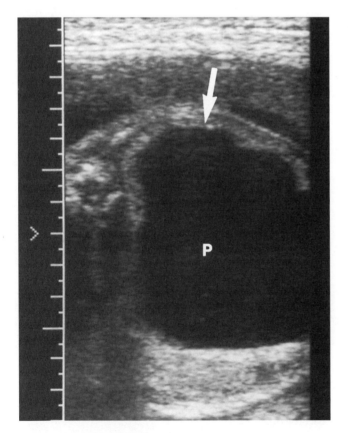

Fig. 16.25 Severe hydronephrosis. There is massive enlargement of the renal pelvis (P) in this case of unilateral pelvi-ureteric junction obstruction in a Down's syndrome fetus. The calyceal shape is lost and the parenchyma is thin (arrow).

dilatation occurs on more than one occasion, post-natal follow-up is advised.

The time of onset of the ultrasonic signs of this condition appears to be variable. A significant number of cases have been reported as first recognisable later than 24 weeks,[147] but this is not our experience, nearly all being apparent at the routine mid-trimester scan. Only one out of four cases of hydronephrosis in a screening study in the first trimester was diagnosed at early scan.[94]

In severe pelvi-ureteric junction obstruction calyceal rupture may occur resulting in only minimal dilatation of the pelvicalyceal system but a large perinephric urinoma (Fig. 16.26).

Differential diagnosis

The main differential diagnosis is multicystic dysplastic kidney.[86] In hydronephrosis the reniform shape is usually present and renal parenchyma is present peripherally. The 'cysts' of calyceal dilatation are orderly and aligned around and communicate with the renal pelvis (Figs 16.27 and 16.28). In addition, bilateral reflux may mimic true obstruction and be impossible to distinguish, although in many cases hydro-ureter will be seen in this condition.

Associated abnormalities

The incidence of other renal tract abnormalities (vesico-ureteric reflux, obstructive mega-ureter and contralateral abnormalities such as multicystic dysplastic kidney) is approximately 27%.[172] Associated extrarenal abnormalities occur in about 19% of cases,[109] Hirschsprung's disease, cardiovascular abnormalities, neural tube defects,

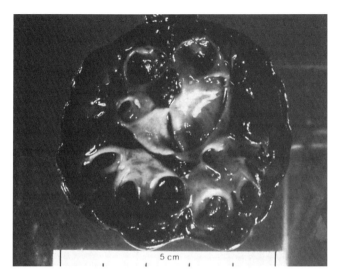

Fig. 16.27 Moderate hydronephrosis. The dilated calyces are seen to be enlarged in an orderly fashion around the pelvis. (Courtesy of Dr Jane Zuccollo, Queens Medical Centre, Nottingham.)

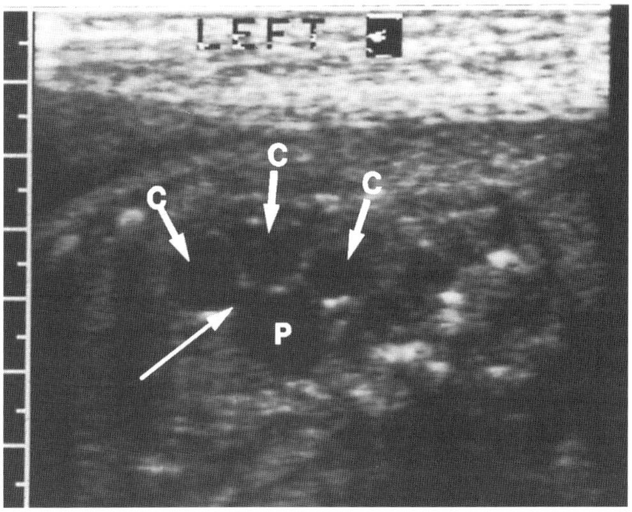

Fig. 16.28 Moderate hydronephrosis. Longitudinal scan of moderate hydronephrosis. The 'cystic structures' (C) are arranged around and communicate with (long arrow) the dilated renal pelvis (P).

oesophageal atresia and imperforate anus being common. Chromosomal abnormalities also occur.[77]

Prognosis

This is generally good for isolated unilateral lesions, even when the degree of dilatation is considerable.[173] Even in bilateral disease the prognosis appears favourable: in one report following surgical correction of such lesions within 6 months of age there were no postoperative deaths and renal function was generally good.[174]

Obstetric management

In unilateral pelvi-ureteric junction obstruction obstetric management should be normal, provided the abnormality appears isolated and the other kidney is normal. In the case of a very large hydronephrosis the pelvis may require decompression antenatally[175] and if polyhydramnios results[168] this may need careful management. There are no data to suggest that early delivery for surgical correction improves outcome.

In bilateral pelvi-ureteric junction obstruction the management depends on the severity of the abnormality and the gestational age. The severity is difficult to quantify. The degree of renal damage is approximately proportional to the severity of the dilatation, but this is not invariable[176] and hydronephrosis may not be present in a fetus with chronic urinary tract obstruction.[177] Assessment of amniotic fluid volume has been suggested as a helpful guide to prognosis,[62] but again is not entirely reliable as polyuria rather than oliguria may occur in failing renal function.[111]

As previously discussed, peripheral cortical dysplasia poses difficulty in diagnosis.

The best method available to date of assessing renal function is chemical analysis of fetal urine taken from each renal pelvis, or the bladder if the kidneys appear identically affected. Sodium, calcium, urea and creatinine levels have been used to evaluate renal function, the values that correlate with good and bad outcomes being firmly established.[106] If the assessment suggests a poor prognosis (urinary sodium greater than 100 mmol/l, low urinary urea less than 6 mmol/l, and creatinine greater than 150 µmol/l[178,179]), termination should be considered.

In the absence of poor prognostic signs management should be expectant. Serial scans are required, as occasionally in the third trimester the dilatation may progress markedly (presumably as fetal urinary output increases) and therefore the planned post-natal management may need to be modified.

Prenatal urinary diversion procedures have been developed and may be indicated in cases of bilateral pelvi-ureteric junction obstruction though here the results do not support *in utero* surgery, and such invasive procedures are not without mortality and morbidity. Severe, potentially life-threatening chorio-amnionitis has been reported after diagnostic or therapeutic fetal bladder catheterisation.[167] Until techniques improve management should be expectant.

Recurrence risk

The condition is usually sporadic and therefore the recurrence risk is low. However, both familial cases[180] and dominant inheritance[181] have been reported.

Ureterovesical junction obstruction

Obstruction at this level has been considered uncommon for many years,[109] being reported in only 8% of cases of urinary tract obstruction. However, more recently it has been suggested that it accounts for 23% of cases and is the second most common cause of hydronephrosis.[182]

Aetiology and incidence

Distal obstruction of the ureter is primarily functional, resulting from a narrow segment of the ureter at the lower end which does not transmit the normal peristaltic waves.[183] Less commonly, ureteral atresia is responsible. In duplex anomalies obstruction is common, affecting the upper pole moiety, with an ectopic ureterocele (Figs 16.29 and 16.30).[184] The incidence is unknown.

Diagnosis

The normal fetal ureter is too small to define antenatally with ultrasound and therefore, if it is imaged it is dilated, being seen as an echo-free intra-abdominal tubular structure[185] that can be traced back to the renal pelvis (Fig 16.31). If obstruction is the cause the ureter lengthens, and so is more serpiginous than in primary mega-ureter, where the course is much straighter. The bladder should be normal in size and the wall not hypertrophic – otherwise urethral outflow obstruction must be considered. In the majority of cases of obstruction a degree of hydronephrosis is seen.

Associated abnormalities

Duplex systems are a common association. Their diagnosis depends on the recognition of asymmetrical hydro-

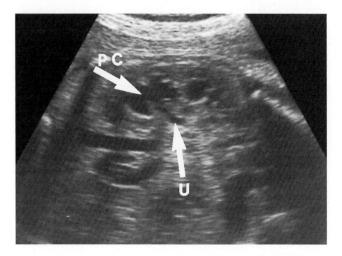

Fig. 16.29 Ureterovesical junction obstruction. In this duplex kidney the pelvicalyceal system (PC) of the upper moiety is dilated and the upper part of the dilated ureter (U) can be seen.

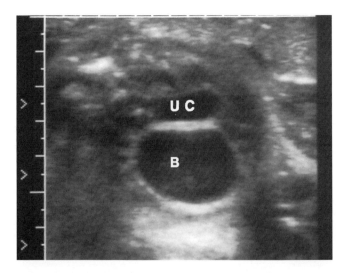

Fig. 16.30 Ureterovesical junction obstruction. A ureterocele (UC) is seen adjacent to the bladder (B).

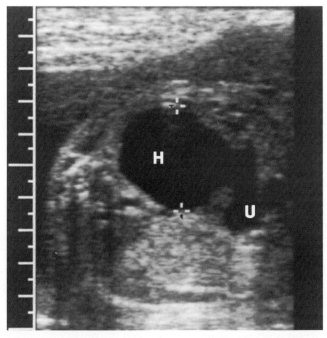

Fig. 16.31 Dilated ureter. A dilated obstructed ureter (U) can be seen pursuing a serpiginous course, and can be traced back to the hydronephrotic renal pelvis (H).

nephrosis between the dilated and non-dilated moieties.[186] Also in this abnormality there is often an element of dysplasia.[184] Other associations are with horseshoe and ectopic kidneys.

Differential diagnosis

Ureterovesical obstruction is easily confused with other causes of mega-ureter and differentiation antenatally is often impossible, though in the presence of a duplex system, ectopic or horseshoe kidney, obstruction is most likely.

Prognosis

In general the prognosis is good provided the condition is isolated.

Obstetric management

Normal management should be pursued, with post-natal assessment and follow-up planned.

Other causes of megaureter

Primary refluxing ureter

Primary vesico-ureteric reflux is the commonest cause of renal failure in childhood and results from an abnormality of the normal antireflux mechanisms at the level of the ureterovesical junction (Fig. 16.32). This commonly results in hydronephrosis and peripheral cortical dysplasia may occur. *In utero* the hydronephrosis is usually mild and non-progressive (Fig. 16.33), but on occasions can be severe.[146] Amniotic fluid is usually present in normal volumes.[105]

Family studies have suggested that primary vesico-ureteric reflux (VUR) has an autosomal dominant inheritance pattern, although this is still an area of debate. Nevertheless, the VUR phenotype is associated with shortness of the submucosal segment of the ureter owing to congenital lateral ectopia of the ureteric orifice.[187]

Some investigators have reported spontaneous resolution of apparently significant fetal hydronephrosis,[105] although such cases may represent spontaneous resolution of obstruction, temporary ureterovesical reflux would seem a more likely cause. Spontaneous neonatal resolution of congenital reflux may also occur. The degree of reflux decreases and may disappear in more than 50% of affected children.[188] Some boys with reflux have a large, sacculated posterior urethra, suggesting that reflux could be secondary to transient obstruction which has been overcome.

Recently one group of researchers has classified VUR based upon its severity and discovered two distinct, although not exclusive, groupings. Mild reflux with normal kidneys predominantly affected females, whereas severe reflux combined with renal damage, which was most likely fetal in origin, was almost exclusively a male disorder.[189]

Secondary refluxing ureter

This occurs when there is bladder neck obstruction or a neuropathic bladder (Fig. 16.34). In the former the thick-walled bladder is obvious. A neuropathic bladder

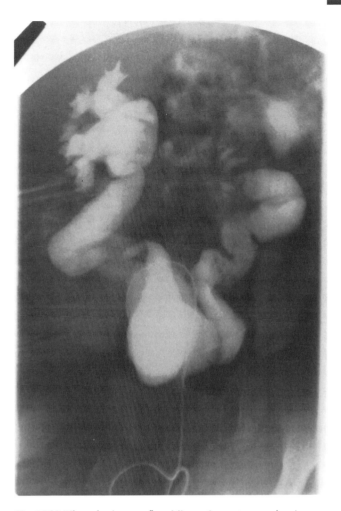

Fig. 16.32 Bilateral primary reflux. Micturating cystogram showing bilateral ureteric reflux resulting in bilateral hydronephrosis and hydroureter.

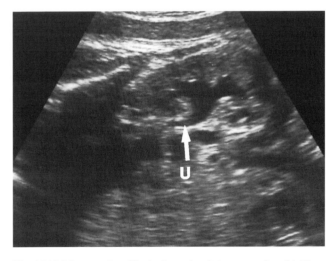

Fig. 16.33 Primary reflux. The hydronephrosis is commonly mild. Here slightly dilated calyces can be seen along with the upper end of the dilated ureter (U).

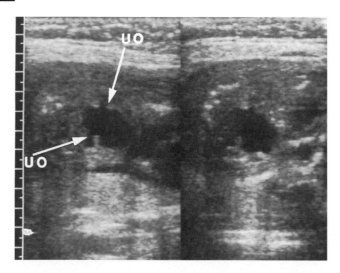

Fig. 16.34 Secondary refluxing ureter. In this case of the VACTERL association the bladder was neuropathic owing to a sacral spinal abnormality. The wide-open ureteric orifices (UO) are demonstrated in the bladder.

may be the result of the vertebrospinal abnormality of the VACTERL association. This condition should be borne in mind, as many of the abnormalities (such as tracheo-oesophageal fistula) are subtle or unlikely to be diagnosed by ultrasound. A dilated ureter may be the only manifestation.

Secondary non-refluxing ureter

Secondary non-refluxing non-obstructive ureteric dilatation is found where there are high rates of urine formation, such as in diabetes insipidus or infection, and in ureters that remain widened after spontaneous cessation of vesico-ureteric reflux.

Bladder outflow obstruction

The most severe degree of obstructive uropathy is seen with obstruction at urethral level.[190] Bladder outflow obstruction may be partial or complete, the usual cause being posterior urethral valves, which have been described as the second most common cause of hydronephrosis (19%).[109] However, data based on prenatal ultrasound examination suggest that the urethra is a less common site of fetal urinary obstruction, accounting for 10% of cases.[182] Posterior urethral valves occur exclusively in males. Urethral obstruction in females is complete, caused by urethral atresia or major cloacal abnormalities.

Posterior urethral valves

A membranous structure in the posterior urethra constitutes the 'valve'. A classification based on gross anatom-

ical characteristics has been proposed.[191] There are three types, of which 1 and 3 are clinically significant. In type 1 the valves are folds that insert into the lateral walls of the urethra. Type 3 valves consist of a diaphragm-like structure with only a small perforation.

Aetiology and incidence

The exact incidence is unknown. Type 1 is thought to result from an exaggerated development of persisting urethral/vaginal folds, with an abnormal insertion of the distal ends of the Wolffian ducts. Type 3 develops because of abnormal persistence and poor canalisation of the urogenital membrane.

Diagnosis

The major features of urethral obstruction by urethral valves are dilatation of the fetal urinary bladder and proximal urethra (Fig. 16.35) with thickening of the bladder wall (Fig. 16.36).[192] The urinary bladder fills the true pelvis and frequently also the false pelvis and abdomen, and does not empty. A dilated posterior urethra can be visualised as a focal outpouching of the urinary bladder extending towards the perineum. The bladder wall is considered hypertrophied if it is thick enough to be measured (Fig. 16.37).[192] The ureters are usually also dilated and hydronephrosis of variable degrees may be present (Figs 16.38 and 16.39), but lack of upper tract dilatation does not exclude urethral valves.[177] Minor degrees of obstruction may not produce much dilatation, whereas severe obstruction may result in dysplasia and hence diminished urine output.

The urinary tract may be decompressed by bladder rupture, and the problem may present as fetal ascites

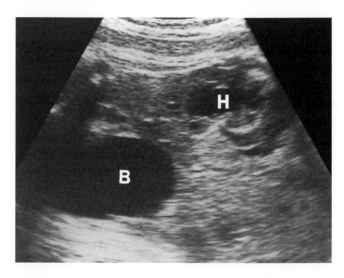

Fig. 16.35 Posterior urethral valves. The bladder (B) is dilated and there is hydronephrosis (H).

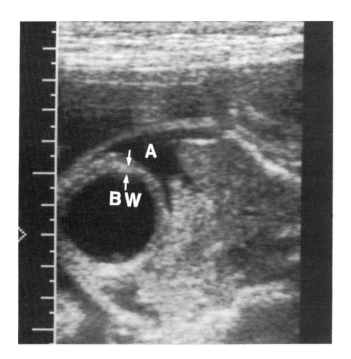

Fig. 16.36 Posterior urethral valves. Note the thick wall of the bladder (BW). There has been spontaneous decompression resulting in urinary ascites (A).

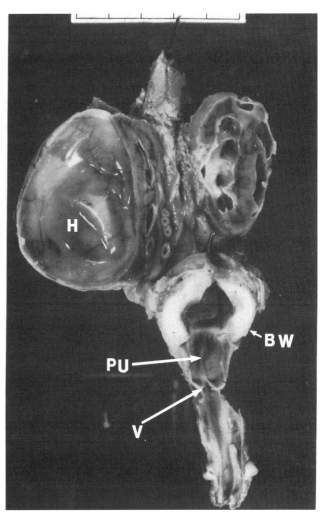

Fig. 16.37 Posterior urethral valves. Note the severe hydronephrosis (H), the thick bladder wall (BW), the dilated posterior urethra (PU) and the valves (V). (Courtesy of Dr Jane Zuccollo, Queens Medical Centre, Nottingham.)

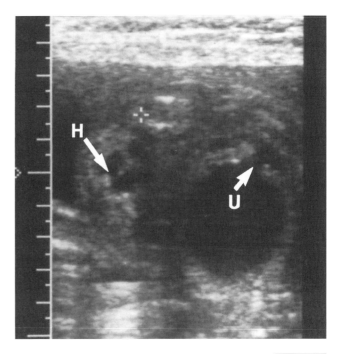

Fig. 16.38 Posterior urethral valves. The dilated ureter (U) can be seen. There is moderate hydronephrosis (H).

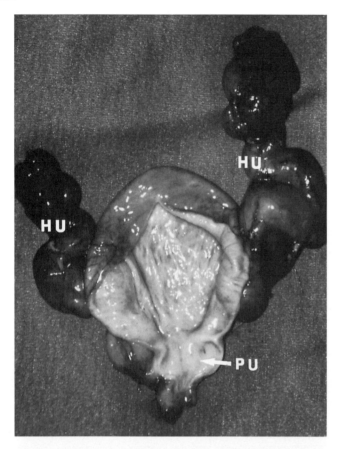

Fig. 16.39 Posterior urethral valves. There is marked bilateral hydro-ureter (HU) and a dilated posterior urethra (PU). (Courtesy of Dr Jane Zuccollo, Queens Medical Centre, Nottingham.)

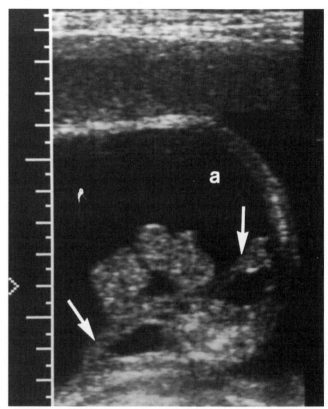

Fig. 16.40 Posterior urethral valves. The fetal kidneys (arrows) are hydronephrotic. Urinary ascites (a) is present owing to rupture of the bladder.

(Fig. 16.40) or as perinephric urinoma resulting from rupture of the calyces.[177] Examination of the urinary tract reveals the underlying cause. Renal dysplasia gives increased cortical reflectivity and cortical cysts but, as previously discussed, the ultrasound appearance of the kidneys does not correlate well either with the presence of dysplasia or its degree.

The volume of liquor should be noted, as oligohydramnios may occur and is related to the severity and duration of the obstruction. Severe oligohydramnios is a poor prognostic sign; conversely, normal amniotic fluid carries a good prognosis.[1,193]

When the degree of obstruction is major the diagnosis is usually made at the routine mid-trimester scan. With more minor degrees of partial obstruction it may not be apparent until later. There are now numerous reports of diagnosis of bladder outflow obstruction from 11 weeks.[194–197]

Differential diagnosis

Other obstructive uropathies (namely pelvi-ureteric junction obstruction or ureterovesical junction obstruction and primary mega-ureter) must be considered, the bladder wall thickening being the distinguishing feature. Massive vesico-ureteric reflux may be difficult to differentiate.[198] Megacystis–microcolon syndrome may be mistaken for posterior urethral valves. In this condition there is usually polyhydramnios and a dilated stomach.

Associated abnormalities

Posterior urethral valves are associated with duplication of the urethra, megalo-urethra, cryptorchidism and hypospadias. Abnormalities outside the urinary tract are tracheo-oesophageal fistula, total anomalous pulmonary venous drainage, mitral stenosis, skeletal abnormalities and imperforate anus.[108,109] Chromosomal abnormalities, including trisomies 13 and 18, have been reported.[162]

Prune belly syndrome, in which there is a hypotonic abdominal wall, a large hypotonic bladder with dilated ureters and cryptorchidism, was originally considered as a separate specific entity[199] but is now considered to be secondary to fetal abdominal distension of various causes, one of the most common being urethral obstruction. This accounts for its male predominance.[200] The condition spans a wide range of severity, from death due to pulmonary hypoplasia in the neonatal period or renal insufficiency in infancy to long-term survival, though extensive cosmetic surgery may be required. A case of bladder outflow obstruction where termination was not wanted apparently resolved (at least ultrasonically) during the remainder of the pregnancy. The liquor volume was slightly reduced. The neonate had prune belly syndrome and died of renal failure within the first few months.

Prognosis

Neonates with urethral obstruction have a high mortality (up to 50%).[201,202] The incidence of chronic renal failure in infants diagnosed in the first 3 months of life is 39%.[203] Most of the data regarding the prognosis, particularly in the long term, are based on disease diagnosed post-natally, and this does not necessarily represent the same spectrum as disease diagnosed antenatally. In general the prognosis seems much worse when diagnosed *in utero*. In the majority of survivors renal function improves following surgery, but this is not always the case. The development of renal failure may be delayed for 9–10 years.[204]

Obstetric management

When the diagnosis of urethral valves is made, management depends on the presence of other serious abnormalities, the gestational age at diagnosis, the parents' wishes and renal function. A careful search for other abnormalities must be made and a rapid karyotyping procedure performed. This may prove difficult with oligohydramnios, though, as in cases of suspected renal agenesis, warm saline instilled into the intra-uterine cavity may help. In any pregnancy, even in a case of isolated posterior urethral valves, if obstruction is virtually complete the prognosis of the condition is such that termination seems a reasonable option if the parents wish it.

Once other abnormalities are excluded, if the parents wish to continue with the pregnancy the presence of dysplasia and renal function should be assessed by careful examination of the kidneys, assessment of amniotic fluid volume and fetal urine aspiration, if possible from both kidneys or, if equally affected, the bladder. One poor prognostic sign is oligohydramnios. Approximately 95% of fetuses with severely reduced liquor will not survive the neonatal period.[192] Other poor prognostic signs are dysplasia of the kidneys (present in a high percentage of cases[205]) and abnormal urinary biochemistry, as previously discussed in pelvi-ureteric junction obstruction.[178,179]

If the prognostic criteria are good it must still be remembered that as yet these cannot be confidently extrapolated from the prenatal period to the long-term outlook. Caution must be exercised when counselling parents. Follow-up management of the baby should be planned ahead, probably with delivery in a paediatric surgical centre. If the prognosis is poor, options are termination of pregnancy in the early weeks and non-interventional management later on.

In experiments in fetal lambs, timely decompression of obstructive uropathy was shown to prevent renal dysplasia[22] and this led to interest in *in utero* decompression of the urinary tract, with variable success.[14,106,206] Nakayama *et al.*[207] compared a group of neonates in whom posterior valves were diagnosed at birth and active management given, with a similar group treated *in utero*. There was a significant difference in mortality: 45% in the neonatally diagnosed group compared to 22.8% in the group treated *in utero*. These data are encouraging but great care must go into the selection of cases to decide suitability for *in utero* surgery[208] which, as previously discussed, carries a high risk. At gestations where delivery is contraindicated, decompression should only be considered in the presence of oligohydramnios once other abnormalities have been excluded and the urine biochemistry has been found to be satisfactory.[209] The choices for fetal intervention include ultrasound-guided percutaneous vesico-amniotic shunt, fetoscopic vesicostomy or open fetal vesicostomy, shunting being most commonly used.[210–212] *In utero* decompression with restoration of amniotic fluid can prevent the development of pulmonary hypoplasia, but it is not yet certain whether it will arrest or reverse renal dysplastic changes and damaged renal function.

Recurrence risks

The condition is usually sporadic but familial cases have been reported.[213]

Urethral atresia and cloacal abnormalities

In these conditions the bladder outflow obstruction is complete.

Diagnosis

Urethral atresia is characterised by anhydramnios. The fetal abdomen is completely filled and distended by an enormous symmetrical cystic structure and the chest circumference is extremely small in relation to the abdominal circumference (Fig. 16.41). Because of the severity of the oligohydramnios and the massive bladder dilatation, identification of other abnormalities is difficult if not impossible.

If the atresia is due to a persistent cloaca the cystic structure may be more complex, with two or three 'loculations' and some solid content on their posterior wall (Fig. 16.42). Spontaneous decompression of the urinary tract results in ascites (Fig. 16.43).

Prognosis

This condition is lethal and termination should be offered.

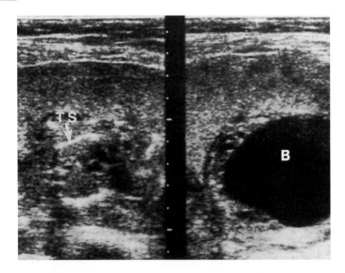

Fig. 16.41 Urethral atresia. There is anhydramnios. Note the massive centrally placed cystic structure, the completely obstructed bladder (B). The transverse section of the thorax (TS) is very small.

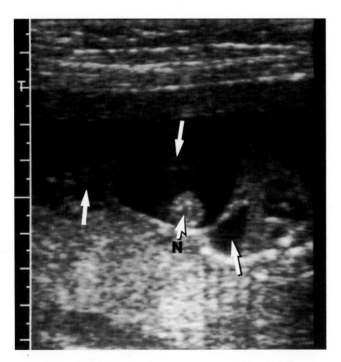

Fig. 16.42 Cloacal atresia. There are three cystic structures (arrows) in the lower abdomen in this fetus, one containing a solid nodule (N) of embryonic tissue.

Megacystis–microcolon–intestinal hypoperistalsis syndrome

This consists of the association of a distended and un-obstructed bladder with a dilated small bowel and distal microcolon. Motility of the stomach and intestine is impaired, leading to malnutrition. The small bowel is

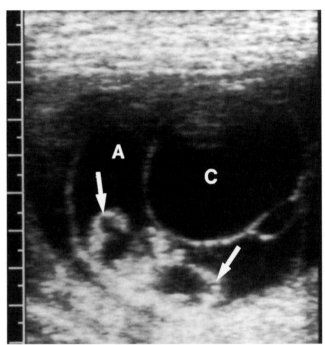

Fig. 16.43 Cloacal atresia. The kidneys (arrows) are hydronephrotic, with highly reflective renal parenchyma indicating dysplasia. (C) indicates the massively dilated persistent cloaca. There is urinary ascites (A).

short and fixed. The condition is rare, predominantly affecting females.[214,215]

Diagnosis

Antenatal visualisation of this syndrome has been reported.[216,217] The condition should be suspected in the presence of a distended bladder with a normal or increased amount of amniotic fluid in a female fetus when no other lower body abnormality can be seen.

Prognosis

The condition is usually lethal.

Obstetric management

It is unlikely that the diagnosis could be made with certainty antenatally and therefore management must be expectant.

Recurrence risk

Although usually sporadic, some familial cases have been reported.[214]

Bladder exstrophy and exstrophy of the cloaca

Bladder exstrophy occurs when midline closure of the anterior abdominal wall is incomplete. The defect involves not only the abdomen but also the anterior wall of the urinary bladder. The posterior wall of the bladder is therefore exposed, along with the trigone and ureteric orifices, and urine dribbles intermittently from the everted bladder. Bladder exstrophy may be isolated or form part of a major maldevelopment: exstrophy of the cloaca. In this there may be complete breakdown of the cloacal membrane with exstrophy of a persistent cloaca, failure of fusion of the genital tubercles and pubic rami and, often, exomphalos.[218]

Incidence and aetiology

Bladder exstrophy results from failure of mesenchymal cells to migrate between the ectoderm of the abdomen and the cloaca during the fourth week of development.[28] As a result no muscle or connective tissue forms in the anterior abdominal wall over the urinary bladder. Later the thin epidermis and the anterior wall of the bladder rupture, exposing the mucous membrane of the bladder. Defective development of the mesenchymal cells prior to the fourth week results in the more extensive cloacal exstrophy.

Bladder exstrophy is a rare condition, occurring once in 10 000–50 000 births,[28] and is more common in males. Most cases are sporadic but familial cases have been reported.[219] Exstrophy of the cloaca has an incidence of one in 200 000 live births without a sex preponderance[220] and is sporadic.

Diagnosis

Bladder exstrophy is not easy to diagnose and should be considered in the list of differential diagnoses when the bladder is absent on repeated scans, despite the liquor volume being normal. Along with the absent bladder four other features have been associated with bladder exstrophy: often a bulge or mass is seen on or protruding from the anterior abdominal wall;[173,221] the penis is small and the scrotum displaced anteriorly; the insertion of the umbilicus is sometimes set lower than normal and finally there can be abnormal widening of the iliac crests.[222]

In cloacal exstrophy the most obvious findings may be those of the associated problems, mainly the vertebral abnormalities or the exomphalos. In one patient, a severe case examined at 17 weeks gestation, there was a large exomphalos; below this no abdominal wall could be identified and no bladder was seen. Bilateral hydronephrosis was present, with moderately reduced liquor. Kyphoscoliosis of the lumbar spine was obvious. In another case of lesser degree a small exomphalos was present and below this a semi-solid mass protruded from the anterior abdominal wall. Again no bladder was present. The liquor was normal. In this case separation of the pubic rami was seen at pathological examination.

Differential diagnosis

Other conditions which appear similar to cloacal exstrophy are the caudal regression syndrome and body stalk abnormality. In the former, limb abnormalities are likely to be present. In the latter the short umbilical cord ensures that the anterior part of the fetus touches the placenta.

Associated abnormalities

These are rare in bladder exstrophy but common in cloacal exstrophy,[223] of which the majority of associated problems are a direct result of the underlying maldevelopment process. These are largely skeletal defects, which are present in 72% of cases, the majority being incomplete development of the lumbosacral vertebral column, leading to herniation of a grossly dilated central canal of the spinal cord and separation of the pubic bones.[224] Exomphalos, also resulting directly from the maldevelopment, occurs in the majority of cases. Renal abnormalities are common. Some of these, such as urethral tract dilatation, may be secondary to obstruction at the ureterovesical junction, or neurological due to the spinal cord abnormalities. Renal agenesis and multicystic kidneys have also been reported. Cardiovascular problems may occur.[223,225] It should be remembered that, as both these conditions are essentially part of a spectrum, when an apparently isolated bladder exstrophy is seen great care must be taken to exclude other abnormalities, particularly of the sacral spine, before counselling parents.

Prognosis

The problems of bladder exstrophy are chiefly incontinence of urine and the abdominal wall defect, with maldevelopment of the genitalia. Primary bladder closure or urinary diversion and abdominal wall closure have been performed with reasonable success, although there may be recurrent problems of urinary tract infections, calculi formation and incontinence. Surgical correction of female genitalia is reasonably successful but male genital defects are difficult to correct and so gender reassignment is practised,[186] with all its associated problems. Fertility is decreased. Morbidity is generally low and the majority of adults adjust to their problems.[226]

Cloacal exstrophy has a mortality rate of 55%.[227] Surgical correction requires a series of operations with variable results. Morbidity in the survivors is very high.

Obstetric management

If these conditions are diagnosed, termination should be offered following counselling regarding the condition. If this is not required normal obstetric management should be pursued. Care must be taken with the exposed bladder mucosa after delivery, as it is extremely friable and should be covered with a non-adherent dressing.[186] Mode or place of delivery seems to have no bearing on outcome.

Recurrence risk

The majority of cases are sporadic but as familial cases have been reported the risk of recurrence is given as 1%.[219] If the parent has bladder exstrophy then the chance of an affected offspring is 1 in 70.[228]

Renal tumours

Renal tumours in the neonate, and therefore in the antenatal period, are extremely rare. The most common is the mesoblastic nephroma (fetal renal hamartoma) derived from secondary mesenchyme, which has a limited capacity to differentiate. The cells are predominantly fibroblasts or intermediate between fibroblast and smooth muscle.[229]

Diagnosis

If a solid unilateral mass is seen in the renal area and no normal renal outline can be identified on that side, mesoblastic nephroma should be considered.[230,231] Typically it stretches the kidney, and careful imaging may show a rim of normal renal tissue surrounding the tumour. It must be remembered that ultrasound cannot give a histological diagnosis, although mesoblastic nephroma is the most likely renal tumour in this age group. The earliest diagnosis has been made at 26 weeks.[230] Polyhydramnios is invariably present, the reason being unknown.[232]

Associated abnormalities

14% of cases are reported as being associated with other abnormalities, chiefly of the gastrointestinal tract, hydrocephaly and other genitourinary problems.

Prognosis

Intra-uterine growth retardation appears to be an associated feature.[233] Nephrectomy is almost always curative,[234] although there are isolated reports of local recurrence and a case of malignant mesenchymal nephroma with pulmonary metastases in a 7-month-old child.[235,236]

Obstetric management

As the outcome is generally good normal obstetric management may be pursued, with careful monitoring and treatment for polyhydramnios.

Renal malposition and abnormalities of shape

Ectopic kidney

Congenital renal ectopia is characterised by an abnormally located kidney supplied by arteries in its immediate vicinity. The ectopic kidney may be located ipsilateral to its normal location (simple ectopia) or contralateral (crossed ectopia). Examples of a simple ectopia with contralateral renal agenesis and crossed ectopia have also been reported.[237,238]

Aetiology and incidence

The most frequent type of renal ectopia is simple, found in 1 per 800 autopsies.[239] All the other types are extremely rare. The majority of all ectopic kidneys, whether simple or crossed, are located more caudally in the fetal abdomen than the normal kidney. The migration of the kidney from its point of origin in the renal pelvis to its usual site, which normally occurs during the second month of gestation, may become arrested at any point. The cause of this migratory inhibition is unknown. Conversely, in rare instances the ascending kidney apparently overshoots and migrates into the thorax.[238]

Diagnosis

A pelvic kidney has been diagnosed antenatally as early as 18 weeks but is more usually identified after 26 weeks.[240,241] An echo-poor mass was seen above the bladder. In addition, on that side the kidney could not be visualised in the renal bed, although the kidney on the other side appeared normal in every respect. Post-natally this proved to be a horseshoe kidney.

Considering the apparent commonness of this variant it is surprising it is not more extensively documented in prenatal ultrasound literature.

Differential diagnosis

In general echo-poor masses seen in the pelvis on ultrasound represent an abnormality of the urinary tract or bowel, or in the female an ovarian cyst. Most of these can be ruled out by the presence of normal amniotic fluid volume, normality of the rest of the renal tract and the appearance of otherwise normal bowel, the important diagnostic feature being the inability to see two kidneys in their correct position.

Associated abnormalities

Some types of ectopia, particularly the crossed, are associated with an increase in the frequency of associated congenital abnormalities of the genitourinary, skeletal and cardiovascular systems.[238]

Prognosis

Ectopic kidney, especially a simple type, may be without clinical significance, being detected only at the time of postmortem as an incidental finding. Pelvic kidneys and the various forms of crossed ectopia are associated with recurrent urinary tract infections, pyelonephritis and renal calculi formation.[238] A study of 26 cases of prenatally diagnosed pelvic kidneys found that if there were no other associated ultrasound abnormalities then kidney function is likely to be normal and the outcome good. However, the children do need neonatal follow-up.[241]

Obstetric management

Normal obstetric management should be pursued. Knowledge of the presence of an ectopic kidney may aid in prophylaxis against calculus formation and infection in later life.

Horseshoe kidney

Horseshoe kidney is a common congenital anomaly. In 90% of cases the fusion involves the lower poles and prevents normal rotation of the kidney, which in turn requires the ureter to rise anterior to it and pass over the fused lower renal poles. The ultimate position of the fused kidneys tends to be lower than normal.[242]

Aetiology and incidence

The anomaly results from the fusion of the left and right metanephric blastema during the second month, prior to their cephalic migration. The cause is unclear. The frequency has been variously estimated to be from 1 in 350 to 1 in 1800.[242] There is a male preponderance.

Diagnosis

At the normal level of scanning for kidneys renal tissue is seen on both sides but, scanning more caudally, the renal tissue could be seen to be continuous across the abdomen.[243] Considering its reported frequency horseshoe kidney is rarely diagnosed, perhaps because the fused part lies lower than the usual level of scanning for kidneys and the upper poles seen in the usual place are taken to be the kidneys.

Associated abnormalities

Horseshoe kidney occurs in a number of chromosome abnormalities, namely Turner's syndrome, trisomy 18 and the 18q syndrome. It is also found in the iris coloboma and anal atresia syndrome. The associated abnormalities are therefore the ones associated with these conditions, including IUGR, microcephaly, facial dysplasias, hemivertebrae and cardiac abnormalities.

Prognosis

Generally the prognosis is good, but urinary tract infection and renal calculus formation are common[244] and tumours, including renal cell carcinoma, transitional cell carcinomas and Wilms' tumours, may develop.[245,246] Another problem is that of pain related to compression of the isthmus of the fused kidneys by the vena cava and aorta, accentuated by hypertension and associated with a sensation of fullness and nausea. Surgical procedures are commonly required to treat the complications.[247]

Obstetric management

Normal obstetric management should be pursued.

Supernumerary kidney

This term describes a free accessory organ which is distinct, encapsulated and may be large or small and closely related to but not attached to the usual kidney. The majority are in fact smaller and lower than the ipsilateral normal kidney and located on the left side.[247–249] Approximately one-third have a completely duplicated ureter but more commonly a bifid ureter is shared with the ipsilateral kidney.

Aetiology and incidence

This is an extremely rare abnormality.

Diagnosis

To date there is no reported diagnosis of a supernumerary kidney *in utero*, but the finding of another smaller echo-poor mass just below a kidney should be examined carefully for further typical renal appearances.

Prognosis

The prognosis is good but secondary development of hydronephrosis and pyelonephritis is common.[247]

Associated abnormalities

When the supernumerary kidney has been diagnosed in children multiple non-genitourinary and genitourinary malformations have been observed.[249,250]

Prognosis

The presence of other abnormalities alters the prognosis but otherwise in the isolated supernumerary kidney this is good.

Obstetric management

Management of an isolated supernumerary kidney should be normal. When other abnormalities coexist the management should be altered according to the prognosis conferred by the other abnormalities.

Conclusion

Many of the conditions that affect the urinary tract are not clinically obvious at birth. Delay in diagnosis and treatment has been shown to have a deleterious effect on outcome. The fetal urinary tract is very amenable to ultrasound diagnosis and investigation. Although the diagnosis and definition of the degree of the disorder are sometimes difficult, much useful information can be gained by a combination of ultrasound examination and fetal urine sampling, when appropriate. There is little doubt that antenatal ultrasound examination contributes greatly to the management of urinary tract abnormalities.

REFERENCES

1 Garrett W J, Grunwald G, Robinson D E. Prenatal diagnosis of fetal polycystic kidney by ultrasound. Aust NZ J Obstet Gynaecol 1970; 10: 7–9

2 Garrett W J, Kossoff G, Osborn R A. The diagnosis of fetal hydronephrosis, megaureter, and urethral obstruction by ultrasonic echography. Br J Obstet Gynaecol 1975; 82: 115–120

3 Bellinger M F, Cornstock C H, Grosso D, Zaino R. Fetal posterior urethral valves and renal dysplasia at 15 weeks gestational age. J Urol 1983; 129: 1238–1239

4 Diamond D A, Sanders R, Jeffs R D. Fetal hydronephrosis. Consideration regarding urologic intervention. J Urol 1984; 131: 1155–1159

5 Pachi A, Giancotti A, Torcia V, De Prosperi V, Maggi E. Meckel–Grüber syndrome: ultrasonographic diagnosis at 13 weeks gestational age in an at-risk case. Prenat Diagn 1989; 9: 187–190

6 Ceccherini I, Lituania M, Cordone M S et al. Autosomal dominant polycystic kidney disease: prenatal diagnosis by DNA analysis and sonography at 14 weeks. Prenat Diagn 1989; 9: 751–758

7 Stiller R J, Pinto M, Heller C, Hobbins J C. Oligohydramnios associated with bilateral multicystic dysplastic kidneys: prenatal diagnosis at 15 weeks gestation. JCU 1988; 16: 436–439

8 Souka A P, Nicolaides K H. Diagnosis of fetal abnormalities at the 10–14 week scan. Ultrasound Obstet Gynaecol 1997; 10: 429–442

9 Watson A R, Readett D, Nelson C S, Kapilar L, Mayell M J. Dilemmas associated with antenatally detected urinary tract abnormalities. Arch Dis Child 1988; 63: 719–722

10 Gunn T R, Mora J D, Pease P. Outcome after antenatal diagnosis of upper tract dilatation by ultrasonography. Arch Dis Child 1988; 63: 1240–1243

11 Livera L N, Brookfield D, Egginton J A, Hawnaur J M. Antenatal ultrasonography to detect fetal renal abnormalities: a prospective screening programme. BMJ 1989; 298: 1421–1423

12 Duval J M, Milon J, Coadou Y. Ultrasonographic anatomy and diagnosis of fetal uropathies affecting the upper urinary tract. I. Obstructive uropathies. Anat Clin 1985; 7: 301

13 Warkany J. The kidney. In: Congenital malformations. Chicago: Year Book Medical Publisher, 1972

14 Harrison M R, Golbus M S, Filly R A. Postpartum evaluation of fetal hydronephrosis: optimal timing for follow-up sonography. Radiology 1984; 152: 423–424

15 Turnock R R, Shawis R. Management of fetal urinary tract anomalies detected by prenatal diagnosis. Arch Dis Child 1984; 59: 962–965

16 Guaderer M W L, Jassan M N, Izant R J. Ultrasonographic antenatal diagnosis: will it change the spectrum of neonatal surgery? J Paediatr Surg 1984; 19: 404–407

17 Dubbins P A, Kurtz A B, Wapner R J, Goldberg B B. Renal agenesis: spectrum of in utero findings. JCU 1981; 9: 189–193

18 Kramer S A. Current status of fetal intervention for congenital hydronephrosis. J Urol 1983; 130: 641–646

19 Sanders R, Graham D. Twelve cases of hydronephrosis in utero diagnosed by ultrasonography. J Ultrasound Med 1982; 1: 341–348

20 Grupe W E. The dilemma of intrauterine diagnosis of congenital renal dilatation. Pediatr Clin North Am 1987; 34: 629–638

21 Mahoney B S, Filly R A, Callen P W, Hricak H, Golbus M S, Harrison M R. Fetal renal dysplasia: sonographic evaluation. Radiology 1984; 152(1): 143–146

22 Glick P L, Harrison M R, Adzick N S, Noall R A, Villa R L. Correction of congenital hydronephrosis in utero IV: in utero decompression reprevents renal dysplasia. J Pediatr Surg 1984; 19(6): 649–657

23 Wladimiroff J W, Campbell S. Fetal urine-production rates in normal and complicated pregnancy. Lancet 1974; i: 151–154

24 Wladimiroff J W. Effect of frusemide on fetal urine production. Br J Obstet Gynaecol 1975; 82: 221–224

25 Laing F C, Burke V D, Wing V W, Jeffrey R B, Hashimoto B. Postpartum evaluation of fetal hydronephrosis: optimal timing for follow-up sonography. Radiology 1984; 152: 423–424

26 Nicolaides K H, Cheng H H, Snijders R J M, Moniz C F. Fetal urine biochemistry in the assessment of obstructive uropathy. Am J Obstet Gynecol 1992; 166: 932–937

27 Johnson M P, Bukowski T P, Reitlman C, Isada N B, Pryde P G, Evans M I. In utero surgical treatment of fetal obstructive uropathy a new comprehensive approach to identify appropriate candidates for vasoamniotic shunt therapy. Am J Obstet Gynecol 1994; 170: 1770–1779

28 Moore K L. The urogenital system. In: Moore K L, ed. The developing human: clinically orientated embryology, 4th edn. Philadelphia: WB Saunders, 1988: 246–285

29 Parmley T H, Seeds A E. Fetal skin permeability to isotopic water (THO) in early pregnancy. Am J Obstet Gynecol 1970; 108: 128–131

30 Fairweather D V I, Eskes T K A B. Amniotic fluid: research and clinical application. Amsterdam: Excerpta Medica, 1978

31 Baker M E, Rosenberg E R, Bowie J D, Gall S. Transient in utero hydronephrosis. J Ultrasound Med 1985; 4(1): 51–53

32 Patten R M, Mack L A, Wang K Y, Cyr D R. The fetal genitourinary tract. Radiol Clin North Am 1990; 28(1): 115–130

33 Lawson T L, Foley W D, Berland L L, Clark K E. Ultrasonic evaluation of fetal kidneys. Radiology 1981; 138: 153–156

34 Rosati P, Guarilia L. Transvaginal sonographic assessment of the fetal urinary tract in early pregnancy. Ultrasound Obstet Gynecol 1996; 7: 95–100

35 Gonzales J, Gonzales M, Mary J Y. Size and weight of human kidney growth velocity during the last three months of pregnancy. Eur Urol 1980; 6: 37–44

36 Casey M L, Carr B R. Growth of the kidney in the normal human fetus during early gestation. Early Hum Dev 1982; 6: 11–14

37 Bertagnoli L, Lalatta F, Gallicchio R et al. Quantitative characterisation of the growth of the fetal kidney. JCU 1983; 11(7): 349–356

38 Grannum P, Bracken M, Silverman R, Hobbins J C. Assessment of fetal kidney size in normal gestation by comparison of ratio of kidney circumference to abdominal circumference. Am J Obstet Gynecol 1980; 136: 249–254

39 Jeanty P, Dramaix-Wilmet M, Elkhazen N, Hubinont C, Van Regemorter N. Measurement of fetal kidney growth on ultrasound. Radiology 1982; 144: 159–162

40 Kurjak A, Kirkinen P, Latin V, Ivankovic D. Ultrasonic assessment of fetal kidney function in normal and complicated pregnancies. Am J Obstet Gynecol 1981; 141(3): 266–269

41 Fagerquist M, Sillen U, Oden A, Hokegard K H, Blomber S G. Fetal urine production estimated with ultrasound. The lower limit of normality is illustrated in a case with severe hypoplasia of the kidneys. Ultrasound Obstet Gynecol 1996; 7: 268–271

42 Carter C O, Evans K. Birth frequency of renal agenesis. J Med Genet 1981; 18: 158–159

43 Wilson R D, Baird P A. Renal agenesis in British Columbia. Am J Med Genet 1985; 21: 153–165

44 Hack M, Jaffe J, Blankstein J, Goodman R M, Brish M. Familial aggregation in bilateral renal agenesis. Clin Genet 1974; 5: 173–177

45 Schinzel A, Homberger C, Sigrist T. Renal agenesis in 2 male sibs born to consanguineous parents. J Med Genet 1978; 15: 314–316

46 Pashayan H M, Dowd T, Nigro A V. Bilateral absence of the kidneys and ureters: 3 cases reported in one family. J Med Genet 1977; 14: 205–209

47 Buchta R M, Viseskul C, Gilbert E F, Sarto G E, Opitz J M. Familial bilateral renal agenesis and hereditary renal dysplasia. Zeitschr Kinder 1973; 115: 111–129

48 Carter C O, Evans K, Pescia G. A family study of renal agenesis. J Med Genet 1979; 16: 176–188

49 Yunis E, Uribe J G. Full trisomy 7 and Potters syndrome. Hum Genet 1980; 84: 13–18

50 Ferrandez A, Schmid W. Potter syndrome (Nirenagenesie) mit chromosamaler aberation beim patient und mosaik beim vater. Helv Paediatr Acta 1971; 26: 210–214

51 Mikelsaar A V, Lazjuk C J, Lurie J W et al. A 4p-syndrome. A case report. Humangenetik 1973; 19: 345–347

52 Prevs M, Kaplan P, Kirkham T H. The renal anomalies and oligohydramnios in the cerebro-oculofacio-mandibular syndrome. Am J Dis Child 1977; 131(1): 62–64

53 Halal F, Desgranges M F, Leduc B, Théoré G, Bettez P. Acro-renal-mandibular syndrome. Am J Med Genet 1980; 5(3): 277–284

54 Carmi R, Binshtock M, Abeliovich D, Bar-Ziv J. The brachio-oto-renal (BOR) syndrome: report of bilateral renal agenesis in three sibs. Am J Med Genet 1983; 14(4): 625–627

55 Biedel C W, Pagon R A, Zapata J O. Müllerian anomalies and renal agenesis: autosomal dominant urogenital dysplasia. J Pediatr 1984; 104(6): 861–864

56 Grix A Jr, Curry C, Hall B D. Patterns of multiple malformations in infants of diabetic mothers. Birth Defects 1982; 18: 55–77

57 Balfour R P, Laurence K M. Raised serum AFP levels and fetal renal agenesis. Lancet 1980; i: 317

58 Barss V A, Benacerraf B R, Frigoletto F D Jr. Second trimester oligohydramnios, a predictor of poor fetal outcome. Obstet Gynecol 1984; 16(5): 608–610

59 Koontz W L, Seeds J W, Adams N J, Johnson A M, Cefalo R C. Elevated maternal serum alpha-fetoprotein second trimester oligohydramnios and pregnancy outcome. Obstet Gynecol 1983; 62(3): 301–304

60 Mercer L J, Brown L G. Fetal outcome with oligohydramnios in the 2nd trimester. Obstet Gynecol 1986; 67(6): 840–842

61 Raghavendra B N, Young B K, Greco M A et al. Use of frusemide in pregnancies complicated by oligohydramnios. Radiology 1987; 165: 455–458

62 Hellstrom W J G, Kogan B A, Jeffrey Jnr R B, McAninch J W. The natural history of prenatal hydronephrosis with normal amounts of amniotic fluid. J Urol 1984; 132: 947–950

63 Chamberlain P F, Climming M, Torchia M G, Biehl D, Manning F A. Ovine fetal urine production following maternal intravenous furosemide administration. Am J Obstet Gynecol 1985; 151: 815–819

64 Beerman B, Groschinsky-Grind M, Fahraens L, Lindstrom B. Placental transfer of frusemide. Clin Pharmacol 1978; 24: 560–562

65 Grannum P. Fetal urinary tract anomalies. Diagnosis and management. Clin Diagn Ultrasound 1986; 19: 53–57

66 Potter E L. Bilateral absence of ureters and kidneys: report of 50 cases. Obstet Gynecol 1965; 25: 3–12

67 Curry C J R, Jensen K, Holland J, Miller L, Hall B D. The Potter sequence: a clinical analysis of 80 cases. Am J Med Genet 1984; 19: 679–702

68 Potter E. Facial characteristics of infants with bilateral renal agenesis. Am J Obstet Gynecol 1946; 41: 855–858

69 Thomas I, Smith D W. Oligohydramnios, cause of the non renal features of Potter's syndrome, particularly pulmonary hypoplasia. J Pediatr 1974; 84: 811–814

70 Fantel A, Shepherd T. Potters syndrome – non renal features induced by oligohydramnios. Am J Dis Child 1975; 129: 1346–1347

71 Hislop A, Hey E, Reid L. The lungs in congenital bilateral renal agenesis and dysplasia. Arch Dis Child 1979; 54(1): 32–38

72 Roodhooft A M, Birnholz J C, Holmes L B. Familial nature of congenital absence and severe dysgenesis of both kidneys. N Engl J Med 1984; 310: 1341–1345

73 Robson W L, Thomason M A, Minette L J. Cystic dysplasia of the testis associated with multicystic dysplasia of the kidney. Urology 1988; 51: 477–479

74 Rudnik-Schoeborn S, Schuler H M, Schwanitz G, Hansmann M, Zerres K. Further arguments for non-fortuitous association of Potter sequences with XYY males. Ann Genet 1996; 39: 43–46

75 Ratten J, Beischer N A, Fortune D W. Obstetric complications when the fetus has Potter's syndrome. Am J Obstet Gynecol 1973; 115(7): 890–896

76 Emanuel B, Nachmar R, Aronson N, Weiss H. Congenital solitary kidney: a review of 74 cases. J Urol 1974; 111: 394–397

77 Nicolaides K H, Campbell S. Diagnosis and management of fetal malformations. In: Rodeck C, ed. Fetal diagnosis of genetic defects. London: Baillière Tindall, 1987; 591–622

78 Osathanondh V, Potter E L. Pathogenesis of polycystic kidneys. Type I due to hypoplasia of interstitial portions of collecting tubules. Arch Pathol 1964; 77: 466–473

79 Osathanondh V, Potter E L. Pathogenesis of polycystic kidneys. Type 2 due to inhibition of ampullary activity. Arch Pathol 1964; 7: 474–484

80 Osathanondh V, Potter E L. Pathogenesis of polycystic kidneys. Type 3 due to multiple abnormalities of development. Arch Pathol 1964; 77: 485–501

81 Osathanondh V, Potter E L. Pathogenesis of polycystic kidneys. Type 4 due to urethral obstruction. Arch Pathol 1964; 77: 502–512

82 Bernstein J. The morphogenesis of renal parenchymal maldevelopment. Pediatr Clin North Am 1971; 18(2): 395–407

83 Hartman D S, Davis C J. Multicystic dysplastic kidneys. In: Hartman D S, ed. Renal cystic disease. Philadelphia: WB Saunders, 1989: 127–145

84 Potter E L. Early ampullary inhibition. In: Normal and abnormal development of the kidney. Chicago: Year Book Medical, 1972

85 Felson B, Cussen L J. The hydronephrotic type of unilateral congenital multicystic disease of the kidney. Semin Roentgenol 1975; 10(2): 113–123

86 Sanders R C, Hartman D S. The sonographic distinction between neonatal multicystic kidney and hydronephrosis. Radiology 1984; 151: 621–625

87 Resnick J, Vernier R L. Cystic disease of the kidney in the newborn infant. Clin Perinatol 1981; 8(2): 375–390

88 Griscom N T, Vawter G F, Fellers F X. Pelvicofundibular atresia: the usual form of multicystic kidney: 44 unilateral and two bilateral cases. Semin Roentgenol 1975; 10(2): 125–131

89 Petersen R O. Congenital anomalies. In: Urologic pathology. Philadelphia: J B Lippincott, 1986

90 Hashimoto B E, Filly R A, Callen P W. Multicystic dysplastic kidney in utero: changing appearances. Radiology 1986; 159: 107–109

91 Sty J R, Babbitt D P, Oechler H W. Evaluating the multicystic kidney. Clin Nucl Med 1980; 5: 457–461

92 Rouse G A, Kaminsky C K, Saaty H P, Grube G L, Fritzsche P J. Current concepts in sonographic diagnosis of fetal disease. Radiographics 1988; 8(1): 119–132

93 Avni E F, Thoua Y, Lalmand B, Didier F, Droulle P, Schulman C C. Multicystic dysplastic kidney: evolving concepts. Natural history from in utero diagnosis and post-natal follow-up. J Urol 1987; 138: 1420–1424

94 Hernadi L, Torocsik M. Screening for fetal anomalies in the 12th week of pregnancy by transvaginal sonography in an unselected population. Prenat Diagn 1997; 17: 753–759

95 Bronshtein M, Yoffe N, Brandes J M, Blumenfeld Z. First and early second trimester diagnosis of fetal urinary tract anomalies using transvaginal sonography. Prenat Diagn 1990; 10: 653–666

96 Kleiner B, Filly R A, Mack L, Callen P W. Multicystic dysplastic kidney: observations of contralateral disease in the fetal population. Radiology 1986; 161: 27–29

97 Rizzo N, Gabrielli S, Pilu G et al. Prenatal diagnosis and obstetrical management of multicystic dysplastic renal disease. Prenat Diagn 1987; 7: 109–118

98 Gill B, Bennett R T, Barnhard Y, Bar-Hava I, Girz B, Divon M. Can fetal renal artery Doppler studies predict postnatal renal function in morphologically abnormal kidneys? A preliminary report. J Urol 1996; 156: 190–192

99 D'Alton M, Romero R, Grannum P, De Palma L, Jeanty P, Hobbins J C. Antenatal diagnosis of renal anomalies with ultrasound. IV. Bilateral multicystic kidney disease. Am J Obstet Gynecol 1986; 154(3): 532–537

100 De Klerk D P, Marshall F F, Jeffs R D. Multicystic dysplastic kidneys. J Urol 1977; 118: 306–308

101 Robson W L, Thomason M A, Minette L J. Cystic dysplasia of the testis associated with multicystic dysplasia of the kidney. Urology 1998; 51: 477–479

102 Warkany J. Congenital cystic disease of the kidney. Chicago: Year Book Publications, 1981

103 Beck A D. The effect of intra-uterine urinary obstruction upon the development of the fetal kidney. J Urol 1971; 105: 784–789

104 Baert L. Cystic kidneys, renal dysplasia, and microdissection data in 5 children with congenital valvular urethral obstruction. Eur Urol 1978; 4(5): 383–387

105 Sanders R C, Nussbaum A R, Solez K. Renal dysplasia: sonographic findings. Radiology 1988; 167: 623–626

106 Harrison M R, Golbus M S, Filly R A et al. Management of the fetus with congenital hydronephrosis. J Pediatr Surg 1982; 17(6): 728–742

107 Mahoney B S. The genitourinary system. In: Callen P W, ed. Ultrasonography in obstetrics and gynecology, 2nd edn. Philadelphia: WB Saunders, 1988; 254–275

108 Glick P L, Harrison M R, Golbus M S et al. Management of the fetus with congenital hydronephrosis II; prognostic criteria and selection for treatment. J Pediatr Surg 1985; 20(4): 376–387

109 Lebowitz R L, Griscom N T. Neonatal hydronephrosis. Radiol Clin North Am 1977; 15(1): 49–59

110 Sibley R K, Dehener L P. The kidney. In: Dehener L P, ed. Paediatric surgical pathology, 2nd edn. Baltimore: Williams & Wilkins, 1987; 589–692

111 Manning F A, Harrison M R, Rodeck C. Members of the International Fetal Medicine and Surgery Society. Catheter shunts for fetal hydronephrosis and hydrocephalus. Report of the International Fetal Surgery Registry. N Engl J Med 1986; 315(5): 336–340

112 Newman L B, McAlister W H, Kissane J. Segmental renal dysplasia associated with ectopic ureteroceles in childhood. Urology 1974; 3: 23–26

113 Abuhamad A Z, Horton C E, Jr. Horton S H, Evans A T. Renal duplication anomalies in the fetus: clues for prenatal diagnosis. Ultrasound Obstet Gynecol 1996; 7: 174–177

114 Fisher C F S J. Renal dysplasia in nephrectomy specimens from adolescents and adults. J Clin Pathol 1975; 28(11): 879–890

115 Montemarano H, Bulas D I, Chandra R, Tifft C. Prenatal diagnosis of glomerulocystic kidney disease in short rib polydactyly syndrome type II, Majewski type. Paediatr Radiol 1995; 25: 469–471

116 Braithwaite J M, Economides D L. First trimester diagnosis of Meckel–Grüber syndrome by transabdominal sonography in a low-risk case. Prenat Diagn 1995; 15: 1168–1170

117 Lieberman E, Salinas-Madrical L, Gwinn J L, Brennan L P, Fine R N, Landing E H. Infantile polycystic disease of the kidneys and liver: clinical pathological and radiological correlations and comparison with congenital hepatic fibrosis. Medicine 1971; 50: 277–318

118 Blythe H, Ockenden B G. Polycystic disease of the kidney and liver. J Med Genet 1971; 8: 257–284

119 Potter E L. Type I cystic kidney: tubular gigantism. In: Normal and abnormal development of the kidney. Chicago: Year Book Publishing, 1972: 141–153

120 Eggli K D, Hartman D S. Autosomal recessive polycystic kidney disease. In: Hartman D S, ed. Renal cystic disease. Philadelphia: WB Saunders, 1989: 73–87

121 Grantham J J. Clinical aspects of adult and infantile polycystic kidney disease. Contries Nephrol 1985; 48: 178–188

122 Luthy D A, Hirsch J H. Infantile polycystic kidney disease: observations from attempts at prenatal diagnosis. Am J Med Genet 1985; 20: 505–517

123 Melson G L, Shackelford G D, Cole B R, McClennan B L. The spectrum of sonographic findings in infantile polycystic kidney disease with urographic and clinical correlations. Clin Ultrasound 1985; 13: 113–119

124 Stapleton F B, Hilton S, Wilcox J. Transient nephromegaly simulating infantile polycystic disease of the kidneys. Pediatrics 1982; 67: 554–559

125 Zerres K, Hansmann M, Mallmann R, Gembruch U. Autosomal recessive polycystic kidney disease: problems of prenatal diagnosis. Prenat Diagn 1988; 8: 215–229

126 Bronshtein M, Bar-Hana I, Blumenfeld Z. Clues and pitfalls in the early prenatal diagnosis of late onset infantile polycystic kidney. Prenat Diagn 1992; 12: 293–298

127 Simpson J L, Sabbagha R E, Elias S, Talbot C, Tamura R K. Failure to detect polycystic kidneys in utero by second trimester ultrasonography. Hum Genet 1982; 60(3): 295

128 Argubright K F, Wicks J D. Third trimester ultrasonic presentation of infantile polycystic kidney disease. Am J Pediatr 1987; 4(1): 1–4

129 Reuss A, Waldimiroff J W, Niermeijer M E. Prenatal diagnosis of renal tract abnormalities by ultrasound. Prog Clin Biol Res 1989; 305: 13–18

130 Townsend R R, Goldstein R B, Filly R A, Callen P W, Anderson R L, Golbus M. Sonographic identification of autosomal recessive polycystic kidney disease associated with increased maternal serum/amniotic fluid alpha-fetoprotein. Obstet Gynecol 1988; 71(2): 1008–1012

131 Sumner T E, Volberg F M, Martin J F, Resnick M I, Shertzer M E. Real-time sonography of congenital cystic kidney disease. Urology 1982; 20(1): 97–101

132 Romero R, Pilu G, Jeanty P, Ghidini A, Hobbins J C. The urinary tract and adrenal glands. In: Prenatal diagnosis of congenital abnormalities. Norwalk: Appleton and Lange, 1988: 255–299

133 Jain M, LeQuesne G W, Bourne A J, Henning P. High-resolution ultrasonography in the differential diagnosis of cystic diseases of the kidney in infancy and childhood: preliminary experience. J Ultrasound Med 1997; 16: 235–240

134 Reeders S T, Brenning M H, Davies K E et al. A highly polymorphic DNA marker linked to adult polycystic disease on chromosome 16. Nature 1985; 317: 542–544

135 Milutinovic J, Agodoa L C, Cutler R E, Striker G E. Autosomal dominant polycystic kidney disease: early diagnosis and data for genetic counselling. Lancet 1980; i: 1203–1206

136 Bear J C, McMannon P, Morgan J et al. Age at clinical onset and sonographic detection of adult polycystic kidney disease. Am J Med Genet 1984; 18: 45–48

137 Dalgaard O Z. Bilateral polycystic disease of the kidneys: a follow-up study of two hundred and eighty four patients and their families. Acta Med Scand 1957; 158 (Suppl. 328): 1–255

138 Zerres M, Hansmann M, Knupple G, Stephan M. Prenatal diagnosis of genetically determined early manifestation of autosomal dominant polycystic kidney disease. Hum Genet 1985; 71: 368–369

139 Main D, Mennuti M T, Cornfield D, Coleman B. Prenatal diagnosis of adult polycystic kidney disease. Lancet 1983; ii: 337–338

140 Journel H, Guyott C, Barc R M, Belbeoch P, Quemener A, Jouan H. Unexpected ultrasonographic prenatal diagnosis of autosomal dominant polycystic kidney disease. Prenat Diagn 1989; 9: 663–671

141 McHugo J M, Shafi M I, Rowlands D, Weaver J B. Prenatal diagnosis of adult polycystic disease. Br J Radiol 1988; 61: 1072–1074

142 Novelli G, Frontali M, Bladini D et al. Prenatal diagnosis of adult polycystic kidney disease with DNA markers on chromosome 16 and the genetic heterogeneity problem. Prenat Diagn 1989; 9: 759–767

143 Breuning M H, Verwest A, Ijdo J et al. Characterization of new probes for diagnosis of polycystic kidney disease. Proceedings of the 5th International Clinical Genetics Seminar in Progress in Clinical and Biological Research, vol. 305. Alan R Liss, New York, 1989; 69–75

144 Gabow P A, Ikle D W, Holmes J H. Polycystic kidney disease. Prospective analysis of nonazotemic patients and family members. Ann Intern Med 1984; 101: 238–247

145 Ross D G, Travers H. Infantile presentation of adult-type polycystic kidney disease in a large kindred. J Pediatr 1975; 87(5): 760–763

146 Fryns J P, Vandenberghe K, Moerman F. Mid-trimester ultrasonographic diagnosis of early manifesting 'adult' form of polycystic kidney disease. Hum Genet 1986; 74: 461

147 Arger P H, Coleman B G, Mintz M C et al. Routine fetal genitourinary tract screening. Radiology 1985; 156: 485–489

148 Grignon A, Filion R, Filiatrault D et al. Urinary tract dilatation in utero: classification and clinical applications. Radiology 1986; 160: 645–647

149 Blane C E, Koff S A, Bowermann R A, Barr M Jr. Non-obstructive fetal hydronephrosis: sonographic recognition and therapeutic implications. Radiology 1983; 147: 95–99

150 Walsh G, Dubbins P A. Antenatal renal pelvis dilatation: a predictor of vesicoureteral reflux? AJR 1996; 167: 897–900

151 Hoddick W K, Filly R A, Mahony B S, Callen P W. Minimal fetal renal pyelectasis. J Ultrasound Med 1985; 4: 85–89

152 Ghidini A, Sirtori M, Vergani P, Orsenigo E, Tagliabue P, Parravicini E. Ureteropelvic junction obstruction in utero and ex utero. Obstet Gynecol 1990; 75(5): 805–808

153 Anderson N G, Abbott G D, Mogridge N, Allan R B, Maling T M, Wells J E. Vesicoureteric reflux in the newborn: relationship to fetal pelvic diameter. Paediatr Nephrol 1997; 11: 610–616

154 Grignon A, Filiatrault D, Homsy Y et al. Ureteropelvic junction stenosis: antenatal ultrasonographic diagnosis, post-natal investigation and follow-up. Radiology 1986; 160: 649–651

155 Quintero R A, Johnson M P, Arias F et al. In utero sonographic diagnosis of vesicoureteral reflux by percutaneous vesicoinfusion. Ultrasound Obstet Gynecol 1995; 6: 386–389

156 Anon. Vesicoureteric reflux: all in the genes? Report of a meeting of physicians at the Hospital for Sick Children, Great Ormond Street, London. Lancet 1996; 348: 725–728

157 Mayor G, Genton N, Torrado A, Guignard J, Renal function in obstructive nephropathy: long-term effect of reconstructive surgery. Pediatrics 1975; 56: 740–747

158 Madarikan B A, Hayward C, Roberts G M, Lari J. Clinical outcome of fetal uropathy. Arch Dis Child 1988; 63: 961–963

159 Clarke N W, Gough D C S, Cohen S J. Neonatal urological ultrasound: diagnostic inaccuracies and pitfalls. Arch Dis Child 1989; 64: 578–580

160 Steele B T, De Maria J, Toi A, Stafford A, Hunter D, Caco C. Neonatal outcome of fetuses with urinary tract abnormalities diagnosed by prenatal ultrasonography. CMAJ 1987; 137: 117–120

161 Scott J E, Swallow V, Coulthard M G, Lambert H J, Lee R E. Screening of newborn babies for familial ureteric reflux. Lancet 1997; 350: 396–400

162 Nicolaides K H, Rodeck K H, Gosden C M. Rapid karyotyping in non-lethal fetal malformations. Lancet 1986; i: 283–287

163 Nicolaides K H. Personal communication. 1991

164 Schwoebl M G, Sacher P U B H, Hirsig J, Stauffer U G. Prenatal diagnosis improves the prognosis of children with obstructive uropathies. J Pediatr Surg 1984; 19(2): 187–190

165 Bukowski T P, Betrus G G, Aquilina J W, Perlmutter A D. Urinary tract infections and pregnancy in women who underwent antireflux surgery in childhood. J Urol 1998; 159: 1286–1289

166 Kelalis P P, Culp O S, Stickler G B, et al. Ureteropelvic obstruction in children: experience with 109 cases. J Urol 1971; 106: 418–422

167 Manning F A. Common fetal urinary tract anomalies. In: Hobbins J C, Benacerraf B R, eds. Clin Diagn Ultrasound. Edinburgh: Churchill Livingstone, 1989: Vol 25, 139–161

168 Seeds J W, Mandell J. Congenital obstructive uropathies. Pre- and postnatal treatment. Urol Clin North Am 1986; 13(1): 155–165

169 Johnston J H, Evans J P, Glassberg K I, Shapiro S R. Pelvic hydronephrosis in children: a review of 219 personal cases. J Urol 1977; 117(1): 97–101

170 Antonakopoulos G N, Fuggle W J, Newman J, Considine J, O'Brien J M. Idiopathic hydronephrosis. Arch Pathol Lab Med 1985; 109: 1097–1101

171 Hanna M K, Jeffs R D, Sturgess J M, Barkin M. Urethral structure and ultrastructure. Part II. Congenital ureteropelvic junction obstruction and primary obstructive megaureter. J Urol 1976; 116: 725–730

172 Drake D P, Stevens P S, Eckestein H B. Hydronephrosis secondary to ureteropelvic obstruction in children: a review of 14 years of experience. J Urol 1978; 119: 649–651

173 Jaffe R, Schoenfield A, Ovadia J. Sonographic findings in prenatal diagnosis of bladder exstrophy. Am J Obstet Gynecol 1990; 162: 675–678

174 Robson W J, Rudy S M, Johnston J H. Pelviureteric obstruction in infancy. J Pediatr Surg 1976; 11(1): 57–61

175 Jaffe R, Abramovicz J, Feigin M, Ben-Aderet N. Giant fetal abdominal cyst. J Ultrasound Med 1987; 6: 45–47

176 Kleiner B, Callen P W, Filly R A. Sonographic analysis of the fetus with ureteropelvic obstruction. AJR 1987; 148: 359–363

177 Glazer G M, Filly R M, Callen P W. The varied sonographic appearance of the urinary tract in the fetus and newborn with urethral obstruction. Radiology 1982; 144: 563–568

178 Nicolaides K H, Cheng H H, Snijders R J M, Moniz C F. Fetal urine biochemistry in the assessment of obstructive uropathy. Am J Obstet Gynecol 1992; 166: 932–937

179 Crombleholme T N, Harrison M R, Golbus M S et al. Fetal intervention in obstructive uropathy, prognostic indicators and efficacy of intervention. Am J Obstet Gynecol 1990; 162: 1239–1244

180 Atwell J D. Familial pelviureteric junction hydronephrosis and its association with a duplex pelvicalyceal system and vesicoureteric reflux. A family study. Br J Urol 1985; 57(4): 365–369

181 Buscemi M, Shanske A, Mallet E, Ozoktay S, Hanna M K. Dominantly inherited ureteropelvic junction obstruction. Urology 1985; 26(6): 568–571

182 Brown T, Mandell J, Lebowitz R L. Neonatal hydronephrosis in the era of sonography. AJR 1987; 148: 959–963

183 Tokunaka S, Koyanagi T. Morphologic study of primary non reflux megaureters with particular emphasis on the role of urethral sheath and ureteral dysplasia. J Urol 1982; 128(2): 399–402

184 Share J C, Lebowitz R L. Ectopic ureterocele without ureteral and calyceal dilatation (ureterocele disproportion): findings on urography and sonography. AJR 1989; 152: 567–571

185 Montana M A, Cyr D R, Lenke R R, Shuman W P, Mack L A. Sonographic detection of fetal ureteral obstruction. AJR 1985; 145: 595–596

186 Jeffs R D, Lepor H. Management of the extrophy-hypospadias complex and vulval anomalies. In: Walsh P C, ed. Cambell's urology, 5th edn. Philadelphia: W B Saunders, 1986: 1882–1921

187 Eccles M R, Bailey R R, Abbott G D, Sullivan M J. Unravelling the genetics of vesicoureteric reflux: a common familial disorder. Hum Mol Genet 1996; 5: 1425–1429

188 Kessler R M, Altman D H. Real time sonographic detection of vesicoureteral reflux in children. AJR 1982; 138: 1033–1036

189 Yeung C K, Godley M L, Dhillon H K, Gordon I, Duffy P G, Ransley P G. The characteristics of primary vesico-ureteric reflux in male and female infants with pre-natal hydronephrosis. Br J Urol 1997; 80: 319–327

190 Mack L A, Davies P F, Cyr D R et al. Ultrasonic diagnosis of fetal abnormalities. Perinatol Neonatol 1986; 10: 29–31

191 Young H H, Frentz W A, Baldwin J C. Congenital obstruction of the posterior urethra. J Urol 1919; 3: 289–291

192 Mahoney B S, Callen P W, Filly R A. Fetal urethral obstruction: US evaluation. Radiology 1985; 157: 221–224

193 Dean W M, Bordeau E J. Amniotic fluid alpha-fetoprotein in fetal obstructive uropathy. Pediatrics 1980; 66(4): 537–539

194 Sebire N J, Van Kaisenberg C, Rubio C, Snijders R J M, Nicolaides K H. Fetal megacystis at 10 to 14 weeks of gestation. Ultrasound Obstet Gynecol 1996; 8: 387–390

195 Bulic M, Podobnik M, Korenic I, Bistricki J. First trimester diagnosis of low obstructive uropathy: an indicator of initial renal function in the fetus. JCU 1987; 15: 537–541

196 Zimmer E Z, Bronshtein M. Fetal intraabdominal cysts detected in the first and early second trimester by transvaginal sonography. JCU 1991; 19: 664–667

197 Cullen M T, Green J, Wetham J, Salafia G, Gabrielli S, Hobbins J C. Transvaginal ultrasonographic detection of congential abnormality in the first trimester. Am J Obstet Gynecol 1990; 163: 466–476

198 Reuter K L, Lebowitz R L. Massive vesicoureteral reflux mimicking posterior urethral valves in a fetus. JCU 1985; 13(8): 584–587

199 Bruton O C. Agenesis of abdominal musculature associated with genito-urinary and gastrointestinal tract anomalies. J Urol 1951; 66(4): 607–611

200 Pagon R A, Smith D W, Shepard T H. Congenital abnormalities of the urinary system. Pediatrics 1979; 94(6): 900–906

201 Tsingoglou S, Dickson J A S. Lower urinary obstruction in infancy. A review of lesions and symptoms in 165 cases. Arch Dis Child 1972; 47: 215–217

202 Egami K, Smith E D. A study of the sequelae of posterior urethral valves. J Urol 1982; 127: 84–87

203 Adzick N S, Harrison M R, Flake A W, deLorimer A A. Urinary extravasation in the fetus with obstructive uropathy. J Pediatr Surg 1985; 20(6): 608–615

204 Warshaw B L, Edelbrock H H, Ettenger R B et al. Progression to end-stage renal disease in children with obstructive uropathy. J Pediatr 1982; 100(2): 183–187

205 Hayden S A, Russ P D, Pretorius D H, Manco-Johnson M L, Clewell W H. Posterior urethral obstruction. J Ultrasound Med 1988; 7: 371–375

206 Shalev E, Weiner E, Feldman E, Sudarsky M, Shmilowitz L, Zuckerman H. External bladder-amniotic fluid shunt for fetal urinary tract obstruction. Obstet Gynecol 1984; 63(Suppl): 31S–34S

207 Nakayama D K, Harrison M R, de Lorimer A A. Prognosis of posterior urethral valves presenting at birth. J Pediatr Surg 1986; 21(1): 43–45

208 Johnson M P, Bukowski T P, Reitleman C, Isada N B, Pryde P G, Evans M I. In utero surgical treatment of fetal obstructive uropathy: a new comprehensive approach to identify appropriate candidates for vesicoamniotic shunt therapy. Am J Obstet Gynecol 1994; 170: 1770–1779

209 Vanderwall K J, Harrison M R. Fetal Surgery. In: Chervenak F A, Kurjak A, eds. The fetus as a patient. Parthenon, 1996; 265

210 Manning F A, Harrison M R, Rodeck C H. Special report: catheter shunt for fetal hydronephrosis and hydrocephalus. N Engl J Med 1986; 315: 336–340

211 MacMahan R A, Renou P M, Shelton P A, Paterson R J. In utero cystostomy. Lancet 1991; 40: 1234

212 Crombleholme T M, Harrison M R, Langer J C, Adzick N S. Early experience with open fetal surgery for congenital hydronephrosis. J Paediatr Surg 1988; 23: 1114–1121

213 Grajewski R S, Glassberg K I. The variable effect of posterior urethral valves as illustrated in identical twins. J Urol 1983; 130: 1188–1190

214 Berdon W E, Baker D H, Blanc W A, Gay B, Santulli T V, Donovan C. Megacystis–microcolon–intestinal hypoperistalsis syndrome: a new cause of intestinal obstruction in the newborn. Report of radiologic findings in five newborn girls. AJR 1976; 126(5): 957–964

215 Young L W, Yunis E J, Girdany B R, Sieber W K. Megacystis–microcolon–intestinal hypoperistalsis syndrome: additional clinical, radiologic, surgical and histopathologic aspects. AJR 1981; 137(4): 749–755

216 Vezina W C, Morin F R, Winsberg F. Megacystismicrocolon–intestinal hypoperistalsis syndrome: antenatal ultrasound appearance. AJR 1979; 133(4): 749–750

217 Manco L G, Osterdahl P. The antenatal sonographic features of megacystis–microcolon–intestinal hypoperistalsis syndrome. JCU 1984; 12(9): 595–598

218 Verco P W, Khor B H, Barbary J, Enthoven C. Ectopia vesicae in utero. Australas Radiol 1986; 30(2): 117–120

219 Ives E, Coffey R, Carter C O. A family study of bladder extrophy. J Med Genet 1980; 17(2): 139–141

220 Graivier L. Exstrophy of the cloaca. Ann Surg 1968; 34: 387–390

221 Mirk P, Calisti A, Fileni A. Prenatal sonographic diagnosis of bladder exstrophy. J Ultrasound Med 1986; 5(5): 291–293

222 Gearhart J P, Ben-Chaim J, Jeffs R D, Sanders R C. Criteria for the prenatal diagnosis of classic bladder exstrophy. Obstet Gynecol 1995; 85: 961–964

223 Muecke E L. Exstrophy, epispadias and other anomalies. In: Walsh P C, ed. Campbell's urology, 5th edn. Philadelphia. W B Saunders, 1981; 1856–1880

224 Soper R T, Kilger K. Vesico-intestinal fissure. J Urol 1964; 92: 490–501

225 Caddedu J A, Benson J E, Silver R I, Lakshmanan Y, Jeffs R D, Gearhart J P. Spinal abnormalities in classic bladder exstrophy. Br J Urol 1997; 79: 975–978

226 Lattimer J K, Beck L, Yeaw S, Puchner P J, Macfarlane M T, Krisiloff M. Long-term follow-up after exstrophy closure: late improvement and good quality of life. J Urol 1978; 119(5): 664–666

227 Howell C, Caldamone A, Snyder H, Ziegler M, Duckett J. Optimal management of cloacal exstrophy. J Pediatr Surg 1983; 18(4): 365–369

228 Shapiro E, Lepor H, Jeffs R D. The inheritance of the exstrophy–epispadias complex. J Urol 1984; 132(2): 308–310

229 Wigger H J. Fetal mesenchymal hamartoma of kidney. A tumour of secondary mesenchyme. Cancer 1975; 36(3): 1002–1008

230 Appuzio J J, Unwin W, Adhate A, Nichols R. Prenatal diagnosis of fetal renal mesoblastic nephroma. Am J Obstet Gynecol 1986; 154: 636–637

231 Ehman R L, Nicholson S F, Machin G A. Prenatal sonographic diagnosis of congenital mesoblastic nephroma in a monozygotic twin pregnancy. J Ultrasound Med 1983; 2(12): 555–557

232 Walter J P, McGahan J P. Mesoblastic nephroma: prenatal sonographic detection. JCU 1985; 13(9): 686–689

233 Blank E, Neerhout R C, Burry K A. Congenital mesoblastic nephroma and polyhydramnios. JAMA 1978; 240(14): 1504–1505

234 Sotelo-Avila C, Gooch W M III. Neoplasms associated with the Beckwith–Wiedemann syndrome. Perspect Pediatr Pathol 1976; 3: 255–272

235 Gonzalez-Crussi F, Sotelo-Avila C, Kidd J M. Malignant mesenchymal nephroma of infancy: report of a case with pulmonary metastases. Am J Surg Pathol 1980; 4(2): 185–190

236 Walker D, Richard G. Fetal hamartoma of the kidney; recurrence and death of patient. J Urol 1973; 110: 352–353

237 Tanenbaum B, Silverman N, Weinberg S R. Solitary crossed renal ectopia. Arch Surg 1970; 101: 616–618

238 Malek R S, Kelalis P P, Burke E C. Ectopic kidney in children and frequency of association with other malformations. Mayo Clin Proc 1971; 46: 461–467

239 Ward J N, Nathanson B, Draper J W. The pelvic kidney. J Urol 1965; 94: 36–39

240 Colley N, Hooker J G. Prenatal diagnosis of pelvic kidney. Prenat Diagn 1989; 9: 361–363

241 Meizner I, Yitzhak M, Levi A, Barki Y, Barnhard Y, Glezerman M. Fetal pelvic kidney: a challenge in prenatal diagnosis. Ultrasound Obstet Gynecol 1995; 5: 391–393

242 Lowsley O S. Surgery of horseshoe kidney. J Urol 1952; 67: 565–578

243 Sherer D M, Cullen J B, Thompson H O, Metlay L A, Woods J R Jr. Prenatal sonographic findings associated with a fetal horseshoe kidney. J Ultrasound Med 1990; 9(8): 477–479

244 Culp O S, Winterringer J R. Surgical treatment of horsehoe kidney; comparison of results after various types of operations. J Urol 1955; 73: 747–756

245 Ware S M, Shulman Y. Transitional cell carcinoma of renal pelvis in horsehoe kidney. Urology 1983; 21(1): 76–78

246 Weiner M, Sarma D, Rao M. Renal cell carcinoma in a horseshoe kidney. J Surg Oncol 1984; 26: 77–79

247 Carlson H E. Supernumerary kidney; summary of 51 reported cases. J Urol 1950; 64: 224–229

248 Tada Y, Kokado Y, Hashinaka Y et al. Free supernumerary kidney; a case report and review. J Urol 1981; 126(2): 231–232

249 N'Guessan G, Stephens F D. Supernumerary kidney. J Urol 1983; 130(4): 649–653

250 Antony J. Complete duplication of female urethra with vaginal atresia and supernumerary kidney. J Urol 1977; 118(5): 877–878

Gastrointestinal tract abnormalities

David R Griffin and Lyn S Chitty

Introduction

Detailed visualisation of the fetal abdominal wall and contents forms part of the routine survey in the second trimester. The liver, gallbladder and spleen are detected in most fetuses from mid-pregnancy onwards, in addition to portions of the hollow intestinal organs. Abnormalities of the abdominal wall and the gastrointestinal tract are usually readily demonstrated with ultrasound, and form the third largest group of detected anomalies after renal and central nervous system abnormalities.

Anterior abdominal wall defects

Omphalocele

Definition and aetiology

Omphalocele is an anterior abdominal wall defect characterised by the herniation of intra-abdominal contents into the base of the umbilical cord. The contents, which may include bowel, liver, spleen and pancreas, are covered with a layer of amnion and peritoneum, into which the umbilical cord inserts (Fig. 17.1). The size of these defects is variable, ranging from a small hernia containing a few loops of bowel to a very large one containing most of the abdominal viscera (see Ch. 6) Omphalocele is estimated to occur in between 1/4000 and 1/5800 live births.[1,2]

Associated abnormalities

Omphalocele may be an isolated lesion but is also frequently associated with other abnormalities, syndromes and autosomal trisomies. An overall incidence of associated defects of between 17% and 82% has been reported.[1,3–5] The frequency of abnormal karyotypes varies between 6% and 54%.[1,3,4,6–8] The most common abnormality reported is trisomy 18, but there have been reports of triploidy, 47 XXY, trisomy 13 and trisomy 21. Cardiac anomalies (ventricular and atrial septal defects and tetralogy of Fallot) are found in up to 36% of cases,[1,3,4,6,9] neural tube defects (anencephaly, encephalocele and myelomeningocele) in up to 39%,[5,6] and genitourinary abnormalities in up to 40%.[3] Gastrointestinal anomalies, either primary or secondary (e.g. bowel obstruction), are also a frequent association. Intra-uterine growth retardation has been reported in 20% of cases.[2]

Omphalocele may occur as part of a syndrome,[10] the most common being Beckwith–Wiedemann, which may account for a significant proportion of all cases of omphalocele.[3,9,11] Other features include hemihypertrophy, macroglossia, generalised organomegaly (particularly nephromegaly) and polyhydramnios.[11,12]

Most cases of omphalocele are sporadic and the recurrence risk for isolated cases appears to be less than 1%.

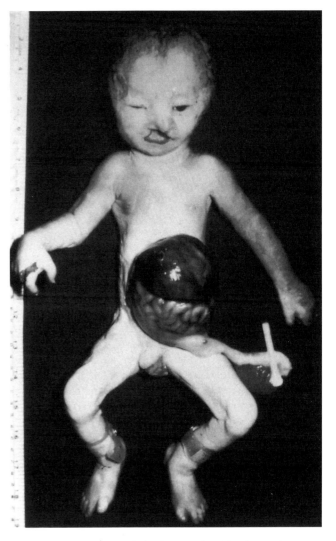

Fig. 17.1 Fetus with an omphalocele. Note the cleft palate in this case, where the underlying pathology was trisomy 18.

Few familial cases have been reported.[13–15] When occurring as part of a syndrome the recurrence risk is that of the syndrome.

Diagnosis

The sonographic diagnosis of omphalocele is made by the demonstration of a mass adjacent to the anterior abdominal wall (Figs 17.2 and 17.3). The hernia should be in the midline and be covered with a membrane continuous with the umbilical cord, which inserts into the hernia (Fig. 17.2B). The main differential diagnosis is gastroschisis, which lacks a surrounding membrane and is separate from the cord insertion. These findings permit an accurate diagnosis in most cases, except those rare instances where rupture of the amnioperitoneal sac occurs *in utero*.[16] Diagnosis of an omphalocele is possible from around 12

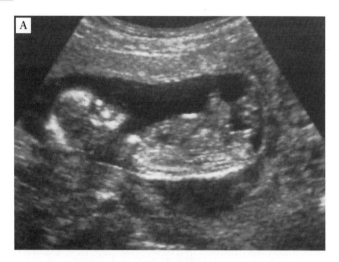
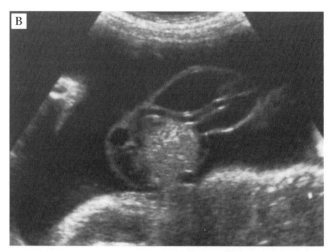

Fig. 17.2 Omphalocele at 14 and 32 weeks. A: Longitudinal scan showing a small omphalocele at 14 weeks, which is about the earliest time the diagnosis can be made because of the physiological herniation seen prior to this. B: Same patient at 32 weeks gestation, showing detail of the umbilical vessels entering the sac of the omphalocele.

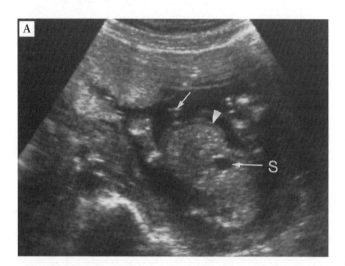
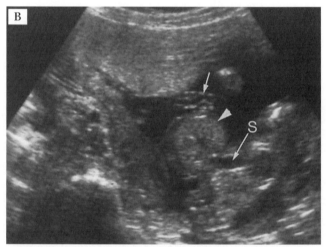

Fig. 17.3 Omphalocele at 18 weeks. A: Longitudinal and B: transverse scans of an omphalocele (arrowhead) at 18 weeks gestation showing the typical features. S – stomach, cord – arrow.

weeks gestation. However, prior to this the diagnosis should be made with caution to avoid confusion with the physiological herniation of the gut which occurs normally.

Management and prognosis

Any fetus with an omphalocele should undergo careful sonographic examination for associated anomalies, fetal echocardiography and karyotyping. It has been suggested that the ultrasound appearances can help determine the risk of a chromosomal anomaly in a fetus with an omphalocele. In most cases with an abnormal karyotype there will be an additional major malformation, or marker such as a digital, facial or renal anomaly. Cases without liver in the sac, which are usually the smaller defects, have

been found to have a higher incidence of karyotypic abnormalities.[17] If Beckwith–Wiedmann is suspected karyotyping should be performed and the laboratory asked to exclude abnormalities of 11p or uniparental disomy.[18] In cases with a normal karyotype but other abnormalities the prognosis will depend on the nature of those abnormalities. In all cases where the pregnancy continues serial ultrasonography should be performed to monitor fetal growth.

In cases where the lesion is isolated the prognosis is very good. A small defect can usually be closed in a single operation; larger ones may require a two-stage procedure and the infant may suffer some respiratory compromise. The majority will survive surgery and the long-term prognosis is good.

The mode of delivery for fetuses with this abnormality is still a subject for debate as there has been no good randomised study comparing the outcome of vaginal versus abdominal delivery. In two retrospective uncontrolled studies there was no obvious benefit gained from caesarean section.[2,19]

Gastroschisis

Definition and aetiology

Gastroschisis is a prenatal evisceration of abdominal contents through a full-thickness para-umbilical defect in the anterior abdominal wall, usually to the right of the umbilical cord, which has a normal insertion (Fig. 17.4). There is no covering membrane and the defect is usually small. Loops of bowel are most commonly herniated through the defect. These often become thickened and matted together because of inflammation induced by contact with amniotic fluid, or as a result of ischaemia following torsion of the bowel. Occasionally stomach or liver may herniate through the defect. Gastroschisis occurs in about 1 in 12 000 live births,[1] but has increased in incidence over recent years.[20]

Associated abnormalities

Gastroschisis is usually an isolated lesion, reports of associated anomalies (excluding intestinal atresias etc.) varying from 2.5% to 24%.[1,3,4,9] Congenital heart defects have been noted in up to 8.5% of cases.[4] Other associated malformations include diaphragmatic defects,[1] neural tube defects[6] and mild abnormalities of the renal tract, particularly hydronephrosis and horseshoe kidney.[9,22] It may be associated with amyoplasia[23] and it has also been seen as part of the amnion rupture sequence.[22,24] Association with an abnormal karyotype appears to be exceedingly rare.[25]

However, in up to 25% of cases there may be gastrointestinal problems owing to vascular impairment and adhesions. These include bowel malrotation, intestinal atresias and stenosis.[4,26]

Most cases of gastroschisis are sporadic and the recurrence risk is less than 1%.

Diagnosis

Sonographically a gastroschisis is characterised by an irregular mass, which has been likened to a cauliflower or a bunch of grapes, in front of the fetal abdomen. It has no membranous covering and frequently loops of bowel may be seen floating outside the abdominal wall attached to mesentery (Figs 17.5 and 17.6). The umbilical cord inserts normally, close to and usually to the left of the defect (Fig. 17.7). The diagnosis may be made from 12 weeks

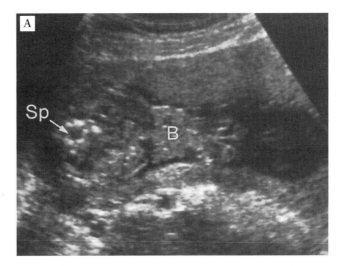

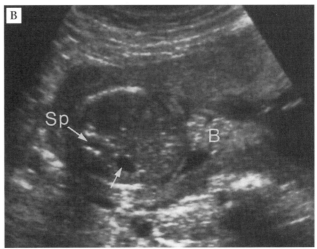

Fig. 17.5 Gastroschisis. A and **B:** Cross-sectional views of a 17-week fetus with a gastroschisis demonstrating the herniated bowel (B), spine (Sp) and stomach (arrow).

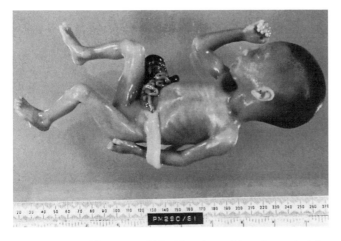

Fig. 17.4 Fetus with a gastroschisis. Note the cord insertion to the left of the defect in the anterior abdominal wall.

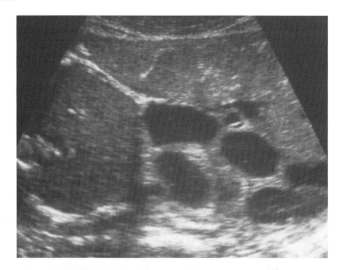

Fig. 17.6 Gastroschisis with dilated loops of bowel. A 37-week fetus with a gastroschisis, showing the liver, placenta and dilated loops of herniated bowel with thickened walls.

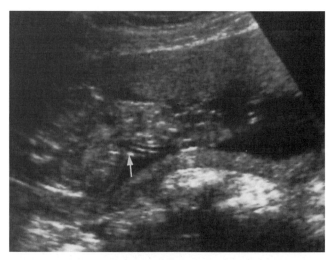

Fig. 17.7 A 17-week fetus with a gastroschisis showing the spine, herniated bowel and cord insertion (arrow) to the side of the hernia.

gestation onwards. False-negative and false-positive prenatal diagnoses of gastroschisis have been reported.[27] Two false negatives have been described, one in which the diagnosis was considered but rejected (the abnormal structure seen was thought to be an oedematous cord) and the other where the diagnosis was missed on a routine scan for fetal growth at 29 weeks. One of two false-positive cases was found (at subsequent caesarean section) to have an abruption of the placenta, matted cord and blood clot having caused the confusion. In the other case oligohydramnios following premature rupture of the membranes impaired imaging.

Prognosis and management

A fetus found to have a gastroschisis should have a detailed anomaly scan and echocardiography. In cases where the pregnancy continues serial scans should be performed to monitor fetal growth. Where the lesion is isolated the prognosis is good, although premature delivery may result in death from respiratory distress syndrome. Sepsis may also be life threatening. In a recent series reported from University College Hospital 86% of neonates who underwent surgical repair of a gastroschisis survived. Two of those who died had multiple congenital abnormalities, two of the others died from sepsis and two had short bowel syndrome. Elective delivery around 37 weeks may be advisable to prevent increased matting of the bowel wall, which can theoretically result in further complications.

As with omphalocele, the mode of delivery for neonates with a gastroschisis is open to debate, with no clear advantage to either abdominal or vaginal delivery.[2,19]

Body stalk anomaly

Definition and aetiology

Body stalk anomaly is an extensive defect in the anterior abdominal wall due to failed formation of the body stalk. Absence of the umbilicus and umbilical cord causes adherence of the placenta to the herniated viscera (Fig. 17.8). The incidence is about one in 14 000 births.[6]

Associated abnormalities

These are common and generally severe. They include defects of the intestinal and genitourinary tracts, heart, lungs and skeletal system. A marked scoliosis is one of the most frequent and characteristic associations. Neural tube defects are particularly common.[28]

Diagnosis

Prenatal diagnosis has been reported using maternal serum α-fetoprotein (MSAFP) and ultrasound.[6,29,30] Sonographically the fetus is particularly immobile and apparently attached to the placenta at the site of the abdominal wall defect (Fig. 17.9). No free loops of umbilical cord are visible.[29,30] This diagnosis may also be made from around 12 weeks gestation.

Prognosis and management

This condition is invariably fatal[6,28] and, if detected before viability, the option of termination should be discussed.

Anterior abdominal wall defects cause elevation in the MSAFP[6] and therefore examination of the ventral wall is

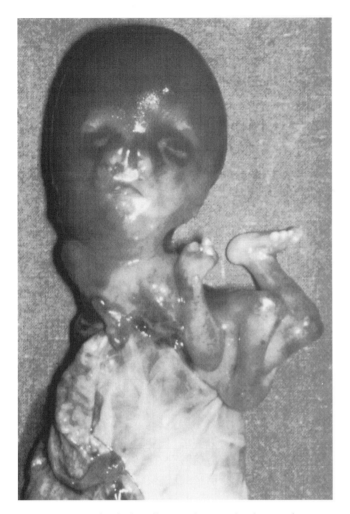

Fig. 17.8 Fetus with a body stalk anomaly. Note the absence of umbilical cord and membranes adherent to the anterior abdominal wall at the site of the defect. Figure courtesy of D. Donnai.

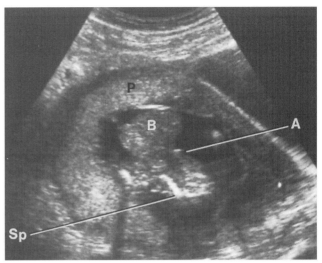

Fig. 17.9 Fetus with a body stalk anomaly. Note the acutely curved spine (Sp), the defect in the anterior abdominal wall (A) and the herniated contents (B), which are attached to the placenta (P).

a prerequisite part of the sonographic examination in all pregnancies complicated by raised MSAFP.

Bladder and cloacal exstrophy

Definition and aetiology

These anomalies are caused by the maldevelopment of the caudal fold of the anterior abdominal wall (see Ch. 6). In bladder exstrophy the anterior wall of the bladder is absent, exposing the posterior wall. Cloacal exstrophy is a more complex anomaly, where the posterior bladder wall protrudes through the anterior abdominal wall as with bladder exstrophy, but in addition to the ureters opening into the protruded mucosa, the ileum opens at the umbilical end and the blind-ending colon at the caudal end of the defect. The anus is absent.

Bladder exstrophy occurs in between 1/10 000 and 1/50 000 births, and is twice as common in males as in females.[31] Exstrophy of the cloaca is very rare and only occurs once in 200 000 births.[32] Most cases of exstrophy are sporadic and the recurrence risk in a family is 1%.[33,34]

Associated abnormalities

Associated abnormalities are rare in bladder exstrophy but common in cloacal exstrophy.[35] Renal anomalies occur in 60%, skeletal defects (spina bifida in particular) in 72%, omphalocele in 87%, cardiovascular abnormalities in 16%, and other gastrointestinal abnormalities in 10.5% of cases with cloacal exstrophy.[35–37]

Diagnosis

Prenatal diagnosis of both forms of exstrophy has been reported.[38,39] The diagnosis of bladder exstrophy was suspected[38] because of a solid mass in the lower part of the fetal abdomen and the inability to demonstrate a bladder despite the presence of normal amounts of amniotic fluid (Fig. 17.10). There was excessive mobility of the fetal pelvic girdle when pressure was exerted with the ultrasound transducer because of failed development of the pubic bones. The differential diagnosis of cloacal exstrophy includes omphalocele and gastroschisis. Visualisation of a normal bladder and the relationship of the mass to the anterior abdominal wall are helpful features in the precise delineation of the defect.

Management and prognosis

The main problems associated with bladder exstrophy are urinary incontinence, the anterior abdominal wall defect

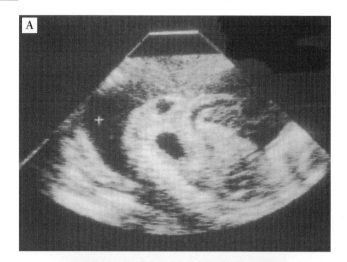

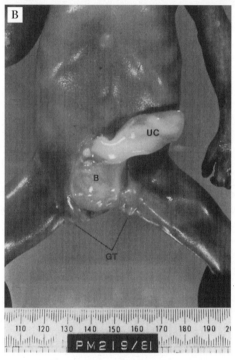

Fig. 17.10 Bladder exstrophy. A: Ultrasound findings in a fetus subsequently shown to have bladder exstrophy. B: Shows the fetus with bladder (B) exposed, umbilical cord (UC) and the genital tubercles (GT). Note the wide spacing of the pelvic bones.

and variable deformities of the external genitalia, which can be serious enough in the male to require sex reassignment in up to 2% of cases.[31] In the female genital defects are more easily repaired, although vaginal dilatation and perineoplasty may be required for satisfactory sexual function. Urinary incontinence can be treated surgically by primary bladder closure and reconstruction of the bladder neck, or by urinary diversion and cystectomy.[31] Fertility is reduced in both males and females and the risk of their having an affected offspring is increased to 1 in 70.[34]

Cloacal exstrophy is a much more serious problem, often with a high risk of mortality. However, a recent report has suggested that this can be reduced by optimal surgical management.[37] Untreated infants die from sepsis, short bowel syndrome, renal or central nervous system defects. The surgical approach to repair consists of a series of operations in the first few years of life, including early closure of the anterior abdominal wall defect and the bladder, continence surgery in early childhood, and vaginal reconstruction in the teenage years. There is usually considerable difficulty in creating a functional penis, and sex reassignment may be required in affected males.[40] The ultimate prognosis in cases where there is successful surgical repair depends also on the presence of other abnormalities which may confer considerable disability.

If the diagnosis of exstrophy is made before viability then termination of pregnancy is an option that should be considered. After this time no alteration in obstetric care is required, although delivery in a centre with neonatal surgical facilities is advisable. Following delivery the exposed bladder should be covered by an impermeable wrap and fluid and electrolyte balance carefully monitored. Full assessment of the gastrointestinal and urinary systems is needed prior to surgery.

Intestinal obstructions

Oesophageal atresia

Definition and aetiology

Oesophageal atresia is the congenital absence of a segment of the oesophagus. In most cases there is an associated tracheo-oesophageal fistula. The major variations seen in tracheo-oesophageal fistula are shown in Figure 17.11, the first variant (a) being the most common, occurring in about 80% of cases. Oesophageal atresia (with or without tracheo-oesophageal fistula) occurs in about 2/10 000 live births.[41]

Associated abnormalities

In infants with oesophageal atresia the incidence of associated abnormalities ranges from 40% to 57%.[42] Cardiovascular abnormalities (29%) are the most common association, with anorectal (14%), other gastrointestinal and genitourinary problems (14%) also occurring frequently. Several syndromes are associated with oesophageal atresia. These include the VATER (vertebral defects, anorectal malformation, tracheo-oesophageal fistula, renal anomaly and radial dysplasia) and schisis associations (cleft lip and palate, omphalocele and hypogenitalism).[42,43] Oesophageal atresia has been reported in association with aneuploidy, in particular trisomy 18,[42,44] Down's syndrome and other karyotypic

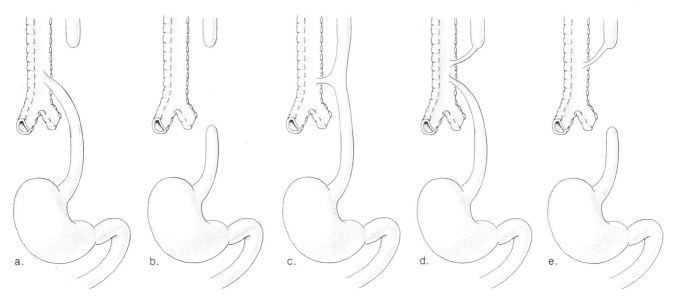

Fig. 17.11 Oesophageal atresia and tracheo-oesophageal fistula. Diagram showing the major variations seen in tracheo-oesophageal fistula. The first (a) is the most common. Only in types (b) and (e) will ultrasound be able to establish the diagnosis because of an empty stomach.

abnormalities.[42,44] Most cases of isolated oesophageal atresia with or without tracheo-oesophageal fistula are sporadic and the recurrence risk to siblings is very low.[44]

Diagnosis

The diagnosis of oesophageal atresia is suspected when, in the presence of polyhydramnios, repeated examinations fail to demonstrate a fetal stomach. These signs are almost invariably absent if there is a tracheo-oesophageal fistula, as the stomach will fill passively via the trachea. Thus relatively few cases of oesophageal atresia are amenable to prenatal diagnosis. In the few cases reported in the literature prenatal diagnosis has been made in the third trimester, when ultrasonography has been performed because of polyhydramnios.[45–47] However, it should be possible to make the diagnosis earlier following persistent failure to demonstrate a fetal stomach.

Management and prognosis

In cases where oesophageal atresia is suspected a detailed anomaly scan, echocardiography and fetal karyotyping should be performed to exclude associated anomalies. Survival depends on the presence of coexisting anomalies and karyotypic abnormalities. The prognosis in those with an isolated lesion born at term is excellent following postnatal surgery. Primary repair or bowel interposition generally result in good long-term survival. In the remainder, where there are other abnormalities or prematurity, the outlook is poorer. Chittmittrapap *et al.*[42] report a survival of 70% in such cases, the major cause of death being cardiac complications.

Duodenal obstruction

Definition and aetiology

Duodenal atresia or stenosis occurs in about 2/10 000 births and is the most common form of small bowel obstruction.[48] The blockage is usually caused by a membrane or web across the lumen of the bowel. Less commonly it results from a blind-ending loop of bowel, or atresia of large portions of intestine. In about 20% of cases an annular pancreas coexists.[49]

Associated abnormalities

Duodenal obstruction is an isolated abnormality in 30–50% of cases.[49,50] In the remainder the condition may be associated with congenital heart disease (8–20%), vertebral and skeletal deformities (37%), other intestinal anomalies (26%) and genitourinary malformations (8%). One-third of cases of duodenal obstruction are associated with trisomy 21,[48–52] but in these there are usually other sonographic abnormalities detected.

Diagnosis

Duodenal obstruction may be diagnosed on a transverse abdominal scan by demonstration of the typical 'double-bubble' (Fig. 17.12) appearance of the dilated stomach and proximal duodenum. A connection between the two structures must be demonstrated at the pylorus (Fig. 17.13). This abnormality is not usually evident at a routine 18–20-week scan but is more often detected later in pregnancy, when the patient presents for an anomaly scan because of polyhydramnios. There are, however, a

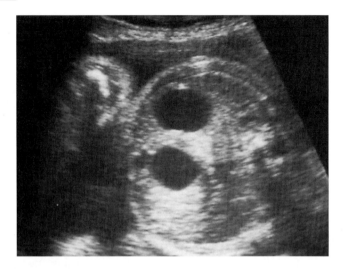

Fig. 17.12 A 32-week fetus with duodenal atresia demonstrating the typical 'double-bubble' appearance and proximal duodenum.

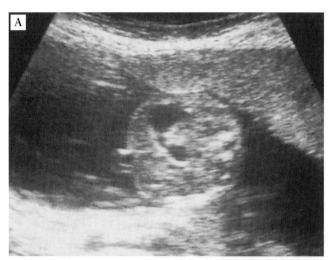

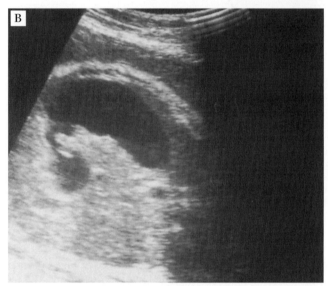

Fig. 17.13 Duodenal atresia at 24 and 36 weeks. A: Fetus at 24 weeks and **B:** again at 36 weeks, demonstrating the pylorus connecting the stomach and proximal duodenum. Note the associated polyhydramnios.

few reports of the diagnosis being made between 19 and 23 weeks.[25,53] The main differential diagnosis is that of an abdominal cyst, where two fluid structures may also be seen, one corresponding to the normal stomach and the other to the cyst. However, in these cases there is usually no polyhydramnios and no connection can be demonstrated between the two fluid-filled spaces.

Management and prognosis

The management of any fetus found to have duodenal atresia should include a detailed scan to detect associated abnormalities, echocardiography and karyotyping. When the duodenal atresia is isolated the prognosis is excellent. In the recent GOS series there was a 97% survival rate, of the 30 cases. The one death occurred in a child who had multiple anomalies. Duodenal atresia may be associated with prematurity because of the polyhydramnios, which may cause preterm labour, and the resultant prematurity may worsen the prognosis. Prenatal diagnosis may decrease morbidity from vomiting, aspiration pneumonia, electrolyte imbalance and stomach perforation by alerting the neonatologist to the increased risks.[54] Some would argue that delivery in a specialised centre is desirable in order to expedite surgical repair; however, in the series reported here from GOS all infants were *ex utero* transfers.

Other small bowel obstructions

Incidence and aetiology

Jejunal and ileal atresia and stenosis are less common than duodenal atresia and occur in less than 1/10 000 births. The most common sites are in the distal ileum (36%), proximal jejunum (31%), distal jejunum (20%) and prox-

imal ileum (13%). They are thought to be due to fibrosis following an intra-uterine vascular accident.[43,55] Small bowel obstruction can also result from meconium ileus, in which viscid, thick meconium accumulates and obstructs the distal ileum.

Associated abnormalities

Small bowel atresias and stenosis are usually isolated but may be seen in association with other intestinal anomalies.[56,57] Association with an abnormal karyotype is rare but has been reported.[44,57] Cases secondary to meconium ileus have a significant association with cystic fibrosis, and babies who are small for dates because of placental insufficiency.[58,59] Cystic fibrosis is an autosomal recessive disorder and therefore parents who have had one child with this condition have a 25% chance of a recurrence in future pregnancies, although not all recurrences will present with meconium ileus. Accurate diagnosis for most parents can now be performed using molecular biological techniques.

In uncomplicated cases of small bowel atresia the recurrence risk is small;[60,61] however, where multiple atresias are present there may be a significant risk of recurrence.

Diagnosis

Small bowel obstructions may be suspected when multiple fluid-filled spaces are seen within the fetal abdomen (Figs 17.14 and 17.15). The differential diagnosis includes other conditions capable of causing multiple echo-free areas in the fetal abdomen (duodenal atresia, hydronephrosis, multicystic kidney etc.). Usually the 'cysts' can be recognised as distended loops of bowel because of peristaltic activity and floating particles within the lumen.[62]

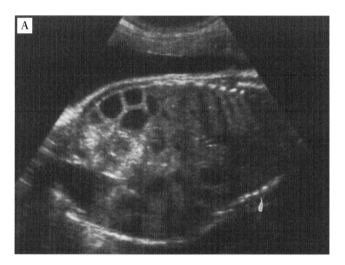
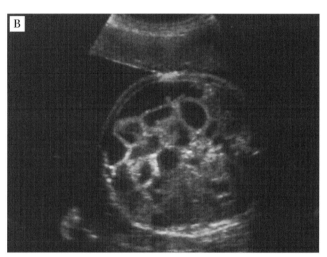

Fig. 17.14 Small bowel atresia. A: Longitudinal and **B:** cross-sectional views of a fetus with small bowel atresia, showing multiple echo-free areas corresponding to loops of dilated bowel. Note the associated polyhydramnios.

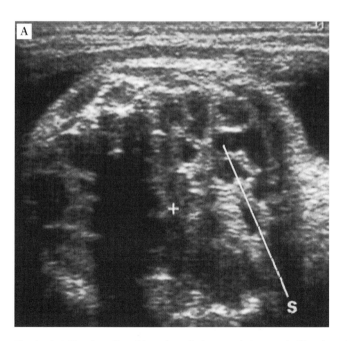
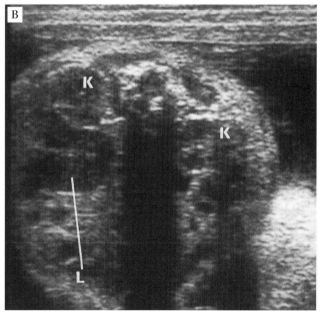

Fig. 17.15 Dilated small and large bowel. A 32-week fetus with dilated small (S) and large (L) bowel. K – kidneys.

Furthermore, careful examination will demonstrate a normal stomach and renal tract. As with the other intestinal atresias the diagnosis is usually not made until late in the second or third trimester, when the fetus is scanned for some obstetric reason. Polyhydramnios may occur in cases of jejunal atresia but is less common when the obstruction is more distal.[62,63] Meconium ileus has been diagnosed at 18 weeks in cases known to be at risk of cystic fibrosis. Increased reflectivity of the intra-abdominal (intestinal) contents is found[58] or, later in pregnancy, classic signs of small bowel obstruction may be observed.[64]

Prognosis and management

The prognosis for infants with isolated intestinal atresia is good. However, if multiple atresias are present short bowel syndrome may result, requiring parenteral nutrition with its concomitant complications.[57] Neonates with meconium ileus have a variable prognosis, depending on the gestational age at delivery and the underlying pathology.

Large bowel obstruction

Incidence and aetiology

Atresia and stenosis of the large bowel occur very rarely and account for less than 10% of all intestinal atresias.[65] Most cases of large bowel atresia are thought to be the result of a vascular accident, volvulus or intussusception.[55] The reported incidences for anal atresia vary from 1/2500 to 1/3300 live births.[66] Hirschsprung's disease, caused by varying lengths of aganglionic bowel, can also give the appearance of bowel obstruction.[67] This condition occurs in 1/8000 births and affects males more commonly than females.[68]

The recurrence risk for large bowel atresia is usually quoted as about 1%. Isolated anal atresia also carries a low risk of recurrence, but where it occurs as part of a syndrome the recurrence risk is as for the syndrome. For Hirschsprung's disease the risk depends on whether the index case was male or female, and whether it was long- or short-segment disease.[68]

Associated abnormalities

Colonic atresias are usually isolated lesions. Up to 70% of anal atresias and stenoses are associated with other anomalies, particularly those involving the vertebrae, trachea, oesophagus and renal tract (VATER association). There are also many syndromes that include anal atresia.[69] Trisomy 21 occurs in 2% of cases of Hirschsprung's disease.

Diagnosis

In contrast to small bowel obstruction the diagnosis of large bowel obstruction may be difficult in that, as a result of fluid absorption by the colonic mucosa, there may be little or no proximal dilatation. Furthermore, because obstruction of either the small or the large intestine may result in grossly enlarged loops of bowel, prenatal identification of the precise site of obstruction may not be possible. In some cases the haustral pattern may help to localise the obstruction to the large bowel (Fig. 17.15). Polyhydramnios, on the other hand, usually indicates small bowel obstruction. It must be remembered that there is considerable variability in the appearance of the bowel in the third trimester, such that in some cases suspicion of obstruction may arise in a perfectly normal fetus (Fig. 17.16).

Prenatal diagnosis of anal atresia has been reported in the third trimester.[70] Fluid-filled loops of bowel were seen in the lower abdomen in the absence of polyhydramnios. We have recently made the diagnosis in a fetus at 22 weeks gestation (Fig. 17.17). A fluid-filled lesion was seen arising from the perineal region behind the bladder and extending up into the abdomen in the position of the sigmoid colon. Peristalsis could be seen and there was no polyhydramnios.

A precise diagnosis of Hirschsprung's disease in a fetus is difficult in the absence of a positive family history. In a case with progressive dilatation of the large bowel late in the third trimester, the differential diagnosis was between Hirschsprung's disease, colonic atresia and imperforate anus.[67]

Management and prognosis

These abnormalities are rarely detected before viability. A careful search for other abnormalities should be made in order to try to define the prognosis more precisely.

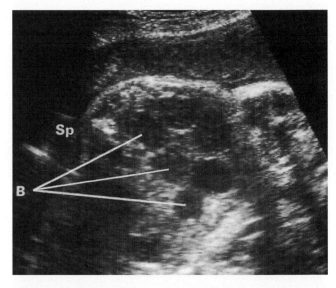

Fig. 17.16 Normal bowel. A normal 37-week fetus, showing the bowel (B) and spine (Sp).

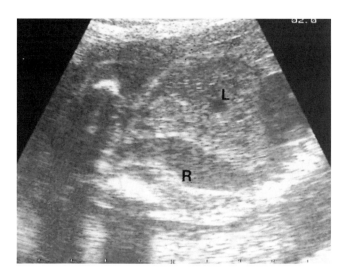

Fig. 17.17 Anal atresia. A longitudinal view of a 22-week fetus with anal atresia, showing liver (L), thorax and dilated rectosigmoid colon (R).

However, in most cases the definitive diagnosis must await delivery and the results of post-natal investigations. Usually there is no reason to depart from normal obstetric practice, but delivery in a centre where there is easy access to paediatric surgical facilities may be advised.

The prognosis for isolated large bowel or anal atresia is excellent. The outcome in cases of imperforate anus associated with other abnormalities or syndromes will depend on the severity of these associations. The prognosis in cases of Hirschsprung's disease depends on the length of bowel involved. Mortality rates of up to 20% in infancy have been reported, but these figures do not include cases where the diagnosis is suspected prenatally. In these cases some of the complications secondary to delay in diagnosis could be avoided (enterocolitis, caecal perforation, malnutrition etc.), thereby possibly improving the prognosis.

Meconium peritonitis

Definition and aetiology

Meconium peritonitis occurs as a result of peritoneal inflammation following intra-uterine bowel perforation. Although it is rare, several cases have been diagnosed prenatally.[71,72] In 25–40% of cases it is secondary to the meconium ileus of cystic fibrosis.[73,74] In some cases the aetiology is unclear, and in others the perforation occurs proximal to an intestinal atresia or stenosis. Two types of fetal meconium peritonitis have been described: the fibro-adhesive and the cystic varieties. In the former there is an intense inflammatory reaction of the peritoneum leading to the formation of a dense calcified mass, which seals off the perforation. In the other type the perforation is not sealed and loops of bowel become fixed around the perforation site, forming a cystic cavity into which meconium continues to leak.

Associated abnormalities

The only significant extra-abdominal associations are those of cystic fibrosis.[73,74] The other major associations are the underlying cause of the bowel obstruction which has resulted in perforation, e.g. intestinal atresia, volvulus.

Diagnosis

The presence of a highly reflective intra-abdominal mass is suggestive of meconium peritonitis, particularly if associated with ascites and polyhydramnios, though the diagnosis should still be suspected in their absence. The differential diagnosis includes intra-abdominal haemorrhage, early ascites, fetal hypoxia, cystic fibrosis, tumour (haemangioma, teratoma, ovarian dermoid, hepatoblastoma, metastatic neuroblastoma) and fetal gallstones, but these are not usually associated with polyhydramnios.

Management and prognosis

The main diagnosis to be excluded is that of cystic fibrosis. Measurement of amniotic fluid intestinal isoenzymes and alkaline phosphatase can assist in this,[75] but with the identification of the gene for cystic fibrosis[76] and mutations within this gene it is more accurate to screen first the parents and then the fetus, if appropriate, for abnormalities in the gene. Delivery in a tertiary centre is advisable, as neonates with meconium peritonitis require immediate surgical care.

Meconium peritonitis is a serious condition with a mortality rate as high as 62% reported for those neonates who undergo surgery.[73] However, this figure does not include cases diagnosed prenatally, and it is clear that early diagnosis and treatment improves the survival. Of eight prenatally diagnosed cases, five survived, one pregnancy was electively terminated and deaths occurred in two premature neonates.[71,72,77–81]

Intra-abdominal cystic lesions

Abdominal cystic masses are frequent findings on fetal ultrasound examination. Dilated bowel or renal tract anomalies are the most common explanation, although cystic structures may arise from most abdominal or pelvic organs. It may not be possible to make a precise diagnosis prenatally, but the most likely diagnosis is usually suggested by the position of the cyst, its relationship to other structures and the normality of other organs.

Choledochal cyst

Definition and aetiology

A choledochal cyst is a cystic bile duct dilatation, usually single, but in rare instances multiple. It is usually found in the common bile duct, but can involve the intrahepatic or extrahepatic portions of the biliary tree. It is a rare disorder in the western world, with the majority of cases being reported in Japan.[82] It is a sporadic occurrence and there are no reported cases of recurrence within a family. The cause of the dilatation is controversial and may be due to weakness in the duct wall, distal obstruction causing increased pressure and hence proximal dilatation, or a combination of both.

Associated anomalies

No specific associations have been described.

Diagnosis

There are several reports of prenatal diagnosis of choledochal cyst.[83–86] The diagnosis was suggested by the visualisation of an echo-free non-pulsatile area in the right of the fetal abdomen near the portal vein. In two cases the diagnosis was confirmed by defining dilated hepatic ducts near or leading to the cyst.[84,86]

The differential diagnosis includes duodenal atresia and cysts in other intra-abdominal organs, such as the liver, mesentery, omentum and ovary.

The definition of normal abdominal organs together with the absence of polyhydramnios, peristalsis in the cyst or a connection with the stomach, helps exclude other diagnoses, but a definitive diagnosis is dependent on the visualisation of a tubular structure arising from the cyst and passing into the liver parenchyma.

Management and prognosis

Choledochal cysts are usually detected in the third trimester and there seems to be no indication to alter standard obstetric practice. If the findings are confirmed in the neonate then surgery is indicated, as untreated cysts can lead to progressive biliary cirrhosis and portal hypertension.[87]

Ovarian cysts

Definition and aetiology

Ovarian cysts are quite rare. They are usually unilateral and vary in size from a few millimetres in diameter to a large cyst that fills the entire abdomen. The majority are benign simple cysts such as theca lutein cysts or corpus luteal cysts, although granulosa cell tumours and teratomas have been reported in neonates.[87]

Associated abnormalities

There is one case reported with associated hydrocephalus and agenesis of the corpus callosum.[88] In other cases hypo-

thyroidism has been diagnosed in children with ovarian cysts.[89]

Diagnosis

This diagnosis has been reported several times, usually late in the second or third trimester, and may be suspected when a female fetus has an intra-abdominal cystic lesion which is separate from the renal or gastrointestinal tracts.[88,90–93] They may be septate or unilocular, and typically arise from the pelvis or lower abdomen. They are usually unilateral, although bilateral cases have been reported, and may measure up to several centimetres in diameter (Fig. 17.18). Resolution *in utero* has been reported.[93] The differential diagnosis includes urachal and

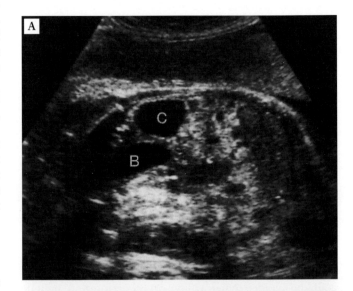

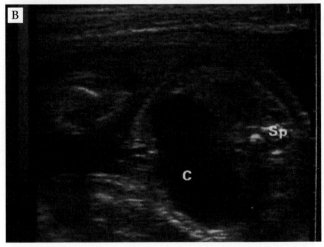

Fig. 17.18 Ovarian cyst. A: Longitudinal view of a fetus with an ovarian cyst showing normal bladder (B) with a large ovarian cyst (C) arising from the pelvis. **B:** Transverse scan in another case showing a large central lower abdominal cyst. Sp – spine.

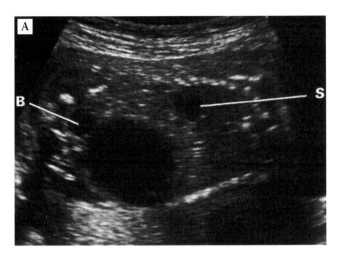
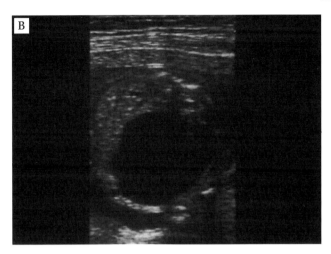

Fig. 17.19 Duplication cyst. A: Longitudinal and **B:** transverse views of a 20-week female fetus with what was thought prenatally to be an ovarian cyst and which was drained several times during pregnancy. Post-natally at laparotomy this was found to be a duodenal duplication cyst, thus demonstrating the difficulty in correctly identifying some intra-abdominal cystic lesions with ultrasound. Note the normal stomach (S) and bladder (B).

mesenteric cysts, duodenal atresia and duplication cysts and dilated bowel. Absence of peristaltic movements helps exclude dilated bowel, and absence of the typical 'double bubble' makes duodenal atresia an unlikely diagnosis. A urachal cyst is single and lies in the anterior part of the fetal abdomen, extending from the bladder to the umbilicus. It may be impossible to exclude the diagnosis of other intra-abdominal cystic lesions prenatally (Fig. 17.19).

Management and prognosis

Serial ultrasound examinations are recommended to monitor the growth of the cyst. Provided it remains small standard obstetric practice can be followed, but where the cyst grows to very large proportions there is a risk of dystocia or rupture during vaginal delivery. In such a case an elective caesarean section is a reasonable approach. Alternatively, ultrasound-guided aspiration of the cyst can be undertaken, despite the remote risk of spillage of an irritant or malignant fluid into the abdominal cavity.

The overall prognosis for a fetus with an ovarian cyst is good, as the majority are benign and many will resolve spontaneously. In the neonate large cysts can infarct, undergo torsion, cause ascites, rupture, bleed or cause intestinal obstruction. Torsion *in utero* has been reported in the case of a large cyst.[93]

Other intra-abdominal cysts

Definition and aetiology

These include cysts which are found in the mesentery of the large or small bowel (mesenteric cysts), cysts of the omentum (omental cysts) and cysts which are located in the retroperitoneal space (retroperitoneal cysts). They are all rare, with mesenteric cysts occurring more commonly than omental cysts, which are more frequent than retroperitoneal cysts.[94] The cause of these cysts is unclear: they are generally considered to be lymphatic hamartomas. They are usually single and multilocular, and can vary in size from a few millimetres to several centimetres. The fluid they contain may be serous, chylous or haemorrhagic.

Associated abnormalities

There are no recognised associations reported.

Diagnosis

These cysts should be considered in the differential diagnosis of any intra-abdominal cystic lesion. Other potential diagnoses include ovarian, pancreatic, choledochal and hepatic cysts, and duodenal atresia. In a female the most likely diagnosis is that of an ovarian cyst. Other diagnoses can be excluded by careful delineation of abdominal organs, but it may prove impossible to make a precise diagnosis prenatally. A mesenteric cyst may cause unilateral hydronephrosis by obstructing the ureter.

Management and prognosis

These cysts are often asymptomatic and found incidentally at surgery for some other indication. The clinical manifestation depends on their size and location. Most are benign, but malignant degeneration has been described in adulthood.[95] Retroperitoneal cysts have a high tendency to recur, as complete excision is difficult owing to their close proximity to major blood vessels.[95]

Serial ultrasound examinations should be performed to monitor the size of the cysts prenatally. Unless they grow to such proportions that there is a danger of rupture during vaginal delivery, standard obstetric practice should be followed. Aspiration may be considered to avoid caesarean section.

Hepatosplenomegaly

Incidence and aetiology

Isolated hepatomegaly or splenomegaly are rare and they more commonly occur together in a variety of conditions. Some of the more common causes in the neonate are given in Table 17.1. These include immune and non-immune hydrops, haemolytic anaemias, congenital infections, metabolic disorders and neoplastic conditions. Hepatosplenomegaly also occurs as part of the Beckwith–Wiedemann and Perlman syndromes.

Associated abnormalities

The associated abnormalities vary according to the underlying pathology.

Diagnosis

Hepatosplenomegaly is diagnosed when their sizes lie outside the 95th percentile on the nomograms that exist for evaluation of their size (see Appendix).[96,97]

Tumours can cause diffuse enlargement or a change in the sonographic appearance of all or part of the liver. Calcification within the liver suggests congenital infection or hepatoblastoma. In the latter case the MSAFP is raised in over 80% of cases. Congenital infections may also cause other structural abnormalities in the fetus (microcephaly, congenital heart defects), which can be detectable with ultrasound. An isolated echo-poor area within the liver may be a solitary cyst or an hepatic haemangioma, a benign tumour which can also give the appearance of a well circumscribed homogeneous intrahepatic mass.

Hepatosplenomegaly when found in conjunction with enlarged kidneys, a generally macrosomic fetus, and particularly if associated with polyhydramnios, suggests the diagnosis of an overgrowth syndrome such as Beckwith–Wiedemann, Perlman or Simpson–Golabi–Behmel syndromes. However, in low-risk cases it will rarely be possible to make a definitive diagnosis based on ultrasound findings alone.

Management and prognosis

Definitive diagnosis will often have to await the results of post-natal investigations. Haemolytic anaemias can be diagnosed either by cordocentesis or by analysis of the bilirubin content of amniotic fluid. Congenital infections can be detected by performing the appropriate tests on maternal serum or fetal blood. Where there is a positive family history many of the metabolic disorders can be diagnosed by analysis of amniotic fluid or fetal blood. In low-risk cases examination of white cell enzymes may prove useful.

The prognosis will depend on the aetiology of the hepatosplenomegaly.

Situs inversus

Situs inversus can be detected *in utero* if the left and right sides of the fetus are established by reference to the positions of the head and spine. If situs inversus abdominis is identified, special attention should be given to the cardiovascular anatomy (see Ch. 18).

Table 17.1 Causes of neonatal hepatosplenomegaly

Cause	Hepatomegaly	Splenomegaly
Bacterial infection	+	+
Viral infection	+	+
Toxoplasmosis	+	+
Syphilis	+	+
Congenital haemolytic anaemia	+	+
Isoimmunisation	+	+
Congestive heart failure	+	+
Leukaemia	–	+
Lymphoma	–	+
Haemangioma	+	+
Hamartoma	+	+
Hepatoblastoma	+	–
Metastatic tumour	+	–
Benign cyst	+	+
Galactosaemia	+	+
Zellweger syndrome	+	+
Other metabolic disorders	+	+
Beckwith–Weidemann syndrome	+	+
Perlman syndrome	+	–

REFERENCES

1 Baird P A, MacDonald E C. An epidemiologic study of congenital malformations of the anterior abdominal wall in more than half a million consecutive live births. Am J Hum Genet 1981; 33: 470–478

2 Carpenter M W, Curci M R, Dibbins A W, Haddow. Perinatal management of ventral wall defects. Obstet Gynecol 1984; 64: 646–651

3 Grosfield J L, Dawes L, Weber T R. Congenital abdominal wall defects: current management and survival. Surg Clin North Am 1981; 61: 1037–1049

4 Mayer T, Black R, Matlak M E, Johnson D G. Gastroschisis and omphalocele: an eight year review. Ann Surg 1980; 192: 783–787

5 Hauge M, Bugge M, Nielson J. Early prenatal diagnosis of omphalocele constitutes indication for amniocentesis. Lancet 1983; ii: 507

6 Mann L, Ferguson-Smith M A, Desai M, Gibson A A M, Raine P A M. Prenatal assessment of anterior abdominal wall defects and their prognosis. Prenat Diagn 1984; 4: 427–435

7 Gilbert W M, Nicolaides K H. Fetal omphalocele: associated malformations and chromosomal defects. Obstet Gynecol 1987; 70: 633–635

8   Nivelon-Chevallier A, Mavel A, Michels R et al. Familial Beckwith–Wiedemann syndrome: prenatal echography diagnosis and histologic confirmation. J Hum Genet 1983; 5: 397

9   Mabogunie O A, Mahour G H. Omphalocele and gastroschisis. Trends in survival across two decades. Am J Surg 148: 679–686

10   Winter R M, Knowles S A S, Bieber F R, Baraitser M (eds) Body wall defects. In: The malformed fetus and stillbirth: a diagnostic approach. Chichester: John Wiley, 1980; 134–143

11   Koontz W L, Shaw L A, Lavery J P. Antenatal sonographic appearance of Beckwith–Wiedemann syndrome. JCU 1986; 14: 57–59

12   Elliott M, Maher E R. Beckwith–Wiedemann syndrome. J Med Genet 1994; 31(7): 560–564.

13   Rott H D, Truckenbrodt H. Familial occurrence of omphalocele. Hum Genet 1974; 24: 259–260

14   Havalad S, Noblett H, Spiedel B D. Familial occurrence of omphalocele, suggesting sex-linked inheritance. Arch Dis Child 1979; 54: 142–151

15   Osuna A, Lindham S. Four cases of omphalocele in two generations of the same family. Clin Genet 1976; 9: 354–356

16   Harrison M R, Golbus M S, Filly R A. Management of the fetus with an abdominal wall defect. In: Orlando F L, ed. The unborn patient. Prenatal diagnosis and treatment. New York: Grune & Stratton, 1984; 217–234

17   Nyberg D A, Fitzsimmons J, Mack L A et al. Chromosomal abnormalities in fetuses with omphalocele. Significance of omphalocele contents. J Ultrasound Med 1989; 8(6): 299–308

18   Reik W, Brown K W, Schrend M. Imprinting mutations in the Beckwith–Wiedemann syndrome suggested by an altered imprinting pattern in the IGF^2-M domain. Hum Mol Genet 1995; 4: 2379–2385

19   Kirk E P, Wah R M. Obstetric management of the fetus with omphalocele or gastroschisis: a review and report of one hundred and twelve cases. Am J Obstet Gynecol 1983; 146: 512–518

20   Chitty L, Iskaros J. Congenital anterior abdominal wall defects. BMJ 1996; 313(7062): 891–892.

21   Reid COMV, Hall J G, Anderson C; Association of amyoplasia with gastroschisis, bowel atresia and defects of the muscle layers of the throat. Ann J Med Genet 1986 24: 701–710

22   Bair J H, Russ P D, Pretoious D H, Manchester D, Manco-Johnson M L. Fetal omphalocele and gastroschisis: a review of 24 cases. AJR 1986; 147: 1047–1051

23   Reid C O, Hall J G, Anderson C et al. Association of amyoplasia with gastroschisis, bowel atresia, and defects of the muscular layer of the trunk. Am J Med Genet 1986; 24(4): 701–710

24   Davidson J M, Johnson T R B, Rigdon D T, Thompson B H. Gastroschisis and omphalocele: prenatal diagnosis and perinatal management. Prenat Diagn 1984; 4: 355–363

25   Romero R, Pilu G, Jeanty P, Ghidini A, Hobbins J C. Prenatal diagnosis of congenital anomalies. Norwalk: Appleton and Lange, 1988

26   Gryboski J, Walker W A. Gastrointestinal problems in the infant. Philadelphia: W B Saunders, 1983: 284–287

27   Lindfors K K, McGahan J P, Walter J P. Fetal omphalocele and gastroschisis: pitfalls in sonographic diagnosis. AJR 1986; 147: 797–800

28   Potter E L, Craig J M. Diaphragmatic and abdominal hernias. In: Pathology of the fetus and infant. Chicago: Year Book Publishers, 1975: 374–392

29   Lockwood C J, Scioscia A L, Hobbins J C. Congenital absence of the umbilical cord resulting from maldevelopment of the embryonic body folding. Am J Obstet Gynecol 1986; 155: 1049–1051

30   Jauniaux E, Vyas S, Finlayson C, Moscoso G, Driver M, Campbell S. Early sonographic diagnosis of body stalk anomaly. Prenat Diagn 1990; 10: 127–132

31   Jeffs R D, Lepor H. Management of the exstrophy–epispadias complex and urachal anomalies. In: Walsh P C ed. Campbell's urology, Vol 2. Philadelphia: Saunders, 1986; 1882–1921

32   Graivier L. Extrophy of the cloaca. Am Surg 1968; 34: 387–390

33   Ives E, Coffey R, Carter C O. A family study of bladder exstrophy. J Med Genet 1980; 17: 139–141

34   Shapiro E, Lepor H, Jeffs R D. The inheritance of the exstrophy-epispadias complex. J Urol 1984; 132: 308–310

35   Muecke E C. Exstrophy, epispadias and other anomalies of the bladder. In: Walsh P C, ed. Campbell's urology, Vol 2. Philadelphia: W B Saunders, 1986; 1856–1880

36   Soper R T, Kilger K. Vesico-intestinal fissure. J Urol 1964; 92: 490–501

37   Howell C, Caldamone A, Snyder H, Ziegler M, Duckett J. Optimal management of cloacal exstrophy. J Pediatr Surg 1983; 18: 365–369

38   Mirk P, Calisti A, Fileni A. Prenatal sonographic diagnosis of bladder exstrophy. J Ultrasound Med 1936; 5: 291–293

39   Kutzner D K, Wilson W G, Hogge W A. OEIS complex (cloacal exstrophy); prenatal diagnosis in the second trimester. Prenat Diagn 1988; 8: 247–253

40   Tank E S, Lindenauer S M. Principles of management of exstrophy of the cloaca. Am J Surg 1980; 119: 95–98

41   David T J, O'Callaghan S E. Oesophageal atresia in the South-West of England. J Med Genet 1975; 12: 1–11

42   Chittmittrapap S, Spitz L, Kiely E M, Brereton R J. Oesophageal atresia and associated anomalies. Arch Dis Child 1989; 64: 364–368

43   Winter R M. Knowles S A S, Bieber F R, Baraitser M (eds). Abnormalities of the gastrointestinal tract. In: The malformed fetus and stillbirth. Chichester: John Wiley, 1988; 140–143

44   Smith F G, Berg J M, eds. Down's anomaly. Edinburgh: Churchill Livingstone, 1986; 14–41

45   Eyheremendy E, Pfister M. Antenatal real-time diagnosis of esophageal atresias. JCU 1983; 11: 395–397

46   Zemlyn S. Prenatal detection of esophageal atresia. JCU 1981; 9: 453–454

47   Rahmani M R, Zalev A H. Antenatal detection of esophageal atresia with distal tracheoesophageal fistula. JCU 1986; 14: 143–145

48   Fonkalsrud E W. Duodenal atresia or stenosis. In: Bergsma D, ed. Birth defects compendium. New York: Alan R. Liss, 1979; 350

49   Fonkalsrud E W, DeLorimier A A, Hays D N. Congenital atresia and stenosis of the duodenum. A review compiled from members of the surgical section of the American Academy of Pediatrics. Pediatrics 1969; 43: 79–83

50   Young D G, Wilkinson A W. Abnormalities associated with neonatal duodenal obstruction. Surgery 1968; 63: 832–836

51   Aubrespy P, Derlon S, Seriat-Gautier B. Congenital duodenal obstruction: a review of 82 cases. Prog Pediatr Surg 1982; 11: 109–123

52   Arwell J D, Klijian A M. Vertebral anomalies and duodenal atresia. J Pediatr Surg 1982; 17: 237–240

53   Nicolaides K H, Campbell S. Diagnosis and management of fetal malformations. Baillière's Clin Obstet Gynaecol 1: 1987; 591–622

54   Romero R, Ghidini A, Costigan K, Touloukian R, Hobbins J C. Prenatal diagnosis of duodenal atresia: does it make any difference? Obstet Gynecol 1988; 71: 739–741

55   Louw J H. Investigations into the etiology of congenital atresia of the colon. Dis Colon Rectum 1964; 7: 471–478

56   Bernstein J, Vawter G, Harris G B C, Young V, Hillman L S. The occurrence of intestinal atresia in newborns with meconium ileus. Am J Dis Child 1960; 99: 804–818

57   De Lorimier A, Fonkalsrud E W, Hays D M. Congenital atresia and stenosis of the jejunum and ileum. Pediatr Surg 1969; 65: 819–827

58   Muller F, Aubry M C, Gasser B, Duchatel F, Boue J, Boue A. Prenatal diagnosis of cystic fibrosis. II. Meconium ileus in affected fetuses. Prenat Diagn 1985; 5: 109–117

59   Blott M, Greenough A, Gamsu H R, Nicolaides K N, Campbell S. Antenatal factors associated with obstruction of the gastrointestinal tract by meconium. BMJ 1988; 296: 250

60   Guttman F M, Braun P, Garance P H et al. Multiple atresias and a new syndrome of hereditary multiple atresias involving the gastrointestinal tract from stomach to rectum. J Pediatr Surg 1973; 8: 633–640

61   Kao K J, Fleischer R, Bradford W D, Woodward B H. Multiple congenital septal atresias of the intestine: histomorphologic and pathogenic implications. Pediatr Pathol 1983; 1: 443–448

62   Kjoller M, Holm-Nielson G, Meiland H, Mauritzen K, Berget A, Hancke S. Prenatal obstruction of the ileum diagnosed by ultrasound. Prenat Diagn 1985; 5: 427–430

63   Lloyd I R, Chatsworth H W. Hydramnios as an aid to the early diagnosis of congenital obstruction of the alimentary tract. A study of the maternal and fetal factors. Pediatrics 1958; 24: 903–909

64   Shalev J, Navon R, Urbach D, Mashiach S, Goldman B. Intestinal obstruction and cystic fibrosis: antenatal ultrasound appearance. J Med Genet 1983; 20: 229–233

65   Freeman N V. Congenital atresia and stenosis of the colon. Br J Surg 1966; 53: 595–599

66   Ravitch M M, Barton B A. The need for pediatric surgeons as determined by the volume of work and the mode of delivery of surgical care. Surgery 1974; 76: 754–763

67 Vermesch M, Mayden K L, Confino E, Giglia R V, Gleicher N. Prenatal sonographic diagnosis of Hirschprung's disease. J Ultrasound Med 1986; 5: 37–39

68 Carter C O, Evans K, Hickman V. Children of those treated surgically for Hirschsprung's disease. J Med Genet 1981; 18: 87–90

69 Winter R M, Knowles S, Bieber F R, Baraitser M (eds). Genital and anal malformations. In: The malformed fetus and stillbirth: a diagnostic approach. Chichester: John Wiley, 1988; 160–165

70 Bean W J, Calonje M A, Aprill C N, Geshner J. Anal atresia: a prenatal ultrasound diagnosis. JCU 1978; 6: 111–112

71 Blumenthal D H, Rushovich A M, Williams R K, Rochester D. Prenatal sonographic findings of meconium peritonitis with pathologic correlation. JCU 1982; 10: 350–352

72 Schwimer S R, Vanley G T, Reinke R T. Prenatal diagnosis of cystic meconium peritonitis. JCU 1984; 12: 37–39

73 Bergsmans M G M, Merkus J M W, Baars A M. Obstetrical and neonatal aspects of a child with atresia of the small bowel. J Perinat Med 1984; 12: 325

74 Finkel L I, Solvis T L. Meconium peritonitis, intraperitoneal calcifications and cystic fibrosis. Pediatr Radiol 1982; 12: 92–93

75 Brock D J H, Bedgood D, Barron L, Hayward C. Prospective prenatal diagnosis of cystic fibrosis. Lancet 1985; i: 1175–1178

76 Riordan J R, Rommens J M, Kaerem B et al. Identification of the cystic fibrosis gene: cloning and characterisation of complementary DNA. Science 1989; 245: 1066–1072

77 Baxi L V, Yeh M N, Blanc W A, Schillinger J N. Antepartum diagnosis and management of in utero intestinal volvulus with perforation. N Engl J Med 1983; 308: 1519–1521

78 Clair M R, Rosenberg E R, Ram P C, Bowie J D. Prenatal sonographic diagnosis of meconium peritonitis. Prenat Diagn 1983; 3: 65–68

79 Garb M, Red F F, Riseborough J. Meconium peritonitis presenting as fetal ascites on ultrasound. Br J Radiol 1980; 53: 602–604

80 Lauer J D, Cradock T V. Meconium pseudocyst: Prenatal sonographic and radiologic correlation. J Ultrasound Med 1982; 1: 333–335

81 McGahan J P, Hanson F. Meconium peritonitis with accompanying pseudocyst; prenatal sonographic diagnosis. Radiology 1983; 148: 125–126

82 Gryboski J, Walker W A. Gastrointestinal problems in the infant. Philadelphia: W B Saunders, 1983; 309–312

83 Dewbury K C, Aluwihare A P R, Chir M, Birch S J, Freeman N V. Case reports. Prenatal ultrasound demonstration of a choledochal cyst. Br J Radiol 1980; 53: 906–907

84 Elrad H, Mayden K L, Ahart S, Giglia R, Gleicher N. Prenatal ultrasound diagnosis of choledochal cyst. J Ultrasound Med 1985; 4: 553–555

85 Frank J L, Hill M C, Chirathivat S, Sfakianakis G N, Marchildon M. Antenatal observation of a choledochal cyst by sonography. AJR 1981; 137: 166–168

86 Howell C G, Templeton J M, Weiner S. Glassman M, Betts J M, Witzleben. Antenatal diagnosis and early surgery for choledochal cyst. J Pediatr Surg 1983; 18: 387–393

87 Carlson D H, Griscom N T. Ovarian cysts in the newborn. AJR 1972; 116: 664–672

88 Sandler M A, Smith S J, Pope S G, Madrazo B L. Prenatal diagnosis of septated ovarian cysts. JCU 1985; 13: 55–57

89 Evers J L, Rolland R. Primary hypothyroidism and ovarian activity: evidence for an overlap in the synthesis of pituitary glycoproteins. Case report. Br J Obstet Gynaecol 1981; 88: 195–202

90 Tabsh K M A. Antenatal sonographic appearance of a fetal ovarian cyst. J Ultrasound Med 1982; 1: 329–331

91 Preziosi P, Fariello G, Maiorana A, Malena S, Ferro F. Antenatal sonographic diagnosis of complicated ovarian cysts. JCU 1986; 14: 196–198

92 Holzgreve W, Winde B, Willital G H, Beller F K. Prenatal diagnosis and perinatal management of a fetal ovarian cyst. Prenat Diagn 1985; 5: 155–158

93 Rizzo N, Gabrielli S, Perolo A et al. Prenatal diagnosis and management of fetal ovarian cysts. Prenat Diagn 1989; 9: 97–104

94 Vanek V W, Phillips A K. Retroperitoneal, mesenteric and omental cysts. Arch Surg 1984; 119: 838–842

95 Kurtz R J, Heinmann T M, Beck A R, Holt J. Mesenteric and retroperitoneal cysts. Ann Surg 1986; 203: 109–112

96 Schmidt W, Yarkoni S, Jeanty P et al. Sonographic measurements of the fetal spleen: clinical implications. J Ultrasound Med 1985; 4: 667

97 Vintzileos A M, Neckles S, Campbell W A et al. Fetal liver ultrasound measurements during normal pregnancy. Obstet Gynecol 1985; 66: 47

Heart abnormalities

John L Gibbs

Introduction

The antenatal diagnosis of major cardiac abnormalities is an important step forward in the management of congenital heart disease. Whereas some parents choose to terminate a pregnancy after a major anomaly is detected, many elect to continue. Advance knowledge that a child has a cardiac abnormality is extremely valuable, as appropriate treatment may be planned early and instituted immediately after delivery. This may have a dramatically beneficial effect on morbidity for the child, particularly in the presence of duct-dependent circulation. It is rare nowadays for a child with, for instance, a major aortic arch anomaly to die peri-operatively, yet some of these patients (who have an excellent long-term outlook from the cardiac point of view) suffer morbidity, such as long-term handicap from cerebral ischaemia. Cerebral damage in neonates with heart disease is usually related to rapid-onset severe hypoxaemia and metabolic acidosis, most often resulting from ductal closure in a duct-dependent circulation – the damage is often done before the child arrives at a specialist cardiac centre. Such babies usually appear well initially, with few, and often subtle, clinical signs. Their heart disease only becomes recognised when they abruptly become desperately ill. Treatment of the newborn with prostaglandin E is extremely effective in maintaining ductal patency and, at least in theory, their current commonly moribund condition at presentation with cardiac disease is almost entirely avoidable if antenatal detection of heart disease can be perfected. The great majority of cardiac anomalies that cause either the pulmonary or the systemic circulation to be dependent on the duct are recognisable by any ultrasonographer with a little specialist training, although more than the simple four-chamber view is required if screening is to be effective.

Congenital heart disease occurs in approximately 8 per 1000 live births, but many of these infants have relatively minor lesions. As a very rough guide, major cardiac anomalies, which should be detectable antenatally, occur in 2–3 per 1000 fetuses, and therefore an obstetric unit dealing with 5000 deliveries a year should be able to detect 10 or more major fetal cardiac abnormalities per annum.

Timing

At 18 weeks gestation it is almost always possible to see the fetal cardiac chambers, valves and great arteries sufficiently well to exclude most major anomalies. Thus the currently popular obstetric practice of performing a routine fetal anomaly screening scan at between 18 and 20 weeks is convenient from the cardiac point of view. In thin mothers who are easy to scan it may be possible to obtain high-quality images of the fetal heart at 16 weeks gestation using traditional equipment. In our unit we offer a 16-week scan to ectomorphs with pregnancies known to be high risk for heart disease, and early studies of trans-vaginal scanning of the heart at even earlier gestations have shown some promise.[1-4] For routine scans at both general obstetric units and specialist cardiac centres 18 weeks remains the timing of choice.

Referral to a specialist cardiac centre

Specialist cardiac departments do not have the resources to offer a service to all comers, and it is therefore clearly appropriate that screening should be the responsibility of the same obstetric ultrasonographer who undertakes the general fetal anomaly scan.

The major indication for referral to a cardiologist is the suspicion of an abnormality at the routine screening scan. It is wise to have a low threshold to ask for help: it is not acceptable to patients to delay referral by arranging repeat screening appointments just to make sure that there is a problem. It is not necessary for an obstetric ultrasonographer to become an expert in congenital heart disease: all that is required is the ability to recognise that the heart is not normal.

Most pregnant women who have previously had a child with congenital heart disease, or who have had congenital heart disease themselves, know that their fetus has an increased risk of a cardiac anomaly, and most prefer to return to a specialist cardiac unit for a detailed fetal echocardiogram, in addition to having a general fetal anomaly screening scan at their local hospital. The risk of recurrence of congenital heart disease, if there is a single previous child affected, is roughly 2–3%, but this rises to about 10% if a parent is affected (depending, to some extent, on the exact abnormality). These parents require a different approach to those with no previous experience of congenital heart disease. The fetal heart is highly likely to be normal, yet the parents are often extremely anxious, particularly if their experiences in the past have been of death or major morbidity. It is relatively easy to recognise major heart disease but extremely difficult to be truly confident that there is no significant cardiac anomaly. For this reason it is probably wise for obstetric ultrasonographers to devolve responsibility for these echocardiograms to a cardiologist. However, it is simply not possible to be absolutely certain that the fetal heart is normal. Relatively minor defects, such as ventricular septal defects, may be undetectable if they are small (or even if they later prove large enough to require surgical treatment). Atrial septal defects may be easily missed; mild valvar or subvalvar stenosis may be missed; and rare but major anomalies such as abnormal pulmonary venous drainage or coronary artery anomalies may be very difficult to detect at any stage of pregnancy. It is good policy never to tell a mother that her fetus has a normal heart, but to give reassurance that no major abnormality has been detected and that it is rare to miss an abnormality that would carry a high risk of death or major morbidity.

Other groups which may benefit from specialist fetal echocardiography are fetuses with chromosomal abnormalities, oesophageal atresia or multiple anomalies, as all of these are often associated with congenital heart disease.[5] Maternal diabetes carries an increased risk of anomalies generally (perhaps as high as 2% risk for heart disease)[6] and the fetus may have a generously proportioned heart,[7,8] but routine referral of diabetics for detailed fetal echocardiography is controversial. The view in my own department is that routine obstetric anomaly screening is probably adequate.

A practical approach to scanning

It is useful from an academic point of view to know the approximate orientation of the heart in the fetal chest, as well as the planes in which various views of the heart may be obtained (Figs 18.1 and 18.2),[9,10] but it is important to remember that in practice one very rarely uses detailed fetal surface anatomy when scanning the heart. Most fetal echocardiographers approach the heart in a similar manner to other organs. After finding the organ and seeing a recognisable anatomical feature the scanning plane and transducer position are finely tuned to improve the image, and if one manoeuvre does not work another manipulation usually will.

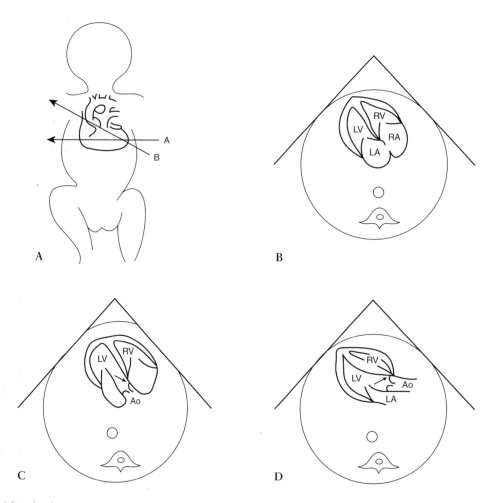

Fig. 18.1 Four- and five chamber views. A: Approximate scanning planes for obtaining the standard four- and five-chamber views. **B:** Because the heart lies more horizontally in the fetus than in the neonate the four-chamber view is obtained in a transverse plane (line A). **C:** As the transducer plane is angled cranially (line B) the aortic valve (Ao) comes into view in its 'wedged' position between the mitral valve and the right ventricle. **D:** As the transducer is angled further cranially the right ventricular cavity becomes foreshortened and the ascending aorta (the 'fifth' chamber) as well as the aortic valve becomes visible. The great value of imaging the aortic valve or ascending aorta arising from the left ventricle lies in demonstrating the joining (arrowed) of the ventricular septum to the front of the aortic valve. This excludes the presence of a variety of major abnormalities of the outlet pole of the heart which may be missed completely if only the four-chamber view is obtained. There are many different fetal positions in which these features may be seen, and it is important not to rely too much on surface anatomy; it is the images themselves that are important, rather than the orientation in which they are obtained. LV – left ventricle, RV – right ventricle, LA – left atrium, RA – right atrium.

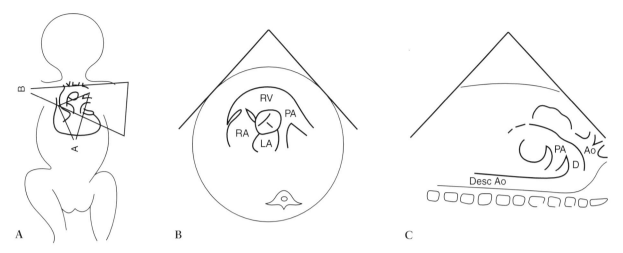

Fig. 18.2 The great arteries. A: Approximate scanning planes for obtaining the standard views of the great arteries. **B:** The pulmonary artery, its bifurcation and its origin from the right ventricle may be seen using a scanning plane between the xiphisternum and the upper thoracic spine (plane A). It is an important feature of normal great artery relationship that the pulmonary artery wraps around the aorta, so that when the aorta is seen in short axis the pulmonary trunk is seen in long axis and vice versa. **C:** The aortic arch and duct may be seen in a plane approximately between the right shoulder tip and the left scapula (plane B). PA – pulmonary artery, D – arterial duct, desc Ao – descending aorta; remainder as for Figure 18.1.

Ultrasound mode and choice of transducer

Cross-sectional echocardiography alone is adequate for the analysis of the great majority of fetal cardiac scans, as anatomy is of prime importance. However, M-mode imaging, because of its fast sampling rate, is ideally suited to assessment of heart rate and rhythm, and is particularly useful if the M-mode cursor can be passed through both the right ventricle and the left atrium (or vice versa), such that both atrial and ventricular contractions (and their relationships to each other) may be recorded. Pulsed-wave Doppler is also useful in assessing rate and rhythm, but colour flow mapping is of relatively little value, being most helpful in differentiating venous from arterial flow or as a rapid means of detecting valve regurgitation.

The choice of transducer depends to a large extent on the machine manufacturer and to a small extent on operator preference. Cardiologists tend to prefer phased-array transducers, using the highest frequency (7.5 MHz at 18–20 weeks, if possible) compatible with the distance of the fetal heart from the abdominal wall. None the less, high-quality images can often be obtained with linear, curvilinear or even mechanical transducers. At later gestations it may be necessary to reduce the frequency to 3.5 MHz, but lower frequencies naturally result in lower resolution.

Sequential segmental analysis

Congenital heart disease can involve complex and multiple structural abnormalities, but even complex disease may be evaluated relatively easily by treating the heart as a series of structures and connections. This simple, logical approach is known as sequential segmental analysis and involves initial analysis of the great veins, followed by the atria, the atrioventricular connections, the ventricles, the ventriculo-arterial connections, and finally the great arteries. This approach naturally has to be modified for the fetus: the ultrasonographer should not necessarily keep to this order, but should be opportunist and prepared to look at whichever structures the fetus obliges by showing at any particular stage of the examination. Because only a certain number of abnormalities can occur at each stage of analysis, this approach allows a complete picture of even the most complex congenital heart disease to be built up in fairly simple stages. The first stage of sequential analysis is to establish the viscero-atrial situs. With normal situs (situs solitus) the abdominal organs are in their usual positions, the right-sided lung has three lobes, the left lung two lobes, the morphological right atrium is on the right side, and the morphological left atrium on the left (the atria are morphologically different). Normal connections are referred to as 'concordant', that is, the right atrium is connected to the right ventricle, the right ventricle to the pulmonary artery, the left atrium to the left ventricle, and the left ventricle to the aorta. When abnormal the atrioventricular connections may be absent (for example tricuspid atresia), discordant (for example right atrium connecting to left ventricle), or double inlet (both atrioventricular valves connecting to one ventricle) or common (as in complete atrioventricular septal defect). Similarly, the ventriculoarterial connections may be absent, discordant, double outlet or common (as in truncus arteriosus, where both the aorta and pulmonary artery arise from a common arterial trunk).

It has been suggested that a simple measurement of the rotational axis of the fetal heart may be a reliable indicator of the presence of important cardiac abnormalities.[11-14] Although it is clear that with many important structural abnormalities the long axis of the heart may be rotated, this simple measurement cannot be regarded as an adequate substitute for screening by proper anatomical assessment of the four- and five-chamber views.

The normal heart

The great veins

The superior and inferior caval veins lie anteriorly and to the right of the fetal spine and can usually be easily identified as they join the right atrium (Fig. 18.3), and it is normally possible to see a hepatic vein draining to the inferior vena cava just before it joins the atrium. The pulmonary veins may be difficult to image clearly, partly because they are poorly filled and therefore small, especially at early gestations. One pulmonary vein from each side may none the less often be identified on a slightly modified four-chamber view (Fig. 18.4).

The atria, atrioventricular connections and the ventricles

The four-chamber view

The four-chamber view is popular for screening purposes because so much information concerning cardiac anatomy

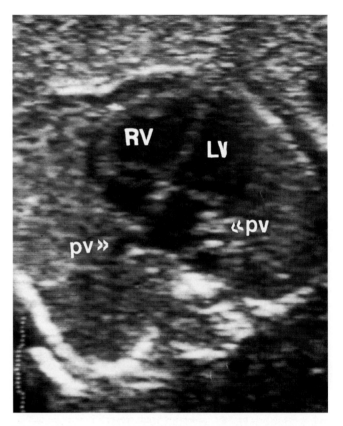

Fig. 18.4 Pulmonary veins. At least one pulmonary vein (pv, arrowed) from each lung can usually be visualised as the veins join the left atrium. The veins are often best seen in a slightly modified four-chamber view (the scan plane is rotated so that the right atrium is cut almost tangentially, giving the false impression that it is smaller than the left atrium).

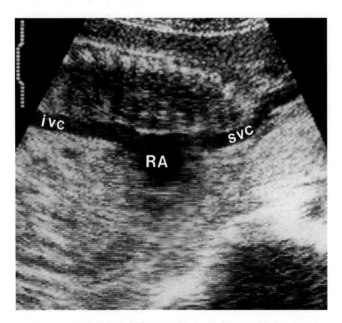

Fig. 18.3 Long-axis view with the fetal spine at the top of the picture, showing the superior (SVC) and inferior (IVC) venae cavae joining the right atrium (RA).

and function can be seen, and it is usually the easiest view to obtain. Because the fetal heart and ribs are more horizontal than they are post-natally after the lungs have expanded, the four-chamber view is obtained in transverse plane through the fetal thorax. Correct orientation is vital and can usually be guided by simultaneous imaging of a full-length rib (Fig. 18.5). If multiple ribs are seen it is likely that a tangential cut through one ventricle will be taken, giving a false impression that one ventricle is smaller than the other.

In the normal four-chamber view the heart should occupy one-third to one-half of the thorax and the right and left sides of the heart should appear equal in size during the second trimester (although at later gestations in the normal fetus the right ventricle may appear slightly larger than the left). While imaging the four chambers the heart rate, to some extent the heart rhythm, and the myocardial function should all be apparent, in addition to the cardiac anatomy. It is usually sufficient to make crude estimates of heart size, rate and rhythm, rather than detailed measurements, although ranges of normal cardio-

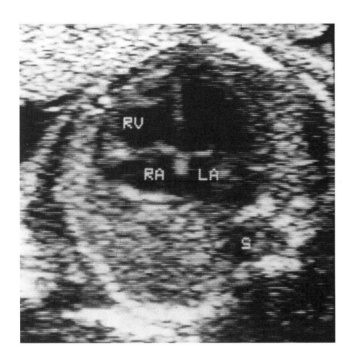

Fig. 18.5 The four-chamber view. The ribs are imaged almost in their full length; the heart should take up a third to a half of the thorax and the right and left sides of the heart are equal in size. The right ventricle (RV) is immediately behind the sternum and directly opposite the fetal spine (s). It is identifiable as the right ventricle not only by its position but by the muscle bar (the moderator band) crossing its apex. In this normal heart the septal leaflet of the tricuspid valve may be seen to join the septum slightly more towards the apex of the heart than the insertion of the septal leaflet of the mitral valve. One of the right pulmonary veins is seen joining the left atrium.

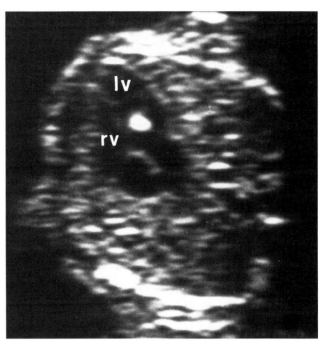

Fig. 18.6 Ventricular golf balls. Reflective masses ('peas' or 'golf balls') in the left ventricle are common and, as in this case, may be very prominent. The masses are entirely benign, although some claim a loose association with chromosomal abnormalities. The masses are most commonly seen in the region of the mitral papillary muscles.

thoracic ratio, chamber and vessel sizes and normal flow velocities across the cardiac valves at different gestations are available for reference.[9,15–20]

The tricuspid and mitral valves are also of equal diameter in the normal heart, and both valves should be seen to open. If imaging the valve leaflets is difficult, colour flow mapping will usually allow immediate confirmation of laminar flow across the valves. Valve regurgitation is very rarely seen in the normal fetal heart (although very mild tricuspid regurgitation may be seen in some normal neonates). Doppler measurement of mitral and tricuspid flow is of limited value in routine fetal cardiac assessment, although it may be useful in the analysis of arrhythmias.

Peak flow velocities across the mitral and tricuspid valves are fairly constant throughout gestation, the normal values being about 50 cm/s for both valves (see section on arrhythmias).[9]

It is common in the normal fetal heart to see a small, highly reflective mass in the left ventricle. These are often sited at the junction of the mitral valve supporting apparatus with the papillary muscles on the free wall of the left ventricle. However, they may sometimes appear to be within the left ventricular cavity itself, or adjacent to the

ventricular septum. These masses, often referred to as 'golf balls' or 'left ventricular peas', sometimes appear very strikingly bright (Fig. 18.6). When the masses appear adjacent to the septum or within the left ventricular cavity they are usually related to left ventricular bands (often referred to as false tendons), which cross the ventricular cavity and may vary from delicate thin fibrous cords to muscular strands. Careful scanning of the ventricle will usually reveal the full length of the band (Fig. 18.7). Bands may occasionally be multiple and are entirely normal (some species, such as cats, have numerous ventricular bands). When the mass is associated with one of the papillary muscles of the mitral valve it is most often sited at the apex of the papillary muscle. Autopsy studies of these masses (when they occur in structurally abnormal hearts) have shown a small area of fibrosis in the papillary muscle, but no clue as to the cause of the fibrotic area. Follow-up of babies with left ventricular peas have shown that the mass is often still present post-natally (although less reflective), but there seems to be no interference with cardiac function. They usually disappear within a few months. The more one looks, the more common left ventricular peas appear to be. It is the author's view that they are entirely benign and have no sinister connotations at all, but others have suggested that they might have a loose association with chromosomal anomalies.[21–27]

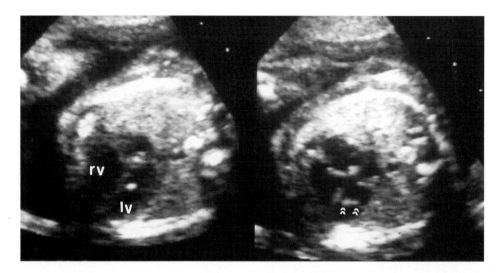

Fig. 18.7 Ventricular bands. Some reflective foci in the heart are due to left ventricular bands (otherwise known as false tendons), a common finding in the normal heart. If a mass is seen adjacent to the ventricular septum (as shown on the left) adjustment of the scanning plane (as shown on the right) may reveal the full length of the band (arrowed) crossing the ventricular cavity. There is no suggestion of any association between left ventricular bands and chromosomal abnormalities.

The ventricular outlets

The 'five-chamber' view

After finding the four-chamber view a very slight manipulation of the transducer, usually involving cranial angulation and rotation of the scan plane a few degrees to the left of the fetal thorax, will enable imaging of the aorta (the 'fifth chamber') as it arises from the left ventricle. In the normal heart the ventricular septum should be seen to join the anterior leaflet of the aortic valve and the anterior wall of the aorta, often appearing as a gentle 'S' bend (Fig. 18.8). It is the junction of the ventricular septum with the aorta that is important; it is not necessary to see all five chambers at once – indeed, often the right atrium will disappear as the aorta comes into view. This view of the origin of the aorta is essential if so-called conotruncal abnormalities (those involving the outlet of the heart) are to be excluded. Such abnormalities are often major yet may occur with a completely normal four-chamber view.[28–31] Therefore, if screening for major cardiac abnormalities is to be effective, this view of the aorta arising from the left ventricle must be sought in addition to the standard four-chamber view. The aortic valve and the proximal ascending aorta may also be inspected at this stage, but it should be borne in mind that mild or even moderate abnormalities of the valve may not be apparent at 18–20 weeks gestation. The pulmonary artery and the right ventricular outflow tract are imaged at right-angles to the plane in which the left ventricular outflow and proximal aorta are seen. In the normal heart the great arteries never arise in parallel, but cross over each other. Thus if the aorta is seen in short axis the pulmonary artery

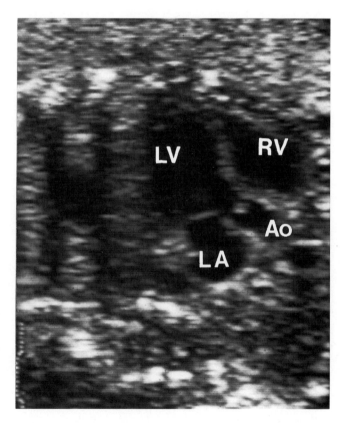

Fig. 18.8 The 'five-chamber' view. The scanning plane has been rotated so that the right atrium has disappeared from view but the outlet of the left ventricle has opened up to show the attachment of the ventricular septum to the anterior wall of the aorta (Ao). It is this junction of the septum and anterior aorta (or anterior aortic valve) that is so vital to visualise to exclude many of the major anomalies that affect the outlet of the heart.

is seen anteriorly in long axis, and vice versa. This cross-over is an important feature of normal anatomy, and when the great arteries are seen to cross over each other it is highly likely that the arteries are normally related (that is, the aorta posterior and arising from the left ventricle, the pulmonary artery anterior and arising from the right ventricle). However, the most reliable way to determine great artery identity is to seek the pulmonary artery bifurcation (or trifurcation if the arterial duct (ductus arteriosus) is also included in the plane of view) (Fig. 18.9). In case of difficulties in identifying a great artery it may also be possible to identify the aorta by showing the head and neck vessels arising from the aortic arch (Fig. 18.10). As a practical guide the aortic arch is most easily imaged by following the ascending aorta using fine transducer adjustment. In the normal fetus the aorta and pulmonary artery should be approximately equal in diameter: an obvious inequality in size is an indicator of important structural disease and should prompt referral to a specialist centre.[9,32] Visualisation of a great artery arch is not a reliable means of identifying the aorta as there are two arches in the normal fetus, one the aortic arch and the second the arch of the pulmonary artery, the arterial duct and the descend-

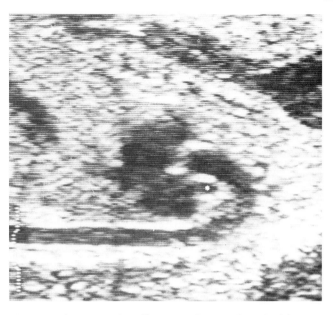

Fig. 18.10 The aortic arch. Differentiation between the arch of the aorta and the arch formed by the pulmonary artery, the arterial duct and the descending aorta may sometimes be difficult, but in this example the origins of the head and neck vessels are clearly seen, confirming that this is the aortic rather than the ductal arch. When the aorta is seen in long axis the pulmonary artery (in this case the right pulmonary artery, marked with a small asterisk) should be seen in short axis beneath the arch of the aorta.

ing aorta. In the normal fetus the two arches can be seen to be different shapes, the aortic arch having a tight curve similar to the handle of a walking stick, and the ductal arch being much wider (Fig. 18.11). The arterial duct is of similar diameter to the aorta and the pulmonary trunk in the normal fetus, although ductal constriction may rarely be induced by maternal drug administration whether the fetal heart is structurally normal or not.[33–35]

Doppler interrogation of pulmonary artery and aortic flow is of limited value in routine fetal cardiac assessment and is most useful in the measurement of heart rate and rhythm. Normal peak flow velocities across the aortic and pulmonary valves are fairly constant throughout gestation, both values being around 50–60 cm/s.[9]

Normal cardiac rhythm

The normal fetal heart rate is about 140 beats/minute (bpm). It is normal for the heart to show abrupt (and sometimes very dramatic) changes of rate for short periods of time. The most striking normal changes are sudden bradycardias, where the heart rate may fall briefly to very slow rates (30/min or so), with recovery occurring after a few seconds. Ectopic beats, causing the rhythm to be irregular, are so frequently seen in the fetus (particularly in the third trimester) that they can be considered normal (see section on arrhythmias). Sinus tachycardias rarely exceed a rate of

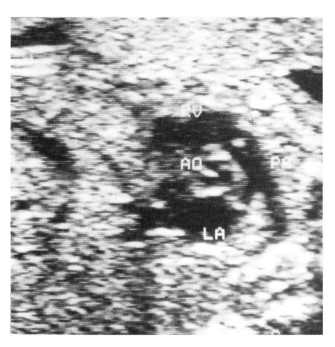

Fig. 18.9 Pulmonary artery. The only certain way to identify the pulmonary artery is to see its bifurcation. This is possible in a variety of different views, but is most easily achieved using this short axis view of the aorta (AO), when the pulmonary artery may be seen wrapping around the aorta, the bifurcation and the proximal right and left pulmonary arteries having an appearance much like a pair of trousers. The closed leaflets of both the aortic and pulmonary valves are clearly visible. An important feature of normal great arteries is that they do not run in parallel: the pulmonary artery is seen here in long axis and the aorta appears in short axis.

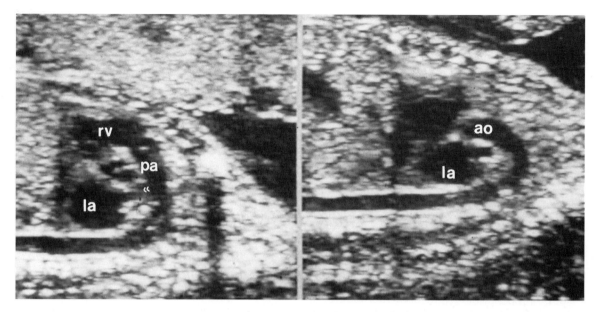

Fig. 18.11 The two arterial arches; on the left the ductal arch, and on the right the aortic arch in the same fetus. The ductal arch is wider and the right pulmonary artery (arrowed) can be seen arising from it. The aortic arch is 'tighter', with an appearance similar to the handle of a walking stick. The important hallmark of the normal 'wrapping around' relationship of the great arteries is well demonstrated; when one artery is seen in long axis the other appears in short axis.

around 180 bpm and sustained rates of over 180 or below 100 for a period of more than 5 minutes are almost always abnormal.[9] The fetal heart rate may be measured accurately using either M-mode or Doppler (see section on arrhythmias).

Structural abnormalities

Veins and their connections

Abnormalities of the systemic veins are rare and when they do occur are almost always associated with complex congenital heart disease, which is apparent on the four-chamber view. They are most often associated with abnormal viscero-atrial situs. In situs inversus the heart, great vessels and abdominal organs are in positions which are the mirror image of normal and the heart may or may not be structurally normal. In ambiguous situs[36] (either left atrial isomerism or right atrial isomerism) the heart may be on the right or the left and the most common intracardiac anomaly is atrioventricular septal defect. The inferior vena cava often connects to the heart via an azygos or hemiazygos vein, and anomalies of pulmonary venous drainage are also common (Fig. 18.12). Abnormal situs may be associated with other anomalies: situs inversus may be part of Kartagener's syndrome, in which there is a congenital abnormality of cilial function which may affect respiratory function and fertility; situs ambiguous may be associated with foregut malrotation; and both may be associated with biliary atresia.

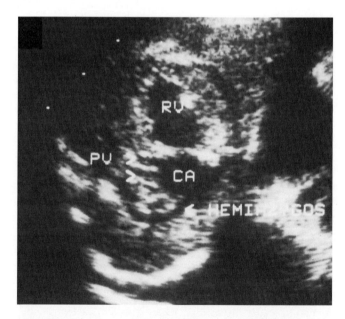

Fig. 18.12 Anomalous systemic and pulmonary venous drainage in association with complex congenital heart disease. Only two cardiac chambers are identifiable. The inferior vena cava is connected to the common atrium (CA) via a hemiazygos connection which has a typically curved appearance (arrowed), in contrast to the normal vena cava (see Fig. 18.3). Two pulmonary veins (arrowed) are also seen joining the common atrium.

Anomalous drainage of the pulmonary veins may be partial or total and the site of return of the veins is very variable. Partial anomalous pulmonary venous drainage is

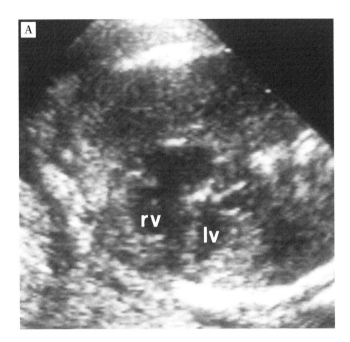
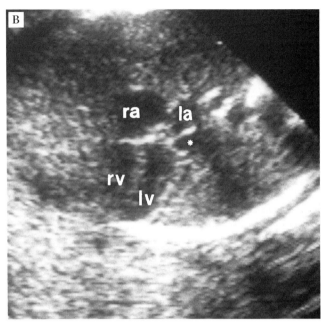

Fig. 18.13 Total anomalous pulmonary venous drainage. A: The four-chamber view shows that the right ventricle appears larger than the left ventricle. **B:** Closer inspection of the left atrium reveals that the left atrial cavity is small. Posterior to the left atrium and separate from it is a second chamber (marked with an asterisk), the anomalous common pulmonary vein. In this case the anomalous vein joined the innominate vein and thence the superior vena cava, but the exact site of drainage may be difficult to ascertain until after delivery.

unlikely to be detected antenatally, and even total anomalous drainage may be easily missed. When all the pulmonary venous drainage returns to the right side of the heart (most frequently to the innominate vein superiorly or the portal vein infradiaphragmatically) the right side of the heart becomes markedly dilated early in neonatal life. However, in the fetus pulmonary blood flow is low and the right heart may therefore appear normal or only mildly dilated, even late in pregnancy. When the fetal right ventricle and pulmonary artery are seen to be dilated total anomalous pulmonary venous drainage should be considered as a possible cause (Fig. 18.13).

The atria and atrioventricular connections

Atrial septal defects, one of the commonest forms of congenital heart disease, may be difficult to detect in the fetus because the foramen ovale is normally widely patent (Fig. 18.14). Even if the flap of the foramen ovale is seen to wave about normally in the left atrium[37,38] it is not possible to be certain that the atrial septum will be intact postnatally. It is occasionally possible to detect secundum defects antenatally when the flap appears deficient and when there are bright margins (often called the 'T sign') to the foramen (Fig. 18.15). Most atrial septal defects remain undetected until infancy. Primum atrial septal defect, or (more properly) partial atrioventricular septal defect, is

easier to detect as the inferior part of the atrial septum is involved and is usually obviously deficient on a standard four-chamber view.

Right or left atrial enlargement is usually related to tricuspid or mitral regurgitation, respectively. Colour Doppler may prove valuable as a very quick means of confirming the presence of regurgitation. Bilateral atrial enlargement with normal ventricular dimensions is very rare and is likely to be due to restrictive cardiomyopathy.

Atrioventricular septal defect

The most common anomaly of the atrioventricular junction is the atrioventricular septal defect. In its partial form ('primum' atrial septal defect) it appears as an atrial septal defect affecting the septum immediately adjacent to the atrioventricular junction (the crux of the heart). In its complete form there is also a ventricular septal defect in continuity with the atrial septal defect. Abnormal development of the atrioventricular valve is an inherent part of this anomaly, with the superior and inferior leaflets of the right and left components of the valve bridging the septal defect, effectively producing a common atrioventricular valve. This anomaly is usually obvious on a four-chamber view (Fig. 18.16). It is of particular importance because of its strong association with trisomy 21, and it is usual practice in the UK to offer fetal karyotyping to mothers of a fetus with a complete atrioventricular septal defect. Some

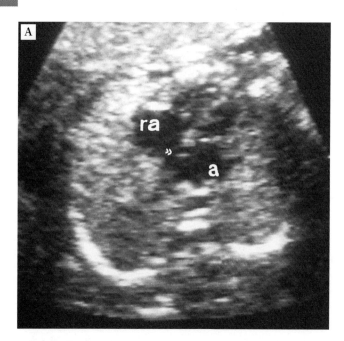

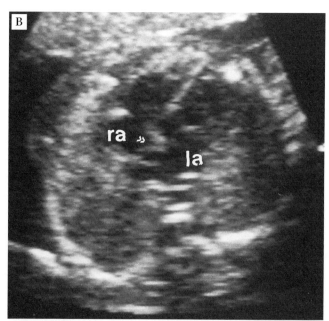

Fig. 18.14 The normal atrial septum. A: The oval foramen has a very variable appearance: because it is thin it may be difficult to image, often giving the false impression that there is a defect in the atrial septum and making it almost impossible to exclude confidently the presence of a genuine atrial septal defect. **B:** When visible, the normal flap of the foramen should bulge from right to left (arrowed). The flap is often very mobile and normal blood flow across the foramen may push the flap of the valve well across into the left atrium.

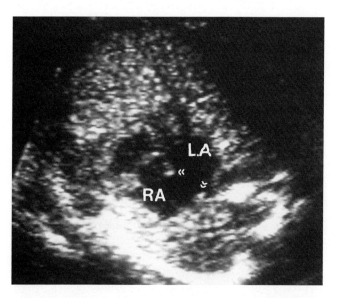

Fig. 18.15 A genuine secundum (or oval foramen) atrial septal defect. The flap of the foramen is absent and the edges of the defect appear bright (arrowed). This bright appearance of the edges of a septal defect (whether atrial or ventricular, and often referred to as the 'T' sign) is a useful indicator that the defect is genuine rather than artefactual.

authors have reported that an antenatal diagnosis of uncomplicated atrioventricular septal defect carries a 90% risk of Down's syndrome, with an even higher risk if any other fetal anomaly (such as nuchal thickening) is present.

Atrioventricular septal defects which occur in association with situs ambiguous, however, do not have particular associations with chromosomal abnormalities.

Tricuspid valve

The most frequently detected tricuspid valve abnormality is atresia. It is usually clearly visible on a standard four-chamber view, when the tricuspid valve is seen to be replaced by a thick wedge of tissue (or very rarely the valve is present but imperforate because of fused commissures) and there is no forward flow from the right atrium into the right ventricle. Because of this lack of right ventricular filling the right ventricular cavity is usually hypoplastic, and may be so small that it is difficult to identify. In most cases there is a ventricular septal defect, which allows some filling of the right ventricle from the left (Fig. 18.17). Tricuspid atresia may be associated with other defects, such as transposition of the great arteries or coarctation of the aorta.

Tricuspid regurgitation, if severe, may lead to fetal hydrops and intra-uterine death. The most obvious feature, however, is cardiomegaly, which may be so marked that the heart acts as a space-occupying lesion, encroaching on the lungs and sometimes resulting in pulmonary hypoplasia. The most frequent cause of tricuspid regurgitation is Ebstein's anomaly, where the septal leaflet of the valve is displaced towards the apex of the right ventricle, rendering the valve incompetent and also

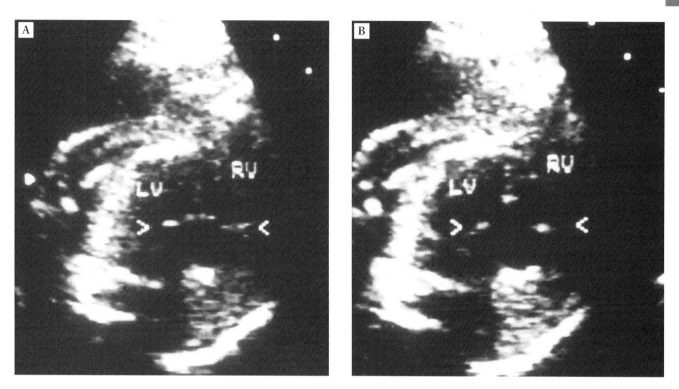

Fig. 18.16 A complete atrioventricular septal defect. A: in systole when the atrioventricular valve is closed, and **B:** in diastole when the valve is open. When the valve is closed it is apparent that the usual offset of the atrioventricular valves is absent, and when the valve is open the extent of the atrial and ventricular components of the septal defect are seen, the crux of the heart appearing to be absent. Note again the 'T' sign (see Fig. 18.15) at the crest of the ventricular septum. These defects have a very strong association with Down's syndrome.

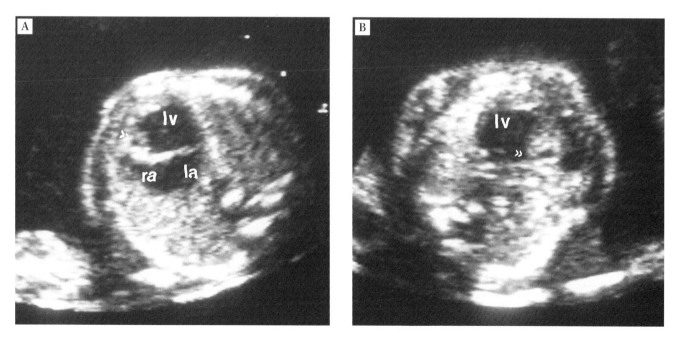

Fig. 18.17 Tricuspid atresia. A: The tricuspid valve is replaced by a thick wedge of immobile tissue and the right ventricular cavity (arrowed) is diminutive. **B:** Fine adjustment of the scanning plane will usually enable visualisation of a ventricular septal defect allowing some blood to enter the tiny right ventricular cavity. In many cases, as here, the VSD is very small (arrowed) and will lead to restricted flow from the left ventricle to the pulmonary artery, and to ductal dependency after birth.

sometimes causing obstruction to right ventricular filling. The diagnosis is usually evident with simple imaging of the heart, but if the cause of cardiomegaly is in doubt colour Doppler provides an instant means of recognition of the tricuspid regurgitant jet (Fig. 18.18). Ebstein's anomaly of the tricuspid valve may be associated with maternal lithium therapy during the first trimester. Occasionally severe tricuspid regurgitation occurs with normal attachments of the tricuspid valve. This is usually due to dysplasia of the valve,[39-42] the leaflets being thickened and unable to coapt in ventricular systole. Rarely severe tricuspid regurgitation may occur with a structurally normal tri-

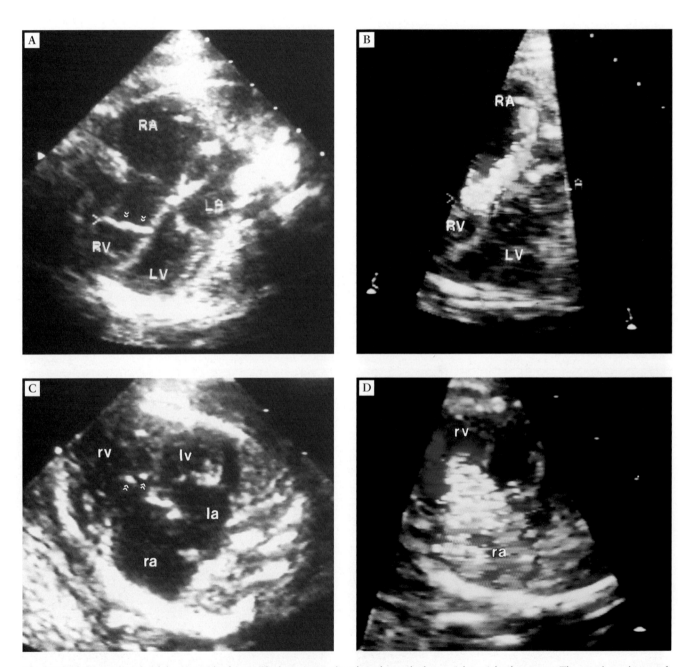

Fig. 18.18 Ebstein's anomaly of the tricuspid valve. A: The heart is grossly enlarged, mostly due to right atrial enlargement. The septal attachment of the tricuspid valve (arrowed) is displaced towards the apex of the right ventricle. **B:** Colour flow Doppler shows a jet of severe tricuspid regurgitation extending from the mid-cavity of the right ventricle to the far wall of the right atrium. **C:** In milder forms it may be difficult to differentiate Ebstein's anomaly from dysplasia of the tricuspid valve using cross-sectional imaging alone. Colour flow Doppler in tricuspid dysplasia shows tricuspid regurgitation with a jet origin at the usual level of the tricuspid valve. **D:** In this case the jet origin is well within the right ventricular cavity, confirming Ebstein's anomaly.

cuspid valve in the presence of pulmonary atresia with an intact ventricular septum. In this situation the only escape route from the right ventricle in systole is through the tricuspid valve.

Mitral valve

Mitral atresia, the most frequent mitral valve abnormality detected antenatally, usually occurs as part of the spectrum of hypoplastic left heart syndrome. In almost all cases the mitral valve is replaced by a wedge of tissue, similar in appearance to the atrioventricular junction in tricuspid atresia. The left atrium is usually small and the left ventricle often severely hypoplastic, sometimes so much so that it is difficult to identify the left ventricular cavity. In such cases the aortic valve is usually also atretic, with the ascending aorta therefore also being markedly hypoplastic (Fig. 18.19). If there is a ventricular septal defect some filling of the left ventricle from the right ventricle occurs, and in these cases the left ventricle may be only mildly hypoplastic and the aortic valve and ascending aorta may be normally developed. Coarctation of the aorta may occur in association with this combination of abnormalities. Despite the major disturbance to cardiac structure the overall fetal heart size is often normal in mitral atresia, and prenatal heart failure or intra-uterine death is unusual. In the majority of cases symptoms only appear some time after delivery, as the systemic circulation is dependent on the presence of the arterial duct.

Mitral stenosis is rarely detectable in the fetus unless the valve is markedly hypoplastic, when the appearances are very similar to hypoplastic left heart syndrome. It is usually associated with other cardiac abnormalities, such as coarctation of the aorta, which are more likely to be detected during routine anomaly screening. Mitral regurgitation is very rare in fetal life, and when it does occur is usually secondary to other abnormalities, such as severe left ventricular outflow obstruction or poor myocardial function.

Discordant atrioventricular connections

When the atrioventricular connections are discordant the right atrium connects with the mitral valve and left ventricle, and the left atrium connects with the tricuspid valve and right ventricle. This almost always occurs in association with other abnormalities, most commonly with discordant ventriculo-arterial connections, in which the left ventricle gives rise to the pulmonary artery and the right ventricle to the aorta. This combination is often referred to as 'congenitally corrected transposition'. Ventricular septal defects, pulmonary stenosis and dextrocardia are also commonly associated. When congenitally corrected transposition occurs without other cardiac abnormalities

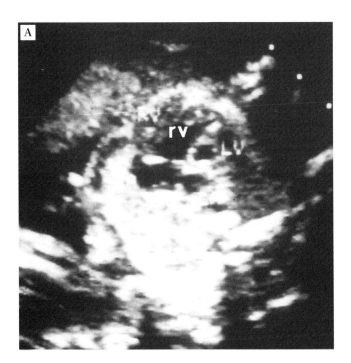 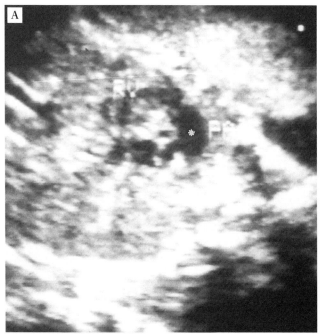

Fig. 18.19 Mitral atresia. A: The left atrium and left ventricle are strikingly smaller than the right heart chambers, although the overall heart size is normal. The mitral valve is replaced by a thick wedge of tissue. In many cases of mitral atresia the aortic valve is also atretic or severely hypoplastic. **B:** In this case short-axis imaging of the heart shows a dilated pulmonary artery (marked with an asterisk) wrapping around a grossly hypoplastic aorta and giving the classic appearance of the full spectrum of hypoplastic left heart syndrome.

the findings on the fetal scan may be relatively subtle. The normal offset of the origins of the tricuspid and mitral valve is reversed, the left-sided valve being attached nearer to the apex, and the moderator band appears in the left-sided ventricle.

Double-inlet left ventricle

In this rare anomaly both mitral and tricuspid valves connect to the left ventricle (Fig. 18.20). As a result the right ventricle is usually markedly hypoplastic and may not be evident at all. The appearances are those of a single ventricular chamber, although there is usually a rudimentary right ventricle identifiable post-natally. Double-inlet left ventricle may be associated with other anomalies, for example transposition of the great arteries or coarctation.

The ventricles

Primary abnormalities of the ventricular myocardium are rare in fetal life: the majority of abnormalities detected antenatally are secondary to defects of the atrioventricular or ventriculo-arterial valves or the aorta.

Ventricular hypertrophy

Hypertrophic cardiomyopathy is rarely detected antenatally but may cause ventricular hypertrophy, particularly

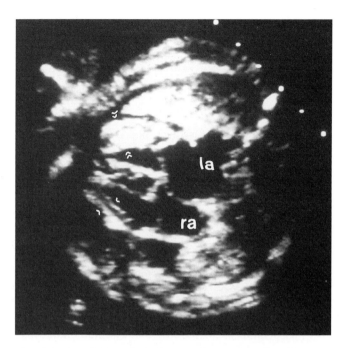

Fig. 18.21 **Gross left ventricular hypertrophy** (compare the wall thicknesses, arrowed, of the right and left ventricles) due to severe aortic stenosis. The left atrium is enlarged, the atrial septum is bulging from left to right (always an indicator of major left heart pathology), and there are bilateral pleural effusions due to heart failure.

at later stages of gestation. As in post-natal life it may predominantly affect the ventricular septum, or extend to the whole of the myocardium. Because the condition is autosomal dominant mothers with a family history often ask for fetal cardiac assessment. It is important to be aware of the limitations of fetal echocardiography in this setting. Normal appearances of the myocardium are obviously reassuring to some extent but do not exclude the possibility of later development of cardiomyopathy, and so parents must be counselled appropriately. Fetuses of diabetic mothers frequently have some degree of myocardial hypertrophy.[7,8] This may be manifested as just mild ventricular wall thickening, but occasionally gross hypertrophy occurs such that myocardial function (particularly ventricular filling) becomes impaired. In severe cases the appearance of the heart may be difficult to distinguish from hypertrophic cardiomyopathy.

Hypertrophy of one or other ventricle is usually secondary to severe aortic or pulmonary stenosis (Fig. 18.21). Biventricular hypertrophy may occur with fetal renal anomalies (presumably due to hypertension).

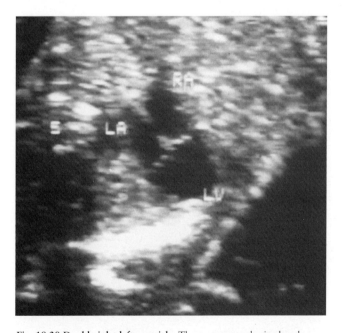

Fig. 18.20 **Double-inlet left ventricle.** There are normal mitral and tricuspid valves opening into a single ventricular chamber. In this condition there is usually a tiny rudimentary right ventricle, which may only be identifiable post-natally. Rarely, very large ventricular septal defects with 'almost absent' ventricular septum will give a similar appearance.

Ventricular dilatation and poor function

Myocarditis or dilated cardiomyopathy may present *in utero* and it is likely that myocarditis is one cause of 'idiopathic' non-immune fetal hydrops. The heart is usually enlarged with poor ventricular contractility (Fig. 18.22),

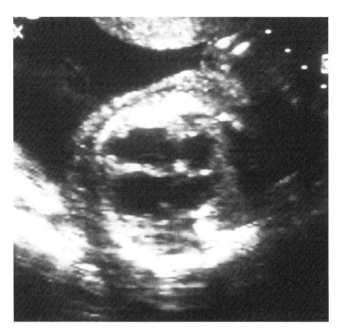

Fig. 18.22 Hydrops with bilateral pleural effusions. The heart is markedly enlarged but structurally normal. No cause was found in this particular case. Similar appearances may occur with twin–twin transfusion.

structural defect. Virology occasionally reveals evidence of infection (such as coxsackie or parvovirus), but often no cause for the myocardial failure is found. Alcohol has been found to have some effect on the fetal heart[43] but does not appear to be a major cause of fetal cardiomyopathy. Twin-to-twin transfusion may cause cardiomegaly and hydrops in the recipient twin, and the donor may also develop heart failure due to severe anaemia.

An important treatable cause of myocardial failure is sustained supraventricular tachycardia (SVT). Most cases are seen to have a tachycardia at the time hydrops is detected, but even prolonged supraventricular tachycardia sufficient to produce heart failure may be intermittent. If a hydropic fetus is seen to be in sinus rhythm this does not completely exclude the possibility of SVT being the cause of hydrops. Frequent ectopic beats may sometimes provide a clue to diagnosis, and frequent serial scans may be necessary to detect the arrhythmia.

Masses in the ventricles

Tumours within the myocardium are most frequently benign rhabdomyomas (Fig. 18.23). Even when large they seldom interfere with cardiac function, and although they may increase in size during gestation it is common for the tumours to regress spontaneously post-natally. Such tumours present considerable difficulties when counselling parents as they rarely seem to cause major cardiac prob-

and there may be functional mitral and/or tricuspid regurgitation. Myocarditis should be considered in cases of cardiomegaly where detailed assessment fails to identify any

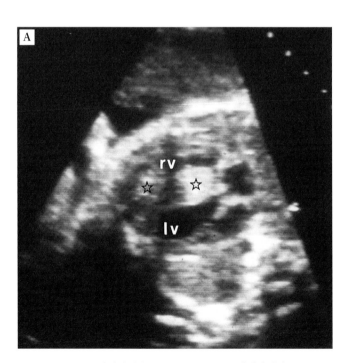

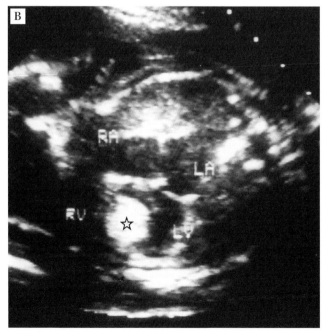

Fig. 18.23 Myocardial rhabdomyomas. A: Myocardial rhabdomyomas most commonly occur in the ventricular septum and are frequently multiple (marked with asterisks). Very large tumours may occur in some cases. **B:** The right ventricular cavity is almost obliterated by a huge rhabdomyoma (marked with an asterisk). Despite the size of this the fetus remained well at term and the tumour slowly became smaller after delivery. Both these fetuses proved to have tuberous sclerosis.

lems but they do have a strong association with tuberous sclerosis, which may cause developmental delay and epilepsy, sometimes with severe handicap. Cardiac rhabdomyoma appears to be the only reliable antenatal marker for tuberous sclerosis, making fetal echocardiography a useful tool in detection of the disease in mothers known to have a family history. However, as rhabdomyomas may also occur as an isolated anomaly with a generally good prognosis, decision making for parents can be particularly difficult. There are insufficient data at present to give parents an accurate assessment of the risk of tuberous sclerosis in a fetus with a single rhabdomyoma, but the risk does seem to be much higher if the tumours are multiple or are lobulated. Not all tumours in the myocardium are rhabdomyomas and not all apparent masses are genuine tumours. Dystrophic calcification of the fetal heart may have a very similar appearance to multiple rhabdomyomas (Fig. 18.24), raising further difficulties with parental counselling. This phenomenon is caused by calcification of areas of ischaemic or otherwise damaged myocardium, which in turn may be related to placental insufficiency or intra-uterine infection (such as cytomegalovirus). The prognosis for a fetus with areas of dystrophic

myocardial calcification is unknown. Benign fibromas of the myocardium may give a similar appearance. Malignant tumours of the fetal myocardium are as exceedingly rare as they are post-natally.

Ventricular septal defects

The four-chamber view of the heart will detect the few ventricular septal defects (VSDs) that involve the inlet part of the ventricular septum or the trabecular septum, but will miss the many that are localised to the perimembraneous outlet septum (Fig. 18.25). The five-chamber view is necessary in most cases to detect VSDs; small defects may be missed even when high-quality images of the heart are obtained, but larger defects will be apparent when searching for the normal attachment of the ventricular septum to the anterior wall of the aortic root. With uncomplicated VSDs colour flow Doppler rarely helps with the diagnosis as there is little or no shunting through the defect antenatally.

Ventricular septal defects in association with a great artery overriding the crest of the ventricular septum are rarely isolated and may be seen with tetralogy of Fallot, double-outlet right ventricle, pulmonary atresia or common arterial trunk.

Ventriculo-arterial valves and connections

Pulmonary stenosis and atresia

Pulmonary valve stenosis may easily be missed at any gestation unless it is severe enough to cause a detectable degree of right ventricular hypertrophy or the valve is markedly thickened. It is very rare for isolated infundibular stenosis to present in fetal life. When pulmonary stenosis is severe or the valve is atretic the right ventricle is hypertrophied (Fig. 18.26). In this condition the appearance of the right ventricular cavity is enormously variable. It may appear normal, dilated or reduced in size, and there is often tricuspid regurgitation detectable with colour flow Doppler. The valve abnormality is usually visible and the pulmonary trunk and its branches are usually hypoplastic (Fig. 18.27). In extreme cases it may be very difficult to differentiate between 'critical' pulmonary stenosis and pulmonary atresia. Colour flow Doppler may sometimes help by revealing a narrow jet through the valve, but the absence of a jet does not necessarily indicate atresia (this may be equally difficult post-natally). Pulmonary stenosis may become more severe as gestation progresses, and occasional cases have been reported where valve stenosis detected in the second trimester has become complete atresia by term. An important part of the assessment of right ventricular outflow obstruction is the size of the pulmonary arteries, as this will to a large extent dictate the

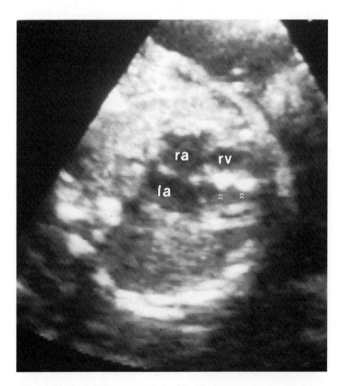

Fig. 18.24 Dystrophic calcification of the ventricular septum. This may give very similar appearances to single or multiple tumours. In this case there appear to be two large, distinct masses (arrowed) in the septum. The parents chose to terminate the pregnancy. Autopsy showed the majority of the ventricular septum to be infarcted, with localised areas of dystrophic calcification giving the appearances of masses. No cause was evident and there were no other features to suggest a generalised ischaemic insult to the fetus.

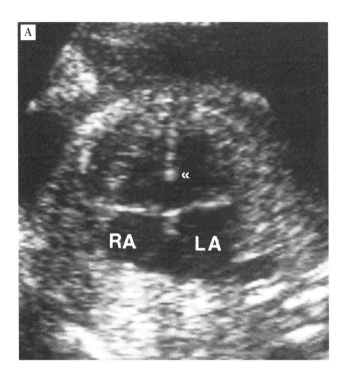

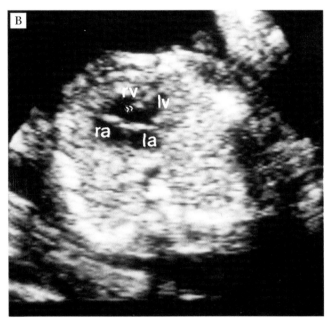

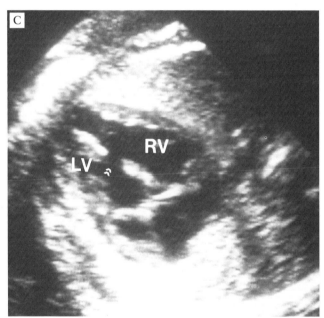

Fig. 18.25 Ventricular septal defects. A: Care must be taken in assessing the integrity of the ventricular septum when it is imaged along its long axis, as 'dropout' of the echo signal in the part of the septum furthest away from the transducer may give a false impression of a septal defect. The 'T' sign, seen here (arrowed) is a useful indicator that this defect is genuine. Ideally, the septum should be imaged at 90° to its long axis to avoid false-positive diagnosis of a defect, but **B:** even an angle of 45° or so will allow much clearer definition of the defect (the 'T' sign is present again). **C:** Defects in the thicker, muscular (or trabecular) part of the septum usually present fewer problems and significant defects are usually easily seen (mid-muscular ventricular septal defect arrowed).

type and success of post-natal surgical treatment. Pulmonary atresia in the presence of an intact ventricular septum may be associated with coronary artery anomalies, the commonest being fistulae between the coronary arter-

ies and the right ventricular cavity. There may be 'interruption' (a missing segment) of major coronary artery branches, with the distal vessel supplied only by the fistulous connection with the right ventricle. Dilated coronary

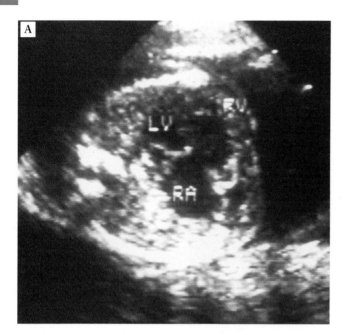

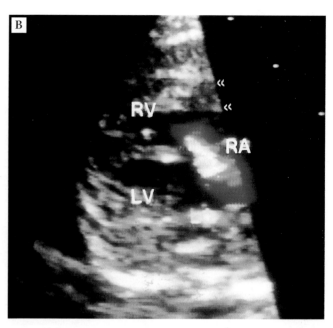

Fig. 18.26 Pulmonary atresia with intact ventricular septum. A: The right atrium (RA) is enlarged. **B:** The right ventricle (RV) is very thick walled (arrows) due to hypertrophy, and colour flow Doppler reveals the tricuspid regurgitant jet responsible for the atrial enlargement. Very severe pulmonary stenosis may cause a similar appearance.

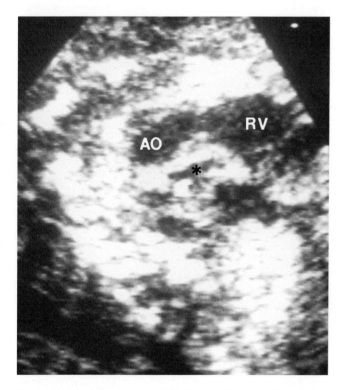

Fig. 18.27 Pulmonary atresia. A dilated aorta arises anteriorly and the posterior pulmonary artery, identifiable by its bifurcation, is tiny (marked with an asterisk) owing to atresia of the pulmonary valve (a case of complex transposition, with ventricular septal defect as well as pulmonary atresia).

arteries or unusual flow patterns within the right ventricular wall are a clue to the presence of such fistulae which, particularly when large, are often associated with the poorer end of the spectrum of post-natal prognosis.

Tetralogy of Fallot and pulmonary atresia with ventricular septal defect

The principal abnormalities in tetralogy of Fallot are a ventricular septal defect with some degree of aortic override and infundibular pulmonary stenosis (Fig. 18.28). Because the right ventricle may decompress through the VSD right ventricular hypertrophy is not a feature in the fetus, although in some cases the infundibular myocardium may be seen to be thickened, causing the right ventricular outflow tract to be narrow. Pulmonary atresia with ventricular septal defect has anatomical findings very similar to the tetralogy, but with complete atresia of the right ventricular outflow tract. The four-chamber view is usually normal. The size of the pulmonary arteries is a major factor in later choice of treatment, and it is important to take this into account when counselling parents on the likely prognosis.

The aortic valve

Like pulmonary stenosis, mild to moderate degrees of aortic stenosis may be missed even with good-quality

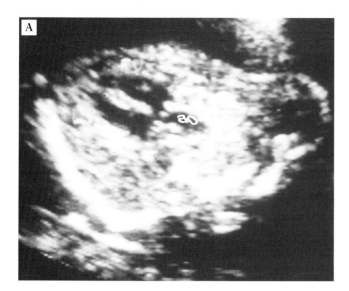

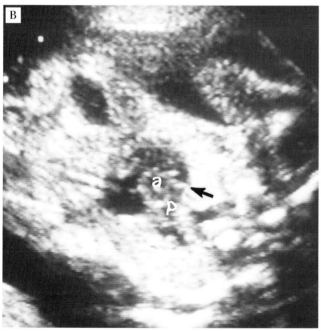

Fig. 18.28 Tetralogy of Fallot. A: Ventricular septal defect with aortic override in a case of tetralogy of Fallot. The four-chamber view is usually normal and the ventricular septal defect will only be seen when the 'fifth' chamber, the aorta (ao), is seen. Aortic override may occur in anomalies other than tetralogy (such as pulmonary atresia with ventricular septal defect or common arterial trunk), so the finding should provoke a detailed assessment of the great arteries. **B:** In this case of tetralogy a short-axis view of the heart shows the pulmonary artery (p) to be smaller than the aorta (a), and the pulmonary valve (arrowed) is thickened and stenosed.

imaging. In more severe cases the left ventricular wall is thickened because of hypertrophy, and in very severe cases the ventricle becomes dilated, function becomes progressively impaired, there is often functional mitral regurgitation detectable on colour Doppler, and the fetus may

become hydropic (see Fig. 18.21). In some cases of severe left ventricular outflow obstruction the endocardium may appear thickened and abnormally reflective owing to endocardial fibroelastosis. Endocardial fibroelastosis (EFE) may rarely occur in the fetus in the absence of outflow obstruction ('primary' EFE), when atrial enlargement may be a prominent feature because of impaired ventricular filling. Aortic stenosis may, like pulmonary stenosis, become more severe as gestation progresses, and there are rare occasions when it may progress to aortic atresia with hypoplasia of the left heart elements (part of the spectrum of the hypoplastic left heart syndrome).[44–46]

The pulmonary arteries

Isolated pulmonary artery anomalies are very rare in the fetus. Hypoplasia of the right or left pulmonary artery may occur in association with hypoplasia of one lung, but in such cases the pulmonary hypoplasia is usually obvious, the heart is usually shifted towards the hypoplastic lung, and assessment of the size of the pulmonary artery is of limited diagnostic or prognostic value. Diffuse pulmonary artery hypoplasia is almost always a consequence of severe right ventricular outflow obstruction. A pulmonary artery larger than the aorta usually indicates obstructed flow in the left side of the heart.[47]

In the rare 'absent pulmonary valve syndrome' (a misnomer, as the pulmonary valve is present but is severely dysplastic and incompetent) the pulmonary trunk and its major branches are dilated. This may occur in isolation but is more commonly associated with tetralogy of Fallot. The pulmonary arteries may be so hugely dilated that the pulmonary trunk appears as large as the ventricles, causing considerable confusion and difficulty in interpretation of the anatomy (Fig. 18.29). The right ventricle is usually dilated to some degree because of the pulmonary regurgitation, and colour flow Doppler will usually provide a rapid guide to the diagnosis, showing turbulent to-and-fro flow through the pulmonary valve. The dilated pulmonary arteries may compress the major airways, causing tracheomalacia and bronchomalacia, which may sometimes prove fatal post-natally.

The aorta

Coarctation of the aorta is the commonest cause of heart failure in the first few weeks of life, yet is very difficult to diagnose reliably antenatally.[48,49] The obstruction to the aortic arch may be very discrete and is therefore frequently impossible to image directly, even with the best equipment, a thin mother and a cooperative fetus. The antenatal diagnosis of coarctation therefore rests upon indirect signs. The major indicator is right ventricular dilatation, the pulmonary artery usually being dilated too (particularly when compared to the size of the ascending aorta) (Fig. 18.30).

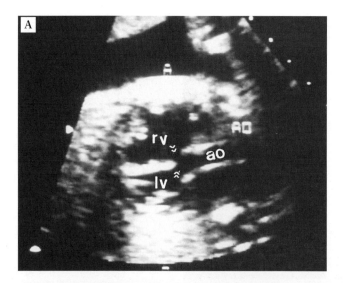

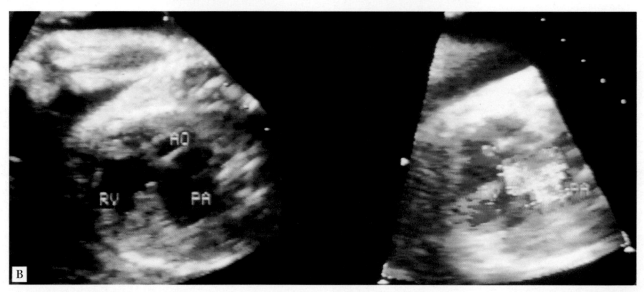

Fig. 18.29 Tetralogy of Fallot with absent pulmonary valve. In this combination of abnormalities the cardiac anatomy is often confusing due to gross dilatation of the pulmonary trunk and pulmonary arteries. As in this case, the pulmonary artery may be so dilated that it appears to be an additional chamber of the heart rather than a great artery. **A:** In contrast to simple tetralogy, the right ventricle is usually larger than the left ventricle. **B:** The hugely dilated pulmonary artery (PA) appears larger than the cardiac chambers; colour flow Doppler is useful in this situation as it will show turbulent 'to-and-fro' flow in the pulmonary artery owing to the combination of pulmonary stenosis and severe regurgitation.

The pathophysiology of coarctation *in utero* is still very poorly understood. The popular theory to explain dilatation of the right ventricle is that the right heart is required to provide a greater percentage of systemic cardiac output (through the duct to the descending aorta) than in the normal heart. Newer hypotheses involve restricted flow across the foramen ovale, possibly related to functional abnormalities of the foramen itself. Such indirect methods of diagnosis of coarctation are inevitably inaccurate and, even with the levels of expertise currently available in large specialist centres, false-negative and false-positive diagnoses remain one of the major limitations of fetal echocar-

diography. There may be additional indirect clues to the presence of coarctation. It is associated with other abnormalities in about 40% of cases. These may be minor and difficult to detect in the fetus (such as bicuspid aortic valve), but more important aortic stenosis may be recognisable. The aortic root may be mildly hypoplastic, and therefore a rather small aortic root associated with right ventricular dilatation should lead to a strong suspicion of coarctation. Mitral stenosis may be associated with coarctation but is also difficult to recognise unless severe. Coarctation may occur in the presence of many other important anomalies, particularly ventricular septal

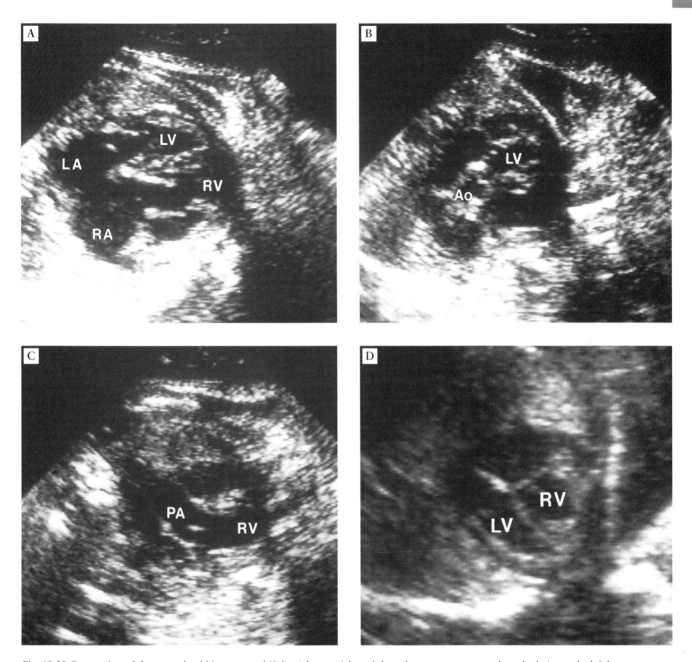

Fig. 18.30 Coarctation of the aorta should be suspected if the right ventricle and the pulmonary artery are enlarged relative to the left heart elements. **A:** This may be very obvious. **B:** Comparison of the size of the aorta and **C:** the pulmonary artery will usually help; in this case the pulmonary artery is almost twice the size of the aorta. The degree of right ventricular dilatation may be misleading: even severe coarctation may occur post-natally with minor degrees of right heart dilatation, as in the case shown in **D:** where the circulation was duct dependent after delivery.

defect. If the ventricular septal defect is of significant size the right ventricular dilatation seen with isolated coarctation often does not occur, but the pulmonary artery is almost always clearly seen to be larger than the aorta, and this simple sign – a substantial difference in the sizes of the two arteries – is the mainstay of diagnosis of coarctation in the presence of complex heart disease.

The indirect signs of interruption of the aortic arch (an absent segment, usually between the origins of the left common carotid and the left subclavian arteries) are similar to those of coarctation: the pulmonary artery is usually strikingly larger than the aortic root, the aortic root is usually small in absolute terms, and there is almost always an associated ventricular septal defect.

Transposition of the great arteries

In simple transposition of the great arteries the four-chamber view is usually normal. The 'five-chamber' view oftens reveals that the two great arteries arise in parallel, in contrast to the usual arrangement of one artery appearing in short axis when the other is seen in long axis. When clear images are difficult to obtain colour flow Doppler may highlight the parallel courses of the two arteries. Confirmation of the identity of each great artery is by visualisation of the pulmonary artery bifurcation or the origin of the head and neck vessels arising from the aorta (Fig. 18.31).

Common arterial trunk

Common arterial trunk, a single arterial trunk giving rise to both aorta and pulmonary arteries, is one of the major anomalies that may be associated with a normal standard four-chamber view. The 'five-chamber' view will reveal a ventricular septal defect with a large, single great artery overriding the crest of the ventricular septum. It is usually possible to follow the course of the common trunk to reveal the origin of the pulmonary arteries from the ascending common trunk (Fig. 18.32).

Pericardial abnormalities

Pericardial effusion

Pericardial effusion is most commonly seen with fetal hydrops in association with pleural effusions (Fig. 18.33) and ascites. In this setting antenatal treatment of the pericardial effusion is rarely, if ever, indicated. If the underlying cause of the hydrops can be treated, or resolves

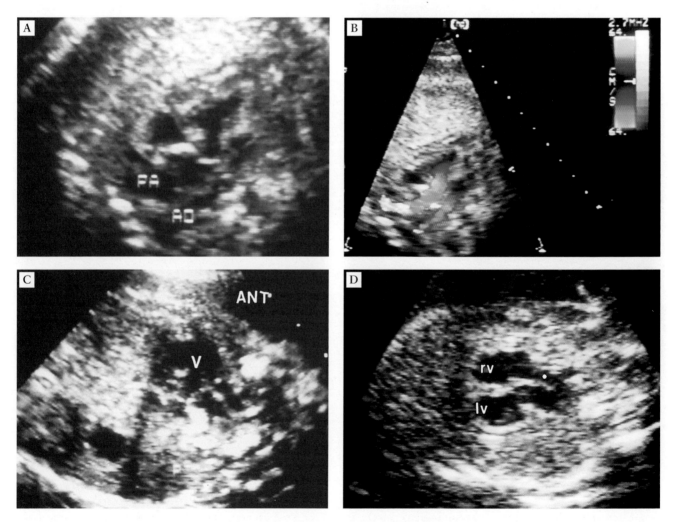

Fig. 18.31 Transposition of the great arteries. A: In the majority of cases of transposition the aorta and the pulmonary artery are seen in parallel, in contrast to the normal relationship of the two vessels 'wrapping around' each other with the aorta anterior. **B:** When image quality is poor colour flow Doppler may highlight the course of the parallel vessels. Note that in this case the pulmonary artery is larger than the aorta; this fetus also had a coarctation of the aorta. **C:** Although parallel courses of the great arteries strongly suggest the presence of transposition, confirmation that the posterior great artery bifurcates and **D:** that the anterior artery gives rise to the head and neck vessels is important.

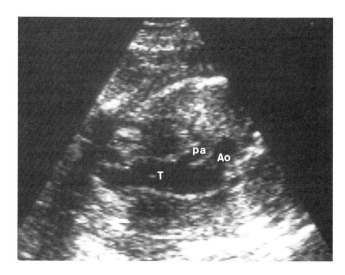

Fig. 18.32 Common arterial trunk. A single large great artery, the common trunk (T), arises from the heart to give rise to both the aorta and the pulmonary trunk. This is just one of the anomalies in which a ventricular septal defect with an overriding great vessel is seen in the 'five-chamber' view (see section on tetralogy of Fallot and its related abnormalities).

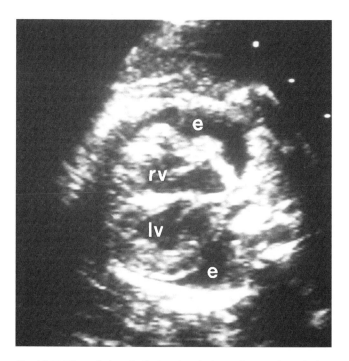

Fig. 18.33 Bilateral pleural effusions in a hydropic fetus with marked cardiomegaly. No cause was found in this case. Similar appearances may be seen in twin–twin transfusion.

tion or, if very large, may inhibit lung development. In such cases drainage of the pericardium may be rewarding, but repeated drainage procedures may be required. Such effusions are often idiopathic (possibly related to congenital abnormalities of lymphatic drainage), but may require formal surgical drainage post-natally. Small amounts of pericardial fluid (a thin rim around the heart) can often be seen in the normal fetus.

Cardiac causes of fetal hydrops

Fetal heart failure leading to hydrops is relatively unusual. It may be due to arrhythmias, either prolonged episodes of supraventricular tachycardia or sustained severe bradycardia with congenital complete heart block. Structural cardiac abnormalities such as severe aortic stenosis with secondary mitral regurgitation, or severe tricuspid regurgitation (as may occur with Ebstein's anomaly of the tricuspid valve or pulmonary atresia with intact ventricular septum) may also cause progressive cardiomegaly and hydrops. Treatment for sustained supraventricular tachycardia may be effective, but for all other fetuses with a cardiac cause for hydrops the prognosis is very poor.

Chromosomal abnormalities

It is probably wise for all fetuses with suspected or proven chromosomal abnormalities to have a detailed echocardiogram. Post-natally some 40% of babies with Down's syndrome, 35% of those with Turner's syndrome and over 90% of those with Edward's (trisomy 18) and Patau's (trisomy 13) syndromes will have some kind of congenital heart disease, and it seems likely that these figures are even higher in the fetus. Down's syndrome has a strong association with atrioventricular septal defects (so strong that antenatal diagnosis of AV septal defect should prompt an offer of karyotyping), although other anomalies such as ventricular septal defect, atrial septal defect, tetralogy and the like also occur. Coarctation is particularly common with Turner's syndrome, although other anomalies such as septal defect, aortic stenosis and aortic root dilatation may also occur. The great majority of fetuses with trisomies 13 or 18 have ventricular septal defects, and rarer chromosomal anomalies are also frequently associated with cardiac malformations.

Screening for familial cardiac disease

Families with a history of hereditary conditions associated with heart abnormalities, such as hypertrophic cardiomyopathy, Marfan's syndrome, Noonan's syndrome, muscular dystrophies and tuberous sclerosis, frequently request detailed fetal echocardiography. It is relatively rare to find

spontaneously, the pericardial fluid is usually resorbed. Pericardial effusions may occur without generalised hydrops in the absence of other cardiac disease, or may be secondary to a pericardial or mediastinal tumour. They may become sufficiently large to compromise cardiac func-

fetal cardiac abnormalities in such cases. Parents often feel greatly reassured by the finding of an apparently normal fetal heart, but it is important to recognise and explain the limited reassurance that can be given in these circumstances. A normal appearance of the heart in fetal life does not exclude the possibility of the development of a cardiac abnormality post-natally, in later childhood or in adult life.

Arrhythmias

M-mode and Doppler are invaluable in the assessment of arrhythmias. Both modalities allow accurate measurement of heart rate. An M-mode recording with the cursor positioned to pass through a ventricular wall as well as an atrial wall often allows assessment of the relationship between atrial and ventricular contractions, and this may also be possible in some cases using pulsed Doppler recording of mitral or tricuspid flow. Assessment of this relationship usually allows differentiation between sinus bradycardia and second- or third-degree heart block, and usually also permits differentiation of atrial flutter from re-entrant supraventricular tachycardia (the latter may be important when deciding upon treatment).

Irregularity

Irregularity of the fetal heart rhythm is common, particularly in the third trimester, and is usually due to atrial ectopic beats. Although these may be apparent on the cross-sectional image, M-mode or Doppler (Fig. 18.34) make the ectopic beats immediately apparent. Bigeminal rhythm (alternating normal beats and ectopics, usually atrial) is not uncommon in the fetus, is harmless, requires no treatment, and will settle spontaneously given time. Despite its benign nature bigeminal rhythm can cause difficulties in obstetric management, and may even precipitate unnecessary early delivery because of failure of monitoring devices to detect the ectopic beats. Because ectopic beats are early the ventricles have not had time to fill normally and there is little blood ejected from the heart. The normal beats are detected by standard monitoring but the fetal heart sounds related to the ectopic beat are not, resulting in the monitor reading the heart rate as half its real value. If monitoring suggests fetal bradycardia but all other parameters suggest a contented rather than a distressed fetus, an echocardiogram is well worth while before proceeding to emergency delivery. In cases where there are difficulties in assessing fetal wellbeing in the presence of arrhythmias (whether perceived or real), direct fetal ECG monitoring[50] or fetal pulse oximetry[51] may be helpful during labour.

Bradycardia

Fetal distress remains the most common cause of genuine sustained sinus bradycardia, but there is a variety of more benign causes of bradycardia that must be borne in mind if unnecessary early delivery is to be avoided. Sinus node disease may rarely cause sustained bradycardia; the fetal heart is usually structurally normal and there are usually no other signs of distress.[52] Even with rates as low as 60 there may be no significant haemodynamic embarrassment and early delivery is contraindicated unless there is heart failure, merely serving to add the problems of prematurity to those of the existing cardiac abnormality. It is worth bearing in mind that maternal anti-arrhythmic medication may produce sinus bradycardia in the fetus.[53] Mild sinus bradycardia with rates close to 100 may occur in fetuses who later prove to have a congenital long QT syndrome.[54,55] These patients have sinus bradycardia and are prone to paroxysmal ventricular tachycardia later in life, and may exhibit a family history of syncope or sudden death. In such cases it is wise to arrange formal cardiac assessment post-natally. Fetuses with left atrial isomerism (usually associated with complex structural abnormalities) do not have a normal sinus node and usually have a pacemaker sited low in the atrial mass, set at a lower rate than the normal sinus node and producing mild degrees of sinus bradycardia (sometimes as low as the 80s). The finding of a sinus bradycardia with, say, a complete atrioventricular septal defect should therefore prompt careful assessment of viscero-atrial situs, including pulmonary and systemic venous anatomy, which may be of major prognostic importance.

Second-degree heart block may cause intermittent or sustained bradycardia of variable rate. It is rare for second-degree block to occur as an isolated event and most fetuses have associated structural cardiac abnormalities, for example congenitally corrected transposition of the great arteries. With complete (third-degree) heart block the heart rate is usually in the 60s, and M-mode or Doppler shows no fixed relationship between atrial and ventricular contraction (Fig. 18.35). Complete heart block is often well tolerated but hydrops and fetal death may occur, the risk generally being greater the lower the heart rate. Complete heart block may occur in the presence of structural abnormalities of the heart, and in such cases the prognosis is usually poor. More frequently, however, it is an isolated abnormality, although the fetal heart may be somewhat enlarged because of the large stroke volume resulting from the slow rate. There is a strong association with maternal lupus antibodies (anti-Ro and anti-La),[56] but there are often no maternal symptoms of connective tissue disease. Occasionally serial scans in a fetus apparently tolerating heart block well will reveal the development of hydrops. The mechanism of heart failure in this setting is poorly understood, but there seems little doubt that maternal lupus antibodies may cause a fetal myocarditis as well as immune-mediated damage to the fetal conducting system. There are anecdotal reports of maternal steroid therapy resulting in an improvement in

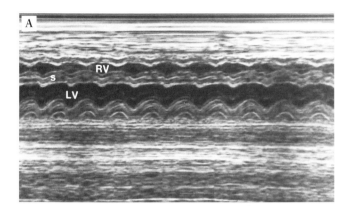

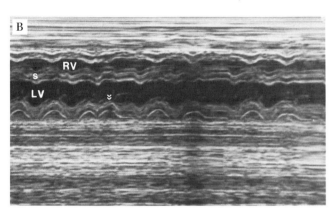

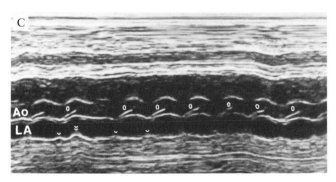

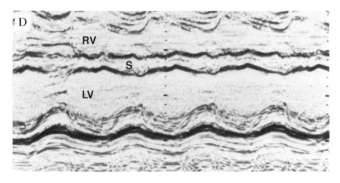

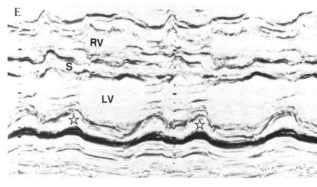

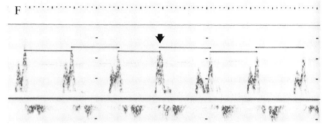

Fig. 18.34 M-mode recordings can be invaluable in the assessment of heart rate and rhythm. The distance between the vertical dotted lines in each of these traces represents 1 second. **A:** The cursor is positioned through the right ventricle, the ventricular septum (s) and the left ventricle showing normal, regular sinus rhythm. **B:** An ectopic beat (arrowed) is seen, followed by a short compensatory pause and resumption of regular sinus rhythm. Most fetal ectopic beats are supraventricular in origin. They are very common, are almost invariably harmless, and are a frequent cause of irregularity of the fetal heart rhythm. **C:** The M-mode cursor has been positioned through the aortic root (ao) and the left atrium. Atrial contraction can be identified by movement of the posterior left atrial wall (single arrows), and the aortic valve leaflets can be seen to open (marked with an o) following each normal atrial systole. An atrial ectopic beat occurs (double arrows) followed by a compensatory pause. The aortic valve does not open following the ectopic beat, either because the ventricle is inadequately filled to open the valve or because the ectopic beat has failed to conduct to the ventricles. **D** and **E:** A near-continuous recording from the same fetus in sinus rhythm (**D**) followed by an episode of bigeminal rhythm (**E**), where each normal beat is followed by an ectopic beat (star) followed in turn by a compensatory pause. Fetal heart rate monitoring is likely to fail to detect the ectopic beats, falsely suggesting the fetus has marked bradycardia. Bigeminal rhythm is entirely benign and requires no intervention. **F:** If M-mode recordings are difficult to record or interpret pulsed Doppler recordings of atrioventricular or semilunar valve flow may be useful. In this example of mitral flow regular sinus rhythm with the usual two waveforms of mitral flow (e and a waves) is followed by an atrial ectopic, where the a wave has occurred early and is superimposed on the e wave (arrowed). The resulting irregularity of the heart rate can be appreciated by the horizontal lines drawn between each a wave: lines 1 and 2 are of equal length, 3 is shorter as the ectopic beat has occurred early, 4 is longer than 1 and 2 because of the compensatory pause, and 5 returns to the same length as lines 1 and 2.

myocardial function in such cases,[57] but so far there is no concrete evidence of a beneficial effect. Similarly there are anecdotal reports of improvement in heart failure in fetuses with complete heart block following maternal administration of sympathomimetic agents such as salbutamol, although our experience in Leeds suggests that doses of salbutamol sufficient to produce even a small increase in fetal heart rate are often poorly tolerated by the

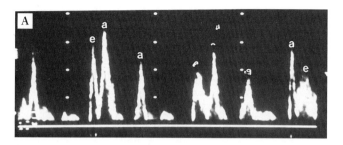
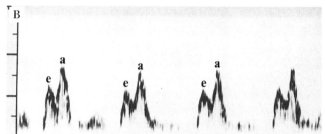

Fig. 18.35 Mitral flow. A: M-mode recording of mitral flow in complete heart block. The overall heart rate is about 60 bpm and the e and a waves are dissociated from each other. **B:** The normal pattern for comparison.

mother. Attempts at intra-uterine fetal heart pacing[58] have met with little success, partly because of difficulty in maintaining a stable pacing wire position. As with most cardiac abnormalities early delivery is best avoided unless there is imminent fear of fetal loss.[59] Symptomatic heart block is difficult to manage in the term neonate but much more difficult in a tiny baby, who also has the problems associated with prematurity. Fortunately the majority of fetuses surviving to term have a good prognosis.[60,61]

Tachycardia

Tachyarrhythmias in the fetus are almost invariably supraventricular in origin and the heart rate is usually around 240 bpm. Most are re-entrant tachycardia;[62] M-mode recording shows the atrial and ventricular rates to be the same. Atrial flutter also occurs[63] but is much rarer and is identifiable on the M-mode recording, which shows the atrial rate to be much faster (usually between 300 and 400 bpm) than the ventricular rate (Fig. 18.36). Most fetal supraventricular tachycardia occurs in a structurally normal heart, but accessory conduction pathways may occur in the presence of structural abnormalities. For example, in Ebstein's anomaly of the tricuspid valve and in tuberous sclerosis pre-excitation may occur. Supraventricular tachycardia may resolve spontaneously[64] and may be benign if it is paroxysmal and of short duration,[65] but tachycardia sustained for days or weeks may result in increasing impairment of myocardial function, leading ultimately to hydrops and fetal death. Opinion is divided on the optimum drug treatment. In the UK most cardiologists now try maternal digoxin if the fetus appears well, aiming for maternal blood levels at the upper end of the usual adult therapeutic range, and changing to flecainide[66] if there is no fetal response within a week or so. Other drugs such as procainamide[67] and quinidine[68] have also been used, with some success. If the fetus is hydropic most UK cardiologists would choose flecainide as first-line therapy, as it crosses the placenta to the fetal circulation more effectively than does digoxin. However, flecainide is a powerful drug with potentially major side effects for the mother, and therefore careful maternal monitoring with

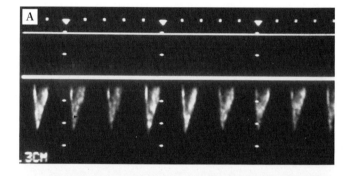
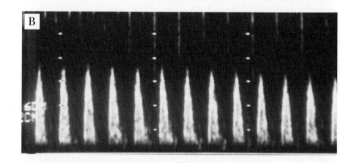
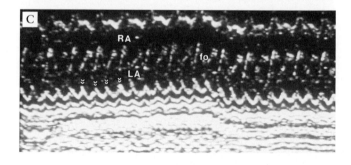

Fig. 18.36 Aortic waveforms. A: Pulsed Doppler recording from the aorta in sinus rhythm and **B:** in supraventricular tachycardia. The distance between the vertical dotted lines represent 1 second. The ventricular rate in **B** is approximately 240 bpm. **C:** An M-mode recording in this fetus, taken with the cursor positioned through the atria and the atrial septum, shows that the left atrial wall contractions (marked with double arrows) are occurring at twice the ventricular rate, representing atrial flutter with 2:1 block. The rapid motion of the foramen ovale (fo) also reflects the rate of atrial contraction.

electrocardiography and blood flecainide levels is essential. In cases resistant to flecainide there are anecdotal reports of the use of a variety of different anti-arrhythmic drugs, given either to the mother or directly into the umbilical cord or intramuscularly to the fetus,[69,70] but it is not yet clear which drug or combination of drugs offers the best chance of a return to stable sinus rhythm. As a general rule it is wise to avoid early delivery,[71] treating *in utero* even if hydrops is present. However, such decisions may be difficult in practice as both early delivery and intra-uterine treatment carry some risk of fetal death.

Pregnancy outcome following antenatal diagnosis of cardiac abnormalities

In the early days of fetal echocardiography cardiologists used to assume that the outlook for antenatally detected cardiac abnormalities would be similar to that for postnatal diagnosis. It is clear now that this is not the case for certain anomalies (Ebstein's anomaly of the tricuspid valve, for instance), and that fetal diagnosis may be associated with a worse prognosis.[72–74] This is partly because the less favourable end of the spectrum of anomalies is more likely to be detected antenatally, and partly because fetal attrition was sometimes not recognised as being related to cardiac anomalies until fetal echocardiography became widely available.

Antenatal treatment of heart disease

Antenatal treatment of supraventricular tachycardia may be very rewarding, but treatment for structural heart disease in the fetus has met with little success. Ultrasound-guided balloon dilatation of severe aortic valve stenosis has been attempted in a few cases,[75] but technical difficulties with the development and use of the tiny balloon catheters required have been considerable and at present the technique cannot be recommended. Exciting research on fetal sheep suggests that antenatal treatment for some major cardiac abnormalities might soon be on the horizon.[76] Further development of other, more advanced imaging technologies, such as three-dimensional fetal echocardiography,[77–79] may prove to be a stimulus to more adventurous attempts at antenatal intervention for life-threatening abnormalities.

Counselling

Any well educated doctor is probably capable of describing congenital cardiac malformations to parents. However, it is not possible to counsel accurately on matters of treatment and prognosis unless the counsellor is actively involved in the medical and surgical treatment of congenital heart disease, and for this reason it is a widely held view in Europe that effective counselling can only be undertaken by a specialist in the field, usually a paediatric cardiologist. Litigation is becoming increasingly frequent after parents have been told that the fetal echocardiogram is 'normal'. An important part of counselling parents is an explanation of the limitations as well as the benefits of fetal echocardiography.

REFERENCES

1 Bronshtein M, Zimmer E Z, Milo S, Ho S Y, Lorber A, Gerlis L M. Fetal cardiac abnormalities detected by transvaginal sonography at 12–16 weeks gestation. Obstet Gynecol 1991; 78: 374–378

2 Achiron R, Weissman A, Rostein Z, Lipitz S, Mashiach S, Hegesh J. Transvaginal echocardiographic examination of the fetal heart between 13 and 15 weeks gestation in a low risk population. J Ultrasound Med 1994; 13: 783–789

3 Allan L D, Santos R, Pexieder T. Anatomical and echocardiographic correlates of normal cardiac morphology in the late first trimester fetus. Heart 1997; 77: 68–72

4 Bronshtein M, Siegler E, Eshcoli Z, Zimmer E Z. Transvaginal ultrasound measurements of the fetal heart at 11 to 17 weeks of gestation. Am J Perinatol 1992; 9: 38–42

5 Fogel M, Copel J A, Cullen M T, Hobbins J C, Kleinman C S. Congenital heart disease and fetal thoracoabdominal anomalies: associations in utero and the importance of cytogenetic analysis. Am J Perinatol 1991; 8: 411–416

6 Meyer-Wittkopf M, Simpson J M, Sharland G K. Incidence of congenital heart defects in fetuses of diabetic mothers: a retrospective study of 326 cases. Ultrasound Obstet Gynecol 1996; 8: 8–10

7 Veille J C, Hanson R, Sivakoff M, Hoen H, Ben-Ami M. Fetal cardiac size in normal, intrauterine growth retarded, and diabetic pregnancies. Am J Perinatol 1993; 10: 275–279

8 Rizzo G, Arduini D, Romanini C. Accelerated cardiac growth and abnormal cardiac flow in fetuses of type 1 diabetic mothers. Obstet Gynecol 1992; 80: 369–376

9 Allan L D. Manual of fetal echocardiography. Lancaster: MTP Press, 1989

10 Allan L D, Sharland G, Cook A. Color atlas of fetal cardiology. London: Mosby-Wolfe, 1994

11 Shipp T D, Bromley B, Hornberger L K, Nadel A, Benacerraf B R. Levorotation of the fetal cardiac axis: a clue for the presence of congenital heart disease. Obstet Gynecol 1995; 85: 97–102

12 Smith R S, Comstock C H, Kirk J S, Lee W. Ultrasonographic left cardiac axis deviation: a marker for fetal anomalies. Obstet Gynecol 1995; 85: 187–191

13 Crane J M, Ash K, Fink N, Desjardins C. Abnormal fetal cardiac axis in the detection of intrathoracic anomalies and congenital heart disease. Ultrasound Obstet Gynecol 1997; 10: 90–93

14 Bork M D, Egan J F, Diana D J et al. A new method for on-screen ultrasonographic determination of fetal cardiac axis. Am J Obstet Gynecol 1995; 173: 1192–1195

15 Shime J, Gresser C D, Rakowski H. Quantitative two-dimensional echocardiographic assessment of fetal cardiac growth. Am J Obstet Gynecol 1986; 154: 294–300

16 Tan J, Silverman N H, Hoffman J I, Villegas M, Schmidt K G. Cardiac dimensions determined by cross-sectional echocardiography in the normal human fetus from 18 weeks to term. Am J Cardiol 1992; 70: 1459–1467

17 Siddiqi T A, Meyer R A, Korfhagen J, Khoury J C, Rosenn B, Midovnik M. A longitudinal study describing confidence limits of normal fetal cardiac, thoracic and pulmonary dimensions from 20 to 40 weeks' gestation. J Ultrasound Med 1993; 12: 731–736

18 Beeby A R, Dunlop W, Heads A, Hunter S. Reproducibility of ultrasonic measurement of fetal cardiac haemodynamics. Br J Obstet Gynaecol 1991; 98: 807–814

19 Schmidt K G, Silverman N H, Hoffman J I. Determination of ventricular volumes in human fetal hearts by two-dimensional echocardiography. Am J Cardiol 1995; 76: 1313–1316

20 Tulzer G, Khowsathit P, Gudmunsson S et al. Diastolic function of the fetal heart during second and third trimester: a prospective longitudinal Doppler echocardiographic study. Eur J Pediatr 1994; 153: 151–154

21 Brown D L, Roberts D J, Miller W A. Left ventricular echogenic focus in the fetal heart: pathologic correlation. J Ultrasound Med 1994; 13: 613–616

22 Petrikovsky B M, Challenger M, Wyse L J. Natural history of echogenic foci within ventricles of the fetal heart. Ultrasound Obstet Gynecol 1995; 5: 92–94

23 Sepulveda W, Cullen S, Nicolaidis P, Hollingsworth J, Fisk N M. Echogenic foci in the fetal heart: a marker for chromosomal abnormality. Br J Obstet Gynaecol 1995; 102: 490–492

24 Simpson J M, Cook A, Sharland G. Significance of echogenic foci in the fetal heart: prospective study of 228 cases. Ultrasound Obstet Gynecol 1996; 8: 225–228

25 Bronshtein M, Jacobi P, Ofir C. Multiple fetal intracardiac echogenic foci: not always a benign sonographic finding. Prenat Diagn 1996; 16: 131–135

26 Dildy G A, Judd V E, Clark S L. Prospective evaluation of the antenatal incidence and postnatal significance of the fetal echogenic cardiac focus: a case control study. Am J Obstet Gynecol 1996; 175: 1008–1012

27 Petrikovsky B, Challenger M, Gross B. Unusual appearances of echogenic foci within the fetal heart: are they benign? Ultrasound Obstet Gynecol 1996; 8: 229–231

28 Vergani P, Mariani S, Ghidini A et al. Screening for congenital heart disease with the four-chamber view of the fetal heart. Am J Obstet Gynecol 1992; 167: 1000–1003

29 Wigton T R, Sabbagha R E, Tamura R K, Cohen L, Minogue J P, Strasburger J F. Sonographic diagnosis of congenital heart disease: comparison between the four-chamber view and multiple cardiac views. Obstet Gynecol 1993; 82: 219–224

30 Tegnander E, Eik-Nes S H, Johansen O J, Linker D T. Prenatal detection of heart defects at the routine fetal examination at 18 weeks in a non-selected population. Ultrasound Obstet Gynecol 1995; 5: 372–380

31 Kirk J S, Riggs T W, Comstock C H, Lee W, Yang S S, Weinhouse E. Prenatal screening for cardiac anomalies: the value of routine addition of the aortic root to the four-chamber view. Obstet Gynecol 1994; 84: 427–431

32 Benacerraf B R. Sonographic detection of fetal anomalies of the aortic and pulmonary arteries: value of four-chamber view vs direct images. AJR 1994; 163: 1483–1489

33 Tulzer G, Gudmunsson S, Sharkey A M, Wood D C, Cohen A W, Huhta J C. Doppler echocardiography of fetal ductus arteriosus constriction versus increased right ventricular output. J Am Coll Cardiol 1991; 18: 532–536

34 Rasanen J, Jouppila P. Fetal cardiac function and ductus arteriosus during indomethacin and sulindac therapy for threatened preterm labor: a randomised study. Am J Obstet Gynecol 1995; 173: 20–25

35 DiSessa T G, Moretti M L, Khoury A, Pulliam D A, Arheart K L, Sibai B M. Cardiac function in fetuses and newborns exposed to low dose aspirin during pregnancy. Am J Obstet Gynecol 1994; 171: 892–900

36 Phoon C K, Villegas M D, Ursell P C, Silverman N H. Left atrial isomerism detected in fetal life. Am J Cardiol 1996; 77: 1083–1088

37 Wilson A D, Rao P S, Aeschlimann S. Normal fetal foramen flap and transatrial Doppler velocity pattern. J Am Soc Echocardiogr 1990; 3: 491–494

38 Kachalia P, Bowie J D, Adams D B, Carroll B A. In utero sonographic appearance of the atrial septum primum and septum secundum. J Ultrasound Med 1991; 10: 423–426

39 Lang D, Oberhoffer R, Cook A et al. Pathologic spectrum of malformations of the tricuspid valve in prenatal and neonatal life. J Am Coll Cardiol 1991; 17: 1161–1167

40 Sharland G K, Chita S K, Allan L D. Tricuspid valve dysplasia or displacement in intrauterine life. J Am Coll Cardiol 1991; 17: 944–949

41 Hornberger L K, Sahn D J, Kleinman C S, Copel J A, Reed K L. Tricuspid valve disease with significant tricuspid insufficiency in the fetus: diagnosis and outcome. J Am Coll Cardiol 1991; 17: 167–173

42 Oberhoffer R, Cook A C, Lang D et al. Correlation between echocardiographic and morphological investigations of lesions of the tricuspid valve diagnosed during fetal life. Br Heart J 1993; 68: 580–585

43 Richards I S, Kulkarni A, Brooks S M, Lathrop D A, Bremner W F, Sperelakis N. A moderate concentration of ethanol alters cellular membrane potentials and decrease contractile force of human fetal heart. Dev Pharmacol Ther 1989; 13: 51–56

44 Allan L D, Sharland G, Tynan M J. The natural history of the hypoplastic left heart syndrome. Int J Cardiol 1989; 25: 341–343

45 Hornberger L K, Sanders S P, Rein A J, Spevak P J, Parness I A, Colan S D. Left heart obstructive lesions and left ventricular growth in the mid trimester fetus. A longitudinal study. Circulation 1995; 92: 1531–1538

46 Simpson J M, Sharland G K. Natural history and outcome of aortic stenosis diagnosed prenatally. Heart 1997; 77: 205–210

47 Comstock C H, Riggs T, Lee W, Kirk J. Pulmonary-to-aorta diameter ratio in the normal and abnormal fetal heart. Am J Obstet Gynecol 1991; 165: 1038–1044

48 Sharland G K, Chan K Y, Allan L D. Coarctation of the aorta: difficulties in prenatal diagnosis. Br Heart J 1994; 71: 70–75

49 Hornberger L K, Sahn D J, Kleinman C S, Copel J, Silverman N H. Antenatal diagnosis of coarctation of the aorta: a multicenter experience. J Am Coll Cardiol 1994; 23: 417–423

50 Thorp J M, Guidry A M. A technique for intrapartum monitoring of fetuses with congenital bradycardias. Am J Perinatol 1994; 11: 353–355

51 van den Berg P P, Nijland R, van den Brand S F, Jongsma H W, Nijhuis J G. Intrapartum fetal surveillance of congenital heart block with pulse oximetry. Obstet Gynecol 1994; 84: 683–686

52 Tyrell S N, Gibbs J L. Sinus node disease in the fetus. Int J Cardiol 1988; 19: 382–384

53 Magee L A, Downar E, Sermer M, Boulton B C, Allen L C, Koren G. Pregnancy outcome after gestational exposure to amiodarone in Canada. Am J Obstet Gynecol 1995; 172: 1307–1311

54 Vigliani M. Romano-Ward syndrome diagnosed as moderate fetal bradycardia. A case report. J Reprod Med 1995; 40: 725–728

55 Hofbeck M, Ulmer H, Beinder E, Sieber E, Singer H. Prenatal findings with prolonged QT interval in the neonatal period. Heart 1997; 77: 198–204

56 Scott J S, Maddison P J, Taylor P V, Esscher E, Scott O, Skinner R P. Connective tissue disease, antibodies to riboneucleoprotein and congenital heart block. N Engl J Med 1983; 390: 209–212

57 Watson W J, Katz V L. Steroid therapy for hydrops associated with antibody-mediated congenital heart block. Am J Obstet Gynecol 1991; 165: 553–554

58 Carpenter R J, Strasburger J F, Garson A et al. Fetal ventricular pacing for hydrops secondary to complete atrioventricular block. J Am Coll Cardiol 1986; 8: 1434–1436

59 Deloof E, Devlieger H, Van Hoestenberghe R, Van den Berghe K, Daenen W, Gewillig M. Management with a staged approach of the premature hydropic fetus due to complete congenital heart block. Eur J Paediatr 1997; 156: 521–523

60 Julkunen H, Kaaja R, Wallgren E, Teramo K. Isolated congenital heart block: fetal and infant outcome and familial incidence of heart block. Obstet Gynecol 1993; 82: 11–16

61 Groves A M, Allan L D, Rosenthal E. Outcome of isolated congenital complete heart block diagnosed in utero. Heart 1996; 75: 190–194

62 van Engelen A D, Weijtens O, Brenner J I, Copel J A, Stoutenbeek P, Meijboom E J. Management outcome and follow up of fetal tachycardia. J Am Coll Cardiol 1994; 24: 1371–1375

63 Chao R C, Ho E S, Hsieh K S. Fetal atrial flutter and fibrillation: prenatal echocardiographic detection and management. Am Heart J 1992; 124: 1095–1098

64 Simpson L L, Marx G R, D' Alton M E. Supraventricular tachycardia in the fetus: conservative management in the absence of haemodynamic compromise. J Ultrasound Med 1997; 16: 459–464

65 Simpson J M, Milburn A, Yates R W, Maxwell D J, Sharland G K. Outcome of intermittent tachyarrhythmias in the fetus. Pediatr Cardiol 1997; 18: 78–82

66 Frohn-Mulder I M, Stewart P A, Witsenburg M, Den Hollander N S, Wladimiroff J W, Hess J. The efficacy of flecainide versus digoxin in the management of fetal supraventricular tachycardia. Prenat Diagn 1995; 15: 1297–1302

67 Dumesic D A, Silverman N H, Tobias S et al. Transplacental cardioversion of fetal supraventricular tachycardia with procainamide. N Engl J Med 1982; 307: 1128

68 Spinnato J A, Shaver D C, Flinn D S, Sibai B M, Watson D L, Marin-Garcia J. Fetal supraventricular tachycardia: in utero therapy with digoxin and quinidine. J Am Coll Cardiol 1984; 64: 730–735

69 Blanch G, Walkinshaw S A, Walsh K. Cardioversion of fetal tachyarrhythmia with adenosine. Lancet 1994; 344: 1646

70 Parilla B V, Strasburger J F, Socol M L. Fetal supraventricular tachycardia complicated by hydrops fetalis: a role for direct fetal intramuscular therapy. Am J Perinatol 1996; 13: 483–486

71 Guntheroth W G, Cyr D R, Shields L E, Nghiem H V. Rate based management of fetal supraventricular tachycardia. J Ultrasound Med 1996; 15: 453–458

72 Davis G K, Farquhar C M, Allan L D, Crawford D C, Chapman M G. Structural cardiac abnormalities in the fetus: reliability of prenatal diagnosis and outcome. Br J Obstet Gynaecol 1990; 97: 27–31

73 Montana E, Khoury M J, Cragan J D, Sharma S, Dhar P, Fyfe D. Trends and outcomes after prenatal diagnosis of congenital cardiac malformations by fetal echocardiography in a well defined birth population. J Am Coll Cardiol 1996; 28: 1805–1809

74 Sharland G K, Lockhart S M, Chita S K, Allan L D. Factors influencing the outcome of congenital heart disease detected prenatally. Arch Dis Child 1991; 66: 284–287

75 Maxwell D, Allan L, Tynan M J. Balloon dilatation of the aortic valve in the fetus: a report of two cases. Br Heart J 1991; 65: 256–258

76 Kohl T, Stelnicki E J, VanderWall K J et al. Transoesophageal echocardiography in fetal sheep. A monitoring tool for open and fetoscopic cardiac procedures. Surg Endosc 1996; 10: 820

77 Zosmer N, Jurkovic D, Jauniaux E, Gruboeck K, Lees C, Campbell S. Selection and identification of standard cardiac views from three-dimensional volume scans of the fetal thorax. J Ultrasound Med 1996; 15: 25–32

78 Deng J, Gardener J E, Rodeck C H, Lees W R. Fetal echocardiography in three and four dimensions. Ultrasound Med Biol 1996; 22: 979–986

79 Sklansky M S, Nelson T R, Pretorius D H. Usefulness of gated 3 dimensional fetal echocardiography to reconstruct and display structures not visualized with two-dimensional scanning. Am J Cardiol 1997; 80: 665–668

Skeletal abnormalities

David R Griffin and Lyn S Chitty

Introduction

A description of the normal ultrasound examination of the fetal musculoskeletal system is contained in Chapter 8. Figure 19.1 shows the normal appearances of the fetal limb bones for comparison with the commoner skeletal dysplasias and malformations to be described.

Patient selection for detailed skeletal survey

There are several groups of women who are at increased risk of carrying a fetus with a skeletal abnormality. They can be classified into four main categories:

1　Those with a positive family history;
2　Women who have been exposed to certain drugs in the first trimester;
3　Insulin-dependent diabetics;
4　Cases where another fetal abnormality has been detected on ultrasound examination.

Family history of deformity

Many of the syndromes described in this chapter are single gene disorders inherited in an autosomal dominant (AD), autosomal recessive (AR) or X-linked fashion. Dominantly inherited conditions may either occur as a new mutation or show a typical family history with one parent affected. As a result of variable expression of the gene not all affected members may manifest the disease to the same extent. Examples of conditions showing dominant inheritance are cleidocranial dysostosis, achondroplasia and Holt–Oram syndrome. Lethal dominant conditions will obviously not occur in other generations and are usually new mutations unlikely to recur in the family. Lethal conditions with

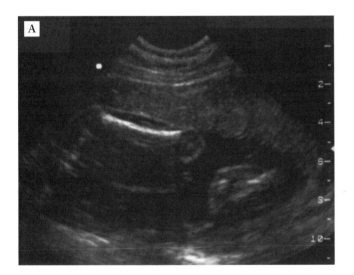
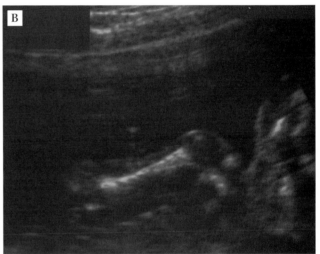
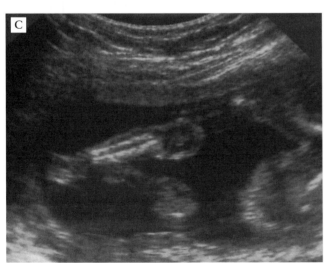
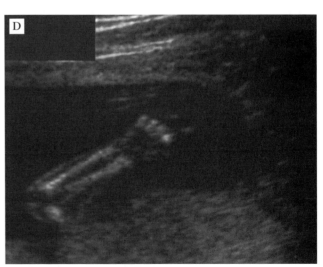

Fig. 19.1 Scans of normal fetal limb bones. A: Femur, **B:** humerus; **C:** tibia and fibula and **D:** radius and ulna at 18 weeks.

recessive inheritance, on the other hand, will only occur in the homozygous offspring of heterozygous unaffected parents. With autosomal recessive inheritance, following the first affected child those parents run a 25% risk of having another and a 67% risk of passing the gene on to their unaffected children. Fortunately the gene frequency of these conditions is very low and the chance of two carriers meeting is extremely remote. However, if members of the same family (particularly first cousins) marry, the likelihood of both parents carrying the same recessive gene is considerably increased. Many of the lethal and crippling deformities described here are recessive.

Drugs in early pregnancy

It is as well to perform a skeletal survey on any patient who has taken significant quantities of medication in the first trimester, as this time is critical for organogenesis. The devastating effects of the hypnotic thalidomide are well recorded. Other drugs that have been specifically implicated in skeletal dysmorphism are warfarin, which may produce a syndrome identical to chondrodysplasia punctata, phenytoin (digital hypoplasia), alcohol, known teratogens such as methotrexate and aminopterin, and some anaesthetic agents. A comprehensive list of drug-associated malformations has been published by Koren *et al*.[1]

Diabetics

Insulin-dependent diabetics, particularly those with poor control (elevated HbAIC) at the time of conception, have a tenfold increase in the risk of fetal malformation, especially congenital heart disease, renal anomalies and skeletal anomalies (caudal regression syndrome) (Fig. 19.2).

The finding of any fetal anomaly during scanning

The following abnormalities are particularly associated with skeletal malformations:

- Polyhydramnios/oligohydramnios
- Fetal hydrops
- Small thorax
- Facial clefting
- Short femur found on routine examination.

Aids to diagnosis of skeletal dysplasias

The skeletal dysplasias are a heterogeneous group of over 100 rare disorders, the distinction between them in many cases being subtle. It is therefore helpful for those particularly interested in the differential diagnosis of these conditions to have access to a comprehensive reference of fetal

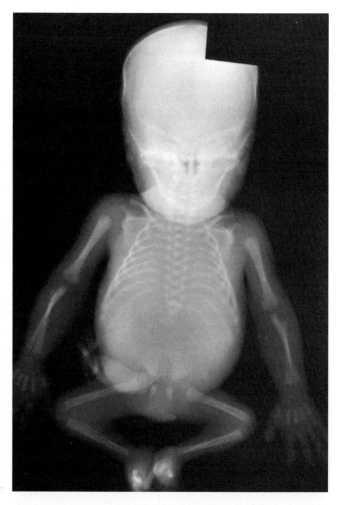

Fig. 19.2 Caudal regression syndrome. Radiograph of the 26 week fetus of a diabetic mother. It shows agenesis of the lumbar and sacral spine typical of caudal regression syndrome.

and neonatal pathology.[2] It is also important to collaborate closely with the geneticists, who may have access to a dysmorphology computer database.

Before a patient at known risk of a skeletal dysplasia is scanned as much information on affected family member(s) as possible should be obtained in order to confirm the diagnosis. This may include photographs, radiographs, detailed pathology reports and reports of any genetic consultations.

Skeletal malformations

Osteochondrodysplasias

These skeletal dysplasias are rare, with an incidence of less than 1/30 000 (Table 19.1). The list of syndromes and subgroups continues to increase. The degree of limb shortening (Fig. 19.3) and deformity is variable between (and sometimes within) syndromes.[3]

Table 19.1 Approximate incidence of 'common' lethal skeletal dysplasias

Thanatophoric dysplasia	1 in	30 000
Osteogenesis imperfecta (type II)	1 in	55 000
Achondrogenesis (all types)	1 in	75 000
Chondrodysplasia punctata	1 in	85 000
Hypophosphatasia (severe form)	1 in	110 000
Campomelic dysplasia	1 in	150 000

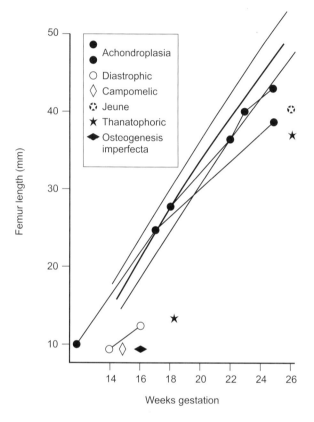

Fig. 19.3 Nomogram of fetal femur length (O'Brien et al[3]) showing measurements of femur length in fetuses confirmed as having achondrogenesis type II, achondroplasia, osteogenesis imperfecta type IIa, diastrophic dysplasia, campomelic dysplasia, Jeune thoracic dystrophy and thanatophoric dysplasia. Note the late deviation from normal growth in two fetuses with achondroplasia and one with Jeune thoraic dystrophy.

In families at high risk of a skeletal abnormality because of a previous affected individual, the diagnosis or exclusion of a relevant dysplasia is facilitated by prior knowledge of the pattern of malformations expected. By contrast, accurate diagnosis of an unexpected case discovered at routine scanning is a challenge which demands expert knowledge and diligent attention to detail. Some of the features to note before making a diagnosis are listed below.

Long bones   Note the degree of shortening in relation to nomograms (see Appendix). Is the shortening greater in the proximal long bones (rhizomelic), e.g. femur and humerus, or distal long bones (mesomelic), e.g. radius/ulna and tibia/fibula, or equal in all? Do the bones appear straight, bowed or crumpled? Is there a normal accoustic shadow?

Joints   Note the attitude and movement or fixation of joints, with particular attention to the lower limbs and talipes equinovarus (Fig. 19.4).

Spine   Examine the spine for deformities, hemivertebrae, disorganisation, normal ossification of the vertebral bodies and platyspondyly (flattened vertebrae).

Ribs and thorax   The heart should normally fill about one-third of the thoracic cavity. If the ribs are short the thorax will be small and narrow and bell-shaped and the abdomen will be protuberant ('champagne cork' appearance). The ribs themselves can be examined in a parasagittal view, which may show anomalies of the ribs such as absence, fusion (Jarcho–Levin) or beading (osteogenesis imperfecta type IIa or c). The transverse view through the thorax may also demonstrate short ribs (Figs 19.5 and 19.6) and a small thorax with diminished circumference.

Skull   A poorly ossified skull will be virtually echo free or only weakly reflective, casting little or no acoustic shadow. The intracranial contents will be more than usually clear and the cerebral hemispheres may appear echo free (pseudohydrocephaly) (Fig. 19.7). In later pregnancy the skull will deform easily under pressure from the transducer (Fig. 19.8).

Note any brachycephaly, clover leaf deformity or other abnormality.

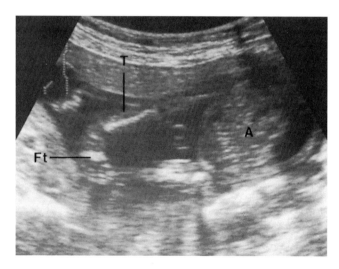

Fig. 19.4 Congenital muscular dystrophy. Scan of the leg of a fetus with congenital muscular dystrophy showing severe talipes. Note that the plantar view of the foot (Ft) is seen in the same plane as the tibia (T). A – abdomen.

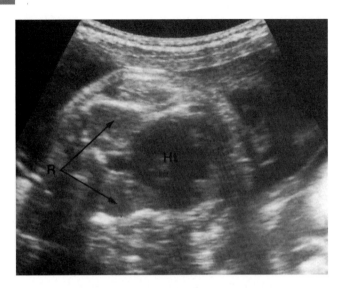

Fig. 19.5 Osteogenesis imperfecta Type IIb at 32 weeks. Small, distorted rib cage (R) and heart (Ht) projecting anteriorly.

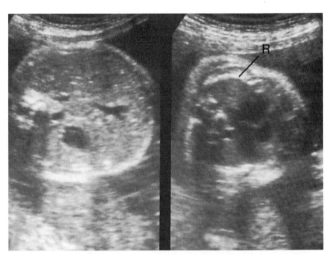

Fig. 19.6 Asphyxiating thoracic dystrophy. Axial scans of abdomen and thorax from a 32 week fetus with asphyxiating thoracic dystrophy. Note small thorax, short ribs (R) and protruding heart.

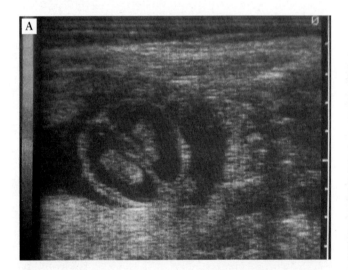

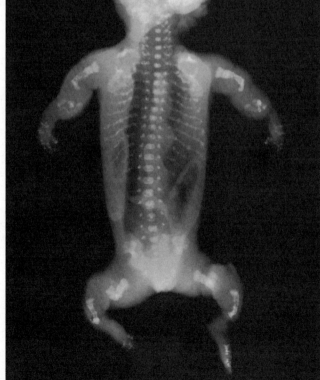

Fig. 19.7 Osteogenesis imperfecta. A: Fetal head in a case of osteogenesis inperfecta type IIa at 17 weeks. The skull shows severe under-mineralisation giving the impression of ventriculomegaly. **B:** Radiograph of this case.

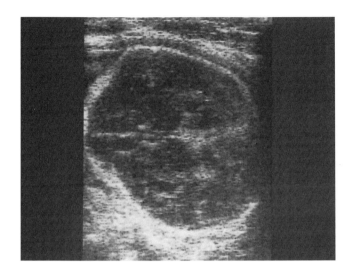

Fig. 19.8 Scans from a 31 week fetus with osteogenesis imperfecta type IIa. The head shows an under-mineralised skull distorted by transducer pressure and casting no acoustic shadow.

Hands and feet Count the fingers and toes to exclude polydactyly/syndactyly and ectrodactyly.

Extra fingers are usually found next to the fifth finger (postaxial) (Fig. 19.9A), but thumbs or big toes may be split or duplicated (pre-axial) (Fig. 19.9B and C). Note the position of wrists and fingers and the length of the fingers.

Limb girdles There are few data on normal fetal limb girdle dimensions, but some osteochondrodystrophies are characterised by short clavicles and hypoplastic ilia and scapulae.

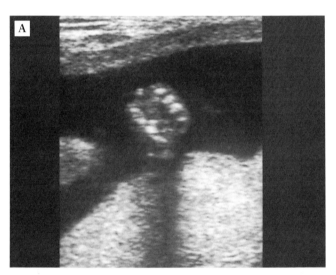

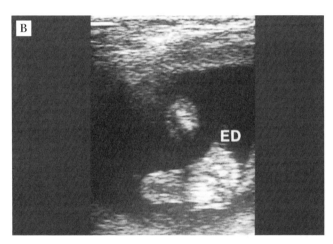

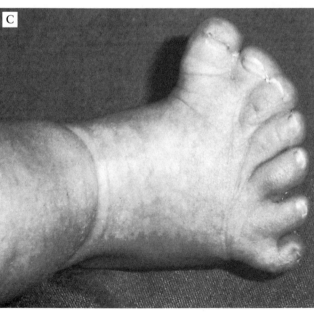

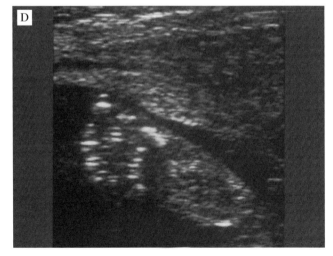

Fig. 19.9 Cephalopolysyndactyly syndrome. Scan and photograph from a fetus and infant with Greig cephalopolysyndactyly syndrome with dominant inheritance. **A:** Clenched hand showing post-axial extra digit. **B:** Plantar view of foot showing pre-axial polysyndactyly. ED – extra digit. **C:** Photograph of foot after birth. **D:** Scan of normal foot for comparison.

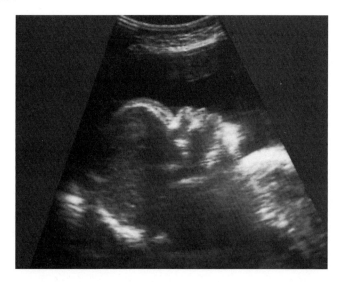

Fig. 19.10 Thanatophoric dysplasia at 31 weeks. Facial profile showing frontal bossing and depressed nasal bridge.

Face   A facial profile (sagittal plane) may show a depressed nasal bridge or prominent forehead (frontal bossing) (Fig. 19.10), flat face, a receding chin (micrognathia) (see Ch. 21, Fig. 21.10) or other features helpful in a differential diagnosis.

A full facial view in the coronal plane (Fig. 19.11) will show cleft lip.

Non-skeletal features   A full examination of the rest of the fetus, including the heart, kidneys, cerebral ventricles and amniotic fluid, may uncover further anomalies to narrow down the differential diagnosis.

Table 19.2 shows syndromes associated with specific malformations. Tables 19.3 and 19.4 are rapid diagnostic

Table 19.2 Clues to the differential ultrasound diagnosis of skeletal dysplasia

Polyhydramnios	Achondrogenesis type I or II Thanatophoric dysplasia Short rib-polydactyly syndrome
Fetal hydrops	Achondrogenesis type I SRP syndromes
Undermineralised skull	Osteogenesis imperfecta (IIa) Achondrogenesis type I Hypophosphatasia
Clover leaf skull	Thanatophoric dysplasia
Small thorax	Achondrogenesis Hypochondrogenesis Thanatophoric dysplasia SRP syndromes Chondroectodermal dysplasia Champomile dysplasia
Marked femoral bowing	Campomelic dysplasia Osteogenesis imperfecta Hypophosphatasia
Talipes equinovarus	Campomelic dysplasia Diastrophic dysplasia
Polydactyly	Chondroectodermal dysplasia SRP syndromes Gerbe syndrome Jeune thoracic dystrophy
Short clavicles	Campomelic dysplasia Cleidocranial dysostosis Kniest syndrome

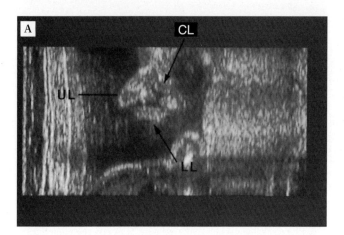

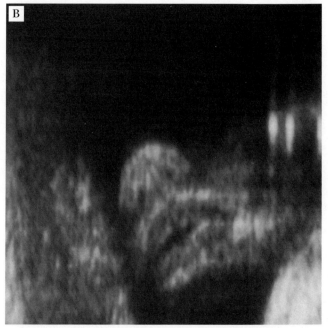

Fig. 19.11 Cleft lip. A: Coronal scan of lips to show a paramedian cleft (CL) of the upper lip (UL). LL – lower lip. **B:** Normal for comparison.

Table 19.3 Skeletal dysplasias characterised by poor mineralisation

Type & Inheritance		Long bones	Spine	Ribs	Other features	Prognosis	References
Achondrogenesis type I	(AR)	Extreme micromelia	Poorly mineralised Short	Short	Polyhydramnios, hydrops, very poor cranial ossification	Lethal	Golbus et al (1977) Smith et al (1981) Glen & Teng (1985) Muller et al (1985a) Donnenfeld (1987)
Achondrogenesis type II	(AR)	Severe micromelia	Unossified spine and sacrum	Short	Polyhydramnios Micrognathia Good cranial ossification	Lethal	Griffin et al (1985)
Osteogenesis imperfecta (type II)	VAR	V short, crumpled multiple fractures	Vertebrae may be flattened	Beaded +/– short	Polyhydramnios Unossified skull Brachycephaly	Lethal	Hobbins et al (1982) milsom et al (1982) Shapiro et al (1982) Dinno et al (1982) Elejalde et al (1983) Brons et al (1988)
Hypophosphatasia (lethal form)	(AR)	Short, bowed	May show deformity	Thin +/– short +/– beaded	Poorly ossified skull	Lethal	Wladimiroff et al (1985)

Table 19.4 Skeletal dysplasia characterised by short ribs

Type & Inheritance		Long bones	Spine	Other features	Prognosis	References
Achondrogenesis type I	(AR)	Extreme micromelia	Poorly mineralised Short	Polyhydramnios, hydrops, very poor cranial ossification	Lethal	Golbus et al (1977) Smith et al (1981) Glen & Teng (1985) Muller et al (1985a) Donnenfeld (1987)
Achondrogenesis type II	(AR)	Severe micromelia	Unossified spine and sacrum	Polyhydramnios Micrognathia Unossified spine/sacrum	Lethal	Griffin et al (1985)
Hypochondrogenesis (Mainly sporadic)	(?AR)	moderate shortening Flared metaphyses	Flat vertebral bodies	Poor ossification of cervical and sacral spine	Lethal	Stoll et al (1985) Griffin (1990)
Thanatophoric dysplasia	(sporadic)	Severe micromelia Thick diaphysis +/– bowing	flat vertebral bodies	Polyhydramnios Megalocephaly Ventriculomegaly +/– Cloverleaf skull Renal & cardiac anomalies Trident hand	Lethal	Chervenak et al (1983) Beetham Reeves (1984) Burrows et al (1984) Camera et al (1984) Elejalde et al (1985) Weiner t al (1986)
Jejune thoracic dystrophy	(AR)	Variable/moderate (especially mesomelic) shortening	Normal	+/– Postaxial polydactyly Hypoplastic lungs Renal dysplasia	70% lethal	Little D (1984) Elejalde et al (1985) Griffin & Chitty (see text)
Short rib-polydactyly syndromes Saldino-Noonan (type I) Majewski (type II)	(AR)	Moderate shortening Spikey metaphyses Tibia hypoplastic	Normal	Postaxial polydactyly Hydrops, anal atresis Median cleft lip Cardiac & renal anomalies	Lethal	Wladimiroff et al (1984) Meizner & Bar-Ziv (1985)
Ellis-Van Creveld syndrome (Chondroectodermal dysplasia)	(AR)	Variable shortening Hypoplastic tibia	Normal	Postaxial polydactyly 50% cardiac anomaly (ASD)	50% lethal Normal IQ	Mahoney & Hobbins (1977) Filly & Golbus (1982) Muller et al (1985)
Campomelic dysplasia	(AR)	Moderate shortening Bowed femulr/tibia Hypo/aplastic fibula	Flat vertebrae	Short clavicles, micrognathia, talipes eq. varus Sex reversal	Usually lethal	Fryns et al (1981) Hobbins et al (1982) Redon et al (1984) Winter et al (1985) Griffin (1990)

guides to some of the commoner skeletal dysplasias. These will be described in diagnostic groups, but it must be remembered that many conditions will fall into more than one category. Those described below include only the more common ones. A comprehensive list would be impossible to produce as new variants continue to be described. The information given below should aid diagnosis, but in cases where there is no positive family history a definitive diagnosis may have to await postnatal radiological and pathological investigations.

Conditions characterised by under-mineralisation

Achondrogenesis types I and II are characterised by under-mineralisation. Both result in stillbirth or neonatal death and are characterised by severe micromelia with a relatively large head and short trunk. Radiologically ossification of the skull, spine and pelvis is more deficient in type I than in type II, and the long bones are shorter in type I. Occurrence is approximately 1/75 000.

Achondrogenesis type I (5q31–5q34) DTST (Parenti–Fraccaro) is characterised by extreme micromelia (very short limbs), with poor modelling, a short, poorly mineralised spine, short ribs and almost absent ossification of the calvarium. Glen and Teng[5] noted femur lengths of 10 mm at 19 weeks. As a result of poor skull mineralisation details of the brain structure will be unusually clear. The skull is soft, so that the head may be deformed by depressing the transducer on the maternal abdomen.

Achondrogenesis type II (12q13–12q14) COL2AI (Langer–Saldino) shows micromelia but to a lesser degree

than in type I,[6–8] with better modelling, and is usually a sporadic occurrence. It probably represents the severe end of the spectrum of the group of conditions that includes hypochondrogenesis (Fig. 19.12) and spondylo-epiphyseal dysplasia congenita (SEDC).

It is likely that most cases of achondrogenesis type I are caused by new dominant mutations, and defects of type II collagen have been observed in some cases. The characteristic sonographic feature is absent mineralisation of the vertebral bodies. The limb bones are short (Fig. 19.13A). The definitive diagnostic feature is the finding of an echo-free column extending from the sacrum to the base of the skull (Fig. 19.13B), which represents the unossified vertebral bodies (Fig. 19.13C). The skull may appear normal. Prenatal diagnosis of achondrogenesis type II has been reported using trans-vaginal ultrasound at 12 weeks gestation.[9]

Hypochondrogenesis (12q13–12q14) COL2AI is another form of neonatally lethal short-limbed dwarfism which is now thought to be part of the same spectrum of disease as achondrogenesis type II, with hypochondrogenesis representing the milder end of the spectrum.[10–13] Inheritance is still uncertain, but so far all cases reported have been sporadic. Mutations in the type II collagen gene have been reported, and it is therefore likely that this condition represents a new dominant mutation. Radiologically the condition is characterised by flared metaphyses and poor mineralisation of the cervical and sacral vertebral bodies.

Osteogenesis imperfecta is subdivided into four main groups. Only types IIa and IIc are characterised by significant under-mineralisation. Type I is often, but not always, manifest in childhood and is rarely amenable to antenatal

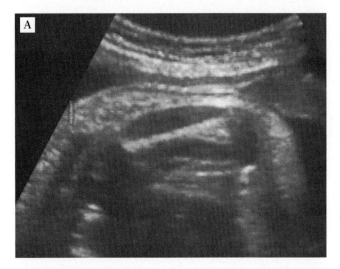
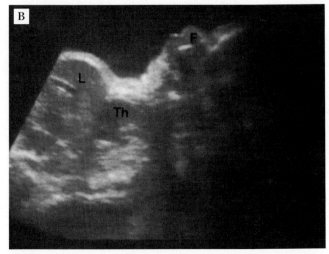

Fig. 19.12 Hypochondrogenesis. Scans of a 31 week fetus found on post-natal radiography to have hypochondogenesis. **A:** Short femur with thickened metaphysis. **B:** Sagittal section of the trunk and face (F) to show 'champagne cork' appearance due to small thorax (Th) and protuberant liver (L).

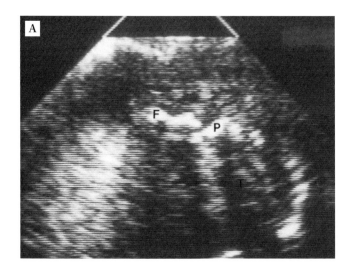

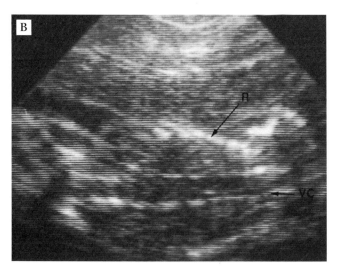

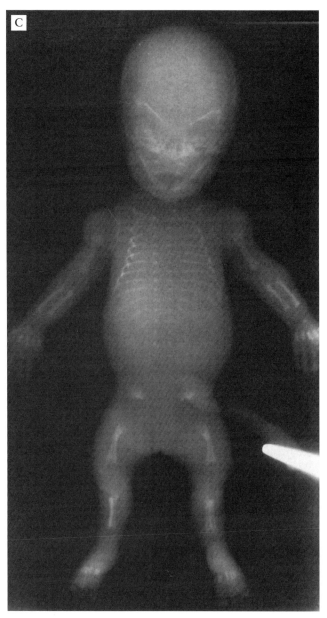

Fig. 19.13 Achondrogenesis. Scans of an 18 week fetus with achondrogenesis type II. **A:** Extremely short but modelled femur (F) with a length of 18 mm. P – pelvis, T – trunk. **B:** Coronal section of the trunk showing cartilaginous, unossified vertebral column (VC). R – ribs. **C:** Radiograph of the fetus showing unossified vertebral bodies and severe micromelia.

diagnosis. Individuals affected by osteogenesis imperfecta type IIB, III or III/IV are usually born with fractures, and there is progressive deformity in childhood. In the more severely affected cases these types may be lethal in the perinatal period or early childhood. Diagnosis *in utero* has been reported for both osteogenesis imperfecta type IIb and type III, neither of which is associated with sufficient hypomineralisation to be a reliably diagnostic feature, but they are described below for convenience.

Osteogenesis imperfecta types IIa and IIc are perinatally lethal and have been the subject of many reports of early antenatal diagnosis with ultrasound.[14–19] The long bones are short, deformed and crumpled because of multiple intra-uterine fractures (Figs 19.14A and 19.15A). The posi-

tional deformity of the lower limbs may be similar to that in campomelic dysplasia and distrophic dysplasia. Fetal movement is reduced. The ribs appear thin, short and beaded (Fig. 19.15B) and the thorax may be small. All reported cases have shown marked under-mineralisation of the skull (Figs 19.14B and 19.16). In later pregnancy the gyri may be clearly seen and the skull can easily be distorted by the pressure of the ultrasound transducer (Fig. 19.8). The appearance of the spine is usually normal but the vertebrae may be flattened (Fig. 19.15C). There may be associated polyhydramnios.

The prognosis for fetuses with types IIa and IIc is invariably fatal, death resulting from pulmonary hypoplasia. It is believed that the majority of cases of type IIa

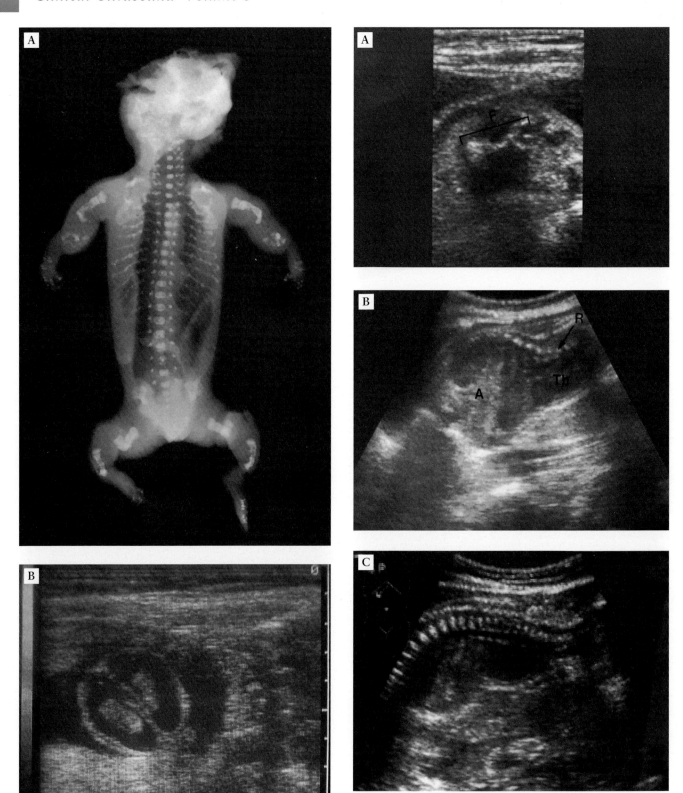

Fig. 19.14 Osteogenesis imperfecta. A: Radiograph of this case.
B: Fetal head in a case of osteogenesis imperfecta type IIa at 17 weeks.
The skull shows severe under-mineralisation giving the impression of
ventriculomegaly.

**Fig. 19.15 Scans from a 31 week fetus with osteogenesis imperfecta
type IIa. A:** The femur (F) is short, under-mineralised and crumpled.
B: Coronal section of the trunk showing small thorax (Th) relative to
the abdomen (A) ('champagne cork' appearance). R – ribs. **C:** Spine
with flattened vertebrae (V).

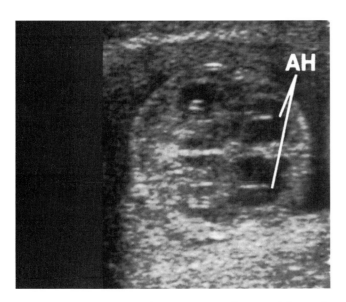

Fig. 19.16 Osteogenesis imperfecta. Axial scans of a 20 week fetus with osteogenesis imperfecta type IIA showing under-mineralised skull and echo-poor cerebral hemisphere (pseudohydrocephalus). The normally placed anterior horns (AH) show normal ventricular anatomy.

are sporadic, but occasional recurrences have been reported in type IIc, where the recurrence risks have been estimated at around 7%, as several affected siblings have been reported as well as a higher incidence of parental consanguinity.[20,21] Most cases of osteogenesis type IIa are caused by new dominant mutations in one of the type I collagen genes, and any recurrences that have been reported are thought to be caused by gonadal mosaicism in one parent[22] (Fig. 19.17A).

Osteogenesis imperfecta types IIB and III These conditions are characterised by generalised mild shortening of all limbs in association with bowing of the lower limbs, in particular the femora and tibiae (Fig. 19.17B). Mineralisation usually appears normal, although on occasions the skull may seem slightly hypomineralised, particularly in type IIB. The facial profile may appear flat. Prenatal diagnosis of these conditions has been reported, but in some cases the features were not sufficient for diagnosis until around 23 weeks gestation. Differential diagnosis from campomelic dysplasia may be difficult. The recurrence risk is estimated at around 7%, as above for IIc. In general, therefore, the recurrence risks for osteogenesis imperfecta will depend on the type of osteogenesis and the presence or absence of parental consanguinity.[20]

Hypophosphatasia (1p34–1p36) presents several different clinical pictures and is classified according to the age of onset. It seems that there are at least two forms of this condition: one is the severe lethal form where the bones are undermineralised, and it is this form that is most likely to present to the prenatal diagnostic sonographer. Although its

occurrence (1/100 000) is said to be about half that of osteogenesis imperfecta type II, reports of ultrasound diagnosis are few.[23,24] Measurement of amniotic fluid alkaline phosphatase may be helpful in confirming a diagnosis, although this has been reported to be unreliable in some cases.[25] There are reports of successful diagnosis from the measurement of cellular alkaline phosphatase activity in amniocytes or chorionic villus cells.[26] The gene location for this condition has now been identified and a prenatal diagnosis has been successfully attempted. Identification of heterozygous gene carriers is possible, as these individuals have low serum levels of bone alkaline phosphatase and phosphoethanolamine is present in their urine.

The ultrasonographic appearance is of an undermineralised skull, similar to that of osteogenesis imperfecta, with short, bowed long-bone diaphyses. In the case reported by Wladimiroff[24] the femur length (14 mm) was below the fifth centile at 16 weeks. Marked angulation of the femur may also occur (Fig. 19.18). Inheritance of the perinatal lethal form is usually autosomal recessive. There is a high incidence of stillbirths and neonatal deaths secondary to respiratory insufficiency.

Conditions characterised by a hypoplastic thorax

Achondrogenesis   see above.

Asphyxiating thoracic dystrophy (Jeune syndrome)   is a short-ribbed limb reduction syndrome inherited in an autosomal recessive fashion. The gene for this condition has been localised to 12p11–p12. There is only minimal to moderate diaphysial shortening and measurements of the long bones may not fall below normal ranges until late in the second trimester, if at all (Fig. 19.19). There may be severe rib shortening and thoracic reduction. The diagnosis can be suspected prenatally on finding a hypoplastic thorax with moderately short long bones.[27,28] Liquor volume is often increased. Postaxial polydactyly is an occasional finding. There is a high (70%) perinatal and infant mortality from respiratory failure secondary to pulmonary hypoplasia. The kidneys frequently show cystic changes, and associated liver and pancreatic dysplasias can cause complications (cirrhosis) in survivors. In many cases these can result in death in early childhood.[29]

Campomelic dysplasia (17q24–17q25) SOX9   is typified by variable shortening and bowing of the femur and tibia, which show angulation in the mid-shaft. The upper limbs are usually normal or only mildly affected. Associated skeletal deformities include macrocephaly (often with associated ventriculomegaly), micrognathia, short clavicles, talipes, and small scapulae and ilia. Most of these features are detectable on careful ultrasonic survey.[14,30–32] The ribs are usually short and the thorax small. Congenital heart

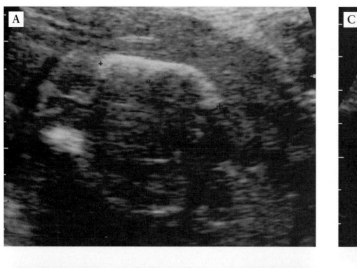

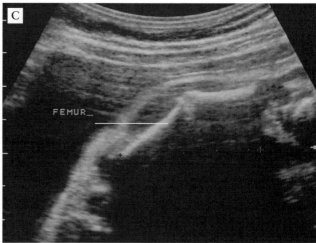

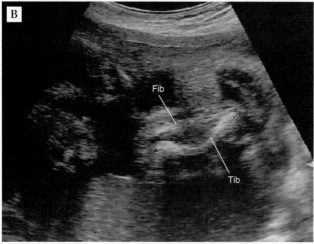

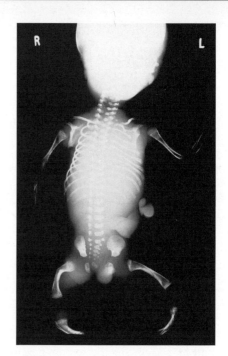

Fig. 19.17 19-week fetus with osteogenesis inperfecta type 11B/111 showing **A:** femur with low reflectivity and bowing. **B:** tibia and fibula, showing bowed tibia. **C:** Same fetus at 30+ weeks with a mid-shaft femoral fracture. **D:** Radiograph of a fetus with OI type 11B/111. Note bowing of femur (without fracture) and tibia, but straight humeri.

disease (VSD, ASD, tetralogy of Fallot) and hydronephrosis each occur in about one-third of cases. Phenotypic sex reversal of male fetuses is common. In about 95% of cases the condition is lethal in the first year of life. There is a birth prevalence of 1/200 000, and although inheritance has been suggested to be autosomal recessive, sibling recurrence is only about 5%.[33] Inheritance is therefore uncertain, and many cases may be caused by new dominant mutations.[34] Figure 19.20 shows a case which was diagnosed on the basis of femoral bowing, short and deformed tibiae and relatively normal upper limbs. The differential diagnoses of campomelic dysplasia and osteo-genesis imperfecta types IIB/III may be difficult (see below).

Ellis–van Creveld syndrome (chondro-ectodermal dysplasia) is inherited in an autosomal recessive fashion, being particularly prevalent among the inbred Amish community in Pennsylvania. The gene has been mapped to 4p16 in some Amish pedigrees and in other families from South American countries.[35] Affected fetuses may show variable degrees of shortening of the long bones, which is more pronounced in the forearm and lower leg (mesomelic). There is postaxial polydactyly of the hands and feet and the ribs are short and horizontal, causing a reduced thoracic cavity and lethal pulmonary hypoplasia in about half of affected infants; 50% of cases have congenital heart disease (ASD). Survivors reach adulthood

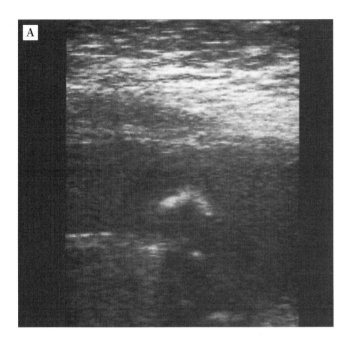

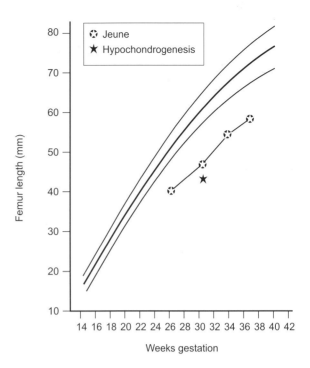

Fig. 19.19 **Asphyxiating thoracic dystrophy.** Nomogram of femur length showing femur growth in a case of asphyxiating thoracic dystrophy (adapted from O'Brien[3]).

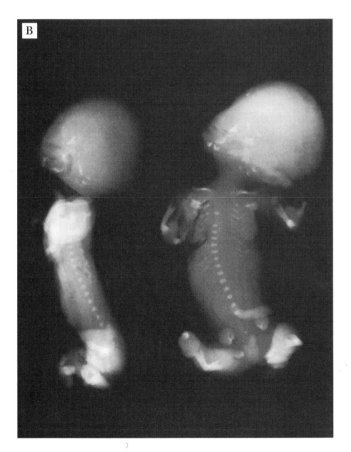

Fig. 19.18 **Hypophosphatasia. A:** Scan from a fetus with hypophosphatasia showing a severely bowed femur measuring 15 mm at 19 weeks. **B:** Radiograph of fetus in A (after rib biopsy) showing marked angulation of femora and humeri, short distal extremities, under-mineralised skull and neural arch and thin, fractured ribs.

with moderate to severe short stature (40–63 inches) being the major problem. The main differential diagnosis is Jeune syndrome. Prenatal diagnosis has been reported.[36,37]

Homozygous achondroplasia can present with severe micromelia and a small thorax,[38] and may be lethal. This condition is caused by a new dominant mutation and the gene has been located to 4p16 in the FGFR3 (fibroblast growth receptor gene 3) gene.[39]

Thanatophoric dysplasia (types I and II) (4p16) F9FR3 is caused by distinct mutations in FGFR3. This is the commonest of the lethal dysplasias, occurring in about 1/30 000 births. Most cases are sporadic. There is severe micromelia, the femora are extremely short, thickened and bowed, and have been likened to a telephone receiver handle (Fig. 19.21). The ribs are very short and thick (Fig. 19.21A) and the thoracic cavity constricted. The combination of small chest and normal abdominal size gives the torso a 'champagne cork' appearance in a longitudinal anteroposterior view (Fig. 19.21B). The vertebrae are flat (platyspondyly), making the spine short. The skull tends towards brachycephaly and in some cases may show the clover leaf deformity.[40–45] There may be associated megalencephaly and cerebral ventriculomegaly. Polyhydramnios is a common presenting sign in the late second or early third trimester. Several authors have reported femur lengths

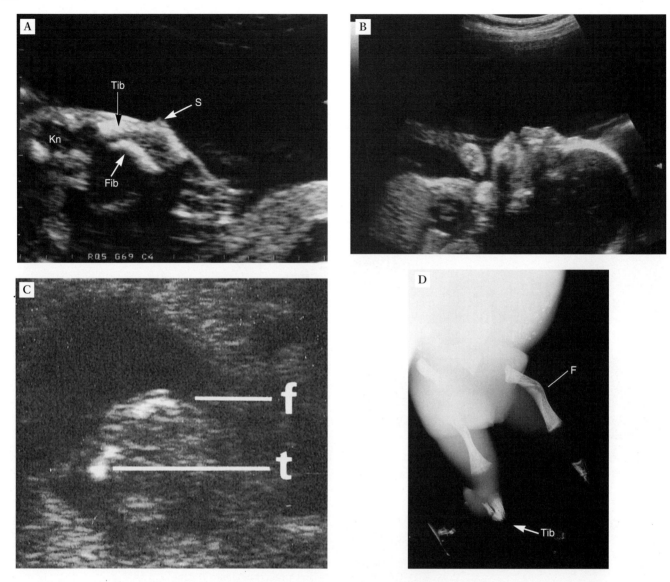

Fig. 19.20 A 19-week fetus with campomelic dysplasia. **A:** Tibia (Tib) and fibula (Fib) showing tibial hypoplasia with marked angulation (S), Kn – Knee. **B:** Facial profile showing flat face and micrognathia. **C:** 17-week femur and tibia showing mid-shaft bowing of the femur. f – fibia, t – tibia. **D:** Radiograph of the lower limbs of fetus with campomelic dysplasia.

of between 18 and 21 mm at 19–20 weeks, 23 mm at 22 weeks and only 26–27 mm at 32 weeks. It is thus apparent that very little growth of the long bones occurs from the middle of the second trimester onwards (Fig. 19.22). The condition may be associated with cardiac and renal anomalies. Other dysmorphic features of the condition such as frontal bossing, depressed nasal bridge, short splayed fingers (trident hand [Fig. 19.21C]) and, in later pregnancy, excessive skin folds may be evident.

Short rib–polydactyly syndromes (SRPS) are characterised by varying degrees of micromelia and short ribs, with a narrow thorax and postaxial polydactyly. There are

many of these conditions, but the most common include Saldino–Noonan (SRPS type I) and Majewski (SRPS type II). Orofacial–digital syndrome type 4 is now thought synonymous with Majewski syndrome (Fig. 19.23). Saldino–Noonan typically has shortened long bones with pointed metaphyses. Urogenital and anorectal anomalies are common, including imperforate anus, vaginal atresia and other renal anomalies. Many cases also have cardiac anomalies. Majewski may be distinguished from Saldino–Noonan by the finding of a median cleft lip or palate and disproportionately short and ovoid tibiae. Affected infants may have ambiguous genitalia, cardiac malformations and central nervous system abnormalities,

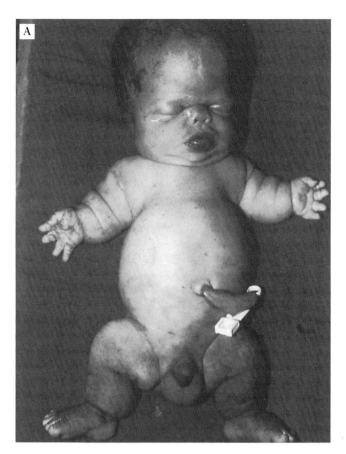

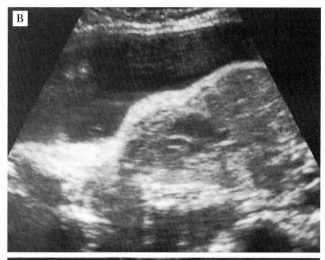

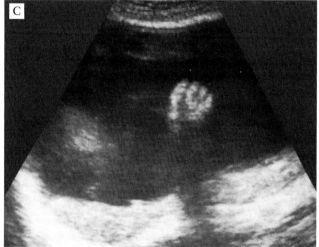

Fig. 19.21 Thanatophoric dysplasia at 31 weeks. A: Photograph of a term infant following neonatal death showing typical features of thanatophoric dysplasia. **B:** Small thorax and normal liver giving 'champagne cork' appearance. **C:** Short, stubby fingers of 'trident hand' and polyhydramnios.

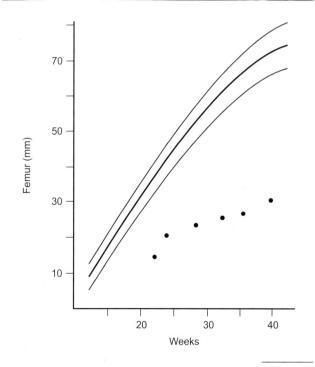

Fig. 19.22 Growth chart for thanatophoric dysplasia. Serial femur measurements from a fetus with thanatophoric dysplasia showing severely impaired growth compared to nomogram. Other long bones showed even lower (almost static) growth velocity.

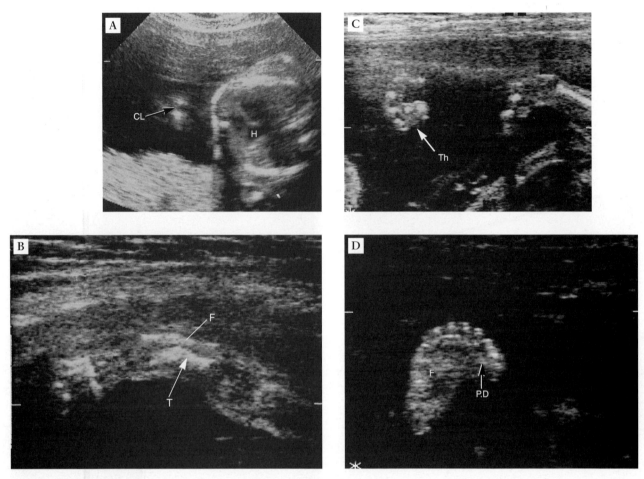

Fig. 19.23 Fetus at 23+ weeks with confirmed prenatal diagnosis of OFD Type IV showing: A: median cleft lip (CL), H – Heart. **B:** Tibial (T) hypoplasia with mid-shaft bowing (F – fibula). **C:** Hand with bifid thumb (Th) and postaxial polydactyly (PD). **D:** Foot (F) with pre-axial polydactyly.

including posterior fossa anomalies and agenesis of the corpus callosum. These conditions are inherited in an autosomal recessive fashion and there are several reports of prenatal diagnosis using ultrasound for both types.[46–48]

Conditions characterised by rhizomelic shortening

Chondrodysplasia punctata (rhizomelic type) is a condition characterised by rhizomelic shortening, particularly of the humerus, joint contractures and stippling of the epiphyses, which may be detected *in utero* during the second trimester. This rhizomelic form of chondrodysplasia punctata is inherited in an autosomal recessive fashion and should not be confused with the other forms, where both the genetics and the prognosis are different. The prognosis for the rhizomelic form is bad, with death usually occurring within the first 2 years of life. All affected children have severe microcephaly and global developmental delay. Around two-thirds of children die within the first year of life, with others dying late in infancy; survival beyond 5 years is rare. This condition is associated with abnormal peroxisomes in the liver, resulting in a reduction in phytanic acid oxidation, such that chorionic villus and amniotic fluid dihydroxyacetone phosphate acyltransferase (DHAP-AT) levels are reduced. This can form the basis of prenatal diagnosis by measurement of the DHAP-AT level in chorionic villi or amniotic fluid.

A recent case occurring *de novo* in a primigravida mother showed short fetal humeri and femora at routine 18-week scan. More detailed examination revealed the typical splayed metaphyses and disorganised echoes around the epiphyses (stippled epiphyses) (Fig. 19.24). The limbs were flexed and showed severe limitation of movement. Fetal radiography performed *in utero* gave no useful additional information. The pregnancy was terminated and the diagnosis confirmed by fetal radiography (Fig. 19.24C) and biochemistry.[49]

X-linked chondrodysplasia punctata may show similar fractures and spinal disorganisations. Facial features are flat and coarse.

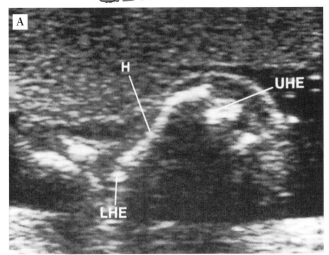

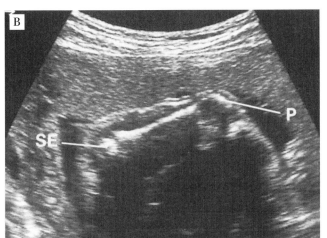

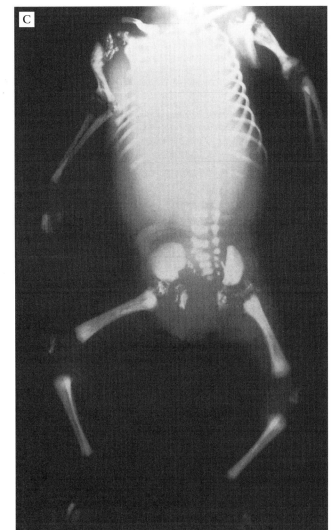

Fig. 19.24 Rhizomelic chondrodyplasia punctata. Scans from the upper arm and leg of a 19 week fetus with rhizomelic chondrodysplasia punctata. **A:** The humerus (H) is thick, short and bowed and shows disorganised upper humeral (UHE) and lower humeral (LHE) epiphyses. **B:** Mineralised stippled epiphysis at the upper femur (SE) and mineralised patella (P). **C:** Radiograph showing marked shortening of the humerus and disorganised, stippled epiphyses at upper and lower humerus, upper femur and patella. Note also fixed flexion deformity of the elbow.

Diastrophic dysplasia (5q21–5q34) DTST is characterised by rhizomelic shortening of the limbs, severe talipes, 'hitch-hiker' thumbs (Fig. 19.25) and, in many cases, a cleft palate and characteristic swelling of the pinnae. Reports of prenatal diagnosis are mainly in high-risk pregnancies and are based on the finding of short, flexed limbs and severe talipes. 'Hitch-hiker' thumbs have been recognised on ultrasound in the first and second trimesters.[50–53] This condition is inherited in autosomal recessive fashion and the gene has been localised to 5q21–5q34. The spectrum of abnormality is broad and prenatal diagnosis, based on ultrasound findings, may not be possible before around 20 weeks. There is an increased neonatal mortality, usually secondary to respiratory insufficiency. The majority of

infants who survive are intellectually unimpaired, but may suffer progressive kyphoscoliosis and orthopaedic problems which may lead to severe physical handicap. Pregnancy is possible in surviving females but caesarean section delivery will generally be required.

Non-lethal dysplasias

Heterozygous achondroplasia has been diagnosed by ultrasound in the late second trimester of pregnancy. Considerable caution should be exercised before making a definitive diagnosis before 24 weeks gestation, as limb measurements in this condition may not deviate from the normal range until 24 weeks or so (see Fig. 19.3). This

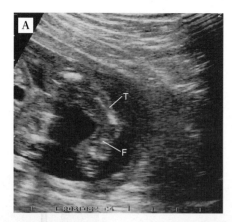

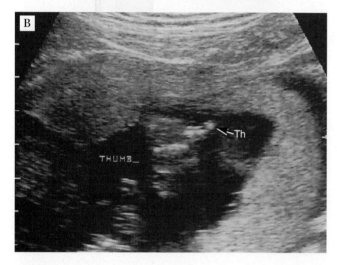

Fig. 19.25 19-week fetus with diastrophic dysplasia. A: Lower leg demonstrating talipes (T – tibia; F – foot). **B:** Hand demonstrating adducted 'hitch-hiker' thumb (Th).

experience is confirmed by other reports of ultrasonographic diagnosis.[23,37] Achondroplasia is inherited in an autosomal dominant fashion, although many cases may be new mutations. The condition is caused by mutation in the FGFR3 gene at 4p16.3. Other sonographic features of this condition include the finding of short stubby fingers and mild frontal bossing, together with increased liquor volume. The chest may occasionally appear small. The finding of these features together with shortened long bones in the third trimester may point to the diagnosis of achondroplasia, but other aetiologies, such as early intra-uterine growth retardation or chromosomal anomaly should be excluded. Doppler studies may help to detect growth retardation. Definitive diagnosis using molecular techniques is possible, as the majority of cases are due to a single mutation in the FGFR3 gene.[54]

Cleidocranial dysostosis (6p21) is inherited in an autosomal dominant fashion and is characterised by shortened or absent clavicles and under-mineralisation of the skull, but not usually of sufficient degree for prenatal detection. The cranial sutures may also be wide and this, together with abnormalities of the clavicles, are features that may be detected with ultrasound prenatally. The gene has been located to 6p21. The prognosis is good and intellect normal.

Conditions associated with spinal abnormalities

Jarcho–Levin (spondylothoracic dysplasia) is a skeletal disorder characterised by disorganisation of the spine and multiple abnormalities of the vertebrae, including fusion and hemivertebrae and an abnormal rib cage. The long bones are unaffected. The vertebral anomalies can cause a short neck and the spine is often foreshortened and has a kyphosis and/or scoliosis. As a result of the vertebral changes there is often posterior fusion of the ribs with anterior flaring, resulting in a 'crab-chest' deformity. It is inherited in an autosomal recessive fashion and usually results in death from respiratory failure within the first year of life, although there are occasional survivors beyond this time. Clinically there is some overlap with spondylocostal dysplasia, where there are similar abnormalities but usually much milder in form.

Prenatal diagnosis of Jarcho–Levin syndrome based on the finding of disorganisation of the spine (particularly in the thoracic region), in association with normal limb biometry, has been made in both high- and low-risk cases.[55–59]

Dyssegmental dysplasia is a lethal syndrome characterised by marked shortening of the extremities and a deformed, under-mineralised spine. It has been diagnosed by antenatal ultrasonography at 18 weeks.[60] The inheritance is autosomal recessive.

There are many other skeletal dysplasias, some of which may show features amenable to prenatal diagnosis, for example Kneist syndrome, kyphomelic dysplasias etc. however, many do not show sufficient limb shortening or other features for second-trimester diagnosis.[61] With the rapid advances of molecular biology many of these conditions are now being mapped, and therefore in high-risk cases prenatal molecular diagnosis may be appropriate.

Limb reduction deformities

This group of deformities is characterised by the absence or reduction of limbs or segments of limbs. In general this is a heterogeneous group of disorders, many of which are not genetic in origin. The deformity may involve the absence of all limbs (amelia) or the reduction (phocomelia) of one, more or all limbs (tetraphocomelia). There may also be reduction of a longitudinal segment of a limb (hemimelia), such as the radius. In the absence of associated abnormalities the prognosis is generally good, as technological advances in limb prostheses are such that excellent functional and cosmetic results can be obtained, even in apparently severe reduction (Fig. 19.26). However, a detailed general examination of the fetus is indicated, as a limb reduction deformity may be part of a spectrum of abnormalities which will increase the risk of an underlying chromosomal defect (Fig. 19.27) or genetic syndrome.

Amniotic band syndrome (ABS) This group of disorders shows a great variation in severity, from minor digital constriction rings or amputations to major structural disruption of the head (encephalocele) and face, trunk (ventral wall defects) and limbs (deformity and amputations). The lesions are asymmetrical. Careful ultrasonic examination may reveal bands of amnion attached to and immobilising deformed fetal parts.[62]

If multiple asymmetrical abnormalities are found ABS should be considered and bands sought. Bands or ridges in

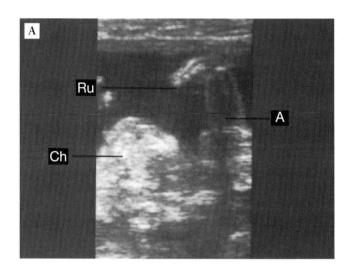

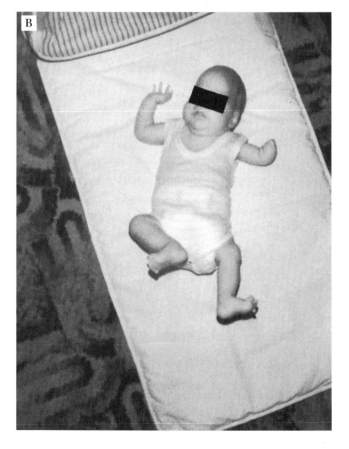

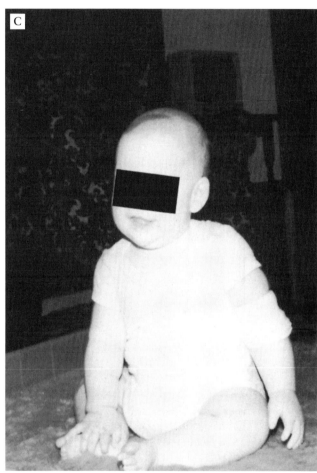

Fig. 19.26 Reduction defect. A: Scan of an isolated amputation-like reduction defect of the forearm showing shortened radius and ulna (RU) and absent hand. A – upper arm, Ch – chin. **B:** Photograph of infant at 8 weeks of age without prosthesis; **C:** with prosthesis at 6 months.

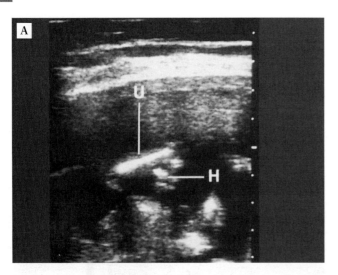

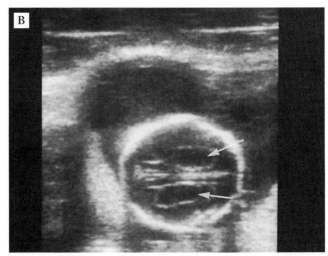

Fig. 19.27 Trisomy 18. Scan at 18 weeks showing: **A:** Radial aplasia and wrist deformity. U – ulna, H – hand. **B:** Large bilateral choroid plexus cysts (arrows).

the amnion may be seen in normal pregnancies. If these are not attached to the fetus and a careful search reveals no deformity they should be regarded as harmless.

The aetiology of the amniotic band syndrome is a source of continuing debate. It may be due to early amnion rupture, vascular occlusion during embryonic or fetal development, or result from a gene mutation.

Associated genetic syndromes

Roberts syndrome (pseudo-thalidomide syndrome) is inherited in an autosomal recessive fashion and is characterised by severe tetraphocomelia, with median facial clefting associated with marked growth retardation. Other features of the syndrome are syndactyly, talipes and microcephaly. Many infants are stillborn or die in infancy, and mental retardation is a common complication in the few that survive. An affected individual presents features similar to those associated with the teratogenic effects of the drug thalidomide, hence the alternative name pseudo-thalidomide syndrome. Premature separation of the centromeres (chromosome puffing) may be seen in many cases on cytogenetic examination.[63] This may be of use prenatally when trying to confirm the diagnosis.

Hypoglossia–hypodactyly syndrome is the main differential diagnosis for Robert syndrome and presents with very similar features, although the clinical expression is very variable. In this condition the jaw is usually small and there are variable transverse defects, affecting any or all limbs. Limb anomalies can vary from absence of the digits to absence of the distal part of a whole limb. The tongue is usually small. The syndrome has been associated with early chorionic villus sampling carried out at 8–9 weeks gestation.[64] The prognosis for intellectual development is good: the inheritance is uncertain as most cases are sporadic.

Thrombocytopenia – absent radius syndrome (TAR) is a condition inherited in an autosomal recessive fashion with variable degrees of limb reduction deformity, predominantly in the upper limbs. The defects are usually bilateral radial aplasia or variable degrees of hypoplasia. The thumbs are always present. Ulnar or humeral reduction is seen in some cases. These deformities are diagnostic markers for the underlying haemopoietic defect of hypomegakaryocytic thrombocytopenia, which may be recognised on fetal blood sampling. In about one-third of cases there is coexistent congenital heart disease. Malformations of the lower limbs, ribs and cervical spine may also be seen. Successful ultrasonographic diagnosis in the second trimester has been reported.[14,65,66]

The prognosis depends on the severity of the cardiac lesion rather than the bleeding diathesis. The majority survive infancy and the thrombocytopenia improves with age. In severely affected cases support with platelet transfusions may be necessary.[67,68]

Fanconi pancytopenia syndrome is an autosomal recessive syndrome associated with bone marrow failure and severe anaemia. Nearly 80% of affected individuals have aplasia or hypoplasia of the thumb and radius. These anomalies may be unilateral. The anaemia tends to be progressive, usually presenting later in the first decade of life. Other abnormalities, including supernumerary thumbs, renal anomalies and CNS anomalies, have been reported. The prognosis is poor, with microcephaly, mental retardation and growth retardation occurring in infancy. There are a number of genes responsible for Fanconi anaemia, and prenatal diagnosis in families at increased risk is possible using molecular methods or chromosome breakage studies, but a sample from the index case is required.[69,70]

Blackfan–Diamond (Aase) congenital anaemia is also associated with radial defects in a significant proportion of cases.[67] The inheritance is uncertain, with some dominant and some recessive forms reported. Prenatal diagnosis has been reported in a high-risk family.[71]

Holt–Oram syndrome is an autosomal dominant syndrome of upper limb/girdle deformity and congenital heart disease of very variable degrees. Limb reduction deformities vary considerably in severity and may involve any part of the upper limb and shoulder girdle. The thumbs may be absent, hypoplastic or triphalangeal (finger-like), or associated with syndactyly. ASD and VSD are the commoner cardiac abnormalities. Successful diagnosis in the second and third trimesters of high-risk pregnancies has been based on the ultrasonographic demonstration of both limb and cardiac deformities.[72,73] The expression of this disorder within a family is extremely variable, and a gene carrier may only have the minimum signs (e.g. difficulty in pronation of the forearm or minor abnormalities of the thumb).[73,74]

Polysyndactyly

Abnormalities of the fingers are best seen in a fully fanned hand (see Ch. 21, Fig. 4). The fetus is not always obliging enough to give this view and a section across the clenched hand in the axial plane will suffice to detect extra (or a deficiency of) bones. A full plantar view of the foot should display polydactyly (Fig. 19.9D).

Polydactyly may be pre-axial (see Fig. 19.9) (duplicate or bifid thumbs or big toes) or postaxial (on the ulnar side of the index finger or the lateral aspect of the foot). Syndactyly denotes fusion of either the bones (osseous syndactyly) or soft tissues (cutaneous syndactyly) of the fingers or toes.

There are many syndromes with these abnormalities as a feature (see Fig. 19.9). The commoner ones are listed in Table 19.5. For a more detailed list and description of the syndromes the reader is referred to Smith[67] and Winter *et al.*[2] As the syndromes have differing prognostic significance it behoves the ultrasonologist to make a detailed search for other fetal abnormalities before reaching a diagnosis. Fetal karyotyping should also be considered. Isolated polysyndactyly occurs as an autosomal dominant condition in some families.

Ectrodactyly

Ectrodactyly, or split hands or feet (Fig. 19.28), can occur as part of the ectrodactyly ectodermal dysplasia clefting syndrome (EEC) or as an isolated abnormality. Both con-

Table 19.5 Some syndromes associated with polysyndactyly

Polydactyly	Syndactyly
Meckel Gruber	Apert (acrocephalosyndactyly)
Ellis-van-Creveld	Oral facial digital
Greig cephalopolysyndactyly	Roberts (pseudothalidomide)
Grebe	Carpenter
SRP	
Oral facial digital	
Carpenter (acrocephalopolysyndactyly)	
Jeune (asphyxiating thoracic dystrophy)	
Jouberts	
Trisomy 13	

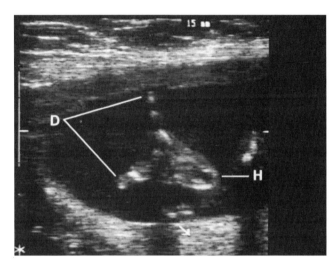

Fig. 19.28 Ectrodactyly. Scan of the foot of a fetus with bilateral ectrodactyly of the feet ('lobster claw' deformity). The hands appeared normal. H – heel, D – two digits. (Figure courtesy of Professor S. Campbell).

ditions are inherited as autosomal dominant traits, but ectrodactyly may be associated with other syndromes with variable inheritance. EEC is associated with difficulty in sweating, sparse hair, abnormal teeth and facial clefts. The degree of penetrance within families can be very variable. Isolated ectrodactyly can affect one or more limbs to variable degrees. Isolated cases are new dominant mutations but before counselling low recurrence risks for apparently normal parents careful examination is mandatory as they may have very minimal signs (e.g. extra longitudinal skin creases on feet or hands).[75] A case of ectrodactyly diagnosed in a low-risk pregnancy is shown in Figure 19.28. Both feet had complete ectrodactyly. The diagnosis in severe cases such as this should not be a problem. However, more minor degrees may not be amenable to prenatal detection with ultrasound.

Positional deformities

Talipes (club foot) In this condition the foot is plantar-flexed and internally rotated. The condition may be detected on ultrasound by observing the relationship between the shaft of the tibia and the axis of the toes or plantar surface of the foot (Fig. 19.29). The views of the leg used to detect abnormalities are shown in Chapter 8, Figures 8.50–8.52. Talipes may occur as an isolated malformation in about 1/1200 births, as a result of asymmetrical intra-uterine environmental pressures (oligohydramnios, amniotic bands or intra-uterine tumours), as a marker of chromosomal abnormality, or as an integral part of a multitude of genetic syndromes (see Fig. 19.4).[67] Fetal karyotyping should be considered if talipes is present with another structural abnormality.

Rocker-bottom feet are a feature of trisomy 18 (Edwards' syndrome [Fig. 19.29]), 18q syndrome, trisomy 13 (Patau syndrome) and Pena–Shokeir type II syndrome. The deformity is characterised by a prominent heel, and replacement of the normal concavity of the plantar arch by convexity. The finding of this deformity should be a stimulus to detailed fetal examination for other defects and fetal karyotyping.

Multiple congenital contractures (arthrogryposis multiplex congenita) is a heterogeneous group of disorders all of which have multiple joint contractures present at birth. These are a result of limitation of fetal joint mobility and may be secondary to neurological (central or peripheral), muscular, connective tissue or skeletal abnormalities. Intra-uterine crowding, as with oligohydramnios, may also cause multiple joint contractures. Hageman *et al.*[76] reviewed 75 newborns with multiple congenital contractures and found abnormalities in the central nervous system in 55%, the peripheral neuromuscular system in 8% and connective tissues and skin in 11%. Oligohydramnios was associated in 7%.

These conditions should be recognised on ultrasound examination in the second trimester, when fixed, immobile limbs are found in bizarre positions (Figs 19.4 and 19.30–19.31). Polyhydramnios and fetal hydrops or nuchal thickening are frequent accompanying features. Specific syndromes, such as Pena–Shokeir syndrome type I,[77,78] lethal multiple pterygium syndrome[79] and congenital muscular dystrophy, have been described. These are mainly autosomal recessive. Kirkinen *et al.*[80] describe ultrasonic observation of six high-risk pregnancies from the first trimester. Although apparently normal at between 8 and 12 weeks, by the 16 week all six fetuses showed severe generalised subcutaneous oedema with restricted fetal movement. In two there was ascites or hydrothorax, which are common accompaniments to these syndromes.[81–87] The prognosis in these cases is usually poor, with a high incidence of stillbirth and neonatal deaths secondary to pulmonary hypoplasia.

The distal arthrogryposes are a group of milder conditions affecting peripheral joints such as hands, feet and

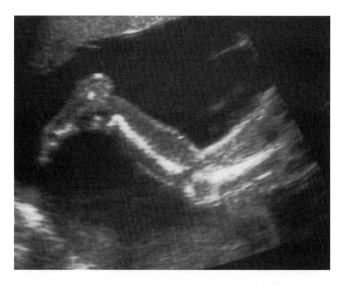

Fig. 19.29 Rocker-bottom foot. Sagittal scan of the foot of a fetus with trisomy 18 showing prominent heel suggestive of 'rocker-bottom' feet. This deformity was found in association with omphalocele and cleft lip and palate.

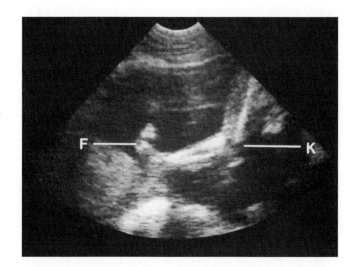

Fig. 19.30 Arthrogryposis. Scan of a fetal leg in a case of arthrogryposis multiplex congenita. The hips were adducted and the knee (K) hyperextended so that the foot (F) pointed directly at the face. There were also marked fixed positional deformities of the upper limb.

the jaw.[88] The deformities may be corrected with surgery, and life expectancy and neurological function are normal. These conditions are autosomal dominant. Prenatal ultrasound diagnosis in an affected family has been described on the detection of flexed fingers and extended wrists.[89,90]

Counselling and follow-up

Some of the characteristic features of a wide spectrum of skeletal and postural deformities have been described.

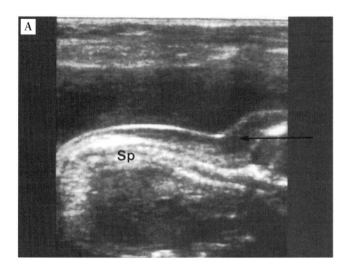

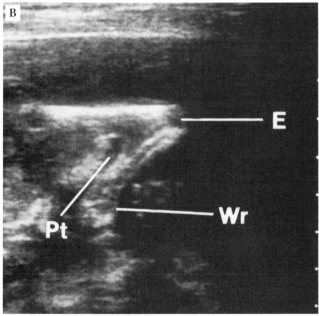

Fig. 19.31 Multiple pterygium syndrome. Scans from a fetus with fethal multiple pterygium syndrome. **A:** Posterior sagittal section of the spine (Sp) and occipital region showing nuchal oedema (arrow). **B:** The arm is in fixed flexion at the elbow (E). There is a skin web of pterygium (Pt) in the antecubital fossa. The wrist (Wr) shows a flexion deformity. Similar pterygia were apparent in the popliteal fossae.

Diagnostic accuracy will be improved if time is spent examining the fetus in detail. A reference textbook may be very helpful in reaching an accurate diagnosis of many of the lethal dysplasias. In cases where the diagnosis or prognosis is in doubt it may be prudent to consult a geneticist or paediatrician before finally counselling a couple, who may themselves wish a further specialist consultation before they come to a final decision on management.

On delivery of the affected fetus anteroposterior and lateral photographs and detailed radiographs should be taken. If the fetus is dead but fresh fetal blood or skin should be sent for cytogenetic studies. In many cases consultation with a geneticist may be appropriate to discuss storage of DNA, which may be useful for future early diagnosis. It is also important that, where appropriate, the post-mortem examination is performed by a perinatal pathologist interested in skeletal dysplasias. Only when all this information has been gathered should the definitive diagnosis be made and the couple finally counselled by a geneticist as to the risk of recurrence in future pregnancies, and the implications for other family members. The possibilities for subsequent prenatal diagnosis should be covered in discussion.

REFERENCES

1 Koren G, Edwards M B, Miskin M. Antenatal sonography of fetal malformations associated with drugs and chemicals: a guide. Am J Obstet Gynecol 1987; 176: 79

2 Winter R M, Knowles S A S, Bieber F R, Baraitser M. The malformed fetus and stillbirth; a diagnostic approach. Chichester: John Wiley, 1988; 166–201

3 O'Brien G D, Queenan J T, Campbell S. Assessment of gestational age in the second trimester by real-time ultrasound measurement of the femur length. Am J Obstet Gynecol 1981; 139: 540–545

4 Orioli I M, Castilla E E, Barbosa-Neto J G. The birth prevalence rates for the skeletal dysplasias. J Med Genet 1986; 23: 328–332

5 Glenn L W, Teng S S K. In utero sonographic diagnosis of achondrogenesis. JCU 1985; 13: 195–198

6 Golbus M S, Hall B D, Filly R A, Poskanzer L B. Prenatal diagnosis of achondrogenesis. J Pediatr 1977; 91: 464

7 Donnenfeld A E, Mennuti M T. Second trimester diagnosis of fetal skeletal dysplasias. Obstet Gynecol Surv 1987; 42: 199–217

8 Muller L M, Cremin B J. Ultrasonic demonstration of fetal skeletal dysplasia. S Afr Med J 1985; 65: 222–226

9 Soothill P W, Vuthiwong C, Rees H. Achondrogenesis type 2 diagnosed by transvaginal ultrasound at 12 weeks' gestation. Prenat Diagn 1993; 13(6): 523–528

10 Griffin D, Campbell S, Allan L, Roberts A, Little D. Fetal anomalies. In: Barnet E, Morley P, eds. Clinical diagnostic ultrasound. Oxford: Blackwell Scientific Publications, 1985: 559–580

11 Borochowitz Z, Ornoy A, Lachman R, Rimoin D L. Achondrogenesis II – hypochondrogenesis: variability versus heterogeneity. Am J Med Genet 1986; 24: 273–288

12 Stoll C, Manini P, Bloch J, Roth M-P. Prenatal diagnosis of hypochondroplasia. Prenat Diagn 1985; 5: 423–426

13 van der Harten J J, Brons J T J, Dijkstra P F et al. Paediatr Pathol 1988; 8: 233–252

14 Hobbins J C, Bracken M B, Mahoney M J. Diagnosis of fetal dysplasias with ultrasound. Am J Obstet Gynecol 1982; 142: 306–312

15 Milsom I, Mattsson L-A, Dahlen-Nilsson I. Antenatal diagnosis of osteogenesis imperfecta by real-time ultrasound: two case reports. Br J Radiol 1982; 55: 310–312

16 Shapiro J E, Phillips J A, Byers P H et al. Prenatal diagnosis of lethal osteogenesis imperfecta (OI type II). J Pediatr 1982; 100: 127–133

17 Dinno N D, Yacuob U S, Kadlec J F, Garver K L. Midtrimester diagnosis of osteogenesis imperfecta, type II. Birth Defects 1982; 18: 125–132

18 Elejalde B R, de Elejalde M M. Prenatal diagnosis of perinatally lethal osteogenesis imperfecta. Am J Med Genet 1983; 14: 353–359

19 Brons J T J, van der Harten J J, Wladimiroff J W, van Geijn H P. Prenatal ultrasonographic diagnosis of osteogenesis imperfecta. Am J Obstet Gynecol 1988; 159: 176–181

20 Young I D, Thompson E M, Hall C M, Pembrey M E. Osteogenesis imperfecta type IIA: evidence for dominant inheritance. J Med Genet 1987; 24: 386–389

21 Thompson E M, Young I D, Hall C M, Pembrey M E. Recurrence risks and prognosis in severe sporadic osteogenesis imperfecta. J Med Genet 1987; 24: 390–405

22 Byers P H, Steiner R D. Osteogenesis imperfecta. Ann Rev Med 1992; 43: 269–282

23 Kurtz A B, Wapner R J. Ultrasonographic diagnosis of second trimester skeletal dysplasias: a prospective analysis in a high risk population. J Ultrasound Med 1983; 2: 99–106

24 Wladimiroff J W, Niermeijer M F, Van der Harten J J, Stewart F G A, Bloms W, Huijmans J G M. Early prenatal diagnosis of congenital hypophosphatasia: case report. Prenat Diagn 1985; 5: 47–52

25 Mulivor R A, Mennuti M, Zackai E H, Harris H. Prenatal diagnosis of hypophosphatasia: genetic, biochemical and clinical studies. Am J Hum Genet 1978; 30: 271–282

26 Warren R C, McKenzie C F, Rodeck C H, Moscoso G, Brock D J, Barron L. First trimester diagnosis of hypophosphatasia with a monoclonal antibody to the liver/bone/kidney isoenzyme of alkaline phosphatase. Lancet 1985; ii: 856

27 Little D. Prenatal diagnosis of skeletal dysplasias. In: Rodeck C H, Nicolaides K H, eds. Prenatal diagnosis. London: Royal College of Obstetricians and Gynaecologists, 1984: 301–306

28 Elejalde B R, de Elejalde M M, Pansch D. Prenatal diagnosis of Jeune Syndrome. Am J Med Genet 1985; 21: 433–438

29 Donaldson M D C, Warner A A, Trompeter R S, Haycock G B, Chantler C. Familial juvenile nephronophthisis, Jeune's syndrome and associated disorders. Arch Dis Child 1985; 60: 426–434

30 Fryns J P, van den Berghe K, van Assche A, van den Berghe H. Prenatal diagnosis of campomelic dwarfism. Clin Genet 1981; 19: 199–201

31 Redon J Y, Le Grevellec J Y, Marie F, Le Coq E, Le Guern H. Un diagnostic antenatal de dysplasie campomelique. J Gynecol Obstet Biol Reprod 1984; 13: 437–441

32 Winter R, Rosenkranz W, Hofmann H, Zierler H, Becker H, Borkenstein M. Prenatal diagnosis of campomelic dysplasia by ultrasonography. Prenat Diagn 1985; 5: 1–8

33 Lynch S A, Gaunt M L, Minford A M. Campomelic dysplasia: evidence of autosomal dominant inheritance. J Med Genet 1993; 30(8): 683–686

34 Mansour S, Hall C M, Pembrey M E, Young I D. A clinical and genetic study of campomelic dysplasia. J Med Genet 1995; 32(6): 415–420

35 Polymeropoulos M H, Ide S E, Wright M et al. The gene for the Ellis–van Creveld syndrome is located on chromosome 4p16. Genomics 1996; 35(1): 1–5

36 Mahoney M J, Hobbins J C. Prenatal diagnosis of chondroectodermal dysplasia (Ellis-van-Creveld syndrome) with fetoscopy and ultrasound. N Engl J Med 1977; 297: 258–260

37 Filly R A, Golbus M S, Cary J C, Hall J G. Short limbed dwarfism: ultrasonographic diagnosis by mensuration of fetal femoral length. Radiology 1981; 138: 653–656

38 Filly R A, Golbus M S. Ultrasonography of the normal and pathologic fetal skeleton. Radiol Clin North Am 1982; 20: 311–323

39 Tavormina P L, Shiang R, Thompson L M et al. Thanatophoric dysplasia (types I and II) caused by distinct mutations in fibroblast growth factor receptor 3. Nature Genet 1995; 9(3): 321–328

40 Elejalde B R, de Elejalde M M. Thanatophoric dysplasia: fetal manifestations and prenatal diagnosis. Am J Med Genet 1985; 22: 669–683

41 Weiner C P, Williamson R A, Bonsib S M. Sonographic diagnosis of cloverleaf skull and thanatophoric dysplasia in the second trimester. JCU 1986; 14: 463–465

42 Chervenak F A, Blakemore K J, Isaacson G, Mayden K, Hobbins J C. Antenatal sonographic findings of thanatophoric dysplasia with cloverleaf skull. Am J Obstet Gynecol 1983; 146: 984–985

43 Beetham F G T, Reeves J S. Early ultrasound diagnosis of thanatophoric dwarfism. JCU 1984; 12: 43–44

44 Burrows P E, Stannard M W, Pearrow J, Sutterfield S, Baker M L. Early antenatal sonographic recognition of thanatophoric dysplasia with cloverleaf skull deformity. AJR 1984; 143: 841–843

45 Camera G, Dodero D, De Pascale S. Prenatal diagnosis of thanatophoric dysplasia at 24 weeks. Am J Med Genet 1984; 18: 39–43

46 Wladimiroff J W, Niermeijer M F, Laar J, Jahoda M, Stewart P A. Prenatal diagnosis of skeletal dysplasia by real-time ultrasound. Obstet Gynecol 1984; 63: 360–364

47 Meizner I, Bar-Ziv J. Prenatal ultrasonic diagnosis of short-rib polydactyly syndrome (SRPS) type 3: a case report and a proposed approach to the diagnosis of SRPS and related conditions. JCU 1985; 13: 284–287

48 Gembruch U, Hansmann M, Frodisch H J. Early prenatal diagnosis of short rib-polydactyly (SRP) syndrome type 1 (Majewski) by ultrasound in a case at risk. Prenat Diagn 1985; 5: 357–362

49 Hoefler S, Hoefler G, Moser A B, Watkins P A, Chen W W, Moser H W. Prenatal diagnosis of rhizomelic chondrodysplasia punctata. Prenat Diagn 1988; 8: 571–576

50 Mantagos S, Weiss R W, Mahoney M, Hobbins J C. Prenatal diagnosis of diastrophic dwarfism. Am J Obstet Gynecol 1981; 139: 111–113

51 Gembruch U, Niesen M, Kehrberg H, Hansmann M. Diastrophic dysplasia: a specific prenatal diagnosis by ultrasound. Prenat Diagn 1988; 8: 539–545

52 O'Brien G D, Rodeck C, Queenan J T. Early prenatal diagnosis of diastrophic dwarfism by ultrasound. BMJ 1980; 280: 1300

53 Kaitila I, Ammala P, Karjalainen O, Liukkonen S, Rapola J. Early prenatal detection of diastrophic dysplasia. Prenat Diagn 1983; 3: 237–244

54 Bellus G A, Hefferon T W, Ortiz de Luna R I et al. Achondroplasia is defined by recurrent G380R mutations of FGFR3. Am J Hum Genet 1995; 56(2): 368–373

55 Campbell S, Griffin D, Roberts A, Little D. Early prenatal diagnosis of abnormalities of the fetal head, spine, limbs and abdominal organs. In: Orlandi P, Polani P, Bovicelli L, eds. Recent advances in prenatal diagnosis. Chichester: John Wiley, 1981: 41–59

56 Tolmie J T, Whittle M J, McNay M B, Gibson A A M, Connor J M. Second trimester prenatal diagnosis of the Jarcho–Levin syndrome. Prenat Diagn 1987; 7: 129–134

57 Apuzzio J J, Diamond N, Ganesh M S, Despostio F. Difficulties in the prenatal diagnosis of Jarcho-Levin syndrome. Am J Obstet Gynecol 1987; 156: 916–918

58 Romero R, Ghidini A, Eswara M S, Seashore M R, Hobbins J C. Prenatal findings in a case of spondylocostal dysplasia type I (Jarcho–Levin syndrome). Obstet Gynecol 1988; 71: 988–991

59 Marks M, Hernanz-Schulman M, Horii S et al. Spondylothoracic dysplasia. Clinical and sonographic diagnosis. J Ultrasound Med 1989; 8: 1–5

60 Kim H J, Costales F, Bouzouki M, Wallach R C. Prenatal diagnosis of dyssegmental dwarfism. Prenat Diagn 1986; 6: 143–150

61 Benacerraf B R, Greene M F, Barss V A. Prenatal sonographic diagnosis of congenital hemivertebra. J Ultrasound Med 1986; 5: 257–259

62 Mahony B S, Filly R A, Callen P W, Golbus M S. Amniotic band syndrome: antenatal sonographic diagnosis and potential pitfalls. Am J Obstet Gynecol 1985; 152: 63–68

63 Parry D M, Mulvihill J J, Tsai S, Kaiser-Kupfer M I, Cowan J M. SC phocomelia syndrome, premature centromere separation, and congenital nerve paralysis in two sisters, one with malignant melanoma. Am J Med Genet 1986; 24: 653–672

64 Firth H V, Boyd P A, Chamberlain P, MacKenzie I Z, Lindenbaum R H, Huson S M. Severe limb abnormalities after chorion villus sampling at 56–66 days' gestation. Lancet 1991; 337(8744): 762–763

65 Luthy D A, Mack L, Hirsch J, Cheng E. Prenatal diagnosis of thrombocytopenia with absent radii. Am J Obstet Gynecol 1981; 141: 350–351

66 Filkins K, Russo J, Bilinki I. Prenatal diagnosis of thrombocytopaenia absent radius syndrome using ultrasound and fetoscopy. Prenat Diagn 1984; 4: 139

67 Smith D W. Recognizable patterns of human malformations: genetic, embryologic and clinical aspects. Philadelphia: W B Saunders, 1982

68 Hall J G. Thrombocytopenia and absent radius (TAR) syndrome. J Med Genet 1987; 24: 79–83

69 Alter B P. Fanconi's anaemia and its variability. Br J Haematol 1993; 85(1): 9–14

70 Taylor A M, McConville C M, Byrd P J. Cancer and DNA processing disorders. Br Med Bull 1994; 50(3): 708–717

71 McLennan A E, Chitty L S, Rissik J, Maxwell D J. Prenatal diagnosis of Blackfan–Diamond syndrome: case report and review of the literature. Prenat Diagn 1996; 16: 349–353

72 Muller L M, de Jong G, van Heerden K M M. The antenatal ultrasonographic detection of the Holt-Oram syndrome. S Afr Med J 1985; 68: 313–315

73 Brons J T J, Van Geijn H P, Wladimiroff J W et al. Prenatal ultrasound diagnosis of the Holt–Oram syndrome. Prenat Diagn 1988; 8: 175–181

74 Newbury-Ecob R A, Leanage R, Raeburn J A, Young I D. Holt–Oram syndrome: a clinical genetic study. J Med Genet 1996; 33(4): 300–307

75 Penchaszadeh V B, Negrotti T C. Ectrodactyly–ectodermal dysplasia–clefting (EEC) syndrome: dominant inheritance and variable expression. J Med Genet 1976; 13: 281–284

76 Hageman G, Ippel E P F, Beemer F A, de Pater J M, Lindhout D, Willemse J. The diagnostic management of newborns with congenital contractures: a nosologic study of 75 cases. Am J Med Genet 1988; 30: 883–904

77 Pena S D J, Shokeir M H K. Syndrome of camptodactyly, multiple ankyloses, facial anomalies and pulmonary hypoplasia: a lethal condition. J Pediatr 1974; 85: 373–375

78 Hall J G. Invited editorial comment: analysis of Pena–Shokeir phenotype. Am J Med Genet 1986; 25: 99–117

79 Hall J G. The lethal multiple pterygium syndromes. Am J Med Genet 1984; 17: 803–807

80 Kirkinen P, Herva R, Leisti J. Early prenatal diagnosis of a lethal syndrome of multiple congenital contractures. Prenat Diagn 1987; 7: 189–196

81 Shenker L, Reed K, Anderson C, Hauck L, Spark R. Syndrome of camptodactyly ankyloses, facial anomalies and pulmonary hypoplasia (Pena–Shokeir syndrome): obstetric and ultrasound aspects. Am J Obstet Gynecol 1985; 152: 303–307

82 Chen H, Immken L, Lachman R et al. Syndrome of multiple pterygia, camptodactyly, facial anomalies, hypoplastic lungs and heart, cystic hygroma and skeletal anomalies: delineation of a new entity and review of lethal forms of multiple pterygium syndrome. Am J Med Genet 1984; 17: 809–823

83 Jeanty P, Romero R, D'Alton M, Venus I, Hobbins J. In utero sonographic detection of hand and foot deformities. J Ultrasound Med 1985; 4: 595–601

84 MacMillan R, Harbart G, Davis W, Kelly T. Prenatal diagnosis of Pena-Shokeir syndrome type I. Am J Med Genet 1985; 21: 279–284

85 Muller L M, de Jong G. Prenatal ultrasonic features of the Pena–Shokeir I syndrome and the trisomy 18 syndrome. Am J Med Genet 1986; 25: 119–129

86 Goldberg J D, Chervenak F A, Lipman R A, Berkowitz R L. Antenatal sonographic diagnosis of arthrogryposis multiplex congenita. Prenat Diagn 1986; 6: 45–49

87 Zeitune M, Feigin M D, Abramowicz I, B-Aderet N, Goodman R. Prenatal diagnosis of the pterygium syndrome. Prenat Diagn 1988; 8: 145–149

88 Hall J G, Reed S D, Green G. The distal arthrogryposes: delineation of new entities – review and nosological discussion. Am J Med Genet 1982; 11: 185–239

89 Baty B J, Cubberley D, Morris C, Cary J. Prenatal diagnosis of distal arthrogryposis. Am J Med Genet 1988; 29: 501–510

90 Griffin D R. Detection of congenital abnormalities of the limbs and face by ultrasound. In: Chamberlain G, ed. Modern antenatal care of the fetus. Oxford: Blackwell Scientific, 1990; 389–427

Thoracic abnormalities

Lyn S Chitty and David R Griffin

Introduction

Congenital abnormalities of the fetal lungs that can be recognised on ultrasound examination include congenital diaphragmatic hernia, congenital cystic adenomatoid malformation of the lung, pulmonary sequestrations, bronchogenic cysts, pleural effusions, and tracheal or laryngeal atresias and other rarer tumours. Space-occupying lesions within the chest can result in pulmonary hypoplasia, and in general terms it is this that dictates the ultimate outcome for a fetus with a lesion within the chest. Attempts have been made to determine the maturity of the fetal lungs and the presence or absence of pulmonary hypoplasia by comparing the reflectivity with that of the liver, but the method was found to be too inaccurate to be useful in clinical practice. Likewise, nomograms for thoracic dimensions do not successfully predict pulmonary hypoplasia, but recent reports suggest that there may be some benefit in using the lung-to-head ratio or pulmonary artery Dopplers.

In all cases where a fetal abnormality that might require post-natal surgical intervention is identified, early consultation with paediatric surgeons and neonatologists is helpful. There have been rapid advances in management in these areas, and such specialists are best placed to discuss potential management and prognosis with the parents.

Bronchogenic cyst

Definition and aetiology   A bronchogenic cyst is a cystic structure which is lined with bronchial epithelium and may contain cartilage, muscle and mucous glands. The incidence is unknown, as many are asymptomatic in early life.[1,2] These cysts arise from an abnormal budding of the foregut and can remain attached to the tracheo-bronchial tree, in the mediastinum or within the pulmonary parenchyma. Bronchogenic cysts vary in size and location. They may become separated from their origin during development and migrate into the mediastinum, neck, pericardium and other sites.[3]

Associated abnormalities   Bronchogenic cysts arise as a result of a bronchopulmonary foregut anomaly and are therefore associated with other abnormalities which have a common embryological origin. These include oesophageal duplications, diverticulum and cysts, tracheo-oesophageal fistula, neuro-enteric cysts and lung sequestrations.[4,5] Vertebral anomalies may be associated with bronchogenic cysts.[6] Association with aneuploidy is very rare.

Diagnosis   There are very few reports of the prenatal diagnosis of bronchogenic cysts.[5,7–9] The earliest was at 17 weeks gestation, when a unilocular cystic lesion was identified. The neonate was also found to have extrapulmonary sequestration and a duplication of the oesophagus. In general a definitive diagnosis is rarely made prenatally and the final diagnosis will depend on the post-natal, surgical and histological examination (Fig. 20.1). The differential diagnosis of a bronchogenic cyst includes other mediastinal and pulmonary masses, as listed in Table 20.1.

Management and prognosis   Many bronchogenic cysts are asymptomatic and are only discovered as an incidental finding on a chest radiograph later in life,[1,10,11] whereas others may cause airway compression, recurrent respiratory tract infections later in life,[1–3] or a significant degree of pulmonary hypoplasia secondary to compression of the developing lung. Delivery in a unit with neonatal intensive care and paediatric surgical facilities is recommended if the lesion is large and there is mediastinal shift. Treatment is by surgical excision if the lesion is symptomatic. The long-term prognosis for those who survive surgery is good.[1,2,10,11]

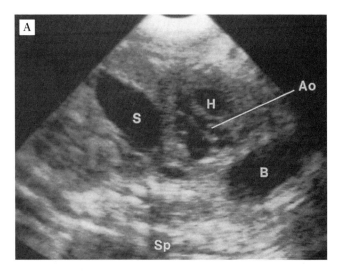

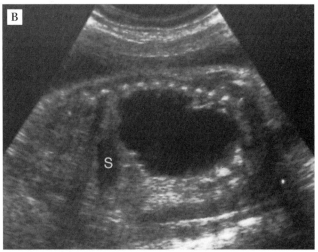

Fig. 20.1 Bronchogenic cyst. A: Longitudinal view through the fetal thorax and abdomen showing a bronchogenic cyst (B). **B:** A very large cyst filling the chest. Heart (H) with aortic root (Ao), S – stomach, Sp – spine.

Table 20.1 Differential diagnosis of intrathoracic abnormalities

Solid lesions
Cystic adenomatoid malformation, microcystic type III
Pulmonary sequestration
Mediastinal teratoma
Rhabdomyoma
Right-sided diaphragmatic hernia
Tracheal/laryngeal atresia

Cystic lesions
Cystic adenomatoid malformation types I and II (macrocystic)
Bronchogenic cyst
Mediastinal encephalocele
Congenital diaphragmatic hernia
Pericardial and pleural effusions

Occasionally thoracic cysts may be demonstrated antenatally (Fig. 20.2) which are not substantiated by postnatal imaging. Both of the infants shown were well at birth

and their chest radiographs showed minimal abnormalities, and so further investigations were not thought to be justified. The first infant remained asymptomatic at 2½ years. However, it is now recognised that a plain chest radiography may not be sufficient to demonstrate all lesions, and more sophisticated imaging, such as CT or MRI may be required.

Pulmonary sequestration

Definition and aetiology   Pulmonary sequestration is a rare congenital abnormality of bronchopulmonary foregut origin in which some pulmonary parenchyma is separated from normal lung. The sequestrated lobe does not usually communicate with an airway and it has an independent blood supply directly from the systemic circulation.[12–14] Two types of lung sequestration are recognised: intra- and extralobar. In the intralobar type the

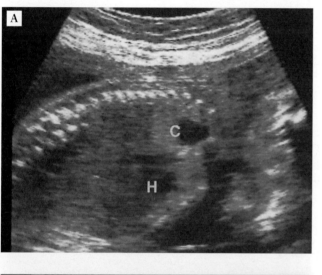

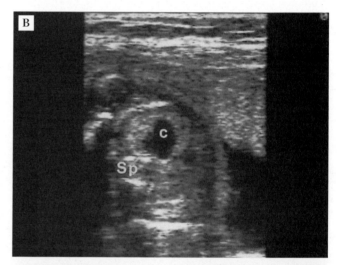

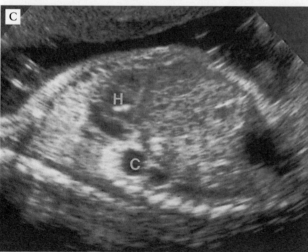

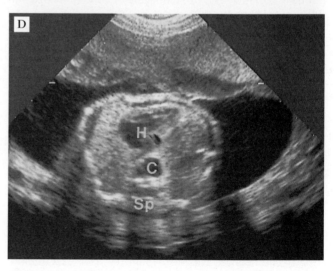

Fig. 20.2 Intrathoracic cystic lesions. A: Longitudinal and **B:** transverse views showing the cystic lesion (C) at the apex with the heart (H) and spine (Sp). **C:** The cyst (C) at the lung base is shown in longitudinal and **D:** transverse section.

sequestrated and normal lung share a common pleura, whereas in the commoner extralobar variety the sequestrated lobe is covered by its own layer of visceral pleura. They are usually unilateral and include only a part of the lung,[15] although cases with bilateral lesions have been reported.[16] The most common location is between the lower lobe and the diaphragm. Other locations include paracardiac, mediastinal and abdominal sites. The sequestrated lobe is variable in size and has arterial and venous communication with systemic vessels.

In the majority of cases of intralobar sequestration the lower lobes are affected. The arterial supply arises most commonly from the thoracic or abdominal aorta, with venous drainage into the pulmonary veins.

Associated anomalies   As lung sequestration is one of the bronchopulmonary foregut malformations it has associations similar to those of bronchogenic cysts.[17–19] It is often found in association with cystic adenomatoid malformation.[1,20] Extrapulmonary abnormalities are reported in patients with intralobar sequestration.[15] These include skeletal deformities, diaphragmatic hernia, congenital heart disease, renal and intracranial anomalies.[15,21,22] The incidence of extrapulmonary abnormalities in extralobar pulmonary sequestration is reported to be higher, diaphragmatic hernia being the most common.[1,12,15,20]

Pulmonary sequestration may be associated with fetal hydrops and pleural effusions, which are poor prognostic indicators.[23]

Diagnosis   In the fetus this condition is most often discovered as a mass of uncertain origin in the chest and a definitive diagnosis is not possible without histology,[7,24–28] unless an independent blood supply is demonstrated using Doppler ultrasound. The sequestrated lobe appears as a highly reflective, intrathoracic (Fig. 20.3) or intra-abdominal mass. It may be associated with hydrops and polyhydramnios.[24,26,27] The differential diagnosis includes other solid lesions found in the chest (Table 20.1). Extralobar sequestration[29] may simulate the pyramidal shape of the lower lung (Fig. 20.4).

Prenatal diagnosis of intralobar pulmonary sequestration has been reported,[5,29] but a definitive diagnosis is rarely made prenatally. Even in the perinatal period a preoperative diagnosis is only made in around 40% of cases.[15]

Management and prognosis   If the diagnosis is made before viability and there is associated hydrops, then termination of the pregnancy should be considered. In other cases, detected later in pregnancy, or where the decision to continue the pregnancy has been made, standard obstetric management should be followed. Delivery in a centre with neonatal intensive care and surgical facilities is advised if the lesion is large and causes significant mediastinal shift

towards term, as respiratory support and early surgery may occasionally be required. Parents should be offered an early consultation with a paediatric surgeon, who will be best placed to discuss current management.

The spectrum of these conditions is wide. Some cases may be discovered as an incidental finding on a routine chest radiograph. Many infants are asymptomatic until later in life, when recurrent pulmonary infections or haemorrhage, gastrointestinal symptoms or heart failure from a left-to-right shunt occur.[12,18,22,23,29,30] However, the anomalous blood supply to the sequestrated lung can cause a sufficiently severe left-to-right shunt to cause cardiac failure soon after birth.[30,31] The prognosis for extralobar sequestration presenting in infancy is reported to be poor, as many cases have associated abnormalities.[15] In one report of four cases detected antenatally only one survived. The three who died had extralobar sequestration and hydrops. The survivor had intra-abdominal sequestration with no hydrops.[25] When the condition presents as an isolated prenatal finding with no associated hydrops, or later in life, the prognosis is good. Spontaneous improvement *in utero* has been reported.[32]

Cystic adenomatoid malformation

Definition and aetiology   Congenital cystic adenomatoid malformation of the lung (CCAML) is a rare congenital cystic malformation characterised by excessive overgrowth of the terminal respiratory structures, resulting in the formation of variously sized intercommunicating cysts. Histologically CCAML has been classified into three subgroups according to the size of the cysts.[33] The type I lesion is composed of single or multiple large cysts greater than 2 cm in diameter. Type II is composed of multiple small cysts less than 1 cm in diameter, and type III is a large, bulky microcystic lesion. Any of these may cause mediastinal shift. The lesion is usually unilateral. Differentiation between the types can be difficult sonographically and it is best to classify them as either microcystic (which presents as a uniformly highly reflective area in the chest) or macrocystic (a mixture of high and low reflectivity within the lung).

Associated anomalies   CCAML is usually an isolated finding. In many cases sonographic findings may resolve spontaneously *in utero*, whereas in others the findings persist; in only a few is there progression and development of polyhydramnios and hydrops. These are poor prognostic signs, particularly when the second trimester is the time of initial presentation. It has been suggested that the hydrops may result from venous obstruction by the expanding mass, which compresses the inferior vena cava. In cases of macrocystic CCAML, where there has been a large unilocular cyst, hydrops may decrease after surgical decompression of the cyst.[34]

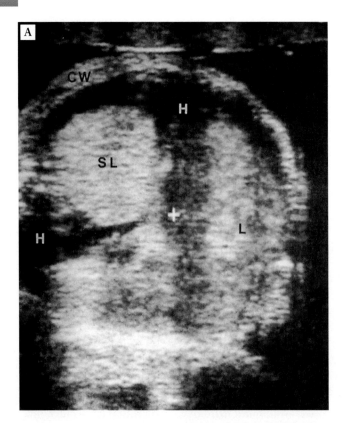

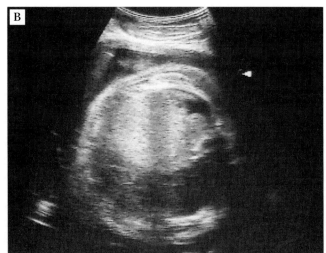

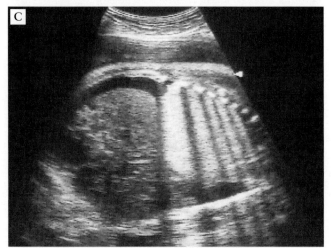

Fig. 20.3 Sequestrated lobe. A: Transverse view through the fetal chest demonstrating a sequestrated lobe (SL). Note the hydrothorax (H), chest wall (CW) and liver (L) which is visible in this section owing to depression of the liver by the intrathoracic mass. **B:** Transverse and **C:** longitudinal view through the fetal chest at 30 weeks in a different case, demonstrating the rounded mass occupying most of the left side of the chest. There was mild hydrops, with ascites, pleural effusions and skin oedema in this case, and there was a neonatal death secondary to pulmonary hypoplasia at 31 weeks.

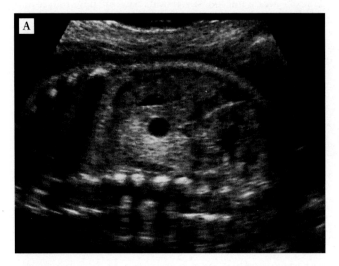

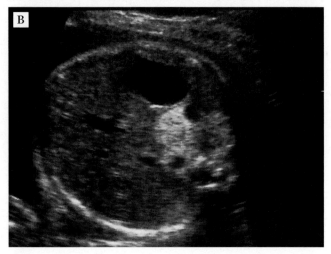

Fig. 20.4 Extrapulmonary sequestration. Note the highly reflective mass below the diaphragm in **A:** the parasagittal view and **B:** the transverse view, where the mass is seen behind the stomach. The neonate was asymptomatic at birth. The nature of the mass was confirmed by biopsy and management is conservative at present.

Associated bronchial abnormalities have been reported in a number of cases[1,20,35] and include pulmonary sequestration and congenital diaphragmatic hernia. Extrapulmonary anomalies have also been reported, including renal anomalies, bowel atresias, hydrocephaly, spinal anomalies and cardiac abnormalities.[36,37] In one study 11% of cases had additional malformations,[37] but there does not seem to be a significant association with aneuploidy.

Diagnosis The diagnosis of CCAML depends on the demonstration of an intrathoracic mass which may contain large cysts (macrocystic) (Figs 20.5 and 20.6), or which may have the appearance of a uniformly reflective area (microcystic type, Figs 20.7 and 20.8). Mediastinal shift can occur in all types and this is manifested as displacement of the heart within the chest. The differential diagnosis includes other intrathoracic lesions (Table 20.1). When considering macrocystic CCAML the main differential diagnosis is diaphragmatic hernia, which can usually be distinguished by observation of bowel peristalsis within the chest or of paradoxical visceral movement with breathing. Intra-abdominal location of the fetal stomach is also a very useful sign (compare Fig. 20.5C with Fig. 20.10A).

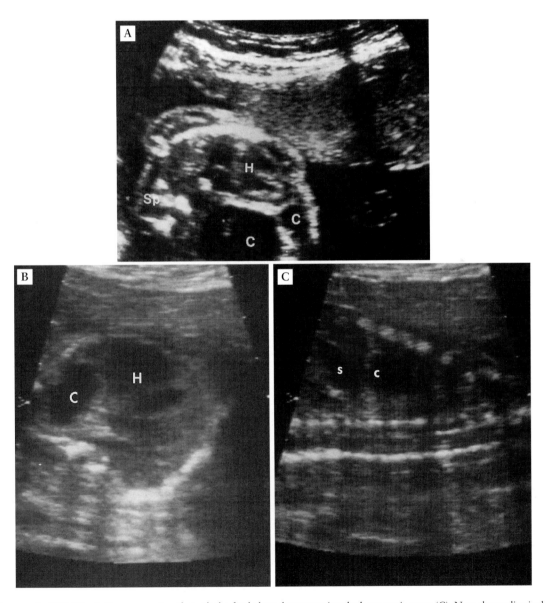

Fig. 20.5 Macrocystic CCAML. A: Transverse view through the fetal chest demonstrating the large cystic areas (C). Note the mediastinal shift with displacement of the heart (H). **B:** Transverse and **C:** longitudinal views through the fetal thorax, showing the cystic space (C) in the chest with stomach (S) below the diaphragm, with minimal displacement of the heart (H). Sp – spine.

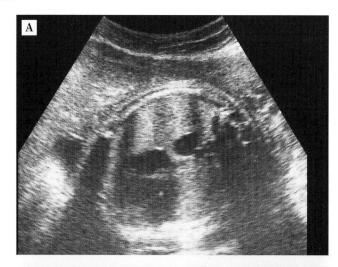

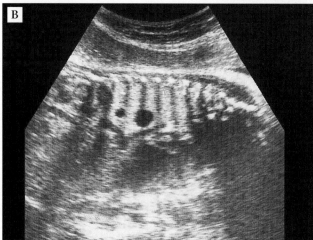

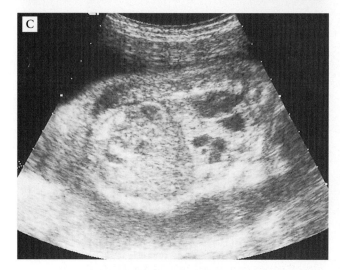

Fig. 20.6 Macrocystic CCAML. A: Transverse and **B:** longitudinal views through the fetal chest of a fetus with a mixed lesion. Note the highly reflective area in the chest with the echo-free cystic space and displacement of the heart. **C:** Longitudinal view though fetal chest showing an extensive lesion. This persisted until birth and neonatal surgery was required to relieve the respiratory difficulties.

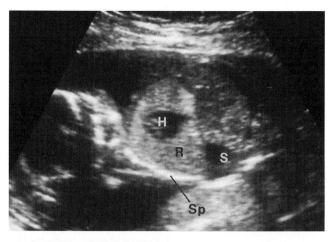

Fig. 20.7 Microcystic CCAML. Longitudinal view demonstrating the highly reflective appearance of CAM III (R) which is involving the entire lung. The heart (H), spine (Sp) and stomach (S) can be seen.

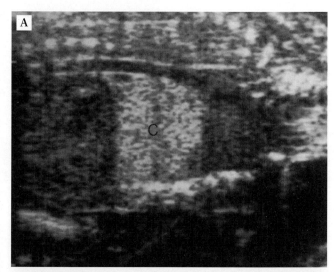

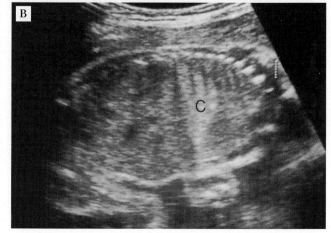

Fig. 20.8 Resolving microcystic CCAML. Apparent CAM III (C) confined to the right lower lobe. **A:** Shows the early appearances. **B:** Note the apparent diminution.

There are many reports of the prenatal diagnosis of CCAML in the literature.[7,34,38–47] Many are diagnosed in the second trimester at the time of a routine anomaly scan, but may also be diagnosed later in pregnancy when a scan is performed for another reason.[34,46,47]

Management and prognosis The diagnosis of CCAML should stimulate a careful search for other anomalies. In the macrocystic type where there is a unilocular large cyst with associated hydrops or polyhydramnios, decompression of the cyst(s) has been reported, with good results.[39,42,46] Resolution of the hydrops may then be seen.[34] Spontaneous *in utero* improvement of CCAML is often observed[48] (Figs 20.8 and 20.9). These observations make it difficult to predict the outcome of CCAML diagnosed prenatally. However, in general the prognosis for a fetus with CCAML is good.[47] In the authors' recent experience of 40 cases seen in the prenatal period, one pregnancy was terminated because of the presence of early hydrops, two required intrathoracic shunting with good results, and only one fetus died following early delivery at 29 weeks because of an abruption of the placenta. All other babies are alive and well. Three required surgery in the early newborn period and a few others had transient respiratory difficulties. This is compatible with some of the recent series reported in the literature.[47,49,50] However, when hydrops, polyhyramnios or mediastinal shift occurs the prognosis has been reported to be poor, with nearly 50% of cases resulting in stillbirth.[39,50] However, in our experience even the presence of mediastinal shift did not predict poor outcome: indeed, in many cases the degree of mediastinal shift lessened as the pregnancy continued (Fig. 20.9).

Cases undetected prenatally may present in the neonatal period with acute progressive respiratory distress because of mediastinal displacement and pulmonary compression by the expanding cystic lesion. Others may develop recurrent respiratory infections in infancy and childhood, but many remain asymptomatic for years.

The management of CCAML in the newborn period is debated. Surgical removal is recommended in symptomatic neonates. However, when a child is found to be asymptomatic management policies vary. There are many reports of complete resolution of these lesions *in utero*,[51,52] with apparently no abnormalities seen on a post-natal plain radiograph. However, there are now several reports of lesions not being detected on plain radiography, but large lesions are seen when more sophisticated imaging (CT, MRI or VQ scans) is performed.[49] We observed this phenomenon in four of the cases seen in our unit. Obstetric management should include delivery in a centre with neonatal intensive care and surgical facilities for those cases where the lesion has persisted or increased in size and mediastinal shift persists at term. In other cases the risk of significant neonatal difficulties is probably small, and delivery in local units may well be acceptable.

Congenital diaphragmatic hernia

Incidence and aetiology Congenital diaphragmatic hernia has an incidence of approximately 1/2000 births.[53] It occurs when a defective fusion or formation of the pleuroperitoneal membrane allows herniation of the abdominal contents into the thoracic cavity. Congenital diaphragmatic hernias are classified according to the location of the defect and occur most commonly in the posterior part of the diaphragm through the foramen of Bochdalek. The majority (75%) are left sided, with only 3% being bilateral.[53]

Associated anomalies Congenital diaphragmatic hernia is associated with a wide variety of abnormalities, the most common of which are malrotation of the gut and pulmonary hypoplasia, occurring as secondary phenomena. Normal lung development begins at about 5 weeks gestation. The full adult number of bronchioles is developed by the 16th week, but alveoli continue to develop up to and beyond birth. Abdominal contents within the chest inhibit normal lung development, reducing the number of conducting airways and alveoli and resulting in pulmonary hypoplasia.[54] The severity of the hypoplasia depends on the stage of pulmonary development when herniation takes place and the volume of viscera herniated into the chest.

Other structural abnormalities or aneuploidy occur in 24–57% of all cases.[53,55–58] However, the incidence of associated anomalies is much lower in infants who survive the perinatal period. It is rare for a neonate with a diaphragmatic hernia and another significant abnormality to survive. Neural tube defects, other central nervous system anomalies and cardiac malformations are the most frequent extrathoracic findings. Cardiac malformations may occur in up to 23% of cases,[59] and renal and skeletal abnormalities may also be found in the presence of a congenital diaphragmatic hernia. Congenital diaphragmatic hernia may also be found as a component of a number of syndromes,[60] in particular Fryns syndrome, which is inherited in an autosomal recessive fashion.

Chromosomal abnormalities, in particular trisomy 18, but also trisomies 13 and 21 and tetraploidy, have been reported in cases of diaphragmatic hernia.[53,55,58–60] The precise risk of an associated karyotypic abnormality in the presence of a diaphragmatic hernia is difficult to assess, and reports of the incidence vary from 5% to 21%.[55,61] However, in the majority of cases with an abnormal karyotype there are likely to be other malformations in addition to the diaphragmatic hernia.

Diagnosis The diagnosis of a diaphragmatic hernia can be made if abdominal organs are visualised within the thorax (Figs 20.10 and 20.11). However, bowel loops may be difficult to distinguish from other cystic lesions,[61] and

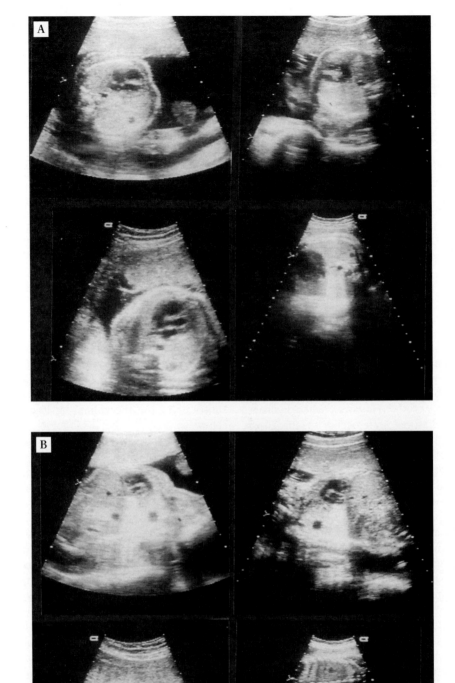

Fig. 20.9 Resolving macrocystic CCAML. A: Transverse and **B:** longitudinal views through the fetal chest at 20, 24, 29 and 35 weeks gestation, showing regression of the cystic lung lesion with time. Note the resolution of the mediastinal shift as the area of affected lung decreases.

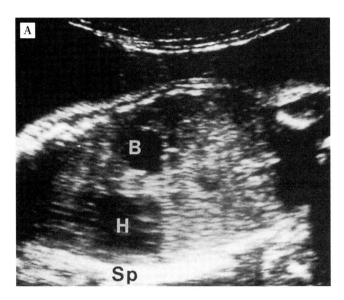

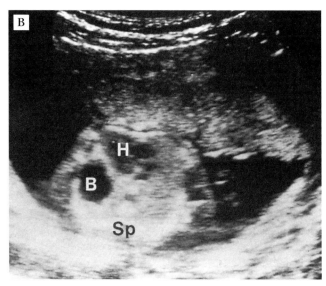

Fig. 20.10 Congenital diaphragmatic hernia. A: Longitudinal and **B:** transverse views through the chest in a fetus with a congenital diaphragmatic hernia. Note the bowel (B) in the chest, the absence of the normally situated stomach, spine (Sp) and heart (H).

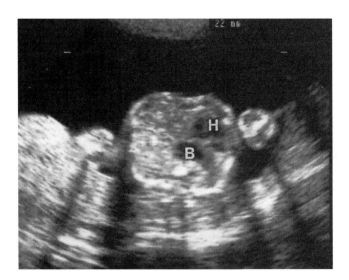

Fig. 20.11 Congenital diaphragmatic hernia. Transverse view through the chest of a fetus with a congenital diaphragmatic hernia demonstrating the mediastinal shift as indicated by the displacement of the heart (H). Note the bowel (B) in the chest.

the differential diagnosis therefore includes all causes of cystic lesions in the chest (Table 20.1). Inability to locate an intra-abdominal stomach is a useful aid to diagnosis in cases of left-sided hernia. Paradoxical movement of the viscera in the chest with fetal respiration may also be a useful discriminatory sign. In later pregnancy peristalsis of the bowel may also be seen in the chest.[62] Other features include mediastinal shift (Fig. 20.11) and polyhydramnios.[61] Prenatal diagnosis of a right-sided hernia has been reported,[62] but these may be more difficult to detect prenatally as in these cases the stomach normally maintains its normal position within the abdomen and it is the liver that herniates into the chest. The reflectivity of liver and lung is similar in mid-pregnancy, making the diagnosis difficult.

The diagnosis of congenital diaphragmatic hernia can be made at the time of a routine second-trimester scan,[61–63] but is also commonly made in later pregnancy (usually in the third trimester), when scanning for other indications.[64] Some authors have reported the presence of polyhydramnios as being a poor prognostic sign,[61] but others have not confirmed this observation.[63,65]

Not all cases of diaphragmatic hernia can be detected *in utero*, because although the defect may be present at an early stage of development, herniation of abdominal contents need not necessarily occur *in utero*. Approximately 5% of all cases present after the neonatal period, even in adulthood.[66,67] Harrison *et al.*[61] report a case where a diaphragmatic hernia was clearly visible at 26 weeks but had not been detected at a routine 20-week scan. They also refer to three other cases where the diagnosis had not been made at an earlier scan. They suggest that either small defects are not amenable to early detection, or that late herniation of the viscera occurs. All four of these cases survived. They postulate that non-survivors have large defects and early visceral herniation, resulting in more severe pulmonary hypoplasia and, incidentally, easier prenatal detection. This hypothesis is supported by data from others, who report improved survival for fetuses with an isolated diaphragmatic hernia detected after 24 weeks gestation.[63,65]

Management and prognosis The overall prognosis for neonates with a diaphragmatic hernia is poor, the major causes of death being pulmonary hypoplasia and/or the associated anomalies. Many fetuses with major extra-thoracic anomalies are stillborn or die in the neonatal period,[57,58,61] as do those with cardiac malformations.[59,61,63] Many who have an isolated diaphragmatic hernia die in the neonatal period from respiratory insufficiency prior to surgery. In cases diagnosed *in utero*, overall survival rates for those with an isolated diaphragmatic hernia range from 20% to 66%,[55,63,65] although survival in those with an isolated left-sided lesion may exceed 50%.[68] In those who survive to undergo surgical repair, survival will usually exceed 80%.[58,65] With continued improvements in neonatal intensive care this figure may improve.

There is much debate as to which prenatal features are useful prognostic indicators. It is clear that the presence of associated anomalies or an abnormal karyotype is a bad sign. Some authors report that in isolated cases polyhydramnios predicts a poor outcome,[61] whereas others do not find this association.[63,65] Poor prognostic factors include evidence of liver in the chest, evidence of cardiac ventricular disproportion before 24 weeks,[63] and an early diagnosis. Favourable prognostic factors include congenital diaphragmatic herniae that are left sided and isolated, an intra-abdominal stomach, and diagnosis after 24 weeks gestation.

The management of cases diagnosed prenatally should include fetal karyotyping and a detailed search for other structural abnormalities which may influence the prognosis. In particular women should be referred for expert fetal echocardiography, as cardiac lesions may be very difficult to detect and classify in the presence of a distorted mediastinum.[63] The parents should be offered a consultation with a paediatric surgeon with experience in the management of congenital diaphragmatic hernia. As the prognosis is so variable, even when the lesion is isolated, termination of pregnancy is a reasonable option and should be discussed.

In ongoing pregnancies delivery should be in a unit with neonatal intensive care and paediatric surgical facilities. Current post-natal management includes stabilisation of the infant and then transfer of care to the paediatric surgeon. Recent experimental data suggest that exogenous surfactant given before the first breath is taken may be useful.

Family studies have shown that the recurrence risk for an isolated diaphragmatic hernia is about 2%.[53,69] When it occurs as part of a syndrome, the recurrence risk is that of the syndrome. In view of the significant risk of a genetic aetiology (11% in complex cases in the North Thames West series) expert perinatal pathology and a genetic opinion is recommended in all cases ending in fetal demise.

The prospects of open fetal surgery

Harrison[54,70–72] has developed an animal model of diaphragmatic hernia by inserting a balloon into the thorax of fetal lambs and Rhesus monkeys. His group initially demonstrated that inflation of the balloon caused fatal pulmonary hypoplasia. Deflating the thoracic balloon but inflating an intra-abdominal balloon allowed sufficient lung development to allow survival after birth.

After devising an appropriate surgical technique which avoids impeding umbilical blood flow, Harrison[73] has now reported the outcome of the first six pregnancies. These women all had poor prognostic indicators and therefore underwent hysterotomy between 21 and 30 weeks, with the fetus being externalised while the umbilical circulation was maintained. The diaphragmatic defect was repaired and an abdominoplasty performed to prevent the returned bowel from impairing umbilical blood flow. There were three fetal deaths at the time of surgery, one immediate neonatal death, and the two remaining infants died after birth from non-pulmonary causes. Post-mortem appeared to demonstrate that relative normal lung growth was possible after such a repair. None of the mothers suffered significant morbidity and four of the six have had further pregnancies without complication. The group has recently reported a further nine cases resulting in four living children.[74]

More recently the procedure of tracheal occlusion *in utero* has been developed. This results in the expansion of the fetal lung, pushing the viscera back into the abdomen and producing lungs that are larger and functionally better at birth than in untreated controls. This development has occurred in parallel with the development of the EXIT technique, which is an *ex-utero* intrapartum treatment developed to unplug the trachea at birth. To date there has been relatively little experience of these techniques, and further study is required before knowing whether or not this will improve the survival of fetuses with a diaphragmatic hernia.

Tracheal atresia

Incidence and aetiology   Tracheal or laryngeal atresia may be found as an isolated anomaly or as part of a genetic syndrome, the most common of which is Fraser's syndrome. These are very rare anomalies.

Diagnosis   The diagnosis of tracheal or laryngeal atresia or obstruction should be suspected when enlarged, uniformly highly reflective lungs are seen sonographically. The heart often appears compressed, the mediastinum seeming smaller than normal. In most cases the diaphragm is flattened or may be convex in shape, protruding into the abdomen (Fig. 20.12). These appearances can be seen in the mid-second trimester, and one report describes the detection of a dilated fluid-filled upper trachea in the third trimester.

The differential diagnosis of these findings includes tracheal atresia/obstruction, laryngeal atresia/obstruction,

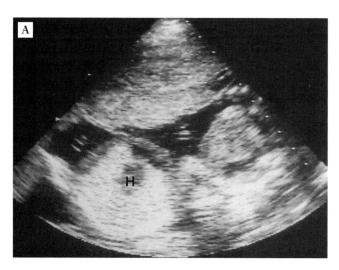 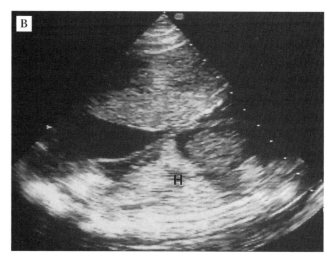

Fig. 20.12 Tracheal agenesis. A: Transverse and **B:** longitudinal views through a fetus with tracheal agenesis. Note how the heart (H) is compressed and the associated pleural effusions and ascites. The lungs appear uniformly highly reflective.

subglottic stenosis and bilateral microcystic congenital cystic adnomatoid malformation.

Associated abnormalities This finding is often associated with ascites and generalised hydrops, together with polyhydramnios. Genetic syndromes may be associated, in particular Fraser syndrome, in which case the association with severe renal anomalies makes it likely that there will be oligohydramnios rather than polyhydramnios.

Management and prognosis When tracheal/laryngeal obstruction is suspected, detailed anomaly scanning should be performed. As the prognosis is poor it is reasonable to discuss the option of termination of pregnancy. Some fetuses will die *in utero*; others succumb in the neonatal period when adequate ventilation cannot be established. Prior knowledge of the potential diagnosis has been reported to result in prompt post-natal treatment, and in one case a tracheostomy was performed prior to cord clamping. In all cases the parents should have the opportunity to discuss the prognosis with paediatric surgeons and, when the pregnancy is continued, delivery should take place in a unit with neonatal intensive care and paediatric surgical facilities.

Pleural effusion

Incidence and aetiology Pleural effusions often occur as part of generalised fetal hydrops, but may be isolated. Only isolated pleural effusions are considered here: they are either idiopathic or due to chylothorax.[13] The incidence is not known.

Associated abnormalities Pleural effusions may be found in association with other bronchopulmonary abnor-malities, including sequestrated lobes, bronchogenic cysts, CCAML and tracheo-oesophageal fistula. Chylothorax has been found in association with pulmonary lymphang-iectasia, with trisomy 21,[75] Noonan's syndrome,[76] and other genetic syndromes.[77] Polyhydramnios is a frequent association.[8,75]

Diagnosis The diagnosis of a pleural effusion is easily made when the mediastinal contents and lungs are found to be displaced towards the centre of the thorax, surrounded by an anechoic area (Fig. 20.13). The lesion may be uni- or bilateral. A specific diagnosis of the nature of the fluid cannot be made by ultrasound, as the lymph appears serous and therefore echo free until after the commencement of oral feeding.

Management and prognosis When a pleural effusion is detected the rest of the fetus should be carefully examined to exclude other abnormalities. Skilled fetal echocardiography should be performed, as pleural effusions may be the first manifestation of hydropic changes secondary to a congenital cardiac lesion.[78] Other causes of fetal hydrops should be excluded as far as possible, and fetal karyotyping and virology studies performed.

In the absence of any other abnormality the prognosis for a fetus with pleural effusions is difficult to assess. There is the theoretical risk of pulmonary hypoplasia secondary to compression, as with all other intrathoracic space-occupying lesions, and death due to pulmonary hypoplasia has been reported in cases diagnosed prenatally.[8] In addition, if left untreated the fetus may develop generalised hydrops.[79] In an attempt to prevent these problems *in utero* thoraco-centesis has been performed, with reports of varying success rates.[79] Pijpers *et al.*[80] report a series of eight cases of isolated bilateral hydrothorax diagnosed prenatally at

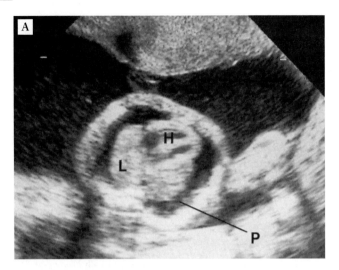
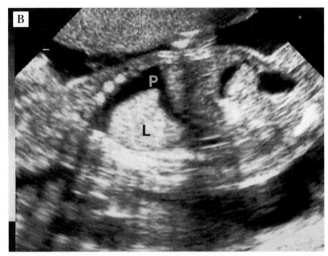

Fig. 20.13 Pleural effusions. A: Transverse and **B:** longitudinal views in a fetus with pleural effusions. Note the hydrothorax (P), compressed lungs (L) and the heart (H).

between 25 and 33 weeks gestation. No attempts at thoracocentesis were made and all infants were alive and well at the age of 1 month. However, it may be that diagnosis in later pregnancy is associated with a more favourable outcome. These authors conclude that a prospective study should be carried out to compare survival with and without pleuro-amniotic shunting. This may well be relevant, as there are reports of spontaneous resolution of hydrothorax *in utero*.

The recurrence risk for hydrothorax in future pregnancies depends on the aetiology. There are some families where X-linked inheritance of idiopathic hydrothorax seems possible.

REFERENCES

1 Bailey P V, Tracy T, Connors R H, deMello D, Lewis J E, Weber T R. Congenital bronchopulmonary malformations. Diagnostic and therapeutic considerations. J Thorac Cardiovasc Surg 1990; 99: 557–560

2 Eraklis A J, Griscom N T, McGovern J B. Bronchogenic cysts of the mediastinum in infancy. N Engl J Med 1969; 281: 1150–1155

3 Ramenofsky M L, Leape L L, McCauley R G K. Bronchogenic cyst. J Paediatr Surg 1979; 14: 219–224

4 O'Connell D J, Kelleher J. Congenital intrathoracic bronchopulmonary foregut malformations in childhood. Can Assoc Radiol J 1979; 30: 103–108

5 Vergnes P, Chateil J F, Boissinot F et al. Malformations pulmoaires de diagnostic antenatal. Chir Pediatr 1989; 30: 185–192

6 Fallon M, Gordon A R G, Lendrum A C. Mediastinal cysts of foregut origin associated with vertebral anomalies. Br J Surg 1954; 41: 520–533

7 Mayden K L, Tortora M, Chervenak F A, Hobbins J C. The antenatal sonographic detection of lung masses. Am J Obstet Gynecol 1984; 148: 349–351

8 Reece E A, Lockwood C J, Rizzo N, Pilu G, Bovicelli L, Hobbins J C. Intrinsic intrathoracic malformations of the fetus: sonographic detection and clinical presentation. Obstet Gynecol 1987; 70: 627–632

9 Young G, L'Heureux P R, Krueckeberg S T, Swanson D A. Mediastinal bronchogenic cyst: prenatal sonographic diagnosis. AJR 1989; 152: 127

10 Nobuhara K K, Gorski Y C, La Quaglia M P, Shamberger R C. Bronchogenic cysts and esophageal duplications: common origins and treatment. J Pediatr Surg 1997; 2(10): 1408–1413

11 Ribet M E, Copin M C, Gosselin B H. Bronchogenic cysts of the lung. Ann Thorac Surg 1996; 61(6): 1636–1640

12 Buntain W L, Woolley M M, Mahour G H et al. Pulmonary sequestration in children: a twenty-five year experience. Surgery 1977; 81: 413–420

13 Ryckman F C, Rosenkrantz J G. Thoracic surgical problems in infancy and childhood. Surg Clin North Am 1985; 65: 1423–1454

14 Carter R. Pulmonary sequestration. Ann Thorac Surg 1969; 7: 68–89

15 Savic B, Birtel F J, Tholen W et al. Lung sequestration: report of seven cases and review of 540 published cases. Thorax 1979; 34: 96–101

16 Wimbish K J, Agha F P, Brady T M. Bilateral pulmonary sequestration: computerised tomographic appearance. AJR 1983; 140: 689–690

17 Demos N J, Teresi A. Congenital lung malformations: a unified concept and case report. J Thorac Cardiovasc Surg 1975; 70: 260–264

18 Gerle R D, Jaretzki A, Ashley C A, Berne A S. Congenital bronchopulmonary-foregut malformation: pulmonary sequestration communicating with the gastrointestinal tract. N Engl J Med 1968; 278: 1413–1419

19 Heithoff K B, Sane S M, Williams H J et al. Bronchopulmonary foregut malformations. A unifying etiological concept. AJR 1976; 126: 46–55

20 Stocker J T, Kagan-Hallet K. Extralobar pulmonary sequestration. Analysis of 15 cases. Am J Clin Pathol 1979; 72: 917–925

21 Iwa T, Watanabe Y. Unusual combination of pulmonary sequestration and funnel chest. Chest 1979; 76: 314–316

22 White J J, Donahoo J S, Ostrow P T et al. Cardiovascular and respiratory manifestations of pulmonary sequestration in childhood. Am Thorac Surg 1974; 18: 286–294

23 Dolkart L A, Reimers F T, Helmuth W V, Porte M A, Eisinger J Antenatal diagnosis of pulmonary sequestration: a review. Obstet Gynecol Surv 1992; 47(8): 515–520

24 Jouppila P, Kirkinen P, Herva R et al. Prenatal diagnosis of pleural effusions by ultrasound. JCU 1983; 11: 516–519

25 Mariona F, McAlpin G, Zador I et al. Sonographic detection of fetal extrathoracic pulmonary sequestration. J Ultrasound Med 1986; 5: 283–285

26 Romero R, Chervenak F A, Kotzen J et al. Antenatal sonographic findings of extralobar pulmonary sequestration. J Ultrasound Med 1982; 1: 131–132

27 Weiner C, Varner M, Pringle K et al. Antenatal diagnosis and palliative treatment of non-immune hydrops secondary to pulmonary extralobar sequestration. Obstet Gynecol 1986; 68: 275–280

28 Choplin R H, Siegel M J. Pulmonary sequestration: six unusual presentations. AJR 1980; 134: 695–700

29 Maulik D, Robinson L, Dailey D K et al. Prenatal sonographic depiction of intralobar pulmonary sequestration. J Ultrasound Med 1987; 6: 703–706

30 Goldblatt E, Vimpani G, Brown L H et al. Extralobar pulmonary sequestration. Presentation as an arteriovenous aneurysm with cardiac failure in infancy. Am J Cardiol 1971; 29: 100

31 Ransom J M, Norton J B, Williams G D. Pulmonary sequestration presenting as congestive heart failure. J Thorac Cardiovasc Surg 1978; 76: 378–380

32 Benya E C, Bulas D I, Selby D M, Rosenbaum K N. Cystic appearance of extralobar pulmonary sequestration. Pediatr Radiol 1993, 23: 605–607

33 Stocker J T, Madewell J E, Drake R M. Congenital adenomatoid malformation of the lung. Classification and morphologic spectrum. Hum Pathol 1977; 8: 155–171

34 Clark S L, Vitale D J, Minton S D, Stoddard R A, Sabey P L. Successful fetal therapy for cystic adenomatoid malformation associated with second trimester hydrops. Am J Obstet Gynecol 1987; 157: 294–295

35 Cachia R, Sobonya R E. Congenital adenomatoid malformation of the lung with bronchial atresia. Hum Pathol 1981; 12: 947–950

36 Miller R K, Sieber W K, Yunis E J. Congenital adenomatoid malformation of the lung. Ann Pathol 1980; 15: 387–407

37 Thorpe-Beeston J G, Nicolaides K N. Cystic adenomatoid malfunction of the lung: prenatal diagnosis and outcome. Prenat Diagn 1994; 14: 677–688

38 Rempen A, Feige A, Wunsch P. Prenatal diagnosis of bilateral cystic adenomatoid malformation of the lung. JCU 1987; 15: 3–8

39 Adzick N S, Harrison M R, Glick P L et al. Fetal cystic adenomatoid malformation: prenatal diagnosis and natural history. J Pediatr Surg 1985; 20: 483–488

40 Fitzgerald E J, Toi A. Antenatal ultrasound diagnosis of cystic adenomatoid malformation of the lung. Can Assoc Radiol J 1986; 37: 48–49

41 Petit P, Bossens M, Thomas D, Moerman P, Fryns J P, Van den Berghe H. Type III congenital cystic adenomatoid malformation of the lung: another cause of elevated alpha fetoprotein? Clin Genet 1987; 32: 172–174

42 Nugent C E, Hayashi R H, Rubin J. Prenatal treatment of type I congenital cystic adenomatoid malformation by intrauterine fetal thoracocentesis. JCU 1989; 17: 675–677

43 Pezzuti R T, Isler R J. Antenatal ultrasound detection of cystic adenomatoid malformation of the lung: report of a case and review of the recent literature. JCU 1983; 11: 342–346

44 Carles D, Serville F, Mainguene M, Glycos E, Herfaut G, Naya L. Prenatal diagnosis of type III congenital cystic adenomatoid malformation of the lung. J Hum Genet 1986; 34: 339–341

45 Vesce F, Garutti P, Grandi E, Perri G, Altavilla G. Prenatal diagnosis of cystic adenomatoid malformation of the lung. Clin Exp Obstet Gynecol 1989; 16: 121–125

45 Wolf S A, Hertzler J H, Philippart A I. Cystic adenomatoid malformation of the lung. J Pediatr Surg 1980; 15: 925–930

46 Nicolaides K H, Blott M, Greenough A. Chronic drainage of fetal pulmonary cyst. Lancet 1987; i: 618

47 Sapin E, Lejeune V, Barbet J P et al. Congenital adenomatoid disease of the lung: prenatal diagnosis and perinatal management. Pediatr Surg Int 1997; 12(2–3): 126–129

48 Budorick N E, Pretorius D H, Leopold G R, Stamm E R. Spontaneous improvement of intrathoracic masses diagnosed in utero. J Ultrasound Med 1992; 11: 653–662

49 Winters W D, Effmann E L, Nghiem H V, Hyberg D A. Congenital masses of the lung: changes in cross-sectional area during gestation. JCU 1997; 25(7): 372–377

50 Miller J A, Corteville J E, Langer J C. Congenital cystic adenomatoid malformation in the fetus: natural history and predictors of outcome. J Pediatr Surg 1996; 31(6): 805–808

51 Fine C, Adzick N S, Doubilet P M. Decreasing size of a congenital cystic adenomatoid malformation in utero. J Ultrasound Med 1988; 7: 405–408

52 Saltzmann D H, Adzick N S, Benacerraf B R. Fetal cystic adenomatoid malformation of the lung: apparent improvement in utero. Obstet Gynecol 1988; 71: 1000–1002

53 David T J, Illingworth C A. Diaphragmatic hernia in the southwest of England. J Med Genet 1976; 13: 253–262

54 Harrison M R, Jester J A, Ross N A. Correction of congenital diaphragmatic hernia *in utero*. I. The model: intrathoracic balloon produces fetal pulmonary hypoplasia. Surgery 1980; 88: 174–182

55 Benacerraf B R, Adzick N S. Fetal diaphragmatic hernia: ultrasound diagnosis and clinical outcome in 19 cases. Am J Obstet Gynecol 1987; 156: 573–576

56 Nakayama D K, Harrison M R, Chinn D H et al. Prenatal diagnosis and natural history of the fetus with a congenital diaphragmatic hernia: initial clinical experience. J Pediatr Surg 1985; 20: 118–124

57 Butler N, Claireaux A E. Congenital diaphragmatic hernia as a cause of perinatal mortality. Lancet 1962; i: 659–663

58 Hansen J, James S, Burrington J, Whitfield J. The decreasing incidence of pneumothorax and improving survival of infants with congenital diaphragmatic hernia. J Pediatr Surg 1984; 19: 385–388

59 Greenwood R D, Rosenthal A, Nadas A S. Cardiovascular abnormalities associated with congenital diaphragmatic hernia. Pediatrics 1976; 57: 92–97

60 Winter R M, Knowles S A S, Bieber F R, Baraitser M (eds). Respiratory tract anomalies. In: The malformed fetus and stillbirth – a diagnostic approach. Chichester: John Wiley, 1988; 121–129

61 Harrison R H, Adzick N S, Nakayama D K, deLorimier A A. Fetal diaphragmatic hernia: fatal but fixable. Semin Perinatol 1985; 9: 103–112

62 Chinn D H, Filly R A, Callen P W, Nakayama D K, Harrison M R. Congenital diaphragmatic hernia diagnosed prenatally by ultrasound. Radiology 1983; 148: 119–123

63 Crawford D C, Wright V M, Drake D P, Allan L D. Fetal diaphragmatic hernia: the value of fetal echocardiography in the prediction of postnatal outcome. Br J Obstet Gynaecol 1989; 96: 705–710

64 Chitty L S. Ultrasound screening for fetal abnormalities. Prenat Diagn 1995; 15: 1241–1257

65 Geary M P, Chitty L S, Morrison J J, Wright V, Pierro A, Rodeck C H. Perinatal outcome and prognostic factors in prenatally diagnosed congenital diaphragmatic hernia. Ultrasound Obstet Gynaecol 1998; 12: 107–111

66 Comstock C H. The antenatal diagnosis of diaphragmatic anomalies. J Ultrasound Med 1986; 5: 391–396

67 Ruff S J, Campbell J R, Harrison M W et al. Pediatric diaphragmatic hernia: an 11 year experience. Am J Surg 1980; 139: 641–645

68 Geary M, Chitty L, Morrison J J, Rodeck C H. prenatal diagnosis of congenital diaphragmatic hernia: prognostic factors and perinatal outcome. J Obstet Gynecol 1997; 17: 1: 30

69 Norio R, Kaariainen H, Rapola J, Herva R, Kekomaki M. Familial congenital diaphragmatic defects: aspects of aetiology, prenatal diagnosis and treatment. Am J Med Genet 1984; 17: 471–483

70 Harrison M R, Ross N A, deLorimier A A. Correction for congenital diaphragmatic hernia in utero. III. Development of a successful surgical technique using abdominoplasty to avoid compromise of umbilical blood flow. J Paediatr Surg 1981; 16: 934

71 Harrison M J, Golbus M S, Filly R A. The unborn patient. In: Orlando F, ed. Prenatal diagnosis and treatment. Grune & Stratton, 1984: 257–275

72 Harrison M R, Bressack M A, Churg A M et al. Correction of congenital diaphragmatic hernia in utero. II. Simulated correction permits fetal lung growth with survival at birth. Surgery 1980; 88: 260

73 Harrison M R, Langer J C, Adzick N S et al. Correction of congenital diaphragmatic hernia in utero. V. Initial clinical experience. J Pediatr Surg 1990; 25: 47–55

74 Harrison M R, Adzick N S, Longaker M T et al. Successful repair in utero of a fetal diaphragmatic hernia after removal of herniated viscera from the left hemithorax. N Engl J Med 1990; 322: 1582–1584

75 Alonso C R P, Lozano G B, Andres M C B, Puerto M J M, Lopez M C, Posadas A S. Quilotorax espontaneo: siete casos de diagnostico prenatal. An Esp Pediatr 1989; 30: 19–22

76 Nisbet D L, Griffin D R, Chitty L S. Prenatal features of Noonan's syndrome. Prenat Diagn 1999; (in press)

77 Maymon R, Ogle R F, Chitty L S. Smith–Lemli–Opitz syndrome presenting with persisting nuchal oedema and non-immune hydrops. Prenat Diagn 1999; 19: 105–107

78 Allan L D, Crawford D C, Sheridan R, Chapman M G. Aetiology of non-immune hydrops: the value of echocardiography. Br J Obstet Gynaecol 1986; 93: 223–225

79 Benacerraf B R, Frigoletto F D, Wilson M. Successful midtrimester thoracocentesis with analysis of the lymphocyte population in the pleural effusion. Am J Obstet Gynecol 1986; 155: 396–399

80 Pijpers L, Reuss A, Stewart P A, Wladimiroff J W. Noninvasive management of isolated bilateral fetal hydrothorax. Am J Obstet Gynecol 1989; 161: 330–332

Chromosomal markers

Peter Twining

Introduction

The incidence of chromosomal disease in conceptuses has been estimated to be approximately 8%. However, this figure falls to only 0.7% (1/160) in the newborn period, owing to the very high loss rate in chromosomally abnormal pregnancies, with up to 94% of cases ending in spontaneous abortion.

Chromosomally abnormal fetuses account for 50% of all spontaneous abortions.[1] Given that the overall spontaneous abortion rate is approximately 15%, and the fact that the overall incidence of specific chromosome defects in abortuses and their incidence in live births are known, one can estimate the proportion of all conceptuses of a given karyotype that are lost by spontaneous abortion.[1] Table 21.1 outlines the outcome of 10 000 conceptuses with regard to loss rates for specific chromosomal abnormalities.

It is seen that the more severe chromosomal abnormalities, such as triploidy, trisomy 13 and trisomy 18, demonstrate high early loss rates, presumably due to the presence of multiple abnormalities, but it is of interest to note that only 1% of conceptuses with Turner's syndrome and 25% of conceptuses with trisomy 21 are liveborn (Table 21.1). Some of this loss will occur later, as some 30% of fetuses with trisomy 21, 74% of cases of trisomy 18 and 71% of trisomy 13 fetuses will be lost between 16 weeks gestation and term.[2,3]

It is clear therefore that the liveborn rates for chromosomal disease represent only a small proportion of the total; however, in the late first and early second trimesters there are sufficient numbers of cases to produce a major challenge in prenatal ultrasound diagnosis.

There are a number of reasons for making a prenatal diagnosis of chromosomal disease, not least of which is the option of pregnancy termination if the diagnosis is made prior to viability. Even if the diagnosis is made late, the mode of delivery can be discussed and the possibility of conservative management considered. It is well established that certain chromosomal abnormalities, particularly trisomy 18, are associated with high rates of caesarean section for fetal distress, and so prenatal diagnosis may avoid this complication.[4]

In certain situations, as in non-lethal conditions such as trisomy 21, a prenatal diagnosis either early or late can give the parents time to come to terms with the diagnosis and prepare themselves for the possibility of neonatal surgery on the baby.

Prenatal diagnosis therefore provides the parents with the information on which to base decisions on the continuation of pregnancy, the mode of delivery, and also the likely outcome for an affected pregnancy. The ultrasound findings are an extremely important part of the prenatal diagnosis of chromosomal disease, as it is often an ultrasound-detected abnormality that prompts a karyotype procedure. In addition it is the meticulous assessment of complex abnormalities using ultrasound, where the full extent of the disease can be assessed and this information passed on to the parents prior to the decision-making process.

The most important aspect of the ultrasound diagnosis of chromosomal disease is the detection of fetal structural abnormalities. Some of the common chromosomal syndromes have fairly specific phenotypes, such as trisomy 13 and trisomy 18.[5,6] There is also a direct correlation between the number of abnormalities and the risk of chromosomal disease.[7] It can be seen from Table 21.2 that the frequency of trisomies 13 and 18 increases with the increase in number of fetal abnormalities detected with ultrasound. In the case of Turner's syndrome and triploidy the frequency remains fairly static, whereas in trisomy 21 the frequency of the syndrome decreases as the number of abnormalities detected increases.

Specific rates for chromosomal disease have also been estimated for isolated abnormalities, and these are outlined in Table 21.3. The presence of associated abnormalities dramatically increases the risk for chromosomal disease.[9] In practice, isolated abnormalities with a high incidence of chromosomal disease usually indicate a

Table 21.1 Outcome of 10 000 conceptions (Reproduced with permission from Thompson M W, McInnes R R, Willard H F. Genetics in medicine, 5th edn. W B Saunders, 1991)

Outcome	Conceptions	Spontaneous abortions Number	%	Livebirths
Total	10 000	1500	15	8500
Normal chromosomes	9200	750	8	8450
Abnormal chromosomes				
Total	800	750	94	50
Trisomy 13	9	8	90	1
Trisomy 18	19	17	90	2
Trisomy 21	45	33	75	12
Trisomy other	312	311	99.7	1
Turner's syndrome	140	138	99	2
Triploidy	170	170	100	–
Others	105	73	74	32

Table 21.2 Frequency of chromosomal abnormalities and number of ultrasound-detected defects. (Reproduced with permission from Nicolaides K, Snijders R J M, Gosden C M et al. Ultrasonographically detectable markers of fetal chromosomal abnormalities. Lancet 1992; 340: 704–707)

Number of defects	Percentage of fetuses with a chromosomal abnormality	Type of chromosomal abnormality (%)					
		Trisomy			Turner's	Tripoidy	Other
		21	18	13			
>2	29	21	30	11	13	15	8
>3	48	16	35	13	8	15	5
>4	62	12	42	15	12	12	6
>5	70	5	54	20	9	10	5
>6	72	–	62	20	14	16	9
>7	82	–	79	15	–	3	3
>8	92	–	77	18	–	–	3

Table 21.3 Prevalence of fetal chromosomal defects in fetuses with isolated and multiple abnormalities. (Reproduced with permission from Snijders R J M, Nicolaides K, eds. Ultrasound markers for fetal chromosomal defects. London: Parthenon Publishing, 1996[8])

Abnormality	Isolated (%)	Multiple (%)
Ventriculomegaly	2	17
Holoprosencephaly	4	39
Choroid plexus cysts	<1	48
Posterior fossa cyst	0	52
Facial cleft	0	51
Micrognathia	–	62
Cystic hygroma	52	71
Nuchal oedema	19	45
Diaphragmatic hernia	2	49
Heart defects	16	66
Duodenal atresia	38	64
Exomphalos	8	46
Talipes	0	33
Growth retardation	4	38

Table 21.4 Fetal abnormalities with a low prevalence of chromosomal abnormalities

Gastroschisis
Jejunal atresia
Large bowel obstruction
Unilateral multicystic kidney
Ovarian, duplication, mesenteric cysts
Hemivertebra
Fetal tumours
Cystic adenomatoid malformation of lung
Sequestrated segment of lung
Porencephaly
Schizencephaly

specific syndrome, such as cystic hygroma with Turner's syndrome, and duodenal atresia and nuchal oedema with trisomy 21.

In contrast, it is known that certain abnormalities have a low incidence of chromosomal disease if isolated, for example facial clefting and talipes. Further examples of conditions known to have a low incidence of chromosomal disease are described in Table 21.4.

The demonstration of a fetal abnormality with ultrasound should always prompt a meticulous search for other anomalies. In particular, the hands, feet, face and heart should be carefully scrutinised in order to detect further signs of chromosomal disease. Sometimes it may be very difficult to exclude associated anomalies, particularly when there is maternal obesity, oligohydramnios, unfavourable fetal lie, or gestational age below 16 weeks. These factors should always be taken into account when a full fetal assessment is being carried out.

In some specific abnormalities there is evidence to suggest that the severity of the defect is inversely related to the risk of chromosomal disease. A number of studies have shown that smaller omphaloceles have a higher risk of chromosomal disease than larger defects.[10,11] A similar situation is seen in cases of mild ventriculomegaly and mild dilatation of the renal pelves, which may well have a higher incidence of chromosomal disease than more marked hydrocephalus or hydronephrosis.[12–14]

There are also a number of secondary or non-specific features that provide additional clues to the presence of chromosomal disease. The two most important additional features are intra-uterine growth retardation and polyhydramnios[15] and, if seen together, these carry a high risk of a chromosomal defect. The time of onset and type of growth retardation is also important, as early second-trimester growth retardation is a common finding in triploidy,[16] whereas late growth retardation is seen in the trisomic syndromes. Umbilical artery Doppler studies are often normal in growth retardation secondary to chromosomal disease, and symmetrical growth retardation is common prior to 30 weeks gestation, whereas asymmetrical growth retardation is usual after 30 weeks.[17]

Most anomaly scanning is carried out at 18–20 weeks gestation, and in routine clinical practice this is undoubtedly the best time to detect fetal abnormality, as it produces high detection rates.[18–20] The detection rates for chromosomal disease vary from syndrome to syndrome and depend to a certain extent on the severity of the condition. In trisomies 13 and 18, up to 98% and 83% of fetuses, respectively, will demonstrate abnormalities detectable on ultrasound.[21,22] In contrast, only 33% of fetuses with trisomy 21 are detected using ultrasound at 18–20 weeks.[9,23]

The introduction of nuchal thickness assessment scanning at 10–14 weeks gestation may well improve the detection rate of trisomy 21, with recent reports indicating an 80% detection rate and a false-positive rate of 5%.[24] This exciting new development is discussed in more detail in the section on trisomy 21.

The ultrasound diagnosis of chromosomal disease is normally confirmed using an invasive karyotype procedure. Amniocentesis has for many years been the most commonly used means of obtaining a karyotype. Carried out at 16 weeks gestation and with a loss rate of approximately 1%, it has gained general acceptance. The main disadvantage, however, is the 2–3 week delay before the result is available. This problem can be overcome with the use of chorion villus sampling or placental biopsy where, for a similar loss rate at 18–20 weeks, a karyotype result can be obtained in 2–3 days.[25]

Trisomy 13

Bartholin first described this condition in 1657, but its trisomic aetiology was not recognised until 1960, when reported by Patau.[5,26] The incidence is reported as 1/5000 births. The extra chromosome usually arises from new disjunction in maternal meiosis, but about 20% of cases are caused by an unbalanced translocation.[1]

The outlook is extremely poor, with 82% of babies dying within the first month of life; only 5% survive the first 6 months.[27]

There is a fairly specific phenotype associated with trisomy 13 and the most important features are seen within the brain, face, hands and heart (Fig. 21.1).

Cranial findings

The most common abnormality of the brain seen in trisomy 13 is holoprosencephaly (Fig. 21.2), and in one series of antenatally diagnosed holoprosencephaly trisomy 13 occurred in 40% of cases.[28] The head is often microcephalic and other, less common findings include the Dandy–Walker syndrome and ventriculomegaly. Enlargement of the cisterna vena magna has also been reported.[21] Neural tube defects may occasionally be seen.

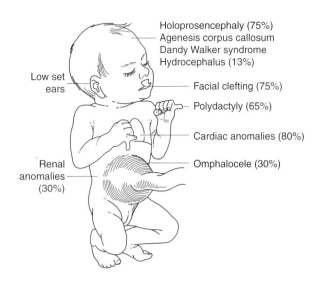

Fig. 21.1 Abnormalities detected by ultrasound in trisomy 13 (frequency in brackets).

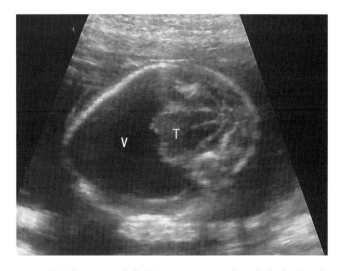

Fig. 21.2 Holoprosencephaly. Transverse section through the fetal head showing fused thalami (T) and single ventricular cavity (V).

Facial findings

Facial clefting is a common finding in trisomy 13, occurring in 60–80% of cases.[5] One antenatal series recorded facial clefting in 48% of cases.[21] The form of clefting is usually either median (midline) (Fig. 21.3) or bilateral cleft lip and palate. The facial abnormalities associated with holoprosencephaly, such as cyclopia, cebocephaly and hypotelorism, may also be seen.[29] Microphthalmia may be demonstrated in up to 50% of cases and the ears may have abnormal helices and be low set.[5]

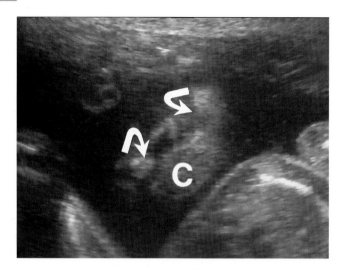

Fig. 21.3 Median cleft lip. Coronal section through chin (C) and upper lip, showing a large midline defect on the upper lip. The lateral margins of the cleft are indicated by the curved arrows.

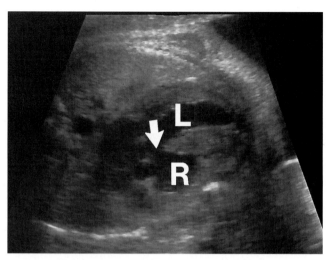

Fig. 21.5 Ventricular septal defect. Transverse section through fetal thorax with four chamber view. (L – left ventricle, R – right ventricle, arrow points to large ventricular septal defect).

Hands and feet

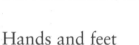

In up to 60% of fetuses the hands and feet show polydactyly (Fig. 21.4).[21] Less frequent observations include fixed flexion and overlapping of the fingers, as seen in trisomy 18, and talipes or rocker-bottom feet.

Cardiac findings

Cardiac abnormalities are an important feature of chromosomal disease, and in trisomy 13 are seen in up to 80% of cases. The commonest findings are ventricular septal

defect (Fig. 21.5), atrioventricular septal defect and hypoplastic left heart.[30,31] An additional feature of the hypoplastic left heart syndrome which may be fairly specific for trisomy 13 is the presence of an echogenic focus within the hypoplastic left ventricle.[21]

Abdominal findings

Omphalocele is the finding of greatest significance within the abdomen, and this often contains bowel only. An omphalocele may be seen in up to 30% of fetuses with trisomy 13. Renal dysplasia and hydronephrosis may also be seen in up to 30% of cases.

Other findings

Generalised hydrops can be seen in up to 24% of trisomy 13 fetuses[21] and should always prompt a karyotype procedure.

Growth retardation, either symmetrical (before 30 weeks) or asymmetrical (after 30 weeks), is seen in over 80% of third-trimester fetuses with trisomy 13.[21] Umbilical artery Doppler traces are likely to be normal,[17] and the presence of polyhydramnios is an ominous sign and highly suggestive of a chromosomal abnormality.[21]

A single umbilical artery is a common finding in trisomy 13; other cord abnormalities are rare, but include umbilical cord cysts.[32] The author has also observed a fetus with trisomy 13 demonstrating persistence of the right umbilical vein in association with highly reflective hepatic foci, representing focal areas of hepatic necrosis with calcification. A similar case not associated with chromosomal disease has also been reported.[33]

Cholecystomegaly has also been described in association with trisomy 13.[5,34]

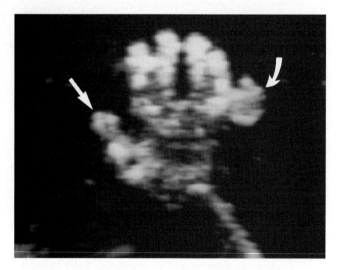

Fig. 21.4 Postaxial polydactyly. Coronal section through the hand showing the thumb (straight arrow) and extra digit (curved arrow). (Reproduced with permission from Twining and Zuccollo, Ultrasound markers of chromosomal disease. Br J Radiol 1993; 66: 408–414.)

Differential diagnosis

The main differential diagnosis of trisomy 13 is the Meckel–Grüber syndrome, as there are a number of overlapping features in both syndromes. Meckel–Grüber syndrome generally presents as renal dysplasia, polydactyly and occipital encephalocele, often associated with posterior fossa abnormalities.[35] The main differentiating factor on ultrasound is likely to be normal cardiac anatomy in the Meckel–Grüber syndrome, whereas cardiac anomalies are almost always present in trisomy 13. In practical terms this highlights the importance of obtaining confirmation of the ultrasound diagnosis with a karyotype procedure.

The outcome for both syndromes is poor, but an important reason for differentiating the two is the differing recurrence risks. The Meckel–Grüber syndrome has an autosomal recessive inheritance, whereas the empirical recurrence risk for trisomy 13 is less than 2%.[1]

Trisomy 18

The first description of trisomy 18 was made in 1960 by Edwards, following the discovery of the extra 18 chromosome.[36] It has an incidence of 1/3000 births and a female-to-male ratio of 3:1. The great majority of cases have full 18 trisomy as a result of faulty chromosomal distribution. The recurrence risk is likely to be less than 1%.[5]

The outlook is extremely poor, with 50% of babies dying within the first week of life and most of the remaining cases succumbing within the first year. Only 5% survive the first year, as severely mentally retarded infants.[27,37]

As in trisomy 13 there is a fairly specific phenotype which can be detected using ultrasound. Once again the major features are seen in the hands, feet, face, heart and head (Fig. 21.6).

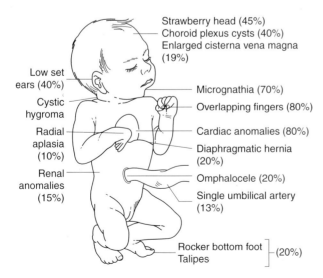

Fig. 21.6 Abnormalities detected by ultrasound in trisomy 18. (frequency in brackets).

Findings in hands and feet

The typical appearances in the hands are fixed flexion of the fingers with overlapping of fingers (Fig. 21.7). The characteristic configuration is overlapping of the index over the third finger and the fifth finger over the fourth. There are, however, many variations of these appearances, and occasionally one may see fixed flexion of some fingers in association with fixed extension of one or more others (Fig. 21.8). More severe abnormalities may also be seen, such as radial aplasia (Fig. 21.9), which can be unilateral or affect both hands.[38] Less common findings include hypoplasia or absence of the thumb, syndactyly of the third and fourth fingers, and a shortened fifth finger.[5]

There is often bilateral talipes or rocker-bottom feet.[22]

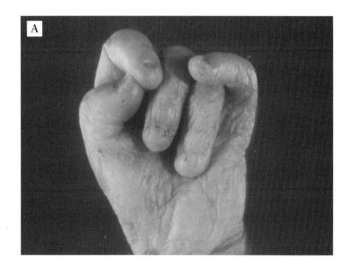

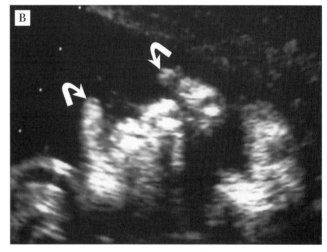

Fig. 21.7 Overlapping fingers in trisomy 18. **A:** A neonate with the classic configuration of fifth finger over the fourth and second finger over the third. **B:** Coronal scan through a fetal hand demonstrating the same overlapping (curved arrows point to overlapping fingers.) (Reproduced with permission from Reed, Claireux and Cockburn. Diseases of fetus and newborn. Chapman and Hall, 1995.)

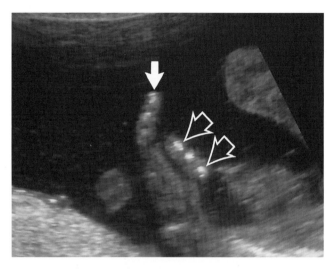

Fig. 21.8 Pointing finger. Coronal scan through a fetal hand showing flexion of the third, fourth and fifth fingers (open arrows) and fixed extension of the second finger (straight arrow).

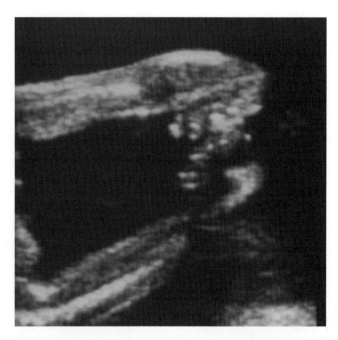

Fig. 21.9 Bilateral radial aplasia. Coronal section through both forearms showing bilateral radial aplasia. (Reproduced with permission from Twining and Zuccollo, Ultrasound markers of chromosomal disease. Br J Radiol 1993; 66: 408–414.)

Facial findings

Micrognathia is the commonest facial abnormality and is seen in up to 70% of cases (Fig. 21.10).[9] Facial clefting is seen in less than 15% of cases. Low-set 'pixie-type' ears are also a feature, but are often difficult to demonstrate on ultrasound.

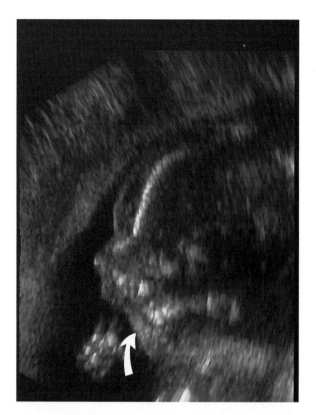

Fig. 21.10 Micrognathia. Sagittal section through face (profile view), showing marked micrognathia (curved arrow).

Cardiac findings

Cardiac abnormalities are seen in up to 80% of fetuses with trisomy 18. The most common is a ventricular septal defect (Fig. 21.5), followed by atrioventricular septal defect[39] and double-outlet right ventricle.[30] Less common cardiac abnormalities include pulmonary stenosis, coarctation of the aorta and tetralogy of Fallot.[5]

Cranial findings

There are a number of important findings in the head which are useful in the antenatal diagnosis of trisomy 18. The initial evaluation should include an assessment of head shape, as the characteristic 'strawberry skull' (Fig. 21.11) can be seen in 45% of fetuses with trisomy 18.[40] The appearance, however, is not totally specific for trisomy 18, as it has also been reported in association with skeletal dysplasias[41] and may also be a normal variant.

The major intracranial abnormalities seen in fetuses with trisomy 18 include enlargement of the cisterna vena magna,[42] agenesis of the corpus callosum and hydrocephalus.[43,44] The Dandy–Walker malformation may also be demonstrated.[42] Neural tube defects occur in less than 10% of cases.[22] The other important finding is choroid plexus cysts, and these are discussed in more detail below.

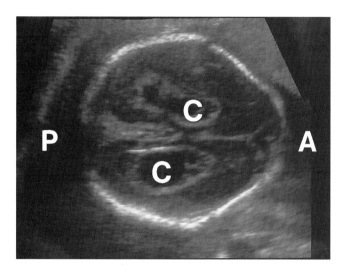

Fig. 21.11 Strawberry-shaped skull and choroid plexus cysts.
Transverse section through fetal head showing flattened occiput and pointed frontal bones (strawberry skull). Also note large choroid plexus cysts (C). A – anterior, P – posterior.

Choroid plexus cysts

Choroid plexus cysts are seen in 25–42% of fetuses with trisomy 18,[22,45] but also occur in approximately 1% of normal fetuses (Fig. 21.11). Chudleigh *et al.*[46] first described choroid plexus in 1984, but there is still controversy as to the significance of isolated choroid plexus cysts. Most occur at 14–16 weeks gestation and the vast majority have resolved by 22 weeks.[21,47,48] The size varies between 3 and 16 mm in diameter, and although early reports suggested a greater risk of trisomy 18 with larger cysts,[49] later studies have not confirmed this finding.[45,50]

It is now well established that the majority of fetuses with choroid plexus cysts and trisomy 18 also have other abnormalities;[22,45] however, it has been estimated that in approximately 4% of fetuses with trisomy 18 apparently isolated choroid plexus cysts may be the only ultrasound finding.[45] In view of this certain groups have advocated karyotyping all fetuses with choroid plexus cysts, whether other abnormalities are present or not.[50,51] It is, however, clear that many of the cases of apparently isolated choroid plexus cysts that are subsequently found to have trisomy 18 often have other abnormalities present at post-mortem, which, although subtle, can be detected on detailed ultrasound scanning.[22,45] The level of scanning expertise available to assess fetuses with choroid plexus cysts is extremely important, as what may appear to be a case of isolated choroid plexus cysts at routine scanning may on detailed scanning turn out to have subtle associated malformations, many of which are described above.

At present, therefore, one would certainly offer a karyotype if choroid plexus cysts are seen in association with other abnormalities, as the fetus has at least a 50% chance of having trisomy 18.[45] The risk of a fetus with isolated choroid plexus cysts having trisomy 18 has been calculated to be in the range of 1/150–1/374.[52,53] More recently a review by Gupta *et al.* estimated that the presence of isolated choroid plexus cysts increased a patient's age-specific risk by a factor of 9 (95% confidence intervals between 4.16 and 19.1) (Table 21.5).[45] The review also stated that centres with high-quality antenatal ultrasound should calculate the risk of trisomy 18 using a likelihood ratio at the lower end of the quoted confidence intervals (Fig. 21.12). Where high-quality obstetric ultrasound is available the detection of choroid plexus cysts is an indication for detailed scanning to look for ultrasound markers of trisomy 18, rather than a karyotype procedure.[45,52] If the detailed scan is normal the patient can be reassured that the fetus has a relatively low risk of trisomy 18. This author also recommends a repeat scan at 22 weeks gestation to demonstrate resolution of the cysts, but also to reassess the fetus, and in particular the heart, to exclude a small ventricular septal defect. One further important reason for repeating the scan is that although demonstration of resolution of the choroid cysts does not decrease the inherent (albeit low) risk of trisomy 18, it does produce a significant reduction in maternal anxiety levels (Fig. 21.13).[54]

Table 21.5 Estimates of maternal age-specific risk for trisomy 18 at mid-trimester in fetuses with and without choroid plexus (CP) cysts and additional anomalies. (Reproduced with permission from Gupta et al. Management of fetal choroid plexus cysts. Br J Obstet Gynaecol 1997; 104: 881–886)

Maternal age (years)	Overall (prior risk)	CP cysts absent	CP cysts present Apparently isolated	CP cysts present Additional abnormalities
20	1/4576	1/8474	1/506	1/3
21	1/4514	1/8359	1/499	1/3
22	1/4435	1/8213	1/491	1/3
23	1/4333	1/8024	1/479	1/2
24	1/4204	1/7785	1/465	1/2
25	1/4045	1/7491	1/447	1/2
26	1/3850	1/7130	1/426	1/2
27	1/3619	1/6702	1/400	1/2
28	1/3351	1/6206	1/371	1/2
29	1/3050	1/5648	1/337	1/2
30	1/2724	1/5044	1/301	1/2
31	1/2385	1/4417	1/264	>1/2
32	1/2046	1/3789	1/226	>1/2
33	1/1721	1/3187	1/190	>1/2
34	1/1420	1/2630	1/157	>1/2
35	1/1152	1/2133	1/127	>1/2
36	1/921	1/1706	1/102	>1/2
37	1/727	1/1346	1/80	>1/2
38	1/567	1/1050	1/63	>1/2
39	1/439	1/813	1/49	>1/2
40	1/338	1/626	1/37	>1/2
41	1/258	1/478	1/29	>1/2
42	1/197	1/365	1/22	>1/2
43	1/149	1/276	1/16	>1/2
44	1/113	1/209	1/13	>1/2
45	1/85	1/157	1/9	>1/2

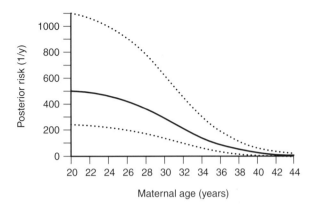

Fig. 21.12 Estimates of maternal age-specific risk for trisomy 18 at mid-trimester in fetuses with apparently isolated choroid plexus cysts (between 4.16 and 19.1 = 95% confidence intervals). (Reproduced with permission from Gupta et al. Management of fetal choroid plexus cysts. Br J Obstet Gynaecol 1997; 104: 881–886.)

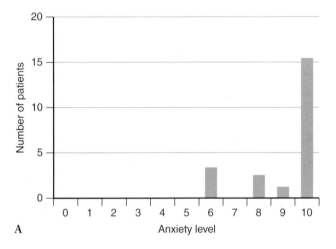

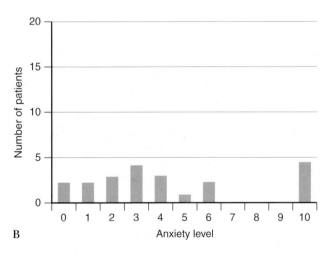

Fig. 21.13 Anxiety levels in patients with fetal choroid plexus cysts. A: Anxiety levels at initial diagnosis. **B:** Shows how anxiety levels fall following the 22 week repeat scan.

One further point of note is that the presence of isolated choroid plexus cysts does not increase the risk of the fetus having trisomy 21.[45,55]

Chest and abdominal findings

Diaphragmatic hernia is a frequent finding in the chest, occurring in up to 30% of cases.[55] Abdominal abnormalities include omphalocele and renal anomalies such as renal dysplasia, hydronephrosis and horseshoe kidney.[11,22,56]

Other findings

As in trisomy 13, growth retardation is often seen in the third trimester and follows a similar pattern (symmetrical before 30 weeks and asymmetrical after 30 weeks). Polyhydramnios may also be associated.[17,57]

Cystic hygroma with or without hydrops can be seen in up to 20% of fetuses with trisomy 18,[22] and should always be considered a potential sign of chromosomal disease.

Umbilical cord cysts have also been described in association with trisomy 18.[32] Other less common findings include hemivertebrae, scoliosis, cataracts, microphthalmia and hypertelorism.[5]

Differential diagnosis

The main differential diagnosis is between the arthrogryposis syndromes, which can produce similar appearances of clenched fists and overlapping fingers together with bilateral talipes. However, there are usually no other abnormalities present, and in particular the fetal heart is normal in most cases of arthrogryposis. In addition there is a so-called pseudo-Edwards syndrome, which has the same phenotype as Edwards syndrome but a normal karyotype.

Trisomy 21

Down's syndrome is the commonest chromosomal abnormality and was first described by Langdon Down in 1866.[58] Although a chromosomal aetiology was suggested in the early 1930s[59,60] it was not until 1959 that Lejeune confirmed the presence of an extra chromosome 21 in affected individuals.[61]

The average incidence of trisomy 21 is 1/800, but this increases significantly with increased maternal age (Table 21.6). In about 95% of cases there is a true trisomy of chromosome 21, which probably occurs during maternal meiosis. In 4% of cases the patient has 46 chromosomes, one of which is a Robertsonian translocation between chromosome 21q and the long arm of either 14 or 22.[1]

The recurrence risk for true trisomy 21 is estimated to be 1%, but for a Robertsonian translocation this can be as high as 15%.[1]

Table 21.6 Trisomy 21: risk by maternal age and gestation. Estimated risk (11/number given in the table). (Reproduced with permission from Snijders R J M, Nicolaides K H, eds. Ultrasound markers for fetal chromosomal defects. London: Parthenon Publishing, 1996)

Age (yrs)	Gestation (wks)									
	10	12	14	16	18	20	25	30	35	Birth
20	804	898	981	1053	1117	1175	1294	1388	1464	1527
21	793	887	968	1040	1103	1159	1277	1370	1445	1507
22	780	872	952	1022	1084	1140	1256	1347	1421	1482
23	762	852	930	999	1060	1114	1227	1317	1389	1448
24	740	827	903	969	1029	1081	1191	1278	1348	1406
25	712	795	868	933	989	1040	1146	1229	1297	1352
26	677	756	826	887	941	989	1090	1169	1233	1286
27	635	710	775	832	883	928	1022	1097	1157	1206
28	586	655	715	768	815	856	943	1012	1068	1113
29	531	593	648	695	738	776	855	917	967	1008
30	471	526	575	617	655	688	758	813	858	895
31	409	457	499	536	568	597	658	706	745	776
32	347	388	423	455	482	507	559	599	632	659
33	288	322	352	378	401	421	464	498	525	547
34	235	262	286	307	326	343	378	405	427	446
35	187	210	229	246	261	274	302	324	342	356
36	148	165	180	193	205	216	238	255	269	280
37	115	128	140	150	159	168	185	198	209	218
38	88	98	107	115	122	129	142	152	160	167
39	67	75	82	88	93	98	108	116	122	128
40	51	57	62	67	71	74	82	88	93	97
41	38	43	47	50	53	56	62	66	70	73
42	29	32	35	38	40	42	46	50	52	55
43	21	24	26	28	30	31	35	37	39	41
44	16	18	20	21	22	23	26	28	29	30

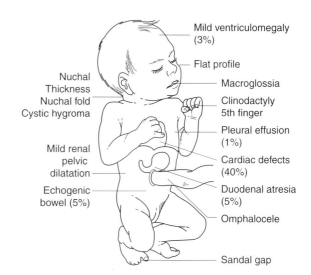

Fig. 21.14 Abnormalities detected by ultrasound in trisomy 21 (frequency in brackets).

The most specific ultrasound findings for trisomy 21 are duodenal atresia, atrioventricular septal defects and an increased nuchal thickness. Nuchal thickness scanning is discussed later in the chapter.

Figure 21.14 outlines the ultrasound features of trisomy 21.

Duodenal atresia

It has been estimated that duodenal atresia (Fig. 21.15) occurs in 5% of trisomy 21 babies; however, its antenatal detection carries a 30% risk of the condition.[66] The value of this finding is limited, as it is not generally detected with confidence before 24 weeks gestation and so is often not

The prenatal loss rate is high, with 75% of trisomy 21 conceptuses lost from spontaneous abortion (Table 21.1). Post-natal survival depends on the presence of cardiac abnormalities, as a quarter of affected babies die before their first birthday; 50% of patients survive to over 50 years of age, and 1/7 is still alive at age 68. There is an increased risk of leukaemia, and also of premature senility.[1]

There is a fairly typical phenotype (Fig. 21.14), but many of the features are subtle and difficult to demonstrate on ultrasound. In the best hands scanning at 18–20 weeks gestation will reveal abnormalities in only 33% of affected fetuses.[9,23]

Using age as a screening test detects only 15% of affected pregnancies, but the introduction of serum screening has meant that up to 60% of Down's syndrome fetuses may be detected.[62] Serum screening has also been advocated in the first trimester of pregnancy,[63] but the development of nuchal thickness scanning has meant that up to 80% of Down's syndrome fetuses may be detected.[64]

Although there are major limitations to the ultrasound diagnosis of trisomy 21 at mid-second trimester scanning there are a number of important findings which should suggest the diagnosis. In addition, over recent years a number of 'soft markers' have been reported which may be associated with an increased risk of trisomy 21.[65]

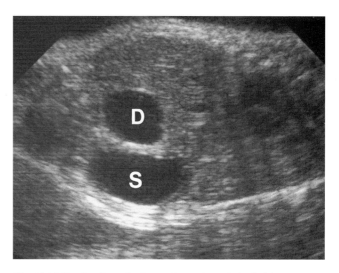

Fig. 21.15 Duodenal atresia. Coronal scan through fetal abdomen showing fluid in stomach (S) and distended duodenum (D).

picked up until the third trimester, when the patient usually presents with polyhydramnios.[66]

Atrioventricular septal defects

Cardiac abnormalities are seen in 40% of neonates with Down's syndrome and the most common anomaly seen is atrioventricular septal defect (Fig. 21.16).[29]

It has been found that up to 62% of fetuses demonstrating an atrioventricular septal defect have Down's syndrome.[67] The other important associated cardiac anomalies are ventricular and atrial septal defects. In addition, the presence of an isolated pericardial effusion should also raise the possibility of Down's syndrome, as Sharland *et al.* reported trisomy 21 in 26% of fetuses with an isolated pericardial effusion.[68]

Nuchal thickness

Loose folds of skin on the back of the neck are a common finding in neonates with trisomy 21,[5] and thickening of the soft tissues at the back of the neck is a useful ultrasound sign in Down's syndrome,[69,70] occurring in approximately 16% of Down's syndrome fetuses.[23]

The position for the nuchal thickness measurement is found by scanning through the posterior fossa in the transverse plane. Both the cerebellum and the cavum septum pellucidum should be visible (Fig. 21.17). The measurement of the soft tissue is made from the outer edge of the occipital bone to the outer skin surface. A thickness of 6 mm or more is considered abnormal at 16–20 weeks gestation, and trisomy 21 is present in 20–40% of fetuses demonstrating this finding.[69–75]

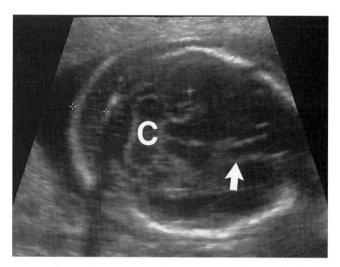

Fig. 21.17 Increased nuchal fold. Transverse section through fetal head showing increased nuchal fold. Caliper measurement 8.7 mm; C – cerebellum; arrow points to cavum septum pellucidum.

An increased nuchal thickness may also be seen in other conditions, such as skeletal dysplasias, early hydrops, and in 2–8.5% of the normal population.[71,72] Careful detailed scanning should always be carried out in cases of increased nuchal thickness in order to look for other markers of Down's syndrome, and to exclude other causes of nuchal oedema. Fetuses with isolated nuchal thickening and a normal karyotype have a good outcome.[76]

Cystic hygroma and hydrops

Although cystic hygroma is much more common in fetuses with Turner's syndrome it is well established that up to 5% of fetuses with cystic hygroma and 12% of fetuses with hydrops may have Down's syndrome.[6,76]

Facial findings

The dysmorphic facial appearance of Down's syndrome is well documented, but these findings are often very difficult to demonstrate with ultrasound. A number of appearances have been documented, and these include a flat profile,[8,77] macroglossia[78] and a shortened ear length.[79]

Cranial findings

Intracranial abnormalities are uncommon in trisomy 21, although mild ventriculomegaly may be seen in up to 3% of affected fetuses.[23] Another reported finding is reduced frontal lobe dimensions.[80]

Other findings

There are a number of less common findings seen in trisomy 21, and these include omphalocele, oesophageal

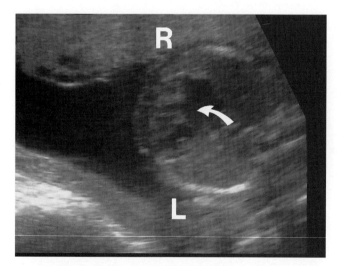

Fig. 21.16 Atrioventricular septal defect. Transverse section through fetal thorax showing four-chamber view. R – right, L – left; curved arrow points to large atrioventricular septal defect.

atresia and anal atresia.[23] There have also been reports of increased iliac bone lengths[81] and reduced breast size in Down's fetuses.[82] Pleural effusions have also been demonstrated in fetuses with trisomy 21.[5]

Soft markers for Down's syndrome

There are a number of minor ultrasound findings that have been reported as markers for Down's syndrome. They include a short femur or humerus, echogenic bowel, mild renal pelvic dilatation, echogenic foci in the fetal heart, clinodactyly of the fifth finger and a sandal gap (between the first and second toes).

The significance of an isolated soft marker is difficult to determine, as many of the data reported involve studies from high-risk groups. Furthermore, as each marker is present in 1–5% of all pregnancies, more and more fetuses will have at least one such marker.[83]

Various authors have proposed scoring systems and likelihood ratios in an attempt to overcome the difficulties of quantifying risk. This section will deal with each finding in turn and outline the sonographic approach to these soft markers.

Short femur

Lockwood and colleagues were among the first authors to report a link between a short femur and trisomy 21,[84] and early studies seemed to confirm this finding.[85] There has, however, been considerable debate in the literature, and later reports have revealed a considerable overlap with the normal population, so that its value as an isolated finding is questionable.[86–88] On the available data one would not routinely recommend a karyotype on the basis of an isolated short femur in a low-risk patient. If other abnormalities are present or the patient is at high risk of carrying a fetus with Down's syndrome, then a karyotype should be considered.

An alternative approach is to use likelihood ratios, as reported by Snijders and Nicolaides (Table 21.7).[89] In this situation, with a likelihood ratio of 2.3 the presence of a short femur approximately doubles the background age-specific risk of Down's syndrome (Table 21.6).

Table 21.7 Likelihood ratios for isolated soft markers for Down's syndrome. The likelihood ratio should be multiplied by the maternal age-specific risk (Table 21.6) to produce the modified Down's syndrome risk. (Reproduced with permission from Snijders R J M, Nicolaides K H, eds. Ultrasound markers for fetal chromosomal defects. London: Parthenon Publishing 1996)

Sonographic finding	Likelihood ratio
Nuchal fold 6 mm or more	19
Echogenic bowel	5.5
Short femur	2.3
Mild renal pelvic dilatation	1.5

Short humerus

Benaceraff *et al.* have incorporated a short humerus and a short femur into the scoring system for the detection of trisomy 21 and found it a useful marker (Table 21.8).[15,65] Nyberg *et al.* found significant humeral shortening in 24% of Down's fetuses, and suggested that fetuses with both a short femur and a short humerus carried an 11-fold greater risk of Down's syndrome.[90] Johnson *et al.* using the ratio of humerus plus femur length divided by the foot length, detected 53% of Down's syndrome fetuses.[91] Larger studies are, however, required to confirm these findings.

Echogenic bowel

Echogenic bowel was first reported by Lince *et al.*[92] and was for many years considered a normal variant.[92,93] Many workers have attempted to grade the degree of echogenicity of bowel with regard to liver texture or other intra-abdominal structures, but the most reliable definition is when the echogenic bowel has the same reflectivity as bone (Fig. 21.18).[94,95] Another approach is to reduce the

Table 21.8 Sonographic scoring system for the detection of trisomy 21. (Reproduced with permission from Benacerraf B. The second trimester fetus with Down's syndrome: detection using sonographic features. Ultrasound Obstet Gynecol 1996; 7: 147–155)

Sonographic finding	Score
Major defect	2
Nuchal fold 6 mm or more	2
Short femur	1
Short humerus	1
Mild renal pelvic dilatation	1
Echogenic bowel	1

Fetuses with a score of 2 or more are considered at high risk for Down's syndrome.

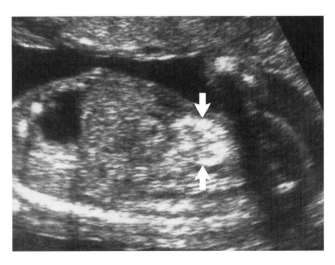

Fig. 21.18 Echogenic bowel. Sagittal section through fetal abdomen showing echogenic bowel (arrows).

Table 21.9 Incidence of chromosomal abnormality and associated abnormalities in studies of fetuses with echogenic bowel. (Reproduced with permission from Carroll S G, Maxwell D J. Significance of echogenic areas in the fetal abdomen. Ultrasound Obstet Gynecol 1996; 7: 293–298)

Reference	Study population (HR – high risk U – unselected)	Number	Incidence of trisomy 21	Incidence of all chromosomal abnormalities	Incidence of associated malformations
94	HR	30	0	1	1
102	HR	19	5	6	4
103	HR	15	2	2	2
96	HR	95	11	24	17
95	HR	50	6	8	8
93	U	10	0	0	0
104	U	32	2	2	1
105	U	7	0	1	1
97	U	182	7	9	?
99	U	14	0	3	?
106	U	145	8	8	5
Total	HR + U	599	39 (6.6%)	64 (11%)	39/52
High risk	HR	209	24 (11%)	41 (20%)	32
Unselected*	U	194	8 (4%)	11 (5%)	7
Unselected† and isolated echogenic bowel	U	189	3 (1.6%)	11 (6%)	7

* Unselected studies with exclusion of studies 97 and 98 because of insufficient data on associated anomalies.
† Isolated echogenic bowel calculated by subtracted known cases of chromosomal disease with associated abnormalities.

gain setting until the image of bone is lost before that of the echogenic bowel.[106]

The incidence of echogenic bowel has been reported as ranging between 0.2% and 0.6%, and more recent studies have revealed associations with chromosomal disease, particularly Down's syndrome, cystic fibrosis, intra-uterine growth retardation, congenital infection and fetal demise.[96,98] The aetiology of echogenic bowel is obscure, but various groups have suggested differing causes, including hypoperistalsis or decreased fluid content of meconium,[98] swallowed blood following intra-amniotic bleeding,[99] and possibly gut ischaemia.[100]

Carrol and Maxwell[101] recently reviewed 599 cases of echogenic bowel and found chromosomal disease present in 64 (11%), of which 39 (6.6%) were trisomy 21 (Table 21.9). As can be seen from the data, five of the 11 studies comprise high-risk patients (i.e. over 35 years of age, or with a raised biochemical screening result) and so it is difficult to apply these results to the low-risk population. Analysis of the studies using unselected populations reveals an incidence of 4% for Down's syndrome, but these include fetuses with other abnormalities. By subtracting out those fetuses with associated anomalies one obtains a crude figure of 1.6% for the incidence of Down's syndrome in fetuses with isolated echogenic bowel from unselected populations. This figure suggests that one probably should offer a karyotype to patients whose fetus demonstrates echogenic bowel, even in the low-risk population. In addition, Snijders and Nicolaides have calculated a likelihood ratio of 5.5 for echogenic bowel

(Table 21.7), which would suggest that the presence of echogenic bowel carries a significant risk of trisomy 21 above the age of 20 years (Table 21.6). These data would tend to support the view that echogenic bowel is a significant finding in the diagnosis of trisomy 21.

Carrol and Maxwell[101] also found overall rates of 11% for growth retardation, 8% for intra-uterine fetal death and 0.8% for neonatal deaths in fetuses with echogenic bowel. It was noted that 50% of cases were associated with raised serum α-fetoprotein, and it may well be that bleeding in early pregnancy may explain the raised serum α-fetoprotein, the echogenic bowel (swallowed blood) and the intra-uterine growth retardation (secondary to placental damage following bleeding).

The other main association appears to be cystic fibrosis, and parental carrier testing can be considered if the karyotype is normal.[102–103] Screening for fetal infection should also be carried out.[104-106]

Further ultrasound scans also need to be carried out to assess fetal growth and exclude intra-uterine growth retardation later in pregnancy.[101] Most cases of echogenic bowel resolve by about 28 weeks gestation.

Mild renal pelvic dilatation

This is a relatively common antenatal finding, occurring in 1.6–2.8% of fetuses.[14,107–110] The renal pelves are best measured on a transverse section with the spine uppermost (Fig. 21.19). Measurements are made in the anteroposterior direction and have been reported as up to 4 mm to 20

ation progresses then this significantly increases the risk of post-natal structural renal disease.[109,112]

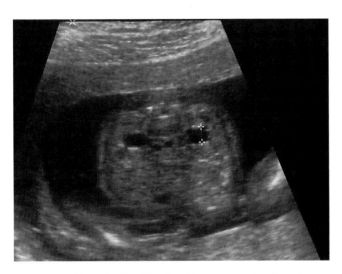

Fig. 21.19 Mild renal pelvic dilatation. Transverse section through lower fetal abdomen with spine uppermost. (Calipers measuring anteroposterior diameter of renal pelvis).

Table 21.10 Incidences of trisomy 21 in fetuses with isolated mild renal pelvic dilatation

Author	Reference	Incidence
Benaceraff 1990	14	1:33
Wickstrom 1996	109	1:121
Corteville 1992	108	0:116
Chitty 1992	110	1:150
Nicolaides 1996	111	1:161
Dudley 1997	112	1:100

weeks gestation, up to 5 mm from 20 to 30 weeks, and up to 7 mm from 30 to 40 weeks.[14] Table 21.10 outlines the reported incidences of trisomy 21 in fetuses with apparently isolated mild renal pelvic dilatation. It is seen that these range from 1:33 to 1:161, and this to a certain extent reflects the fact that most series are from high-risk populations. Courteville *et al.* reported 127 fetuses with mild renal pelvic dilatation and calculated the predictive value of isolated renal pelvic dilatation for Down's syndrome to be 1:340.[108] In addition, Snijders and Nicolaides reported 805 fetuses with mild renal pelvic dilatation and found five with trisomy 21.[111] The difference between the observed and the expected frequency for trisomy 21 in the group of 805 was not significant based on the maternal age-specific rates. The estimated likelihood ratio for isolated mild renal pelvic dilatation is only 1.5 (Table 21.7).

The demonstration of mild renal pelvic dilatation should therefore prompt careful detailed scanning to look for other markers of trisomy 21, rather than a karyotype procedure.[111] If other abnormalities are seen then a karyotype should be considered.

Further follow-up scans should be carried out to detect any possible progression to a true hydronephrosis. If dilat-

Echogenic foci in the heart

Echogenic foci in the fetal heart were first described by Schechter *et al.* in 1987,[113] and are thought to represent microcalcification within papillary muscle.[114] The vast majority are seen in the left ventricle (Fig. 21.20), but they are occasionally seen on the right and may occur in both ventricles. The majority are single, but they may be multiple and most resolve by the third trimester.[115] Echogenic foci have an incidence ranging between 2% and 5% of all pregnancies.[114–116]

There is debate within the literature as to the significance of echogenic foci, and although some series have shown an association with trisomy 21[117–119] most of these reports are from the high-risk group. Studies from unselected populations, or where age-specific risk has been included, show no increased risk of trisomy 21 following the detection of echogenic foci.[115,116,120,121] Echogenic foci should therefore be considered a normal variant in the low-risk population, but may well represent a marker for trisomy 21 in the high risk patient.[121]

Clinodactyly

Hypoplasia of the middle phalanx (clinodactyly) of the fifth finger (Fig. 21.21) is common in patients with trisomy 21 and is thought to occur in 60% of affected neonates.[122] However, it also occurs in up to 3% of the normal population.[123]

Benaceraff *et al.* have described this sign in fetuses with trisomy 21[124] and, by refining the diagnosis, have reported

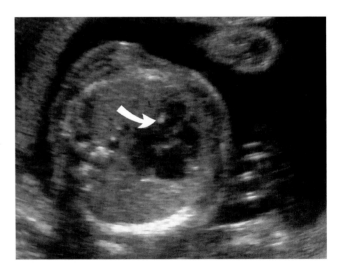

Fig. 21.20 Echogenic focus in the left ventricle. Transverse section through fetal thorax showing four-chamber view. (Arrow points to echogenic focus in the left ventricle.)

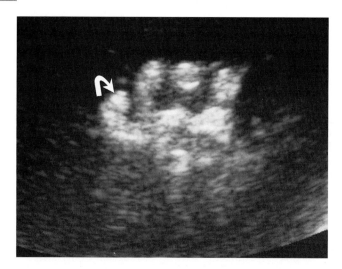

Fig. 21.21 Clinodactyly fifth finger. Coronal section of fetal hand showing clinodactyly of the fifth finger (curved arrow). (Reproduced with permission from Reed, Claireux and Lockburn. Diseases of fetus and newborn. Chapman and Hall, 1995.)

a 75% detection rate.[125] Unfortunately, the same paper revealed an incidence of 18% in the normal population, which makes its value as a marker for trisomy 21 extremely doubtful with such a high false-positive rate.[125] However, taken together with other markers of trisomy 21 it may serve as a useful confirmatory sign.

A simian crease has also been described in fetuses with trisomy 21.[126]

Sandal gap

Separation of the first and second toes (sandal gap) occurs in 45% of children with Down's syndrome[5] and has been described antenatally.[7,65] Wilkins *et al.* described two fetuses at high risk of trisomy 21 that demonstrated a wide gap between the first and second toes. Both also demonstrated other anomalies and both were found to have trisomy 21 following a karyotype procedure.[127]

Once again this sign should be reserved as a marker for the high-risk population.

Sonographic approach to trisomy 21

It is clear from the previous section that there are a number of important ultrasound findings which are useful in making a diagnosis of trisomy 21. The main ultrasound markers are an atrioventricular septal defect, duodenal atresia, an increased nuchal fold and echogenic bowel. There are also a number of minor signs for soft markers which, when present, do not significantly increase the risk of trisomy 21 if seen in isolation in the low-risk population. These include a short femur, short humerus, mild renal pelvic dilatation, echogenic foci in the heart, clin-

odactyly of the fifth finger and a sandal gap. These minor markers may be useful in the high-risk group, i.e. women over 35 years of age or with a raised risk on biochemical screening. In this group of women, who are often unsure as to whether to opt for a karyotype procedure, the presence of a minor marker could be a useful factor in the decision to carry out an invasive test.

Benaceraff *et al.* have proposed a scoring system which uses both major and minor ultrasound findings (Table 21.8), and although this approach is popular in the USA it has not gained universal acceptance in Europe.

A more recent system is the development of likelihood ratios, which can be multiplied by the patient's background age-specific Down's syndrome risk and a modified risk obtained (Tables 21.6 and 21.7). This is an attractive approach, as an absolute figure can be offered to the patient as to her new risk with regard to her background risk. The main drawback to this system is that accurate prevalence rates for various minor markers are difficult to obtain and the data are based on relatively small numbers of cases. It is, however, a step in the right direction.

The significance of a normal scan has also been investigated, and it has been suggested that following a normal detailed ultrasound scan the background age-specific Down's syndrome risk can be reduced. Data from several studies suggest that the background risk can be reduced by about 28–45%.[111,128–130] This approach may, however, result in up to 15% of trisomy 21 fetuses being missed.[31] In view of this, caution is urged when attempting to reduce background age-specific risks based on a normal detailed ultrasound scan.

Nuchal thickness scanning

The association of first-trimester nuchal fluid and trisomy 21 was first described by Szabo and Gellen in 1990.[132] Since then there have been many studies documenting the use of nuchal thickness scanning in the diagnosis of Down's syndrome (Table 21.11). The cause of increased nuchal fluid in fetuses with Down's syndrome is not clear, but may be due to a combination of altered extracellular matrix in the nuchal skin,[133] together with the high rate of heart defects,[134,135] which may predispose fluid to accumulate at this site. It is well known that neonates with Down's syndrome exhibit loose folds of skin in the neck which may be a result of previous fetal nuchal fluid that has resolved.[5]

The nuchal thickness measurement is carried out at 10–14 weeks gestation, scanning the fetus in a sagittal plane with the spine lowermost (Fig. 21.22). The measurement is made such that the anteroposterior depth of fluid is assessed, care being taken to ensure that the measurement calipers do not encroach on the fluid space. In addition, the amnion should not be confused with the nuchal membrane. Most studies use a cut-off of 3 mm as

Table 21.11 Data from nuchal thickness (NT) studies

Author	Number in study	High risk (HR) or low risk (LR)	Number with increased NT	Gestational age (wks)	NT thickness (mm)	Sensitivity for trisomy 21 (%)	False-positive rate (%)	Percentage measured (%)	Type of scan TA – transabdominal TV – Trans-vaginal
Schulte-Vallentin et al. 1992	632	HR	8	10–14	>4	100	0.1	100	—
Salvodelli et al. 1993	1400	HR	24	9–12	>4	54	0.35	100	TA
Brambati et al. 1995	1819	HR	70	8–15	>3	30	4	100	TA/TV
Comas et al. 1995	481	HR	51	9–13	>3	57	0.7	100	TV
Szabo et al. 1995	3380	HR/LR	96	9–12	>3	90.0	1.2–5.4	100	TV
Bewley et al. 1995	1127	LR	70	8–13	>3	33	6	62	TA
Hafner et al. 1995	1972	LR	26	10–13	>2.5	50	7.7	100	TA
Nicolaides et al. 1996	20543	HR	3302	10–14	*	86	11	100	TA
Nicolaides et al. 1996	22076	LR	1316	10–14	*	84	6	100	TA
Kornman et al. 1996	923	HR	36	<13	>3	24	5	58	TA
Thilaganathan et al. 1997	2920	LR	147	10–14	*	71	5	91	TA
Kadir et al. 1997	1302	LR	22	10–13	†	83	1–3	100	TA/TV

* Risk calculated using a cut-off risk of 1/300 estimated from maternal age and nuchal thickness.
† Screen positive when nuchal thickness measurement above 99th centile.

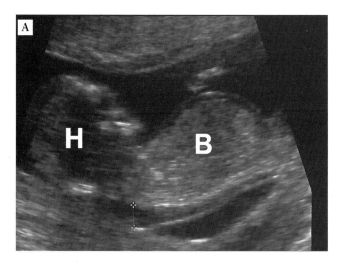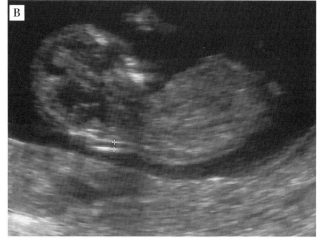

Fig. 21.22 Increased nuchal translucency measurement. A: Sagittal scan through a 12-week fetus showing increased nuchal translucency (H – head, B – body, caliper measurements 5.6 mm). **B:** Normal nuchal thickness.

the upper limit of normal, but this measurement should be correlated with maternal age, as it is known that values below 3 mm can be associated with a significant increased risk of Down's syndrome in older women.[111] A number of investigators have looked into the reproducibility of nuchal thickness measurements, and although Roberts *et al.* found discrepancies in up to 18% of cases,[36] Pandya *et al.* found good reproducibility in 95% of patients[137] and stressed the importance of well-trained operators carrying out the measurements.

Analysis of the studies involving nuchal thickness scanning reveal that many of them involve the high-risk population (Table 21.11). Sensitivities for the detection of

trisomy 21 range from 24% to 100%. Two of the studies demonstrating low sensitivities also demonstrated incomplete measurement data, with only 58% and 62% of nuchal thickness measurements carried out on the study population.[130,138] This is likely to have a significant effect on sensitivity results. Most studies demonstrated at least a 50% detection rate for trisomy 21, with a mean false-positive rate around 5%.[139–145] The largest low-risk study is made up of over 22 000 pregnancies and, by using an algorithm based on maternal age, gestational age at the time of scan and a cut-off risk of 1:300, 84% of Down's syndrome fetuses were detected, with a false-positive rate of 6%. The results indicate that early nuchal thickness scanning is a useful screening test for trisomy 21; however, careful attention must be placed on training and meticulous attention to detail when carrying out the measurement. In addition, an algorithm using maternal age and gestational age at scan should be incorporated into the calculation of risk.

One criticism that has been made of nuchal thickness scanning, but which applies equally to other forms of early prenatal diagnosis, such as biochemical screening, is that a number of the fetuses diagnosed as having trisomy 21 may well abort prior to delivery. It is well established that up to 75% of trisomy 21 conceptuses do not survive to term,[1] and so a proportion of the fetuses diagnosed at 10–14 weeks gestation will end in spontaneous abortion. Hyett *et al.* reported an 11.4% loss rate for trisomy 21 fetuses with increased nuchal thickness between 12 and 14 weeks gestation, which was almost double the background rate.[146] In contrast, Pandya *et al.* followed six Down's syndrome fetuses with increased nuchal thickness to term and all were liveborn.[147] On balance, the natural loss rate for trisomy 21 fetuses will affect and reduce the overall detection rates at 10–14 weeks gestation, but the fact that the majority will survive to term following this period indicates that the test still has enormous importance.

The importance of using fetal heart rate to aid in the early diagnosis of trisomy 21 is unclear at present. Hyett *et al.* found a significant increase in heart rate in first-trimester Down's syndrome fetuses.[148] Martinez *et al.*, in contrast, found that fetuses with Down's syndrome had decreased heart rates.[149] Martinez *et al.* have, however, suggested using umbilical artery Doppler together with nuchal thickness scanning, and have found that an increased nuchal thickness measurement together with an abnormally high umbilical artery pulsatility index produced a detection rate of 89%.[150]

The addition of first-trimester biochemical screening to nuchal thickness measurements appears to increase the sensitivity of nuchal thickness screening by about 5%.[151] The relationship of nuchal thickness scanning to biochemical screening at 16 weeks gestation has also been investigated, and it would seem that the high pick-up rate for trisomy 21 in the first trimester reduces the positive predictive value of biochemical screening in the second trimester. In the study by Thulaganathan *et al.* nuchal thickness scanning detected five out of seven fetuses with trisomy 21, and sequential serum biochemical screening only detected a further single case of trisomy 21.[152] Similar findings were demonstrated by Kadir and Economides.[153]

Although an increased nuchal thickness measurement is a valuable marker for chromosomal disease, particularly trisomy 21, if the chromosome studies are normal in the affected fetus there are a number of other abnormalities and syndromes that may be present. The most important of these are cardiac abnormalities, and in a recent study major cardiac abnormalities were seen in 24 of 1427

fetuses (1.7%) with an increased nuchal thickness and normal chromosomes.

A number of other conditions appear to have a higher incidence in fetuses with an increased nuchal thickness: these include diaphragmatic hernia, omphalocele and body stalk anomaly. Rare syndromes have also been reported in association with an increased nuchal thickness, and include arthrogryposis syndromes, skeletal dysplasias, Meckel–Grüber syndrome, VATER syndrome, Roberts syndrome and Smith–Lemli–Opitz syndrome.[154]

The significance of finding fetuses with increased nuchal thickness and a normal karyotype is that careful detailed scanning is required, including fetal echocardiography in the second trimester to exclude cardiac and other anomalies.

Turner's syndrome

Turner's syndrome is characterised by short stature, webbed neck, cubitus valgus, broad chest with widely spaced nipples and ovarian dysgenesis.[5] However, neonates may appear normal and the diagnosis may not be made until short stature or delayed puberty becomes apparent.[5]

The incidence of Turner's syndrome is approximately 1/5000 live births, but the vast majority are lost as spontaneous abortions.[1]

The most important ultrasound finding in the antenatal diagnosis of Turner's syndrome is the presence of a cystic hygroma. The typical appearance is of a large multiseptate fluid collection in the posterior nuchal region (Fig. 21.23). An important diagnostic point is the presence of a midline nuchal septum, which should always be present. These cystic hygromata are often associated with generalised hydrops.[155]

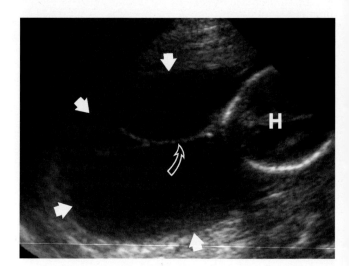

Fig. 21.23 Cystic hygroma. Transverse scan through head and neck of an 18-week fetus showing a large cystic hygroma (straight arrows). Curved arrow points to midline nuchal septum. H – head.

Karyotyping should always be carried out, as although 70% of fetuses with a cystic hygroma will be found to have Turner's syndrome, approximately 5% will have trisomy 21, 5% trisomy 18, and 20% a normal karyotype.[156] Cystic hygromata occurring at other sites in the body, and usually in the third trimester, have a low incidence of chromosomal disease.

Associated anomalies seen in Turner's syndrome include coarctation of the aorta (15%) and renal anomalies, including horseshoe kidney, hydronephrosis and renal agenesis.[157]

Cystic hygromata should always be differentiated from encephalocele, in which the diagnosis is based on an abnormal head shape, a calvarial defect and intracranial abnormalities.[158]

Triploidy

This condition occurs when there is an extra set of chromosomes present. The extra set may come from either parent. The frequencies of the different combinations are:- 69XXY (60%), 69XXX (37%) and 69XYY (3%).[159] It has been estimated that triploidy accounts for 16% of all spontaneous abortions,[1] and the majority of triploidy conceptuses abort spontaneously (Table 21.1). Of the fetuses that survive to the early second trimester the most important finding is growth retardation, often associated with oligohydramnios.[16,17,160] The placenta may show hydropic change, and this is more common when the extra set of chromosomes has a paternal origin.[161,162]

There is no specific phenotype to triploidy, but intracranial abnormalities such as holoprosencephaly, agenesis of the corpus callosum and mild ventriculomegaly may be seen. Other findings of note include syndactyly of the third and fourth fingers (Fig. 21.24) and a wide gap between the first and second toes.

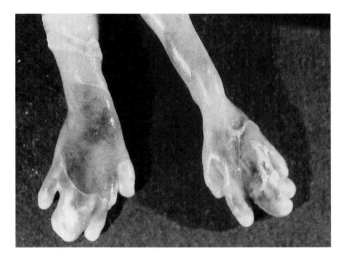

Fig. 21.24 Triploidy fetus showing syndactyly of third and fourth fingers.

The outlook is very poor overall, although a few fetuses occasionally survive into the third trimester.

REFERENCES

1 Thompson M W, McInnes R R, Willard M F. Clinical cytogenetics: general principles and autosomal abnormalities. In: Genetics in medicine, 5th edn. Philadelphia: W B Saunders, 1991

2 Hook E B. Chromosome abnormalities and spontaneous fetal death following amniocentesis: further data and associations with maternal age. Am J Hum Genet 1983; 35: 100–116

3 Ferguson-Smith M A, Yates J R W. Maternal age specific rates for chromosomal aberrations and factors influencing them: report of a collaborative European study on 52,965 amniocenteses. Prenat Diagn 4: 5–44

4 Schneider A S, Mennut M T, Zackai E M. High caesarean section rate in trisomy 18 births: a potential indication for late prenatal diagnosis. Am J Obstet Gynecol 1981; 140: 367–370

5 Jones K L. Smith's recognisable patterns of human malformation, 4th edn. Eastbourne: Saunders, 1988

6 Nicolaides K H, Shawa L, Brizot M, Snijders R. Ultrasonographically detectable markers of fetal chromosomal defects. Ultrasound Obstet Gynecol 1993; 3: 56–69

7 Nicolaides K H, Snijders R J M, Gosdon C M et al. Ultrasonographically detectable markers of fetal chromosomal abnormalities. Lancet 1992; 340: 704–707

8 Snijders R J M, Nicolaides K M. Ultrasound markers for fetal chromosomal defects. London: Parthenon Publishing, 1996

9 Twining P, Zuccollo J. The ultrasound markers of chromosomal disease: a retrospective study. Br J Radiol 1993; 66: 408–414

10 Getachew M M, Goldstein R B, Edge V et al. Correlation between omphalocele contents and karyotypic abnormalities: sonographic study in 37 cases. AJR 1991; 158: 133–136

11 Nyberg D A, Fitzsimmons J, Mack L A et al. Chromosomal abnormalities in fetuses with omphalocele: significance of omphalocele contents. J Ultrasound Med 1989; 8: 299–308

12 Nicolaides K H, Berry S, Snijders R J M et al. Fetal lateral cerebral ventriculomegaly: associated malformations and chromosomal defects. Fetal Diagn Ther 1990; 5: 5–14

13 Nicolaides K H, Cheng H, Abbas A et al. Fetal renal defects: associated malformations and chromosomal defects. Fetal Diagn Ther 1992; 7: 1–11

14 Benacerraf B R, Mandell J, Estroff J A et al. Fetal pyelectasis: a possible association with Down's syndrome. Obstet Gynecol 1990; 76: 58–60

15 Benacerraf B R. Prenatal sonography of autosomal trisomies. Ultrasound Obstet Gynecol 1991; 1: 66–75

16 Edwards M T, Smith W L, Hanson J, Abu Yousef M. Prenatal sonographic diagnosis of triploidy. J Ultrasound Med 1986; 5: 279–281

17 Snijders R J M, Sherod C, Gosden C M, Nicolaides K H. Fetal growth retardation: associated malformations and chromosomal abnormalities. Am J Obstet Gynecol 1993; 168: 547–555

18 Royal College of Obstetricians and Gynaecologists. Working party report on routine ultrasound examination in pregnancy. London: RCOG, 1984

19 Chitty L S, Hunt G H, Moore J, Lobb M O. Effectiveness of routine ultrasonography in detecting fetal structural abnormalities in a low risk population. BMJ 1991; 303: 1165–1169

20 Luck C A. Value of routine ultrasound scanning at 19 weeks: a four year study of 8849 deliveries. BMJ 1992; 304: 1474–1478

21 Lehman C D, Nyberg D A, Winter T C et al. Trisomy 13 syndrome, prenatal ultrasound findings in a review of 33 cases. Radiology 1995; 194: 217–222

22 Nyberg D A, Kramer D, Resta R G, Kapur R. Prenatal sonographic findings of trisomy 18. J Ultrasound Med 1993; 2: 103–113

23 Nyberg D A, Resta R G, Luthy D A et al. Prenatal sonographic findings of Down's syndrome, review of 94 cases. Obstet Gynecol 1990; 76: 370–377

24 Snijders R J M, Johnson S, Sebire N J et al. First trimester ultrasound screening for chromosomal defects. Ultrasound Obstet Gynecol 1996; 7: 216–226

25 Ledbetter D H, Martin A O, Verlinsky Y et al. Cytogenetic results of chorionic villus sampling. High success rate and diagnostic accuracy in the United States collaborative study. Am J Obstet Gynecol 1990; 162: 495–501

26 Patau K, Smith D W, Therman E. Multiple congenital anomaly caused by an extra chromosome. Lancet 1960; i: 790–793

27 Baty B J, Blackburn B L, Carey J C. Natural history of trisomy 18 and trisomy 13: I. Growth, physical assessment, medical histories, survival and recurrence risk. Am J Med Genet 1994; 49: 175–188

28 Greene M F, Benacerraf B R, Frigoletto F D. Reliable criteria for the prenatal sonographic diagnosis of alobar holoprosencephaly. Am J Obstet Gynecol 1987; 156: 687–689

29 Benacerraf B R, Frigoletto F D, Greene M F. Abnormal facial features and extremities in human trisomy syndromes: prenatal US appearance. Radiology 1986; 159: 243–246

30 Brown D L, Emerson D S, Shulman L P et al. Predicting aneuploidy in fetuses with cardiac anomalies. J Ultrasound Med 1993; 3: 153–161

31 Paladini D, Calabro R, Palmieri S, D'andrea T. Prenatal diagnosis of congenital heart disease and fetal karyotyping. Obstet Gynecol 1993; 81: 679–682

32 Sepulveda W, Pryde P G, Greb A E et al. Prenatal diagnosis of umbilical cord pseudocyst. Ultrasound Obstet Gynaecol 1994; 4: 147–150

33 Achiron R, Seidman D S, Afek A et al. Prenatal ultrasonographic diagnosis of fetal hepatic hyperechogenicities, clinical significance and implications for management. Ultrasound Obstet Gynecol 1996; 7: 251–255

34 Sepulveda W, Nicolaidis P, Hollingsworth J, Fisk N. Fetal cholecystomegaly: a prenatal marker of aneuploidy. Prenat Diagn 1995; 15: 193–197

35 Meckel S, Passarge E. Encephalocele, polycystic kidneys and polydactyly as an autosomal recessive trait simulating certain other disorders: the Meckel syndrome. Ann Genet 1971; 14: 97–103

36 Edwards J H. A new trisomic syndrome. Lancet 1960; i: 787

37 Baty B J, Jorde L B, Blackburn B L, Carey J C. Natural history of trisomy 18 and trisomy 13 II. Psychomotor development. Am J Med Genet 1994; 49: 189–194

38 Twining P, Zuccollo J, Clewes J, Swallow J. Fetal choroid plexus cysts: a prospective study and review of the literature. Br J Radiol 1991; 64: 98–102

39 Copel J, Cullen M, Green J S et al. The frequency of aneuploidy in prenatally diagnosed congenital heart disease: an indication for fetal karyotype. Am J Obstet Gynecol 1988; 158: 409–413

40 Nicolaides K H, Salveston D R, Snijders R J M, Gosden C M. Strawberry shaped skull in fetal trisomy 18. Fetal Diagn Ther 1992; 7: 132–137

41 Seymour R, Jones A. Strawberry shaped skull in fetal thanatophoric dysplasia. Ultrasound Obstet Gynecol 1994; 4: 434–436

42 Nyberg D A, Mahoney B S, Heggs F N et al. Enlarged cisterna vena magna and the Dandy Walker malformation: factors associated with chromosome abnormalities. Obstet Gynecol 1991; 77: 436–442

43 Twining P, Zuccollo J, Jaspan T. The outcome of fetal ventriculomegaly. Br J Radiol 1994; 67: 26–31

44 Nicolaides K H, Berry S, Snijders R J M et al. Fetal lateral cerebral ventriculomegaly: associated malformations and chromosomal defects. Fetal Diagn Ther 1990; 5: 5–14

45 Gupta J K, Klan K S, Thornton J G, Lilford R J. Management of fetal choroid plexus cysts. Br J Obstet Gynaecol 1997; 104: 881–886

46 Chudleigh P, Pearce J M, Campbell S. The prenatal diagnosis of transient cysts of the fetal choroid plexus. Prenat Diagn 1984; 4: 135–137

47 Nadel A S, Bromley B S, Frigoletto F D et al. Isolated choroid plexus cysts in the second trimester fetus: is amniocentesis really indicated? Radiology 1992; 185: 545–548

48 Ostlere S J, Irving H C, Lilford R J. Fetal choroid plexus cysts: a report of 100 cases. Radiology 1990; 175: 753–755

49 Furness M E. Choroid plexus cysts and trisomy 18. Lancet 1987; ii: 693

50 Shields L E, Ulrick S B, Easterling T R et al. Isolated fetal choroid plexus cysts and karyotype analysis: is it necessary? J Ultrasound Med 1996; 15: 389–394

51 Walkinshaw S, Pilling D, Sprigg A. Isolated choroid plexus cysts: the need for routine offer of karyotyping. Prenat Diagn 1994; 14: 663–667

52 Gross S J, Shulman L P, Tolley E A et al. Isolated fetal choroid plexus cysts and trisomy 18: a review and meta analysis. Am J Obstet Gynecol 1995; 172: 83–87

53 Gupta J K, Cave M, Lilford R J et al. Clinical significance of fetal choroid plexus cysts. Lancet 1995; 346: 724–729

54 Twining P, Clewes J S. The emotional impact of the antenatal detection of choroid plexus cysts at 18–20 weeks. Fourth World Congress of Ultrasound in Obstetrics and Gynaecology, Budapest. Ultrasound Obstet Gynecol 1994; 4 (Suppl 1): 200

55 Thorpe-Beeston G, Gosden C M, Nicolaides K H. Congenital diaphragmatic hernia, associated malformations and chromosomal defects. Fetal Ther 1989; 4: 21–28

56 Nicolaides K H, Snijders R J M, Cheng H et al. Fetal abdominal wall and gastrointestinal tract defects: associated malformations and chromosomal defects. Fetal Diagn Ther 1992; 7: 102–115

57 Dicke J M, Crane J P. Sonographic recognition of major malformations and aberent growth in trisomic fetuses. J Ultrasound Med 1991; 10: 433–438

58 Down J L M. Observations on an ethnic classification of idiots. Clinical Lecture Reports, London Hospital 1866; 3: 259

59 Bleyer A. Indication that mongoloid imbecility is a gametogenic mutation of degenerating type. Am J Dis Child 1934; 47: 342–347

60 Waardenburg P J. Das Menschliche Auge Und Seine Erbanlagen. The Hague: Martinus Nijhoff, 1932

61 Lejeune J, Gautier M, Turpin R. Etude des chromosomes somatiques de neuf enfants mongoliens. C R Acad Sci Paris 1959; 248: 1721

62 Wald N J, Kennard A, Densem J W et al. Antenatal maternal serum screening for Down's syndrome: results of a demonstration project. BMJ 1992; 305: 391–394

63 Wald N J, George L, Smith D et al. Serum screening for Down's syndrome between 8 and 14 weeks of pregnancy. Br J Obstet Gynaecol 1996; 103: 407–412

64 Nicolaides K H, Sebire N J, Snijders R J M, Johnson S. Down's screening in the United Kingdom. Lancet 1996; 347: 906–907

65 Benacerraf B R. The second-trimester fetus with Down's syndrome: detection using sonographic features. Ultrasound Obstet Gynecol 1996; 7: 147–155

66 Nelson L H, Clark C E, Fishburne J I et al. Value of serial sonography in the *in utero* detection of duodenal atresia. Obstet Gynecol 1982; 59: 657–660

67 Allan L D, Sharland G K, Chita S K. Chromosomal abnormalities in fetal congenital heart disease. Ultrasound Obstet Gynecol 1991; 1: 8–11

68 Sharland G, Lockhart S. Isolated pericardial effusion: an indication for fetal karyotyping? Ultrasound Obstet Gynecol 1995; 6: 29–32

69 Nicolaides K H, Azar G, Snijders R J M, Gosden C M. Fetal nuchal oedema, associated malformations and chromosomal defects. Fetal Diagn Ther 1992; 7: 123–131

70 Benacerraf B R, Laboda L A, Frigoletto F D. Thickened nuchal fold in fetuses, not at risk for aneuploidy. Radiology 1992; 84: 239–242

71 Grandjean H, Sarramon M F. Sonographic measurement of nuchal skinfold thickness for detection of Down's syndrome in second trimester fetus: a multicentre prospective study. Obstet Gynecol 1995; 86: 103–106

72 Watson W J, Miller R C, Menard K et al. Ultrasonographic measurement of fetal nuchal skin to screen for chromosomal abnormalities. Am J Obstet Gynecol 1994; 170: 583–586

73 Devore G R, Alfi O. The association between an abnormal nuchal skin fold, trisomy 21 and ultrasound abnormalities identified during the second trimester of pregnancy. Ultrasound Obstet Gynecol 1993; 3: 387–394

74 Toi A, Simpson G F, Filly R A. Ultrasonically evident fetal nuchal skin thickening: is it specific for Down's syndrome? Am J Obstet Gynecol 1987; 156: 150–153

75 Borrell A, Costa M B, Martinez J et al. Early mid trimester fetal nuchal thickness: effectiveness as a marker of Down's syndrome. Obstet Gynecol 1996; 175: 45–49

76 Boyd P A, Anthony M Y, Manning N et al. Antenatal diagnosis of cystic hygroma or nuchal pad – report of 92 cases with follow up of survivors. Arch Dis Child 1996; 74: 38–42

77 Turner G, Twining P. The facial profile in the diagnosis of fetal abnormalities. Clin Radiol 1993; 47: 389–395

78 Nicolaides K H, Salvesen D R, Snijders R J M, Gosden C M. Fetal facial defects: associated malformations and chromosomal abnormalities. Fetal Diagn Ther 1993; 8: 1–9

79 Lettieri L, Rodis J F, Vintzileos A M et al. Ear length in second trimester aneuploid fetuses. Obstet Gynecol 1993; 81: 57–60

80 Bahado-Singh R O, Wyse L, Dorr M A et al. Fetuses with Down's syndrome have disproportionately shortened frontal lobe dimensions on ultrasonographic examination. Am J Obstet Gynecol 1992; 167: 1009–1014

81 Abuhamad A Z, Kolm P, Mari G et al. Ultrasonographic fetal iliac length measurement in the screening for Down's syndrome. Am J Obstet Gynecol 1994; 171: 1063–1067

82 Petrikovsky B M, Schneider E P, Klin V R et al. Fetal breasts in normal and Down's syndrome fetuses. JCU 1996; 24: 507–511

83 Nicolaides K H. Screening for fetal chromosomal abnormalities: need to change the rules. Ultrasound Obstet Gynecol 1994; 4: 353–354

84 Lockwood C, Benacerraf B R, Krinsky A et al. A sonographic screening for Down's syndrome. Am J Obstet Gynecol 1987; 157: 803–808

85 Benacerraf B R, Galman R, Frigoletto F D. Sonographic identification of second trimester fetuses with Down's syndrome. N Engl J Med 1987; 317: 1371–1376

86 Lynch L, Berkowitz G S, Chitkara U et al. Ultrasound detection of Down's syndrome: is it really possible? Obstet Gynecol 1989; 73: 267–270

87 Nyberg D A, Resta R G, Hickok D. Femur length shortening in the detection of Down's syndrome: is prenatal screening feasible? Am J Obstet Gynecol 1990; 162: 1247–1252

88 Twining P, Whalley D, Lewin E, Foulkes K. Is a short femur length a useful marker for Down's syndrome? Br J Radiol 1991; 64: 990–992

89 Snijders R J M, Nicolaides K H. Ultrasound markers for fetal chromosomal defects. Frontiers in medicine series. London: Parthenon Publishing, 1996

90 Nyberg D A, Resta R G, Luthy D A et al. Humerus and femur length shortening in the detection of Down's syndrome. Am J Obstet Gynecol 1993; 168: 534–538

91 Johnson M P, Michaelson J E, Barr M et al. Combining humerus and femur length for improved ultrasonographic identification of pregnancies at increased risk for trisomy 21. Am J Obstet Gynecol 1995; 172: 1229–1235

92 Lince D M, Pretorius D H, Manco-Johnson M L et al. The clinical significance of increased echogenicity in the fetal abdomen. AJR 1985; 145: 683–686

93 Bromley B, Doubilet P, Frigoletto F et al. Is fetal hyperechoic bowel on second trimester sonogram an indication for amniocentesis? Obstet Gynecol 1994; 83: 647–651

94 Fakhry J, Reisner M, Shapiro L R et al. Increased echogenicity in the lower fetal abdomen: a common normal variant in the second trimester. J Ultrasound Med 1986; 5: 489–492

95 Dicke J M, Crane J P. Sonographically detected hyperechogenic fetal bowel: significance and implications for pregnancy management. Obstet Gynecol 1992; 80: 778–782

96 Nyberg D A, Dubinsky T, Resta R G et al. Echogenic bowel during the second trimester: clinical importance. Radiology 1993; 188: 527–531

97 Muller F, Dommergues M, Aubry M C et al. Hyperechogenic fetal bowel: an ultrasonographic marker for adverse fetal and neonatal outcome. Am J Obstet Gynecol 1995; 173: 508–513

98 Stringer M D, Thornton J G, Moran G C. Hyperechogenic fetal bowel. Arch Dis Child 1996; 74: F1–F2

99 Sepulveda W, Reid R, Nicolaidis P et al. Second trimester echogenic bowel and intra-amniotic bleeding: association between fetal bowel echogenicity and amniotic fluid spectrophotometry at 410 nm. Am J Obstet Gynecol 1996; 174: 834–842

100 Ewer A K, McHugo J M, Chapman S, Neuvell S J. Fetal echogenic gut: a marker of intrauterine gut ischaemia? Arch Dis Child 1993; 69: 510–513

101 Carroll S G, Maxwell D J. The significance of echogenic areas in the fetal abdomen. Ultrasound Obstet Gynecol 1996; 7: 293–298

102 Sciosa A L, Pretorius D M, Budorick N E et al. Second trimester echogenic bowel and chromosomal abnormalities. Am J Obstet Gynecol 1992; 167: 889–894

103 Gollin J, Gollin G, Shaffer W, Copel J. Increased abdominal echogenicity *in utero*: a marker for intestinal obstruction? Am J Obstet Gynecol 1993; 168: 349

104 Hill L M, Fries J, Hecker J, Grzybec P. Second trimester echogenic small bowel: an increased risk of adverse prenatal outcome. Prenat Diagn 1994; 14: 845–850

105 Sipes S L, Weiner C P, Wenstram K D et al. Fetal echogenic bowel on ultrasound: is there clinical significance? Fetal Diagn Ther 1994; 9: 38–43

106 Slotnick R N, Abuhamad A Z. Prognostic implications of fetal echogenic bowel. Lancet 1996; 347: 85–87

107 Wickstrom E A, Thangavelu M, Parilla B V et al. A prospective study of the association between isolated fetal pyelectasis and chromosomal abnormality. Obstet Gynecol 1996; 88: 379–382

108 Corteville J E, Dicke J M, Crane J. Fetal pyelectasis and Down's syndrome: is genetic amniocentesis warranted? Obstet Gynecol 1992; 79: 770–772

109 Wickstrom E, Maizels M, Sabbagha R et al. Isolated fetal pyelectasis assessment of risk for postnatal uropathy and Down's syndrome. Ultrasound Obstet Gynecol 1996; 8: 236–240

110 Chitty L, Chudleigh T, Campbell S, Pembray M. Incidence, natural history and clinical significance of mild fetal pyelectasis. Br J Radiol 1992; 65: 636

111 Snijders R J M, Nicolaides K H. Ultrasound markers for fetal chromosomal defects. Frontiers in medicine series. London: Parthenon Publishing, 1996

112 Dudley J A, Haworth J M, McGraw M E, Frank J D, Tizard E J. Clinical relevance and implications of antenatal hydronephrosis. Arch Dis Child 1997; 76: F31–F34

113 Schechter A G, Fakhry J, Shapiro L R, Gewitz M H. *In utero* thickening of the *chordae tendinae*: a cause of intracardiac echogenic foci. J Ultrasound Med 1987; 6: 691–695

114 Roberts D J, Genest D. Cardiac histologic pathology characteristic of trisomies 13 and 21. Hum Pathol 1992; 23: 1130–1140

115 Petrikovski B M, Challenger M, Wyse L J. Natural history of echogenic foci within ventricles of the fetal heart. Ultrasound Obstet Gynecol 1995; 5: 92–94

116 Merati R, Lovotti M, Norchi S et al. Prevalence of fetal left ventricular hyperchogenic foci in a low risk population. Br J Obstet Gynecol 1996; 103: 1102–1104

117 Bromley B, Lieberman E, Laboda L, Benaceraff B. Echogenic intracardiac focus: a sonographic sign for fetal Down's syndrome. Obstet Gynecol 1995; 96: 998–1001

118 Sepulveda W, Cullen S, Nicolaidis P et al. Echogenic foci in the fetal heart: a marker of chromosomal abnormality. Br J Obstet Gynaecol 1995; 102: 490–492

119 Simpson J M, Cook A C, Sharland G K. The significance of echogenic foci in the fetal heart: a prospective study of 228 cases. Ultrasound Obstet Gynecol 1996; 8: 225–228

120 How H Y, Villafane J, Parihus R R, Spinnato J A. Small hyperechoic foci of the fetal cardiac ventricle: a benign sonographic finding? Ultrasound Obstet Gynecol 1994; 4: 205–207

121 Achiron R, Lipitz S, Gabbay U, Yagel S. Prenatal ultrasonographic diagnosis of fetal heart echogenic foci: no correlation with Down's syndrome. Obstet Gynecol 1997; 89: 945–948

122 Hall B. Mongolism in newborn infants. Clin Pediatr 1966; 5: 4

123 Greulich W W. A comparison of the dysplastic middle phalanx of the fifth finger in mentally normal caucasian, mongoloids, and negroes, with that of individuals of the same racial groups who have Down's syndrome. AJR 1973; 118: 259–281

124 Benaceraff B R, Osathanond R, Frigoletto F D. Sonographic demonstration of hypoplasia of the middle phalanx of the fifth finger: a finding associated with Down's syndrome. Am J Obstet Gynecol 1988; 159: 181–183

125 Benaceraff B R, Harlow B L, Frigoletto F D. Hypoplasia of the middle phalanx of the fifth finger. a feature of the second trimester fetus with Down's syndrome. J Ultrasound Med 1990; 9: 389–394

126 Jeanty P. Prenatal detection of simian crease. J Ultrasound Med 1990; 9: 131–136

127 Wilkins I. Separation of the great toe in fetuses with Down's syndrome. J Ultrasound Med 1994; 13: 229–231

128 Vintzileos A M, Egan J F. Adjusting the risk for trisomy 21 on the basis of second trimester ultrasonography. Am J Obstet Gynecol 1995; 72: 837–844

129 Nyberg D A, Luthy D A, Cheng E Y et al. Role of prenatal ultrasonography in women with positive screen for Down's syndrome

on the basis of maternal serum markers. Am J Obstet Gynecol 1995; 173: 1030–1035

130 Bewley S, Roberts L J, Mackinson A M, Rodeck C H. First trimester fetal nuchal thickness: problems with screening the general population 2. Br J Obstet Gynaecol 1995; 102: 386–388

131 Nadel A S, Bromley B, Frigoletto F, Benaceraff B R. Can the presumed risk of autosomal trisomy be decreased in fetuses of older women following a normal sonogram? J Ultrasound Med 1995; 1"14: 297–302

132 Szabo J, Gellen J. Nuchal fluid accumulation in trisomy 21 detected by vaginosonography in first trimester. Lancet 1990; iii: 1133

133 Brand-Saberi B, Epperlein H H, Romanos G E, Christ B. Distribution of extracellular matrix components in nuchal skin from fetuses carrying trisomy 18 and trisomy 21. Cell Tissue Res 1994; 277: 465–475

134 Hyett J, Moscoso G, Papapanagiotou G et al. Abnormalities of the heart and great arteries in chromosomally normal fetuses with increased nuchal thickness thickness at 11–13 weeks of gestation. Ultrasound Obstet Gynecol 1996; 7: 245–250

135 Hyett J, Moscoso G, Nicolaides K H. First trimester nuchal thickness and cardiac septal defects in fetuses with trisomy 21. Am J Obstet Gynecol 1995; 172: 1411–1413

136 Roberts L J, Bewley S, Mackinson A M, Rodeck C H. First trimester fetal nuchal thickness: problems with screening the general population 1. Br J Obstet Gynaecol 1995; 102: 381–385

137 Pandya P P, Altman D G, Brizot M L et al. Repeatability of measurement of fetal nuchal thickness thickness. Ultrasound Obstet Gynecol 1995; 5: 334–337

138 Kornman L H, Morssink L P, Beekhuis J R et al. Nuchal thickness cannot be used as a screening test for chromosome abnormalities in the first trimester of pregnancy in a routine ultrasound practice. Prenat Diagn 1996; 16: 747–806

139 Schulte Vallentin M, Schindler H. Non-echogenic nuchal oedema as a marker in trisomy 21 screening. Lancet 1992; 339: 1053

140 Salvodelli G, Binkert F, Achermann J, Schmid W. Ultrasound screening for chromosomal anomalies in the first trimester of pregnancy. Prenat Diagn 1993; 13: 513–518

141 Brambati B, Cislaghi C, Tului L et al. First trimester Down's syndrome screening using nuchal thickness: a prospective study in patients undergoing CVS. Ultrasound Obstet Gynecol 1995; 5: 9–14

142 Comas C, Martinez J M, Ojuel J et al. First-trimester nuchal edema as a marker of aneuploidy. Ultrasound Obstet Gynecol 1995; 5: 26–29

143 Szabo J, Gellen J, Szemere G. First-trimester ultrasound screening for fetal aneuploides in women over 35 and under 35 years of age. Ultrasound Obstet Gynecol 1995; 5: 161–163

144 Hafner E, Schuchter K, Philipp K. Screening for chromosomal abnormalities in an unselected population by fetal nuchal thickness. Ultrasound Obstet Gynecol 1995; 6: 330–333

145 Snijders R J M, Johnson S, Sabire N J et al. First trimester ultrasound screening for chromosomal defects. Ultrasound Obstet Gynecol 1996; 7: 216–276

146 Hyett J A, Sebire N J, Snijders R J M, Nicolaides K H. Intrauterine lethality of trisomy 21 fetuses with increased nuchal thickness thickness. Ultrasound Obstet Gynecol 1996; 7: 101–103

147 Pandya P P, Snijders R J M, Johnson S, Nicolaides K H. Natural history of trisomy 21 fetuses with increased nuchal thickness thickness. Ultrasound Obstet Gynecol 1995; 5: 381–383

148 Hyett J A, Noble P L, Snijders R J M et al. Fetal heart rate in trisomy 21 and other chromosomal abnormalities at 10–14 weeks of gestation. Ultrasound Obstet Gynecol 1996; 7: 239–244

149 Martinez J M, Comas C, Ojuel J et al. Fetal heart rate patterns in pregnancies with chromosomal disorders and subsequent fetal loss. Obstet Gynecol 1996; 87: 118–121

150 Martinez J M, Borrell A, Antohn E et al. Combining nuchal thickness with umbilical artery Doppler velocimetry for detecting fetal trisomies in the first trimester of pregnancy. Br J Obstet Gynaecol 1997; 104: 11–14

151 Noble P L, Abraha H D, Snijders R J M, Sherwood P, Nicolaides K H. Screening for fetal trisomy 21 in the first trimester of pregnancy: maternal serums free B HCG and fetal nuchal thickness thickness. Ultrasound Obstet Gynecol 1995; 6: 390–396

152 Thilaganathan B, Slack A, Wathen N C. Effect of first trimester nuchal thickness on second-trimester maternal serum biochemical screening for Down's syndrome. Ultrasound Obstet Gynecol 1997; 10: 261–264

153 Kadir R A, Economides D L. The affect of nuchal thickness measurement on second-trimester biochemical screening for Down's syndrome. Ultrasound Obstet Gynecol 1997; 9: 244–247

154 Souka A P, Snijders R J M, Novakov A, Soares W, Nicolaides K H. Defects and syndromes in chromosomally normal fetuses with increased nuchal thickness at 10–14 weeks of gestation. Ultrasound Obstet Gynecol 1998; 11: 391–400

155 Obrien W F, Cefalo R C, Bair D G. Ultrasonographic diagnosis of fetal cystic hygroma. Am J Obstet Gynecol 1980; 138: 464–466

156 Azar G B, Snijders R J M, Gooden C, Nicolaides K H. Fetal nuchal cystic hygromata: associated malformations and chromosomal defects. Fetal Diagn Ther 1991; 6: 46–57

157 Nyberg D A, Crane J P. Chromosome abnormalities in diagnostic ultrasound in fetal anomalies. In: Nyberg D A, Mahoney B S, Pretorius D M, eds. St Louis: Mosby Year Book, 1990; 676–724

158 Goldstein R, Lapidus A S, Filly R A. Fetal cephaloceles: diagnosis with ultrasound. Radiology 1991; 180: 803–808

159 Trauffer P M L, Anderson C E, Johnson A et al. The natural history of euploid pregnancies with first trimester cystic hygromas. Am J Obstet Gynecol 1994; 170: 1279–1284

160 Lockwood C, Sciosa A, Stiller R. Sonographic features of the triploid fetus. Am J Obstet Gynecol 1987; 157: 285–287

161 Szulman A E, Philipp E, Bone J G, Bone A. Human triploidy: association with partial hydatidiform moles and non molar conceptuses. Hum Pathol 1982; 12: 1016

162 Rubenstein J B, Swayne L C, Dise C A et al. Placental changes in fetal triploidy syndrome. J Ultrasound Med 1986; 5: 545–550

22

Miscellaneous abnormalities

Peter Twining

Facial abnormalities

Introduction

Abnormalities of the face are among the most common congenital abnormalities[1] and are important not only because there is a high association with chromosomal and genetic conditions[2] but also because facial abnormalities have a major psychological and social impact on an individual.[3] Pruzansky[4] has observed that: 'The face of man is his window on the world, it is the façade by which others perceive and judge him. That which affects the face of man, strikes at the most visible part of his body'. Clifford,[5] commenting on the stigma associated with facial abnormalities, suggests that 'Such a person is marked, not because he fails to achieve the ideal state of "being beautiful" but because he has failed to achieve an unstated minimal standard of acceptability'.

The antenatal diagnosis of facial abnormalities is important, therefore, as it gives the parents time to come to terms with the abnormality and to plan a management strategy which will involve both paediatricians and plastic surgeons. Where other abnormalities are present and a chromosomal or genetic syndrome is suspected, then further investigation such as karyotyping can be considered, or more detailed counselling may be offered by clinical geneticists.

Although standard two-dimensional ultrasound imaging is the mainstay of obstetric anomaly scanning, three-dimensional imaging may add further information, particularly for parents where visualisation of the abnormality may be very difficult.[6] The production of a 'picture' demonstrating the defect has proved to be of particular benefit to some patients (Fig. 22.1). In addition it may also provide paediatric and plastic surgeons with a better idea of the type and extent of the anomaly, and so improve patient counselling and surgical planning. In the UK routine anomaly scanning is offered to all pregnant women, but because of differences in scanning protocols between centres it has been estimated that the fetal face is routinely assessed in only 50% of examinations. Detection rates for fetal facial anomalies range between 25% and 43% in unselected populations.[7–9]

Embryology of the face

The human face is formed between the fourth and 10 weeks of pregnancy by the fusion of five facial swellings: an unpaired frontonasal process, a pair of maxillary swellings and a pair of mandibular swellings. The maxillary and mandibular swellings give rise to the upper and lower jaws (Fig. 22.2A).[10]

During the fifth week the medial and lateral nasal processes appear (Fig. 22.2B) and by the seventh week have fused to form the nose. The maxillary swellings

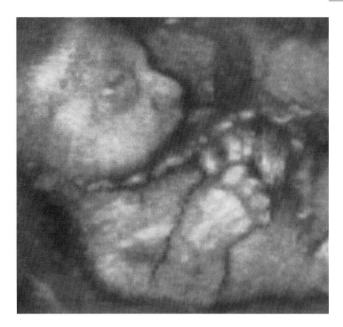

Fig. 22.1 Micrognathia. 3D ultrasound image of a 28-week fetus with marked micrognathia. (Reproduced with permission from ??? P, Methugo J, Pilling D eds Textbook of Fetal Abnormalities. Churchill Livingstone, 1990)

migrate medially and fuse in the midline to form the upper lip and the primary (anterior) palate (Fig. 22.2C, D). The posterior or secondary palate forms from two bands of tissue which arise from the medial walls of the maxillary swellings and fuse in the midline (Fig. 22.3). Thus by 10 weeks the basic facial anatomy is formed.

Normal anatomy

A full assessment of the fetal face requires detailed scanning in the transverse, coronal and sagittal planes; however, routine exclusion of major facial abnormalities can be carried out using a combination of transverse and coronal scanning.

Transverse scanning is useful in assessing the orbits (Fig. 22.4). These are best demonstrated by starting from the standard biparietal diameter section and then rotating the transducer through the anterior cranial fossa to the orbits and nose. Orbital diameters can be assessed subjectively, or reference can be made to standard tables (Figs 22.5 to 22.7).[11] Scanning below the orbits reveals the lips, maxilla and mandible (Fig. 22.8) in transverse section.

The coronal plane is best for demonstrating the lips and nostrils. Once again, starting from the standard biparietal diameter section and rotating through 90° produces the coronal plane. Advancing the transducer anteriorly will provide demonstration of the orbits. In this plane it is important to visualise the lens within the eye (Fig. 22.9). By following the curve of the face, the lips and nose can then be demonstrated (Fig. 22.10).

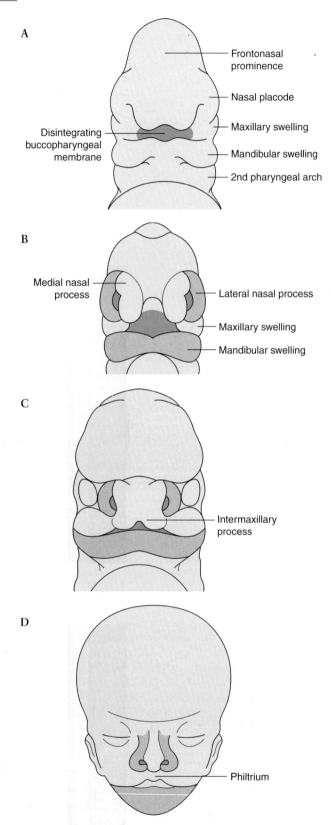

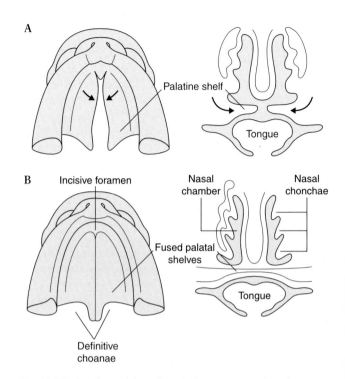

Fig. 22.3 Embryology of the palate. A: Appearances at 8 weeks.
B: Appearances at 10 weeks. (Reproduced with permission from Larsen
W J, Human embryology. Churchill Livingstone, 1993.)

Fig. 22.2 Embryology of the face. A: 5-week fetus; **B:** 6-week fetus;
C: late 7th week; **D:** 10th week. (Reproduced with permission from
Larsen W J, Human embryology. Churchill Livingstone, 1993.)

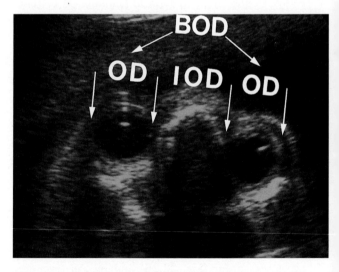

Fig. 22.4 Transverse scan through the orbits. OD – ocular diameter,
IOD – interocular diameter, BOD – binocular diameter.

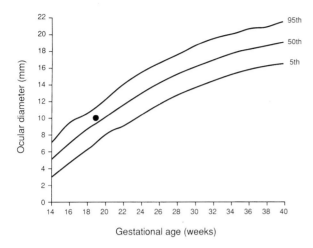

Fig. 22.5 Growth of the ocular diameter. (Reproduced with permission from Jeanty et al. Fetal ocular biometry by ultrasound. Radiology 1982; 143: 513–516.)

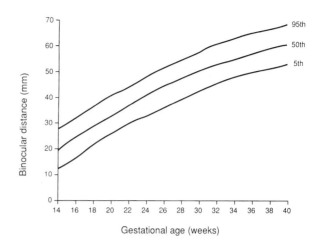

Fig. 22.7 Growth of the binocular distance. (Reproduced with permission from Jeanty et al. Fetal ocular biometry by ultrasound. Radiology 1982; 143: 513–516.)

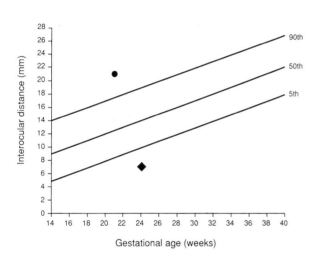

Fig. 22.6 Growth of the interocular distance. (Reproduced with permission from Jeanty et al. Fetal ocular biometry by ultrasound. Radiology 1982; 143: 513–516.)

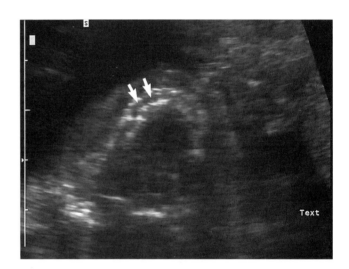

Fig. 22.8 Tooth buds. Transverse scan through the mandible showing tooth buds (arrows).

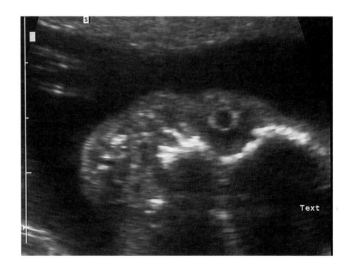

Fig. 22.9 Lens. Coronal scan through the orbit demonstrating the lens.

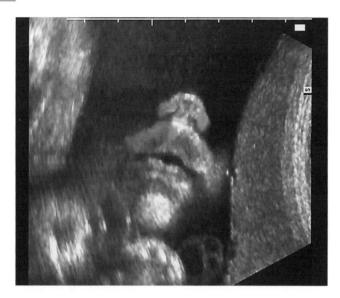

Fig. 22.10 Upper lip and nostrils. Coronal scan through the lips showing the upper lip and nostrils.

The sagittal or profile view is most easily obtained when the fetus is facing the transducer. By scanning from the side of the uterus the profile view can be obtained even when the fetus faces laterally (Fig. 22.11). Turner and Twining were able to produce profile views in 95% of fetuses at 16–20 weeks gestation.[12] The profile view is particularly useful as it gives a global view of the face and is valuable in detecting micrognathia and frontal bossing.

The sagittal plane is also useful for visualising the fetal ears (Fig. 22.12), but the relationship to the head is best

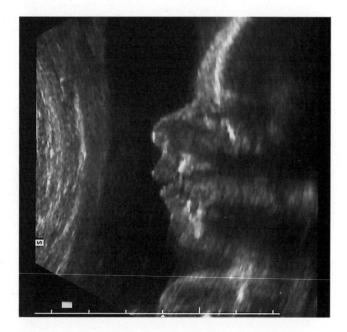

Fig. 22.11 A face in profile. Mid-sagittal section of the face.

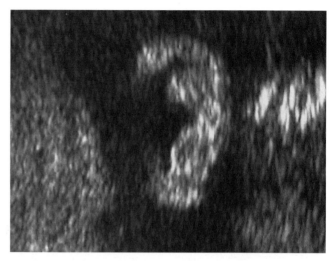

Fig. 22.12 An ear. A sagittal scan through the fetal ear.

assessed by using the coronal plane, which is most appropriate for demonstrating low-set ears (Fig. 22.13).

Facial clefting

Facial clefting was first diagnosed antenatally by Christ and Meininger in 1981,[13] and subsequent reports have confirmed their findings.[14–16]

The incidence of facial clefting is approximately 1 per 1000, but ranges between 0.5 per 1000 for blacks and 2 per 1000 for Asians.[17] Cleft lip is commoner in males, and unilateral cleft lip is seen twice as frequently on the left side than on the right.[18] The recurrence risks for cleft lip and/or palate are outlined in Table 22.1. It should be noted that cleft lip with or without cleft palate and isolated cleft palate are different entities, and that the presence of one does not increase the recurrence risk of the other.[17] Most cases of facial clefting are idiopathic; however, there are a number of causes and associations, including chromosomal and various syndromes, some of which are outlined in Table 22.2.

Table 22.1 Recurrence risks for idiopathic cleft lip with or without cleft palate and cleft palate alone

Affected person	Risk (%)
Cleft lip with or without cleft palate	
One parent	2
One child	4–7
One parent plus one child	11–14
Two children	10
Cleft palate only	
One parent	7
One child	2–5
One parent plus one child	14–17

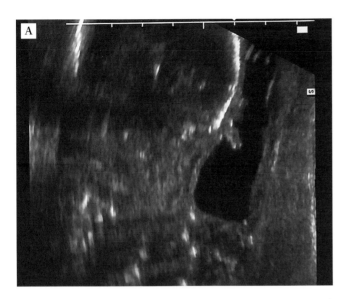 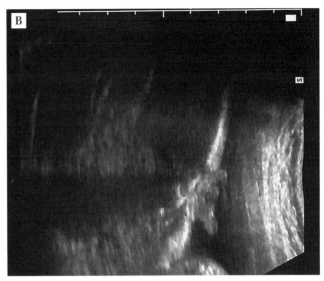

Fig. 22.13 Ears. Coronal scan through the ear and shoulder showing relationship of ear to head and shoulder. **A:** Normal appearances. **B:** Low-set ears.

Table 22.2 Conditions associated with cleft lip with or without cleft palate

Drugs
    Phenytoin
    Carbamazepine
    Steroids
    Diazepam

Chromosomal defects
    Trisomy 13 (65%)
    Trisomy 18 (15%)
    Trisomy 21 (0.5%)
    Triploidy (30%)

Syndromes and malformations
    Amniotic band syndrome
    Holoprosencephaly
    Electrodactyly ectodermal dysplasia syndrome
    Roberts syndrome*
    Miller syndrome*
    Mohr syndrome*
    Frontonasal dysplasia*

*Associated with micrognathia.

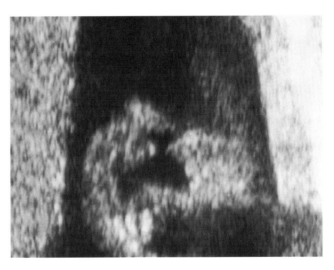

Fig. 22.14 Unilateral cleft lip and palate. Coronal scan showing unilateral cleft lip and palate. (Reproduced with permission from Turner and Twining. The facial profile in the diagnosis of fetal abnormalities. Clinical Radiology 1993; 47: 389–395.)

The diagnosis of facial clefting is based on the demonstration of a vertical defect within the upper lip on scanning in the coronal plane. In unilateral cleft lip the defect is just to the left or right of the midline (Fig. 22.14). In bilateral cleft lip two vertical clefts may be seen, one on either side (Fig. 22.15). In median cleft lip the defect is central and large and is often associated with other facial anomalies and the holoprosencephaly sequence (Fig. 22.16).

Involvement of the palate in unilateral cleft lip can be assessed by scanning into the nose, where a palatal defect is demonstrated (Fig. 22.14). In bilateral cleft lip and palate a central, highly reflective mass of tissue known as premaxillary protrusion may be seen between the clefts, and occasionally obscuring them, (Fig. 22.17).[19] Premaxillary protrusion represents hypertrophied alveolar and gingival tissue between the two clefts and is best visualised on coronal and sagittal scanning. Isolated cleft palate is difficult to demonstrate as the clefting usually involves the posterior or secondary palate. Indirect signs include polyhydramnios and a small stomach bubble.[20] Recent reports indicate that colour Doppler may be of value in demonstrating the flow of liquor across a palatal cleft during fetal breathing (Fig. 22.18).[21]

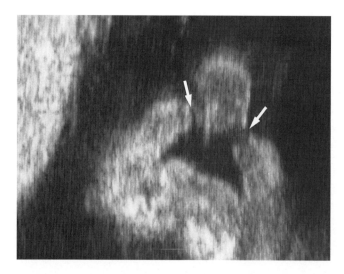

Fig. 22.15 Bilateral cleft lip. Coronal scan showing bilateral clefting (arrows).

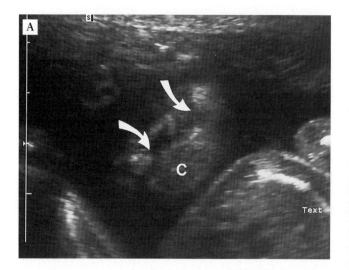

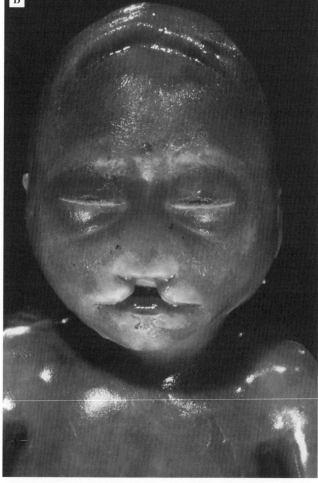

Fig. 22.16 Median facial clefting. A: Coronal scan through the upper lip showing a median cleft lip. C – chin; arrows – edge of cleft. **B:** Post-mortem photograph of affected fetus showing medial clefting. (Courtesy of Dr J. Zucollo, Department of Paediatric Pathology, Nottingham.)

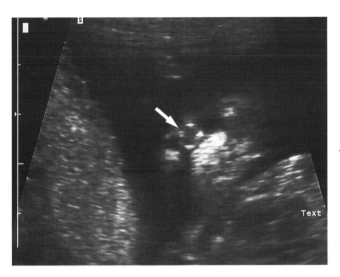

Fig. 22.17 Bilateral cleft lip and palate. Transverse scan showing clefts with central premaxillary protrusion (arrow).

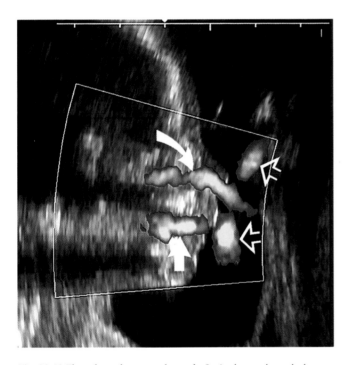

Fig. 22.18 Flow through nose and mouth. Sagittal scan through the fetal face showing flow through the nose (curved arrow) and mouth (straight arrow) demonstrated by colour flow Doppler. (Open arrows point to umbilical cord.)

Once a diagnosis of facial clefting has been made a detailed scan should be carried out looking for other abnormalities, in particular signs of chromosomal disease though if these are normal, other syndromes should be considered (Table 22.2).[22]

Amniotic band syndrome and limb–body wall complex

The incidence of amniotic band syndrome has been estimated to be between 1 in 1200 and 1 in 1500 live births, but accounts for up to 1 in 50 spontaneous abortions.[23,24]

The syndrome is related to early amnion rupture, which allows the embryo to enter the chorionic cavity and become entangled in the fibrous septa that cross the chorionic space. The septa or bands produce amputation defects and very specific forms of facial clefting. The most typical finding is a vertical cleft involving the orbit, or a lateral cleft.[25,26] Others include lateral encephalocele, limb amputation defects and abdominal wall defects which may involve the chest wall (gastropleuroschisis).[27] The spine is often involved with a marked kyphoscoliosis and the association with an abdominal wall defect is almost diagnostic of the amniotic band syndrome.[26] The prognosis is extremely poor.

Ectrodactyly ectodermal dysplasia syndrome

This syndrome combines facial clefting with characteristic hand and foot abnormalities.[28] The most frequent finding is a cleft hand or foot, with wide separation of the fingers and toes (Fig. 22.19). The features can be variable and occasionally mild, so exclusion of the syndrome may be difficult. Renal abnormalities may be seen, including hydronephrosis and reflux. The syndrome is inherited in an autosomal dominant mode.

Roberts syndrome

This autosomal recessive condition combines facial clefting and micrognathia with major limb reduction abnormalities, which are more severe in the arms.[29] These range from

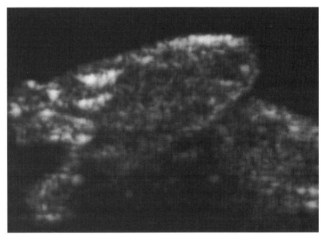

Fig. 22.19 Ectrodactyly–ectodermal dysplasia clefting syndrome. Scan showing cleft foot.

phocomelia through to radial or humeral aplasia. Associated abnormalities include congenital heart disease and renal dysplasia.[30] The prognosis is very poor and most affected babies do not survive the neonatal period.

Micrognathia

Micrognathia is seldom an isolated finding unless mild, in which case it is likely to be a normal variant. More severe forms are almost always part of a chromosomal, skeletal or genetic syndrome. Jones[31] lists 54 syndromes in which micrognathia may be a feature. Table 22.3 outlines some of the commoner associations.[32]

Micrognathia is best demonstrated using the profile view, where the relationship of the mandible to the maxilla can be clearly seen (Fig. 22.20). An important associated finding is polyhydramnios, which should always prompt a detailed assessment of the face and mandible.

The most common association is with chromosomal disease and trisomy 18 in particular. Nicolaides *et al*.[2]

Table 22.3 Causes of micrognathia

Idiopathic	Mild form
Chromosomal disease	Trisomy 18, triploidy
Skeletal dysplasias	Camptomelic dysplasia Diastrophic dysplasia Short rib polydactyly syndrome Achondrogenesis
Genetic syndromes	Treacher–Collins syndrome Goldenhars syndrome Hemifacial microsomia Pierre–Robin syndrome Seckel syndrome Pena–Shokeir syndrome

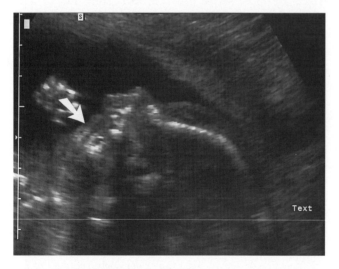

Fig. 22.20 Micrognathia. Sagittal scan through a fetus with trisomy 18 showing micrognathia (arrow points to hypoplastic mandible).

reported 56 cases of micrognathia, 66% of which were associated with chromosomal disease. The other main group of associated abnormalities are the skeletal dysplasias. Turner and Twining[12] found four cases of skeletal dysplasias in nine fetuses with micrognathia, and the conditions included diastrophic dysplasia, camptomelic dysplasia and the short rib polydactyly syndrome.

There are also a number of rare genetic syndromes associated with micrognathia: these include the Treacher-Collins syndrome, Goldenhars' syndrome, hemifacial microsomia and Seckel syndrome.

The Treacher-Collins syndrome has an autosomal dominant inheritance, so there is often a family history of the condition. The main features are micrognathia associated with absent or low-set ears.[33] There is often polyhydramnios; however, the syndrome may be mild and produce subtle ultrasound findings and so it may not be excluded on detailed ultrasound scanning.[34]

Goldenhars' syndrome and hemifacial microsomia are similar to the Treacher-Collins syndrome, but the micrognathia is often asymmetrical and there is a high association with cardiac defects, mainly ventricular septal defects and Fallot's tetralogy.[35,36] The inheritance is also different, as most cases of Goldenhars' and hemifacial microsomia are sporadic.

The Pierre-Robin syndrome (Robin anomalad) usually presents as fairly marked micrognathia associated with polyhydramnios.[37] As in other forms of micrognathia, paediatric support at delivery is important in the management of these babies.[38]

The Seckel syndrome is a rare autosomal recessive syndrome with a characteristic appearance on ultrasound scanning. The main features are micrognathia associated with growth retardation and microcephaly, producing a receding forehead and large beaked nose (Fig. 22.21).[39] There is moderate shortening of the long bones and long-term outcomes indicate moderate to severe mental retardation.[40]

Severe micrognathia has a poor outlook and Bromley and Benaceraff reported only four survivors in their series of 20 cases.[32] Nicolaides[2] also stressed the poor prognosis and reported only one survivor in the group of 19 fetuses with a normal karyotype.

The major cause of death in the neonatal period is related to respiratory insufficiency and also to the high rate of associated malformations. It is essential to have paediatric support present at delivery in order to expedite endotracheal intubation should it be required.

Macroglossia

Macroglossia is an uncommon finding but usually indicates either trisomy 21 or Beckwith–Wiedemann syndrome. In their series of 146 fetuses with facial anomalies, Nicolaides *et al*.[2] documented 13 cases of macroglossia,

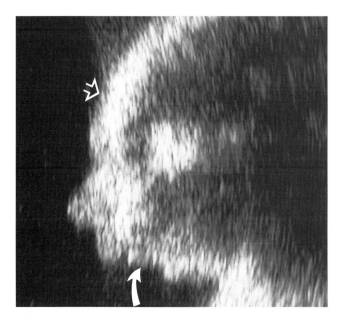

Fig. 22.21 Seckel syndrome. Profile view showing severe micrognathia (curved arrow) and small forehead secondary to microcephaly (open arrow). (Reproduced with permission from Twining P, McHugo J, Pilling D, eds. Textbook of fetal abnormalities. Churchill Livingstone, 1999.)

nine of which were found to have trisomy 21 and two the Beckwith–Wiedemann syndrome.

Beckwith–Wiedemann syndrome comprises macroglossia, visceromegaly, macrosomia and omphalocele.[41] Intelligence is usually normal but there is an increased risk of malignancy in childhood, especially Wilms' tumours.[31]

Tumours and masses in the mouth

Nasopharyngeal teratoma accounts for less than 1% of all teratomas, which have an overall incidence of 1 in 20 000–40 000 live births.[42]

Nasopharyngeal teratomas arise from the palate and, as they enlarge, they protrude through the mouth to produce a large mixed cystic and solid mass distorting the mouth and extending into the amniotic fluid (Fig. 22.22). There is often associated polyhydramnios due to reduced fetal swallowing. The outlook is very poor, with most babies succumbing in the early neonatal period because of respiratory insufficiency.

In view of the high neonatal mortality rate aggressive obstetric management has been proposed, with serial amniocentesis, followed by caesarean section when pulmonary maturity has been achieved. Paediatric surgical support should be present at delivery to perform a tracheotomy should it be necessary.[43]

Epulis or congenital gingival granular cleft tumour appears as a homogeneous mass arising from the upper gum. The mass is round and well defined and displaces the lips and tongue.[44] Following surgical excision the outcome is good.

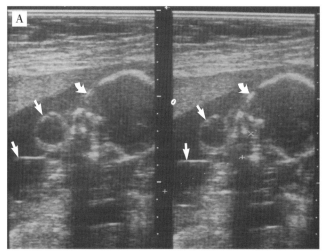

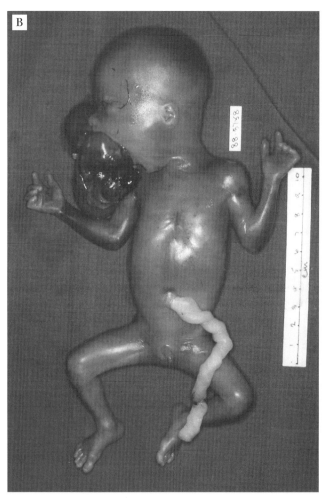

Fig. 22.22 Nasopharyngeal teratoma. A: Scan through the head showing a mixed cystic and solid tumour arising through the mouth (curved arrow points to skull, straight arrows point to tumour). **B:** Post-mortem photograph of the fetus with nasopharyngeal teratoma. (Reproduced with permission from Twining P, McHugo J, Pilling D, eds. Textbook of fetal abnormalities. Churchill Livingstone, 1999.)

Very rarely an encephalocele can involve the skull base and protrude into the mouth, producing a cystic mass within or extending out of the mouth.[45] A useful sign in the diagnosis is the presence of abnormal intracranial anatomy. The main differential diagnosis of a cystic mass within the mouth is a salivary gland cyst. Shipp *et al.*[46] reported a case diagnosed at 22 weeks as a simple intra-oral cyst. The cyst remained unchanged in size during pregnancy and was aspirated in the neonatal period.

The nose and orbits

Holoprosencephaly

Holoprosencephaly has an incidence of 1 in 5000–10 000 live births and is a complex brain abnormality consisting, in its most severe alobar form, of a single ventricular cavity, fused thalami and the absence of the midline structures.[47] It is associated with a number of characteristic facial abnormalities, which prompted De Meyer[48] to state that the face predicts the brain. The most common findings in the face include cyclopia, ethmocephaly, cebocephaly, hypotelorism and facial clefting (Fig. 22.23).

Cyclopia

This is an uncommon finding in holoprosencephaly and represents ocular fusion to produce a single orbit. Usually the ocular fusion is incomplete and two fused eyes can be seen with the single orbit (Fig. 22.24). The nose is situated above the eye in the form of a proboscis (Fig. 22.25).

Ethmocephaly

This facial appearance consists of severe hypotelorism (orbits too close together) associated with a proboscis at the level of the orbits.

Cebocephaly

This is characterised by hypotelorism and a hypoplastic nose with a single nostril. The profile view often reveals an abnormally shaped nose (Fig. 22.26).

Hypotelorism

Hypotelorism is commonly associated with holoprosencephaly and may be the only finding of note. It is rarely seen in other conditions and so is a fairly specific feature of holoprosencephaly.

Facial clefting

The facial clefting in holoprosencephaly is either median (midline) facial clefting or bilateral cleft lip and palate. Median clefting is often associated with nasal hypoplasia and hypotelorism (Fig. 22.27).

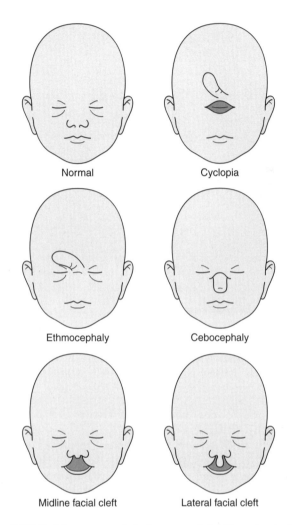

Fig. 22.23 Facial appearances in holoprosencephaly. (Reproduced with permission from Nyberg D A, ed. Diagnostic ultrasound of fetal anomalies: text and atlas. Mosby Year Book, 1990.)

Abnormalities of the orbits

Hypertelorism

Hypertelorism (increased distance between the orbits) may be seen in a number of rare conditions and genetic syndromes, some of which are outlined in Table 22.4.

Frontonasal dysplasia is a rare midfacial syndrome associated with marked hypertelorism, a broad nasal tip which may be cleft and occasionally facial clefting.[49,50] Intelligence is usually normal and plastic surgery can produce good cosmetic results.

A frontal encephalocele can present as severe hypertelorism associated with a large anterior midline skull defect. Associated abnormalities include hydrocephalus and agenesis of the corpus callosum. The outcome is better than for occipital encepholocele and the main disabilities are facial disfigurement, anosmia and visual disturbances.[51,52]

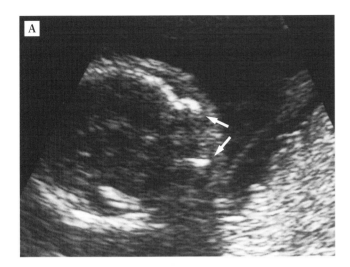

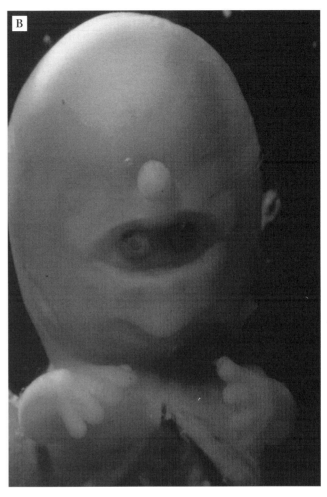

Fig. 22.24 Cyclopia. A: Transverse scan through a single orbit (arrows). **B:** Post-mortem photograph of a fetus showing cyclopia and a proboscis. (Reproduced with permission from Twining P, McHugo J, Pilling D, eds. Textbook of fetal abnormalities. Churchill Livingstone, 1999.)

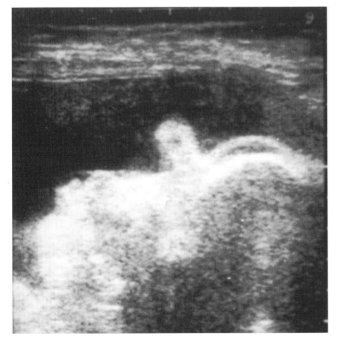

Table 22.4 Syndromes associated with hypertelorism

Frontonasal dysplasia
Frontal encephalocele
Craniosynostosis syndromes
   Apert's syndrome
   Saethre–Chotzen syndrome
   Pfeiffer syndrome
   Crouzon syndrome
Di George syndrome
Hydrolethalus syndrome
Coffin–Lowry syndrome
Noonan syndrome
Larsen syndrome

Fig. 22.25 Proboscis. Midline sagittal view of fetal face demonstrating a proboscis.

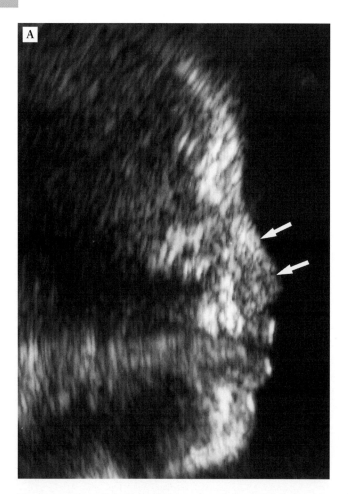
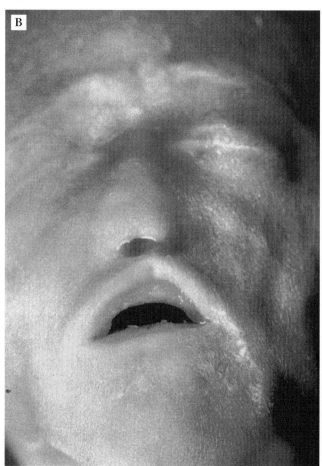

Fig. 22.26 Cebocephaly. A: Sagittal scan through the fetal face showing an abnormal nose (arrows). **B:** Post-mortem of same fetus showing hypotelorism and a single nostril. (Reproduced with permission from Turner and Twining. The facial profile in the diagnosis of fetal abnormalities. Clinical Radiology 1993; 47: 389–395.)

Other causes of hypertelorism include the craniosynostosis syndromes.

Microphthalmia and anophthalmia

Microphthalmia occurs with an incidence of approximately 1 in 5000 live births, whereas anophthalmia is less common, occurring in 1 in 20 000.[53] It may be difficult clinically to differentiate between severe microphthalmia and anophthalmia, but sonographically the distinction may be possible. Both conditions may present with a small orbit; however, if the lens is present then the diagnosis is most likely microphthalmia, as absence of the lens indicates anophthalmia.[54]

Microphthalmia is diagnosed sonographically as asymmetry of the orbits if unilateral (Fig. 22.28), or small orbits bilaterally if both eyes are affected. Charts of the normal ranges of orbital measurements should be referred to (Figs 22.5 to 22.7), as occasionally the appearances may be subtle. Anophthalmia should be suspected if the lens cannot be demonstrated within a small orbit. In addition, it should be noted that anophthalmia may occur later in pregnancy: Brownstein et al.[55] reported two cases of anophthalmia in their series of orbital abnormalities and in both cases orbital measurements were normal in the first trimester. This suggests that scanning should not only be carried out during the second trimester, but also later on in pregnancy in patients with a family history of anophthalmia.

Both anophthalmia and microphthalmia are associated with chromosomal disease, genetic syndromes and intracranial abnormalities. When these orbital abnormalities are found, a careful search should be carried out for other abnormalities and a karyotype examination considered.

The outlook depends to a large extent on the associated abnormalities or syndrome. Reconstructive surgery can be carried out to improve the cosmetic appearance.

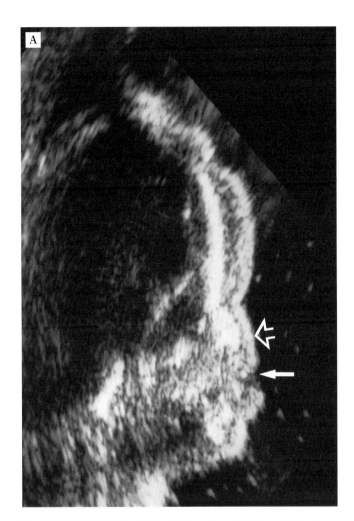

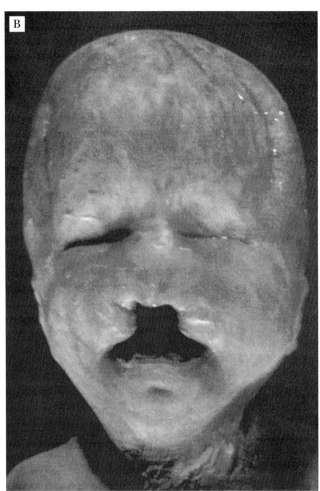

Fig. 22.27 Medial clefting. A: Sagittal scan through a fetus with holoprosencephaly showing a flat profile, nasal hypoplasia and absence of the upper lip, indicating median clefting (straight arrow points to absence of the upper lip, open arrow – hypoplastic nose). **B:** Post-mortem photograph showing medial clefting. (Reproduced with permission from Turner and Twining. The facial profile in the diagnosis of fetal abnormalities. Clinical Radiology 1993; 47: 389–395.)

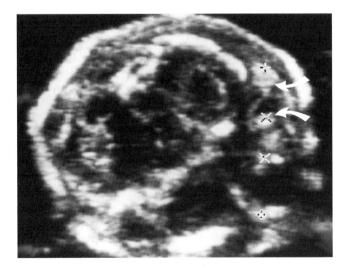

Fig. 22.28 Microphthalmia. Transverse scan through the fetal head showing microphthalmia (arrows). (Published with permission from Twining P, McHugo J, Pilling D, eds. Textbook of fetal abnormalities. Churchill Livingstone, 1999.)

Congenital cataracts

Congenital cataracts have an incidence of approximately 1 in 5000–10 000 births[56] and have many causes, including congenital infection, enzyme disorders and rare genetic syndromes.[57] There are three sonographic appearances. The first is complete opacification of the lens, the second is a double ring appearance, where the cataract appears as a ring within the lens and thirdly as a central highly reflective area within the lens.[56]

Dacrocystocele

Dacrocystoceles are cysts of the lacrimal ducts and are typically located inferomedial to the orbit. They are not generally detected prior to 30 weeks gestation, and are usually no more than 1 cm in diameter.[58] They may resolve spontaneously during pregnancy or during the first few months of life.[46]

Abnormalities of the forehead

Frontal bossing

Frontal bossing has been described in a number of skeletal dysplasias, craniosynostosis syndromes and rare genetic syndromes (Table 22.5). It is best visualised using the profile view or sagittal scan plan (Fig. 22.29). The most common skeletal dysplasias demonstrating frontal bossing are thanatophoric dysplasia and achondroplasia, however, the latter condition may not become apparent until the third trimester.[12]

The flat profile

The most important association with a flat profile is trisomy 21 but a number of rare associations have also been reported.[31] Once again the flat facial profile is best appreciated on the sagittal scan plane.

Table 22.5 Syndromes associated with frontal bossing

Skeletal dysplasias
Achondroplasia
Thanatophoric dysplasia
Achondrogenesis
Craniosynostosis syndromes
Crouzon syndrome
Pfeiffer syndrome
Craniofrontonasal dysplasia
Other syndromes
Russell–Silver syndrome
Robinson syndrome

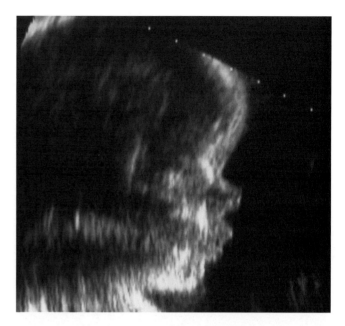

Fig. 22.29 Frontal bossing. Sagittal scan through a fetus with achondroplasia taken at 28 weeks gestation. Note that at 20 weeks the appearances were normal. (Reproduced with permission from Turner and Twining. The facial profile in the diagnosis of fetal abnormalities. Clinical Radiology 1993; 47: 389–395.)

Harlequin ichthyosis

This rare condition is characterised by thickened, fissured skin which resembles the diamond pattern of the harlequin costume. The sonographic features include thickened skin which may slough off.[52] The mouth is held fixed and open and is 'O' shaped owing to eversion of the lips. Cystic masses are seen anterior to the orbits due to the pronounced eversion of the eyelids.[59,60] There may also be flexion deformity of the limbs. The outlook is very poor and most affected neonates die within hours or days of birth. The inheritance is autosomal recessive.

Umbilical cord

Embryology

The umbilical arteries first appear in the fifth week of pregnancy as ventral branches of the paired dorsal aortas. The two dorsal aortas fuse and the definitive umbilical arteries originate as two lateral branches from the caudal end of the descending aorta.[61] Simultaneously, an arterial plexus forms around the allantois to form a single artery extending almost the entire length of the body stalk. As the right and left umbilical arteries advance distally within the body stalk, this allantoic artery shortens relative to the umbilical arteries. Eventually the allantoic artery unites with both umbilical arteries to form the interarterial anastomosis, normally present near the placental insertion.[61]

Abnormalities of cord length and twisting

The mature umbilical cord is made up of two umbilical arteries and a single, larger umbilical vein (Fig. 22.30). The right umbilical artery is usually larger than the left, and this may be a factor in the direction of twisting of the umbilical cord.[62] It is well established that left or counterclockwise twists are seven times more common than right or clockwise twists in the normal three-vessel cord. It has been postulated that the rotational torque resulting from differential blood flow between the left and right umbilical arteries produces preferential twisting to the left.[62] The number of twists present during the first trimester is roughly the same as that seen in term cords (most often between 0 and 40),

indicating that the cord lengthens by an increase in pitch between each turn of its helix, rather than an increase in the number of turns.[62] Indeed, Leonardo da Vinci observed in the 15th century that 'the length of the umbilical cord is equal to the length of the child in every stage of its age'.[63]

Short umbilical cords are seen in multiple abnormality syndromes, such as the amniotic band syndrome and the limb–body wall complex. In addition, fetal akinesia conditions such as the Pena–Shokeir syndrome can be associated with a shortened umbilical cord.[64]

Absence of cord twisting (Fig. 22.31) is seen in 5% of live births, 7% of twin pregnancies and 15% of single umbilical artery cords. The frequency of absent cord twisting in cases of intra-uterine death is 18%, but whether this is a cause or an effect is difficult to determine.[62] Recent work confirms a higher incidence of fetal death, heart rate decelerations, caesarean section for fetal distress and fetal anomalies in cases of absent cord twisting.[65] It would therefore be prudent to carry out follow-up scans to check for fetal growth and well-being if this finding is documented in the second trimester.

Single umbilical artery

Most cases of single umbilical artery probably result from atresia of a previously formed umbilical artery and this abnormality occurs in up to 1% of all pregnancies.[61,66,67] Although occasional absence of an umbilical artery has been observed since Renaissance times, it was not until 1870 that Josef Hyrtle, Professor of Anatomy at Vienna, reported the first series of 14 cases in his monograph on the blood vessels of the human placenta.[68]

A single umbilical artery may be demonstrated either by scanning transversely through the cord (Fig. 22.32) or scanning through the fetal pelvis to demonstrate the

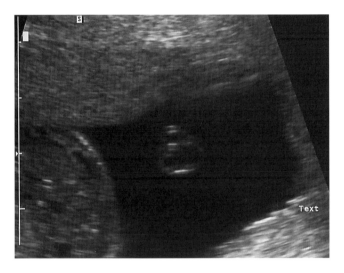

Fig. 22.30 Normal three-vessel cord.

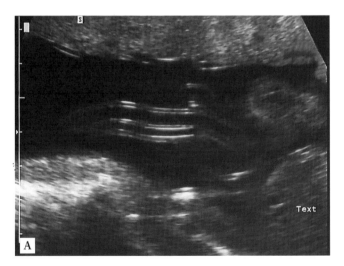
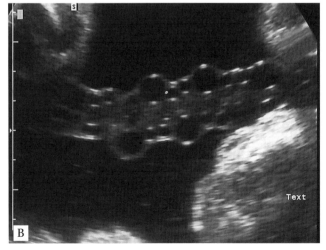

Fig. 22.31 Umbilical cords. A: The straight umbilical cord – absence of normal coiling. B: Normal coiled cord.

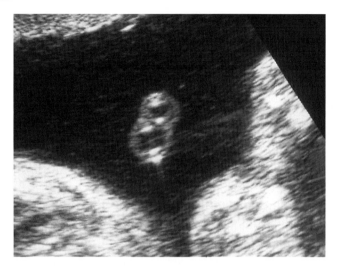

Fig. 22.32 Single umbilical artery.

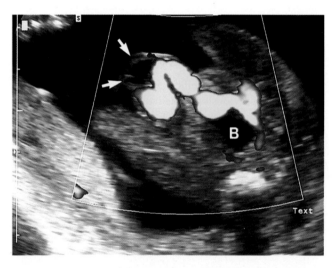

Fig. 22.33 Single umbilical artery. Scan through fetal pelvis showing small omphalocele (arrows) and colour flow demonstrating a single umbilical artery around the bladder (B).

Table 22.6 Ultrasound-detectable abnormalities associated with a single umbilical artery

Abnormality	Approximate incidence (%)
Urinary tract	
Renal dysplasia	19
Renal agenesis	11
Hydronephrosis/hydro-ureter	11
Cardiac	
Ventricular septal defect	21
Atrial septal defect	9
Hypoplastic left heart	3
Truncus arteriosis	7
Fallot's tetralogy	3
Coarctation of the aorta	3
Skeleton	
Cleft lip and palate	13
Talipes	12
Polydactyly	8
Long bone abnormalities	8
Sacral agenesis	1
Gastrointestinal tract	
Omphalocele	13
Gastroschisis	3
Tracheo-oesophageal fistula	8
Gut atresia	4
Imperforate anus	16
Craniospinal defects	
Anencephaly	11
Spina bifida	8
Hydrocephaly	3
Holoprosencephaly	4
Microcephaly	2
Cerebellar abnormalities	2
Miscellaneous	
Diaphragmatic hernia	8
Cystic hygroma	9
Sacrococcygeal teratoma	3

absence of one umbilical artery coursing around the bladder (Fig. 22.33). Demonstration of a single umbilical artery at the fetal end of the cord is probably more important than a single umbilical artery observed near the placental end, as the umbilical arteries may normally fuse for a variable distance before inserting into the placenta.[61,69] A single umbilical artery is commoner in multiple pregnancies and has a higher incidence of absence of cord twisting than does a three-vessel cord.[62]

Associated abnormalities are seen in up to 20% of cases of single umbilical artery, though there seems to be no specific pattern of anomalies.[70] The most common involve the musculoskeletal, genitourinary, cardiovascular, gastrointestinal and central nervous systems (Table 22.6).

Multiple abnormalities raise the possibility of chromosomal disease the commonest being trisomy 18, followed by trisomy 13, Turner's syndrome and triploidy.[61,71,72] The detection of a single umbilical artery should prompt a careful sonographic examination of the fetus to exclude associated abnormalities. If abnormalities are present, a karyotype test should be considered. When a single umbilical artery is an isolated finding it should not affect the clinical outcome.[61]

Persistent right umbilical vein

In the 4-week embryo the chorionic veins unite to form a single umbilical vein which bifurcates in the mid-cord to form the right and left umbilical veins. The right umbilical vein normally regresses and the left umbilical vein persists to form the umbilical vein, which then communicates with the left portal vein (Fig. 22.34). If these communications

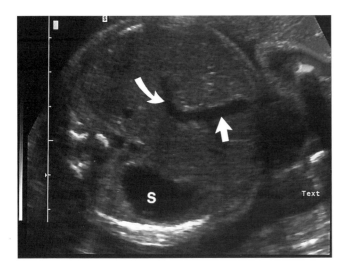

Fig. 22.34 Normal appearances of the umbilical vein. Transverse scan through fetal abdomen showing umbilical vein (straight arrow) joining the portal view (curved arrow). S – stomach.

do not occur, the umbilical veins form aberrant connections, so that they may bypass the liver and communicate directly with the right atrium, inferior vena cava or iliac veins, or drain through a caput medusae (subcutaneous anastomosis) (Fig. 22.35). These aberrant connections are commonly associated with persistence of the right umbilical vein (Table 22.7). Although early reported series of persistence of the right umbilical vein showed a high incidence of associated abnormalities,[73,74] later reports suggest this may be a benign normal variant.[75–77].

The sonographic appearance of a persistent right umbilical vein depends on the structure with which it commun-

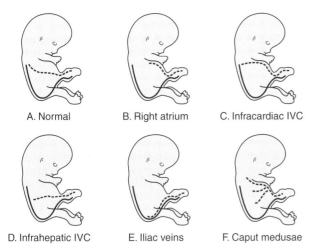

Fig. 22.35 The possible communications of the right umbilical vein. A: Normal, B: right artrium, C: infracardiac IVC, D: infrahepatic IVC, E: iliac veins, F: caput medusae. (Reproduced with permission from Jeanty P. Persistent right umbilical vein: an ominous prenatal finding, Radiology 1990; 177: 735–738.)

Table 22.7 Anomalies associated with persistent right umbilical vein (Reproduced with permission from Jeanty P. Persistent right umbilical vein: an ominous prenatal finding. Radiology 1990; 177: 735–738)

Gastrointestinal
    Anomalies of liver segmentation and the position of the ligamentum teres (to the right of the gallbladder) in all fetuses
    Malrotation of the bowel
    Tracheo-oesophageal fistula
    Annular pancreas
    Duodenal atresia
    Imperforate anus
    Accessory spleen
    Echogenic bowel
    Ascites

Cardiovascular
    Situs inversus
    Atrial septal defect
    Absence of ductus venosus
    Total anomalous pulmonary venous return (infracardiac type)
    Ventricular septal defect
    Aberrant right subclavian artery
    Caput medusae
    Ductal agenesis when vein bypasses the liver
    Mitral atresia
    Coarctation of aorta
    Double-outlet right ventricle
    Hydrops

Musculoskeletal
    Phocomelia
    Hemivertebra
    Sirenomelia
    Moderately short limbs
    Simian crease

Genitourinary
    Unilateral agenesis of kidney
    Bilateral hydronephrosis
    Unicornuate uterus
    Ectopic kidney
    Hypospadias
    Allantoic duct remnant

Miscellaneous
    Polyhydramnios
    Single umbilical artery
    Normal
    Thickened nuchal fold

icates. When this is the right portal vein, the umbilical vein passes lateral to and to the right of the gallbladder, where it connects to the right portal vein. When it is the inferior vena cava, the umbilical vein courses directly across the abdomen to insert into the inferior vena cava (Fig. 22.36). Insertion into the iliac vein is best demonstrated on sagittal scanning, where the umbilical vein can be seen descending into the pelvis and inserting into the iliac vein below the level of the bladder (Fig. 22.37).

The evaluation of a persistent right umbilical vein should include a meticulous search for associated abnormalities which determine fetal outcome. Isolated persistence of the right umbilical vein appears to have a good outcome.

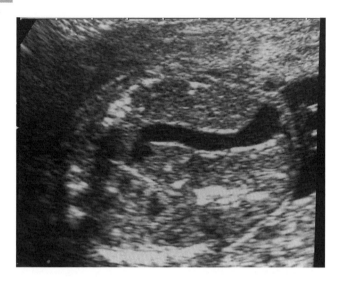

Fig. 22.36 Persistence of the right umbilical vein. Transverse scan through the fetal abdomen showing persistence of the right umbilical vein inserting into the inferior vena cava. Hepatic calcifications represent focal areas of hepatic necrosis. (Reproduced with permission from Twining P, McHugo J, Pilling D, eds. Textbook of fetal anomalies. Churchill Livingstone, 1999.)

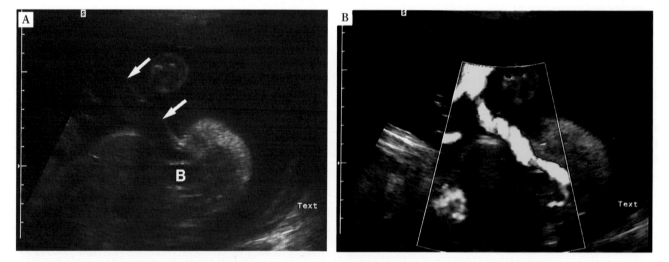

Fig. 22.37 Persistence of the right umbilical vein. A: Sagittal scan through fetal abdomen showing persistence of the right umbilical vein (straight arrows) draining into the right iliac vein. B – bladder. **B:** Colour flow image showing umbilical vein draining into iliac vein.

The small number of cases reported where the umbilical vein inserts into the iliac vein have suggested an association with Noonan's syndrome.[78–80]

Umbilical vein varix

Focal dilatation or varix of the umbilical vein is an uncommon finding, accounting for only 4% of all cord abnormalities.[74] The varix may affect the intra-abdominal portion of the umbilical vein (Fig. 22.38) or the intra-amniotic umbilical vein.

Varix of the intra-abdominal portion of the umbilical vein should be differentiated from other intra-abdominal cysts, such as choledochal cysts, duplication cysts and mesenteric cysts. A varix of the umbilical vein forms a continuation with the umbilical vein and also shows spectral and colour Doppler signals which easily differentiate it from other abdominal cystic lesions. Intra-abdominal varix of the umbilical vein appears to have a good outcome.[81,82]

However, varix of the intra-amniotic portion of the umbilical vein is associated with a high risk of both umbilical venous and arterial thrombosis and subsequent fetal demise.[83–86] In view of this delivery of the fetus as soon as lung maturity is established[87] has been advocated in order to avoid the risk of cord thrombosis. Varix of the intra-amniotic portion of the umbilical cord is differentiated from cord cysts by the presence of venous Doppler signals.

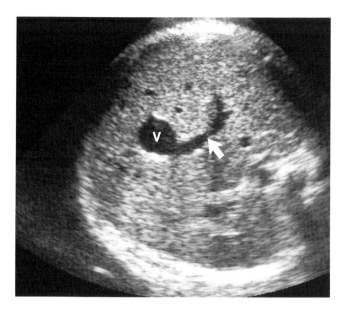

Fig. 22.38 Umbilical vein varix. *Varix of the intra-abdominal portion of umbilical vein. V–varix. Arrow – portal vein.*

Umbilical cord cysts

Umbilical cord cysts are usually classified into either true cysts or pseudocysts. True cysts are derived from the embryological remnants of either the allantois or the omphalomesenteric duct. They have an epithelial lining and are located close to the fetal insertion of the cord.[88] True cord cysts usually measure 1–2 cm in diameter. Pseudocysts are more common than true cysts and may also be located close to the fetal cord insertion. They are thought to represent localised oedema or degeneration of Wharton's jelly (Fig. 22.39).[89]

Umbilical cord cysts appear to be common in the first trimester and can occur in up to 3% of pregnancies.[88] It is

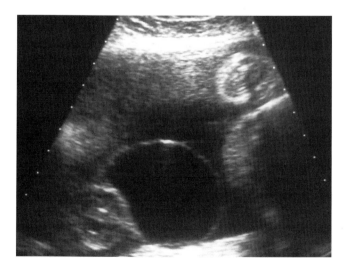

Fig. 22.39 Umbilical cord cyst.

thought that they are pseudocysts as the majority resolve by 20 weeks gestation.

Umbilical cord cysts seen in the second trimester can be associated with omphalocele, patent urachus, Meckel's diverticulum and chromosomal disease.[89–96] The commonest chromosomal abnormality seen is trisomy 18 but in most cases multiple abnormalities are present. The detection of an umbilical cord cyst should therefore prompt a careful assessment of the fetus, with special attention to visualisation of the cord insertion and also signs of chromosomal disease, particularly trisomy 18. When cord cysts are seen in the first trimester, these fetuses should be followed up and detailed scanning carried out at 18–20 weeks gestation.

The differential diagnosis of umbilical cord cysts should include a varix of the intra-amniotic portion of the umbilical cord, an umbilical artery aneurysm[97] and a haemangioma of the cord.[98]

True knots of the cord

True knots of the cord are estimated to occur in 1% of pregnancies but are not usually detected with ultrasound.[74] True knots are usually of no significance but have been associated with fetal demise. They are thought to be more common in long cords, male fetuses and multiparous women.[97] If a true cord knot is detected then it would be prudent to monitor the pregnancy regularly for fetal growth and well-being.[98–100]

Unusual abdominal cysts

Choledochal cysts

Choledochal cysts represent dilatation of part of the extrahepatic biliary tree. Sonographically they appear in the right upper quadrant in a subhepatic location separate from the gallbladder and stomach (Fig. 22.40).[101,102] The differential diagnosis includes a duplication cysts of the duodenum or a mesenteric cyst. Occasionally dilated intrahepatic ducts may be seen in association with the cyst, and this is virtually pathognomonic of the condition.[103,104] Early neonatal surgery is indicated to remove the cyst.

Ovarian cysts

Ovarian cysts are one of the commonest abdominal cysts. They usually present in the third trimester, either as single or multiple cysts in the pelvis or lower abdomen, but may be present anywhere within the abdomen. The cysts are thought to be a result of excessive stimulation of the fetal ovary by both placental and maternal hormones.[105,106]

Most cysts remain unchanged in size and may occasionally decrease prior to delivery. The majority of simple

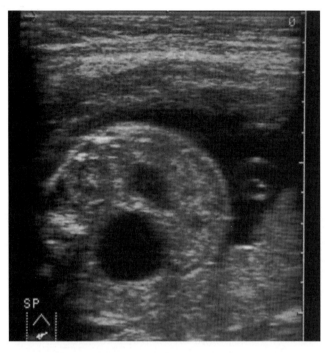

Fig. 22.40 Choledochal cyst. Transverse scan through upper abdomen demonstrating a choledochal cyst.

ovarian cysts resolve within the first few months of life.[106] If they persist then aspiration in the neonatal period has been advocated.[107]

Torsion has been estimated to occur in approximately 27% of ovarian cysts and is more common with large cysts.[107,108] The presence of solid areas (Fig. 22.41A) or layering of debris within a cyst (Fig. 22.41B) should raise the possibility of torsion and most authors recommend surgical excision in the early neonatal period.[106–109]

The main differential diagnoses of ovarian cysts are duplication and mesenteric cysts. Demonstration of the fetal gender is useful in the diagnosis.

Duplication and mesenteric cysts

Duplication cysts can occur anywhere within the abdomen and can mimic many other abdominal cysts and pathologies (Fig. 22.42). Most do not increase in size and can usually be investigated in the neonatal period.

Mesenteric cysts are commonly multiloculated and can be extensive. Other cystic intra-abdominal masses include urinomas, which are closely related to the kidney and are caused by extravasation of urine secondary to obstruction (Fig. 22.43). An uncommon cause of a large cystic mass is a meconium pseudocyst (Fig. 22.44). These usually result from perforation of the bowel, with extrusion of meconium into the peritoneal cavity. Intra-abdominal calcification and dilated bowel loops may also be visible.

Duodenal and oesophageal atresia

The combination of duodenal and oesophageal atresia without a tracheo-oesophageal fistula leads to the formation of a closed loop of bowel involving the distal oesophagus, stomach and duodenum. The result is a characteristic 'C'-shaped fluid collection within the abdomen (Fig. 22.45A).[110,111] This cystic mass may be seen as early as 14 weeks gestation and gradually increases in size during pregnancy.[112] There is a high incidence of associated abnormalities which varies between 53% and 77%, and in view of this the outlook is often poor,[113] with survival rates in the region of 30%. The other main association of importance is trisomy 21,[114] with series reporting incidences varying between 11% and 30%.[112,113]

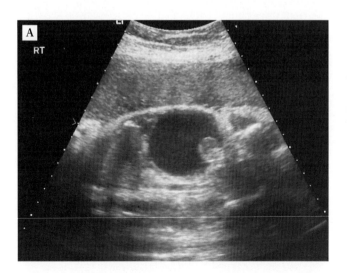

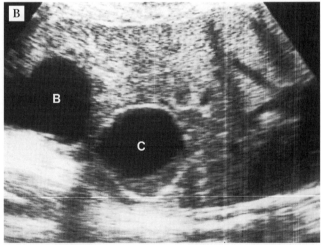

Fig. 22.41 Complicated ovarian cysts. A: An ovarian cyst with a solid area indicating retracting clot; the appearances suggest ovarian torsion. **B:** Debris within a cyst, suggesting possible torsion. B – bladder, C – cyst.

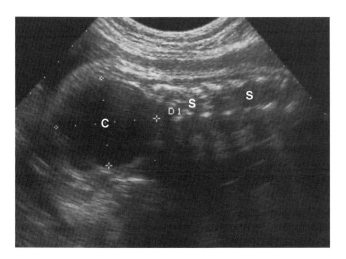

Fig. 22.42 Duplication cyst. Sagittal scan through fetal pelvis showing duplication cyst of the rectum, mimicking a cystic sacrococcygeal teratoma. S – spine, C – cyst.

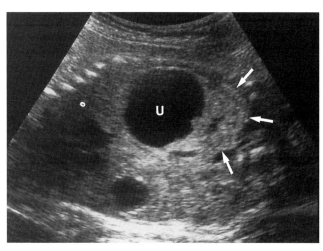

Fig. 22.43 Renal urinoma. Coronal scan through kidney showing renal urinoma (U) with compression of renal tissue (arrows).

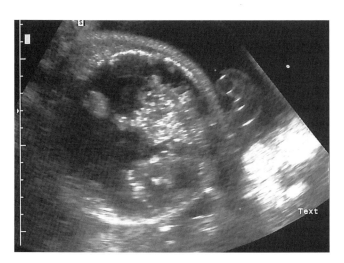

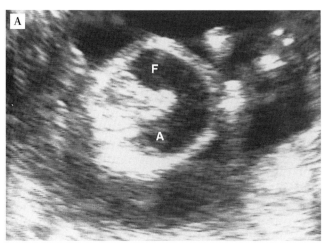

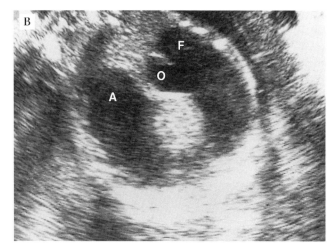

Fig. 22.44 Meconium pseudocyst. Transverse scan through a fetal abdomen at 32 weeks showing a calcified cyst containing debris. At surgery a large meconium pseudocyst was found secondary to perforation of the sigmoid colon. (Reproduced with permission from Twining P, McHugo J, Pilling D, eds. Textbook of fetal anomalies. Churchill Livingstone, 1999.)

Fig. 22.45 Duodenal and oesophageal atresia. A: Coronal scan through a fetal abdomen at 14 weeks gestation, showing typical 'C'-shaped cystic structure. B: Coronal scan through a fetal abdomen at 20 weeks showing 'C'-shaped structure. F – fundus of stomach, A – antrum of stomach, O – dilated part of lower oesophagus.

The demonstration of a 'C'-shaped cystic mass within the abdomen should always prompt the diagnosis of duodenal and oesophageal atresia. It should be noted that the proximal (oesophageal) limb of the 'C' may extend into the thorax and lie behind the heart. The level of this proximal limb depends on the level of the oesophageal atresia (Fig. 22.45B). Because of this finding the condition has often been confused with diaphragmatic hernia.[112,114] The high association with other abnormalities requires a meticulous search for associated anomalies when the diagnosis is suspected and karyotyping is recommended in addition.

Anal atresia and vesicorectal fistula

This condition is a rare cause of oligohydramnios and is a combination of anal atresia associated with either a vesico-rectal or a recto-urethral fistula.[115,116] Sonographically there is oligohydramnios associated with normal kidneys and bladder. Posterior to the bladder is a tubular cystic structure containing reflective material (Fig. 22.46).[115,116] The cystic mass represents the distended rectosigmoid which communicates directly with the bladder. During bladder emptying it appears there is preferential filling of the rectum instead of normal voiding of urine, hence the oligohydramnios. The urine is subsequently absorbed by the colon.

The outlook for this condition is poor owing to the high incidence of pulmonary hypoplasia secondary to severe oligohydramnios. When liquor volume is normal, i.e. the fistula is small, the outlook depends on the extent of associated abnormalities. The VATER syndrome is commonly seen with this combination.[116]

The fetal neck
Cystic hygroma

Cystic hygroma is estimated to occur in approximately 1 in 200 pregnancies but may account for up to 0.5% of spontaneous abortions.[117] It is caused by failure of communication of the jugular lymphatic sacs with the internal jugular vein. The result is a cystic mass in the nuchal region, which may progress to peripheral lymphoedema and the development of hydrops.[118]

The sonographic features of cystic hygroma are a multiseptate cystic mass situated posteriorly on the fetal neck. The mass may be large and there is always a midline septum present which extends to the midline of the neck (Fig. 22.47). Assessment of the remainder of the fetus often reveals generalised hydrops.

The main association of cystic hygroma is with chromosomal disease and Turner's syndrome in particular.[118,119] Turner's syndrome is seen in 75% of fetuses with cystic hygroma. Trisomies 18 and 21 occur in about 5% each and the remainder of the fetuses have a normal karyotype. The overall outlook for fetuses with cystic hygroma is poor because of the high incidence of hydrops and the mortality rate is approximately 80–90%.[119]

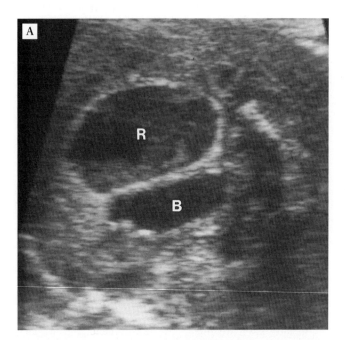
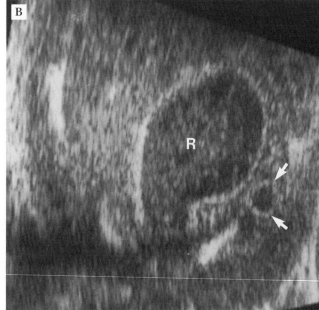

Fig. 22.46 Anal atresia with vesicorectal fistula. A: Oligohydramnios with dilated rectum containing meconium. B – bladder, R – rectum. **B:** Oblique scan showing dilated rectum and some fluid-filled bowel. R – rectum, bowel – arrows.

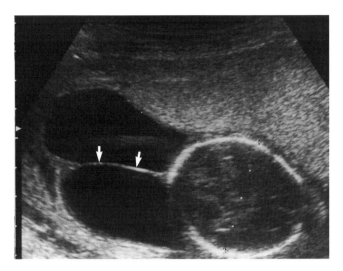

Fig. 22.47 Cystic hygroma. Transverse scan through fetal head showing large cystic hygroma (arrows point to midline nuchal septum).

Cystic hygroma occurring in other sites on the fetus has a low incidence of chromosomal disease but can be difficult to excise completely in the neonatal period.

Occipital encephalocele

Encephaloceles occur when there is a defect in the skull vault and either meninges (meningocele) or brain tissue (encephalocele) herniate through the defect;[120] 80% of encephaloceles occur in the occipital region.[121]

The ultrasound diagnosis is based on demonstrating a midline defect in the skull vault associated with either a cystic or a solid mass posteriorly. The head is often small and abnormal in shape, usually flattened posteriorly. There may be associated hydrocephalus and other intracranial anomalies, such as agenesis of the corpus callosum, the Arnold–Chiari malformation and the Dandy–Walker syndrome. The presence of a lateral encephalocele would always raise the possibility of the amniotic band syndrome.

When extracranial abnormalities are detected, associated chromosomal disease should be suspected and a karyotype test offered. The presence of polydactyly and dysplastic kidneys should indicate the Meckel–Grüber syndrome, which has an autosomal recessive inheritance.

The overall outlook for encephalocele is poor, with only a 55% survival rate and of these 74% will exhibit significant mental retardation. The survival rate for occipital meningocele is better at approximately 80% and up to 48% may have a normal outcome.[121]

Cervical meningocele

Cervical meningocele is rare, but a few cases have been reported in the ultrasound literature.[122,123] As in neural tube defects elsewhere in the spine the classic appearances include splaying of the posterior elements of the spine with an associated meningomyelocele sac. The Arnold–Chiari malformation is often present, as demonstrated by the 'lemon' head and 'banana' cerebellum.[124]

The outcome is thought to be better than for occipital encephalocele but not as good as that for occipital meningocele.[125]

Cervical teratoma

Fetal teratomas are rare tumours and cervical teratomas are even rarer, accounting for only 5% of all teratomas.[126]

Most teratomas are situated anteriorly or anterolaterally and can enlarge markedly during pregnancy, producing hyperextension of the neck (Fig. 22.48). They are predominantly solid on ultrasound but may have cystic components[127,128] and polyhydramnios is seen in up 40% of cases owing to oesophageal compression.[129]

The outlook is generally poor unless immediate neonatal resuscitation is available. Neonatal mortality has been documented at 43% owing to respiratory insufficiency at birth. In view of this full paediatric and surgical support is required at delivery to ensure that an airway can be maintained and outcome improved for the neonate.[130]

Haemangioma

Haemangioma can occur anywhere in the neck and sonographically shows a mixed cystic and solid appearance.[131,132] There have been a few reports in the literature but some authors have documented characteristic Doppler signals which may help with the diagnosis.[132] The main Doppler findings are arterial and venous pulsations within the mass. When the tumours are large, progression to hydrops has been documented.

Goitre

The normal thyroid can usually be demonstrated as two triangular-shaped structures on either side of the trachea on transverse scanning of the fetal neck (Fig. 22.49).

Enlargement of the fetal thyroid, or fetal goitre, is usually caused by maternal treatment with antithyroid drugs for thyrotoxicosis.[133,134]

The ultrasound findings are of a predominantly solid, bilobed mass affecting the anterior neck. Occasionally polyhydramnios is seen and, if the mass is large, the neck may be hyperextended. Other findings include intrauterine growth retardation, bradycardia and delayed appearance of ossification centres.[133]

In most cases treatment can be commenced in the early neonatal period, but some authors have advocated intrauterine therapy with amniotic injections of thyroxine.[135]

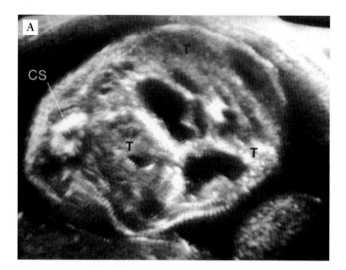

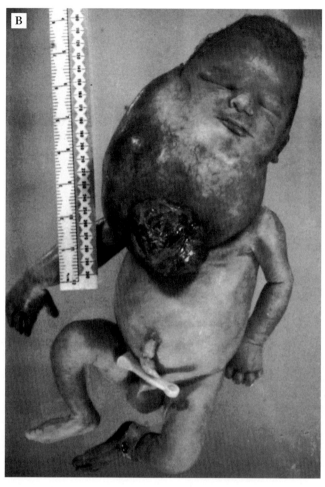

Fig. 22.48 Cervical teratoma. A: Transverse section through the fetal neck demonstrating a mixed cystic and solid mass. T – tumour, CS – cervical spine. **B:** Post-mortem photograph of same fetus.

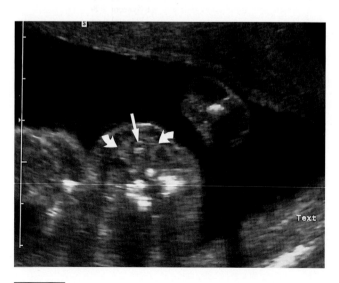

Fig. 22.49 Normal thyroid. Transverse scan through the fetal neck showing trachea (straight arrow) and thyroid (curved arrows).

REFERENCES

1 Pilu G, Reece A, Romero R et al. Prenatal diagnosis of craniofacial malformations with ultrasonography. Am J Obstet Gynecol 1986; 155: 45–50

2 Nicolaides K M, Salvesen D R, Snijders R J, Gosden C M. Fetal facial defects associated malformations and chromosomal abnormalities. Fetal Diagn Ther 1993; 8: 1–9

3 Stewart R E. Craniofacial malformations: clinical and genetic considerations. Pediatr Clin North Am 1978; 25: 485–515

4 Pruzansky S. Clinical investigation of the experiments in nature. In: ASHA Reports No. 8. Orofacial anomalies: clinical and research implications. 1973

5 Clifford E. Psychosocial aspects of orofacial anomalies: speculation in search of data. In: ASHA Reports No. 8. Orofacial anomalies: clinical and research implications. 1973

6 Lee A, Deutinger J, Bernaschek G. Three dimensional ultrasound: abnormalities of the fetal face in surface and volume rendering mode. Br J Obstet Gynaecol 1995; 102: 302–306

7 Anderson N, Boswell O, Duff G. Prenatal sonography for the detection of fetal anomalies. Results of a prospective study and comparison with prior series. AJR 1995; 165: 943–950

8 Chitty L S, Hunt G H, Moore J, Lobb M. Effectiveness of routine ultrasonography in detecting fetal structural abnormalities in a low risk population. BMJ 1991; 303: 1165–1169

9 Shirley I M, Bottomley F, Robinson V. Routine radiographer screening for fetal abnormalities by ultrasound in an unselected low risk population. Br J Radiol 1992; 65: 564–569

10 Larsen W J. Human embryology. London: Churchill Livingstone, 1993

11 Jeanty P, Dramaix-Wilmet M, Van Gansbeke D, Van Regemorter N. Fetal occular biometry by ultrasound. Radiology 1982; 143: 513–516

12 Turner G, Twining P. The facial profile in the diagnosis of fetal abnormalities. Clin Radiol 1993; 47: 389–395

13 Christ J E, Meininger M G. Ultrasound diagnosis of cleft lip and cleft palate before birth. Am Plast Surg 1983; 11(4): 308–312

14 Benaceraff B R, Frigoletto F D, Bieber F R. The fetal face: ultrasound examination. Radiology 1984; 153: 495–497

15 Seeds J W, Cefalo R C. Technique of early sonographic diagnosis of bilateral cleft lip and palate. Obstet Gynecol 1983; 62: 25–75

16 Saltzman D H, Benaceraff B R, Frigoletto F D. Diagnosis and management of fetal facial clefts. Am J Obstet Gynecol 1986; 155: 377–379

17 Nyberg D A, Sickler G K, Hegg F et al. Fetal cleft lip with and without cleft palate: ultrasound classification and correlation with outcome. Radiology 1995; 195: 677–684

18 Das S K, Runnels R S, Smith J C, Cohly H H. Epidemiology of cleft lip and cleft palate in Mississippi. South Med J 1995; 8: 437–442

19 Nyberg D A, Hegge F N, Kramer D et al. Premaxillary protrusion: a sonographic clue to bilateral cleft lip and palate. J Ultrasound Med 1993; 12: 331–335

20 Bundy A L, Saltzman D H, Emerson D, Fine C. Sonographic features associated with cleft palate. JCU 1986; 14: 486–489

21 Monni G, Ibba R M, Olla G, Cao A. Colour Doppler ultrasound and prenatal diagnosis of cleft palate. JCU 1995; 23: 189–191

22 Pashayan H M. What else to look for in a child born with a cleft of the lip and/or palate. Cleft Palate J 1983; 20: 54–82

23 Fiedler J M, Phelan J P. The amniotic band syndrome in monozygotic twins. Am J Obstet Gynecol 1983; 146: 864–865

24 Kalouseck D K, Bamforth S. Amnion rupture in previable fetuses. Am J Med Genet 1988; 31: 63–73

25 Moerman P, Fryns J P, Vandenberghe K, Lauweryns J. Constrictive amniotic bands, amniotic adhesions and limb body wall complex: discrete disruption sequences with pathogenetic overlap. Am J Med Genet 1992, 42: 470–479

26 Burton D J, Filly R A. Sonographic diagnosis of the amniotic band syndrome. AJR 1991; 156: 555–558

27 Mahony B S, Filly R A, Callen P W, Golbus M S. The amniotic band syndrome: antenatal sonographic diagnosis and potential pitfalls. Am J Obstet Gynecol 1985; 152: 63–68

28 Rodini E, Richieri-Costa A. Ectrodactyly–ectodermal dysplasia clefting syndrome: report on 20 new patients, clinical and genetic considerations. Am J Med Genet 1990; 37: 42–53

29 Robins D B, Ladda R L, Thieme G A. Prenatal detection of Roberts S C Phocomelia syndrome, report of two siblings with characteristic manifestations. Am J Med Genet 1989; 32: 390–394

30 Paladini D, Palmieri S, Lecora M et al. Prenatal ultrasound diagnosis of Roberts syndrome in a family with negative history. Ultrasound Obstet Gynecol 1996; 7: 208–210

31 Jones K L. Smith's recognisable patterns of human malformation. London: W B Saunders, 1997

32 Bromley B, Benaceraff B R. Fetal micrognathia: associated anomalies and outcome. J Ultrasound Med 1994; 13: 529–533

33 Crane J, Beaver H. Mid trimester diagnosis of mandibulofacial dysostosis. Am J Med Genet 1986; 25: 251–255

34 Meizner I, Carmi R, Katz M. Prenatal ultrasonic diagnosis of mandibulofacial dysostosis. JCU 1991; 19: 124–127

35 Robinow M, Reynolds J F, Fitzgerald. Hemifacial microsomia, ipsilateral facial palsy and malformed auricle in two families: an autosomal dominant malformation. Am J Med Genet 1986; S2: 129–133

36 Tamas D E, Mahoney B S, Bowie J D. Prenatal sonographic diagnosis of hemifacial microsomia (Goldenhar syndrome). J Ultrasound Med 1986; 7: 163–167

37 Pilu G, Romero R, Reece A et al. The prenatal diagnosis of Robin anomalad. Am J Obstet Gynecol 1986; 154: 630–632

38 Dennison W M. The Pierre Robin syndrome. Paediatrics 1965; 36: 336–342

39 Featherstone L S, Sherman S J, Quigg M M. Prenatal diagnosis of Seckel syndrome. J Ultrasound Med 1996; 15: 85–88

40 Majewski F, Goecke T. Studies of microcephalic dwarfism: approach to delineation of the Seckel syndrome. Am J Med Genet 1982; 12: 7–21

41 Shah J G, Metlay L. Prenatal ultrasound diagnosis of Beckwith–Wiedemann syndrome. JCU 1990; 18: 597–600

42 Teal L N, Angtuaco T L, Jimenez J F, Quirk J G. Fetal teratomas: antenatal diagnosis and clinical management. JCU 1988; 16: 329–336

43 Chervenak F A, Isaacson G, Touloukian R et al. Diagnosis and management of fetal teratomas. Obstet Gynecol 1985; 66: 666–671

44 Hullett R L, Bowerman R A, Marks T, Silverstein A. Prenatal ultrasound detection of congenital gingival granular cell tumour. J Ultrasound Med 1991; 10: 185–187

45 Carlan S J, Angel J L, Leo J, Feeney J. Cephalocele involving the oral cavity. Obstet Gynecol 1990; 75: 494–495

46 Shipp T D, Bromley B, Benaceraff B. The ultrasonographic appearance and outcome for fetuses with masses distorting the fetal face. J Ultrasound Med 1995; 14: 673–678

47 McGahan J P, Hyberg D A, Mack L A. Sonography of facial features of alobar and semilobar holoprosencephaly. AJR 1990; 154: 143–148

48 De Meyer W, Zeman W, Palmer C A. The face predicts the brain: diagnostic significance of medial facial anomalies for holoprosencephaly (arrhinencephaly). Pediatrics 1964; 34: 256–264

49 Chervenak F A, Tortora M, Mayden K, Mesologites T. Antenatal diagnosis of medial cleft face syndrome: sonographic demonstration of cleft lip and hypotelorism. Am J Obstet Gynecol 1984; 149: 94–97

50 Frattarelli J L, Boley T J, Miller R A C. Prenatal diagnosis of frontonasal dysplasia. Median cleft syndrome. J Ultrasound Med 1996; 15: 81–83

51 Goldstein R B, Lapidus A S, Filly R A. Fetal cephaloceles: diagnosis with ultrasound. Radiology 1991; 180: 803–808

52 Brown M, Sheridan-Pereira M. Outlook for the child with a cephalocoele. Pediatrics 1992; 90: 914–919

53 Gilbert R. Clusters of anophthalmia in Britain. BMJ 1993; 307: 340–341

54 Pearce W G, Nigam S, Rootman J Primary anopthalmos: histological and genetic features. Can J Ophthalmol 1974; 9: 141–145

55 Bronshtein M, Zimmer E, Gershoni-Baruch R et al. First and second trimester diagnosis of fetal ocular defects and associated anomalies: report of eight cases. Obstet Gynecol 1991; 77: 443–449

56 Monteagudo A, Timor-Tritch I E, Friedman A H, Santos R. Autosomal dominant cataracts of the fetus: early detection by transvaginal ultrasound. Ultrasound Obstet Gynecol 1996; 8: 104–108

57 Gaary E A, Rawnsley E, Marin-Padilla J M et al. In utero detection of fetal cataracts. J Ultrasound Med 1993; 4: 234–236

58 Battaglia C, Artini P G, D'Ambrogio G, Genazzani A R. Prenatal ultrasonographic evidence of transient dactroscystoceles. J Ultrasound Med 1994; 13: 897–900

59 Mihalko M, Lindfors K K, Grix A W et al. Prenatal sonographic diagnosis of Harlequin ichthyosis. AJR 1989; 153: 827–828

60 Meizner I. Prenatal ultrasonic features in a rare case of congenital ichthyosis (Harlequin fetus). JCU 1992; 20: 132–134

61 Nyberg D A, Mahony B S, Luthy D, Kapur R. Single umbilical artery. Prenatal detection of concurrent anomalies. J Ultrasound Med 1991; 10: 247–253

62 Lacro R V, Jones K L, Benirschke M D. The umbilical cord twist: origin direction and relevance. Am J Obstet Gynecol 1987; 157: 833–838

63 Edmonds M W. The spiral twist of the normal umbilical cord in twins and in singletons. Am J Obstet Gynecol 1954; 67: 102–120

64 Hall J G. Analysis of Pena Shokeir phenotype. Am J Med Genet 1986; 25: 99–117

65 Strong T M, Elliott J P, Radin T G. Non-coiled umbilical blood vessels: a new marker for the fetus at risk. Obstet Gynecol 1993; 81: 409–411

66 Benirschke K, Bourne G L. Incidence and prognostic implication of congenital absence of one umbilical artery. Am J Obstet Gynecol 1960; 79: 251–556

67 Vietinck R F, Thiery M, Orye E, De Clercq A, Vaerenbirch P. Significance of the single umbilical artery. Arch Dis Child 1972; 47: 639–642

68 Bryan E M, Kohler M G. The missing umbilical artery 1. Prospective study based on a maternity unit. Arch Dis Child 1974; 49: 844–852

69 Rosenak D, Meizner I. Prenatal sonographic detection of single and double umbilical artery in the same fetus. J Ultrasound Med 1994; 13: 995–996

70 Heifetz S A. Single umbilical artery: a statistical analysis of 237 autopsy cases and review of the literature. Perspect Pediatr Pathol 1984; 8: 345–352

71 Saller D N, Kenne C L, Sun C J, Schwartz S. The association of single umbilical artery with cytogenetically abnormal pregnancies. Am J Obstet Gynecol 1990; 163: 922–925

72 Byrne J, Blanc W A. Malformations and chromosome anomalies in spontaneously aborted fetuses with single umbilical artery. Am J Obstet Gynecol 1985; 151: 340–342

73 Jeanty P. Persistent right umbilical vein: an ominous prenatal finding. Radiology 1990; 177: 735–738

74 Jeanty P. Fetal and funicular vascular anomalies: identification with prenatal ultrasound. Radiology 1989; 173: 367–370

75 Greiss H B, McGahan J P. Umbilical vein entering the right atrium: significance of in utero diagnosis. J Ultrasound Med 1992; 11: 111–113

76 Krisch C F E, Feldstein V A, Goldstein R, Filly R. Persistent intrahepatic right umbilical vein: a prenatal series without significant anomalies. J Ultrasound Med 1996; 15: 371–374

77 Shen O, Tadmor O P, Yagel S. Prenatal diagnosis of persistent right umbilical vein. Ultrasound Obstet Gynecol 1996; 8: 31–33

78 Leonidas J C, Fellows R. Congenital absence of the ductus venosus: with direct connection between the umbilical vein at the distal inferior vena cava. AJR 1976; 126: 892–895

79 Fliegel C P, Nars P W. Aberrant umbilical vein. Pediatr Radiol 1984; 14: 55–57

80 Currarino G, Stannard M W, Kolni H. Umbilical vein draining into the inferior vena cava via the internal iliac vein, bypassing the liver. Pediatr Radiol 1991; 21: 265–266

81 Estroff J A, Benaceraff B R. Fetal umbilical vein varix: sonographic appearance and postnatal outcome. J Ultrasound Med 1992; 11: 69–73

82 Rizzo G, Ardnini D. Prenatal diagnosis of an intra-abdominal ectasia of the umbilical vein with colour Doppler ultrasonography. Ultrasound Obstet Gynecol 1992; 2: 55–57

83 Leizinger E. Varix thrombosis of the umbilical cord. Zeitschr Geburtshilfe Perinatal 1969; 171: 83–87

84 Heifetz S. Thrombosis of the umbilical cord: analysis of 52 cases and literature review. Pediatr Pathol 1988; 8: 37–42

85 Hoag R W. Fetomaternal haemorrhage associated with umbilical vein thrombosis. Case report. Am J Obstet Gynecol 1986; 154: 1271–1273

86 Ghosh A, Woo J S K, MacHenry C. Fetal loss from umbilical cord abnormalities – a difficult case for prevention. Eur J Obstet Gynecol Reprod Biol 1984; 18: 183–187

87 White S P, Kofinas A. Prenatal diagnosis and management of umbilical vein varix of the intraamniotic portion of the umbilical vein. J Ultrasound Med 1995; 13: 992–994

88 Ross J A, Jurkovic D, Kosmer N, Jauniaux E, Hocket E, Nicolaides K M. Umbilical cord cysts in early pregnancy. Obstet Gynecol 1997; 89: 442–445

89 Sepulveda W, Pryde P G, Greb A E, Romero R, Evans H I. Prenatal diagnosis of umbilical cord pseudocyst. Ultrasound Obstet Gynecol 1994; 4: 147–150

90 Janiaux E, Jurkovic D, Campbell S. Sonographic features of an umbilical cord abnormality combining a cord pseudocyst and a small omphalocoele: a case report. Eur J Obstet Gynecol Reprod Biol 1991; 40: 245–248

91 Sepulveda W, Bower S, Dhillon H K, Fisk N M. Prenatal diagnosis of congenital patent urachus and allantoic cyst: the value of colour flow imaging. J Ultrasound Med 1995; 14: 47–51

92 Heifetz S A, Rueda-Pedraza M E. Omphalomesenteric duct cysts of the umbilical cord. Am J Pediatr Pathol 1983; 1: 325–335

93 Ramirez P, Haberman S, Baxi L. Significance of umbilical cord cyst in a fetus with trisomy 18. Am J Obstet Gynecol 1995; 173: 955–957

94 Janiaux E, Donner C, Thomas C, Francotte J, Rodesh F, Allni F E. Umbilical cord pseudocyst in trisomy 18. Prenat Diagn 1988; 8: 557–563

95 Rizzo G, Ardiuni D. Umbilical cord cyst in trisomy 13. Ultrasound Obstet Gynecol 1994; 4: 438

96 Constantine G, Anderson J, Fowlie A. Umbilical cord pseudocyst in trisomy 18. Prenat Diagn 1990; 10: 274–275

97 Siddiqui T A, Bendon R, Schultz D M, Miodovnik M. Umbilical artery aneurysm: prenatal diagnosis and management. Obstet Gynecol 1992; 80: 530–533

98 Resta R G, Luthy D A, Mahoney B S. Umbilical cord haemangioma associated with extremely high alpha-feto protein levels. Obstet Gynecol 1988; 72: 488–491

99 Blickstein I, Shoham Schwartz Z, Lancet M. Predisposing factors in the formation of true knots of the umbilical cord: analysis of morphometric and prenatal data. Int J Gynecol Obstet 1987; 23: 395–398

100 Collins J H. First report: prenatal diagnosis of a true cord knot. Am J Obstet Gynecol 1991; 165: 1898–1899

101 Dewbury K C, Aluwihare A, Birch S J, Freeman N V. Antenatal ultrasound demonstration of a choledochal cyst. Br J Radiol 1980; 53: 906–907

102 Frank J L, Hill M C, Chirathivat S. Antenatal observation of a choledochal cyst by ultrasound. AJR 1981; 137: 166–167

103 Ecrad M, Mayden K L, Ahart S. Prenatal ultrasound diagnosis of a choledochal cyst. J Ultrasound Med 1985; 4: 553–555

104 Rha S Y, Stovroff M C, Glick P L, Allen J E, Ricketts R R. Choledochal cysts: a ten year experience. Am J Surg 1996; 62: 30–34

105 Nussbaum A R, Sanders R C, Hartman D S, et al. Neonatal ovarian cysts: sonographic–pathologic correlation. Radiology 1988; 168: 817–821

106 Meiznerr I, Levy A, Katz M, Maresh A J, Glezerman M. Fetal ovarian cysts: prenatal ultrasonographic detection and postnatal evaluation and treatment. Am J Obstet Gynecol 1991; 164: 874–878

107 Garel L, Filiatrault D, Brandt M et al. Antental diagnosis of ovarian cysts: natural history and therapeutic implications. Pediatr Radiol 1991; 21: 1–3

108 Preziosi P, Ariello G, Maiorana A, Malena S, Ferro F. Antenatal diagnosis of complicated ovarian cysts. JCU 1985; 14: 196–198

109 Sakala E P, Leon Z A, Rouse G A. Management of antenatally diagnosed fetal ovarian cysts. Obstet Gynecol Surv 1991; 46: 407–414

110 Hayden C K, Schwartz M Z, Davis M. Combined oesophageal and duodenal atresia: sonographic findings. AJR 1983; 140: 225–226

111 Duenholter J H, Rigoberto S R, Rosenfeld C R. Prenatal diagnosis of gastrointestinal obstruction. Obstet Gynecol 1976; 47: 618–620

112 Estroff J A, Parad R B, Shove J C, Benaceraff B R. Second trimester prenatal findings in duodenal and oesophageal atresia without tracheo oesophageal fistula. J Ultrasound Med 1994; 13: 375–359

113 Spitz L, Ali M, Breneton R J. Combined oesophageal and duodenal atresia: experience of 18 patients. J Pediatr Surg 1981; 16: 4–7

114 Chitty L S, Goodman J, Seller M J, Maxwell D. Esophageal and duodenal atresia in a fetus with Down's syndrome: prenatal sonographic features. Ultrasound Obstet Gynecol 1996; 7: 450–452

115 Arulkumaran S, Nicolini U, Fisk N M, Rodeck C. Fetal vesicorectal fistula causing olyohydramnios in the second trimester. Case report. Br J Obstet Gynaecol 1990; 97: 449–451

116 Hearnstebbins B, Sherer D M, Abramowicz J S, Hess H M, Woods J R. Prenatal sonographic features associated with an imperforate anus and recto-urethral fistula. JCU 1991; 19: 508–512

117 Marchese C, Savin E, Dragone. Cystic hygroma: prenatal diagnosis and genetic counselling. Prenat Diagn 1985; 5: 221–227

118 Azar GB, Snijders R J M, Gosden C, Nicolaides K M. Fetal nuchal cystic hygromata: associated malformations and chromosomal defects. Fetal Diagn Ther 1991; 6: 46–57

119 Chervenak F A, Isaacson G, Blakemore K et al. Fetal cystic hygroma. Cause and natural history. N Engl J Med 1983; 309: 833–825

120 Goldstein R B, Lapidus A S, Filly R A. Fetal cephalocoeles: diagnosis with ultrasound. Radiology 1991; 180: 805–808

121 Brown M, Sheridan-Pereira M. Outlook for the child with a cephalocele. Paediatrics 1992; 90: 914–919

122 Sabbagha R E, Depp R, Grasse D. Ultrasound diagnosis of occipitothoracic meningocele at 22 weeks gestation. Am J Obstet Gynecol 1978; 131: 113–114

123 Sabbagha R E, Tamura R K, Dal Compos S. Fetal cranial and craniocervical masses: ultrasound characteristics and differential diagnosis. Am J Obstet Gynecol 1980; 138: 511–517

124 Campbell J, Gilbert W M, Nicolaides K M. Ultrasound screening for spina bifida: cranial and cerebellar signs in a high risk population. Obstet Gynecol 1987; 70: 247–250

125 Lorber J, Schofield J K. The prognosis of occipital meningocele. Zeitschr Kinderchir 1979; 28: 347–351

126 Jordan R B, Ganderer M W. Cervical teratomas: an analysis. Literature review and proposed classification. J Pediatr Surg 1988; 23: 583–591

127 Patel R B, Gibson J Y, D'Cruz C A, Burklafter J L. Sonographic diagnosis of cervical teratoma in utero. AJR 1982; 139: 1220–1222

128 Trecet J C, Clarmunt V, Larraz J. Prenatal ultrasound diagnosis of fetal teratoma of the neck. JCU 1984; 12: 509–511

129 Thurkow A L, Visser G M A, Oosterhuis J W. Ultrasound observations of a malignant cervical teratoma of the fetus in a case of polyhydramnios – case history and review. Eur J Gynecol Reprod Biol 1983; 13: 375–384

130 Longer J C, Tabb T, Thompson P et al. Management of prenatally diagnosed tracheal obstruction: access to the airway in utero, prior to delivery. Fetal Diagn Ther 1992; 7: 12–16

131 Lewis B D, Doubilet P M, Meller V L et al. Cutaneous and visceral haemangiomata in the Klippel–Tenamnary–Weber syndrome: antenatal sonographic detection. AJR 1986; 147: 598–600

132 McGahan J P, Schneider J M. Fetal neck haemangioendothelioma with secondary hydrops fetalis: sonographic diagnosis. JCU 1986; 14: 384–388

133 Abuhamad A Z, Fisher D A, Warsof S L et al. Antenatal diagnosis and treatment of fetal goitrous hypothyroidism: case report and review of the literature. Ultrasound Obstet Gynecol 1995; 5: 368–371

134 Noia G, De Santis M, Tucci A et al. Early prenatal diagnosis and therapy of fetal hypothyroid goitre. Fetal Diagn Ther 1992; 7: 138–143

135 Waner S, Scharf J I, Bolognese R J. Antenatal diagnosis and treatment of a fetal goitre. J Reprod Med 1980; 24: 39–42

23

The placenta

Eric Jauniaux

Introduction

Before the development of prenatal investigation techniques morphological examination of the placenta and the cord was limited to retrospective information and was therefore of epidemiological value only and had little influence on pregnancy management. With the improvement of ultrasound equipment it is now possible to examine the placenta and the cord in detail from the beginning of the first trimester. The sonographic differential diagnoses of the principal placental and cord abnormalities are reviewed in this chapter, as well as their pathophysiological significance. The ultrasound features have been correlated with pathological findings.

Placental development and maturation

The developing placenta can be observed by trans-vaginal ultrasound from 5 weeks gestation.[1] At this time it appears as a reflective ring around the gestational sac. During the third month of gestation the enlarging gestational sac fills the entire uterine cavity, and fusion of the decidua capsularis surrounding the amniotic sac and the decidua parietalis completely obliterates the uterine cavity.[2] From this moment the components of the definitive placenta (chorion frondosum) can be clearly discerned *in vivo* (Fig. 23.1).

The three basic placental structures are the chorionic or fetal plate, the placental villous tissue or substance, and the basal or maternal plate. The placental mass is divided into 20–40 cotyledons or functional units, determined by the branching pattern of the villous tree, and includes the primary villous trunk with its derivatives.[3] The maternal surface is also divided into lobes, of no physiological significance, by septa extending from the basal plate towards the chorionic plate.[2]

The circulation of maternal blood through the intervillous chamber is a dynamic process that requires a continuous adaptation of the individual cotyledon to the blood flow offered to it by the corresponding uteroplacental artery. During the first trimester of pregnancy the growing embryo and its placenta are separated from the maternal circulation.[4] Soon after implantation, placental trophoblastic cells infiltrate the decidua and the superficial myometrial layer of the uterine wall.[5-7] These cells infiltrate not only the arterial wall but also the lumen, and this phenomenon is associated with the structural adaptation of the spiral arteries of the normal pregnancy. Transvaginal sonography (Fig. 23.2), hysteroscopy and chorionic villous sampling are unable to detect a continuous blood flow inside the placenta before 12 weeks of gestation.[4] The early placenta is bathed by a fluid possibly composed of maternal plasma and uterine gland secretions.[4] Between 10 and 12 weeks the trophoblastic plugs in the spiral arteries, still remaining from the early extravillous cytotrophoblastic infiltration, no longer obliterate the uteroplacental arteries and a real intervillous circulation is then established.[4] By the end of the third trimester the placental blood supply is estimated to be around 600 ml/min.[7]

A sonographic classification system for grading placentae *in utero* according to maturational changes was proposed by Grannum and associates,[8] as follows:

Grade 0: The placental tissue and the basal plate are homogeneous without the presence of linear highly reflective foci. The chorionic plate is smooth and well defined.

Grade I: The placental tissue contains a few linear highly reflective areas parallel to the basal plate, which remains unchanged. The chorionic plate presents subtle undulations.

Grade II: The placental tissue contains randomly dispersed echoes and is divided by comma-like reflective structures continuous with the chorionic plate. The marked indentations of the chorionic plate do not reach the basal plate, which is well defined by small linear highly reflective areas.

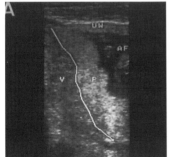 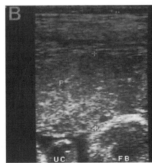 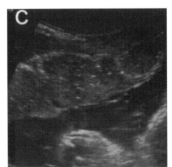 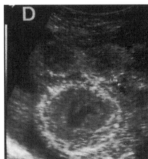

Fig. 23.1 Placental grading. Composite scans of the four placental grades. **A:** Grade 0 at 14 weeks of gestation. **B:** Grade I at 30 weeks of gestation. **C:** Grade II, partially grade III at 38 weeks of gestation. **D:** Premature grade III at 32 weeks in a pregnancy complicated by chronic hypertension.

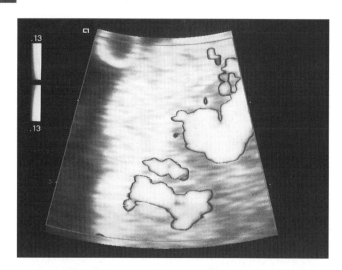

Fig. 23.2 Uteroplacental interface, 8th week. Trans-vaginal sonogram of a gestational sac at 7 weeks and 5 days. No continuous flow is detectable beyond the tip of the spiral vessels.

Grade III: The placental tissue is divided into compartments containing central echo-free areas. The chorionic plate indentations reach the basal plate, which contains almost confluent, very highly reflective areas.

The placentae were graded from 0 to III on the basis of static B-scan changes in the placental structures and the results were correlated with fetal pulmonary maturity evaluated by amniotic fluid lecithin–sphingomyelin (L/S) ratios (Fig. 23.1). Mature L/S ratios were found in 68% of grade I, 88% of grade II and 100% of grade III placentae, suggesting that invasive amniocentesis could be replaced by non-invasive ultrasound grading as a standard test to assess fetal pulmonary maturity.[8] However, subsequent reports did not support these findings and showed that a grade III placenta was associated with an immature L/S ratio in 8–42% of cases, and was therefore not accurate enough to replace amniocentesis in predicting fetal pulmonary maturity.[9–12]

Factors such as chronic hypertension, pre-eclampsia, intra-uterine growth retardation and maternal smoking are associated with accelerated placental maturation,[13,14] whereas diabetes and fetomaternal immunisation are associated with delayed placental maturation.[13] Earlier maturational changes have also been described in twin fetuses compared to singletons.[15] A randomised controlled trial has demonstrated that pregnant women with mature placental appearances (grade III) on ultrasonography between 34 and 36 weeks gestation have an increased risk of problems during labour, and their babies have an increased risk of low birthweight, intrapartum distress and perinatal death.[14]

Therefore, although the placental sonographic grading system is not accurate enough to replace amniocentesis in the assessment of fetal pulmonary maturity, it may be useful as a predictive indicator of potential perinatal problems.

Placental localisation

The importance of accurate localisation of the placenta in patients with antepartum haemorrhage and in those requiring invasive procedures (amniocentesis, cordocentesis or placental biopsy) is well established. Placental localisation by ultrasound was introduced by Donald in 1965, shortly after his first recording of an early gestation sac.[16,17] Placental visualisation by sonography rapidly became standard practice,[18,19] replacing older methods such as soft tissue radiography[20] and radioisotope scanning.[21]

Respiratory distress syndrome associated with premature delivery and severe fetal anaemia related to antepartum maternal haemorrhage are the major causes of neonatal morbidity and mortality associated with placenta praevia.[22] Placenta praevia also causes maternal morbidity due to abruption or post-partum haemorrhage, sometimes requiring therapeutic hysterectomy.[22,23] Thus, an accurate and early diagnosis of placenta praevia is important.

The pathogenesis of placenta praevia is still obscure, but predisposing factors include advancing maternal age, multiparity and prior caesarean sections.[23] A uterine scar in the lower segment predisposes not only to placenta praevia but also to placenta accreta, increasing the overall rate of maternal complications such as uterine rupture or heavy post-partum haemorrhage.[23] The incidence of placenta praevia varies from 1/200 to 1/250 pregnancies, the range probably reflecting differences in definition.[23] The majority of cases of 'low placentae' in early pregnancy have been shown not to be praevia at delivery: 90% of such placentae appear subsequently to move into the upper portion of the uterus.[24,25] Placental 'migration' or 'ascension' due to progressive development of the lower uterine segment has been put forward as the explanation for the difference in the incidence of placenta praevia encountered in the second and third trimesters.[25]

If a low-lying placenta is diagnosed in the second trimester the patient should be examined around 28 weeks to exclude placenta praevia.

Placenta praevia can be divided into four categories:

I   – low-lying placenta positioned close to the os (within 5 cm),

II   – marginal placenta praevia located at the margin of the os,

III   – partial placenta praevia partially covering the internal os,

IV   – total placenta praevia completely covering the internal cervical os.

The prenatal ultrasound diagnosis of total placenta praevia is usually easy because of the large amount of placental tissue overlying the internal os (Fig. 23.3). However, low-lying placentae may not be distinguishable by sonography from marginal or partial placenta praevia (Fig. 23.4). Several conditions, such as maternal obesity,

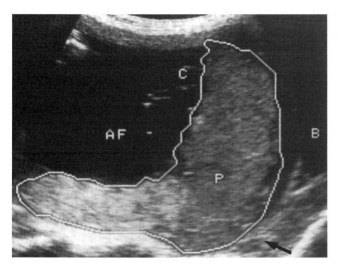

Fig. 23.3 Placenta praevia. Longitudinal sonogram of a total placenta praevia at 28 weeks of gestation. The placenta (P) completely covers the os (arrow) and separates the amniotic fluid (AF) from the bladder (B). Note the marginal insertion of the cord (C).

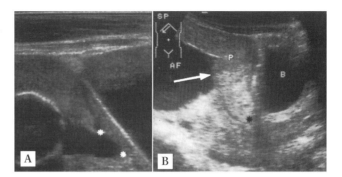

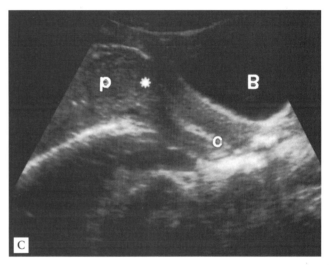

Fig. 23.4 Low-lying placentae. A: Low-lying placenta at 20 weeks of gestation. The distance between the placental edge (*) and the margin edge of the internal cervical os (*) can be estimated by ultrasound. **B:** Spurious placenta praevia at 32 weeks. The placental edge (P) is situated at a distance from the internal os (*). The false impression of placenta praevia is due to focal thickening of the posterior myometrium (arrow). **C:** Posterior placenta praevia (P) at term, partially covering the os (*). The bladder (B) distension can modify the relative position of the placental edge (*).

posterior localisation of the placenta, overdistended bladder, local myometrial thickening or acoustic shadows from the fetal head, can make accurate transabdominal ultrasound diagnosis of the different grades of placenta praevia difficult.[26,27] Asymptomatic low placentae which do not completely cover the internal os in the mid-trimester are not associated with significant increase of maternal or neonatal complications. A conversion to normal position in these cases can always be demonstrated by serial ultrasound examinations. These problems have led to the introduction of trans-vaginal sonography as a more accurate method of diagnosis of placenta praevia. In comparative series this technique appears to be safe and diagnostically superior to transabdominal sonography[26,27] and should now be considered as the gold standard to diagnose posterior placenta praevia (Fig. 23.5). Systematic trans-vaginal sonographic screening for placenta praevia in early pregnancy has shown that the likelihood of placenta praevia at delivery is 5.1% if the placenta extends at least 15 mm over the internal os at 12–16 weeks.[27]

Placental size

Determination of placental size is part of the overall assessment of the intra-uterine environment. Placental growth can be estimated by measuring the thickness or by an estimation of volume.

Placental thickness is measured at the thickest portion of the placenta or beneath the cord insertion.[8] There is a gradual decrease in placental thickness from 32 weeks of gestation until term.[8] Placental thickness is not diagnostic of any particular condition but can contribute to the man-

agement of a fetus at risk.[28] Thick placentae (>4 cm) can be an early sign of developing fetal hydrops of various causes (Fig. 23.6) or of uncontrolled maternal diabetes mellitus (Fig. 23.7). Placentae measuring up to 6 cm can also be found in pregnancies with elevated mid-trimester maternal serum α-fetoprotein (AFP) and an anatomically normal fetus.[29] Thin placentae (less than 2.5 cm) are often seen in patients with intra-uterine growth retardation or fetal death (Fig. 23.8).

Sonographic methods for determining placental volume are usually complex and time consuming; however, these studies have highlighted important pathophysiological information. Longitudinal sonographic studies of the placental volume have shown a wide variation at each stage of gestation from approximately 110–425 ml at 23 weeks to 340–1000 ml at term.[30] As with placental thickness, the growth rate of placental volume decreases after 30 weeks,

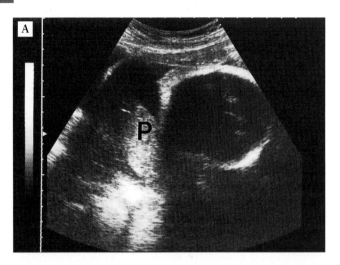

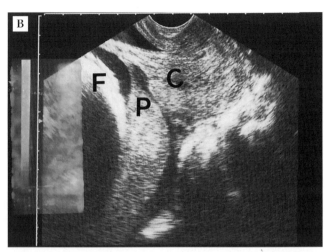

Fig. 23.5 Posterior placental praevia. A: Transabdominal longitudinal sonogram at 32 weeks of gestation of a placenta (P), low-lying at 20 weeks and complicated by vaginal bleeding at 31 weeks. **B:** Trans-vaginal view of the same case showing the placenta (P) clearly crossing above the internal cervical os (C). (F – fetus.)

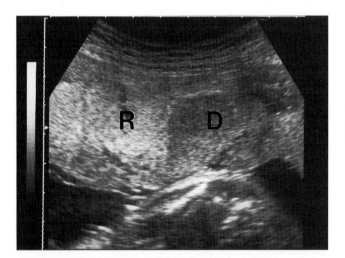

Fig. 23.6 Oedematous placenta. Scans of the placenta in a monochorionic–diamniotic twin pregnancy at 30 weeks complicated by a twin–transfusion syndrome. The hemiplacenta corresponding to the recipient (R) or perfused twin is thicker and highly reflective (oedematous) compared to the placental area corresponding to the transfuser or donor (D).

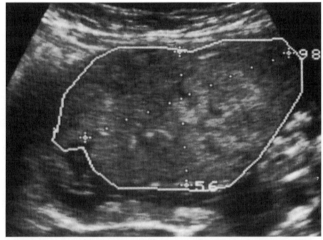

Fig. 23.7 Large placenta in diabetes. Transverse sonogram at 24 weeks showing a thick, heterogeneous placenta in a pregnancy complicated by uncontrolled class A diabetes mellitus.

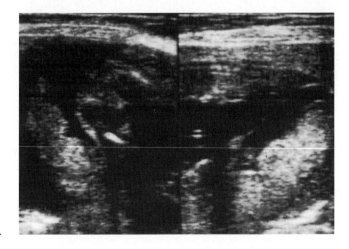

Fig. 23.8 Placental atrophy in a dead twin. Sonograms of a monochorionic–diamniotic twin pregnancy at 21 weeks complicated by the death of one of the twins. The hemiplacenta corresponding to the dead fetus (left) is thinner than the placental area of the living twin (right).

and even falls towards term.[31] There is some evidence that fetal growth retardation is preceded by reduced placental volume growth in the first half of pregnancy.[32] Small placental volumes clearly denote fetal complications.[33] These preliminary results have not been confirmed by larger studies. The development of 3D ultrasound will most certainly improve the clinical value of placental volume measurements.

Major structural abnormalities of the placenta

Abnormalities of placentation

The placenta is normally a circular discoid organ but there are wide variations in its shape which are usually of no clinical significance.[2] However, some unusual shapes are associated with perinatal complications and their diagnosis *in utero* can influence the pregnancy management.[3] For most of these cases there is good evidence that the abnormality develops during implantation of the fertilised ovum or during the early stage of placental development.[3]

Placenta multilobata and accessory lobes

Bilobate placentae consisting of two lobes approximately equal in size are found in less than 4% of pregnancies.[3] Macroscopically and sonographically the placental lobes appear as two well defined masses connected by a thin bridge of chorionic tissue, where the cord is usually inserted (Fig. 23.9). The bilobate placenta is generally of no direct clinical significance, but is often associated with

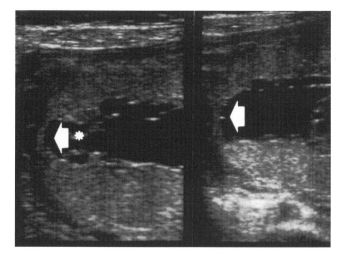

Fig. 23.9 Bilobate placenta. Longitudinal sonograms showing a bilobate fundal placenta at 26 weeks of gestation. The placental lobes are connected by a thin bridge of placental tissue (arrow) where the cord is inserted (*).

velamentous insertion[3] of the cord, which should be excluded before the onset of labour (see p. 551).

Multilobate placentae consisting of three or more lobes are extremely rare and their clinical significance is not well established.[3]

An accessory lobe adjacent to the main placental mass is reported in about 3% of pregnancies.[3] The lobe is often linked to the main placental mass by a thin bridge of chorionic vessels (succenturiata) but it can be entirely separate (spuria) and connected only by the membranes alone.[2] Their clinical significance lies in the risk of vessel rupture during labour, with severe fetal haemorrhage when the accessory lobe is located near the cervical os, or in the retention of the lobe *in utero* after delivery.[2,3] Accessory lobes are usually small and difficult to diagnose antenatally.

Placenta extrachorialis

Placenta extrachorialis is a common abnormality found in about 25% of all placentae and characterised by a transition of membranous to villous chorion at a distance from the placental edge.[2,3] Insertion of the membranes within the placental margin results in placental tissue not covered by the chorionic plate (extrachorialis) and in a smaller than normal amniotic cavity.[2] Two forms can be distinguished:

1   Circum-marginate placenta presents with a flat ring of membranes comprising only amnion and chorion with fibrin, and is practically asymptomatic.[2,3]
2   Circumvallate placenta has a raised, often rolled ring of membranes (Fig. 23.10A), which contains amnion, chorion and decidual tissue.[2] As the uterine wall stretches in the second half of gestation the placenta cannot adapt and there is tearing of membranes and bleeding from the edge of the chorionic plate. Circumvallate placentation is therefore accompanied by a relatively high rate of premature rupture of the membrane, antepartum bleeding and preterm onset of labour.[2,3,34] This form of placentation has also associated with an increased incidence of low birthweight infants, owing to both growth restriction and premature birth.[3]

The 'mamelonated' appearance of the marginal chorionic plate is the main sonographic feature of the circumvallate placenta (Fig. 23.10B). The ultrasound images are of multiple empty subamniotic echo-free areas of various sizes and shapes (Fig. 23.10C), which are strictly limited to the marginal zone of the placenta and persist throughout pregnancy.[34] In contrast, the 'mamelonated' appearance of the marginal chorionic plate is less pronounced in circummarginate placentae (Fig. 23.11). In these cases the abnormal placental sonographic features disappear during the second half of gestation, probably because the placenta can adapt to stretching of the myometrium.

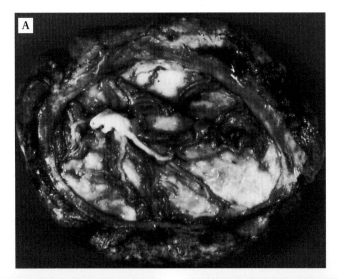

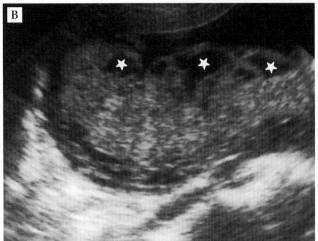 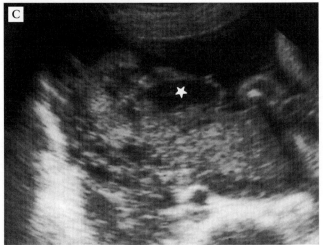

Fig. 23.10 Circumvallate placenta. A: Macroscopic view of a complete circumvallate placenta showing the abnormal membrane insertion away from the placental margin. **B:** Transverse and **C:** longitudinal scan at 20 weeks of the marginal zone of the placenta, demonstrating multiple subamniotic echo-poor areas of various sizes and shape (*). (Reproduced with permission from Jauniaux *et al*. JCU 1989; 16: 126–131.)

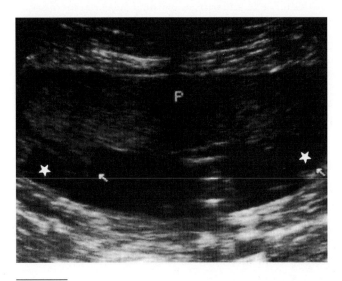

Fig. 23.11 Circum-marginate placenta. Transverse sonogram of the upper part of the amniotic cavity at 17 weeks showing bilateral subamniotic (*) echo-poor areas (arrows). These features could not be identified on the scans from 22 weeks of gestation. Pathological examination demonstrated a circum-marginate placenta. (P – placenta).

Rare abnormalities of placentation

Fenestrate placentae are extremely rare and are characterised by the absence of the central portion of a discoid placenta; there are no prenatal complications.[3]

Placentae membranaceae or placentae diffusae are characterised by persistence of the villous growth over the whole surface of the placental membrane, covering the entire uterine cavity.[2,3,35] This abnormality is extremely rare and is associated in nearly all cases by early antepartum bleeding and either abortion or premature labour, owing to the fact that a part of the placenta is necessarily praevia.[3,35] When the placenta is uniformly distributed over the membranes and of reasonable thickness, the prenatal diagnosis can be made by ultrasound.[35,36]

Placenta accreta has been defined as a placenta with abnormal adherence, either wholly or partly, to the uterine wall.[3,37] This abnormality is characterised by myometrial invasion by the villi and occurs when the decidua basalis is partially or completely absent.[3] According to the degree of myometrial invasion this condition is subdivided into placenta accreta vera, when the villi are simply attached to the myometrium; placenta increta, when the villi invade deeply the myometrium; and placenta percreta, when the villi penetrate the entire thickness of the uterine wall.[3,37] Placenta accreta is a rare but very serious abnormality. All conditions or procedures that affect the integrity of the internal uterine walls, such as caesarean section and other uterine surgery, curettage, sepsis or fibroids, are predisposing factors for abnormal villous penetration.[3] In many patients there is a combination of aetiological factors[3] and the association of a prior uterine scar and a low placental insertion is a particular risk.[23] Placenta accreta has both an overall maternal and a fetal mortality of around 10% due to antepartum or post-partum bleeding, uterine rupture and uterine inversion.[3] Placenta percreta is clearly the most dangerous condition, with a perinatal mortality rate of 96%.[37] On ultrasound the decidual interface between placenta and myometrium is absent at the level of the abnormal villous penetration.[37] Prenatal diagnosis of this condition may allow the obstetrician to demarcate the areas of the placenta that require resection prior to surgery (Fig. 23.12).

Placental vascular lesions

Many inaccurate and misleading expressions have been used by ultrasonographers to describe placental vascular lesions, probably because little attempt has been made to compare ultrasound and pathological findings. The terms most currently used in the literature are placental cyst, thrombotic cyst and intraplacental haemorrhage or bleeding. To avoid confusion, the classic pathological terminology to categorise these placental lesions should be used.

Avillous spaces or placental caverns

Echo-free spaces within the placental tissue vary from small, poorly reflective areas to large echo-free spaces, also called 'maternal lakes'. Large echo-free spaces are found in 67% of placentae examined at any stage of gestation from the first half of pregnancy to term.[38] To some extent careful sonographic examination reveals maternal lakes of different sizes and shapes in virtually all placentae, mainly under the chorionic plate near the umbilical cord insertion or in the marginal zone.

Small spaces in the centre of the cotyledon have been described in mature placentae. These cavities within the cotyledons are secondary to the dispersion of the free-floating terminal villi by maternal arterial jets of blood entering the intervillous space.[2,7] These modifications observed *in utero* by ultrasound correspond anatomically to avillous zones, and can be demonstrated *in vitro* by perfusion of the placenta after delivery.[39]

Large echo-free spaces (maternal lakes) can be found by ultrasound within the placental tissue from the second trimester until the end of pregnancy.[40,41] They contain turbulent blood flow on real-time imaging and their shape can be modified by maternal position or by uterine contractions. Two categories must be distinguished:

1 Stable maternal lakes characterised sonographically by the constancy of their appearance on repeated examinations (Fig. 23.13A). The large lesions are almost unaffected by placental collapse during delivery (Fig. 23.13B). Microscopically they correspond to large avillous areas (caverns) surrounded by normal villous tissue (Fig. 23.13B) and are a non-pathological persistence of the placental anatomical structure from early in pregnancy.[41]
2 Variable maternal lakes which correspond to the first stage of the development of a placental thrombosis. Their size is extremely variable and their reflectivity may change from one examination to another, as blood coagulation and fibrin deposition lead to intervillous, subchorionic or marginal thrombosis (Fig. 23.14), classically described by the pathologists.[2,3,41]

These two categories can only be differentiated by serial ultrasound examinations. Large echo-free spaces may be found in pregnancies with elevated maternal serum α-fetoprotein (MSAFP) if they develop at the time of AFP screening.[29,42] Large spaces can also be observed in excessively thick placentae (Fig. 22.15) and may be associated with fetal growth retardation and premature delivery.[29] The discovery of several of these lesions in the first trimester should prompt early antepartum surveillance.[43]

Thrombosis

Placental thromboses are the result of focal coagulation of blood in the intervillous spaces.[2,3] Intervillous thromboses

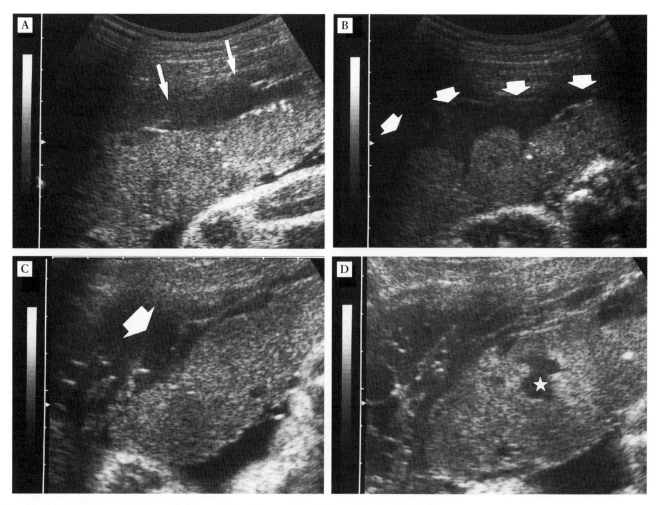

Fig. 23.12 Placenta percreta. Sonograms showing **A:** the absence of decidual interface (arrows); **B:** the area where the myometrium could not be identified and where the placenta appeared to float inside uterine vessels (arrows); **C:** dilated uterine vessels under the placenta with absent decidual interface (arrow); **D:** a centrocotyledonary space (*) above the area of abnormal implantation.

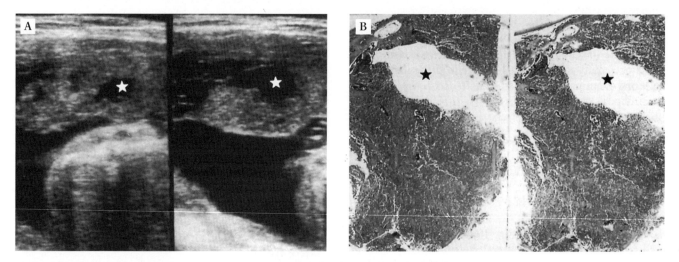

Fig. 23.13 Avillous placental space A: Transverse sonograms at 37 weeks of gestation of a large echo-free space (*), identified at the end of the second trimester. The shape of the lesion and the reflectivity of the surrounding placental tissue remained unchanged until delivery.
B: Histological sections of the lesion showing a large avillous space (*) surrounded by normal placental tissue.

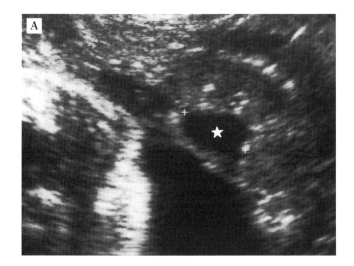

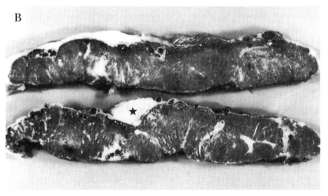

Fig. 23.14 Subchorionic thrombosis. A: Sonogram at 32 weeks showing a large echo-free space (*) beneath the chorionic plate.
B: Macroscopic examination of the placenta at term demonstrating a subchorionic thrombosis (*).

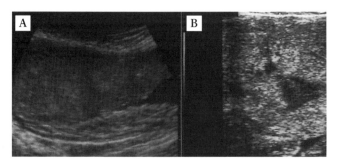

Fig. 23.15 Vascular space in the placenta. Sonograms at 20 weeks of gestation showing a large placenta (thickness >4 cm) with **A:** patchy decreased reflectivity and **B:** large echo-free spaces containing turbulent blood flow. These sonographic features (jelly-like placenta) were associated with elevated MSAFP.

are found in about 40% of placentae[2,3] and contain an admixture of fetal and maternal blood.[44]

Large echo-free spaces containing turbulent flow on real-time imaging are the early stages of the development of

intervillous, subchorionic or marginal placental thromboses.[38,41] Turbulence of maternal blood, with low flow laterally and relatively high flow in the central part, may result from failure of the cotyledon to expand in response to the increasing jet of blood from the corresponding uteroplacental artery.[43] Because of focal overpressure the surrounding villi are pushed away, compressed (Fig. 23.16), and gradually atrophy as fibrin is progressively laid down in the periphery. Finally the maternal blood coagulates in the placental tissue, causing focal obliteration of the intervillous circulation (Fig. 23.17A). This failure to accommodate may be secondary to an inadequate venous drainage from the cotyledon, to alteration of the villous trophoblast with the release of thromboplastic substances,[2] or to villous oedema, as has been described in maternofetal incompatibility.[45,46]

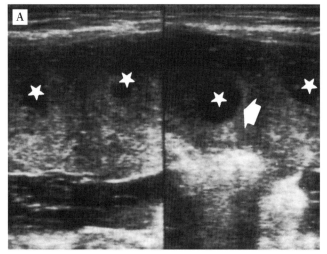

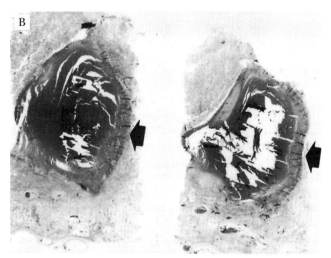

Fig. 23.16 Placental space. A: Sonograms at 35 weeks showing large placental echo-free spaces (*) which contained turbulent blood flow. Note the increased reflectivity of the surrounding villi (arrow).
B: Histological section of the largest lesion. The surrounding villi opposite to the entrance of the maternal blood are compressed and degenerated (arrows).

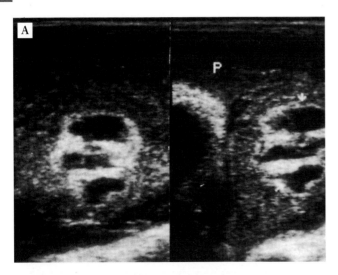

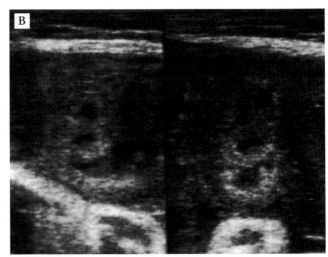

Fig. 23.17 Intervillous thrombosis. A: Sonograms at 39 weeks showing abnormal placental features corresponding to an organised intervillous thrombosis with extensive fibrin deposition in the periphery. B: Sonograms of a placenta at 35 weeks showing small echo-free spaces surrounded by large areas of reflective tissue corresponding to an old intervillous thrombosis.

Placental thrombosis may be detected by ultrasound early in the end of the first trimester[43] and serial ultrasound examinations can demonstrate the evolution of a simple maternal lake to an intervillous thrombosis. A progressive laying down of fibrin and degeneration of the surrounding villi will result in increased reflectivity of the lesion (Fig. 23.17A). Old thrombosis (Fig. 23.17B) may be difficult to differentiate from infarcts if repeated ultrasound examinations are not performed. The sonographic identification of intervillous thrombosis is not only of clinical importance as an indicator of abnormal placental function or of isoimmunisation,[45,46] but also of fetal growth restriction.[43]

Single subchorionic and marginal thromboses are not associated with increased fetal and/or maternal risk.[2,3] However, massive subchorionic thrombosis, also known as 'Breus mole', separating the chorionic plate from the underlying villous tissue is associated with perinatal complications.[3,47] The development of this lesion predisposes to premature onset of labour and can compromise the placental circulation, with fetal distress or death. Sonographically the placenta appears enlarged, with multiple echo-free spaces elevating the fetal plate.[47]

Infarcts

Placental infarcts are similar to infarcts observed in any other organs and are the result of obstruction of the uteroplacental circulation. The relationship between placental infarcts and maternofetal complications has been well documented in pathological studies.[2,3] Small infarcts are found in about 25% of placentae from uncomplicated pregnancies.[3]

The incidence of placental infarction is significantly increased in pregnancies complicated by pre-eclampsia or essential hypertension and is directly related to the severity of the disease.[3] In these maternal hypertensive disorders infarction is usually extensive and involves more than 10% of the placental tissue. These large placental infarcts are associated with an excess of perinatal mortality and intra-uterine growth retardation.[2,3]

Recent or acute infarcts appear macroscopically as red lesions which, on histology, consist of congested villi with widely dilated vessels and narrowed intervillous spaces. Old or chronic infarcts are yellow-white on macroscopic examination and are composed microscopically of necrotic ghost-like villi, often with fibrin deposition in the periphery of the lesion.[2,3]

The sonographic features of placental infarcts have only rarely been reported.[41,48] They appear as large irregular intraplacental areas, with reduced reflectivity in the acute stage and of similar reflectivity to adjacent normal placenta in more advanced stages (Fig. 23.18). They are usually located near the basal plate.

Fibrin deposition

Perivillous fibrin deposition is more often a diffuse and microscopic phenomenon.[2,3] However, large plaques of fibrin are found in 20% of the placentae examined at birth.[1] They are secondary to turbulence of maternal blood in the intervillous space. Perivillous fibrin deposition usually occurs during the second half of pregnancy and large lesions are often found in contact with the fetal plate of the placenta. Subchorionic fibrin deposition is similar sonographically and macroscopically to sub-

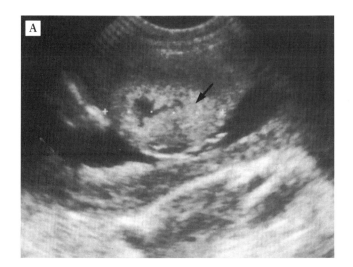

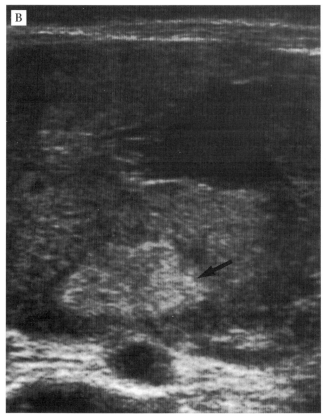

Fig. 23.18 Placental infarct. A: Large highly reflective lesion (arrow) of the placenta at 35 weeks of gestation in a pregnancy complicated by pre-eclampsia, corresponding to an acute infarct. **B:** Large placental area of high reflectivity (arrow) located near the basal plate at 32 weeks in an uncomplicated pregnancy corresponding to a chronic infarct. (Reproduced with permission of the publisher from Jauniaux *et al*. JCU 1990; 9: 419–422.)

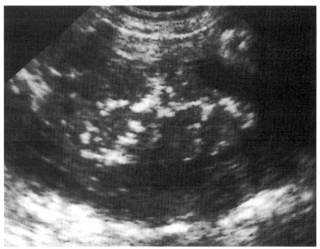

Fig. 23.19 Placental calcification. Sonogram of a third-trimester placenta showing diffuse, intensely reflective foci corresponding histologically to perivillous fibrin and calcium deposits.

sition involving more than 30–40% of the placental tissue is associated with fetal growth retardation.[2,3]

Haematomas

Placental haematomas are localised masses of blood resulting from extravasation of maternal or fetal blood.

Haematomas of fetal origin are secondary to rupture of a chorionic vessel before or during delivery, and are localised under the amniotic layer (subamniotic) covering the fetal plate. Their incidence is unknown, but most of them are found in third-trimester placentae and are thought to occur during delivery, owing to excessive traction on the umbilical cord.[11] However, when haematomas develop earlier in pregnancy they are associated with elevated MSAFP and the lesion can be diagnosed by ultrasound.[29] Early subamniotic haematomas are sometimes complicated by fetal growth retardation and abnormal Doppler traces.[29,49] Sonographically they appear as a single mass protruding from the fetal plate and surrounded by a thin membrane. Whereas the newly formed clot is moderately reflective (Fig. 23.20), the lesion becomes less so as the clot resolves (Fig. 23.21).

Haematomas of maternal origin are the pathological basis of placental abruption, which is recognised as one of the most serious complications of pregnancy.[2,3,50] Vaginal bleeding affects 25% of pregnancies before 20 weeks of gestation[51] and 4% during the third trimester.[50] In this context sonographic examination is important during the first half of gestation. Significant correlation is reported between the size of the haematoma and subsequent pregnancy complications.[52–55] The development of a haematoma is also associated with elevated MSAFP and a positive Kleihauer test, suggesting fetomaternal admixture

chorionic thrombosis. Small diffuse fibrin deposits can be detected by ultrasonography and are frequently mixed with calcium deposits (Fig. 23.19). Extensive fibrin depo-

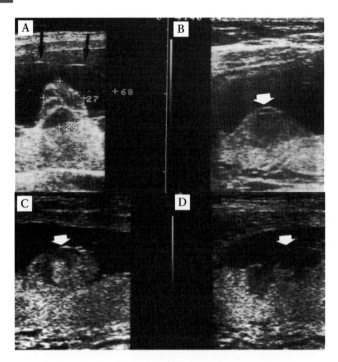

Fig. 23.20 Subamniotic haematoma. A: Subamniotic haematoma containing a newly formed clot on top of the fetal plate and surrounded by a thin membrane (arrow) corresponding to the amnion. **B, C** and **D:** (for comparison). Large echo-free subchorionic spaces (arrows) or maternal lakes elevating the fetal plate. These lesions are secondary to pooling and stasis of maternal blood under the fetal plate.

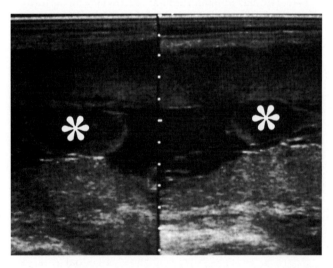

Fig. 23.21 Subamniotic haematoma. Poorly reflective mass protruding from the fetal plate of the placenta (*) corresponding to a subamniotic haematoma due to the rupture of fetal vessels.

of blood in some of these cases.[42,55] By contrast, the value of ultrasound in this condition is limited during the second half of pregnancy. The diagnosis of placental abruption in preterm or term pregnancies is based on the clinical triad (pain, uterine rigidity and vaginal bleeding), and sono-

graphic investigations can only be used in non-acute cases to confirm the clinical diagnosis and to exclude placenta praevia.[50] Placental haematomas produce a wide spectrum of sonographic features, depending on the location of the lesion and the degree of organisation of the blood clot. Acute haemorrhage may be of greater or similar reflectivity to the placenta, whereas resolving haematomas are poorly reflective after 1 week and echo free after 2 weeks.[53] From a pathological point of view placental haematomas are separated into two categories, which can be distinguished on ultrasound findings.

1 Marginal haematomas are found in 1% of all placentae and occur more often[2] in placentae partly implanted in the lower segment of the uterus (Fig. 23.22) or in placenta extrachorialis (Fig. 23.23). Retrospectively, at term these lesions seem to be of no clinical importance.[2,3] However, sonography can detect subchorionic lesions often associated with marginal detachment of the placenta in patients with vaginal bleeding during the first half of pregnancy.[52–55] These subchorionic haematomas probably result from early marginal placental abruption, with collection of blood beneath the chorionic membrane, instead of collecting behind the placenta as happens during the second or third trimester.[52,53] In early pregnancy, much emphasis has been put on the volume of an intra-uterine haematoma or on the presence of vaginal bleeding,[55] but not on the location of the haemorrhage. It is likely that if the bleeding occurs at the level of the definitive placenta (under the cord insertion) it may result in placental separation and subsequent abortion. Conversely, a subchorionic haematoma only detaching the membrane opposite to the cord insertion can probably reach a significant volume before it affects normal pregnancy development.

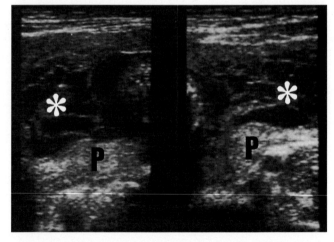

Fig. 23.22 Marginal haematoma. Transverse sonograms at 18 weeks of a heterogeneous mass (*) at the margin of a low inserted placenta (P), corresponding to a marginal placental haematoma.

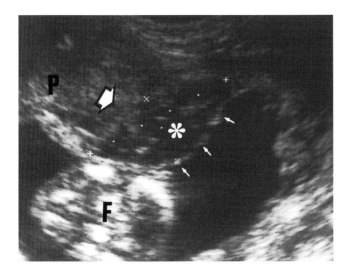

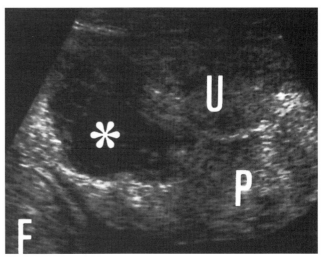

Fig. 23.23 Placental haematoma. Sonogram at 15 weeks showing a poorly reflective lesion (*) between the placental margin (large arrow) and the fetus (F), displacing the chorionic membranes (small arrows). Pathological examination of the placenta demonstrated a marginal haematoma and extrachorialis insertion of the membranes (circumvallate placenta).

Fig. 23.24 Retroplacental haematoma. Sonogram at 32 weeks showing a poorly reflective mass (*) between the uterine wall (U), placenta (P) and fetus (F) 2 weeks after an umbilical cord puncture with passage of the needle through the placenta. Pathological examination demonstrated a large retroplacental haematoma.

2   Retroplacental haematomas are found in 5% of all placentae and 15% of placentae from women with pregnancy-induced hypertension.[3] Retroplacental bleeding with premature placental separation is thought to be due to rupture of a maternal uteroplacental artery.[2,3] Retroplacental haematomas are often accompanied by infarction of the overlying villous tissue and decidual necrosis.[2,3] Pathological evidence of a retroplacental haematoma is found in only 30% of placentae from women with clinical symptoms of placental abruption.[56] These lesions can develop in anteriorly located placentae during or after an invasive procedure, such as amniocentesis or cordocentesis (Fig. 23.24). Acute haematomas are often similar in reflectivity to the surrounding placental tissue, which may explain why they are difficult to diagnose antenatally. Thus negative sonographic examination of the placenta does not exclude the diagnosis of retroplacental haematoma, whereas other intra-uterine abnormalities such as leiomyomas or placental tumours can simulate placental haematomas on sonography.[53] Ultrasound visualisation of a retroplacental haematoma in both acute and non-acute clinical situations is of little value in deciding when to undertake an emergency delivery.[50]

Placental tumours

Placental tumours include a wide range of placental abnormalities with different fetal and maternal implications. Prenatal differential diagnosis of both trophoblastic and non-trophoblastic tumours is based on symptoms, on specific ultrasound features and on biological investigations. The main characteristics of the different placental tumours are summarised below.

1   Trophoblastic tumours
    (a) Classic hydatidiform mole
        (i) Complete mole: diploid (46,XX in 90%; 46,XY in 10%):
            • Generalised swelling of the villous tissue (macroscopic)
            • Diffuse trophoblastic hyperplasia (microscopic)
            • No embryonic or fetal tissue (no gestational sac)
            • High levels of maternal serum human chorionic gonadotrophin (MShCG) and low levels of MSAFP in all cases.
        (ii) Twin pregnancy combining a complete diploid mole and a normal fetus with a normal placenta:
            • Molar mass associated with a normal fetus and placenta
            • High levels of MShCG and normal levels of MSAFP.
    (b) Partial hydatidiform mole
            • Focal swelling and trophoblastic hyperplasia
            • Embryo or fetus
        (i) Triploid (1% of all conceptions)
            • 69,XXX in 70%; 69,XXY in 29%; 69,XYY in less than 1%
            • Abnormal embryo or fetus (fetal growth restriction (100%) + anatomical defects,

including malformed hands, ventriculomegaly and heart anomalies (90%))
- Elevated levels of MShCG and high levels of MSAFP with normal levels of amniotic fluid α-fetoprotein (AFAFP) in most cases.

   (ii) Tetraploidy (very rare)

2 Non-trophoblastic tumours
   (a) Chorioangiomas
- Well circumscribed round mass protruding from the fetal plate
- Large tumours (> 5 cm diameter) associated with IUGR and non-immune hydrops fetalis due to blood shunting
- Elevated levels of MSAFP and AFAFP, with normal levels of MShCG.

   (b) Teratomas
- Isolated mass developing over the chorion with no umbilical cord.

   (c) Metastasis
- From various maternal and fetal origins
- Thick placenta.

Trophoblastic tumours

The principal histopathological finding in this category of placental abnormalities is the presence of microscopic trophoblastic hyperplasia, often associated with enlargement of the placenta and macroscopic hydropic (molar) transformation (swelling) of the villous tissue. These molar changes are not pathognomonic of gestational trophoblastic tumours and can be found in other placental pathologies, such as diffuse mesenchymal hyperplasia[29] or in prolonged placental retention *in utero* after fetal death. Hyperplasia of the trophoblast is associated with elevated levels of human chorionic gonadotrophin (hCG) in the maternal serum[57] and the rise of hCG levels is related to the extent of abnormal trophoblastic development.[57,58] The major prenatal features associated with placental trophoblastic disease are heavy vaginal bleeding, severe vomiting, pregnancy-induced hypertension, a uterus enlarged above the expected size and bilateral ovarian theca-lutein cysts.[58] Pathological examination of the products of conception in these cases is of paramount importance, as patients with trophoblastic tumours may develop persistent trophoblastic disease.[3,57] The placental trophoblastic disorders can be classified into two main categories, classic hydatidiform moles and partial moles.

Classic hydatidiform moles   Complete hydatidiform moles are characterised by generalised swelling of the villous tissue, diffuse trophoblastic hyperplasia and no embryonic or fetal tissue.[3,57] Complete moles are almost always diploid, with 46,XX chromosomal constitution in 90% of cases and a 46,XY karyotype in the remainder.[59] About 10–20% of complete moles can become invasive

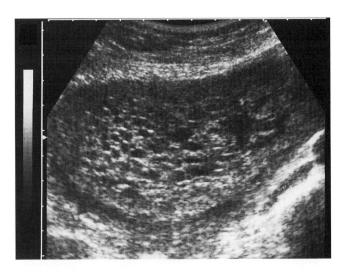

Fig. 23.25 Complete hydatidiform mole. Transverse sonogram at 12 weeks of gestation (calculated from the last menstrual period) showing a uterine cavity filled with heterogeneous central echoes and no gestational sac. The patient presented with bleeding and had a positive pregnancy urine test.

and metastasise.[57] Sonographically the uterus is filled with echo-free spaces of various shapes and sizes (snowstorm appearance).[1] Large echo-free areas or maternal lakes due to stasis of maternal blood in between the molar villi are often found. Theca lutein cysts secondary to the very high β-hCG levels may be diagnosed in up to 50% of cases, producing either soap-bubble or spoke-wheel appearance of the ovaries, which are enlarged. Although the vesicles are present in the first-trimester hydatidiform mole they may be too small to be delineated on sonography, and the tumour appears as homogeneous tissue (Fig. 23.25). Complete moles are associated with high levels of hCG and very low levels of AFP.[57,60] Classic moles may transform to choriocarcinoma (see Ch. 2).

Molar transformation of one ovum in a dizygotic twin pregnancy is a rare entity, comprising a classic hydatidiform mole with a normal pregnancy.[58,61] In these cases the hCG levels are raised, the AFP levels are within the normal range and sonographic or pathological examination shows a molar placental mass, together with a normal placenta and fetus (Fig. 23.26). Colour flow imaging can be helpful in these cases by confirming the avascular nature of the mass.[62]

Partial moles   This type of molar pregnancy refers to the combination of a fetus with localised placental molar degenerations.[62] Histologically it is characterised by focal swelling of the villous tissue, focal trophoblastic hyperplasia, and embryonic or fetal tissue. The abnormal villi are scattered within macroscopically normal placental tissue, which tends to retain its shape. Partial moles are usually triploid and of diandric origin, having two sets of chromosomes of paternal origin and one of maternal

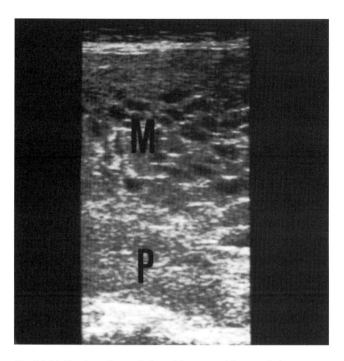

Fig. 23.26 Classic mole coexisting with a normal fetus and placenta. Sonogram at 25 weeks of a molar mass (M) and a normal placenta (P) in a twin pregnancy. Note the vesicular nature of the well developed hydatidiform mole. Colour flow mapping confirmed the avascular nature of the mass.

and cystic changes, irregularity, or increased reflectivity of the materno-embryonic interface, could improve the diagnosis of partial hydatidiform mole (PHM) in first-trimester missed abortion.[65] However, in this retrospective study the authors did not have cytogenetic data. Therefore, the proportion of triploid PHM in their small series cannot be established. In this context, in some cases molar changes may have been secondary to another placental pathology. Less than one-third of second and third-trimester triploidies present with a PHM on ultrasound, suggesting that paternally derived (diandric) triploidies are less common than maternally derived (digynic). Before 15 weeks PHM are also found in about one-third of all triploidies,[66] but gross molar changes are less likely to be detected in early pregnancy (Fig. 23.27). Early prenatal diagnosis therefore demands close and careful ultrasound monitoring of the pregnancy, karyotyping and serial hCG determination.

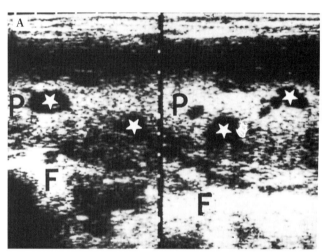

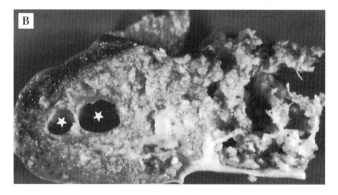

Fig. 23.27 Partial triploid mole. A: Transverse sonograms at 21 weeks of the placenta (P) and the fetus (F). The pregnancy was complicated by severe asymmetrical fetal growth retardation, oligohydramnios and early pregnancy-induced hypertension. The placenta is enlarged and contains echo-free spaces of various sizes and shapes (*). **B:** Pathological and cytological investigations confirmed a partial triploid mole. The placenta was hydropic with focal villous swelling (*).

origin.[63] Most have a 69,XXX or 69,XXY genotype derived from a haploid ovum, with duplication of the paternal haploid set either from a single sperm or, less frequently, from dispermic fertilisation. Triploidy of digynic origin, due to a double maternal contribution, is not associated with placental hydatidiform changes. Vaginal bleeding in the first or second trimester, with a total incidence of 47%, is the most common maternal symptom reported in both types of triploidies.

The phenotypic expression of both diandric and digynic triploidies includes growth restriction and disturbance of organogenesis that becomes obvious in fetuses surviving into the second trimester. From 16 weeks almost all triploid fetuses have a least one measurement below the normal range, and more than 70% present with severe growth restriction.[64] Structural defects are observed antenatally in about 93% of cases. The most common are abnormalities of the hands, bilateral cerebral ventriculomegaly, heart anomalies and micrognathia.[64] Triploid partial moles are not associated with specific fetal anomalies but almost always with symmetrical growth restriction.

Classically, a partial mole presents on ultrasound as an enlarged placenta (thickness > 4 cm at 18–22 weeks) containing multicystic avascular echo-free spaces (Swiss cheese appearance).[62] It has been suggested that the use of ultrasound criteria such as a ratio of transverse to antero-posterior dimension of the gestational sac greater than 1.5

Because they have different perinatal outcome triploid PHM must be distinguished from complete and partial moles with a coexisting fetus and from benign hydropic villous degeneration. Confined placental diploid or triploid mosaicism may appear as triploid partial mole on scanning, but in these cases the fetus is anatomically normal and has a diploid karyotype.[67,68] Ultrasound and pathological examination may in rare cases be complicated by the fact that the molar placental tissue comes from a resorbed twin.[69,70] In these cases the mother remains at risk for the complications of triploid PHM and in particular she may subsequently develop early pregnancy-induced hypertension. Villous hydatidiform transformations can also be found in association with tetraploidy, autosomal trisomy and monosomy X.[71] As the vast majority of tetraploidies abort spontaneously during the first weeks of pregnancy, those resulting from a double or triple paternal contribution and presenting with a partial 'molar' placenta have been rarely described in ongoing pregnancies.[72] In these cases the MShCG is high and the mother is at risk of persistent gestational trophoblastic disease. Finally, hydrops of the stem villi with placentomegaly but a normal trophoblast have also been observed in cases of Beckwith–Wiedemann syndrome, and with a phenotypically normal fetus.[58] This anomaly appears to be a limited malformation of the extra-embryonic mesoderm involving the mesenchyme and the vessels of the stem villi of several cotyledons, and it has therefore been referred to as mesenchymal dysplasia. Apart from a partial mole appearance and increased thickness, the placenta shows no vascular abnormalities until mid-gestation.

Doppler investigation has a limited role in the differential diagnosis or management of PHM. An abnormally high uterine artery resistance index (RI) has been found in about half of the cases of second-trimester triploidy that we investigated.[64] There is no difference in uterine artery RI between triploid pregnancies with and without partial mole, suggesting that the insufficient trophoblastic infiltration of the placental bed is a common feature of both phenotypes of triploidy. By contrast, triploidies presenting with PHM are associated with a higher umbilical artery resistance to flow and a low umbilical vein pH, indicating an impairment of the villous circulation development and trophoblast functions. In these cases abnormal umbilical artery flow velocity waveforms have been reported as early as 12 weeks of gestation.[66]

Non-trophoblastic tumours

This category of placental abnormalities includes tumours arising from any of the non-trophoblastic elements of the placenta.[3]

Chorioangiomas occur in 0.5–1% of the placentae examined at term.[2,3] The microscopic appearance may be that of a capillary angioma (vascular), mesenchymal hyperplasia (cellular), or usually a mixture of the two.[2] Most chorioangiomas are single, encapsulated, small, round and intraplacental.[2,3] Large tumours are variable in shape, divided by fibrous septa, and often protrude from the fetal surface near the cord insertion.[2,3] Degenerative changes such as necrosis, calcification, hyalinisation or myxoid changes are frequently present. A placental tumour combining a vascular chorioangioma and atypical trophoblastic proliferation (chorangiocarcinoma) was recently described, suggesting that in rare cases chorioangiomas could be true neoplasms rather than hamartomas.[73]

Large chorioangiomas are well circumscribed, have a different reflectivity from the rest of the placental tissue (Fig. 23.28) and are easily detectable early in pregnancy by sonography.[3,29,74–76] Chorioangiomas are associated with an increased incidence of polyhydramnios and fetal growth retardation.[3,29] Large vascular tumours (> 5 cm in diameter) can also be complicated by fetal cardiac failure with hydrops owing to the shunting of blood through the tumour.[3,29] Therefore, when a placental mass consistent with a chorioangioma is diagnosed antenatally it is important to perform serial sonographic examinations. An increase in reflectivity of the tumour with gestation has been related to fibrotic degeneration of the lesion,[29] which may reduce the risk of high-output fetal cardiac failure. Placental chorioangiomas can be associated with elevated levels of MSAFP and in the AFAFP.[29] Associated fetal angiomas (cutaneous or hepatic) occur in 10–15% of pla-

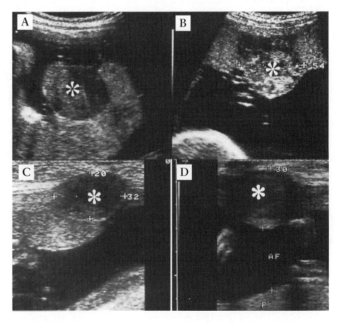

Fig. 23.28 Chorioangiomas. A and **B**: Composite compound sonograms of two placental chorioangiomas and **C** and **D**: two uterine leiomyomas. The chorioangiomas appear as heterogeneous and well circumscribed masses (*), protruding from the fetal plate of the placenta. For comparison, leiomyomas are poorly reflective and involve the uterine wall.

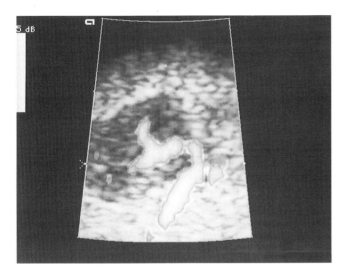

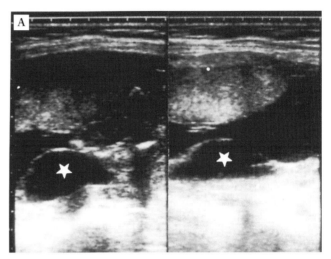

Fig. 23.29 Vascular chorioangioma. Colour flow mapping of a small (3 × 3 × 4 cm) chorioangioma in a pregnancy complicated by polyhydramnios at 24 weeks showing the blood supply to the tumour.

cental chorioangiomas and a detailed examination of the neonate is therefore recommended. The size of the tumour has no impact on the pregnancy if it is purely mesenchymatous. In this context colour flow mapping is of pivotal importance in evaluating the vascular nature of the chorioangioma (Fig. 23.29).[74–76]

Teratomas These extremely rare benign tumours of the placenta lie between the amnion and the chorion.[3] They probably result from an abnormal migration of the primordial germ cells, and can be distinguished from the fetus acardius amorphus by their lack of umbilical cord and polarity.[3] Teratomas have never been described sonographically.

Placental metastases Placental malignant metastases are uncommon, may be of either maternal or fetal origin,[3] and are often microscopic and multifocal. The only placental sonographic feature reported to date is increased thickness in a case of fetal malignant melanoma.[77] Malignant metastases must be differentiated from septic 'metastases' observed in cases of infections *in utero*, such as listerosis, which may create a similar sonographic appearance.

Other placental abnormalities

Placental cysts

Placental cysts (cytotrophoblastic cysts) (Fig. 23.30) are found in 20% of the placentae examined at term.[2,3] They have a round or oval cavity, are isolated from the placental circulation and contain a gelatinous fluid (Fig. 23.30B). These cysts are located within the placental tissue (septal

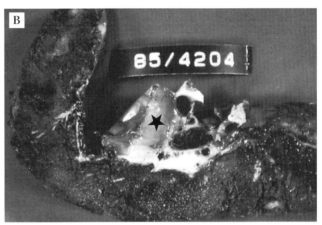

Fig. 23.30 Cytotrophoblastic cyst. A: Transverse scans at 32 weeks showing an echo-free cavity under the fetal plate (*) corresponding to **B:** a subchorionic cytotrophoblastic cyst (*).

cyst) or under the fetal plate (subchorionic cyst) and are the only true placental cysts. Placental cysts occur more frequently in cases of diabetes mellitus or maternofetal rhesus incompatibility.[2,3] Sonographically they appear as single echo-free spaces (Fig. 23.30A) that persist unchanged on serial scans, contain no blood flow on real-time imaging and give no Doppler signal.[41]

Amniotic band disruption complex

Early rupture of the amnion results in mesodermal bands emanating from the chorionic side of the amnion which can tether parts of the developing embryo or fetus, leading to a wide range of malformations.[78] Multiple anomalies, such as limb deformities, craniofacial defects or ventral wall defects, occur in 77% of the cases and the prognosis depends on their severity.[78] Sonographically amniotic bands appear as linear echoes floating in the amniotic fluid and anchored to the chorionic plate but not necessarily connected to the fetal body (Fig. 23.31).

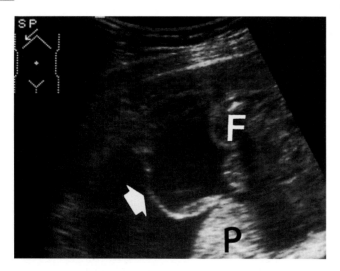

Fig. 23.31 Amniotic bands. Sonogram at 18 weeks of the placenta (P) showing linear echoes floating in the amniotic fluid (arrow) not connected with the fetal body (F). The fetus was born with no abnormalities.

Major structural abnormalities of the umbilical cord

The umbilical cord is derived from the stalk of the yolk sac and the allantois, and normally contains two umbilical arteries and one vein surrounded by a clear gelatinous structure (Wharton's jelly) covered by amnion.[2,3] In transverse sonographic section the arteries and umbilical vein appear as three separate rings, whereas in longitudinal section a portion of the cord will be seen as a series of parallel lines (Fig. 23.32) or as a central vein with the arteries looping around it. The mean umbilical cord circumference at term is 3.6 cm (1.2 cm diameter).[78]

Single umbilical artery syndrome

The absence of one umbilical artery is among the most common congenital fetal malformations, with an incidence of approximately 1% of all deliveries.[79] Associated major fetal anatomical defects are largely responsible for the high fetal and neonatal loss from this pathology.[80] Fetal malformations are present in about 50% of the cases of single umbilical artery (SUA) and can affect any organ system.[79,80] The incidence of intra-uterine growth retardation is significantly elevated among fetuses with an SUA, and is found without other congenital anomalies in 15–20% of cases.[79,80] Table 23.1 summarises the retrospective results of a comparison of sonographic and postnatal findings in 80 cases of SUA syndrome. In this context minor malformations of the musculoskeletal system or the genitourinary tract are often underdiagnosed by ultrasonography, especially if they are isolated.[79]

The prenatal diagnosis of the absence of one umbilical artery was first reported at around 20 weeks of gesta-

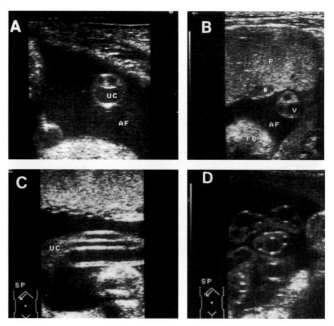

Fig. 23.32 Normal cord. Transverse and longitudinal scans at 28–32 weeks of gestation, showing the normal anatomy of the umbilical cord (UC) with two arteries and one vein.

Table 23.1 Comparison of prenatal sonographic features and post-natal findings in a series of 80 cases of single umbilical artery. (Modified from Jauniaux *et al.* J Gynecol Obstet Biol Reprod 1989).

Comparative data (*n* = 80)	Ultrasound findings	Neonatal findings
Number of fetuses with associated malformation(s)	21 (26.6%)	34 (42.5%)
Incidence of total IUGR	28.3%	36.4%
Incidence of isolated IUGR	15%	20%
Distribution of the different associated fetal malformations		
Musculoskeletal system	15 (28.8%)	32 (32%)
Urogenital system	11 (21.1%)	20 (20%)
Gastrointestinal system	3 (5.8%)	11 (11%)
Central nervous system	12 (23.1%)	11 (11%)
Integument	3 (5.8%)	9 (9%)
Cardiovascular system	4 (7.7%)	8 (8%)
Respiratory system	4 (7.7%)	6 (6%)
Miscellaneous	– (0%)	3 (3%)
Total	52 (100%)	100 (100%)

IUGR = intra-uterine growth retardation.

tion.[81] The umbilical cord anatomy can often be visualised before that time, but a precise diagnosis of a single umbilical artery can be difficult and time consuming. During the second trimester or during the third trimester the umbilical cord anatomy can be examined in detail without difficulty (Fig. 23.33). However, various factors, such as oligohydramnios or multiple loops in the cord, can make accu-

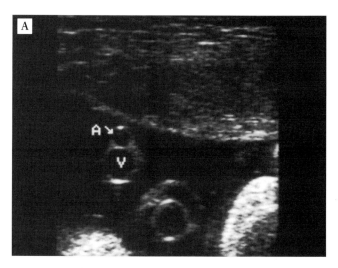
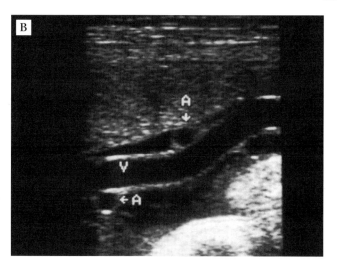

Fig. 23.33 Single umbilical artery. Transverse and longitudinal sonograms at 32 weeks demonstrating **A:** only one artery (A) and **B:** one vein (V). The fetus was growth retarded with no associated malformation.

rate visualisation of the cord vessels impossible, even near term. High-resolution colour Doppler imaging has an important role in early and accurate diagnosis of SUA (Fig. 23.34) and is of clinical value in view of the possible association of a single umbilical artery and intra-uterine growth retardation with no major fetal malformation.[82]

Cord tumours

Embryonic cysts

Remnants of the allantoic duct (urachus) and of the omphalomesenteric duct (vitelline duct) are common findings on microscopic examination of the umbilical cord.[2,3]

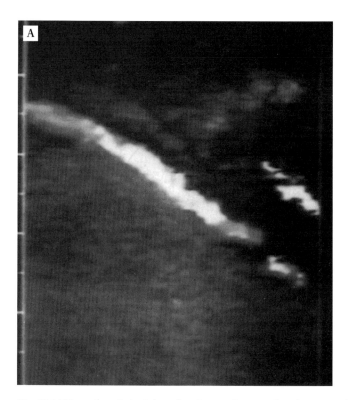
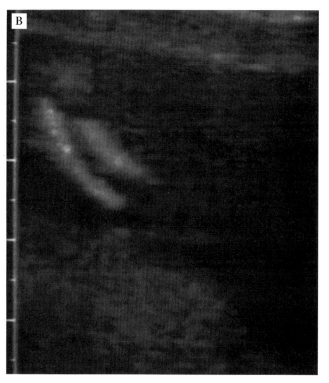

Fig. 23.34 Normal cord. A: Colour flow image of a normal cord at 21 weeks of gestation for comparison with **B:** single umbilical artery. Colour flow image of single umbilical artery cord at 18 weeks associated with multiple fetal malformations and oligohydramnios. (Reproduced with permission from Jauniaux *et al.* Am J Obstet Gynecol 1989; 161: 1195.)

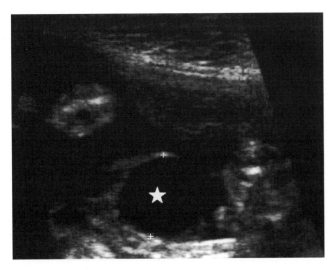

Fig. 23.35 Allantoic duct cyst. Sonogram of the cord near the fetal insertion at 32 weeks showing a poorly reflective round mass corresponding to an allantoic duct cyst (*). Blood flow within the mass was excluded by colour flow imaging.

Traces of the allantoic duct are found in 22.8% of cords examined histologically, located with a similar incidence on both ends of the cord.[83] Remnants of the vitelline duct are found in 2.4%, located mostly on the fetal end of the cord.[83] Cysts originating from these remnants have been reported very occasionally in the literature.

Although most of these cysts are small, some may exceed 5 cm in diameter and can be sonographically detected as a single fluid-filled mass (Fig. 23.35). Allantoic cysts may coexist with an omphalocele[84] or with a patent urachus secondary to a distal genitourinary tract obstruction.[85] Rarely structures arising from vitelline duct remnants differentiate to form gastric mucosa and if ulceration occurs it may cause serious damage to the umbilical vessels. Allantoic and omphalomesenteric cysts having a similar sonographic appearance cannot be distinguished *in utero*. The prevalence of umbilical cord cysts at 7–13 weeks of gestation is 3% and in more than 20% of cases there are fetal chromosomal or structural defects.[86]

Angiomyxomas

The discovery of an umbilical cord angiomyxoma or haemangioma is a rare event. Although the condition was recognised early in the first half of this century, fewer than 30 cases have been recorded in the literature.[87-93] Cord angiomyxomas tend to be in intimate contact with one or more umbilical vessels, from which they probably arise, at both fetal and placental extremities of the cord.[83,87] The majority consist of nodules clearly attached to the cord.[87,93] Potential fetal complications of cord angiomyxomas include compression of the main vessels, with

retarded growth and possible intra-uterine death.[87] Angiomas of the cord may also be associated with non-immune hydrops fetalis.[89] Although 16%–33% of placental chorioangiomas are accompanied by polyhydramnios,[3] only rarely have cases of cord angiomyxomas been complicated in this way.[91] Ultrastructural studies of the umbilical cord amniotic epithelium reveal major differences from the placental amnion, suggesting that passage of fluid occurs with far less ease through the cord amnion.[87] This explains the constant association of oedema and myxomatous degeneration of Wharton's jelly with angiomyxomas, a change that does not occur with placental chorioangiomas.[87] Associated vascular neoplasms at other sites are known to occur in children born with a placental chorioangioma (see p. 544). Two cases of superficial skin angiomas and one case of hepatic angioma out of 30 cases of cord angiomyxomas have been reported.[89,93,94] Therefore, a careful post-natal examination of the neonate is recommended in case of a cord angiomyxoma.

These tumours appear sonographically as focal, highly reflective areas corresponding to myxoid tissue and vascular proliferation (Fig. 23.36), with adjacent poorly reflective (pseudocystic) regions due to focal oedema (myxomatous degeneration) of the Wharton's jelly (Fig. 23.37). Angiomas involving the placental insertion of the cord sometimes extend on to the fetal plate and may be difficult to differentiate sonographically from a classic placental chorioangioma.[90,91] Complete infiltration of the cord by the angiomatous tissue and secondary progressive shortening of the cord have serious implications for vaginal delivery. When such a condition is discovered in the prenatal period a caesarean section is recommended. Serial ultrasound examinations to monitor the enlargement of the lesion must be performed regularly and combined with Doppler measurements to detect the umbilical cord compression. Raised MSAFP may be the earliest prenatal clue to the development of a cord angiomyxoma.[29,88,92] Colour flow Doppler imaging may also help the ultrasonographer (Fig. 23.38) in early prenatal diagnosis of this cord abnormality.[82]

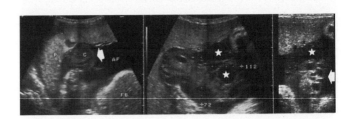

Fig. 23.36 Angiomyxoma of the cord. Heterogeneous multicystic mass involving the entire length of the cord at 36 weeks of gestation. The lesion is made of reflective zones (arrows) surrounded by echo-poor areas (*) and corresponds to an angiomyxoma of the cord (see also Fig. 23.38).

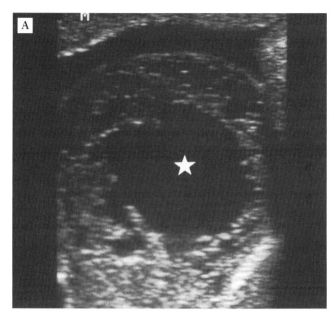

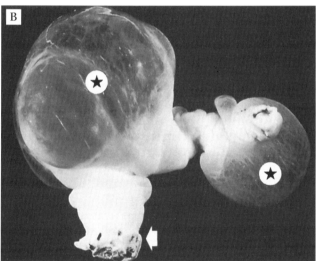

Fig. 23.37 False cyst of the cord. Same case as in Figure 23.36. A: Enlargement of an echo-free area (*) near the fetal insertion of the cord. B: View of the cord after delivery demonstrating two areas of oedema (*), corresponding to the echo-free areas (pseudocyst) described antenatally. The tumour starts near the placental insertion (arrow) and ends 2 cm from the umbilicus (see also Fig. 23.38).

Pseudocysts

Oedema of the Wharton's jelly has been associated with diabetes, maternofetal rhesus incompatibility and stillbirth.[95] Giant focal cord oedema is rare and gives an ultrasound appearance of an echo-free multicystic mass (Fig. 23.39). These pseudocysts are presumably due to the compression of umbilical cord vessels resulting from anterior fetal abdominal defects,[96] or are secondary to the development of a cord angioma (Fig. 23.37).

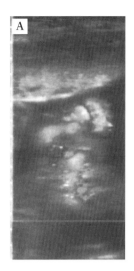
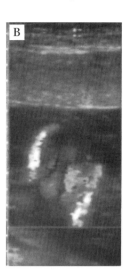

Fig. 23.38 Angiomyxoma of the cord. A: Colour flow image of the cord tumour described in Figures 23.36 and 23.37, showing an abnormal vascular pattern at the placental insertion. **B:** Colour flow image showing the three vessels separated by a reflective structure partially compressing the umbilical vein. (Reproduced with permission from Jauniaux *et al.* Am J Obstet Gynecol 1989; 161: 1195.)

Teratomas

The extremely rare teratoma of the cord is derived from primitive germ cells that aberrantly migrate from the primitive gut wall.[3] The tumour has not yet been documented by ultrasound.

Vascular lesions of the cord

Haematomas

Spontaneous cord haematomas are occasional perinatal findings and are usually located near the fetal umbilicus.[3] Mechanical trauma of the cord, such as prolapse, torsion, strangulation or dissecting aneurysm, are all potential causes of haematoma. The vein appears to be affected more often than the arteries.[3] The implication of a cord haematoma may range from complete occlusion of the cord vessels, with inevitable fetal death, to varying degrees of fetal distress, either acute or chronic.[97–101] Small haematomas will probably not affect fetal umbilical circulation because the blood may be resorbed before delivery. At ultrasound examination the cord appears markedly thickened, sausage-shaped and extremely highly reflective.[98–101] Accidental laceration of the umbilical cord vessels by uncontrolled needle movements was reported during the early days of amniocentesis before ultrasound guidance was used, when the estimated incidence was between 0.3% and 2.3%.[102] Most of the cases were reported after third-trimester amniocentesis, as the relatively small amount of liquor and the large size of the fetus at this stage reduced the possible movement of the cord away

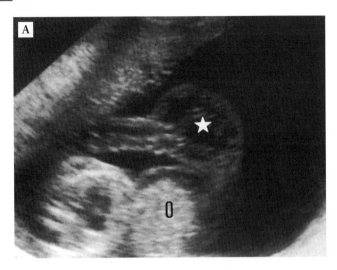

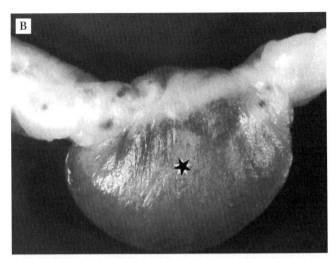

Fig. 23.39 False cyst of the cord. A: Transverse scan of the umbilical cord showing a large poorly reflective mass (*) juxtaposed with an omphalocele (O), corresponding to B: focal oedema (*) of the Wharton's jelly (pseudocyst). (Reproduced with permission from Jauniaux *et al. Prenat Diagn* 1988; 8: 557.)

from the needle tip. Rare observations of haematoma leading to fetal death or cord laceration have been observed *in utero* by sonography during amniocentesis.[103]

Cases of fetal death have also been reported after cordocentesis.[104–106] However, compared to amniocentesis, uncontrolled movements of the needle in cordocentesis are reduced, presumably because in this technique cord puncture is deliberate and precise and is performed under continuous ultrasound guidance. However, increased intravascular pressure, which may be present in the recipient of a twin–twin syndrome[10] or following a top-up fetal blood transfusion, and direct blood injection into the Wharton's jelly during fetal transfusions[98] can result in haematoma (Fig. 23.40) and consequent tamponade of the

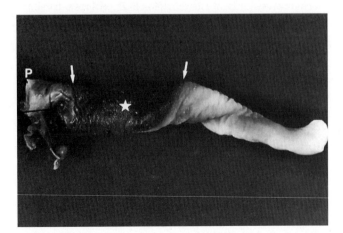

Fig. 23.40 Haematoma of the cord. Macroscopic appearance of the umbilical cord segment proximal to the placenta (P) 1 week after a fetal transfusion *in utero*. The arrows mark the extent of the haematoma (*).

umbilical cord vessels; the complication and mortality rates are higher following intravascular transfusion than after simple fetal blood sampling.[106] This accident should be suspected when fetal bradycardia develops during cordocentesis, and ultrasound can readily detect the development of a potentially harmful haematoma at the site of puncture.

Thrombosis

Thrombosis of one or more umbilical cord vessels is a rare complication with an incidence of approximately 0.08% among placentae examined prospectively at delivery.[107] Thrombosis of the umbilical vein occurs more frequently than thrombosis of one or both arteries, and perinatal morbidity or mortality is more likely with umbilical artery thrombosis than with umbilical vein thrombosis.[107] The prevalence of antenatal and post-natal venous thrombosis is significantly higher in infants born to diabetic mothers.[107] Thrombosis of the umbilical vessels may also be secondary to localised increased resistance in the umbilical circulation in cases of torsion, compression and knotting of the cord.[3,107] It can affect the intra-abdominal portion of the umbilical vein and be associated with non-immune fetal hydrops.[108] Very highly reflective material within the lumen of the umbilical vessels is the main sonographic finding.[108]

Abnormalities of the cord insertion

The umbilical arteries branch off the hypogastric arteries, course lateral to the bladder, on to the anterior abdominal wall, and then through the umbilical cord to the placenta (Figs 23.3 and 23.41). The umbilical vein starts from the

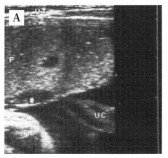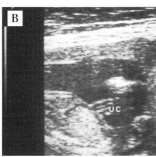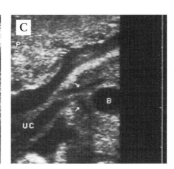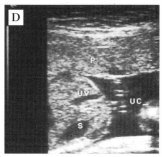

Fig. 23.41 Normal cord. Composite scans of the umbilical cord insertion (UC) showing **A**: the placental (P) insertion of the cord, **B**: the fetal (FB) insertion of the cord, **C**: the two umbilical arteries (arrows) on both sides of the fetal bladder (B), **D**: the umbilical vein (UV) at the level of the fetal liver. S – stomach.

placenta, carrying the oxygenated blood and enters the fetal abdomen inferior to the level of the liver (Fig. 23.41). Both fetal and placental insertions of the cord should be evaluated during sonographic examination. The placental insertion is usually associated with a small echo-free space beneath the chorionic plate (Figs 23.12 and 23.41).

Marginal insertion

Marginal and markedly eccentric insertions of the cord have not been clearly distinguished in the literature. This may explain the wide variation of their incidence in the general population.[3] By measuring the distance between the cord insertion and the closer placental margin one can avoid classification problems. With this method a significantly shorter distance was found in placentae from *in vitro* fertilisation and from the single umbilical artery syndrome compared to controls.[79,109] This form of cord insertion is not associated with an increase of pregnancy complications but may indicate a malrotation of the blastocyst at implantation.[3,109]

Velamentous insertion

Placenta velamentosa (insertion of the umbilical cord into the membranes at the placental margins) is a well defined pathological entity with a frequency around 1% of pregnancies.[2,3] The relation between this abnormal cord insertion and associated developmental defects is a matter of some debate. Some authors have observed a high incidence of fetal malformations associated with extraplacental cord insertions, whereas others have only found an increased number of small for dates neonates but not of malformation.[3] From a clinical point of view, attachment of the cord to the extraplacental membranes is important because of the risk of severe fetal haemorrhage during labour.[110] Antenatal diagnosis of attachment of the cord to the membranes rather than the placental mass can be diagnosed before labour by ultrasonography.[78,110]

Other cord abnormalities

Abnormalities of length

The umbilical cord has an average length of 54 cm at 34 weeks and 60 cm at term.[111] Male fetuses have significantly longer cords than females.[111] A cord less than 35 cm is defined as abnormally short. Short cords are found in fetuses with decreased *in utero* movements from a variety of causes, or are due to a primary defect of umbilical cord and abdominal wall formation.[112,113] Excessive cord length may predispose to true knots or to cord prolapse during labour. It is almost impossible to determine umbilical cord length prior to delivery during routine sonographic examination. In cases of extended cord angiomyxoma the cord is highly reflective and rigid and its length can be estimated by ultrasound.[93]

Prolapse, looping and knots

Prolapse of the umbilical cord through the cervix into the vagina is an obstetric emergency, with an incidence that varies between 0.5% and 0.6% of deliveries.[114–116] Cord prolapses are more likely to occur in premature deliveries, with a long umbilical cord, when the presenting part is unengaged and in pregnancies complicated by polyhydramnios.[78,114] Sonography can easily demonstrate fine parallel linear echoes corresponding to the cord, in the lower segment, below the presenting part.[78,116,117]

Looping of the cord may occur around the fetal neck, body or shoulder[114] and can be diagnosed by sonography (Fig. 23.42). Although in singletons looping of the cord around the neck is an uncommon cause of fetal death, a significant proportion of the high mortality of monoamniotic twins can be attributed to umbilical cord problems.[114]

True knots of the cord are thought to be caused by excessive fetal movements early in pregnancy[117] and must be distinguished from 'false knots', which are caused by focal aggregation of vessels.[3] True knots of the umbilical cord

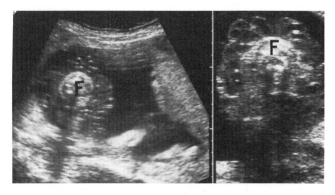

Fig. 23.42 Cord around the neck. Sonograms at 32 weeks showing cord loops surrounding the fetal neck (F).

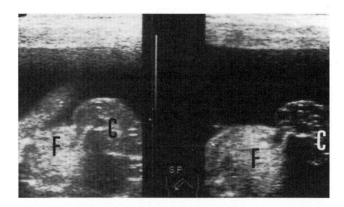

Fig. 23.43 Knot of the cord. Sonograms at 28 weeks showing a homogeneous mass of the cord (C). The appearance of the mass was not modified by fetal (F) movements and persisted on subsequent examination. A true knot of the umbilical cord was found after delivery.

occur in 0.04–1% of pregnancies and are more frequent in monoamniotic twins, in those with a long cord and in pregnancies complicated by polyhydramnios.[78] The umbilical vessels, protected by the Wharton's jelly, are rarely completely occluded. However, tight knots lead to vascular occlusion, with fetal death *in utero*. Sonographically, a true umbilical knot appears as a complex homogeneous mass unmodified by fetal movements and unchanged on subsequent examinations (Fig. 23.43).

Stricture or coarctation

This rare abnormality is characterised by a localised narrowing of the cord with the disappearance of Wharton's jelly, thickening of the vascular walls, and narrowing of their lumina.[78] The site of stricture or constriction is generally close to the fetus, and this abnormality may result from a focal failure of the Wharton's jelly development.[78] Antenatal diagnosis has not as yet been achieved.

Conclusion

The majority of pregnant women used to be scanned between 18 and 22 weeks of gestation for prenatal diagnosis of fetal malformation and placental location. An increasing number of placental and cord abnormalities, including placenta praevia, molar changes, placenta accreta, chorioangioma, cord cyst, single umbilical artery cord and vasa praevia, can be diagnosed between 12 and 16 weeks of gestation. These anomalies have a direct impact on the management of the pregnancy, and the placenta and cord should be examined at the time of the first ultrasound examination.

Most placental and cord lesions occur at an early stage of gestation and may indicate the possibility of late fetal or maternal complications. Placental investigations require close collaboration between sonographers, clinicians and pathologists. Ultrasound/pathological correlation is necessary in cases where the nature of the lesion is not well established *in utero*, but can also help sonographers who are not familiar with placental pathology to improve the accuracy of their diagnoses.

The placenta is a dynamic organ. Depending on the delay between the development of a lesion *in utero* and delivery, the ultrasound features and the pathological findings can be very different. Thus, serial ultrasound examination is recommended in cases where there may be an association between abnormal placental morphology and perinatal complications. Advances in ultrasound equipment, such as computerised sonography and colour Doppler imaging, have enhanced the antenatal diagnosis of many placental and cord abnormalities described in this chapter.

REFERENCES

1 Jauniaux E, Campbell S. Perinatal assessment of placental and cord abnormalities. In: Chervenak F A, Isaacson G, Campbell S, eds. The textbook of obstetrics and gynecologic ultrasound. Boston: Little, Brown and Company, 1993: 327–344

2 Benirschke K, Kaufmann P. Pathology of the human placenta. New York: Springer-Verlag, 1990

3 Fox H. Pathology of placenta, 2nd edn. Philadelphia: W B Saunders, 1997

4 Jauniaux E. Intervillous circulation in the first trimester: the phantom of the color Doppler obstetric opera. Ultrasound Obstet Gynecol 1996; 8: 73–76

5 Brossens I, Robertson W B, Dixon H G. The physiological response of the vessels of the placental bed to normal pregnancy. J Pathol Bacteriol 1967; 93: 569–579

6 Jauniaux E, Zaidi J, Jurkovic D, Campbell S, Hustin J. Comparison of color Doppler features and pathologic findings in complicated early pregnancy. Hum Reprod 1994; 9: 2432–2437

7 Jaffe R, Jauniaux E, Hustin J. Maternal circulation in the first trimester human placenta: myth or reality? Am J Obstet Gynecol 1997; 176: 695–705

8 Grannum P A T, Berkowitz R L, Hobbins J C. The ultrasonic changes in the maturing placenta and their relation to fetal pulmonic maturity. Am J Obstet Gynecol 1979; 133: 915–922

9 Harman C R, Manning F A, Stearns E, Morrison I. The correlation of ultrasonic placental grading and fetal pulmonary maturation in five hundred sixty-three pregnancies. Am J Obstet Gynecol 1982; 143: 941–943

10 Quinlan R W, Cruz A C, Buhi W C, Martin M. Changes in placental ultrasonic appearance. I. Incidence of grade III changes in the placenta in correlation to fetal pulmonary maturity. Am J Obstet Gynecol 1982; 144: 468–470

11 Quinlan R W, Cruz A C. Ultrasonic placental grading and fetal pulmonary maturity. Am J Obstet Gynecol 1982; 142: 110–111

12 Gast M G, Ott W. Failure of ultrasonic placental grading to predict severe respiratory distress in a neonate. Am J Obstet Gynecol 1983; 146: 464–465

13 Hills D, Irwin G A L, Tuck S, Baim R. Distribution of placental grades in high-risk gravidas. AJR 1984; 143: 1011–1013

14 Proud J, Grant A M. Third trimester placental grading by ultrasonography as a test of fetal wellbeing. BMJ 1987; 294: 1641–1644

15 Ohel G, Granat M, Zeevi D et al. Advanced ultrasonic placental maturation in twin pregnancies. Am J Obstet Gynecol 1987; 156: 76–78

16 Donald I. On launching a new diagnostic science. Am J Obstet Gynecol 1968; 103: 609–628

17 Campbell S, Kohorn E I. Placental localization by ultrasonic compound scanning. J Obstet Gynaecol Br Cwlth 1968; 75: 1007–1013

18 Gottesfeld K R, Thompson H E, Holmes J H, Taylor E S. Ultrasonic placentography: a new method for placental localization. Am J Obstet Gynecol 1966; 96: 539–547

19 Donald I, Abdulla U. Placentography by sonar. J Obstet Gynaecol Br Cwlth 1968; 75: 993–1006

20 Dippel A L, Brown W H. Roentgen visualization of the placenta by soft tissue technique. Am J Obstet Gynecol 1940; 40: 986–994

21 Kohorn E I, Walker R H S, Morrison J, Campbell S. Placental localization: a comparison between ultrasonic compound B scanning and radioisotope scanning. Am J Obstet Gynecol 1969; 103: 868–877

22 McShane P M, Heyl P S, Epstein M F. Maternal and perinatal morbidity resulting from placenta praevia. Obstet Gynecol 1985; 65: 176–182

23 Clark S T, Koonings P P, Phelan J P. Placenta previa/accreta and prior cesarean section. Obstet Gynecol 1985; 66: 89–92

24 Rizos N, Doran T A, Miskin M, Benzie B J, Ford J A. Natural history of placenta praevia ascertained by diagnostic ultrasound. Am J Obstet Gynecol 1979; 133: 287–291

25 Kurjak A, Borsic B. Changes of placental site diagnosed by repeat ultrasonic examination. Acta Obstet Gynecol Scand 1977; 56: 161–165

26 Andersen S, Steinke N M S. The clinical significance of asymptomatic mid-trimester low placentation diagnosed by ultrasound. Acta Obstet Gynecol Scand 1988; 67: 339–341

27 Taipale P, Hiilesmaa V, Ylostalo P. Diagnosis of placenta previa by transvaginal sonography at 12–16 weeks in a nonselected population. Obstet Gynecol 1997; 89: 364–367

28 Jauniaux E. Placental ultrasonographic measurements: what can we learn and is it worth doing routinely? Ultrasound Obstet Gynecol 1992; 2: 241–242

29 Jauniaux E, Moscoso G, Campbell S, Gibb D, Driver M, Nicolaides K H. Correlation of ultrasound and pathologic findings of placental anomalies in pregnancies with elevated maternal serum alpha-fetoprotein. Eur J Obstet Gynecol Reprod Biol 1990; 37: 219–230

30 Bleker O P, Kloosterman G J, Breur W, Mieras D J. The volumetric growth of the human placenta: a longitudinal ultrasonic study. Am J Obstet Gynecol 1977; 127: 657–661

31 Geirsson R T, Ogston S A, Patel N B, Christie A D. Growth of the total intra-uterine, intramniotic and placental volume in normal singleton pregnancy measured by ultrasound. Br J Obstet Gynaecol 1985; 92: 46–53

32 Wolf H, Oosting H, Treffers P E. Second-trimester placental volume measurements by ultrasound: prediction of fetal outcome. Am J Obstet Gynecol 1989; 160: 121–126

33 Wolf H, Oosting H, Treffers P E. A longitudinal study of the relationship between placental and fetal growth as measured by ultrasonography. Am J Obstet Gynecol 1989; 161: 1140–1145

34 Jauniaux E, Avni F E, Donner C, Rodesch F, Wilkin P. Ultrasonographic diagnosis and morphological study of placentas circumvallate. JCU 1989; 16: 126–131

35 Hurley V A, Beischer N A. Placenta membranacea. Case reports. Br J Obstet Gynaecol 1987; 94: 798–802

36 Molloy C E, McDowell W, Armour T, Crawford W, Bernstine R. Ultrasound diagnosis of placenta membranacea in utero. J Ultrasound Med 1983; 2: 377–379

37 Jauniaux E, Toplis P J, Nicolaides K H. Sonographic diagnosis of a non-praevia placenta accreta. Ultrasound Obstet Gynecol 1996; 7: 58–60

38 Jauniaux E, Jurkovic D, Campbell S. In vivo investigations of anatomy and physiology of early human placental circulations. Ultrasound Obstet Gynecol 1991; 1: 435–445

39 Vermeulen R C W, Lambalk N B, Exalto N, Arts N F T. An anatomic basis for ultrasound images of the human placenta. Am J Obstet Gynecol 1985; 153: 806–810

40 Jauniaux E, Moscoso G, Vanesse M, Campbell S, Driver M. Perfusion fixation for placental morphologic investigation. Hum Pathol 1991; 22: 442–449

41 Jauniaux E, Avni F E, Elkazen N, Wilkin P, Hustin J. Etude morphologique des anomalies placentaires échographiques de la deuxième moitié de la géstation. J Gynecol Obstet Biol Reprod 1989; 18: 601–613

42 Jauniaux E, Ramsay B, Campbell S. Ultrasonographic investigation of placental morphology and size during the second trimester of pregnancy. Am J Obstet Gynecol 1994; 170: 130–137

43 Jauniaux E, Nicolaides K H. Placental lakes, absent umbilical artery diastolic flow and poor fetal growth in early pregnancy. Ultrasound Obstet Gynecol 1996; 7: 141–144

44 Kaplan C, Blanc W A, Elias J. Identification of erythrocytes in intervillous thrombi: a study using immunoperoxidase identification of hemoglobin. Hum Pathol 1982; 13: 554–557

45 Hoogland H J, De Haan J, Vooys J. Ultrasonographic diagnosis of intervillous thrombosis related to RH isoimmunization. Gynecol Obstet Invest 1979; 10: 237–245

46 Spirt B A, Gordon L P, Kagan E H. Intervillous thrombosis: sonographic and pathologic correlation. Radiology 1983; 147: 197–200

47 Olah K S, Gee H, Rushton I, Fowlie A. Massive subchorionic thrombohaematoma presenting as a placental tumour: case report. Br J Obstet Gynaecol 1987; 94: 995–997

48 Jauniaux E, Campbell S. Sonographic assessment of placental abnormalities. Am J Obstet Gynecol 1990; 163: 1650–1658

49 Deans A, Jauniaux E. Prenatal diagnosis and outcome of subamniotic hematomas. Ultrasound Obstet Gynecol 1998; 11: 319–323

50 Sholl J S. Abruptio placentae: clinical management in nonacute cases. Am J Obstet Gynecol 1987; 156: 40–51

51 Jauniaux E, Jurkovic D. Ultrasound in early pregnancy complications. In: O'Brian P M S, Grudzinskas J G, eds. Problems of early pregnancy – advances in diagnosis and management. London: RCOG, 1997: 137–153

52 Abu-Yousef M M, Bleicher J J, Williamson R A, Weiner C P. Subchorionic hemorrhage: sonographic diagnosis and clinical significance. AJR 1987; 149: 737–740

53 Nyberg D A, Cyr D R, Mack L A, Wilson D A, Shuman W P. Sonographic spectrum of placental abruption. AJR 1987; 148: 161–164

54 Sauerbrei E E, Pham D H. Placental abruption and subchorionic hemorrhage in the first half of pregnancy: US appearance and clinical outcome. Radiology 1986; 160: 190–195

55 Pearlstone M, Baxi L. Subchorionic hematoma: A review. Obstet Gynecol Surv 1993; 48: 65–68

56 Ball R H, Ade C M, Schoenborn J A, Crane J P. The clinical significance of ultrasonographically detected subchorionic hemorrhages. Am J Obstet Gynecol 1996; 174: 996–1002

57 Berkowitz R, Ozturk M, Goldstein D, Bernstein M, Hill L, Wands J R. Human chorionic gonadotropin and free subunits' serum levels in patients with partial and complete hydatidiform moles. Obstet Gynecol 1989; 74: 212–215

58 Jauniaux E, Nicolaides K H. Early ultrasound diagnosis and follow-up of molar pregnancies. Ultrasound Obstet Gynecol 1997; 9: 17–21

59 Kajii T, Ohama K. Androgenic origin of hydatidiform mole. Nature 1977; 268: 633–634

60 Jauniaux E, Gulbis B, Hyett J, Nicolaides K. Biochemical analyses of mesenchymal fluid in early pregnancy. Am J Obstet Gynecol 1998; 178: 765–769

61 Steller M A, Genest D R, Bernstein M R, Lage J M, Goldstein D P, Berkowitz R S. Natural history of twin pregnancy with complete hydatidiform mole and coexisting fetus. Obstet Gynecol 1994; 83: 35–42

62 Jauniaux E Ultrasound diagnosis and follow-up of gestational trophoblastic disease. Ultrasound Obstet Gynecol 1998; 11: 367–377

63 Jacobs P A, Szulman A E, Funkhouser J, Matsuura J S, Wilson C C. Human triploidy: relationship between parental origin of the additional haploid complement and development of partial hydatidiform mole. Ann Hum Genet 1982; 46: 223–231

64 Jauniaux E, Brown R, Rodeck C, Nicolaides K H. Prenatal diagnosis of triploidy during the second trimester of pregnancy. Obstet Gynecol 1996; 88: 983–989

65 Fine C, Bundy A L, Berkowitz R S, Boswell S B, Berezin A F, Doubilet P M. Sonographic diagnosis of partial hydatidiform mole. Obstet Gynecol 1989; 73: 414–418

66 Jauniaux E, Brown R, Snijders R J M, Noble P, Nicolaides K. Early prenatal diagnosis of triploidy. Am J Obstet Gynecol 1997; 176: 550–554

67 Crooij M J, Van Der Harten J J, Puyenbroek J I, Van Geijn H P, Arts N F T. A partial hydatidiform mole, dispersed throughout the placenta coexisting with a normal living fetus. Case report. Br J Obstet Gynaecol 1985; 92: 104–106

68 Sarno A P, Moorman A J, Kalousek D K. Partial molar pregnancy with fetal survival: an unusual example of confined placental mosaicism. Obstet Gynecol 1993; 82: 716–717

69 Steller M A, Genest D R, Bernstein M R, Lage J M, Goldstein D P, Berkowitz R S. Clinical features of multiple conception with partial or complete molar pregnancy and coexisting fetuses. J Reprod Med 1994; 39: 147–154

70 Nugent C E, Punch M R, Barr M, Leblanc L, Johnson M P, Evans M I. Persistence of partial molar placenta and severe preeclampsia after selective termination in a twin pregnancy. Obstet Gynecol 1996; 87: 829–831

71 Jauniaux E, Kadri R, Hustin J. Partial mole and triploidy: screening in patients with first trimester spontaneous abortion. Obstet Gynecol 1996; 88: 616–619

72 Appelman Z, Dgani R, Zalel Y, Elchalal U, Caspi B. Persistent gestational trophoblastic disease following evacuation of a tetraploid partial hydatidiform mole. Gynecol Oncol 1992; 44: 101–103

73 Jauniaux E, Zucker M, Meuris S, Verhest A, Wilkin P, Hustin J. Chorangiocarcinoma: an unusual tumour of the placenta. The missing link? Placenta 1988; 9: 607–614

74 Jauniaux E, Moscoso G, Campbell S. In vivo investigations of placental and umbilical cord anatomy. In: Reed G, Clairaux A, Cockburn F, Connor M, eds. Diseases of the fetus and newborn, 2nd edn. London: Chapman & Hall, 1995: 979–996

75 Jauniaux E, Jurkovic D, Campbell S, Kurjak A, Hustin J. Investigation of placental circulations by color Doppler ultrasound. Am J Obstet Gynecol 1991; 164: 486–488

76 Jauniaux E, Kadri R, Donner C, Rodesch F. Not all chorioangiomas are associated with elevated maternal serum alpha-fetoprotein. Prenat Diagn 1992; 12: 73–74

77 Campbell W A, Storlazzi E, Vintzileos A M, Wu A, Schneiderman H, Nochimson D J. Fetal malignant melanoma: ultrasound presentation and review of the literature. Obstet Gynecol 1987; 70: 434–439

78 Romero R, Pilu G, Jeanty P, Ghidini A, Hobbins J C. Prenatal diagnosis of congenital anomalies. Norwalk, Connecticut: Appleton and Lange, 1988: 385–402

79 Jauniaux E, De Munter C, Pardou A, Elkhazen N, Rodesch F, Wilkin P. Evaluation échographique du sydrome de l'artère ombilicale unique: une série de 80 cas. J Gynecol Obstet Biol Reprod 1989; 18: 341–348

80 Heifetz S A. Single umbilical artery: a statistical analysis of 37 autopsy cases and review of the literature. Perspect Pediatr Pathol 1984; 8: 345–378

81 Persutte W H, Hobbins J. Single umbilical artery: a clinical enigma in modern prenatal diagnosis. Ultrasound Obstet Gynecol 1995; 6: 216–229

82 Jauniaux E, Campbell S, Vyas S. The use of color Doppler imaging for prenatal diagnosis of umbilical cord anomalies: report of three cases. Am J Obstet Gynecol 1989; 161: 1195–1197

83 Jauniaux E, De Munter C, Vanesse M, Hustin J, Wilkin P. Embryonic remnants of the umbilical cord: morphological and clinical aspects. Hum Pathol 1989; 20: 458–462

84 Fink I J, Filly R A. Omphalocele associated with umbilical cord allantoic cyst: sonographic evaluation in utero. Radiology 1983; 149: 473–475

85 Renade R V, Nipladkar K B, Mtsorekar V R. Extraumbilical allantoic cyst: a case report. Indian J Pathol Bacteriol 1960; 9: 87–89

86 Ross J A, Jurkovic D, Zosmer N, Jauniaux E, Hacket E, Nicolaides K H. Umbilical cord cysts in early pregnancy: the prevalence, morphology and natural history. Obstet Gynecol 1997; 89: 442–445

87 Heifetz S A, Rueda-Pedraya M E. Hemangiomas of the umbilical cord. Pediatr Pathol 1983; 1: 385–393

88 Barson A J, Donnai P, Ferguson A, Donnai D, Read A P. Haemangioma of the cord: further cause of raised maternal serum and liquor alpha-fetoprotein. BMJ 1980; 281: 1252

89 Seifer D B, Ferguson J E, Behrens C M, Zemel S, Stevenson D K, Ross J C. Nonimmune hydrops fetalis in association with hemangioma of the umbilical cord. Obstet Gynecol 1985; 66: 283–286

90 Baylis M S, Jones R Y, Hughes M. Angiomyxoma of the umbilical cord detected antenatally by ultrasound. J Obstet Gynecol 1984; 4: 243–244

91 Mishriki Y Y, Vanyshelbaum Y, Epstein H, Blanc W. Hemangioma of the umbilical cord. Pediatr Pathol 1987; 7: 43–49

92 Resta R G, Luthy D A, Mahony B S. Umbilical cord hemangioma associated with extremely high alpha-fetoprotein levels. Obstet Gynecol 1988; 72: 488–490

93 Jauniaux E, Moscoso G, Chitty L, Gibb D, Driver M, Campbell S. An angiomyxoma involving the whole length of the umbilical cord: prenatal diagnosis by ultrasonography. J Ultrasound Med 1990; 9: 419–422

94 Barry F L, McCoy, Callahan W P. Haemangioma of the umbilical cord. Am J Obstet Gynecol 1951; 62: 675–680

95 Coulter J B S, Scott J M, Jordan M M. Oedema of the umbilical cord and respiratory distress in the newborn. Br J Obstet Gynaecol 1975; 82: 453–459

96 Jauniaux E, Donner C, Thomas C, Francotte J, Rodesch F, Avni E. Umbilical cord pseudocyst in trisomy 18. Prenat Diagn 1988; 8: 557–563

97 Schreier R, Brown S. Hematoma of the umbilical cord. Obstet Gynecol 1962; 20: 798–800

98 Ruvinsky E D, Wiley T L, Morrison J C, Blake P G. In utero diagnosis of umbilical cord hematoma by ultrasonography. Am J Obstet Gynecol 1981; 140: 833–834

99 Moise K J, Carpenter R J, Huhta J C, Deter R L. Umbilical cord hematoma secondary to in utero intravascular transfusion for RH isoimmunisation. Fetal Ther 1987; 2: 65–70

100 Sutro W H, Tuck S M, Loesevitz A, Novotny P L, Archbald F, Irwin G L A. Prenatal observation of umbilical cord hematoma. AJR 1984; 142: 801–802

101 Jauniaux E, Donner C, Simon P, Vanesse M, Hustin J, Rodesch F. Pathologic aspects of the umbilical cord after percutaneous umbilical blood sampling. Obstet Gynecol 1989; 73: 215–218

102 Gassner C B, Paul R H. Laceration of umbilical cord vessels secondary to amniocentesis. Obstet Gynecol 1976; 48: 627–630

103 Romero R, Chervenak F A, Coustan D, Berkowitz R L, Hobbins J C. Antenatal sonographic diagnosis of umbilical cord laceration. Am J Obstet Gynecol 1982; 143: 719–720

104 Daffos F, Capella-Paviosky M, Forestier F. Fetal sampling during pregnancy with use of a needle guided by ultrasound: a study of 606 consecutive cases. Am J Obstet Gynecol 1985; 153: 655–660

105 Jauniaux E, Nicolaides K H, Campbell S, Hustin J. Hematoma of the umbilical cord secondary to cordocentesis for intrauterine fetal transfusion. Prenat Diagn 1990; 10: 477–478

106 Ulm M R, Bettelheim D, Ulm B, Frigo P, Bernachek G. Fetal bradycardia following cordocentesis. Prenat Diagn 1997; 17: 919–923

107 Heifetz S A. Thrombosis of the umbilical cord: analysis of 52 cases and literature review. Pediatr Pathol 1988; 8: 37–54

108 Abrams S L, Callen P W, Filly R A. Umbilical vein thrombosis: sonographic detection in utero. J Ultrasound Med 1985; 4: 4: 283–285

109 Jauniaux E, Englert Y, Vanesse M, Hidden M, Wilkin P. Pathologic features of placentas from singleton pregnancies obtained by in vitro fertilization and embryo transfer. Obstet Gynecol 1990; 76: 61–64

110 Gianopoulos J, Carver T, Tomich P G, Kalman R, Gadwood K. Diagnosis of vasa previa with ultrasonography. Obstet Gynecol 1987; 69: 488–491

111 Mills J L, Harley E E, Moessinger A C. Standards for measuring umbilical cord length. Placenta 1983; 4: 423–426

112 Grange D K, Arya S, Opitz J M, Laxova R, Herrmann J, Gilbert E F. The short umbilical cord. Birth Defects 1987; 23: 191–214

113 Jauniaux E, Vyas S, Finlayson C, Moscoso G, Driver M, Campbell S. Early sonographic diagnosis of body stalk anomaly. Prenat Diagn 1990; 10: 127–132

114 Jauniaux E, Mawissa M, Peellarets C, Rodesch F. Nuchal cord in normal third trimester preganancy: a color Doppler imaging study. Ultrasound Obstet Gynecol 1992; 2: 417–419

115 Hales E D, Westney L S. Sonography of occult cord prolapse. JCU 1984; 12: 283–285

116 Johnson R L, Anderson J C, Irsik R D, Goodlin R C. Duplex ultrasound diagnosis of umbilical cord prolapse. JCU 1987; 15: 282–284

117 Chasnoff I J, Fletcher M A. True knot of the cord. Am J Obstet Gynecol 1977; 127: 425–427

Interventional procedures

Janet I Vaughan and Charles H Rodeck

Introduction

Reduction in perinatal mortality and long-term morbidity remains a challenge in modern obstetrics. Ultrasound imaging has enabled ready visualisation of the conceptus and has a unique potential for the diagnosis of fetal problems, so that management policies can be suitably altered. In addition, more subtle diagnoses may be achieved by an extensive range of invasive procedures, all ultrasound guided, which will be reviewed in this chapter. Although it is currently limited, the evolving uses and scope of intra-uterine therapy is an exciting field of medicine which is continually opening new frontiers.

Counselling

All patients undergoing invasive antenatal procedures are entitled to counselling to inform them of the fetal disorder under consideration, the procedures and risks involved for diagnosis or therapy, and the management options. Ideally this should be undertaken before conception, so that the parents can assess the facts objectively without threat to their current pregnancy. If the problem has only arisen during the current pregnancy, counselling must still be optimal and may be given at a time and place separate from that of the procedure. More than one session may be required, as the couple should have the opportunity to consider the issues before deciding on their management plan, which may be not to undergo any procedures. Obstetricians are responsible for ensuring that their patients are adequately informed and, if performing the counselling themselves, must be certain that the information given is accurate, current and non-directional. The skills of a geneticist, fetal medicine specialist or paediatric surgeon will often be required, as the diagnostic and therapeutic options are continually expanding.

Diagnostic procedures

Amniocentesis

Needles have been introduced into the human amniotic sac since at least 1877,[1] but the first clinical use of amniocentesis was reported in 1919 for a case of polyhydramnios.[2] Regular diagnostic amniocentesis began after Bevis reported its usefulness in the management of rhesus isoimmunisation.[3] Diagnostic use remained limited to the third trimester, mainly for the management of rhesus patients, for the next decade. In 1960 fetal gender, established by sex chromatin analysis in amniotic fluid cells, enabled antenatal management of X-linked recessive disorders by termination of male fetuses.[4] This was the first use of amniocentesis in genetic disease. In 1965 Jeffcoate *et al.* used amniotic fluid to diagnose inborn errors of metabolism.[5] They diagnosed the adrenogenital syndrome using amniotic fluid levels of 17-ketosteroid and pregnanetriol. Successful culture of amniocytes to yield a fetal karyotype was reported by Steele and Breg one year later.[6] The relationship between amniotic fluid AFP and open neural tube defects (NTD) was first described in 1972 by Brock and colleagues.[7,8]

Mid-trimester transabdominal amniocentesis remains the most established and widely used antenatal invasive procedure, accounting for 89% of prenatal tests in the UK.[9] In the 12-month period from April 1994 to the end of March 95, 31 887 amniocenteses were performed for karyotyping, representing 4.38% of the pregnant population. Even so, this figure under-represents the high-risk pregnancies eligible for prenatal diagnosis, reflecting such factors as ignorance of the procedure, religious or moral objections, and the unacceptability of late therapeutic abortion.

Technique

Ultrasound examination prior to amniocentesis allows confirmation of gestational age and fetal viability, evaluation of structural abnormalities, placental localisation and exclusion of multiple gestations. The optimal technique is simultaneous ultrasound 'monitoring', which has the advantage of allowing immediate adjustment of needle position as changes in the intra-uterine environment occur, and therefore a higher success rate with reduction in fetal, placental and cord trauma. de Crespigny and Robinson demonstrated a statistically significant reduction in technical difficulties from 9.9% in those with prior ultrasound to 3.7% in the simultaneously monitored group.[10] They also noted a fall in the number of spontaneous abortions from 2.4% to 0.8%. Similarly, in a series of 1300 patients undergoing genetic amniocentesis, Romero *et al.* compared 612 with prior ultrasound to 688 with simultaneous ultrasound monitoring and demonstrated a significant reduction in bloody or dry taps from 12.9% to 3.2%, and in repeat taps from 8.2% to 2%.[11]

Amniocentesis is performed as an outpatient procedure using standard aseptic precautions. A 20–22 G spinal needle is introduced transabdominally. The Canadian Medical Research Council (MRC) study associated needles larger than 19 G with increasing abortion risk.[12] Fifteen to 20 ml are usually aspirated, discarding the first millilitre to reduce maternal contamination.

A prospective randomised controlled trial of genetic amniocentesis in low-risk women reported a significantly increased risk of spontaneous abortion with placental perforation.[13] A more recent comparison of 1487 trans-placental with 3077 non-trans-placental amniocenteses suggested no difference in loss rates, but a reduction in transient rupture of the membranes if performed trans-placentally.[14]

For prenatal diagnosis the traditional timing of amniocentesis has been at 15 weeks or later. At this time the fundus is readily accessible transabdominally and the volume of amniotic fluid is approximately 150–200 ml, enabling aspiration of 15–20 ml without concern. Depending on the indication, a result may take 1–4 weeks, which precludes the termination of an affected fetus much before 20 weeks. In view of this disadvantage associated with mid-trimester amniocentesis, chorionic villus sampling (CVS) and early amniocentesis (EA) developed as alternative prenatal diagnostic procedures (see below).

Experience in performing amniocentesis has been shown to affect the success of the procedure. The UK MRC trial reported that clinicians who had the experience of over 50 procedures had a failure rate of 1.1%, compared to 9.9% for those with experience of fewer than 50.[15] Subsequent fetal loss is also related to the operator's experience, a spontaneous abortion rate of 0.3% with an experience of 50 increasing to 3.7% when this experience was limited to less than 10 in one series.[16]

Indications

Below 20 weeks:

- Chromosome analysis
- Genetic disorders
- Neural tube defects
- Fetal blood grouping
- Viral infection.

After 20 weeks:

- Rhesus alloimmunisation
- Fetal lung maturity
- Preterm premature rupture of the membranes.

Chromosomes   Fetal karyotyping is the most common indication for amniocentesis, the majority being performed to investigate abnormalities associated with increasing maternal age. The age-specific risk figures are higher at the time of amniocentesis than at birth, reflecting the increased abortion and stillbirth rate associated with chromosomally abnormal fetuses.[17,18] However, the reported spontaneous loss rate between amniocentesis and live birth varies from 33%[17] to 18%,[18] and may depend on the level of ascertainment of the live birth data. A recent meta-analysis of published data estimated the spontaneous loss rate of Down's syndrome fetuses between amniocentesis and live birth to be 12% (95% CI 5–18%).[19]

Amniotic fluid contains cells desquamated from fetal skin, body tracts and amnion. Karyotyping is performed on cultured cells and takes 2–3 weeks to obtain a result. Failure to detect an abnormal karyotype at amniocentesis is very unlikely because of the variety of organs contributing to the cell culture. Discordance between the karyotype obtained after amniotic cell culture and the actual fetal karyotype is possible, particularly when mosaicism is

detected. Mosaicism is not rare, with level 2 (multiple cells with the same abnormality in a single flask) and level 3 abnormalities (multiple cells with the same abnormality in multiple flasks) occurring with frequencies of 0.7% and 0.2%, respectively.[20–22] However, only in 20% of level 2 and 60% of level 3 mosaicism will these karyotypes be confirmed in the fetus. Fetal blood sampling (FBS) has been used to investigate this diagnostic dilemma. Gosden *et al.* reported 41 cases of amniotic cell mosaicism, of which 31 fetuses had a normal karyotype on FBS which was confirmed after delivery.[23]

The rate of maternal cell contamination in amniotic fluid cell cultures has been estimated to be 0.34% and the proportion that result in misdiagnosis is 0.11–0.22% of cases.[21,24] Detection using chromosomal heteromorphisms which differ between mother and fetus is possible.

Amniotic fluid cell culture failure rates vary from 0.4 to 1% of cases.[25–27] Recent reports suggest that higher failure rates may occur after 24 weeks gestation[25] and in chromosomally abnormal fetuses.[26,27]

Molecular cytogenetics using fluorescent *in-situ* hybridisation (FISH) with chromosome-specific DNA probes on interphase nuclei of uncultured amniocytes enables rapid targeted prenatal diagnosis (Fig. 24.1). In 7.4% of amniotic fluid samples, interphase FISH may be performed for indications that include abnormal ultrasound, abnormal maternal serum testing and advanced gestations.[28] Multiprobe analysis for chromosomes 13, 18, 21, X and Y

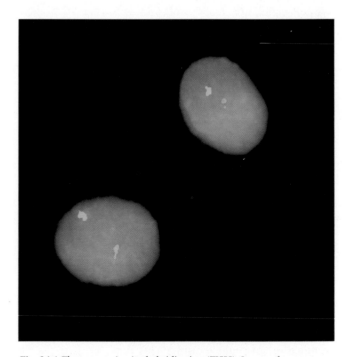

Fig. 24.1 Fluorescent *in situ* hybridisation (FISH). Image of two uncultured amniocytes following a single hybridisation with X (*green*) and Y (*orange*) centromeric probes, indicating a male fetus. (Courtesy of Dr A. Daniel.)

usually takes one day.[29] A recent report of 23 000 cases in the USA revealed that the aneuploidy detection rate was 95%, with a false-positive rate of 0.04% and a false-negative rate of 0.9%.[28] False results may be due to maternal cell contamination, poor hybridisation of probes, probe signal 'splitting' and technologist inexperience.[28,30] Uninformative studies occur in 3–6% of analyses.[28]

Genetic disorders   Amniocentesis enables some genetic conditions to be diagnosed prenatally from biochemical assays of amniotic fluid or cultured cells.[31] For example, Smith–Lemli–Opitz syndrome is an autosomal recessive condition characterised by facial dysmorphism and multiple congenital abnormalities. In 1993 it was first recognised that this condition results from abnormally low cholesterol levels, caused by a defect in the enzyme catalysing the final step in cholesterol biosynthesis.[32,33] Prenatal diagnosis became available by measuring the levels of 7-dehydrocholesterol in amniotic fluid.[34]

DNA analysis was first used in the prenatal diagnosis of the haemoglobinopathies, with the diagnosis of sickle cell anaemia on amniotic cells.[35] However, chorionic villi yield more DNA than amniocytes and, until the routine use of polymerase chain reaction (PCR) enabled amplification of small amounts of DNA, were the preferred tissue for diagnosis. Now amniocytes are as efficient as chorionic villi in DNA analysis.

The use of DNA analysis to diagnose genetic conditions relies on two basic approaches. Fetal diagnosis may be made directly if the genetic mutation is known and a specific gene probe of cloned complementary DNA is available for hybridisation. Alternatively, a disorder for which the mutation has not been identified may be diagnosed using linkage analysis of DNA sequences in close proximity to the gene locus by comparing DNA from the fetus, the proband and other family members. This method involves extensive family studies and is not always informative.

For example, the gene for cystic fibrosis was cloned in 1989, with the specific mutation δF_{508} found to be the most frequently occurring mutation.[36–38] Many other mutant alleles have also been characterised. For prenatal diagnosis using direct DNA analysis, defined mutations must be characterised in both parents. An unknown mutation in one or both parents necessitates the use of linkage analysis. Using both approaches, virtually all families are fully informative unless there is no tissue from the index affected child.[39] In this situation, microvillar enzyme testing on amniotic fluid may be the only option for prenatal diagnosis.[40]

Misdiagnoses may result from inadequate specimens, maternal tissue contamination, non-paternity, recombination, inadequate DNA digestion or inadequate family studies.

Because of the rapidity with which new genes are being identified, collaboration with a clinical geneticist ensures access to centralised databases to obtain accurate up-to-date diagnostic information for specific genetic disorders. Diagnostic work-up is often time-consuming and is best done prior to rather than during the pregnancy.

Neural tube defects   Detailed ultrasound evaluation has an important role in the evaluation of the spine and brain and is now the primary modality used to diagnose neural tube defects (NTD) (see Ch. 15). Amniocentesis is now rarely indicated to confirm this diagnosis.[41]

When it is used to diagnose NTD, amniocentesis is more commonly performed at 16–18 weeks after suspicion has been raised by elevated maternal serum AFP at routine screening. High-risk pregnancies, such as women with spina bifida or with affected children, may also be investigated. Amniotic fluid AFP has detection rates of 90% and false-positive rates of 0.3%. Amniotic fluid acetylcholinesterase (AChE) is more sensitive than amniotic fluid AFP, with a detection rate of 98% and a false-positive rate of 0.3%.[42,43] AChE estimation has the additional advantage that it is independent of gestational age.[44]

Fetal blood group   Determination of fetal blood group is justified in patients with a history of severe disease or with high circulating antibody levels, where the father is heterozygous. A fetus that is found to be antigen negative needs no further investigation. Although the fetal blood group was previously performed by serological testing of fetal blood, this is now accomplished by PCR on amniotic fluid samples[45] (Fig. 24.2), with a sensitivity of 98.7% and a specificity of 100%.[46]

Viral infection   Amniocentesis to detect viral-specific DNA using PCR is more sensitive than IgM antibody detection or viral culture in fetal blood.[47,48] It is now the method of choice for prenatal diagnosis in pregnancies at risk of congenital CMV,[49] toxoplasmosis,[50] rubella[51] and varicella[52] infection. Ultrasound remains the prime modality to assess the fetal condition.

Rhesus alloimmunisation   The severity of fetal red blood cell destruction in alloimmunisation has traditionally been measured indirectly by amniotic fluid bilirubin levels.[53,54] This is achieved by spectrophotometric measurement of the deviation in optical density of amniotic fluid at 450 nm (δ OD 450), and enables the definition of three zones which predict the severity of the anaemia. In the third trimester the accuracy of the prediction of Liley zone III is about 95% correct.[55]

However, extrapolation of these zones backwards into the second trimester gives inaccurate predictions of the severity of the disease, with a 68% false-negative rate for severely affected fetuses.[56] Monitoring by non-invasive ultrasound parameters such as liver length,[57] middle cerebral artery peak velocity[58] and umbilical venous maximal velocities[59] is becoming increasingly popular.

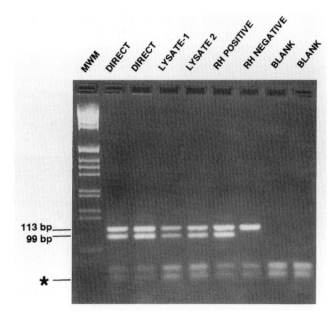

Fig. 24.2 Rh D genotyping. Agarose gel with polymerase chain reaction results for RhD typing using primers specific for exon 7. From left to right, lane *1* is a molecular weight marker (MWM); lanes *2–6* with both 113-base pair (bp) and 99-base pair bands, indicating an RhD-positive genotype; lane *7* with only the 113-base pair band indicative of an RhD-negative genotype; lanes *8* and *9* are blank controls. Asterisk – primer–dimer products. (Reproduced from Van den Veyver and Moise[44] with permission from Elsevier Science Inc; USA.

Fetal lung maturity   The amniotic fluid lecithin/sphingomyelin (L/S) ratio is a good predictor of fetal lung maturity, and its introduction in 1971 revolutionised obstetric management.[60] In current practice its use is declining owing to a combination of improvements in neonatal and obstetric medicine. In particular, antenatal steroid administration and the availability of exogenous neonatal sufactant have diminished the usage of the L/S ratio.

Preterm premature rupture of the membranes Approximately 30–40% of women with preterm prelabour amniorrhexis have evidence of intra-uterine infection, with the consequent risk of preterm delivery and neonatal sepsis.[61] Amniotic fluid culture can detect microbial invasion of the amniotic cavity, but more rapid tests may avoid a delay in diagnosis. The Gram stain of amniotic fluid has the best specificity (98.5%) of the rapid tests, whereas interleukin-6 may have the best sensitivity (80.9%).[62] However, offering amniocentesis to all women with preterm premature rupture of the membranes remains controversial.

Complications

Maternal   There is minimal risk to the mother, with amnionitis occurring in less than 0.1% of cases.[63] At the Montreal Workshop in 1979 there was only one maternal death reported as being due to a direct complication out of 20 000 amniocenteses.[64] Psychological stress, however, is common, owing to the indication for the procedure, the risk of fetal loss and the delay in obtaining the result.[65]

Fetal   The risks to the fetus have been assessed in four major studies (Table 24.1). Of the three collaborative case-controlled studies only the UK MRC trial identified an increased risk (1.4%) of spontaneous abortion following amniocentesis.[15] The National Institute of Child Health and Human Development (NICHD) and the Canadian MRC studies found no complications attributable to the procedure, but had difficulty selecting matched controls.[12,63] In the only prospective randomised controlled trial, 4606 low-risk women were randomised to either MA or no procedure. The post-procedure loss rate in the amniocentesis group was 1.7%, compared to 0.7% in the controls. This significant 1% increment (*P*<0.01%) in the spontaneous abortion rate of the amniocentesis group is the most widely used risk figure quoted in counselling.[13] Using a 20 G needle[66] under continuous ultrasound guidance, an increased risk of abortion was correlated with trans-placental sampling, the withdrawal of discoloured fluid and raised levels of MSAFP prior to the procedure. An increase in the perinatal mortality rate was not demonstrated.

Amniocentesis carries a risk of fetomaternal haemorrhage.[67] This is increased following trans-placental amniocentesis, and if performed by less experienced operators. Unsensitised rhesus-negative patients having amniocentesis should be given prophlactic anti-D immunoglobulin (50 μg up to 20 weeks and 100 μg thereafter). A Kleihauer–Betke test may be performed to quantify the fetomaternal haemorrhage and allow adjustment of the immunoglobulin dose as necessary.

Other less common risks include spontaneous rupture of membranes, fetal trauma and fetal exsanguination.

Neonatal   The UK MRC study in 1978 suggested that there was a higher incidence of postural deformities (talipes) and respiratory difficulties.[15] The former has not been confirmed, but the association of amniocentesis with respiratory distress and pneumonia was also reported by Tabor *et al.* in a randomised trial in 1986.[13] Work in non-human primates supports this finding, but as yet the mechanism is unclear.[68] Fetal trauma is very rare. In the UK MRC study more skin marks and dimples were found in the control neonates than in the subjects.[15]

Table 24.1 Spontaneous abortion rate (%) in amniocentesis

	Subjects	Controls
Canadian MRC[12]	0.9	1.6–1.9
NICHD[63]	2.8	2.4
UK MRC[15]	2.7	1.3
Tabor *et al.*[13]	1.7	0.7

Childhood No adverse consequences have been demonstrated in the two major follow-up studies of infants to one year of age.[69,70] In 1980 Finegan in Canada initiated a longitudinal prospective cohort follow-up study of the infants of 101 women having mid-trimester amniocentesis and 55 women who declined testing as controls. Examination at 6 months and at 4 and 7 years has revealed no difference in behavioural or motor development.[71-73] Nor was intellectual and cognitive development different at 4 and 7 years.[71,73] Physical development has also been similar, except that at 6 months of age 5.5% of the subjects had skin marks from the needle[71] and at 4 years significantly more subjects had reported ear infections.[72] At the 7-year follow-up no physical differences were detected.[73]

Chorionic villus sampling

The concept of diagnostic chorionic villus sampling (CVS) for first-trimester prenatal diagnosis was introduced in 1968 by Hahnemann and Mohr using trans-cervical endoscopy prior to termination of pregnancy.[74] Delayed termination revealed a high complication rate, mainly due to rupture of the amniotic sac and infection, but villi were obtained in 60% of the cases.[75] The success rate of chromosome analysis in these early attempts was low, as difficulties were encountered with culturing the tissue.[76] The effect of these disappointing results, combined with the information that early second-trimester amniocentesis was safe and reliable, inhibited further progress in CVS.

Interest in the west was only rekindled after a report from the Tietung Hospital of the Anshan Iron and Steel Co., China, in 1975 described the successful use of 'blind' trans-cervical needle aspiration of chorionic villi in 100 pregnancies.[77] The aim was to determine fetal gender by chromatin analysis. This was achieved with a 94% success rate and, of the pregnancies that were allowed to continue after CVS, only 6% miscarried. There were no maternal, fetal or neonatal complications.

An additional motivation to develop a successful CVS technique followed advances in laboratory techniques for tissue analysis, in particular the demonstration that villi could be used for gene analysis using recombinant DNA technology. In 1981 Williamson *et al.* performed accurate globin gene hybridisation with DNA extracted from chorionic villi at termination of pregnancy.[78] At the same time Niazi *et al.*[79] described successful fetal karyotyping from pure mesenchymal trophoblast cell cultures also obtained at termination (Fig. 24.3). A year later control studies on enzyme activity in chorionic tissue confirmed the potential for first-trimester detection of metabolic storage disorders.[80] An important advance was a direct cytogenetic analysis on spontaneous mitotic figures in the cytotrophoblast, enabling rapid results in the first trimester (Fig. 24.3).[81]

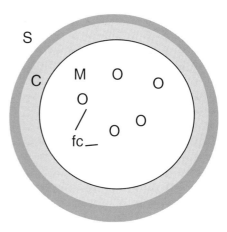

Fig. 24.3 Tertiary stem villus. A transverse section through a tertiary stem villus. M – mesenchymal core with fetal capillaries (fc), C – cytotrophoblast, S – syncytiotrophoblast.

Until 1980 the techniques that had been used for CVS included 'blind' aspiration,[77] endoscopic direct vision biopsy[74-76] and intra-uterine lavage.[82,83] In 1980, Kazy and Stigar from Moscow[84] reported 18 termination patients in whom flexible biopsy forceps were used in conjunction with continuous real-time ultrasound guidance. This was the first reported series with a 100% success rate. In 1982 the same group used ultrasound-guided trans-cervical methods to publish a larger series, including the first diagnostic CVS series for genetic disease.[80] Subsequently diagnostic series were published for the haemoglobinopathies from England,[85] chromosomal and metabolic disorders from Italy[81] and sickle-cell disease from France.[86] All these groups used ultrasound-guided trans-cervical methods, which have become the most widely used.[86-88]

Transabdominal sampling of the placenta was originally performed by Alvarez[89] to diagnose hydatidiform mole in 10–14-week pregnancies. Transabdominal CVS was introduced in Scandinavia[90] in 1984 to reduce the risk of infection and avoid the relative technical contraindications of trans-cervical CVS. It is becoming increasingly popular, both on its own and as a complementary procedure to trans-cervical CVS.

A World Health Organisation-sponsored registry initiated in 1983 has been collating data under the auspices of Laird Jackson at Thomas Jefferson University in Philadelphia, USA. Concern over the introduction of a new prenatal diagnostic technique prior to adequate risk assessment led to several multicentre prospective randomised controlled trials being set up internationally.

Technique

Ultrasonography is an integral part of the CVS technique. A preliminary scan should determine fetal viability, gestational age and the number of gestation sacs. Multiple pregnancy complicates CVS as definitive sampling of each placenta must be feasible. However, the procedure itself carries no greater risk of pregnancy loss than for a single-ton gestation.[91] A routine scan for uterine, adnexal and pelvic pathology should be included. The position of the uterus in the pelvis and in relation to the cervix has a pro-found effect on the success of CVS, and can be manipu-lated to a certain extent by bladder filling. The presence of fibroids may make CVS difficult, and uterine contractions may alter the intra-uterine topography causing transient difficulties.

Ultrasonic location of the placental site is essential to assess the best approach. CVS may be performed trans-cervically (TC) or transabdominally (TA). The choice of technique is usually that preferred by either the operator or the patient, although clinical conditions may support a particular method. For example, in active genital herpes trans-cervical CVS is contraindicated. For maximum flex-ibility it is optimal for operators to be trained in both

techniques. The choice of instruments available for CVS is extensive and depends largely on local availability and operator experience. For trans-cervical CVS they consist of an aspirating cannula, either plastic[85] or metal[88], and a biopsy forceps[86] (Fig. 24.4); for the transabdominal procedure an aspirating cannula, (either a double-needle system[90,92] or a single needle[93]) and a biopsy forceps[94] (Fig. 24.5) are used.

CVS is performed as an outpatient procedure using standard aseptic precautions. The patient is usually draped, but full gowning is not required. Both TC and TA CVS are usually performed as a two-person technique, with one person sampling and one person simultaneously guiding with ultrasound. Alternatively a single-operator technique has been described.[88] Following the CVS, real-time ultrasound is used to check the presence of a fetal heartbeat and to assess complications such as haematoma formation. A follow-up scan is advisable to assess sub-sequent fetal development.

Trans-cervical CVS The patient is positioned in the lithotomy position and the vulva and vagina cleansed with

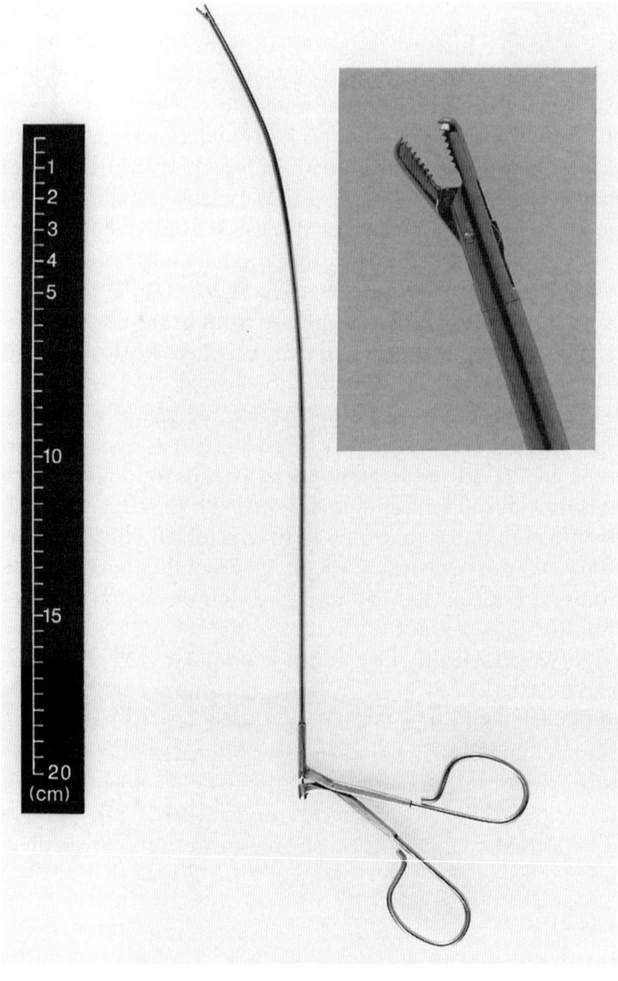

Fig. 24.4 Trans-cervical CVS. Biopsy forceps. (De Elles Instruments, Surrey, UK)

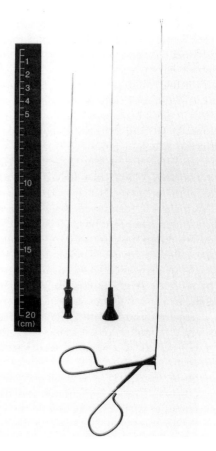

Fig. 24.5 Transabdominal CVS. Biopsy forceps with the trocar and cannula used for insertion. (De Elles Instruments, Surrey, UK)

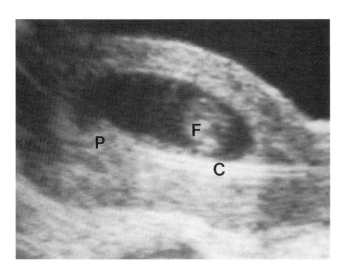

Fig. 24.6 Ultrasound-guided trans-cervical CVS showing an aspiration cannula (C) as a pair of bright lines. P – placenta, F – fetus.

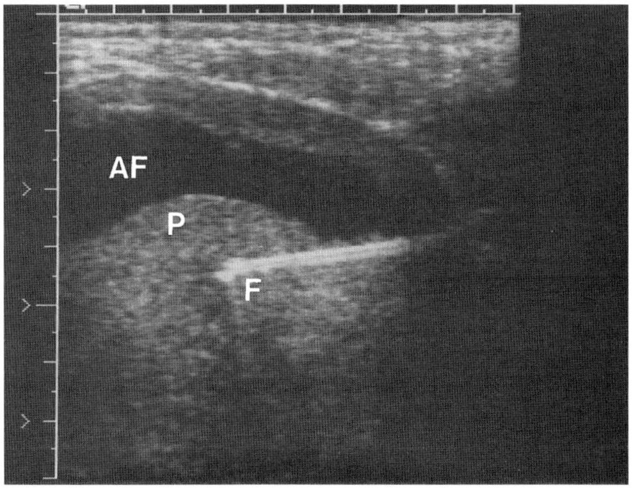

Fig. 24.7 Ultrasound-guided transabdominal CVS showing a pair of biopsy forceps (F) as bright lines within the placenta (P). AF – amniotic fluid.

an antiseptic solution and a speculum inserted to expose the cervix. The cervical os is then meticulously cleaned. A tenaculum may occasionally be required.

The sampling instrument is bent to the optimal shape, depending on the relationship between the cervix, uterus and placental site. It is identified in the cervical canal as a pair of bright lines and is guided from the internal os to the placental site. The correct placement is within the placental tissue parallel to the chorionic plate (Fig. 24.6). The position of the tip should be confirmed prior to sampling.

Aspiration systems require a 20 ml syringe containing 3–5 ml heparinised culture medium to be attached following obturator removal. Suction is applied as the catheter is moved backwards and forwards ('hoovering') and slowly withdrawn. The contents of the catheter and syringe are then flushed into a Petri dish for inspection.

Biopsy systems are simple to use, do not rely on aspiration and are suitable for a single operator. Once they are in the placental substance the jaws are opened, advanced, closed and the forceps withdrawn. Specimens largely uncontaminated with decidua or blood are reliably collected.

Two instrumental insertions may be attempted safely at a single session.[95]

Transabdominal CVS The patient is placed supine and the abdomen cleansed with an antiseptic solution. Sampling is performed under continual ultrasound surveillance. The needle is inserted through the abdomen and advanced so that the tip is just visible within the chorion frondosum and parallel to the chorionic plate (Fig. 24.7). The needle may be guided either free-hand or by means of a needle guide system.

Aspiration may be achieved via a double-needle system,[90,92] consisting of a coaxial 18 gauge guide cannula with a stylet and an inner 20–22 gauge aspirating cannula which is about 1.5 cm longer than the guide. Once in placental tissue the stylet is replaced with the aspirating needle, and a 20 ml syringe attached to aspirate the villi in much the same way as is done trans-cervically. The inner needle is then withdrawn and the sample flushed into a Petri dish for inspection. Additional tissue is collected if necessary. This is achieved simply by reinserting the inner needle and aspirating again. A 19 or 20 G spinal needle can also be used, but, as with the trans-cervical approach, only two insertions should be attempted at a single session.[93]

Transabdominal biopsy uses a coaxial biopsy forceps (Fig. 24.5). The technique is similar to that described previously, except that aspiration is avoided and clean samples are obtained.

In the past immediate microscopy was considered essential following either trans-cervical or transabdominal sampling to distinguish villi from decidua and to assess their quantity and quality. With experience this is no longer found to be necessary, as to the naked eye villi are obviously branching, fluffy and vascular (Fig 24.8), whereas decidua is flat, sheet-like and avascular.

The recommended time to perform CVS for routine prenatal diagnosis is between 10 and 12 weeks gestation. This sampling window avoids the high background spontaneous miscarriage rate present in early pregnancy, but still enables the result to be obtained within the first trimester. In addition, CVS may be associated with teratogenic effects if performed at earlier gestations (see below).

One of the potential advantages of the transabdominal technique is that the method can be used until term, which may be useful for fetal karyotyping.[96]

Experience with CVS improves the success rate for obtaining samples and decreases the fetal loss rate. In

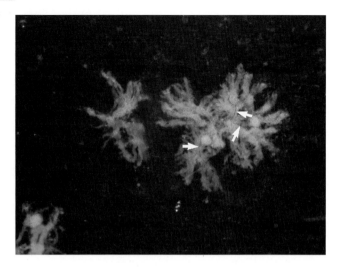

Fig. 24.8 Chorionic villi. Aspirated villi showing branching fronds with central fetal vessels (arrows).

experienced centres over 99% of patients are sampled successfully with one or two insertions.[97] Pregnancy loss rates increase significantly when more than two insertions are required.[95] The NICHD trial documented the loss of a chromosomally normal fetus in 10.8% with three to four attempts, compared to 2.9% with one insertion.[98]

Similarly, the fetal loss rate varies with experience. The average loss rate in 14 centres with fewer than 50 TC procedures is 7.3%, compared to 3.1% in the eight centres with over 1000 cases. The abortion rate after TC CVS is maintained at its lowest level only after 300 cases.[99] Fetal loss rate after TA CVS also declines with experience.[100] The learning curve for TA CVS may be longer and more gradual, with 300 cases being required to equal the TC CVS loss rate and another 1000 to improve the rate further.[99]

Indications

CVS is indicated for fetal karyotyping, DNA analysis, inborn errors of metabolism, and fetal blood group determination.

Karyotyping As with amniocentesis, fetal karyotyping is the most common reason for performing CVS. Of the cases reported to the European collaborative cytogenetic study of first-trimester CVS,[101] 75% were for advanced maternal age, 11.7% for a previous child with a non-inherited chromosome abnormality, and 2.3% for parental rearrangements. The high-risk group of X-linked disorders accounted for 5%, but increasingly these conditions are being diagnosed specifically, using DNA techniques. When advanced maternal age is the indication for first-trimester CVS the risk of detecting a chromosomal abnormality is significantly higher than at amniocente-

sis.[102] Although this is mostly due to false-positive results (see below), true positive aneuploidy is significantly higher at CVS than at amniocentesis.[102] This difference is explained by the increased spontaneous loss rate of chromosomally abnormal fetuses at earlier gestations.[17,20,103]

Structural abnormalities detected on ultrasound have a high incidence of chromosomal abnormality and may be investigated by second- and third-trimester TA CVS as an alternative to fetal blood sampling.[96] This is an increasing indication, now accounting for up to 25% of cytogenetic analyses from CVS.[104]

Karyotyping can be performed on direct/short-term preparations or after tissue culture. For all methods it is essential that villi are meticulously cleansed of maternal cells. A minimum of 10 mg of villi are recommended for cytogenetic analysis.

The **direct method** depends on spontaneous mitoses in the Langerhans' cells of the cytotrophoblast layer of the tertiary stem villi (Fig. 24.3).[81] The advantages include rapid results (1–2 days), and the avoidance of maternal cell overgrowth and bacterial infection. However, the accuracy of the results is jeopardised by too few good metaphase spreads and the poor quality of banding. It is ideal for determining fetal karyotype in X-linked disorders.

The **short-term tissue culture** is based on the same principles as the direct method, except that the villi are cultured for 12–24 hours,[105] improving the quality of the G-banded metaphases.

High-resolution banding for the detection of deletion breakpoints, small translocations and other subtle abnormalities requires long-term tissue culture, as the banding is of better quality. It is the mesenchymal cells of the villi (Fig. 24.3) that are used for long-term culture.[79]

The reliability of the cytogenetic results is crucial to the role of CVS as a first-trimester diagnostic technique. Problems have arisen which are important in this regard, and which should be discussed when counselling patients.

1. Discordance between chorionic villus and fetal karyotypes is termed confined placental mosaicism (CPM) and was first described by Kalousek and Dill in 1983.[104] The clinical consequences of CPM range from normal pregnancy outcome to intra-uterine growth restriction, miscarriage or intra-uterine death of a chromosomally normal fetus.[106] The particular chromosome involved, the type of placental tissue affected and the proportion of abnormal cells are all important in determining outcome.[107] In addition, CPM can have genetic consequences on the fetus, with uniparental disomy (UPD) being the main concern.[108–110]

Since 1986 European collaborative research on mosaicism in CVS (EUCROMIC) has monitored cytogenetic findings in CVS, with emphasis on mosaicism and non-mosaic fetoplacental discrepancies and their effects on interpretation of the CVS.[111] Hahnemann and Vejerslev[111] published 62 865 karyotyped CVS that were reported to EUCROMIC from 1986 to 1992: 94.8% of CVS samples showed a true normal karyotype and 3.7% a true abnormal karyotype compared to the fetus. In 1.5% CVS samples ambiguous cytogenetic results were obtained. These included true positives as seen in true mosaicism (0.12%) and non-mosaic aberration (0.02%), false positives as seen in confined placental mosaicism (1.04%) and false-positive non-mosaic aberration (0.15%), and false-negative CVS (0.03%): 0.15% were unable to be classified.

These figures determined a sensitivity of CVS for prenatal detection of chromosome aberrations of 98.9–99.6% (99% CI), a specificity of 98.5–98.8%, a positive predictive value of 72.6–78.3% and a negative predictive value of 99.95–99.98%.

Several points were highlighted by this report. First, false-positive and false-negative results were rare, but with only a few exceptions occurred after direct preparation alone, providing evidence that cultured cells more accurately reflect the fetal karotype. Secondly, false-negative results occurred most commonly in pregnancies at high risk of chromosomal abnormality, for example structural malformation on ultrasound. This implies that short-term CVS should not be relied upon solely for rapid karyotyping in urgent clinical situations. Thirdly, because of the risk of false-negative amniocentesis in trisomy 8 CVS karyotype, the authors recommend ultrasound to assess fetal malformations and, if necessary, fetal blood sampling for further chromosome analysis.

Phillips *et al.*[112] reviewed 469 cases of placental mosaicism from the literature and found associated fetal mosaicism in 10.7%. Follow-up amniocentesis was found to be predictive of fetal karyotype in 94.4% of mesenchymal core mosaicism and 93.5% of cases with both cytotrophoblast and mesenchymal core mosaicism. A further EUCROMIC report[113] analysed 192 gestations with CVS mosaicism involving single autosomal trisomy to establish which fetuses are at increased risk of true fetal mosaicism or possible uniparental disomy (Table 24.2). Because of the risk of fetal trisomy, follow-up amniocentesis is supported in all gestations involving mosaic autosomal trisomy in the villus mesenchyme (Fig. 24.3). In gestations with mosaic or non-mosaic autosomal trisomy in both cytotrophoblast and villus mesenchyme, DNA testing for UPD in addition to fetal karyotyping is recommended.

2. Failed karyotyping occurred in 1.9% of 62 865 CVS reported from 48 laboratories contributing to EUCROMIC between 1986 and 1992.[111] Similarly, a study from seven laboratories in the USA found that the success rate of obtaining a cytogenetic result varied from 98 to 100%.[114]

3. Maternal cell contamination is negligible in direct and short-term culture as there are no mitoses present in decidua. The USA collaborative study of cytogenetic results from CVS revealed a 1.9% rate of maternal cell contamination in long-term cultures, with one-third having a single maternal cell, one-third having less than 25% maternal cells, and one-third having more than 25% maternal cells.[114] Although in this report there were no cases of incorrect sex prediction or diagnostic errors, the potential for cytogenetic mistakes remains with the culture method, particularly if the sample size is small.

DNA analysis Rapid advances in molecular genetics were a major stimulus to the development of CVS, but it was CVS that really allowed DNA analysis for fetal diagnosis to evolve, as more DNA can be extracted from villi than from amniotic fluid, 20 mg of villi yielding about 20 μg of DNA. Depending on the approach (see amniocentesis), 10–50 mg of villi are required, and a result is usually available in 6–14 days. In 200 pregnancies investigated for haemoglobinopathies there was one misdiagnosis and one failed diagnosis.[115]

Inborn errors of metabolism (IEM) The first chorionic studies of enzymes known to be involved in inborn errors of metabolism were those of Kazy *et al.*[80] Subsequently all enzyme deficiencies expressed in cultured amniotic fluid cells have been shown to be expressed in chorionic villi, but with the advantage that many results can be obtained without cell culture, providing a result in 1–2 days. Depending on the sensitivity and complexity of the assay, between 10 and 50 mg of villi are adequate for diagnosis.[116] It is imperative that the genetic and biochemical disorder, as well as the carrier status of the parents, is confirmed before fetal diagnosis is undertaken.

Fetal blood grouping Rhesus and Kell fetal blood groups may be obtained at CVS using PCR assay of DNA[117] or fetal erythrocytes for red cell grouping, either by microimmunofluorescent or immunogold silver staining techniques.[118–120] Because fetomaternal haemorrhage resulting from the procedure can enhance the disease, this method of fetal grouping should be reserved for women with heterozygous partners and a history of severe disease, who would request termination of an antigenically positive fetus on the grounds that *in utero* treatment is likely to fail.[121]

Table 24.2 Probabilities of mosaic or non-mosaic single autosomal trisomy in the fetus proper according to the combination of cell lineages affected in the placenta[113]

Cytotrophoblast	Villus mesenchyme	Fetus affected (%)
Mosaic	Normal	0
Non-mosaic	Normal	0
Normal	Mosaic	4.1
Normal	Non-mosaic	83.3
Mosaic	Mosaic	23.5
Non-mosaic	Mosaic	18.2
Mosaic	Non-mosaic	100

Complications

Maternal Discomfort is minimal with TC CVS, although the transabdominal approach may cause moderate pain. Abdominal cramping may occur for several hours after either procedure. After TC CVS vaginal spotting occurs in 10–40% of cases,[98] but rarely after TA CVS. Serious immediate post-CVS haemorrhage is rare and is not necessarily associated with fetal loss. Although rarely associated with adverse outcome, post-procedure intra-uterine haematoma has been reported in 4% of patients.[93]

Infection has been a concern from the initial development of trans-cervical CVS,[76] but only two cases of serious maternal infection have been published.[122,123] Methodical aseptic techniques, including using a new sterile catheter for repeat insertions, has ensured a low risk of infection following CVS.[95] In three multicentre prospective controlled trials comparing TC CVS with amniocentesis there were no cases of maternal infection.[98,102,124] Transabdominal CVS has not been associated with maternal infection.

Acute rupture of the membranes is very rare after CVS. Rupture of the membranes days to weeks after the procedure is a potential complication and has been reported with an incidence of 0.3%.[125] Visceral trauma such as uterine perforation has not been reported with the trans-cervical route. Transabdominal uterine puncture should be atraumatic with the methods described, but occasional bleeding and puncture of the bowel or bladder may occur, with resultant peritonism in about 0.3%.[126]

Fetomaternal haemorrhage after both trans-cervical and transabdominal CVS has been documented by demonstrating a rise in MSAFP in the majority of patients.[127–129] Thus the potential for causing rhesus isoimmunisation must be taken seriously and anti-D immunoglobulin prophylaxis is strongly recommended in rhesus D-negative women. Conversely, when anti-D antibodies are already present CVS should be avoided, as enhancement may accelerate the course of the disease.[130] The post-CVS rise in MSAFP is transient and so does not interfere with neural tube screening in the second trimester.[131]

Fetal Determination of the procedure-related loss rate from CVS is confounded by the background loss rate, which varies with both gestational and maternal age. The overall spontaneous fetal loss rate in ultrasonically viable pregnancies is about 2%.[132,133] However, the background fetal loss rate increases with increasing maternal age, being 1.5% before age 30 and 4.5% between 35 and 39 years.[132] Between 2% and 5% of pregnancies shown to be viable at 7–12 weeks are non-viable when rescanned at 18–20 weeks.[132,134]

Therefore, assessment of the procedure-related loss rate from CVS requires a trial comparing the post-procedural loss rates with a non-procedural control group. Alternatively, CVS can be compared to amniocentesis by

Table 24.3 Total fetal loss rate (%) in chorionic villus sampling compared to amniocentesis

	CVS	MA	δ	p
Canadian Collaborative Trial[102]	7.6	7.0	+0.6	ns
NICHD[98]	7.0	5.6	+0.8	ns*
European MRC Trial[124]	13.6	9.0	+4.6	<0.01

*Adjusted for differences in gestational age and maternal age between the two groups.

enrolling all patients prior to the gestational age at which CVS is performed and comparing the total loss rates in each procedural group. Three collaborative trials have evaluated the relative safety of CVS by comparison with amniocentesis.

In 1989 the Canadian Collaborative CVS–Amniocentesis Clinical Trial Group published a prospective randomised controlled trial of 2787 women showing no significant difference in total fetal loss rate between first-trimester TC CVS and mid-trimester amniocentesis (Table 24.3).[102] Similarly, in 1989 a non-randomised prospective trial of 2278 women from the US National Institute of Child Health and Human Development (USNICHD) reported no significant difference in total fetal loss rates between the two procedures[98] (Table 24.3). In 1991 a prospective randomised controlled trial of 3248 women from the European Medical Research Working Party on the Evaluation of Chorion Villus Sampling demonstrated a significant increase of 4.6% in the total fetal loss rate following CVS (Table 24.3).[124] The reason for the discrepancy between the European and North American studies remains uncertain. However, it is probable that operator experience accounts for a large part of the difference, with 31 centres contributing an average of 52 cases, compared to seven centres contributing an average of 325 cases in the NICHD trial, and 11 centres contributing an average of 106 cases in the Canadian trial.[95]

Recent large randomised trials have compared trans-cervical and transabdominal approaches.[97,135,136] The United States collaborative CVS project found no difference in post-procedure loss rates to 28 weeks gestation between the two sampling methods in a prospective randomised trial of 3873 women.[97] The trans-cervical loss rate was 2.5% and the transabdominal rate 2.3% (difference 0.26%; 95% CI –0.5 to 1.0%). In a prospective randomised trial of 3079 women Smidt-Jensen *et al.* found no difference in total pregnancy loss between TA CVS (6.3%) and Mid-trimester amniocentesis (MA) (6.4%), but an increased loss rate in TC CVS of 10.9% (p<0.001).[135] In this centre trans-cervical CVS was not routine practice prior to the trial. It is therefore probable that similar loss rates are achieved once maximum expertise is gained with either approach.

Other fetal complications have not been shown to be increased with CVS. The Canadian trial showed no increase in either intra-uterine growth retardation (IUGR) or preterm labour,[102] and the NICHD study could find no increase in placental abruption or preterm labour.[98] There was a trend towards late stillbirth in the CVS group in the Canadian trial.[102]

Neonatal   There have been no reports of an increase in the neonatal death rate after CVS.

Congenital limb reduction defects (LRD) were first reported in association with CVS by Firth *et al.* in 1991, resulting in ongoing international debate and contradictory information. In their series of 539 transabdominal CVS five babies had severe limb abnormalities, all from a cohort of 289 pregnancies sampled between 56 and 66 days.[137] Four infants had oromandibular–limb hypogenesis syndromes and one a terminal transverse limb reduction defect.

Population-based studies indicate that the risk for LRD and oromandibular–limb hypogenesis syndromes is 1/1690 and 1/175 000 live births, respectively.[138] The occurrence of these abnormalities in more than 1% of CVS-sampled cases implicated CVS in the pathogenesis. Other series supported the data in the initial report[139–141] and suggested that the severity of LRD may be related to the gestational age at the time of CVS, with the earliest exposures being more severe, with more proximal limb deficiencies and orofacial defects.[142]

Conversely, the three largest multicentre trials reported no increase in LRD, but their outcome of interest was fetal loss.[98,102,124] More detailed follow-up of the USNICHD Collaborative CVS Study Group trials indicated that there was no increase in LRD in 9588 CVS, of which 1025 cases were performed prior to 66 days.[143] However, the CVS group was compared to population-based rates, not to the amniocentesis-exposed cohort. Similarly, the report of the WHO International Registry compared population-based birth defect data to 138 996 CVS from 63 centres, concluding that the incidence of LRD after CVS was no different.[144] Reasons for this variability may be explained by different methods of classification of LRD, level of ascertainment of outcomes, or differences between centres in the performance of CVS.[145]

Several case-control studies have used infants with limb deficiencies registered in surveillance systems and control infants with other birth defects to compare exposure rated to CVS.[146–148] The odds ratios for CVS exposure are summarised in Table 24.4.[145]

Placental vascular disruption causing fetal hypoperfusion via vasospasm, fetomaternal haemorrhage or emboli are the current hypotheses for CVS causing LRD.[149,150] Embryoscopic observation of cutaneous haemorrhagic lesions in human pregnancies being terminated after intentionally vigorous CVS supports this concept of placental trauma.[151]

Transabdominal single-needle aspiration has been shown to cause more fetomaternal haemorrhage than

Table 24.4 Risk for limb reduction deficiencies (LRD) and subtypes, by selected case-control studies of limb defects after CVS by selected registries, 1984–1993

Registry	All LRD OR[a] (95%CI)[b]	Transverse LRD OR[a](95%CI)[b]	Subsets of transverse LRD OR[a](95%CI)[b]
US Multistate Case-Control Study[146]	1.7(0.4–6.3)	4.7(0.8–28.4)	digital: 6.4(1.1–38.6)
[c]EUROCAT[148]	1.8(0.7–5.0)	not classified	not classified
[d]IMBDR[147]	not included	12.6(6.2–23.9)	OMLH[e]:223.8 (48.9–1006.8)

[a]Odds ratios
[b]Confidence interval
[c]European Registration of Congenital Anomalies and Twins
[d]Italian Multicentre Birth Defects Registry
[e]Oromandibular–limb hypogenesis

trans-cervical biopsy forceps (Fig. 24.3).[152] Trauma is therefore a major factor, as well as gestational age.

The conclusion from all these data suggests that CVS has an increase in absolute risk from 1/3000 to 1/1000 for all transverse LRD, with a risk of 0.2% at 9 weeks or earlier, 0.1% at 10 weeks, and 0.05% at 11 weeks or more.[153] Counsellors should inform women of this and the controversy prior to having the CVS performed, and procedures should be avoided before 10 weeks gestation.

Early amniocentesis

Early amniocentesis (EA) is defined as an amniocentesis before 14 weeks gestation. Although vaginal aspiration of amniotic fluid as early as 10 weeks gestation was reported in 1973, it was associated with very high complication and failure rates[154] and the introduction of CVS in 1983 overcame the disadvantage of late prenatal diagnosis inherent in mid-trimester amniocentesis. In the late 1980s renewed interest in early amniocentesis arose from the concerns surrounding CVS. The technique was difficult to learn, confined placental mosaicism reduced its accuracy, laboratory processing was time-consuming, the miscarriage rate was thought to be higher than with mid-trimester amniocentesis, and transverse limb abnormalities were a possible complication.

EA was first presented as an alternative to CVS in 1985 by two groups reporting amniocentesis between 12 and 14 weeks.[155,156] The success rate of cell culture was shown to be 100% after 12 weeks,[157] but karyotype results were often prolonged 1–2 days beyond that normal for mid-trimester samples.[155,158] Subsequently, successful diagnoses of inborn errors of metabolism were reported[159] and normal amniotic fluid AFP levels ascertained.[160,161]

Unfortunately, the exact international experience with EA remains unknown because there has never been an active registry and the precise definition is unclear.[162] The introduction of another prenatal diagnostic technique without proper scientific evaluation of its safety and cytogenetic accuracy led several centres to instigate randomised controlled trials to compare EA with either CVS or MA.[163–165]

Technique

An ultrasound scan at the time of the procedure will determine the number of fetuses, gestational age, viability and placental location. Under aseptic conditions a 22 G spinal needle is introduced transabdominally into the amniotic sac under direct ultrasound guidance, avoiding the placenta where possible. The needle and its tip should be visualised throughout the entire procedure. A medium to full bladder is useful to displace the maternal bowel and bring the uterus closer to the anterior abdominal wall, thereby avoiding rescheduling for lack of access.[165] Alternatively, a trans-vesical approach may overcome this technical issue.[165] Similarly, puncturing the amniotic sac with a sharp thrust may overcome tenting of the amnion due to incomplete fusion with the chorion[165] (Fig. 24.9) and avoid the necessity for more frequent needle passes reported in early series.[158] To reduce the risk of miscarriage no more than two insertions are usually attempted per procedure.[166] Approximately 11 ml of fluid are aspirated and the first 0.5–1.0 ml discarded to reduce the risk of maternal contamination.[166] When appropriate, anti-D immunoglobulin should be administered following any attempt at EA.

In the two randomised/semirandomised controlled trials comparing EA with CVS the sampling success of EA has been comparable or better than that of CVS.[164,167]

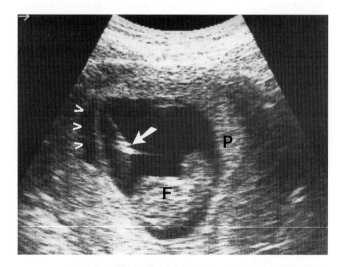

Fig. 24.9 Early amniocentesis. Simultaneous monitoring during early amniocentesis showing the needle passage avoiding the anterior placenta (P) and the extracoelomic cavity (small arrows). Needle tip (large arrow). F – fetus.

Nicolaides *et al.*[167] reported a similar success rate, with 100% for EA and 99.2% for CVS. Sundberg *et al.*[164] reported a better sampling success with EA than with CVS (99.5% vs 97.3%; p< 0.01). If success at first attempt is considered then again EA was reported as being more successful than CVS (98.1% vs 95.9%).[167] In contrast, the randomised controlled trial comparing EA to midtrimester amniocentesis revealed reduced first-attempt success with EA 96.9% versus MA 99.6% (p<0.0001).[166]

The removal of 10 ml of amniotic fluid reduces the volume by 33% at 10 weeks and by 11% at 14 weeks.[168] To avoid this and still increase the cell yield, fetal cells can be trapped by filtering the fluid, which is then returned to the amniotic cavity. Amnifiltration was first reported by Sundberg *et al.*[169] who reduced their mean culture time from 14.3 days for control samples to 8.3 days in the filter samples at gestations of 13–19 weeks. Byrne *et al.* extended the technique to EA between 10 and 14 weeks gestation and obtained a similar number of viable clones as for MA, by removing a total volume of 1 ml of amniotic fluid using a 0.8 µm cellulose acetate membrane and recirculating 20 ml.[170] Subsequent clinical series using this technique have shown fetal loss rates comparable to those of simple EA and CVS.[164,171]

Culture failure rates for EA have varied among the three reported randomised trials. Nicolaides *et al.* had higher failure rates with EA than with CVS at the same gestation (2.0% vs 0.6%; p<0.01)[167] and The Canadian Early and Mid-trimester Amniocentesis Trial (CEMAT) had higher failure rates at EA than with MA (1.7% vs 0.2%; p<0.001).[166] Sundberg *et al.* achieved lower culture failure rates for EA than for CVS (0.2% vs 1.3%; P<0.05),[164] which may reflect the amnifiltration technique used to collect the EA specimens in this trial, or the later gestation at EA sampling.

Early amniocentesis is usually performed at 11–13 weeks gestation.[163] Amniotic fluid may be obtained as early as 8 weeks, but pilot data obtained from women undergoing termination of pregnancy showed reduced cytogenetic success at these very early gestations. Rooney *et al.*[157] obtained a fetal karyotype in 100% of samples at 12–14 weeks, but in only 68% of samples at 8–11 weeks. Similarly, Bryne *et al.*[172] reported successful culture and cytogenetic analyses in all cases where the fetal crown– crump length was more than 37 mm (10 weeks) but in only 61% before this gestation.

In their clinical trial, Nicolaides *et al.*[167] reported increasing culture failure rates with decreasing gestational age at EA. The rate of failure was reported as 4.2%, 2.2%, 1% and 0% at 10, 11, 12 and 13 weeks, respectively.

The effects of removing a relatively large proportion of amniotic fluid in early gestation are unknown. Therefore, to avoid depleting the relatively smaller total volumes of amniotic fluid at earlier gestations Elejalde *et al.* removed 1 ml per week of gestation.[173] This practice has been widely adopted, but with no proven benefit to the fetus.

Although the procedure is similar to mid-trimester amniocentesis, EA is technically more difficult because the uterus is still within the pelvis and the chorion and amnion have not yet fused, complicating access and sac puncture, respectively. Experience is required to overcome these differences. Hanson et al.[158] reported a significant reduction in the rescheduling of patients over 18 months from 14.9% to 7.4% to 2.6% for each 6-month period. Similarly, no retaps were performed after 120 attempts, but 19 of the first 120 (15.8%) procedures required a retap as no fluid was obtained after two attempts.

Indications

The indications for EA are the same as for MA prior to 20 weeks and include chromosome analysis, assessment of neural tube defects, inborn errors of metabolism and DNA analysis.

Chromosomes Chromosomal analysis is the most common indication for EA, with advanced maternal age the usual reason. Karyotyping is performed on cultured cells. Cell culture is successful because the number of cells in the amniotic fluid at 10–14 weeks is almost the same as at MA.[174] Despite the smaller volumes usually aspirated, the interval between sampling and successful result from cell culture is no different to CVS at a median of 12 days (range 8–22).[172]

The maternal age-specific risk figures are also gestational age dependent, as chromosomally abnormal fetuses have a higher rate of miscarriage.[18] Consequently, in the series comparing EA to CVS, both at 10–13 weeks, there was no difference in the incidence of abnormal karyotypes,[167] whereas there were more chromosome abnormalities (2.9% vs 0.7%) in the trial comparing EA at 11–13 weeks with CVS at 10–12 weeks, reflecting the earlier mean sampling gestation.[164]

In contrast, the data on mosaicism at EA indicate that it is significantly lower than with CVS at the same gestation. Nicolaides et al.[167] documented mosaicism at 0.1% for EA and at 1.1% for CVS (p < 0.01).

Maternal contamination resulting in a diagnostic error was reported in one EA in the CEMAT trial.[166] The incidence of maternal cell contamination has not been studied in detail but has been reported at 0.25%.[175]

Neural tube defects Establishment of normal AFP ranges prior to 14 weeks gestation enabled EA to be performed in patients at increased risk of neural tube defects.[160,161,175,176]

Inborn errors of metabolism Diagnosis of a range of metabolic disorders has been reported at EA.[175,177]

DNA analysis Genetic disorders amenable to DNA diagnosis are able to be ascertained successfully from EA,[177] although CVS is a more efficient source of DNA.

Complications

Maternal Two randomised controlled trials have reported an increase in the rate of amniotic fluid leakage at EA (Table 24.5). Sundberg et al.[164] reported that leakage at EA was not related to gestational age at sampling, and suggested that needle size (20 G) or longer procedure time due to amnifiltration may be implicated. However, CEMAT also showed a significantly increased rate of amniotic fluid leakage following EA, and used a 22 G needle and aspirated 11 ml of fluid with no filtration.[166] The CEMAT data indicated no difference between EA and MA in premature rupture of the membranes after 22 weeks.[166] They comment that the increased amniotic fluid leakage prior to 22 weeks may be related to the amnio-chorionic separation present in early gestation.

Fetal The risks to the fetus have been analysed in three randomised controlled trials.[164,166,167] Nicolaides et al.[167] reported an increased total spontaneous loss of 4% after EA compared with CVS performed at the same gestation (Table 24.6). There was no difference in the gestations or birthweights at delivery in the two groups with 100% follow-up. CEMAT[166] found a significant increase of 1.7% in total pregnancy loss when comparing EA to MA. This difference was mainly attributable to the rate of spontaneous post-procedural loss in EA below 20 weeks gestation. However, the total fetal loss rate was used as the outcome variable for the trial to reduce the bias when comparing procedures performed at different gestational ages.[178] These authors concluded that a trial designed to evaluate excess fetal loss after EA would have a 'no procedure' control group. Sundberg et al.[164] found similar total fetal loss rates between EA at 11–13 weeks and CVS at 10–12 weeks but no definite conclusions can be drawn from the data as the trial was stopped early, significantly reducing the power of the safety issue.

Table 24.5 Amniotic fluid leakage (%) associated with early amniocentesis

	n	EA	CVS	MA	δ	p
Sundberg et al.[164]	1103	4.4	0	–	+4.4	<0.001
CEMAT[166]	3691	3.5	–	1.7	+1.8	0.007

Table 24.6 Fetal loss rate (%) at early amniocentesis

	n	EA	CVS	MA	δ	p
Nicolaides et al.[167]	555	5.8	1.8	–	+4	<0.01
CEMAT[166]	4368	7.6	–	5.8	+1.7	0.012

Table 24.7 Rate of talipes equinovarus at EA in randomised controlled trials

	n	EA	CVS	MA	δ	p
Nicolaides *et al.*[167]	519	1.9	0.4	–	+1.5	ns
Sundberg *et al.*[164]	1058	1.7	0	–	+1.7	<0.01
CEMAT[166]	4368	1.3	–	0.1	+1.2	0.0001

Neonatal The Danish trial[164] was abandoned because of a significantly increased occurrence of talipes equinovarus in the EA group (Table 24.7). CEMAT[166] also found an increased incidence of talipes equinovarus in the EA group (Table 24.7). In this trial amniotic fluid leakage after EA increased the incidence of talipes to 15%, with 1.1% incidence if no post-procedural leakage occurred. The incidence of talipes in the MA group was 0.1%, which is similar to that in the general population (1–3 per 1000 live births).[179] Nicolaides *et al.* had a higher frequency of talipes equinovarus in their randomised EA vs CVS subgroups, but the difference was not significant (Table 24.7).[167]

Another particular concern with EA is the respiratory function of the newborn. CEMAT showed no difference in the incidence of ventilation or prolonged oxygen use between EA and MA, but no comparison was made with normal controls.[166] Sundberg *et al.* showed no association between amniotic fluid leakage after EA and respiratory distress syndrome or ventilatory requirements in the neonate.[164] In 1991 Thompson *et al.*[180] demonstrated no difference in functional residual capacity at 2–8 weeks of age in 49 infants following EA, compared with 51 infants after CVS. However, Yuksel *et al.*[181] showed that when a control group of 25 infants not exposed to a first-trimester invasive procedure was compared with 47 infants exposed to EA and 19 exposed to CVS, both first-trimester procedures were independently associated with infants having a high airway resistance. In a retrospective study Greenough *et al.*[179] found increased admissions to neonatal intensive care following EA compared to CVS or controls.

The current consensus on EA is probably that it is not the procedure of choice in the first trimester.[182]

Fetal blood sampling

Fetal blood sampling (FBS) was first performed experimentally in 1973 by Valenti, who aspirated blood from the umbilical cord using a paediatric hysteroscope introduced into the amniotic cavity at hysterotomy.[183] Kan *et al.*[184] described placentocentesis, or 'blind' placental aspiration, which was the first technique to be used clinically to obtain fetal blood for diagnosis.[185] However, samples were usually contaminated with maternal blood and often contained a very low proportion of fetal cells, with 10% or more of patients requiring a repeat procedure. Furthermore, a 10% fetal mortality rate, mainly due to fetal exsanguination, has ensured that this procedure is now obsolete.[186]

Fetoscopy was the first satisfactory method for obtaining samples of fetal blood. In 1974 Hobbins and Mahoney[187] described the percutaneous transabdominal introduction of a 1.7 mm fibre-optic endoscope (Dyonics Inc.) into the amniotic cavity to obtain fetal blood from the vessels on the surface of the chorionic plate. However, these specimens were often diluted with amniotic fluid and contaminated with maternal blood. In 1978, using the same instrument, Rodeck and Campbell[188] sampled the umbilical cord vessels at the placental or fetal insertion and reliably obtained pure fetal blood. This established a precise ultrasound-guided technique enabling a variety of diagnostic and therapeutic procedures to be available from 18 weeks gestation into the third trimester. However, fetoscopy remained a difficult technique to learn and even the most experienced centres had fetal loss rates of about 2–5%[189] and significant risks of amniotic fluid leakage, preterm labour and amnionitis.

Improvements in ultrasound resolution enabled the introduction of ultrasound-guided needling of fetal vessels, the most commonly used being the umbilical vein. This was first reported by Daffos *et al.* in 1983,[190] who successfully obtained fetal blood in 53 cases using a 20 G spinal needle under local anaesthetic. This procedure has become widely adopted and has now entirely displaced fetoscopy for fetal blood aspiration.

Between 1987 and 1991 Ludomirsky collected a multicentre registry of FBS performed in 11 centres in the USA and Canada to determine the current indications and complications.[191] A total of 7462 procedures in 6023 fetuses were recorded.

Technique

As with all invasive ultrasound procedures a preliminary real-time scan should be performed prior to and independent of the procedure. In the case of FBS relevant features include the number of fetuses, viability, gestational age, amniotic fluid volume and the presence or absence of structural anomalies.

Just prior to the procedure the target organ is identified. This may be the placental or umbilical cord insertion,[190] the intrahepatic vein,[192] the heart[193] or a free loop of cord. The most common site of sampling is the umbilical cord at its insertion into the placenta. It should be located in its long axis to allow optimal visualisation for sampling. The optimal real-time transducer to use is probably a curvilinear array, as this combines the advantages of sector and linear probes by allowing a large image field and visualisation of the whole course of the needle, while also being light and easy to manipulate. Use of colour flow imaging may facilitate the location of the umbilical cord insertion.

Holding the transducer wrapped in a sterile plastic bag with the target organ visualised, the abdominal site of entry and direction of the needle are chosen. Using a free-

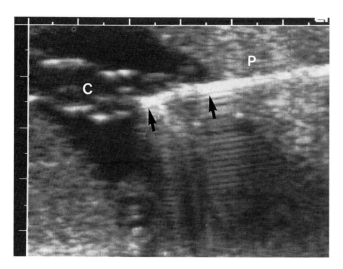

Fig. 24.10 Ultrasound-guided fetal blood sampling. Procedure from an anterior placental cord insertion showing the needle as a bright line (arrows). P – placenta, C – cord.

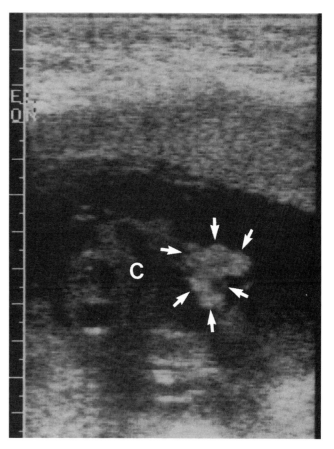

Fig. 24.11 Cord haematoma. Ultrasound image of a cord haematoma (arrows) after fetal blood sampling. C – cord.

hand technique the needle is then guided by simultaneous ultrasound to the chosen site and the needle tip identified as a clearly visible echo (Fig. 24.10). Alternatively, a fixed needle guide may be used. This technique restricts movement to the vertical plane alone and may enable less experienced operators to perform FBS successfully.[194] Once the needle is in the vessel immediate complications may also be monitored ultrasonically. These include alterations in fetal heart rate; intra-amniotic bleeding, seen as turbulent echoes in the amniotic cavity; and haematoma formation, seen as reflective space-occupying lesions (Fig. 24.11).

FBS is performed as an outpatient procedure. A partner or close relative is encouraged to attend for emotional support. Standard aseptic conditions are maintained, including a full scrub. With the patient wedged in a supine position with lateral tilt, the abdomen is washed with antiseptic solution and 1% xylocaine infiltrated at the puncture site. A 20 G spinal needle is then advanced under continuous ultrasound guidance to the appropriate site and 2–5 ml of fetal blood aspirated, depending on the indication.

Confirmation that fetal blood has been aspirated is provided immediately by analysis on a Coulter Channelyzer, which detects the difference in mean cell volume (MCV) between maternal and fetal red blood cells (RBC). Other distinguishing haematological indices include a broad RBC distribution width and a single leukocyte peak in the fetus. Dilution by amniotic fluid occurs in about 1% of procedures but maternal cell contamination is rare.[195]

The different sites of sampling are the placental cord insertion, fetal cord insertion (umbilicus), intrahepatic vein, fetal heart and a free loop of cord.

Placental cord insertion This is the original site described by Daffos *et al.*[190] and is the most widely utilised.

Both the artery and/or vein may be sampled, and each is specifically identified by the direction of flow of the echoes seen when 1 ml sterile saline is injected via the sampling needle. For anterior placentae the route to the umbilical cord is trans-placental and for posterior placentae the route is transamniotic (Fig. 24.12). The vessel is sampled about 1 cm from its placental insertion (Fig. 24.10). Failure to obtain fetal blood occurs in about 3% of cases and a second attempt may be necessary.[196]

Difficulties in sampling from the placental cord insertion may arise in cases of polyhydramnios, maternal obesity, or when the fetus obscures a posterior placental cord insertion. This may be overcome by fetal manipulation, alteration of maternal position, or by postponing the procedure. Alternatively, another site may be chosen for the FBS.

Fetal cord insertion Although possible, this site is not often used as passive mobility of the fetus makes successful sampling difficult.

Fetal intrahepatic umbilical vein This method involves directing a needle through the fetal abdominal

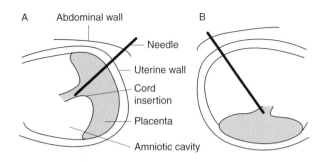

Fig. 24.12 Fetal blood sampling. The approach to fetal blood sampling in **A**: anterior and **B**: posterior placenta.

wall and liver substance into the intrahepatic portion of the umbilical vein (Fig. 24.13). In a transverse abdominal plane the direction of approach is anterior, either midline or via either hypochondrium. Although this method was originally reported by Bang[197] and de Crespigny[198] as a route for intravascular transfusions in fetuses with rhesus isoimmunisation, it was described by Koresawa[192] as the method of choice for second-trimester diagnostic FBS. This approach is useful when difficulties arise, either with access or due to sampling failure at the placental cord insertion. Alternatively this site may be preferentially chosen when visualisation of the placental cord insertion is poor, or to lessen the risks of fetomaternal haemorrhage.[199] Unlike sampling at the placental cord insertion

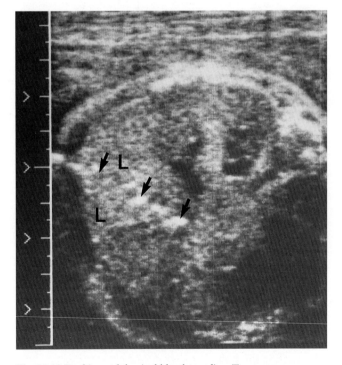

Fig. 24.13 Fetal intra-abdominal blood sampling. Transverse ultrasound section through a fetal abdomen showing the fetal blood sampling needle (arrows) in the intrahepatic portion of the umbilical vein. L – liver.

there is no need to confirm the fetal origin by mean corpuscular volume, nor is infusion of saline needed to assess vessel origin. Nicolini *et al.*[200] report success in obtaining a fetal blood sample in 92% of 214 cases. Analysis of changes in fetal liver enzymes following these procedures indicates that there is usually no hepatic damage.[201]

Fetal heart   Prenatal diagnosis using blood obtained from the fetal heart is possible.[193] The technique described by Bang utilises a 1.2 mm diameter guide needle which is inserted into the fetal thorax. A 0.7 mm needle is then advanced into the fetal ventricle. Puncturing the atrium can be fatal and is best avoided. This method is commonly associated with the potentially severe complications of fetal bradycardia and asystole and is rarely used clinically except in emergencies.

Free loop of umbilical cord   The sampling needle is advanced within the amniotic cavity until it abuts an accessible loop of cord. The vessel is then penetrated with a quick thrust. This method is ideal in cases of oligohydramnios or anhydramnios, as the cord becomes relatively fixed and the placental cord insertion difficult to identify.

Ultrasound-guided FBS is usually performed from 18 to 40 weeks gestation, depending on the indication. At the earlier gestations the procedure seems to be associated with a higher incidence of bradycardia and subsequent fetal death. This may be due to the relatively large size of the needle in relation to the vessel diameter for small fetuses. Also the paucity of Wharton's jelly may prolong traumatic haemorrhage. Very early FBS (prior to 16 weeks) has been reported, with fetal loss rates of 5%.[202]

Excellent results are only achieved after a great deal of experience and training. After 606 procedures, Daffos *et al.* report a 97% success rate at first attempt and failure rate of 0.5%.[196] In a smaller series of 96 procedures, however, rates of 63% and 5%, respectively, were reported.[203]

Indications

Fetal blood sampling was introduced to diagnose genetic haemoglobinopathies but is now used for a wide range of indications (Table 24.8).[191]

Karyotyping   A karyotype can be obtained from cultured fetal lymphocytes within 3 days, which is far more rapid than from amniocytes. This is useful in the further investigation of fetal structural abnormalities identified by ultrasound in the second trimester, as they are associated with a higher incidence of chromosomal aberration than at term.[204] Rapid karyotyping may also be useful for markers of fetal chromosomal abnormality, such as thickened nuchal skinfold and abnormalities of hands and feet.[205] Assessment of fetal structural anomalies now forms the largest group of patients having FBS (Table 24.8).

Table 24.8 Indications for fetal blood sampling[191]

Karyotyping	40%
Fetal red cell alloimmunisation	23%
Intra-uterine fetal infection	8%
Non-immune hydrops fetalis	7%
Fetal acid–base status	6%
Twin–twin transfusion syndrome	5%
Alloimmune thrombocytopenia	4%
Idiopathic thrombocytopenia of pregnancy	3%
Immunological deficiencies	2%
Coagulation factor deficiencies	1%
Haemoglobinopathies	1%
Other	<0.5%

Other indications for fetal blood karyotyping include late booking, failed amniocentesis, or the investigation of mosaicism or pseudomosaicism arising at amniocentesis.[23]

Alloimmunisation In pregnancies affected by red cell alloimmunisation (D, c, Kell) FBS is useful in the assessment of the severity of the disease. Direct measurement of the fetal haematocrit, reticulocyte count and total bilirubin enable the most accurate assessment of the severity of red cell alloimmunisation.[206] The diagnostic FBS can be followed by an intra-uterine intravascular transfusion if necessary.[207] There is a risk that the procedure itself will cause fetomaternal haemorrhage, resulting in a rise in maternal antibody levels and worsening the disease in an affected fetus.[208] This must be considered when offering diagnostic FBS and care must be taken to minimise the risk by avoiding a trans-placental needle passage.

Fetal blood grouping is now usually performed by DNA analysis[44] following amniocentesis, rather than by serological testing of fetal blood (see Amniocentesis)

Because of the risk of antenatal intracranial haemorrhage in alloimmune thrombocytopenia, second- and third-trimester determination of fetal platelet levels is appropriate in at-risk pregnancies.[209]

Non-immune hydrops An integral part of the diagnostic work-up, FBS is used to determine karyotype, viral infection or anaemia, when ultrasound has been unable to demonstrate a cause.

Fetal infections The increased perinatal mortality and long-term sequelae from congenital infection have justified fetal diagnosis. Confirmation of fetal infection usually requires identification of viral-specific IgM antibody or detection of viral-specific DNA in a fetus with suspicious ultrasound features, including hydrops, hydrocephaly, intracranial calcifications, microcephaly, ascites and hepatomegaly, or in a mother at high risk due to recent viral seroconversion.[210]

Congenital toxoplasmosis,[210] cytomegalovirus, rubella,[211] varicella zoster and human parvovirus have all traditionally been diagnosed by FBS after 22 weeks gestation, when the fetus can reliably mount an immune response and produce detectable viral-specific IgM. More recently, detection of viral DNA by PCR techniques has enabled accurate diagnosis following amniocentesis,[212] and fetal blood sampling is rarely indicated unless there is associated hydrops.

Blood gas and acid–base status Analysis of blood from small-for-gestational-age (SGA) fetuses has shown that a substantial proportion are chronically hypoxic, the degree of which correlates with acidosis, hypercapnia, hyperlacticaemia, hypoglycaemia and erythroblastosis.[213] However, the degree of hypoxia and acidosis found at FBS has not been shown to correlate directly with perinatal mortality (Figs 24.14 and 24.15), limiting its usefulness as a clinical test.[214] Non-invasive Doppler measurements of waveform velocities are preferred as they pose no risk to the fetus and correlate with fetal hypoxaemia/acidaemia, and meta-analysis has demonstrated a significantly increased risk of perinatal mortality with abnormal results.[215]

Genetic blood disorders Prenatal diagnosis of haemoglobinopathies is made by measuring globin chain synthesis.[216] The diagnosis of fetal haemophilia A or B is made by quantification of factor VIIIC or factor IX, respectively. Many other coagulopathies and platelet disorders can be diagnosed prenatally as the relevant normal ranges are available.[217] Increasingly first-trimester diagnosis via DNA analysis of chorionic villi is replacing fetal blood analysis for these disorders, provided a family DNA marker has been identified and the pregnancy is sufficiently early.

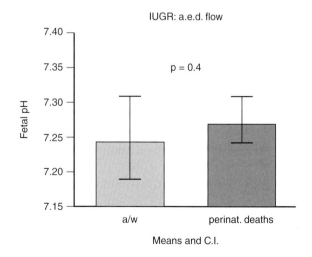

Fig. 24.14 Fetal pH levels in growth-retarded fetuses with absent end-diastolic flow that survived (white) and that died (grey) perinatally: means and confidence intervals.

IUGR: a.e.d. flow

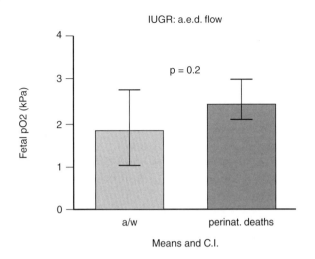

Fig. 24.15 Fetal pO$_2$ levels in growth-retarded fetuses with absent end-diastolic flow that survived (white) and that died (grey) perinatally: means and confidence intervals.

Inherited severe combined immunodeficiencies can be diagnosed by monoclonal anti-T cell lymphocyte antibodies and a fluorescence-activated cell sorter.[218,219]

Other Although a rapid diagnosis of many inborn errors of metabolism can be made on fetal blood, earlier diagnosis is possible on chorionic villi or amniotic fluid.

Complications

Maternal Discomfort at the time of the procedure and for 1–2 days postoperatively is common, but no serious maternal complications have been reported.[190,196,203]

Fetal The largest original series reported spontaneous abortion or intra-uterine death in seven of 606 cases (1.9%), although only two were considered to be due to the procedure.[196] They also reported no increase in preterm delivery or growth retardation. In the multicentre series of Megerian and Ludomirsky[191] the fetal loss rate per procedure was 1.12%, with 0.27% attributed to chorio-amnionitis, 0.22% to ruptured membranes, 0.22% unexplained, 0.18% to severe bradycardia, 0.16% from bleeding at the puncture site and 0.05% from cord thrombosis.

When procedure-related fetal loss rates are analysed according to indication for sampling, significant differences become evident. This information is important when counselling regarding risk. Maxwell *et al.*[220] reported loss rates of 1% for structurally normal fetuses, 7% for structurally abnormal fetuses, 14% for growth-restricted fetuses and 25% for hydropic fetuses. Similarly, Antsakalis *et al.*[221] found loss rates of 1% for structurally normal fetuses, 13% for structurally abnormal fetuses and 9% for growth-restricted fetuses.

Intra-amniotic bleeding is common and usually transient.[196,203] Fetal bradycardia is observed more commonly with arterial samplings[203] and is also usually transient. An uncommon but specific risk of fetal cord sampling is acute bleeding into the Wharton's jelly, producing cord haematoma and tamponade. Although not usually associated with any problems, a recent report has described a case of fetal hepatic necrosis 24 hours following hepatic vein sampling.[222]

Fetal tissue biopsy

Some hereditary disorders are unable to be diagnosed using amniotic fluid or chorionic villus and require specific fetal tissue for prenatal diagnosis. The fetal skin, liver and muscle are the more commonly used sites. The requirement for these procedures may decrease dramatically as genes or chromosome regions linked to the disorders enable probes for DNA diagnosis.

Skin

Unless characterised by a chromosomal abnormality or enzyme defect, prenatal diagnosis of hereditary skin disorders requires histology and ultrastructural studies on fetal skin biopsies[223] obtained either by fetoscopy or by ultrasound-guided techniques.[224,225]

Technique An ultrasound assessment should be performed to confirm gestational age and fetal heart action, to exclude structural anomalies and multiple pregnancy, and to determine fetal lie and placental position.

The preferential site for biopsy depends on the particular condition under investigation. Ultrasound is used to select the abdominal entry point that will allow access to the sampling site, which depends on fetal position and placental location. For example, fetuses at risk of epidermolysis bullosa are best sampled from the buttock or leg, and those at risk of albinism should be biopsied from the eyebrow or scalp.

Performed under local anaesthesia, the procedure is an outpatient technique using standard aseptic precautions. Currently, the most frequently used method is ultrasound guided, performed by introducing a 19-gauge cannula with trocar percutaneously into the uterine cavity under ultrasound surveillance. After withdrawing the trocar fine 20-gauge cupped biopsy forceps (De Elles Instruments, Surrey, UK) are directed to the appropriate site and multiple samples pinched out.

Previously, fetoscopy was used to obtain fetal skin samples, either under direct vision using biopsy forceps passed down the operating side-arm of the fetoscope cannula[224] or by ultrasonically directing larger biopsy forceps down the cannula after removing the fetoscope.[226]

Using direct-vision fetoscopy or ultrasound-guided biopsy in 52 patients at King's College Hospital and

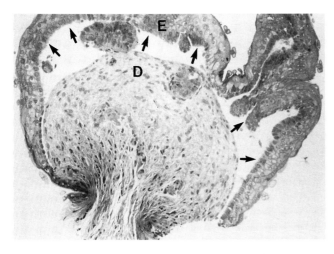

Fig. 24.16 Skin biopsy specimen. Histological diagnosis of epidermolysis bullosa lethalis showing separation (arrows) of the epidermis (E) from the dermis (D).

Queen Charlotte and Chelsea Hospitals between 1980 and 1988 there were no failed procedures.

The biopsy technique causes crush damage, so the specimens are flushed from the forceps using sterile saline and fixed immediately without further handling. The samples can be processed in a matter of hours for analysis by light and electron microscopy (Fig. 24.16).[227]

The majority of skin biopsies are performed at 18–22 weeks gestation, although differentiation of major fetal skin structures is not completed until 24–26 weeks.[228]

Indications Table 24.9 lists the main conditions for which prenatal skin biopsy is indicated.

Complications Following fetal skin biopsy the fetal loss rate is approximately 5% and the preterm birth rate 10%.[231] Review of the 52 skin biopsies performed at King's College Hospital and Queen Charlotte and Chelsea Hospitals between 1980 and 1988 revealed 13 affected fetuses. Of the 40 continuing pregnancies there were no spontaneous abortions, four preterm deliveries and one neonatal death following premature delivery.

Table 24.9 Indications for fetal skin biopsy[229,230]

Disorder	Inheritance
Epidermolysis bullosa lethalis (Fig 24.16)	Autosomal recessive
Epidermolysis bullosa dystrophica	Autosomal recessive
Bullous congenital ichthyosiform erythroderma	Autosomal dominant
Non-ichthyosiform erythroderma	Autosomal recessive
Harlequin ichthyosis	Autosomal recessive
Sjogren–Larsson syndrome	Autosomal recessive
Oculocutaneous albinism	Autosomal recessive
Anhidrotic ectodermal dysplasia	Autosomal recessive
Hypohidrotic ectodermal dysplasia	X-linked recessive

Liver

Prenatal diagnosis of inborn errors of metabolism is usually achieved through an assay of chorion, fetal blood or cultured amniocytes for specific enzyme activity or metabolite detection. In a few rare disorders diagnosis is still only possible on liver tissue, owing to the localised protein expression.[232]

Technique As usual a prebiopsy ultrasound is performed independent of the timing of the biopsy.

Initial experience of liver biopsy was with fetoscopy. More recently ultrasound-guided transabdominal liver biopsies have been performed.[232] Performed under local anaesthesia, the procedure is an outpatient technique using standard aseptic precautions. The route to the fetal liver is selected on ultrasound and, avoiding the placenta, the needle is guided across the amniotic space to the right hypochondrium of the fetus. It is then introduced swiftly into the fetal trunk, as the fetus is likely to withdraw from the needle tip unless rapidly transfixed. This technique is more adaptable than fetoscopy as the needle tip is continuously visualised within the abdomen. It allows more oblique and lateral approaches to the fetal trunk and is particularly advantageous when the fetal spine is anterior. In this regard the technique is similar to needling the intrahepatic portion of the umbilical vein.

For ultrasound-guided liver biopsies a double cannula (17/19 G) (Fig. 24.17) is used similar to that used for transabdominal CVS. The back-and-forth aspirating motion is then confined to the inner cannula, which minimises maternal discomfort from peritoneal irritation and limits the movement of the needle within the fetal liver. The aspiration needle is 19 gauge for its last 8 cm, the rest of the shaft being slightly narrower. A 10 ml syringe is attached to the hub and strong negative pressure exerted after removal. The needle, containing a core of liver tissue, is flushed through with normal saline into a gallipot and the procedure repeated as necessary. Several insertions may be required to obtain the 10–25 mg of tissue required for analysis. A light microscope is useful to confirm that the correct tissue has been sampled.

Following the procedure the fetal heart rate is checked with ultrasound and the fetal peritoneal cavity scanned for evidence of bleeding.

Prior to undertaking liver biopsy for prenatal diagnosis the exact enzyme defect from a previous pregnancy or the maternal carrier status must be identified. Reference ranges for enzyme activities in mid-trimester fetuses have been established.[232,233] Technical failures can be checked against other liver enzymes, which should be normal.[232,234,235] To date no failed procedures or incorrect diagnoses have been reported.

Fetal liver biopsy for any current indication is delayed until 17 weeks gestation, when the enzyme activity is first

Muscle

Prenatal diagnosis of Duchenne (DMD) and Becker (BMD) muscular dystrophies is usually ascertained through molecular analysis of amniotic fluid cells or chorionic villi to detect a deletion in the dystrophin gene.[243] However, 35% of families have no gene deletion and may be uninformative with linkage analysis.[244] As an alternative, these families may undergo fetal muscle biopsy *in utero*, described in 1991 by Evans *et al.*, to obtain a direct histochemical diagnosis.[245]

Technique   A preliminary ultrasound examination is performed for assessment. Fetal muscle is then obtained by ultrasound-guided percutaneous passage of a coring biopsy 'gun' generally used for kidney biopsies. The needle is positioned for entry into the fetal gluteal muscle in a downward fashion over the buttock, pierced into the skin and extended across the gluteal muscle. The trigger is then pulled, drawing the extended piece back and generating a core of muscle.[246] A combined ultrasound and endoscopic approach enables fine-tuning of the position of the biopsy gun.[247]

After sampling the specimens are examined for muscle fibres, and immunoblotting or immunofluorescence is used to determine the presence or absence of dystrophin (Fig. 24.18).[248] An ultrasound examination is done immediately after the procedure for fetal assessment.

Biopsies are usually performed between 18 and 23 weeks gestation.[246] Those attempted prior to 18 weeks have not been successful by ultrasound-guided techniques but may be possible with fine-needle endoscopically assisted ultrasound.[247]

Indications   The current indications for fetal muscle biopsy include male fetuses at risk of DMD with ambiguous DNA studies, female fetuses at risk of DMD because of an X-autosome translocation and male fetuses at risk of BMD and mitochondrial myopathies.[246]

Complications   In the collaborative experience of 12 cases reported by Evans *et al.* 11 biopsies were successful in obtaining tissue for diagnosis.[246] Too few procedures have been performed to assess the safety of the procedure. In the collaborative series two of the 12 cases miscarried within a week of the procedure after spontaneous rupture of membranes, there were no scars or nerve damage, and all live-borns were diagnosed correctly.[246]

Kidney

Kidney biopsy during the second trimester has enabled prenatal diagnosis in a case at risk of congenital Finnish nephrosis, by demonstrating podocyte fusion in the cortical nephrons on electron microscopy.[249]

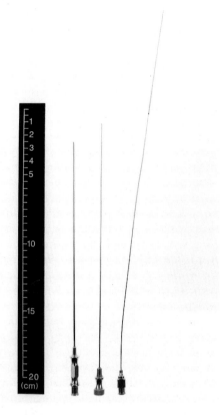

Fig. 24.17 Liver biopsy needle with inserting trocar and cannula. (De Elles Instruments, Surrey, UK.)

expressed. In the future sampling may be performed earlier, as some enzyme activity has been demonstrated in fetal liver from first-trimester terminations.[236,237]

Indications   Fetal liver biopsy has been reported in the prenatal diagnosis of only four conditions: ornithine carbamyl transferase deficiency (OCTD),[232,234] carbamyl phosphate synthetase deficiency (CPSD),[235] glucose 6 phosphatase deficiency[238] and primary hyperoxaluria.[233] The recent availability of DNA analysis for OTCD and CPSD means that liver biopsy is only required in uninformative families.[239–241]

Complications   The risk of fetal loss secondary to ultrasound-guided invasive intra-uterine procedures is 1–2%. General experience suggests that, despite the small numbers, the procedure is safe.[234] Of 14 procedures performed by Nicolini and Rodeck until 1988 there were eight affected fetuses, which were terminated.[238] All six continuing pregnancies delivered live births with no complications.[242] Occasional transient bradycardia was the most common complication. No evidence of intraperitoneal bleeding was found at autopsy following liver biopsy in 18 fetuses,[232,234] but a small skin puncture scar was noted in one neonate.[238]

Ultrasound can provide some prognostic information, but aspiration of fetal urine has also become widely used.[252–258]

Technique

Ultrasound prior to the procedure is essential. The fetus is also screened for other structural abnormalities, which occur in about 30% of cases.[204] The amniotic fluid volume is assessed. Oligohydramnios carries a poor prognosis[259,260] as it is associated with lung hypoplasia. However, it may be related more to the degree of urethral obstruction rather than reduced urine production or renal dysfunction.[258] The gender is determined and the renal tract examined in great detail. The urethra should be evaluated to establish the origin of the obstruction, the bladder assessed for degree of dilation and wall thickening, and the ureters for bilateral involvement and degree of pyelectasis.[257] The kidneys should be examined for degree of hydronephrosis and the degree of cortical thinning, although renal function does not correlate with either. Renal cortical cysts and increased parenchymal reflectivity (see Ch. 16) may be useful in that both have a specificity of 100%, but are only 58% and 66% sensitive, respectively.[252]

Ultrasound is used to locate the sampling site for aspiration and guide the needle to this point using a free-hand technique. Using a sterile technique and local anaesthesia the fetal urine is aspirated using a 20 G spinal needle. Although bladder sampling is more common (Fig. 24.19),

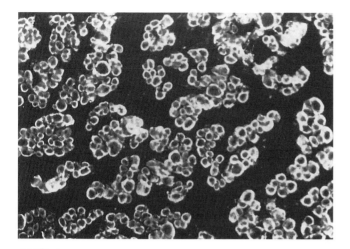

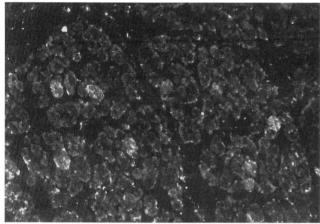

Fig. 24.18 Immunofluorescent stains of fetal muscle. Bright-staining dystrophin reflects normal muscle (top) and non-staining areas from Duchenne muscular dystrophy muscle (bottom). (Reproduced from Evans *et al.*[246] with permission from Elsevier Science Inc., USA.)

A recent preliminary report of 10 fetal renal biopsies in obstructive uropathy indicates a 50% success in obtaining tissue by aspirating with a 19 gauge needle. Renal histopathology altered the prognosis estimated by urinary electrolytes in two cases.[250]

Aspiration of fetal urine

Most urinary tract abnormalities are best corrected after birth, with prenatal diagnosis enabling the delivery to be planned appropriately.[251] Antenatal intervention may be the only chance to improve neonatal survival when life-threatening complications occur in fetal obstructive uropathy. However, one of the most problematic areas in the management is the appropriate selection of the fetus that will benefit from the therapeutic intervention, in that it has an obstruction severe enough to compromise renal and pulmonary development, but not so severe that renal damage is irreversible if the obstruction is relieved.[252]

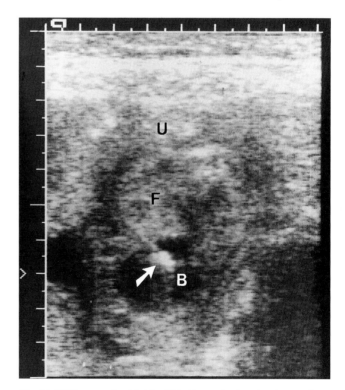

Fig. 24.19 Ultrasound-guided fetal bladder aspiration showing needle tip (arrow) within the fetal bladder (B). F – fetus, U – uterus.

aspiration of dilated renal pelves enables each kidney to be evaluated independently.[261] As with other procedures the approach should be anterior or lateral, with the fetus imaged in transverse section. Once in the amniotic cavity the needle is thrust into the fetus with one movement, as touching the body promotes a reflex withdrawal. Urine is aspirated until the bladder or renal pelvis is seen on ultrasound to be completely empty.

After the procedure the fetal heart rate and sampling site(s) are assessed for any complications. Documented bladder filling 24 hours later is suggestive of subsequent urine production, but may be unreliable if there has been passive filling from a dilated upper urinary tract or if there is polyuric renal failure.

The urine biochemistry is then compared to the normal reference ranges. Values of urinary sodium >100 mmol/l, chloride >90 mmol/l and osmolality >210 mosm/l have been correlated with good renal function,[252,262] but these findings have been challenged,[263] probably because they were derived retrospectively from the outcome of fetuses with obstructive uropathy and because it was falsely assumed that fetal urine biochemistry did not alter with gestation.[258]

References ranges with respect to gestational age indicate sodium (Fig. 24.20) and phosphate decrease, creatinine increases and potassium, calcium and urea are not correlated with gestation.[253,258] In the detection of renal dysplasia, urinary calcium gives the best sensitivity and sodium the best specificity (Table 24.10).[258] More recently β_2-microglobulin[254] and total protein[256] have been included in the prognostic assessment.

Another refinement aimed to reduce the false-positive and false-negative results obtained in the biochemical assessment of fetal obstructive uropathy is the use of sequential urinalysis (Fig. 24.21). This was first per-

Table 24.10 Sensitivity and specificity of urinary sodium (Na$^+$), calcium (Ca^{2+}) and phosphate (PO$_4$$^{2-}$) in the prediction of renal dysplasia within the group of fetuses with obstructive uropathy[258]

	Sensitivity	Specificity
Na$^+$	87% (13/15)	80% (8/10)
Ca^{2+}	100% (15/15)	60% (6/10)
PO$_4$$^{2-}$	53% (8/15)	62% (5/8)

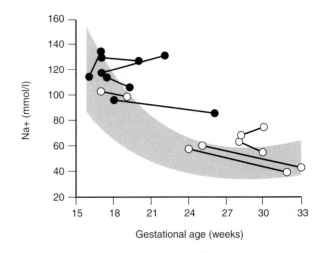

Fig. 24.21 Lower urinary tract obstruction (LUTO). Urinary sodium (Na$^+$) in serial samples from fetuses with LUTO. (●) fetuses with renal dysplasia; (○) fetuses without renal dysplasia. (Reproduced from Nicolini *et al.*[258] with permission from Blackwell Science Ltd, Oxford, UK.)

formed at a 24-hour interval to obtain 'fresh' urine.[255] Subsequently, three vesicocenteses have been proposed, with a significant improvement in the prediction of renal damage with the last sample.[256]

The timing of fetal urinary aspiration to assess renal function in lower urinary tract obstruction depends on the time of onset and the extent of the lesion. Most cases are sampled from 14 to 24 weeks. The aim is to sample the urine prior to the onset of both renal dysplasia due to obstruction and pulmonary hypoplasia due to severe oligohydramnios. However, oligohydramnios is uncommon before the 16th to 17th weeks of gestation, even in the complete absence of fetal micturition, and it may be that in these early cases irreversible kidney damage has already occurred.[264] Alternatively, unless serial ultrasonic scans have proved a short duration of oligohydramnios, this should be regarded as a poor prognostic sign.[259,260]

Indications

The most frequent cause of lower urinary tract obstruction is posterior urethral valves, which occur exclusively in males and, together with prune-belly syndrome, have a good potential for survival.[260,265,266] Urethral atresia and

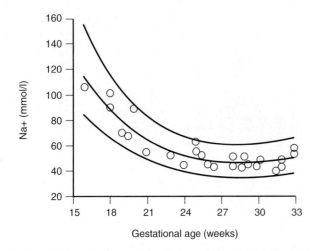

Fig. 24.20 Reference range for fetal urinary sodium (Na$^+$) throughout gestation: mean and 95% data intervals. (Reproduced from Nicolini *et al.*[258] with permission from Blackwell Science Ltd, Oxford, UK.)

cloacal abnormalities are uniformly lethal and unlikely to benefit from investigation.[265]

Complications

The risks of fetal urinary aspiration are similar to those of other fetal invasive procedures.

Fetal diagnostic infusions

In severe oligohydramnios ultrasound visualisation of fetal anatomy is severely restricted owing to the lack of an acoustic window and abnormal fetal posture. Fluid instilled into either the amniotic[267] or the peritoneal[268] cavity can greatly improve the quality of the imaging.

Technique

The finding of severe oligohydramnios necessitates a meticulous ultrasonic fetal examination to establish the aetiology, which is most commonly related to intra-uterine growth retardation or renal tract abnormalities, once preterm premature rupture of the membranes has been excluded. However, even with the improved resolution possible with trans-vaginal ultrasound, anatomical differentiation may still be difficult and false-negative and false-positive diagnoses of renal agenesis have been reported.[269]

Amnio-infusion should be performed under strict aseptic conditions and with antibiotic prophylaxis. Ultrasound is used to identify a suitable entry point into the uterus. Care must be taken, as echo-free areas suggestive of a small pocket of amniotic fluid may be umbilical cord and evaluation with colour Doppler is a prerequisite. A 20 gauge needle is guided into the uterus under continuous ultrasound surveillance and before fluid instillation, aspiration with a 1 ml syringe will exclude the possibility of its being in a vessel. Any fetal blood aspirated can be used to assess karyotype and blood gases. The amount of warm saline instilled depends on the amniotic fluid pressure, the resultant visibility and the gestational age of the fetus.[270] Following the amnio-infusion leakage of fluid from the vagina confirms premature rupture of the membranes.[270]

Following the procedure sonographic visibility is greatly improved and fetal movement facilitates the examination of fetal anatomy. Fetal breathing and swallowing are also commonly observed. As usual, the fetal heart rate should be checked.

Occasionally ultrasound visualisation remains obscured despite amnio-infusion;[271] another technique which may help clarify the fetal intra-abdominal and retroperitoneal anatomy is that of intraperitoneal saline infusion.[268] In particular, renal agenesis may be diagnosed more accurately (Fig. 24.22).

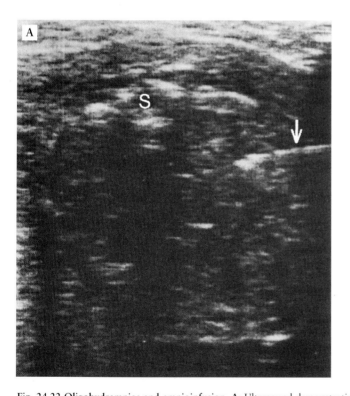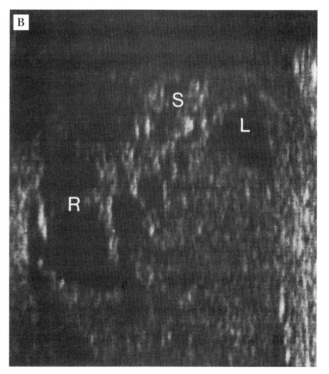

Fig. 24.22 Oligohydramnios and amnioinfusion. A: Ultrasound demonstrating oligohydramnios and the fetal abdomen in cross-section. No renal tissue is seen on either side of the fetal spine (S). The arrow indicates the needle inserted to instil saline. **B:** After the intraperitoneal infusion of saline the right multicystic kidney (R), the liver and fluid in the position of the left kidney (L) are evident. (Reproduced from Nicolini *et al.*[268] with permission from John Wiley and Sons, Chichester, UK.)

Indications

The current indication for performing amnio-infusion and/or peritoneal infusion is severe oligohydramnios or anhydramnios. Gembruch and Hansmann reported 50 such pregnancies in which the final diagnoses included Potter's syndrome, obstructive uropathy, cystic kidneys, Meckel syndrome, Cornelia de Lange syndrome, cytomegaly fetopathy, VATER association, triploidy, severe intra-uterine growth retardation and preterm premature rupture of the membranes.[267] In 92 amnio-infusions Fisk *et al.* reported a change in aetiological diagnosis in 13% of subjects.[270]

Complications

The principal risks associated with amnio-infusion are chorio-amnionitis and spontaneous abortion/preterm labour in those patients in whom the procedure unmasks ruptured membranes.[272] Inadvertent fetal blood sampling at the time of amnio-infusion carries its own risks, such as arterial spasm and cord tamponade.[270]

Intraperitoneal infusion will cause fetal heart rate changes if too much fluid is instilled.

Fetoscopy and embryoscopy

Embryoscopy is the direct examination of the embryo through an intact amniotic membrane.[273] Fetoscopy is the direct endoscopic examination of the intra-amniotic contents, developed in the 1970s as a method for obtaining fetal blood[183,187,188] but evolving into a tool for obtaining fetal skin biopsies and visualising the fetus.[274] Improvements in ultrasound technology enabled the diagnosis of fetal abnormalities early in the second trimester and facilitated percutaneous sampling to obtain fetal blood and tissue.[190] Consequently, second-trimester fetoscopy became obsolete.

The recent development of examining fetal anatomy in the first trimester as an adjunct to ultrasound screening for fetal aneuploidy[275] may have opened a new future for embryofetoscopy.[276,277] In particular, at this gestation accurate diagnoses cannot always be made by ultrasound alone, and rather than waiting for later confirmation embryofetoscopy may allow the earlier choice of continuing or terminating the pregnancy.

Technique

Before performing this procedure genetic counselling and informed consent is mandatory. Fetal viability and gestational age are confirmed by ultrasound examination, as well as a review made of the fetal anatomy and access to the fetus in relation to the placenta.[277] Prophylactic antibiotics and maternal analgesia are recommended. Anti-D prophylaxis should be administered appropriately.

Embryofetoscopy must be performed under continuous ultrasound guidance. Alternative approaches include transcervical embryoscopy, transabdominal embryoscopy and transabdominal fetoscopy.

Trans-cervical embryoscopy The patient is placed in the lithotomy position. The vulva and vagina are cleansed with antiseptic, the bladder is emptied and a tenaculum is applied to manipulate the cervix. A rigid endoscope (1.7 mm) is introduced through the cervical canal and chorionic membrane into the exocoelomic cavity.[278] The chorion must be penetrated at a 90° angle to avoid tenting and subsequent separation from the uterine wall. The success rate in visualising the fetus varies from 95 to 97%.[278,279]

Transabdominal embryoscopy The maternal abdomen is cleansed with antiseptic and draped. Following the administration of local anaesthetic, a 16–19 gauge needle is introduced transabdominally into the extracoelomic space without puncturing the amnion.[280,281] An endoscope of 0.7–0.8 mm in diameter is then introduced to visualise the fetus. Failure rates of 35% have been reported owing to inadvertent puncture of the amniotic membrane.[280]

Transabdominal fetoscopy Using standard aseptic techniques and local anaesthetic, an 18–21 gauge needle is introduced into the amniotic cavity. Flexible or semirigid fibre-optic endoscopes, varying in outer diameter from 0.5 to 1 mm and in field of vision from 55 to 70° are inserted to visualise the fetus.[282,283] Amniotic fluid can be aspirated for testing. Several instruments, including a 22–24 gauge aspirating needle, a 1 mm biopsy forceps or a 400 μm laser fibre can be used through the operating side channel under full endoscopic vision.[277] A xenon light source is used.[277] In 10% of procedures visualisation is obscured by intra-amniotic bleeding from the placenta or uterine wall.[277]

Embryoscopy has to be performed prior to fusion of the amnion and chorion as it utilises the chorionic cavity. It is technically possible from 5 to 12 weeks gestation but is more commonly performed at 9–10 weeks. Fetoscopy is performed from 11 weeks gestation.[277]

Indications

Embryofetoscopy may be performed for pregnancies at risk of recurrence of genetic conditions with external fetal abnormalities.[277] Successful diagnoses include Smith–Lemli–Opitz syndrome,[278] Ellis van Creveld syndrome,[278] Apert syndrome,[278] Meckel–Gruber syndrome,[284] Van der Woude syndrome[285] and Pierre Robin sequence.[277]

Other indications include the further investigation of structural anomalies suspected at first-trimester ultrasound screening, and confirmation of fetal malformations diagnosed by first-trimester ultrasound before proceeding to suction termination of pregnancy.[276,277] Diagnoses confirmed for these reasons include cystic hygroma,[280] omphalocele,[280]

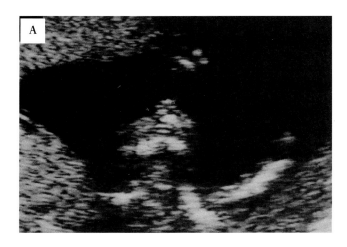

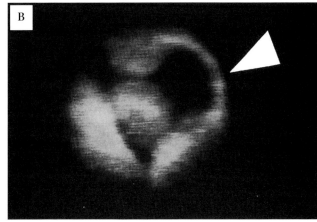

Fig. 24.23 Diagnostic fetoscopy. A: Ultrasound examination of the fetal face at 12 weeks gestation. A lateral facial cleft is suspected (caliper); **B:** Endoscopic vision of a large median cleft of the upper lip and palate (arrowhead); **C:** drawing of the fetoscopic picture. (Reproduced from Ville *et al.*[283] with permission from Parthenon Publishing, UK.)

neural tube defect,[280] midline cleft and palate (Fig. 24.23)[283] and frontal encephalocele.[283] In addition, blood and tissues can be obtained for further testing[277,284] and there is the potential for early fetal therapy.[277]

Complications

The safety of embryofetoscopy is still being evaluated. No data exist to provide estimates of the risk of fetal loss. There is also concern over the effect of white light on the developing fetal retina, but retinal damage could be demonstrated in chickens exposed to embryofetoscopy white light.[286] Human data are still limited, but no infants born following first-trimester embryofetoscopy have demonstrated visual abnormalities.

Therapeutic procedures

Fetal transfusion

The first intra-uterine intravascular fetal blood transfusions were performed in the 1960s for severe rhesus disease, and required hysterotomy and cannulation of the fetal femoral artery,[287] saphenous vein[288] or a chorionic plate vessel.[289] However, the high rates of fetal mortality and maternal morbidity associated with these techniques prohibited their use. Instead, the more acceptable and less invasive technique of percutaneous intraperitoneal transfusion became the accepted method for performing transfusions *in utero*.

The procedure, first described by Liley in 1963,[290] required an amniocentesis to inject urografin into the amniotic cavity, with X-ray follow-up to visualise the fetal bowel containing swallowed contrast medium. An epidural catheter was then inserted into the fetal peritoneal cavity via a 16 gauge Tuohy needle, and further X-ray films were taken to ensure correct placement. Rhesus-negative packed red cells were then transfused, and absorbed into the fetal circulation through the subdiaphragmatic lymphatics and the thoracic duct. Various modifications were introduced to improve the success of the technique, but it was only after the introduction of ultrasound that this was achieved. The risk of malignancy from ionising radiation was also eliminated.

After two decades of intraperitoneal transfusion the survival rates have improved dramatically, from 24–56% in the decade to 1976, to 69–92% in the 1980s.[291-294] The principal factors that continued to limit the survival rates were an early gestational age at initial transfusion and the presence of hydrops fetalis. Thus the advent of fetoscopy fulfilled the continued interest in developing a direct intravascular route for transfusion.

In 1981 Rodeck *et al.* reported on the first intravascular transfusion performed through an umbilical cord vessel using the fetoscope.[295] Three years later the same group published an overall survival rate of 72% in 25 severely affected rhesus fetuses who underwent 77 fetoscopic intrauterine transfusions.[296] In this series a survival rate of 84%

was obtained among fetuses which had their first transfusion before 25 weeks, almost 50% of which had hydrops at this early stage of gestation.

Subsequently the development of ultrasound-guided percutaneous needling has simplified direct intravascular fetal transfusion, and the technique most widely used now is modified from that described by Daffos *et al.*[196] using the umbilical vein at the placental cord insertion.[297,298] Using this technique, Nicolaides *et al.*[298] reported 21 fetuses, including 11 with hydrops, that had a total of 96 transfusions and a survival rate of 95%. Other sites which can be used for transfusion include the intrahepatic portion of the umbilical vein[197,198] and the fetal heart.[299] The advantages of intravascular transfusion include:

1. Measuring pre- and post-transfusion haematocrit;
2. Accurate timing of subsequent transfusions by percentage haematocrit fall per day;
3. Performing before 20 weeks gestation;
4. Avoiding lymphatic transport from the peritoneal cavity and therefore being able to reverse hydrops fetalis *in utero*;
5. Continuing treatment until pulmonary maturity is confirmed.

Technique

Ultrasonic evaluation of the fetus remains an integral part of the management of rhesus isoimmunisation and may detect fetal ascites, which is an early sign in the onset of hydrops (ascites, pericardial effusion, subcutaneous oedema, polyhydramnios and placentomegaly), thus prompting timely intervention. However, in the absence of hydrops ultrasound measurements of abdominal circumference, head circumference, head/abdominal circumference ratio, intraperitoneal volume, extra- and intrahepatic vein diameters and placental thickness >4 cm are not reliable in distinguishing mild from severe fetal haemolytic disease.[300,301]

The role of ultrasound in fetal procedures was described earlier in this chapter.

Intravascular transfusion   Fetal intravascular transfusion (IVT) is usually performed as an outpatient procedure without maternal sedation. Prophylactic antibiotics are often given. A fetal blood sample is taken in the usual manner, using a 20 gauge spinal needle. Fetal analgesia is obtained by intravenous injection of fentanyl at the dose of 1 μg/kg of estimated fetal weight. As fetal movement during the transfusion may cause needle displacement, temporary paralysis may be achieved using intravascular pancuronium bromide.[302]

Once a sample is obtained the fetal haematocrit is determined immediately using a Coulter counter. If this is 2 SD below the normal mean for gestation[207,298] (Fig. 24.24) the needle is kept *in situ* and a transfusion of fresh, concentrated (70–80%) rhesus-negative red cells, cross-matched with maternal blood, is given manually in 5 ml aliquots. Extension tubing connected to a three-way stopcock is attached to the needle (Fig. 24.25) to minimise movement of the needle after it is correctly placed. The fetal heart rate and the flow of the infused blood are monitored continually during the procedure by real-time ultrasound.

The amount of blood transfused depends on the initial haematocrit, the haematocrit of the donor blood and the gestational age. Nomograms have been calculated to provide an estimation of the volume of donor blood required to increase the fetal haematocrit to about 40%[160] (Fig. 24.26). Following the transfusion another fetal sample is aspirated to determine the actual haematocrit, and further blood is given as necessary to bring the final value to 40–50%.

Two methods of IVT are in current use. A 'top-up' or 'bolus' transfusion refers to the intravenous administration of blood into the fetus without removing any blood, and is the most commonly used technique. An 'exchange' transfusion consists of the administration and removal of

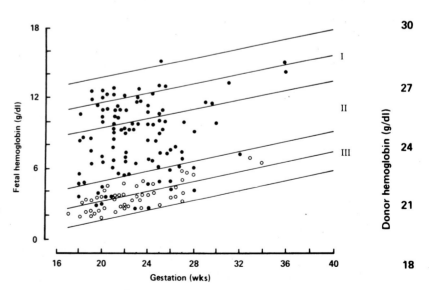

Fig. 24.24 Rhesus alloimmunisation. Fetal haemoglobin concentration in Rh-alloimmunised pregnancies with (○) and without (•) fetal hydrops plotted on the normal range: mean and 95% data intervals. (Reproduced from Nicolaides *et al.*[207] with permission from Lancet Ltd, UK.)

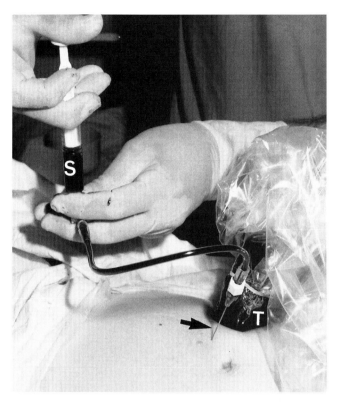

Fig. 24.25 Intravascular transfusion. Set-up for an ultrasound-guided IVT in Rh disease showing needle (arrow) connected to an extension set and three-way stopcock for attaching syringe (S). The transducer is in a sterile plastic bag (T).

approximately equal amounts of blood, the aim being to prevent hypervolaemia and further compromise of an already overburdened fetal myocardium, particularly in a severely hydropic fetus.[303,304] Clinically hypervolaemia has been of little concern, with reports of 'top-up' transfusions of up to 100–150% of fetoplacental blood volume without any change in the fetal heart rate.[298,305] 'Top-up' transfusions have the advantage of being simpler to perform and of being completed in less than half the time it takes to do an 'exchange' transfusion, which reduces the probability of bacterial contamination, needle dislodgement and thrombosis in the umbilical vein. The fetus tolerates 'top-up' transfusions given at a rate of 5–15 ml/min without obvious adverse effects[298] and only minor changes in acid–base and blood gas status.[306]

Intraperitoneal transfusion Percutaneous ultrasound-guided intraperitoneal transfusions are performed in the same way as the intravascular procedures, except that the needle is directed into the fetal abdominal cavity. Correct needle placement is verified in a hydropic fetus by aspirating ascitic fluid or by visualising sterile saline injected into the peritoneal cavity if there is no ascites. The amount of blood transfused is estimated by the empirical formula (gestation in weeks −20) × 10 ml[307] at a rate of 5–15 ml/min with continual monitoring of the fetal heart rate.

Since the development of intravascular transfusions the intraperitoneal approach has become second-line therapy,

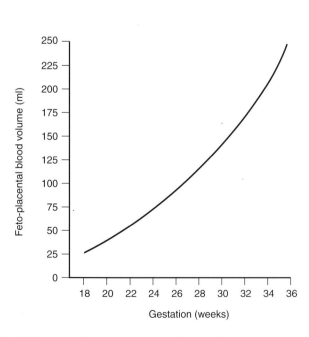

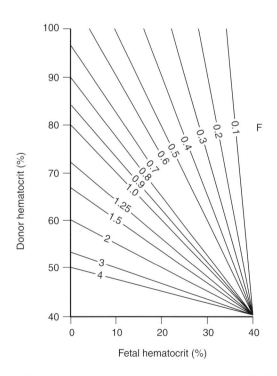

Fig. 24.26 Nomogram for intravascular transfusion. To calculate the volume of donor blood necessary to achieve a fetal haematocrit of 40%, the estimated fetoplacental blood volume (left, e.g. 100 ml at 27 weeks) is multiplied by F (right, e.g. 0.8 for a pretransfusion haematocrit of 10% and a donor haematocrit of 80%). (Reproduced from Nicolaides *et al.*[298] with permission from S Karger AG, Switzerland.)

as inadequate absorption of erythrocytes from the peritoneal cavity precludes treatment in hydropic fetuses.[308] However, it is very effective in the absence of hydrops and may be used in combination with IVT to increase the total blood volume given to the fetus, thereby prolonging the interval between transfusions (up to 4–5 weeks) and reducing the total number of invasive procedures.[308,312]

The first transfusion depends on the gestation at referral and the predicted severity of the disease. In general, for patients with a previous history of RBC alloimmunisation the first FBS and IVT are performed approximately 10 weeks prior to the earliest previous fetal or neonatal death, fetal transfusion, or birth of a severely affected baby, but not before 17–18 weeks gestation.[298] It seems that neither fetal death nor hydrops occurs before this gestation, presumably because the fetal reticuloendothelial system is too immature to destroy antibody-coated red cells. In patients without a previously affected pregnancy the ideal time for the first procedure is after the fetus has become anaemic but before the onset of hydrops. Earlier sampling increases the risk of further maternal antibody production due to a fetomaternal bleed. Therefore, FBS and IVT should be performed if the amniocentesis δ OD 450 nm is worsening, or if there is evidence of fetal hydrops.

The second transfusion is given within 2 weeks of the first because the rate of fall of haematocrit in each fetus is unpredictable.[309] This rate is on average 1% per day but with a range from 0.2% to 3%.[298] The subsequent intervals can be planned depending on the rate of fall in the first interval and the degree of suppression of fetal erythropoiesis, based on the Kleihauer–Betke test. Normally the subsequent transfusion is planned to prevent the development of hydrops by maintaining the fetal haematocrit above the critical level of one-third of the normal mean for gestational age.[310]

Indications

The conditions in which fetal transfusion may be required are red cell alloimmunisation (anti-D, c, Kell); perinatal alloimmune thrombocytopenia; suppression of fetal erythropoiesis (parvovirus); and acute fetomaternal haemorrhage.

Red cell alloimmunisation   The most common cause of severe fetal haemolytic disease is rhesus (Rh) anti-D antibodies developing in an Rh (D)-negative mother with a Rh (D)-positive fetus. Although the incidence of Rh alloimmunisation has been greatly reduced by the use of prophylactic Rh immunoglobulin, there are still 600–700 new Rh (D) immunisations per year in the UK.[311] The perinatal mortality for England and Wales due to Rh alloimmunisation is estimated at 5.0 per 100 000.[312] Once sensitisation has occurred and the fetus has developed severe anaemia and/or hydrops, the prolongation of life *in utero* is dependent on intra-uterine therapy until delivery is safe.

Although generally less serious than anti-D, anti-c antibodies can be associated with an anaemia severe enough to cause hydrops and the principles of management are similar to those in Rh (D) haemolytic disease. With anti-c confusion arises because this is and Rh antibody developing in a Rh D-positive woman. The incidence has been reported as 70 per 100 000 pregnant women.[313]

Anti-Kell antibodies also cause severe anaemia and hydropic changes in the fetus, with an estimated incidence of 10 per 100 000.[314] In this situation the percentage of reticulocytes and normoblasts in the fetal blood and the amniotic fluid bilirubin concentration are much lower for a given haemoglobin level than those associated with anti-D.[315] Anti-Kell antibody causes suppression of effective erythroblastosis in the fetus, rather than haemolysis (Fig. 24.27),[316] and therefore the conventional criteria for management of fetal alloimmunisation should not be applied. Management should focus on Kell genotyping of fetal DNA[317] when the father is heterozygous and monitoring the Kell-positive fetus for the development of anaemia by FBS and serial sonography.[316]

Perinatal alloimmune thrombocytopenia   Perinatal alloimmune thrombocytopenia mediated by PLA-1 antibody causes a high rate of morbidity and mortality through intracranial haemorrhage. The insult may occur during intrauterine life, and in mothers at risk intrauterine intravascular platelet transfusion may be used to prevent neonatal pathology.[209,318]

Suppression of fetal erythropoiesis   Parvovirus B19 infection during pregnancy causes fetal hydrops and subsequent pregnancy loss. Following serologically documented maternal infection 26% of fetuses developed hydrops, which may be subclinical.[319] Fetal infection seems to cause inhibition of erythrocyte precursors, leading to a severe aplastic crisis and subsequent hydrops.[320] Successful *in utero* therapy by serial intravascular blood transfusions has been reported in five cases, with normal neonatal outcome.[319,321]

Acute fetomaternal haemorrhage   Life-threatening fetal anaemia subsequent to massive fetomaternal haemorrhage is uncommon. Successful treatment by intra-uterine transfusion has been reported, suggesting that Kleihauer–Betke stains on maternal blood are useful in the investigation of non-immune hydrops and fetal compromise.[322,323] Intra-uterine death has also occurred following successful transfusion and suggests recurrent haemorrhage.[324]

Complications

At Queen Charlotte's Hospital, London, from 1986 to 1990, 99 fetuses underwent 324 transfusions. The fetal loss rate was 5.6% per transfusion, the greatest risk occurring during the first transfusion. An initial transfusion before 20 weeks carries a risk of fetal loss of 14%,

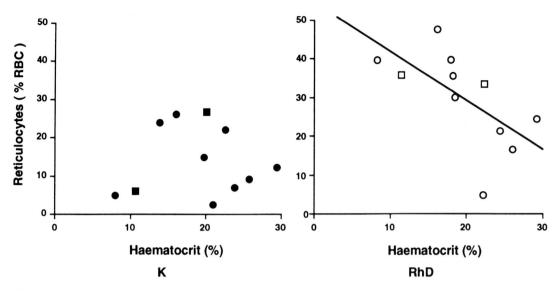

Fig. 24.27 Kell alloimmunisation. Relationship between reticulocytosis and haematocrit in Kell (filled symbols) and RhD (unfilled symbols) fetuses. □ hydropic fetuses, ○ non-hydropic fetuses. Regression line for RhD group (y = 53.2–1.2x) indicates progressive reticulocytosis in response to degree of anaemia. *RBC* – red blood cell (Reproduced from Vaughan *et al.*[315] with permission from Mosby Inc, St Louis, USA.)

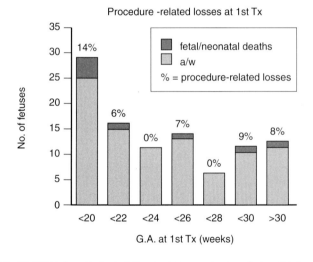

Fig. 24.28 Fetal survival rate following intravascular transfusion. Fetal survival rate (%) following first transfusion in relation to gestational age.

whereas after 30 weeks this falls to 8% (Fig. 24.28). The survival rate of non-hydropic and hydropic fetuses is the same, at 80%.

Chorio-amnionitis or ruptured membranes may result in spontaneous abortion or preterm labour. Fetomaternal haemorrhage complicates 50–75% of treated pregnancies, particularly after trans-placental passage of the needle,[209] and may further compromise this and future pregnancies.

Fetal shunting procedures

Fetal therapy was established with the development of successful *in utero* transfusion to treat life-threatening anaemia. Fetal anomalies exist which are in themselves not lethal but which result in neonatal death or severe impairment owing to the secondary effects of fluid accumulation in the fetus. The concept of chronic drainage of this fluid into the amniotic space gave rise to the use of fetal therapy based on diverting shunt placement. Obstructive uropathy, idiopathic pleural effusions, congenital cystic adenomatoid malformation and hydrocephalus are the conditions which have been considered for treatment with this particular therapy.

In 1982 a group of early investigators in this field met at a conference sponsored by the Kroc Foundation to discuss the management of the fetus with a potentially correctable congenital defect.[325] The resultant guidelines proposed that any fetus being considered for therapy must be a singleton less than 32 weeks, with a normal karyotype and without coexisting anomalies that might worsen the prognosis. Before considering therapy the condition must be accurately diagnosed and there should be evidence, particularly from experimental animal studies, that intervention can improve the outcome. The therapy should be provided by a multidisciplinary team and the patient must be prepared to return for follow-up.

An International Fetal Surgery Registry (IFSR) was established to record the results of fetal surgery and to report on the outcome of all known cases treated.[325] In 1985 a natural history registry was added so that treated and untreated cases could be compared. The last report was in 1993,[326] at which time 28 centres from nine countries had contributed 149 cases; 139 of those cases involved the treatment of either obstructive uropathy (98 cases) or hydrocephalus (41 cases). The number of cases of hydrocephalus contained in the IFSR had not changed from the previous publication in 1986,[266] a reflection of a voluntary moratorium placed on this type of intervention by the International Fetal Medicine and Surgery Society in 1988. This consensus decision was based on the collective evidence that, despite being technically feasible and associated with improved perinatal survival, therapy was associated with a high probability of severe long-term functional impairment.[326] Fetal surgery for hydrocephalus remains highly experimental and will not be discussed further in this chapter.

Obstructive uropathy

In 1982 Golbus *et al.* reported the placement of a suprapubic catheter in a 32-week fetus with lower urinary tract obstruction (LUTO).[327] In the period 1982–1993, 98 shunt placements were reported to the IFSR for treatment of fetal LUTO.[326] The aim of this therapy is primarily to prevent lethal pulmonary hypoplasia and secondarily to prevent renal dysplasia and preserve existing renal function.

Technique   Selection for intra-uterine therapy depends initially on an ultrasound diagnosis of urethral obstruction (see Ch. 16). A specific diagnosis of posterior urethral valves is suggested by determining male genitalia and visualising a dilated proximal urethra (Fig. 24.29). Further evaluation prior to shunt placement consists of three major components:

1. *Confirmation of an isolated bladder outlet obstruction.* Exclusion of associated structural abnormalities may be difficult in the presence of severe oligohydramnios, and intra-amniotic[269] or fetal intra-abdominal[270] fluid instillation, as described in

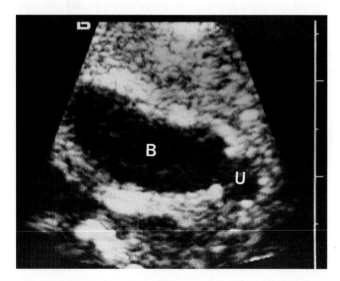

Fig. 24.29 Posterior urethral valves. Ultrasound scan of a 14-week fetus with posterior urethral valves, enlarged bladder (B) and dilated proximal urethra (U).

this chapter, is recommended to improve ultrasound visualisation of fetal anatomy.

2. *Confirmation of a normal male karyotype.* This is usually achieved by fetal blood sampling. The incidence of aneuploidy is increased in lower urinary tract obstructions. Of 98 cases reported to the IFSR seven (7%) were terminated after shunt placement because of an abnormal karyotype.[326] In addition, the karyotypically normal female fetus with a megacystis usually has complex cloacal abnormalities, with a poor prognosis despite shunting. Of the cases recorded by the IFSR the survival rate for males was 47% (39 of 83 continuing pregnancies), but only 17% for females (1 of 6 continuing pregnancies).[326]

3. *Confirmation of normal renal function.* This is accomplished by electrolyte assessment of fetal urine, as already described in this chapter.

Fetal shunt placement is an outpatient technique performed under aseptic conditions with prophylactic antibiotic cover. Local anaesthesia is usually sufficient, although sedation is sometimes required. Anti-D prophylaxis is administered as appropriate. Insertion of vesico-amniotic catheters is generally percutaneous and ultrasound guided. In cases of oligohydramnios catheter introduction is preceded by amnio-infusion to ensure that the fetal external abdominal wall is well visualised. A specially designed 3 mm diameter metal trocar and cannula (RM Surgical Developments) (Fig. 24.30) is then introduced through the maternal abdomen and uterus and directed into the fetal bladder through the anterior abdominal wall. Once the needle tip is seen inside the bladder the trocar is removed and the shunt loaded into the cannula; the technique is illustrated in Figure 24.31. Following successful shunt insertion the catheter is seen as a pair of bright lines within the fetal pelvis and the bladder cannot be identified ultrasonically, as it is continuously empty (Fig. 24.32). The distal end of the shunt is similarly seen protruding from the fetal anterior abdominal wall in the presence of amniotic fluid (Fig. 24.32). Reaccumulation of amniotic fluid is not a specific index of good renal function, it just indicates catheter patency.[264] Thus the concept of a 'diagnostic catheter' is not supported.

Different catheters have been used but the most popular is the Rocket (London, UK). This double-pigtail polyethylene catheter with holes in either end has its coils perpendicular to each other to enable it to lie flat against the fetal anterior wall and minimise the risk of removal by the fetus (Fig. 24.33).

Weekly follow-up is recommended to assess the volume of amniotic fluid, urinary tract dilatation and shunt location, as the catheter may become blocked or dislodged.

Shunt placement is ideally performed as soon as the diagnosis is certain. The mean age at diagnosis of obstructive uropathy reported to the IFSR was 23 weeks (range

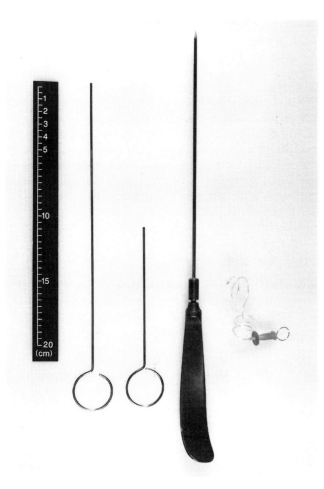

Fig. 24.30 Shunt insertion set (De Elles Instruments, Surrey, UK) showing the cannula and trocar with the short and long introducers.

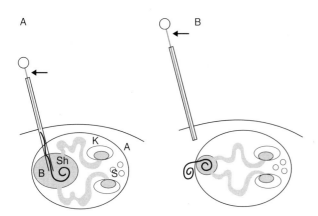

Fig. 24.31 Technique of bladder shunting. A: Cross-section of fetus in amniotic cavity (A), showing spine (S), kidneys (K) and dilated bladder (B). Insertion of proximal end of double-pigtail catheter (Sh) is performed with the short introducer (thin arrow). B: The shunt insertion is completed by withdrawing the cannula into the amniotic cavity and discharging the distal end of the catheter with the long introducer (thick arrow).

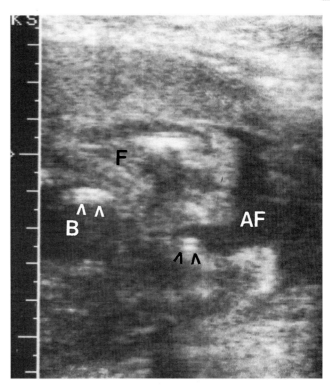

Fig. 24.32 Vesico-amniotic shunt *in situ*. Ultrasound scan of a 22-week fetus (F) with a vesico-amniotic shunt *in situ*. Proximal catheter (white arrow) within the fetal bladder (B), distal catheter (black arrow) in the amniotic cavity (AF).

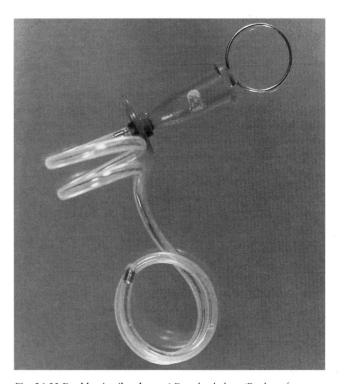

Fig. 24.33 Double-pigtail catheter. 6-Fr polyethylene (Rocket of London, UK) with two curves at right-angles to each other. A guide-wire is used to straighten the catheter for insertion into the cannula.

14–36 weeks), with shunt placement at 24 weeks (range 14–36 weeks).[326]

Experience seems to be important in the number of attempts required for shunt placement. The IFSR reported success at the first attempt in only 17% (17 of 98) of cases, with 10 centres reporting only one case.[236] Bernaschek *et al.*[328] reported a 92% (12 of 13) success at first attempt in the collaborative data from several experienced centres in Europe.

Indications   The underlying condition causing LUTO markedly influences the clinical outcome independent of treatment.[326] For this reason prenatal treatment is only recommended for the condition of posterior urethral valves, which has the potential for a good post-natal outcome. The major drawback is that despite improvements in patient evaluation by advanced ultrasound, karyotyping and sequential urine electrolyte analysis, it remains impossible to diagnose the specific anatomical lesion causing LUTO. Table 24.11 lists the final diagnosis in 55 comprehensively evaluated patients reported by Freedman *et al.* and illustrates the difficulty in selecting appropriate candidates for prenatal therapy.[265] Vesico-amniotic shunting therefore remains controversial.

More recently, Quintero *et al.* have performed percutaneous cystoscopy in a 19-week fetus to confirm the suspected diagnosis of posterior urethral valves. At 22 weeks gestation percutaneous endoscopic fulguration of the valves enabled definitive treatment.[329]

Complications   Percutaneous vesico-amniotic shunt catheter placement has definite risks for both mother and fetus. The procedure-related perinatal loss rate estimated from the IFSR is 5.1% (5 of 98). Four deaths were thought to be related to direct fetal trauma and one following premature labour within 48 hours of shunt placement.[326] Bernaschek *et al.*[328] published an 8% loss rate (1 of 13) following premature labour within 48 hours of shunt placement. Johnson *et al.*[257] reported no procedure-related losses in their series of 15 vesico-amniotic shunts.

Fetal trauma may occur, as trocar insertion into the fetal abdomen may damage the viscera. Gastroschisis has been reported following herniation of the fetal bowel through the iatrogenic abdominal wall defect.[329] Fetal, umbilical or placental haemorrhage may also occur.[262]

Catheter dislodgment is a relatively common complication, with Bernaschek *et al.*[237] reporting a rate of 39% (5 of 13) and Johnson *et al.*[257] 60% (9 of 15). Displacement may be into the fetal abdomen, resulting in vesicoperitoneal urine leakage, or out of the bladder, or out of the fetus altogether. Catheter replacement is the usual remedy.

Obstetric complications include premature rupture of the membranes, preterm delivery and intra-uterine infection.[326]

Fetal pleural effusions

Idiopathic pleural effusions *in utero* are termed primary fetal hydrothorax (PFHT). They may be clinically benign but 50% will cause fetal or neonatal death, usually secondary to pulmonary hypoplasia with or without associated hydrops.[330] Because pleural fluid reaccumulates rapidly after prenatal aspiration, long-term drainage is necessary to prevent pulmonary hypoplasia and reverse hydrops and polyhydramnios, until the fetus is a safe gestational age to be delivered.[331] The insertion of the first pleuro-amniotic shunt was reported by Seeds and Bowes in 1986.[332]

Technique   Pathognomonic in the antenatal diagnosis of fetal pleural effusions is the ultrasonic demonstration of an echo-free space between the lung, chest wall and diaphragm. In large effusions the fetal lung appears highly reflective, with the configuration of a butterfly wing (Fig. 24.34). Polyhydramnios is common. Ultrasonic detection of mediastinal shift and/or subcutaneous oedema indicates progressive pathology. Evaluation prior to pleuro-amniotic shunt placement involves several stages:

1. *Confirmation of an isolated pleural effusion.* Structural malformations associated with pleural effusions include diaphragmatic hernia, extralobar sequestration of lung, mediastinal tumours and cardiac anomalies.[331] Diagnostic thoracocentesis may unmask pathology after decompression has restored normal anatomical relationships. Genetic syndromes and non-immune hydrops may also be associated with pleural effusions. Detailed ultrasound investigation is the key to successful aetiological diagnosis.
2. *Confirmation of a normal karyotype.* Fetal pleural effusions may be associated with aneuploidy, in particular Down's and Turner's syndromes.[333]
3. *Maternal investigations.* Exclusion of maternal infection, haemoglobinopathy and fetomaternal haemorrhage should be considered.[331]

Table 24.11 Aetiology of prenatal lower urinary tract obstruction[265]

Diagnosis	%
Posterior urethral valves	24
Urethral atresia	20
Prune-belly syndrome	16
Cloacal dysgenesis	7
Primary megacystis	4
Megacystis microcolon hypoperistalsis syndrome	2
Resolved post-vesicocentesis	4
Obstructing ureterocele	2
Bilateral reflux	2
Autopsy refused	10
Unknown/lost to follow-up	9
Total	100

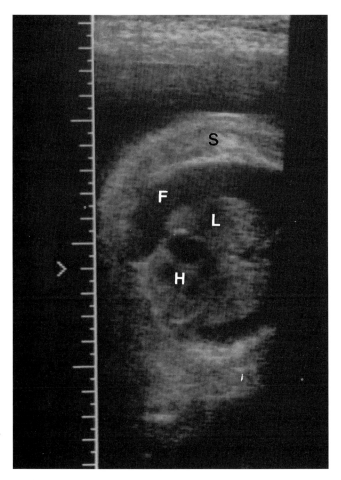

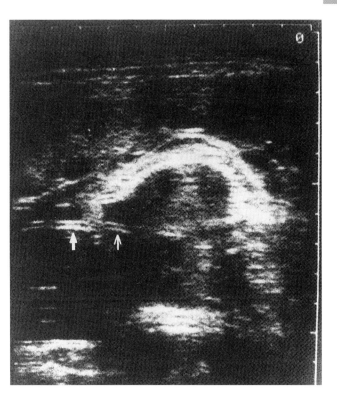

Fig. 24.35 Pleuro-amniotic shunt *in situ*. Ultrasound of a 32-week fetus with a pleuro-amniotic shunt *in situ* showing the intrapleural (thin arrow) and extrapleural (thick arrow) portions. The effusions have drained and the lungs re-expanded. (Reproduced from Rodeck *et al.*[334] with permission from Massachusetts Medical Society.)

Fig. 24.34 Fetal hydrothorax. Ultrasound scan of fetal hydrothorax. F – fluid, L – lung, H – heart, S – subcutaneous oedema.

Preparation and instrumentation are discussed under obstructive uropathy, above. In cases of extreme polyhydramnios the prior removal of amniotic fluid will improve visualisation and facilitate shunt insertion by decreasing the distance traversed.[334] With the fetal thorax in a transverse orientation, the trocar and cannula (Fig. 24.30) are introduced under ultrasound visualisation transabdominally into the amniotic cavity, through the mid-thoracic wall and into the effusion. The trocar is removed and the catheter inserted into the cannula. The proximal end is positioned in the pleural cavity with the short introducer and the distal end in the amniotic space with the long introducer. For bilateral effusions two catheters are inserted. Once inserted, the catheter is seen as a pair of lines extending from the thorax to the pleural space, with the effusion drained, the lung re-expanded and appropriate mediastinal relationships restored (Fig. 24.35).

Weekly ultrasound surveillance is important to assess reaccumulation of the pleural fluid, as catheters may become blocked or dislodged. The resolution or progression of hydrops should also be monitored.

Indications PFHT is the main indication for pleuro-amniotic shunting but is a diagnosis of exclusion. The natural history of isolated pleural effusions suggests spontaneous resolution in 10%, with 100% survival.[331] In the absence of resolution the perinatal mortality varies from 47% in non-hydropic to 62% in hydropic fetuses.[330,331] In a published meta-analysis three significant factors related to poor outcome: delivery at 31 weeks gestation or less; the presence of hydrops and no antenatal therapy. The highest predicted probability of perinatal loss (97%) occurred when all three risk factors were present and the lowest probability when none was present (6%). The chance of loss ranged from 30 to 36% when one risk factor was present to 77–81% when two risk factors were present.[335]

Complications Shunt blockage or dislodgment occurs in about 8% of cases.[333] Preterm labour is not uncommon in these women, as the majority have clinical polyhydramnios. Drainage of amniotic fluid into the maternal peritoneal cavity causing ascites, followed by resolution, has been reported.[336] Other complications have rarely been reported, but potentially include preterm rupture of membranes, infection, fetal or maternal bleeding from punctured vessels, and fetal trauma. Anti-D immunoglobulin should be given appropriately.

Reduction amniocentesis

Polyhydramnios is defined ultrasonically as a deepest vertical pool more than 8 cm in depth; it occurs with an incidence of 0.2–1.6% of all pregnancies[337] and is associated with an increase in perinatal mortality which relates to both the pathology of the underlying condition and the prevalence of prematurity secondary to preterm labour.[338] Fisk *et al.* reported an association between preterm labour and increased intra-amniotic pressure, particularly with vertical pool measurements greater than or equal to 15 cm (Fig. 24.36).[339] The removal of small amounts of fluid rapidly restores the amniotic pressure. Thus, reduction amniocentesis allows normalisation of amniotic pressure with the aim of prolonging the pregnancy to a safer gestation for delivery. The use of maternal prostaglandin synthase inhibitor therapy to treat polyhydramnios is also successful, but may lead to premature closure of the ductus arteriosus or fetal renal or cerebral complications.[340,341]

Technique

When polyhydramnios is diagnosed a detailed ultrasound is necessary to detect structural fetal or placental malformations that may be causative, or complications occurring in multiple pregnancy. Maternal investigations should exclude diabetes mellitus or red blood cell alloimmunisation.

Following aseptic precautions, prophylactic antibiotics and possibly tocolysis, an 18–20 gauge needle is inserted into the polyhydramniotic sac under ultrasound control to avoid the placenta. Fluid is withdrawn until the deepest pool is less than 8 cm. This may vary from 500 ml to

many litres. The optimum speed of removal is not yet determined, but 'rapid removal' has been reported without complication.[342] Reducing needle movement and manipulation by attaching tubing, stopcocks or surgical suction equipment may be beneficial.

Weekly follow-up is essential to assess fetal well-being and liquor volume, as reaccumulation of fluid is common.

Indications

Reduction amniocentesis is indicated in pregnancies complicated by polyhydramnios (>15 cm pool), in which prolongation of gestation may benefit fetal outcome. This arises in congenital malformations requiring post-natal corrective surgery, twin–twin transfusion syndrome (TTTS) and, occasionally, idiopathic polyhydramnios. The perinatal mortality of TTTS approaches 100% in cases managed conservatively,[343] whereas aggressive serial reduction amniocentesis is associated with an overall perinatal survival of 65% from the uncontrolled published series.[342–345] A major concern of reduction amniocentesis in TTTS is that delayed delivery may increase survival at the expense of high perinatal morbidity, including cerebral,[345] cardiac[346] and renal sequelae.

Complications

Preterm rupture of membranes and preterm labour are complications, but with no intervention a similar outcome is inevitable. A recent review of 200 'large-volume' reduction amniocenteses in singleton and twin pregnancies showed a low 1.5% complication rate, with the only case of placental abruption being after the removal of 10 litres of fluid at term in an anencephalic.[347]

Multifetal pregnancy reduction

The widespread use of assisted reproduction technologies has resulted in a doubling of twin and a 10-fold increase in higher multiple births over the last 15 years.[348] Multifetal pregnancy reduction (MFPR) is the term used for the treatment that has emerged solely to reduce fetal numbers, with the aim of decreasing very early preterm labour in the resultant pregnancies.[349–351] Several collaborative reports have been published from data that have been collected internationally since 1988.[351–353] The original method of trans-cervical (TC) suction aspiration under ultrasound control[354] has been superseded by needle-guided techniques because of loss rates as high as 50%.[348]

Technique

Non-directional preprocedure counselling provides detailed information regarding the risks and benefits of MFPR. A preliminary ultrasound should evaluate the fetal

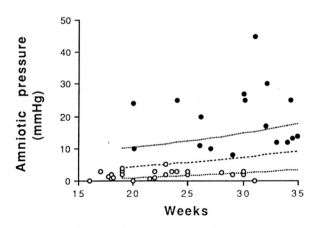

Fig. 24.36 Amniotic pressure. Pregnancies complicated by polyhydramnios (●) or oligohydramnios (○) shown against the normal range for gestation: mean and 95% data intervals. (Reproduced from Fisk *et al.*[339] with permission from Elsevier Science Inc.)

number, viability, relative size and location, chorionicity (see Ch. 12) and procedural accessibility. In addition, nuchal thickness and early fetal anatomy should be assessed for normality (see Chs 7 and 8). Prophylactic antibiotics, aseptic technique and anti-D prophylaxis are recommended.

The two major approaches to MFPR include:

1. Transabdominal (TA) MFPR This is the most common approach and relies on the ultrasound-guided placement of a 20–22-gauge spinal needle above the diaphragm of the fetus to be terminated. Potassium chloride (KCl) is then injected into the thorax or heart. The amount necessary to achieve cardiac asystole is gestational age dependent and ranges from 0.5 ml at 9 weeks to 3 ml at 12 weeks gestation.[348] Asystole should be observed for at least 3 minutes before withdrawing the needle.[349] This procedure is repeated for each fetus to be terminated. The selection of the fetus(es) to terminate is a technical decision based on accessibility, unless there are overriding medical factors, such as significant fetal size discrepancy or malformations evident. Ideally, the fetus in the sac over the internal os is not terminated, as devitalisation of tissue near the cervix may increase the risk of infection and fetal loss.

2. Trans-vaginal (TV) MFPR This ultrasound-guided approach may be adopted for intrathoracic KCl,[355] or for fetal aspiration at 6–7 weeks gestation or mechanical disruption.[348] The fetus in the sac over the os is commonly terminated, with no reported increase in loss rate.[355]

In experienced hands the technical success of these procedures is 100%.[353] The multicentre collaborative study comparing the outcome of 846 TA with 238 TC/TV MFPR procedures revealed that the starting and finishing fetal numbers were higher in the TA group, with only 4.4% of pregnancies reduced to a singleton compared with 12.6% in TC/TV.[353]

Following MFPR serial ultrasound is advisable to monitor fetal growth and development throughout the pregnancy.

The data from the 1993 collaborative report indicate that the optimum gestational age for TA MFPR is between 8 and 12 weeks, with an increase in both fetal losses and very premature delivery if performed at 13 weeks or later.[352] This may relate to the increased remaining tissue mass.

In 1994 the international multicentre collaborative report comparing TA with TC/TV MFPR found a significant difference in timing. The average gestational age for TA was 11.3 weeks (±1.9), compared to 9.2 weeks (±1.8) for TV/TC MFPR. For both techniques the premature delivery rates between 25 and 28 weeks were comparable, at about 5%, as were the loss rate before 24 weeks at 13.1% for TC/TV and 12.5% for TAMFPR.[353]

Decreased loss rates with increased experience indicated a significant learning curve for TA MFPR. The loss rate fell from 16.2% to 8.8% when the TA data from 1988 to 1991 were compared with those from the next two years at the same institutions.[352,353] The most recent report supports a plateauing of risks.[351] There were too few TC/TV cases to assess the learning curve for that approach.

Indications

The prime indication for MFPR is to prevent the very early preterm labour, and its consequent perinatal mortality and morbidity, associated with higher-order multiple pregnancy. This goal has been attained, as the rate of delivery between 25 and 28 weeks gestation following MFPR is 4.5%, which is much lower than in unreduced multiples.[348]

Evidence also supports the reduction of triplets to twins. The rate of delivery has 24 and 32 weeks is 8.2%, compared to 24% in unreduced triplets.[356] Similarly, the mean gestational age at delivery was significantly increased from 31.2 weeks in triplets to 35.6 weeks in triplets reduced to twins.[357] The resultant perinatal mortality rate was 30 per 1000 births in the reduction group and 210 per 1000 births in the non-reduced triplets (p<0.0001).[357] These advantages of triplet reduction to twins are achieved at the expense of higher loss rates up to 24 weeks gestation compared to unreduced triplets, 7.6% vs 2.6%, respectively.[356]

Reduction of triplets and higher-order multiples is ethically acceptable as it reduces the risk of perinatal mortality and morbidity. Although MFPR is not usually justified for reducing twins to a singleton, the recent use of donor oocytes in older women may require more liberal ethical consideration in the future.[348] Also, it is important to appreciate that at present most cases of multiple pregnancy are iatrogenic, and MFPR should be regarded as a provisional approach 'until improved fertility treatment obviates its use'.[348]

Complications

Maternal complications are rare. Disseminated intravascular coagulation has not been reported in over a decade of MFPR.[348] Routine monitoring of maternal coagulation status is therefore not required.

In experienced centres there should be no failed procedures. The overall fetal loss rate up to 24 weeks gestation is 11.7%, which is substantially better than in untreated cases of multifetal pregnancies.[351] There are strong and independent correlations between the starting number (Fig. 24.37) and the finishing number of fetuses with subsequent loss.[351] Reducing to twins has the lowest loss rate irrespective of starting number. Cases reduced to a singleton have a slightly higher loss rate and triplets even higher.

Very early premature delivery between 25 and 28 weeks is also a complication of MFPR. Again, an increased rate

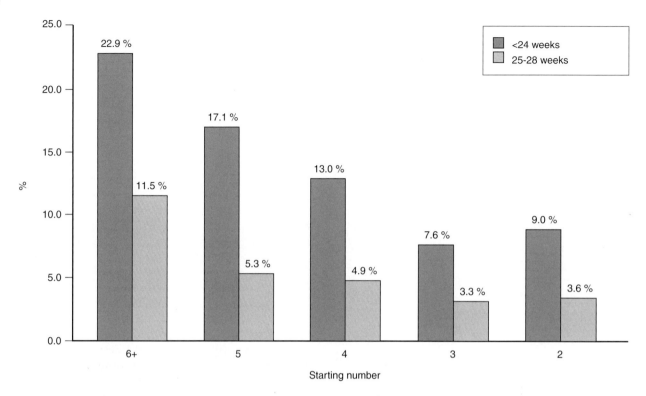

Fig. 24.37 Multifetal pregnancy reduction. Histogram showing the highest rate of pregnancy losses (24 weeks or less) and severe prematurity (25–28 weeks as a function of higher starting numbers. *n* = 1789 (Reproduced from Evans *et al.* with permission from Elsevier Science Inc.)

correlates with the starting (Fig. 24.37) and finishing number of fetuses per pregnancy.[351]

The risk of congenital malformation is unchanged by MFPR. Prenatal diagnosis should be considered as usual. There is no higher risk of pregnancy loss following amniocentesis in MFPR patients.[358] In general, Evans *et al.*[348] prefer to perform MFPR at 10 weeks, followed by CVS at 12 weeks.

Fetal growth following MFPR indicates significantly higher rates of growth restriction, which correlates with increasing starting number.[359]

Selective fetocide

Selective fetocide is the procedure used to terminate the anomalous fetus within a multiple pregnancy. The ethics are complex, but as the intention is to promote the birth of the normal child, ethical approval should be justified as long as it is performed prior to the legal limit for termination and for medical, not social, indications.[360] The first report in 1978 described an induced death *in utero* following cardiac puncture of a twin with Hurler's syndrome at 24 weeks, and successful delivery of the unaffected twin at 33 weeks gestation.[361] In 1994, international collaborative experience showed that in dichorionic twin pregnancies intracardiac injection of potassium chloride (KCl) is the optimal technique, compared to air embolism or

exsanguination.[362] However, this method is unsuitable for monochorionic twins. Occlusion of the circulation of the anomalous monochorial twin is required to avoid the demise of the healthy fetus as well.[363]

Technique

Before the procedure ultrasound is used to identify the abnormal fetus. This is not difficult where the fetuses are of different sexes, or where there is a structural abnormality, but many chromosomal or genetic conditions will rely upon the orientation of the fetal sacs within the uterus. This must be accurately documented at the initial diagnosis, otherwise the correct fetus must be confirmed by repeat invasive testing. Obviously, fetal viability, gestational age and detailed anatomical assessment of the remaining fetus(es) are an integral part of the preprocedural work-up.

Accurate determination of chorionicity is essential as this dictates the availability, method and safety of the selective fetocide procedure. In the first trimester using established criteria (see Ch. 12), ultrasound has a positive predictive value of 100% for dichorionic placentation and 95% for monochorionic placentation.[364] Ultrasound is less accurate in the second trimester. If any uncertainty exists, rapid genetic determination of zygosity by polymerase chain reaction analysis of DNA from amniotic fluid samples is 99.6% accurate.[365]

Dichorionic placentation Maternal preparation is similar to that for multifetal pregnancy reduction (see above). A site on the maternal abdomen is chosen to access the fetal heart or umbilical vein. With ultrasound visualisation a 20–22-gauge needle is inserted and KCl injected. The recommended concentration is 2 mEq/ml,[366] and on average 2 ml is needed for fetuses less than 16 weeks and between 3 and 5 ml at 17 weeks gestation or more.[362] The needle should be left in place until sustained asystole is observed for at least 3 minutes.[367] In all cases of genetic or chromosomal abnormality an amniotic fluid or fetal blood sample should be sent for confirmation that the correct fetus has been terminated. In experienced centres the procedure is 100% successful.[362]

Monochorionic placentation Maternal preparation is standard. Selective fetocide by intracardiac injection of KCl in three monochorial twin pairs in the international collaborative experience resulted in death of the normal fetus within several days of the procedure.[362] This approach has since been abandoned in monochorial twins, because of the acute damage caused to the normal co-twin *via* placental vascular anastomoses. More recently, successful approaches have aimed at vascular occlusion to prevent the normal twin exsanguinating into the terminated twin's circulation. These include the following experimental techniques:

1. Combined intravenous and intracardiac injection of 2 ml of histoacryl via a 20-gauge spinal needle inserted under ultrasound control;[368]
2. Injection of 1 ml 100% alcohol into the intrahepatic portion of the umbilical vein via a 20-gauge needle inserted under ultrasound control.[369] Simultaneous occlusion of both umbilical artery and vein is optimal to separate the two circulations completely;
3. Percutaneous umbilical cord ligation, performed either fetoscopically[370,371] or ultrasonically,[372] has been successful. Unfortunately, at present these procedures usually require more than one abdominal puncture, with a consequent 30% rate of preterm amniorrhexis;[370]
4. Percutaneous fetoscopic umbilical cord laser coagulation may be performed through one abdominal port with an 18-gauge spinal needle. This has been reported successful as early as 16 weeks gestation in an acardiac gestation, with delivery at 41 weeks of a normal co-twin.[373]

Following all these procedures fetal heart motion should be noted in the remaining fetus(es) immediately. After one hour another ultrasound assessment should confirm the demise of the terminated fetus and normal activity in the other(s). Serial ultrasound is recommended to monitor the growth of the remaining twin and resorption of the terminated one.

Second-trimester fetocide must be performed within the legal limits for fetal termination. The international collab-orative group reported a 5.4% miscarriage rate if selective fetocide was performed at or before 16 weeks, but a 14.4% rate if done thereafter.[362]

In 1994, collaborative experience of 183 cases of selective fetocide from nine groups internationally indicated an overall miscarriage rate of 12.6% before 24 weeks.[362] In 1997, Berkowitz *et al.* reported 100 cases from their very experienced group, indicating a 4% total loss rate prior to 24 weeks.[367]

Indications

As described above, selective fetocide has only been routinely indicated in dichorionic placentation, but with improvements in the safety of feto-endoscopic procedures this may change in the near future. Selective fetocide offers the option of delivery of a normal infant without the birth of the affected one, and for some parents avoids the dilemma of terminating the entire pregnancy. The indications for the 183 cases reported from the collaborative experience included 96 (52%) chromosomal, 76 (42%) structural and 11 (6%) genetic disorders.[262]

One of the continuing dilemmas of selective fetocide is its role in the pregnancy discordant for a lethal abnormality. Berkowitz *et al.*[367] stated that there is little justification for the procedure if the abnormal fetus is likely to die *in utero* or shortly after birth, as selective termination may cause the entire pregnancy to miscarry. Their series does include three cases of anencephaly, one of acrania and one thanatophoric dwarf, because the increased risk of poly-hydramnios could lead to preterm labour, which might jeopardise the normal twin. Evans *et al.*[362] believe that the risks of polyhydramnios and preterm labour in abnormal twin pregnancy are higher than the risks of the procedure, and therefore support selective fetocide for lethal conditions. One report addresses the management of twin pregnancies discordant for anencephaly.[374] Of 13 dichorionic twin pregnancies, five underwent selective fetocide at 17–21 weeks. One pregnancy aborted and the rest delivered at a median gestation of 37 weeks. Of the eight managed expectantly, three developed polyhydramnios at 30 weeks. However, all the normal co-twins survived at a median gestation of 35 weeks.

Complications

Maternal No maternal morbidity was reported from the international collaborative experience in 1994.[362] In particular, there were no clinically evident or laboratory-detected coagulopathies. In the 100 cases of selective fetocide reported by Berkowitz *et al.*, three women developed laboratory evidence of coagulopathy but there were no cases of clinically evident disseminated intravascular co-agulation.[367] Fetomaternal haemorrhage does occur, and so anti-D immunoglobulin must be given where appropriate.

Fetal No failed procedures have been reported for dichorionic twins.[362,367] Techniques for selective fetocide in monochorial twins are evolving but there is no recommended procedure available yet.

In dichorial pregnancies fetal loss rates up to 24 weeks vary between 4 and 13%.[362,367] Losses are higher if the procedure is carried out after 16 weeks' gestation.[362] Preterm labour is another complication. Gestational age at delivery is inversely correlated with gestation at the time of the procedure.[362] Fifty-nine percent of procedures performed at or before 20 weeks will result in a term delivery, compared to only 34% in procedures performed after 20 weeks.[362] Lynch *et al.* reported the lowest rates of premature preterm rupture of the membranes, preterm labour and preterm delivery if the selective fetocide was performed in the non-presenting twin before 20 weeks gestation. However, they still offer selective fetocide if the anomalous fetus is discovered after 20 weeks and is in the sac overriding the cervix.[375]

Before performing selective fetocide correct identification of the anomalous fetus is essential. In the international collaborative experience the wrong fetus was terminated in a pregnancy discordant for trisomy 21.[362]

Therapeutic fetoscopy

Although life-saving for a small number of fetal conditions, *in utero* surgery is limited by postoperative premature labour and its extreme invasiveness. More recently, keyhole access to the amniotic cavity has enabled endoscopic fetal surgery ('fetendo').[376] This technique is still in its infancy, with animal models being explored experimentally and limited human experience.[377] However, it does offer new hope for surgical fetal therapy.

Technique

Ultrasound enables the diagnosis of fetal conditions amenable to therapeutic fetoscopy. Preprocedure, the appropriate site of entry on the maternal abdomen is chosen to avoid injury to the placenta and to access the operative field. A percutaneous or laparotomy approach may be used. Standard aseptic preparation is used. Tocolytic therapy and intravenous antibiotics are given, as well as maternal and fetal anaesthesia as appropriate. Under continuous ultrasound surveillance the endoscope is directed into the amniotic cavity. Fibre-optic endoscopes as small as 0.5–2 mm with a resolution of up to 30 000 pixels are available.[377] Continuous irrigation is used to optimise visibility and the fetus is monitored by transabdominal ultrasound. A sideport enables the passage of a laser fibre or other instrumentation. The neodymium–yttrium–aluminium–garnet (Nd: YAG) laser is used as it functions through a fluid medium and is an efficient coagulator. Up to five trocars have been used for fetal procedures, with

each uterine puncture site requiring closure with absorbable sutures plus or minus fibrin glue.[378] The exact operative details vary depending on the indication, but most commonly include procedures on the placenta, cord and membranes (laser coagulation (Fig. 24.38),[373,377,379,380] vessel ligation,[370–372,377] lysis of amniotic bands[381]) and on the fetus (tracheal obstruction,[382] laser ablation or coagulation[328,383–385] or grafting.[386])

Indications

Most human operative fetoscopy experience has been gained with laser coagulation of chorionic plate vessels[379,380] and cord ligation[370–372] for fetofetal transfusion syndromes in monochorionic twins.[377] However, cases have been published on the successful use of endoscopy to treat fetuses for typical indications for *in utero* surgery. Indications are evolving but currently include twin–twin transfusion syndrome; acardiac twin pregnancy; selective fetocide in monochorionic twin pregnancy discordant for anomaly; chorioangioma; amniotic bands; congenital diaphragmatic hernia; posterior urethral valves; congenital cystic adenomatoid malformation of the lung; sacrococcygeal teratoma and myelomeningocele.

Twin–twin transfusion syndrome Monochorionic twin pregnancies presenting in the second trimester with severe twin–twin transfusion syndrome have a high risk of perinatal loss and neurological sequelae in survivors. Amniodrainage may improve survival but is associated with serious handicap in 15–50% of survivors.[387] Fetoscopy with Nd: YAG laser coagulation to separate the placental vascular communications was first described in 1990 by De Lia *et al.* (Fig. 24.38). Fetal survival following this procedure is consistently 55%, with a 5% risk of neurological injury in survivors.[377,380]

Acardiac twin pregnancy These pregnancies have a 50% mortality of the normal twin, either from high-output cardiac failure or as a consequence of prematurity from polyhydramnios.[388] Disruption of perfusion from the normal twin to the acardiac may be achieved by cord obliteration. Fetoscopic cord coagulation is possible but above 21 weeks fails as the cord becomes too large.[389] Fetoscopic cord ligation is the most effective interruption to flow but has a considerable risk of preterm premature rupture of the membranes if more than one port is used to access the amniotic cavity.[377]

Selective fetocide in monochorionic twin pregnancy (see Selective fetocide above)

Chorioangioma Fetal loss rates of 40% may occur with large chorio-angiomas. Ablation of the vascular supply to the tumour has been reported using operative

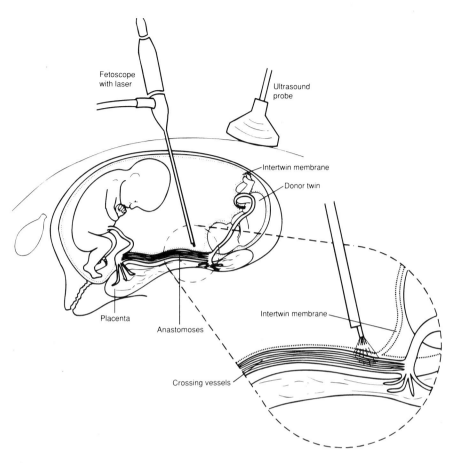

Fig. 24.38 Twin–twin transfusion syndrome. Diagram of the spatial organisation for endoscopic laser coagulation. (Reproduced from Ville *et al.* with permission from Blackwell Science Ltd, Oxford, UK.)

fetoscopy with suture ligation of the arterial supply following subchorionic dissection.[390]

Amniotic bands Lysis of amniotic bands causing isolated limb constriction may avoid spontaneous amputation. Quintero *et al.* have achieved success using two surgical ports into the amniotic cavity to allow the use of scissors under endoscopic guidance.[381]

Congenital diaphragmatic hernia Fetal tracheal occlusion accelerates lung growth and corrects the often fatal pulmonary hypoplasia that complicates congenital diaphragmatic hernia.[382] Successful fetoscopic clipping of the trachea has been reported, with survival in four of the six cases.[391]

Posterior urethral valves The first endoscopic vesicostomy was performed at 17 weeks using fetoscopy and Nd: YAG laser.[383] *In utero* diagnosis of posterior urethral valves is difficult with ultrasound alone (Table 24.11). More recently, Quintero *et al.* have performed *in utero* fetal diagnostic cystoscopy with therapeutic laser ablation of posterior urethral valves.[328]

Congenital cystic adenomatoid malformation of the lung (CCAM) *In utero* fetoscopic Nd: YAG laser coagulation to disrupt the CCAM tumour mass in a hydropic fetus has been successful.[384]

Sacrococcygeal teratoma Laser coagulation of the tumour vasculature has been reported to reduce the effects of the vascular steal that causes hydrops in this condition.[385]

Myelomeningocele Fetoscopic covering of a myelomeningocele by glueing a maternal split skin graft at 23 weeks has been reported in four cases, with 50% success.[386]

Complications

Maternal complications include placental abruption,[385] severe placental haemorrhage[380] and pain following amniotic fluid leakage into the peritoneal cavity.[380] Fetal complications include failure of the procedure,[370] preterm premature rupture of the membranes in up to 47% of cord ligations or fetal procedures,[377] chorio-amnionitis and preterm labour. There is a 25% immediate postoperative fetal loss (mostly donor) following laser coagulation of the placental circulation.[380] The efficacy of fetal surgical intervention requires objective evaluation.

Conclusions

With the advent of high-resolution ultrasound invasive intra-uterine procedures have become readily available. These relatively low-risk techniques allow extensive investigation and occasionally treatment of the fetus. In a society that is continually demanding improvements in perinatal outcome, these procedures will enable further understanding of fetal physiology and pathology. Specialised training is needed to acquire the necessary skills; however, it is the responsibility of every obstetrician to be aware of the scope of prenatal diagnosis and therapy, so that patients can benefit from appropriate referral.

REFERENCES

1 Prochownick L. Beitrage zur leptre vom fruchtwasser und seiner entsehung. Arch Gynäkol 1877; 11: 304–345

2 Henkel M. Akutes hydramnion, leberkompression, enges becken. Punktion des hydramnion. Zentralbl Gynäkol 1919; 43: 841

3 Bevis D C A. The antenatal prediction of haemolytic disease of the newborn. Lancet 1952; i: 395–398

4 Riis P, Fuchs F. Antenatal determination of foetal sex in prevention of hereditary diseases. Lancet 1960; ii: 180–182

5 Jeffcoate T N A, Fliegner J R N, Russel S N, Davis J C, Wade A P. Diagnosis of adrenogenital syndrome before birth. Lancet 1965; ii: 553–555

6 Steele M W, Breg W T. Chromosome analysis of human amniotic fluid cells. Lancet 1966; i: 383–385

7 Brock D J H, Scrimgeour J B. Early prenatal diagnosis of anencephaly. Lancet 1972; ii: 1252

8 Brock D J H, Sutcliffe R G. AFP in the antenatal diagnosis of anencephaly and spina bifida. Lancet 1972; ii: 197–199

9 Lowther G W, Whittle M J, Prenatal diagnosis in the UK - an overview. Eur J Hum Genet 1997; 5: 84–89

10 Ch de Crespigny L, Robinson H P. Amniocentesis: a comparison of 'monitored' versus 'blind' needle insertion technique. Aust NZ J Obstet Gynaecol 1986; 26: 124–128

11 Romero R, Jeanty P, Reece A E et al. Sonographically monitored amniocentesis to decrease intraoperative complications. Obstet Gynecol 1985; 65: 426–430

12 Canadian Medical Research Council. Diagnosis of genetic disease by amniocentesis during the second trimester of pregnancy. A Canadian study. Report No.5 Supply Services, Canada, 1977

13 Tabor A, Philip J, Marsen M, Bang J, Obel E B, Norgaard-Pedersen B. Randomized controlled trial of genetic amniocentesis in 4606 low-risk women. Lancet 1986; i: 1287–1292

14 Giorlandino C, Mobili L, Bilancioni E et al. Transplacental amniocentesis: is it really a higher risk procedure? Prenat Diagn 1994; 14: 803–806

15 Medical Research Council. An assessment of the hazards of amniocentesis. Br J Obstet Gynaecol 1978; 85(Suppl 2): 1–41

16 Verjaal M, Leschot N J. Risk of amniocentesis and laboratory findings in a series of 1500 prenatal diagnoses. Prenat Diagn 1981; 1: 173–181

17 Snijders R J M, Holzgreve W, Cuckle H, Nicolaides K H. Maternal age specific risks for trisomies at 9–14 weeks' gestation. Prenat Diagn 1994; 543–552

18 Halliday J L, Watson L F, Lumley J, Danks D M, Sheffield L J. New estimates of Down syndrome risks at chorionic villus sampling, amniocentesis and livebirth in women of advanced maternal age from uniquely defined population. Prenat Diagn 1995; 15: 455–465

19 Bray I C, Wright D E. Estimating the spontaneous loss of Down syndrome fetuses between the times of chorionic villus sampling, amniocentesis and livebirth. Prenat Diagn 1998; 18: 1045–1054

20 Worton R G, Stern R. A Canadian collaborative study of mosaicism in amniotic fluid cell cultures. Prenat Diagn 1987; 4: 131–144

21 Bui T H, Iselius L, Lindsten J. European collaborative study on prenatal diagnosis: mosaicism, pseudomosaicism and single abnormal cells in amniotic fluid cell cultures. Prenat Diagn 1984; 4: 145–162

22 Hsu L Y F, Perlis T E. United States survey on chromosome mosaicism and pseudomosaicism in prenatal diagnosis. Prenat Diagn 1984; 4: 97–130

23 Gosden C, Nicolaides K H, Rodeck C H. Fetal blood sampling in investigation of chromosome mosaicism in amniotic fluid cell culture. Lancet 1988; i: 613–616

24 Benn P A, Hsu L Y F. Maternal cell contamination of amniotic fluid cell cultures. Results of a US nation wide survey. Am J Med Genet 1983; 14: 361–365

25 Lam Y H, Tang M H Y, Sin S Y, Ghosh A. Clinical significance of amniotic fluid cell culture failure. Prenat Diagn 1998; 18: 343–347

26 Persutte W H, Lenke R P. Failure of amniotic fluid cell growth: is it related to fetal aneuploidy? Lancet 1995; 345: 96–97

27 Reid R, Sepulveda W, Kyle P M, Davies G. Amniotic fluid culture failure: clinical significance and association with aneuploidy. Obstet Gynecol 1996; 87: 588–592

28 Lawce H. A report from: FISH 98 – new technologies and clinical applications. The Third International Clinical FISH Symposium Colorado 1998. J Assoc Genet Technol 1998; 24: 96

29 Eiben B, Trawicki W, Hammans W, Goebel R, Epplen J T. A prospective comparative study on fluorescence in situ hybridisation (FISH) of uncultured amniocytes and standard karyotype analysis. Prenat Diagn 1998; 18: 901–906

30 Bryndorf T, Christensen B, Vad M, Parner J, Brocks V, Philip J. Prenatal detection of chromosome aneuploidies by fluorescence in situ hybridisation: experience with 2000 uncultured amniotic fluid samples in a prospective clinical trial. Prenat Diagn 1997; 17: 333–341

31 Galjaard H. Worldwide experience with first trimester fetal diagnosis by molecular analysis. Proceedings of the 7th International Congress of Human Genetics. Berlin: Springer-Verlag, 1987: 547

32 Irons M, Elias E R, Salen G, Tuint G S, Batta A K. Defective cholesterol biosynthesis in Smith–Lemli–Opitz syndrome. Lancet 1993; 1414

33 Tint G S, Irons M, Elias E R et al. Defective cholesterol biosynthesis associated with the Smith–Lemli–Opitz syndrome. N Engl J Med 1994; 330: 107–113

34 Tint G S, Abuelo D, Till M et al. Fetal Smith–Lemli–Opitz syndrome can be detected accurately and reliably by measuring amniotic fluid dehydrocholesterols. Prenat Diagn 1998; 18: 651–658

35 Kan Y W, Dozy A M. Antenatal diagnosis of sickle cell anaemia by DNA analysis of amniotic fluid cells. Lancet 1978; ii: 910

36 Rommens J M, Iannuzzi M C, Kerem B et al. Identification of the cystic fibrosis gene: chromosome walking and jumping. Science 1989; 245: 1059–1065

37 Riordan J R, Rommens J M, Kerem B et al. Identification of the cystic fibrosis gene: cloning and characterisation of complementary DNA. Science 1989; 245: 1066–1073

38 Kerem B, Rommens J M, Buchanan J A et al. Identification of the cystic fibrosis gene: genetic analysis. Science 1989; 245: 1073–1080

39 Brock D J H. Cystic fibrosis In: Brock D J H, Rodeck C H, Ferguson-Smith M A, eds. Prenatal diagnosis and screening. London: Churchill Livingstone, 1992: 441–460

40 Brock D J H, Clarke H A K, Barron L. Prenatal diagnosis of cystic fibrosis by microvillar enzyme assay on a sequence of 258 pregnancies. Hum Genet 1988; 78: 271–275

41 Richards D S, Seeds J W, Katz V L, Lingley L H, Albright S G, Cefalo R C. Elevated maternal serum alpha-fetoprotein with normal ultrasound: is amniocentesis always appropriate? A review of 26 069 screened patients. Obstet Gynecol 1988; 71: 203–207

42 Milunsky A, Sapirstein V S. Prenatal diagnosis of open neural tube defects using the amniotic fluid acetylcholinesterase assay. Obstet Gynecol 1982; 59: 1–5

43 Wald N, Cuckle H, Nanchatial K. Second report of the acetylcholinesterase study: amniotic fluid acetylcholinesterase measurement in the prenatal diagnosis of open neural tube defects. Prenat Diagn 1989; 9: 813–829

44 Brock D J H, Barron L, van Heyningen V. Prenatal diagnosis of neural tube defects with a monoclonal antibody specific for acetylcholinesterase. Lancet 1985; ii: 5–8

45 Bennett P R, Kim C L, Colin Y, Warwick R M, Cherif-Zahar B, Fisk N M. Prenatal determination of RhD type by DNA amplification following chorionic villus sampling or amniocentesis. N Engl J Med 1993; 329: 607–610

46 Van den Veyver I B, Moise K J. Fetal RhD typing by polymerase chain reaction in pregnancies complicated by rhesus alloimmunization. Obstet Gynecol 1996; 88: 1061–1067

47 Donner C, Liesnard C, Content J, Busine A, Aderca J, Rodesch F. Prenatal diagnosis of 52 pregnancies at risk for congenital cytomegalovirus infection. Obstet Gynecol 1993; 82: 481–486

48 Cazenave J, Forestier F, Bessieres M H, Broussin B, Bebueret J. Contribution of a new PCR assay to the prenatal diagnosis of congenital toxoplasmosis. Prenat Diagn 1992; 12: 119–127

49 Lipitz S, Yagel S, Shalev E, Achiron R, Mashiach S, Schiff E. Prenatal diagnosis of fetal primary cytomegalovirus infection. Obstet Gynecol 1997; 89: 763–767

50 Hohlfeld P, Daffos F, Costa J M, Thulliez P, Forestier F, Vidaud M. Prenatal diagnosis of congenital toxoplasmosis with a polymerase chain reaction test on amniotic fluid. N Engl J Med 1994; 15: 695–669

51 Tanemura M, Suzumori K, Yagami Y, Katow S. Diagnosis of fetal rubella infection with reverse transcriptase and nested polymerase chain reaction: a study of 34 cases diagnosed in fetuses. Am J Obstet Gynecol 1996; 174: 578–582

52 Mouly F, Mirlesse V, Meritet M et al. Prenatal diagnosis of fetal varicella-zoster virus infection with polymerase chain reaction of amniotic fluid in 107 cases. Am J Obstet Gynecol 1997; 177: 894–898

53 Liley A W. Liquor amnii analysis in the management of the pregnancy complicated by rhesus sensitization. Am J Obstet Gynecol 1961; 82: 1359–1370

54 Whitfield C R. A three-year assessment of an action line method of timing intervention in rhesus isoimmunization. Am J Obstet Gynecol 1970; 108: 1239–1244

55 Bowman J M. The management of Rh-isoimmunization. Obstet Gynecol 1978; 52: 1–16

56 Nicolaides K H, Rodeck C H, Mishiban R S, Kemp J R. Have Liley charts outlived their usefulness? Am J Obstet Gynecol 1986; 155: 90–94

57 Roberts A B, Mitchell J M, Pattison N S. Fetal liver length in normal and isoimmunised pregnancies. Am J Obstet Gynecol 1989; 161: 42–46

58 Mari G, Abuhamad A Z, Pirhonen J, Jones D C, Ludomirsky A, Copel J A. Diagnosis of fetal anemia with Doppler ultrasound in the pregnancy complicated by maternal blood group immunization. Ultrasound Obstet Gynecol 1995; 5: 400–405

59 Iskaros J, Kingdom J, Morrison J J, Rodeck C. Prospective non-invasive monitoring of pregnancies complicated by red cell alloimmunisation. Ultrasound Obstet Gynecol 1998; 11: 438–437

60 Gluck L, Kulovich M V. Lecithin/sphingomyelin ratios in amniotic fluid in normal and abnormal pregnancy. Am J Obstet Gynecol 1973; 115: 539–546

61 Carroll S G, Sebire N J, Nicolaides K H. Preterm prelabour amniorrhexis. London: Parthenon Publishing, 1996

62 Romero R, Yoon B H, Mazor M et al. A comparative study of the diagnostic performance of amniotic fluid glucose, white blood cell count, interleukin-6, and Gram stain in the detection of microbial invasion in patients with preterm premature rupture of membranes. Am J Obstet Gynecol 1993; 169: 839–851

63 National Institute of Child Health and Development Amniocentesis Register. The safety and accuracy of midtrimester amniocentesis. US Department of Health, Education and Welfare, 1978: 78–190

64 Prenatal diagnosis – past, present and future. Report of the International Workshop held at Val David, Quebec, Canada, November 1979. London: John Wiley, 1980

65 Farrant W. Stress after amniocentesis for high serum alpha-fetoprotein concentrations [letter]. BMJ 1980; 281: 452

66 Tabor A, Philip J, Bang J, Madsen M, Obel E B, Norgaard-Pedersen B. Needle size and risk of miscarriage after amniocentesis. Lancet 1988; i: 183–184

67 Tabor A, Bang J, Norgaard-Pedersen B. Feto-maternal haemorrhage associated with genetic amniocentesis: results of a randomized trial. Br J Obstet Gynaecol 1987; 94: 528–534

68 Hislop A, Fairweather D V I, Blackwell R J, Howard S. The effect of amniocentesis and drainage of amniotic fluid on lung development in *Macaca fascicularis*. Am J Obstet Gynecol 1984; 91: 835–842

69 NICHD National Registry for Amniocentesis Study Group. Midtrimester amniocentesis for prenatal diagnosis: safety and accuracy. JAMA 1976; 235: 1471–1476

70 Low C, Alexander D, Bryla D, Seigel D. The safety and accuracy of midtrimester amniocentesis. Bethesdea, MD: National Institute of Child Health and Human Development, National Institutes of Health, 1978

71 Finegan J, Quarrington B, Hughes H et al. Infant outcome following mid-trimester amniocentesis: development and physical status at age six months. Br J Obstet Gynaecol 1985; 92: 1015–1023

72 Finegan J, Quarrington B, Hughes H et al. Child outcome following mid-trimester amniocentesis: development, behaviour and physical status at age 4 years. Br J Obstet Gynaecol 1990; 97: 32–40

73 Finegan J, Sitarenios G, Bolan P, Sarabura A. Children whose mothers had second trimester amniocentesis: follow up at school age. Br J Obstet Gynaecol 1996; 103: 214–218

74 Hahnemann N, Mohr J. Genetic diagnosis in the embryo by means of biopsy from extra-embryonic membranes. Bull Eur Soc Hum Genet 1968; 2: 23–29

75 Hahnemann N, Mohr J. Antenatal foetal diagnosis in genetic disease Bull Eur Soc Hum Genet 1969; 3: 47–54

76 Kullander S, Sandahl B. Fetal chromosome analysis after transcervical placental biopsies during early pregnancy. Acta Obstet Gynecol Scand 1973; 52: 355–359

77 Tietung Hospital of Anshan Iron and Steel Co; Department of Obstetrics and Gynaecology. Fetal sex prediction by sex chromatin of chorionic villi cells during early pregnancy. Chin Med J 1975; 1: 117–126

78 Williamson R, Eskdale J, Coleman D V, Niazi N, Loeffler F E, Modell B. Direct gene analysis of chorionic villi, a possible technique for the first trimester diagnosis of haemoglobinopathies. Lancet 1981; ii: 1125–1127

79 Niazi M, Coleman D V, Loeffler F E. Trophoblast sampling in early pregnancy. Culture of rapidly dividing cells from immature placental villi. Br J Obstet Gynaecol 1981; 1: 1081–1085

80 Kazy Z, Rozovsky I S, Bakharev V A. Chorion biopsy in early pregnancy: a method of early prenatal diagnosis for inherited disorders. Prenat Diagn 1982; 2: 39–45

81 Simoni G, Brambati B, Danesino C et al. Efficient direct chromosome analysis and enzyme determinations from chorionic villi samples in the first trimester of pregnancy. Hum Genet 1983; 63: 349–357

82 Rhine S A, Palmer C G, Thompson T. A simple first trimester alternative to amniocentesis for prenatal diagnosis. Birth Defects Orig Art 1977; Ser XII 3D: 231–247

83 Goldberg M F, Chen A T L, Young W A, Reidy J A. First trimester fetal chromosome diagnosis using endocervical lavage: a negative evaluation. Am J Obstet Gynecol 1980; 138: 435–440

84 Kazy Z, Stigar A M. Kozvetlin real-time (ultrahang) kontroll melletti chorion biopsy. Orv Het 1980; 121: 2765–2766

85 Old J M, Ward R H T, Karagozlu F, Petrou M, Modell B, Weatherall D J. First trimester fetal diagnosis for haemoglobinopathies: three cases. Lancet 1982; ii: 1413–1416

86 Goosens M, Dumez Y, Kaplan Y et al. Prenatal diagnosis of sickle cell anaemia in the first trimester of pregnancy. N Engl J Med 1983; 309: 831–833

87 Ward R H T, Modell B, Petriu M, Karagozlou F, Douratsos E. A method of chorionic villus sampling in the first trimester of pregnancy under real-time ultrasonic guidance. BMJ 1983; 286: 1542–1544

88 Rodeck C H, Nicolaides K H, McKenzie C M, Gosden C M, Gosden J R. A single-operator technique for first trimester chorion biopsy. Lancet 1983; ii: 1340–1341

89 Alvarez H. Diagnosis of hydatidiform mole by transabdominal placental biopsy. Am J Obstet Gynecol 1966; 95: 538–541

90 Smidt-Jensen S, Hahnemann N. Transabdominal fine needle biopsy from chorionic villi in the first trimester. Prenat Diagn 1984; 4: 163–169

91 Pergament E, Schulman J D, Copeland K et al. The risk and efficacy of chorion villus sampling in multiple gestations. Prenat Diagn 1992; 12: 377–384

92 Maxwell D, Lilford R, Czepulkowski B, Heaton D, Coleman D. Transabdominal chorionic villus sampling. Lancet 1986; i: 123–126

93 Brambati B, Oldrini A, Ferrazzi E, Lanzani A. Chorionic villus sampling: an analysis of the obstetric experience of 1000 cases. Prenat Diagn 1987; 7: 157–169

94 MacLachlan N A, Rooney D E, Coleman D, Rodeck C H. Prenatal diagnosis: early amniocentesis or chorionic villus sampling. Comtemp Rev Obstet Gynaecol 1989; 1: 173–180

95 Wapner R J. Chorionic villus sampling. Obstet Gynecol Clin North Am 1997; 24: 83–97

96 Nicolaides K H, Soothill P W, Rodeck C H, Warren R C. Why confine chorionic villus (placental) biopsy to the first trimester? Lancet 1986; i: 543–544

97 Jackson L G, Zachary J M, Fowler S E et al. A randomised comparison of transcervical and transabdominal chorionic-villus sampling. N Engl J Med 1992; 327: 594–598

98 National Institute of Child Health and Human Development. The safety and efficacy of CVS for early prenatal diagnosis of cytogenetic abnormalities. N Engl J Med 1989; 320: 609–617

99 Chueh J T, Goldberg J D, Wohlferd M M, Golbus M S. Comparison of transcervical and transabdominal chorionic villus sampling loss rates in nine thousand cases from a single center. Am J Obstet Gynecol 1995; 173: 1277–1282

100 Rosevear S K. Placental biopsy. Br J Hosp Med 1989; 41: 334–348

101 Mikkelsen M, Ayme I. Chromosomal findings in chorionic villi. A collaborative study. Proceedings of the 7th International Congress of Human Genetics. Berlin: Springer-Verlag, 1987

102 Canadian Collaborative CVS–Amniocentesis Clinical Trial Group. Multicentre randomized clinical trial of chorionic villus sampling and amniocentesis. Lancet 1989; i: 1–6

103 Macintosh M C, Wald N J, Chard T et al. Selective miscarriage of Down's syndrome fetuses in women aged 35 years and older. Br J Obstet Gynaecol 1995; 102: 798–801

104 Kalousek D K, Dill F J. Chromosomal mosaicism confined to the placenta in human conceptions. Science 1983; 221: 665

105 Gregson N, Seabright M. Handling chorionic villi for direct chromosome studies. Lancet 1983; ii: 1491

106 Wolstenholme J, Rooney D E, Davison E V. Confined placental mosaicism, IUGR and adverse pregnancy outcome: a controlled retrospective UK collaborative survey. Prenat Diagn 1991; 11: 577

107 Kalousek D K, Vekemans M. Confined placental mosaicism. J Med Genet 1996; 33: 529–533

108 Bennett P, Vaughan J I, Henderson D, Loughna S, Moore G. Association between confined placental trisomy, fetal uniparental disomy and early intrauterine growth retardation. Lancet 1992; 340: 1284–1285

109 Kalousek D K, Langlois S, Barrett I et al. Uniparental disomy for chromosome 16 in humans. Am J Hum Genet 1993; 52: 8–16

110 Vaughan J I, Ali Z, Bower S, Bennett P B, Chard T, Moore G. Human maternal uniparental disomy for chromosome 16 and fetal development. Prenat Diagn 1994; 14: 751

111 Hahnemann J M, Vejerslev L O. Accuracy of cytogenetic findings on chorionic villus sampling (CVS) – diagnostic consequences of CVS mosaicism and non-mosaic discrepancy in centres contributing to EUCROMIC 1986–1992. Prenat Diagn 1997; 17: 801–820

112 Phillips O P, Tharapel A T, Lerner J L, Park V M, Wachtel S S, Shulman L P. Risk of fetal mosaicism when placental mosaicism is diagnosed by chorionic villus sampling. Am J Obstet Gynecol 1996; 174: 850–855

113 Hahnemann J M, Vejerslev L O. European collaborative research on mosaicism in CVS (EUCROMIC) – fetal and extrafetal cell lineages in 192 gestations with CVS mosaicism involving single autosomal trosomy. Am J Med Genet 1997; 70: 179–187

114 Ledbetter D H, Martin A O, Verlinsky Y et al. Cytogenetic results of chorionic villus sampling: high success rate and diagnostic accuracy in the United States collaborative study. Am J Obstet Gynecol 1990; 162: 495–501

115 Old J M, Fitches A, Heath C et al. First trimester fetal diagnosis for haemoglobinopathies: report on 149 cases. Lancet 1986; ii: 763–767

116 Besley G T N. Enzyme analysis. In: Brock D J H, Rodeck C H, Ferguson-Smith M A, eds. Prenatal diagnosis and screening. London: Churchill Livingstone, 1992; 130–131

117 Fisk N M, Bennett P, Warwick R M, Letsky E A, Welch R, Vaughan J I. Clinical utility of fetal RhD typing in alloimmunised pregnancies by means of polymerase chain reaction on amniocytes or chorionic villi. Am J Obstet Gynecol 1994; 171: 50–54

118 Gemke R J B J, Kankai H H H, Overbeeke M A M et al. ABO and rhesus phenotyping of fetal erythrocytes in the first trimester of pregnancy. Br J Haematol 1986; 64: 689–697

119 Furhman H C, Klink F, Grzejszczyk G et al. First trimester diagnosis of RH(D) with an immunofluorescence technique after chorionic villus sampling. Prenat Diagn 1987; 7: 17–21

120 Rodesch F, Lambermont M, Donner C et al. Chorionic biopsy in management of severe Kell alloimmunization. Am J Obstet Gynecol 1987; 156: 124–125

121 Rodeck C H, Letsky E. How the management of erythroblastosis fetalis has changed. Br J Obstet Gynaecol 1989; 96: 759–763

122 Blakemore K J, Mahoney M J, Hobbins J C. Infection and chorionic villus sampling. Lancet 1985; ii: 338

123 Barela A I, Kleinman J G, Golditch I M, Menke D J, Hogge W A, Golbus M S. Septic shock with renal failure after chorionic villus sampling. Am J Obstet Gynecol 1986; 154: 1100–1102

124 MRC Working Party on the Evaluation of Chorion Villus Sampling. Medical Research Council European trial of chorion villus sampling. Lancet 1991; 337: 1491–1499

125 Hogge W A, Schonberg S A, Golbus M S. Chorionic villus sampling: Experience of the first 1000 cases. Am J Obstet Gynecol 1986; 154: 1249–1252

126 Brambati B, Lanzani A, Oldrini A. Transabdominal chorionic villus sampling. Clinical experience of 1159 cases. Prenat Diagn 1988; 8: 609–617

127 Warren R C, Rodeck C H. Experience with a silver cannula for transcervical chorion villus sampling. Contrib Gynaecol Obstet 1986; 15: 32–40

128 Brambati G, Guercilina S, Bonacchi I, Oldrini A, Lanzani A, Piceni L. Feto-maternal transfusion after chorionic villus sampling: clinical implications. Hum Reprod 1986; 1: 37

129 Blakemore K G, Baumgarten A, Schoenfeld-Dimaio M, Hobbins J C, Mason E A, Mahoney M J. Rise in maternal serum α-fetoprotein concentration after chorionic villus sampling and the possibility of isoimmunization. Am J Obstet Gynecol 1986; 155: 988–993

130 Moise K J, Carpenter R J, Wapner R J, Shah D M, Boehm F M. Increased severity of fetal hemolytic disease with known Rhesus alloimmunization after first trimester transcervical chorionic villus biopsy. Fetal Diagn Ther 1990; 5: 76–78

131 Sigler M E, Colyer C R, Rossiter J, Dorfmann A D, Jones S L, Schulman J D. Maternal serum alpha-fetoprotein screening after chorionic villus sampling. Obstet Gynecol 1987; 70: 875–877

132 Wilson R D, Kendrick V, Whittman B K, McGillivray B C. Risk of spontaneous abortion in ultrasonically normal pregnancies. Lancet 1984; ii: 920–921

133 MacKenzie W E, Holmes D S, Newton J R. Spontaneous abortion rate in ultrasonically viable pregnancies. Obstet Gynecol 1988; 71: 81–83

134 Casner K A, Christopher C R, Dysert G A. Spontaneous fetal loss after demonstration of a live fetus in the first trimester. Obstet Gynecol 1987; 70: 827–830

135 Smidt-Jensen S, Permin M, Philip J et al. Randomised comparison of amniocentesis and transabdominal and transcervical chorionic villus sampling. Lancet 1992; 340: 1237–1244

136 Brambati B, Terzian E, Tognoni G. Randomised clinical trial of transabdominal versus transcervical chorionic villus sampling methods. Prenat Diagn 1991; 11: 285–293

137 Firth H V, Boyd P A, Chamberlain P, MacKenzie I Z, Lindenbaum R H, Huson S M. Severe limb abnormalities after chorion villus sampling at 56–66 days' gestation. Lancet 1991; 337: 762–763

138 Foster-Iskenius U G, Baird P A. Limb reduction defects in over one million consecutive livebirths. Teratology 1989; 39: 127–135

139 Hsieh F, Chen D, Tseng L et al. Limb reduction defects and chorion villus sampling [letter]. Lancet 1991; 337: 1092–1093

140 Burton B, Schulz C, Burd L. Limb anomalies associated with chorionic villus sampling. Obstet Gynecol 1992; 79: 726–730

141 Brambati B, Simoni G, Travi M et al. Genetic diagnosis by chorionic villus sampling before 8 gestational weeks: efficiency, reliability and risks on 317 completed pregnancies. Prenat Diagn 1992; 12: 789–799

142 Firth H V, Boyd P A, Chamberlain P F, MacKenzie I Z, Morriss-Kay G M, Huson S M. Analysis of limb reduction defects in babies exposed to chorionic villus sampling. Lancet 1994; 343: 1069–1071

143 Mahoney M. Limb abnormalities and chorionic villus sampling [letter]. Lancet 1991; 337: 1422–1423

144 Kuliev A, Jackson L, Froster U et al. Chorionic villus sampling safety. Am J Obstet Gynecol 1996; 174: 807–811

145 Anonymous. Chorionic villus sampling and amniocentesis: recommendations for prenatal counseling. Morb Mortal Wkly Rep 1995; 44: 1–12

146 Olney R S, Khoury M J, Alo C J et al. Increased risk for transverse digital deficiency after chorionic villus sampling: results of the United States Multi-state Case-Control Study, 1988–1992. Teratology 1995; 51: 20–29

147 Mastroiacovo P, Botto L D. Chorionic villus sampling and transverse limb deficiencies: maternal age is not a confounder. Am J Med Genet 1994; 53: 182–186

148 Dolk H, Bertrand F, Lechat M F, for the EUROCAT Working Group. Chorionic villus sampling and limb abnormalities [letter]. Lancet 1992; 339: 876–877

149 Hoyme H E, Jones K L, Van Allen M I, Saunders B S, Benirschke K. Vascular pathogenesis of transverse limb reduction defects. J Pediatr 1982; 101: 839–843

150 Rodeck C H. Fetal development after chorionic villus sampling. Lancet 1993; 341: 468–469

151 Quintero R A, Romero R, Mahoney M J et al. Embryoscopic demonstration of hemorrhagic lesions on the human embryo after placental trauma. Am J Obstet Gynecol 1993; 168: 756–759

152 Rodeck C H, Sheldrake A, Beattie B, Whittle M J. Maternal serum alphafetoprotein after placental damage in chorionic villus sampling. Lancet 1993; 341: 500

153 Olney R S, Khoury M J, Botto L D, Mastroiacovo P. Limb defects and gestational age at chorionic villus sampling [letter]. Lancet 1994; 344: 476

154 Scrimgeour J B. Amniocentesis: technique and complications. In: Emery EAH, ed. Antenatal diagnosis of genetic disease. London: Churchill Livingstone, 1973: 11

155 Luthardt F W, Luthy D A, Karp L E, Hickok D E, Resta R G. Prospective evaluation of early amniocentesis for prenatal diagnosis. Am J Hum Genet 1985; 37 (Suppl): A 659

156 Henry G, Peakman D C, Winkler W, O'Connor K. Amniocentesis before 15 weeks instead of CVS for earlier prenatal cytogenetic diagnosis. Am J Hum Genet 1985; 37 (Suppl): A835

157 Rooney D E, MacLachlan N, Smith J et al. Early amniocentesis: a cytogenetic evaluation. BMJ 1989; 299: 25

158 Hanson F W, Zorn E M, Tennant F R, Marianos M, Samuels S. Amniocentesis before 15 weeks gestation: outcome, risks and technical problems. Am J Obstet Gynecol 1987; 156: 1524–1531

159 Chadefaux B, Rabier D, Dumez Y, Oury J F, Kamoun P. Eleventh week amniocentesis for prenatal diagnosis of metabolic diseases. Lancet 1989; i: 849

160 Drugan A, Syner F N, Greb A, Evans M I. Amniotic fluid alpha-fetoprotein and acetylcholinesterase in early genetic amniocentesis. Obstet Gynecol 1988; 72: 35–38

161 Crandall B F, Hanson F W, Tennant F, Perdue S T. Alpha-fetoprotein levels in amniotic fluid between 11 and 15 weeks. Am J Obstet Gynecol 1989; 160: 1204–1206

162 Evans M I, Johnson M P, Holzgreve W. Early amniocentesis: what exactly does it mean? J Reprod Med 1994; 39: 77–78

163 Nicolaides K H, Brizot M L, Patel F, Snijders R J M. Comparison of chorionic villus sampling and amniocentesis for fetal karyotyping at 10–13 weeks' gestation. Lancet 1994; 344: 435–439

164 Sundberg K, Bang J, Smidt-Jensen S et al. Randomised study of risk of fetal loss related to early amniocentesis versus chorionic villus sampling. Lancet 1997; 350: 697–703

165 Johnson J-A M, Wilson R D, Winsor E J T, Singer J, Dansereau J, Kalousek D K. The early amniocentesis study: a randomised clinical trial of early amniocentesis versus midtrimester amniocentesis. Fetal Diagn Ther 1996; 11: 85–93

166 The Canadian Early and Mid-Trimester Amniocentesis Trial (CEMAT) Group Randomised trial to assess safety and fetal outcome of early and midtrimester amniocentesis. Lancet 1998; 351: 242–247

167 Nicolaides K H, de Lourdes Brizot M, Patel F, Snijders R. Comparison of chorion villus sampling and early amniocentesis for karyotyping in 1492 singleton pregnancies. Fetal Diagn Ther 1996; 11: 9–15

168 Nelson M M Amniotic fluid volume in early pregnancy. J Obstet Gynaecol Br Cwlth 1972; 70: 50–53

169 Sundberg K, Smidt-Jensen S, Philip J. Amniocentesis with increased cell yield, obtained by filtration and reinjection of the amniotic fluid. Ultrasound Obstet Gynecol 1991; 1: 91–94

170 Byrne D L, Marks K, Braude P R, Nicolaides K H. Amnifiltration in the first trimester: feasibility, technical aspects and cytological outcome. Ultrasound Obstet Gynecol 1991; 1: 320–324

171 Byrne D L, Penna L, Marks K, Offley-Shore B. First trimester amnifiltration: technical, cytogenetic and pregnancy outcome of 104 consecutive procedures. Br J Obstet Gynaecol 1995; 102: 220–223

172 Byrne D, Marks K, Azar G, Nicolaides K. Randomized study of early amniocentesis versus chorionic villus sampling: a technical and cytogenetic comparison of 650 patients. Ultrasound Obstet Gynecol 1991; 1: 235–240

173 Elejalde B R, de Elejalde M M. Early genetic amniocentesis, safety, complications, time to obtain results and contradictions. Am J Hum Genet 1988; 43: A234

174 Byrne D L, Azar G, Nicolaides K H. Why cell culture is successful after early amniocentesis. Fetal Diagn Ther 1991; 6: 84–86

175 Penso C A, Sandstrom M M, Garber M, Ladoulis M, Stryker J M, Benacerrraf B B. Early amniocentesis: report of 407 cases with neonatal follow-up. Obstet Gynecol 1990; 76: 1032–1036

176 Stripparo L, Buscaglia M, Longatti L et al. Genetic amniocentesis: 505 cases performed before the sixteenth week of gestation. Prenat Diagn 1990; 10: 359–364

177 Nevin J, Nevin N C, Dornan J C, Sim D, Armstrong M J. Early amniocentesis: experience of 222 consecutive patients, 1987–1988. Prenat Diagn 1990; 10: 79–83

178 Wilson R D. Safety and fetal outcome of early and midtrimester amniocentesis. Lancet 1998; 351: 1455–1456

179 Greenough A, Yuksel B, Naik S, Cheeseman P, Nicolaides K H. Invasive antenatal procedures and requirement for neonatal intensive care unit admission. Eur J Pediatr 1997; 156: 550–552

180 Thompson P J, Greenough A, Nicolaides K H. Lung function following first-trimester amniocentesis or chorionic villus sampling. Fetal Diagn Ther 1991; 6: 148–152

181 Yuksel B, Greenough A, Naik S, Cheeseman P, Nicolaides K H. Perinatal lung function and invasive antenatal procedures. Thorax 1997; 52: 181–184

182 Whittle M J. Early amniocentesis: time for a rethink [commentary]. Lancet 1998; 351: 226–227

183 Valenti C. Antenatal detection of haemoglobinopathies. A preliminary report. Am J Obstet Gynecol 1973; 115: 851–853

184 Kan Y W, Valenti C, Guidotti R, Carnazza V, Rieder R F. Fetal blood sampling in utero. Lancet 1974; i: 79–80

185 Alter B, Modell B, Fairweather D et al. Prenatal diagnosis of hemoglobinopathies: a review of 15 cases. N Engl J Med 1976; 295: 1437–1439

186 Fairweather D V I, Ward R H T, Modell B. Obstetric aspects of midtrimester fetal blood sampling by needling or fetoscopy. Br J Obstet Gynaecol 1980; 87: 87–99

187 Hobbins J C, Mahoney M J. In utero diagnosis of hemoglobinopathies. Technique for obtaining fetal blood. N Engl J Med 1974; 290: 1065–1067

188 Rodeck C H, Campbell S. Sampling pure fetal blood by fetoscopy in second trimester of pregnancy. BMJ 1978; ii: 728–730

189 Rodeck C H, Nicolaides K H. Fetoscopy. Br Med Bull 1986; 42: 296–300

190 Daffos F, Capella-Pavlovsky M, Forestier F. A new procedure for fetal blood sampling in utero. Prenat Diagn 1983; 3: 271–274

191 Megerian G, Ludomirsky A. Role of cordocentesis in perinatal medicine. Curr Opin Obstet Gynecol 1994; 6: 30–35

192 Koresawa M, Inaba J, Iwasaki H. Fetal blood sampling by liver puncture. Acta Obstet Gynecol Jpn 1987; 39: 395–399

193 Bang J. Ultrasound-guided fetal blood sampling. In: Albertini A. Crosignani P F, eds. Progress in perinatal medicine. Amsterdam: Excerpta Medica, 1983: 223

194   Weiner C P, Okamura K. Diagnostic fetal blood sampling – technique-related losses. Fetal Diagn Ther 1996; 11: 169–175

195   Forestier F, Cox W L, Daffos F, Rainaut M. The assessment of fetal blood samples. Am J Obstet Gynecol 1988; 158: 1184–1188

196   Daffos F, Capella-Pavlovsky M, Forestier F. Fetal blood sampling during pregnancy with the use of a needle guided by ultrasound: a study of 606 consecutive cases. Am J Obstet Gynecol 1985; 153: 655–660

197   Bang J, Bock J E, Trolle D. Ultrasound-guided fetal intravenous transfusion for severe rhesus haemolytic disease. BMJ 1982; 284: 373–374

198   Ch de Crespigny L, Robinson H P, Quinn M, Doyle L, Ross A, Cauchi M. Ultrasound-guided fetal blood transfusion for severe rhesus isoimmunization. Obstet Gynecol 1985; 66: 529–532

199   Nicolini U, Santolaya J, Ojo O E et al. The fetal intrahepatic umbilical vein as an alternative to cord needling for prenatal diagnosis and therapy. Prenat Diagn 1988; 8: 665–671

200   Nicolini U, Nicolaidis P, Fisk N M, Tannirandorn Y, Rodeck C H. Fetal blood sampling from the intrahepatic vein: analysis of safety and clinical experience with 214 procedures. Obstet Gynecol 1990; 76: 47–53

201   Nicolini U, Nicolaidis P, Tannirandorn Y, Fisk N M, Nasrat H, Rodeck C H. Fetal liver dysfunction in Rh alloimmunization. Br J Obstet Gynaecol 1991; 98: 287–293

202   Orlandi F, Damiani G, Jakil C, Lauricella S, Bertolino O, Maggio A. The risks of early cordocentesis (12–21 weeks): analysis of 500 procedures. Prenat Diagn 1990; 10: 425–428

203   Weiner C P. Cordocentesis for diagnostic indications: two years' experience. Obstet Gynaecol 1987; 70: 664–667

204   Nicolaides K H, Rodeck C H, Gosden C M. Rapid karyotyping in non-lethal malformations. Lancet 1986; i: 283–286

205   Benacerraf B R, Frigoletto F D, Laboda L A. Sonographic diagnosis of Down syndrome in the second trimester. Am J Obstet Gynecol 1985; 153: 49–52

206   Weiner C P. Human fetal bilirubin levels and fetal hemolytic disease. Am J Obstet Gynecol 1992; 166: 1449–1454

207   Nicolaides K H, Soothill P W, Clewell W H, Rodeck C H, Mishaban R S, Campbell S. Fetal haemoglobin measurement in the assessment of red cell isoimmunisation. Lancet 1988; i: 1073–1075

208   Nicolini U, Kochenour N K, Greco P et al. Consequences of fetomaternal haemorrhage after intrauterine transfusion. BMJ 1988; 297: 1379–1381

209   Millar D S, Davis L R, Rodeck C H, Nicolaides K H, Mishiban R S. Normal blood cell values in the early midtrimester fetus. Prenat Diagn 1985; 5: 367–373

210   Daffos F, Forestier F, Capella-Pavlovsky M et al. Prenatal management of 746 pregnancies at risk for congenital toxoplasmosis. N Engl J Med 1988; 318: 271–275

211   Morgan-Capner P, Rodeck C H, Nicolaides K H, Cradock-Watson J E. Prenatal detection of rubella-specific IgM in fetal sera. Prenat Diagn 1985; 5: 21–26

212   Torok T J, Wang Q Y, Gary G W, Yang C F, Finch T M, Anderson L J. Prenatal diagnosis of intrauterine infection with parvovirus B19 by the polymerase chain reaction technique. Clin Infect Dis 1992; 14: 149–155

213   Soothill P W, Nicolaides K H, Campbell S. Prenatal asphyxia, hyperlacticaemia, hypoglycaemia, and erythroblastosis in growth retarded fetuses. BM J 1987; 1: 1051–1053

214   Nicolini U, Nicolaidis P, Fisk N M et al. The limited role of fetal blood sampling in prediction of outcome in intrauterine growth retardation. Lancet 1990; ii: 768–772

215   Alfirevic Z, Neilson J P. Doppler ultrasonography in high risk pregnancies: systematic review with meta-analysis. Am J Obstet Gynecol 1995; 172: 1379–1387

216   Weatherall D J, Clegg J B, Naughton M A. Globin synthesis in thalassaemia: an in vitro study. Nature 1965; 208: 1061–1065

217   Mibashan R S, Rodeck C H. Haemophilia and other genetic defects of haemostasis. In: Rodeck C H, Nicolaides K H, eds. Prenatal diagnosis. Proceedings of the XIth Study Group of the Royal College of Obstetricians and Gynaecologists. Chichester: John Wiley, 1984: 179

218   Linch D C, Beverly P C L, Levinsky R J, Rodeck C H. Phenotypic analysis of fetal blood leucocytes: potential for prenatal diagnosis of immunodeficiency disorders. Prenat Diagn 1982; 2: 211–218

219   Levinsky R J. Prenatal diagnosis of severe combined immunodeficiency. In: Rodeck C H, Nicolaides K H, eds. Prenatal diagnosis. Proceedings of the XIth Study Group of the Royal College of Obstetricians and Gynaecologists. Chichester: John Wiley, 1984: 137

220   Maxwell D J, Johnson P, Hurley P, Neales K, Allan L, Knott P. Fetal blood sampling and pregnancy loss in relation to indication. Br J Obstet Gynaecol 1991; 98: 892–897

221   Antsakalis A, Daskalakis G, Papantoniou N, Michalas S. Fetal blood sampling – indication-related losses. Prenat Diagn 1998; 18: 934–940

222   Sturgiss S N, Wright C, Davison J M, Robson S C. Fetal hepatic necrosis following blood sampling from the intrahepatic vein. Prenat Diagn 1996; 16: 866–869

223   Eadý R A J, Rodeck C H. Prenatal diagnosis of disorders of the skin. In: Rodeck C H, Nicolaides K H, eds. Prenatal diagnosis. Proceedings of 11th study group of the Royal College of Obstetricians and Gynaecologists. Chichester: John Wiley, 1984; 147

224   Rodeck C H, Eady R A J, Gosden C M. Prenatal diagnosis of epidermolysis bullosa letalis. Lancet 1980; i: 949–952

225   Bang J. Intrauterine needle diagnosis. In: Holm H H, Kristensen J K, eds. Interventional ultrasound. Copenhagen: Munksgaard, 1985: 122–128

226   Hobbins J C, Mahoney M J, Goldstein L K. New method of intrauterine evaluation by the combined use of fetoscopy and ultrasound. Am J Obstet Gynecol 1974; 118: 1069

227   Eady R A J, Gunner D B, Tidman M J, Nicolaides K H, Rodeck C H. Rapid processing of fetal skin for prenatal diagnosis by light and electron microscopy. J Clin Pathol 1984; 37: 633–638

228   Bakharev V A, Aivazyan A A, Karetnikova N A, Mordovtsev V N, Yantovsky Y R. Fetal skin biopsy in prenatal diagnosis of some genodermatoses. Prenat Diagn 1990; 10: 1–12

229   Cadrin C, Golbus M S. Fetal tissue sampling: indications, techniques, complications and experience with sampling of fetal skin, liver and muscle. West Med J 1993; 159: 269–272

230   Holbrook K A, Smith L T, Elias S. Prenatal diagnosis of genetic skin disease using fetal skin biopsy samples. Arch Dermatol 1993; 129: 1437–1454

231   Eady R A J, Holbrook K A, Blanchet-Bardon C et al. Proceedings: workshop on prenatal diagnosis of skin diseases: dermatology: progress and perspectives. In: Burgdorf W H C, Katz S I, eds. Proceedings of the 18th World Congress of Dermatology. New York: Parthenon Publishing, 1993: 1159–1165

232   Rodeck C H, Patrick A D, Pembrey M E, Tzannatos C, Whitfield A E. Fetal liver biopsy for prenatal diagnosis of ornithine carbamyl transferase deficiency. Lancet 1982; ii: 297

233   Danpure C J, Jennings P J, Penketh R J, Wise P J, Rodeck C H. Fetal liver alanine: glyoxalate aminotransferase and the prenatal diagnosis of primary hyperoxaluria type 1. Prenat Diagn 1989; 9: 271–281

234   Holzgreve W, Golbus M S. Prenatal diagnosis of ornithine transcarbamylase deficiency utilizing fetal liver biopsy. Am J Hum Genet 1984; 36: 320

235   Piceni-Sereni L, Bachmann C, Pfister U, Buscaglia M, Nicolini U. Prenatal diagnosis of carbamyl-phosphate synthetase deficiency by fetal liver biopsy. Prenat Diagn 1988; 8: 307

236   Meisel M, Amon I, Amon K, Huller H. Investigation of glucose-6-phosphatase in the liver of the human fetus. Biol Res Preg 1982; 3: 73

237   Raiha N C R, Suihkonen J. Development of urea-synthesising enzymes in human liver. Acta Pediatr Scand 1968; 57: 121

238   Golbus M S, Simpson T J, Koresawa M, Appelman Z, Alpers C E. The prenatal determination of glucose 6 phosphatase activity by fetal liver biopsy. Prenat Diagn 1988; 8: 401

239   Pembrey M E, Old J M, Leonard J V, Rodeck C H, Warren R, Davies K E. Prenatal diagnosis of ornithine carbamyl transferase deficiency using a gene specific probe. J Med Gen 1985; 22: 462

240   Nussbaum R L, Boggs B A, Beaudet A L, Doyle S, Potter J L, O'Brien W E. New mutation and prenatal diagnosis in ornithine transcarbamylase deficiency. Am J Hum Genet 1986; 38: 149

241   Fox J, Hack A M, Fenton W A et al. Prenatal diagnosis of ornithine transcarbamylase deficiency with the use of DNA polymorphisms. N Engl J Med 1986; 315: 1205

242   Nicolini U, Rodeck C H. Fetal Blood and tissue sampling. In: Brock D J H, Rodeck C H, Ferguson-Smith M A, eds. Prenatal diagnosis. London: Churchill Livingstone, 1992: 39–51

243 Koenig M, Hoffman E P, Bertelson C J et al. Complete cloning of the Duchenne muscular dystrophy (DMD) cDNA and preliminary genomic organisation of the DMD gene in normal and affected individuals. Cell 1987; 50: 509–517

244 Bieber F R, Hoffman E P, Amos J. Dystrophin analysis in Duchenne muscular dystrophy; use in fetal diagnosis and genetic counselling. Am J Hum Genet 1989; 45: 362–367

245 Evans M I, Greb A, Kunkel L M et al. In utero fetal muscle biopsy for the diagnosis of Duchenne muscular dystrophy. Am J Obstet Gynecol 1991; 165: 728–732

246 Evans M I, Hoffman E P, Cadrin C, Johnson M P, Quintero R A, Golbus M S. Fetal muscle biopsy: collaborative experience with varied indications. Obstet Gynecol 1994; 84: 913–917

247 Evans M I, Quintero R A, King M, Qureshi F, Hoffman E P, Johnson M P. Endoscopically assisted, ultrasound-guided fetal muscle biopsy. Fetal Diagn Ther 1995; 10: 167–172

248 Dale B A, Perry T B, Holbrook K A, Hailton E F, Senikas V. Biochemical examination of fetal skin biopsy specimens obtained by fetoscopy: use of the method for analysis of keratin and filaggrin. Prenat Diagn 1986; 6: 37–44

249 Nicolini U, Rodeck C H. Fetal blood sampling. In: Brock D J H, Rodeck C H, Ferguson-Smith M A, eds. Prenatal diagnosis and screening. Edinburgh: Churchill Livingstone, 1992: 39–51

250 Bunduki V, Saldanha L B, Sadek L, Miguelez J, Miyadahira S, Zugaib M. Fetal renal biopsies in obstructive uropathy: feasibility and clinical correlations – preliminary results. Prenat Diagn 1998; 18: 101–109

251 Housley H T, Harrison M R. Fetal urinary tract abnormalities: natural history, pathophysiology and treatment. Urol Clin North Am 1998; 25: 63–72

252 Crombleholme T M, Harrison M R, Golbus M S et al. Fetal intervention in obstructive uropathy: prognostic indicators and efficacy of intervention. Am J Obstet Gynecol 1990; 162: 1239–1244

253 Nicolaides K H, Cheng H H, Snijders R J M, Moniz C F. Fetal urine biochemistry in the assessment of obstructive uropathy. Am J Obstet Gynecol 1992; 166: 932–937

254 Lipitz S, Ryan G, Samuell C et al. Fetal urine analysis for the assessment of renal function in obstructive uropathy. Am J Obstet Gynecol 1993; 168: 174–179

255 Nicolini U, Tannirandorn Y, Vaughan J, Fisk N M, Nicolaidis P, Rodeck C H. Further predictors of renal dysplasia in fetal obstructive uropathy: bladder pressure and biochemistry of 'fresh' urine. Prenat Diagn 1991; 11: 159–166

256 Johnson M P, Corsi P, Bradfield W et al. Sequential urinalysis improves evaluation of fetal renal function in obstructive uropathy. Am J Obstet Gynecol 1995; 173: 59–65

257 Johnson M P, Bukowski T P, Reitleman C, Isada N B, Pryde P G, Evans M I. In utero surgical treatment of fetal obstructive uropathy: a new comprehensive approach to identify appropriate candidates for vesicoamniotic shunt therapy. Am J Obstet Gynecol 1994; 170: 1770–1779

258 Nicolini U, Fisk N M, Beacham J, Rodeck C H. Fetal urine biochemistry: an index of renal maturation and dysfunction. Br J Obstet Gynaecol 1992; 99: 46–50

259 Nakayama D K, Harrison M R, de Lorimer A A. Prognosis of posterior urethral valves presenting at birth. J Pediatr Surg 1986; 21: 43–45

260 Reuss A, Wladimiroff J W, Stewart P A, Scholtmeijer R J. Non-invasive management of fetal obstructive uropathy. Lancet 1988; ii: 949–951

261 Nicolini U, Rodeck C H, Fisk N M. Shunt treatment for fetal obstructive uropathy. Lancet 1987; ii: 1338–1339

262 Glick P I, Harrison M R, Golbus M S et al. Management of the fetus with congenital hydronephrosis II; prognostic criteria and selection for treatment. J Pediatr Surg 1985; 20: 376–387

263 Wilkins I A, Chitkara U, Lynch L, Golberg J D, Mehalek K E, Berkowitz R L. The non predictive value of fetal urinary electrolytes: preliminary report of outcomes and correlations with pathologic diagnosis. Am J Obstet Gynecol 1987; 157: 694–698

264 Nicolini U, Rodeck C H. Fetal urinary diversion. In: Chervenak F, Isaacson G, Campbell S, eds. Textbook of ultrasound in obstetrics and gynecology. New York: Little Brown, 1990

265 Freedman A L, Bukowski T P, Smith C A, Evans M I, Johnson M P, Gonzalez R. Fetal therapy for obstructive uropathy: diagnosis specific outcomes. J Urol 1996; 156: 1786

266 Manning F A, Harrison M R, Rodeck C H and members of the International Fetal Medicine and Surgery Society. Catheter shunts for fetal hydronephrosis and hydrocephalus. N Engl J Med 1986; 315: 336–340

267 Gembruch U, Hansmann M. Artificial instillation of amniotic fluid as a new technique for the diagnostic evaluation of cases of oligohydramnios. Prenat Diagn 1988; 8: 33–45

268 Nicolini U, Santolaya J, Hubinont C, Fisk N M, Maxwell D, Rodeck C H. Visualization of fetal intra-abdominal organs in second trimester severe oligohydramnios by intraperitoneal infusion. Prenat Diagn 1989; 9: 191–194

269 Romero R, Cullen M, Grannum P et al. Antenatal diagnosis of renal anomalies with ultrasound. III. Bilateral renal agenesis. Am J Obstet Gynecol 1985; 151: 38–43

270 Fisk N M, Ronderos-Dumit D, Soliani A, Nicolini U, Vaughan J I, Rodeck C H. Diagnostic and therapeutic transabdominal amnioinfusion in oligohydramnios. Obstet Gynecol 1991; 78: 270–278

271 Hackelöer B J, Waldenfels H V, Martin K, Hamburg D. Treatment and results of oligohidramnios by instillation of artificial amniotic fluid (150 cases). Presented at the 5th Annual Meeting of the International Fetal Medicine and Surgery Society, Bonn, 1988

272 Quetel T A, Mejides A A, Salman F A, Torres-Rodriguez M M. Amnioinfusion: an aid in the ultrasonic evaluation of severe oligohydramnios in pregnancy. Am J Obstet Gynecol 1992; 167: 333–336

273 Cullen M T, Reece E A, Whetham J, Hobbins J C. Embryoscopy: description and utility of a new technique. Am J Obstet Gynecol 1990; 162: 82–86

274 Rodeck C H. Fetoscopy guided by real time ultrasound for pure fetal blood samples, fetal skin samples and examination of the fetus in utero. Br J Obstet Gynaecol 1980; 87: 449–456

275 Blaas, Eikness S, Souka A, Bakalis S. Diagnosis of fetal abnormalities at the 11–14 week scan. In: Nicolaides K H, Sebire N J, Snijders R J M, eds. The 11–14 week scan. The diagnosis of fetal abnormalities. London: The Parthenon Publishing Group, 1999: 115–141

276 Hobbins J C. The future of first-trimester embryoscopy. Ultrasound Obstet Gynaecol 1996; 8: 3–4

277 Ville Y, Khalil A, Homphray T, Moscoso G. Diagnostic embryoscopy and fetoscopy in the first trimester of pregnancy. Prenat Diagn 1997; 17: 1237–1246

278 Dumez Y, Mandelbort L, Dommergues M. Embryoscopy in continuing pregnancies. In: Proceedings of the Annual Meeting of the International Fetal Medicine and Surgery Society, Evian, France, 1992

279 Reece E A, Rotmensch S, Whetham J, Cullen M, Hobbins J C. Embryoscopy: a closer look at first trimester diagnosis. Obstet Gynecol 1992; 166: 775–780

280 Quintero R A, Abumamad A, Hobbins J C, Mahoney M J. Transabdominal thin gauge embryofetoscopy: a technique for early prenatal diagnosis and its use in the diagnosis of a case of Meckel–Gruber syndrome. Am J Obstet Gynecol 1993; 168: 1552–1557

281 Reece E A, Goldstein I, Chatwani A, Brown R, Homko C, Wiznitzer A. Transabdominal needle embryofetoscopy: a new technique paving the way for early fetal therapy. Obstet Gynecol 1994; 84: 634–636

282 Pennehouat G H, Thebault Y, Ville Y, Madelenat P, Nicolaides K H. First-trimester transabdominal fetoscopy. Lancet 1992; 340: 429

283 Ville Y, Bernard J P, Doumerc S et al. Transabdominal fetoscopy in fetal anomalies diagnosed by ultrasound in the first trimester of pregnancy. Ultrasound Obstet Gynecol 1996; 8: 11–15

284 Reece E A, Whetham J, Rotmensch S, Wiznitzer A. Gaining access to the embryonic–fetal circulation via first trimester endoscopy: a step into the future. Obstet Gynecol 1993; 82: 876–879

285 Dommergues M, Lemerrer M, Couly G, Delezoides A L, Dumez Y. Prenatal diagnosis of cleft lip at 11 menstrual weeks using embryofetoscopy in the van der Woude syndrome. Prenat Diagn 1995; 15: 378–381

286 Quintero R A, Crossland W J, Cotton D B. Effect of endoscopic white light on the developing visual pathway: a histologic, histochemical and behavioural study. Am J Obstet Gynecol 1994; 171: 1142–1148

287 Freda V J, Adamsons K J. Exchange transfusion in utero. Am J Obstet Gynecol 1964; 89: 817–821

288 Asensio S H, Figueroa-Longo J G, Pelegrina I A. Intrauterine exchange transfusion. Am J Obstet Gynecol 1966; 95: 1129–1133

289 Seelen J, van Kessel H, van Leusden H et al. A new method of exchange transfusion in utero. Cannulation of vessels on the fetal side of the human placenta. Am J Obstet Gynecol 1966; 95: 872–876

290 Liley A W. Intrauterine transfusion of foetus in haemolytic disease. BMJ 1963; 2: 1107–1109

291 Bock J E. Intrauterine transfusion in the management of pregnant women with severe rhesus immunization. II Results and discussion. Acta Obstet Gynecol Scand 1976; 53 (Suppl): 29–36

292 Clewell W H, Dunne M G, Johnson M L, Bowes W A. Fetal transfusion with real-time ultrasound guidance. Obstet Gynecol 1981; 57: 516–520

293 Scott J R, Kochenour N K, Larkin R M. Changes in the management of severely Rh-immunized patients. Am J Obstet Gynecol 1984; 149: 3361

294 Harman C R, Manning F A, Bowman J M, Lange I R. Severe Rh disease: poor outcome is not inevitable. Am J Obstet Gynecol 1983; 145: 823–829

295 Rodeck C H, Holman C A, Karnicki J, Kemp J R, Whitmore D N, Austin M A. Direct intravascular blood transfusion by fetoscopy in severe rhesus isoimmunization. Lancet 1981; i: 625–628

296 Rodeck C H, Nicolaides K H, Warsof L S, Fysh W J, Gamsu H R, Kemp J R. The management of severe rhesus isoimmunization by fetoscopic intravascular transfusions. Am J Obstet Gynecol 1984; 150: 769–774

297 Berkowitz R L, Chitkara U, Goldberg J D, Wilkins I, Chervenak F A. Intrauterine transfusion in utero: the percutaneous approach. Am J Obstet Gynecol 1986; 154: 622–627

298 Nicolaides K H, Soothill P W, Rodeck C H, Clewell W H. Rhesus disease: intravascular fetal blood transfusion by cordocentesis. Fetal Ther 1986; 1: 185–192

299 Westgren M, Selbing A, Stragenberg M. Fetal intracardiac transfusion in patients with severe rhesus isoimmunization. BMJ 1988; 296: 885–886

300 Nicolaides K H, Fontanarosa M, Gabbe S G, Rodeck C H. Failure of ultrasonographic parameters to detect the severity of fetal anaemia in rhesus isoimmunization. Am J Obstet Gynecol 1988; 158: 920–926

301 Chitkara U, Wilkins I, Lynch L, Mehalek K, Berkowitz R L. The role of sonography in assessing severity of fetal anaemia in Rh- and Kell-isoimmunized pregnancies. Obstet Gynecol 1988; 71: 393–398

302 Grannum P A T, Copel J A. Prevention of Rh isoimmunization and treatment of the compromised fetus. Semin Perinatol 1988; 12: 324–335

303 Berkowitz R L, Chitkara U, Wilkins I A, Lynch L, Plosker H, Bernstein H H. Intravascular monitoring and management of erythroblastosis fetalis. Am J Obstet Gynecol 1988; 158: 783–795

304 Ronkin S, Chayen B, Wapner R J et al. Intravascular exchange and bolus transfusion in the severely isoimmunized fetus. Am J Obstet Gynecol 1989; 160: 407–411

305 Nicolini U, Rodeck C H. A proposed scheme for planning intrauterine transfusion in patients with severe Rh-immunization. J Obstet Gynecol 1988; 9: 162–163

306 Nicolini U, Santolaya J, Fisk N M et al. Changes in fetal acid–base status during intravascular transfusion. Arch Dis Child 1988; 63: 710–714

307 Bowman J M. Rh erythroblastosis. Semin Haematol 1975; 12: 189–207

308 Harman C R, Manning F A, Bowman J M, Lange I R, Menticoglou S M. Use of intravascular transfusion to treat hydrops fetalis in the moribund fetus. Can Med Assoc J 1988; 138: 827–830

309 Nicolini U, Kochenour N K, Greco P, Letsky E, Rodeck C H. When to perform the next intra-uterine transfusion in patients with Rh allo-immunization: combined intravascular and intraperitoneal transfusion allows longer intervals. Fetal Ther 1989; 4: 14–20

310 Nicolaides K H, Rodeck C H. Rhesus disease: the model for fetal therapy. Br J Hosp Med 1985; 34: 141–148

311 Urbaniak S J. Rh(D) haemolytic disease of the newborn: the changing scene. BMJ 1985; 291: 4–6

312 Clarke C A, Whitfield A G W, Mollison P L. Death from Rh haemolytic disease in England and Wales in 1984 and 1985. BMJ 1987; 294: 1001

313 Tovey L A D. Haemolytic disease of the newborn – the changing scene. Br J Obstet Gynaecol 1986; 93: 960–966

314 Caine M E, Mueller-Heubach M D. Kell sensitisation in pregnancy. Am J Obstet Gynecol 1986; 154: 85–90

315 Vaughan J I, Warwick R, Letsky E, Nicolini U, Rodeck C H, Fisk N M. Erythropoietic suppression in fetal anaemia because of Kell alloimmunisation. Am J Obstet Gynecol 1994; 171: 247–252

316 Vaughan J I, Manning M, Warwick R M, Letsky E A, Murray N A, Roberts I A G. Inhibition of erythroid progenitor cells by anti-Kell antibodies in fetal alloimmune anemia. N Engl J Med 1998; 338: 798–803

317 Avent N D, Martin P G. Kell typing by allele-specific PCR (ASP). Br J Haematol 1996; 93: 728–730

318 Nicolini U, Rodeck C H, Kochenour N K et al. In-utero platelet transfusion for alloimmune thrombocytopenia. Lancet 1988; ii: 506

319 Schwarz T F, Roggendorf M, Hottentrager B et al. Human parvovirus B19 infection in pregnancy. Lancet 1988; ii: 566–567

320 Gray E S, Davidson R J L, Anand A. Human parvovirus and fetal anaemia. Lancet 1987; ii: 1144

321 Peters M T, Nicolaides K H. Cordocentesis for the diagnosis and treatment of human fetal parvovirus infection. Obstet Gynecol 1990; 75: 501–504

322 Cardwell M S. Successful treatment of hydrops fetalis by feto-maternal haemorrhage: a case report. Am J Obstet Gynecol 1988; 158: 131–132

323 Fischer R L, Kuhlman K, Grover J, Montgomery O, Wapner R J. Chronic, massive fetomaternal haemorrhage treated with repeated fetal intravascular transfusions. Am J Obstet Gynecol 1990; 162: 203–204

324 Tannirandorn Y, Nicolini U, Nicolaidis P, Nasrat H, Letsky E, Rodeck C H. Intrauterine death due to fetomaternal haemorrhage despite successful treatment of fetal anaemia. J Perinat Med 1990; 18: 233–235

325 Harrison M R, Filly R A, Golbus M S et al. Fetal treatment 1982. N Engl J Med 1982; 306: 1651–1652

326 Albar H, Manning F A, Harman C R. Treatment of urinary tract and CNS obstruction. In: Harman C R, ed. Invasive fetal testing and treatment. Boston: Blackwell Scientific, 1995: 259–314

327 Golbus M S, Harrison M R, Filly R A, Callen P W, Katz M. In utero treatment of urinary tract obstruction. Am J Obstet Gynecol 1982; 142: 383–388

328 Bernaschek G, Deutinger J, Hansmann M, Bald R, Holzgreve W, Bollman R. Feto-amniotic stunting – report of the experience of four European centres. Prenat Diagn 1994; 14: 821–823

329 Quintero R A, Hume R, Smith C et al. Percutaneous fetal cystoscopy and endoscopic fulguration of posterior urethral valves Am J Obstet Gyecol 1995; 172: 206–209

330 Longaker M T, Laberge J-M, Dansereau J et al. Primary fetal hydrothorax: natural history and management. J Pediatr Surg 1989; 24: 573–576

331 Vaughan J I, Fisk N M, Rodeck C H. Fetal pleural effusions. In: Harman C R, ed. Invasive fetal testing and treatment. Boston: Blackwell Scientific, 1995: 219–239

332 Seeds J W, Bowes W A. Results of treatment of severe fetal hydrothorax with bilateral pleuroamniotic catheters. Obstet Gynecol 1986; 68: 577–580

333 Nicolaides K H, Azar G B. Thoraco-amniotic shunting. Fetal Diagn Ther 1990; 5: 153–164

334 Rodeck C H, Fisk N M, Fraser D I, Nicolini U. Long-term in utero drainage of fetal hydrothorax. N Engl J Med 1989; 319: 1135–1138

335 Weber A M, Philipson E H. Fetal pleural effusion: a review and meta-analysis for prognostic indicators. Obstet Gynecol 1992; 79: 281–286

336 Ronderos-Dumit D, Nicolini U, Vaughan J, Fisk N M, Chamberlain P F, Rodeck C H. Uterine–peritoneal uterine leakage: an unusual complication of intrauterine shunting. Obstet Gynecol 1991; 78: 913–915

337 Phelen J P, Martin G I. Polyhydramnios: fetal and neonatal implications. Clin Perinatol 1989; 16: 987–994

338 Chamberlain P F, Manning F A, Morrison I, Harman C R, Lange I R. Ultrasound evaluation of amniotic fluid. II. The relationship of increased amniotic fluid volume to perinatal outcome. Am J Obstet Gynecol 1984; 150: 250–254

339 Fisk N M, Tannirandorn Y, Nicolini U, Talbert D G, Rodeck C H. Amniotic pressure in disorders of amniotic fluid volume. Obstet Gynecol 1990; 76: 210–214

340 Moise K J, Huhta J C, Sharif D S et al. Indomethacin in the treatment of preterm labour: effects on the fetal ductus arteriosus. N Engl J Med 1988; 319: 307–313

341 Cantor B, Tyler T, Nelson R, Stein G H. Oligohydramnios and transient neonatal anuria. A possible complication of the maternal use of prostaglandin synthetase inhibitors. J Reprod Med 1980; 24: 220

342 Elliot J P, Urig M A, Clewell W H. Aggressive therapeutic amniocentesis for treatment of twin–twin transfusion syndrome. Obstet Gynecol 1991; 77: 537–540

343 Saunders N J, Snijders R J, Nicolaides K H. Therapeutic amniocentesis in twin–twin transfusion syndrome appearing in the second trimester of pregnancy. Am J Obstet Gynecol 1992; 166: 820–824

344 Mari G, Abuhamad A, Verpairojkit B et al. Treatment of twin–twin transfusion syndrome. Is the therapeutic amniocentesis still a good management option? SPO Abstracts. Am J Obstet Gynecol 1996; 174: 487

345 Reisner D P, Mahoney B S, Petty C N et al. Stuck twin syndrome: outcome in 37 consecutive cases. Am J Obstet Gynecol 1993; 169: 991–995

346 Zosmer N, Bajoria R, Weiner E, Fisk N. Clinical and echographic features of in utero cardiac dysfunction in the recipient twin in twin-to-twin transfusion syndrome. Br Heart J 1994; 72: 74–79

347 Elliott J P, Sawyer A T, Radin T G, Strong R E. Large volume therapeutic amniocentesis in the treatment of hydramnios. Obstet Gynecol 1994; 84: 1025–1027

348 Evans M I, Littmen L, Richter R, Richter K, Hume R F. Selective reduction for multifetal pregnancy. Early opinions revisited. J Reprod Med 1997; 42: 771–777

349 Berkowitz R L, Lynch L, Stone J, Alvarez M. The current status of multifetal pregnancy reduction. Am J Obstet Gynecol 1996; 174: 1265–1272

350 Committee on Ethics. Multifetal pregnancy reduction and selective fetal termination. Washington: American College of Obstetricians and Gynecologists 191: 1–3, ACOG Committee Opinion No. 94

351 Evans M I, Dommergues M, Wapner R J et al. International collaborative experience of 1789 patients having multifetal pregnancy reduction: a plateauing of risks and outcomes. J Soc Gynecol Invest 1996; 3: 23–26

352 Evans M I, Dommergues M, Wapner R J et al. Efficacy of transabdominal multifetal pregnancy reduction: collaborative experience among the world's largest centers. Obstet Gynecol 1993; 82: 61–66

353 Evans M I, Dommergues M, Timor-Tritsch I E et al. Transabdominal versus transcervical and transvaginal multifetal pregnancy reduction: international collaborative experience of more than one thousand cases. Am J Obstet Gynecol 1994; 170: 902–909

354 Dumez Y, Oury J F. Method for first trimester selective abortion in multiple pregnancy. Contrib Gynecol Obstet 1986; 15: 50–53

355 Timor-Tritsch I E, Peisner D B, Monteagudo M et al. Multifetal pregnancy reduction by transvaginal puncture: evaluation of the technique used in 134 cases. Am J Obstet Gynecol 1993; 168: 799–804

356 Sebire N J, D'Ercole C, Sepulveda W, Hughes K, Nicolaides K H. Effects of embryreduction from trichorionic triplets to twins. Br J Obstet Gynaecol 1997; 104: 1201–1203

357 Macones G A, Schemmer G, Pritts E, Weinblatt V, Wapner R J. Multifetal reduction of triplets to twins improves perinatal outcome. Am J Obstet Gynecol 1993; 169: 982–986

358 Mc Lean L K, Evans M I, Carpenter R J et al. Genetic amniocentesis (AMN) following multifetal pregnancy reduction (MFPR) does not increase the risk of pregnancy loss. Prenat Diagn 1998; 18: 186–188

359 Depp R, Macones G A, Rosenn M F, Turzo E, Wapner R J, Weinblatt V J. Multifetal pregnancy reduction: evaluation of fetal growth in the remaining twins. Am J Obstet Gynecol 1996; 174: 1233–1240

360 Evans M I, Fletcher J C, Rodeck C H. Ethical problems in multiple gestations: selective termination. In: Evans M I, Dixler A O, Fletcher J C, Schulman J D, eds. Fetal diagnosis and therapy. Philadelphia: JB Lippincott, 1989: 266

361 Aberg A, Mitelman F, Cantz M, Gehler J. Cardiac puncture of fetus with Hurler's disease avoiding abortion of unaffected co-twin. Lancet 1978; ii: 990–991

362 Evans M I, Goldberg J D, Dommergues M et al. Efficacy of second trimester selective termination for abnormalities: international collaborative experience among the world's largest centres. Am J Obstet Gynecol 1994; 171: 90–94

363 Golbus M S, Cunningham N, Goldberg J D, Anderson R, Filly R, Callen P. Selective termination in multiple gestations. Am J Med Genet 1988; 31: 339–348

364 Bajoria R, Kingdom J. The case for routine determination of chorionicity and zygosity in multiple pregnancy. Prenat Diagn 1997; 17: 1207–1225

365 Overton T, Leighton A, Bennett P. Polymerase chain reaction and its use in obstetrics. Fetal Maternal Med Rev 1995; 7: 159–173

366 Nicolini U. Invasive testing and opportunities for therapy in multiple pregnancy. In: Harman C R, ed. Invasive fetal testing and treatment. Boston: Blackwell Scientific, 1995: 315–338

367 Berkowitz R L, Stone J L, Eddleman K A. One hundred consecutive cases of selective termination of an abnormal fetus in a multiple gestation. Obstet Gynecol 1997; 90: 606–610

368 Dommergues M, Mandelbrot L, Delezoide A-L et al. Twin–to–twin transfusion syndrome: selective fetocide by embolization of the hydropic fetus. Fetal Diagn Ther 1995; 10: 26–31

369 Denbow M L, Battin M R, Kyle P M, Fogliani R, Johnson P, Fisk N M. Selective termination by intrahepatic vein alcohol injection of a monochorionic twin pregnancy discordant for fetal abnormality. Br J Obstet Gynecol 1997; 104: 626–627

370 Quintero R A, Romero R, Reich H et al. In utero percutaneous cord ligation in the management of complicated monochorionic multiple gestations. Ultrasound Obstet Gynecol 1996; 8: 16–22

371 Crombleholme T M, Robertson F, Marx G, Yarnell R, D'Alton M E. Fetoscopic cord ligation to prevent neurological injury in monozygous twins. Lancet 1996; 348: 191

372 Lemery D J, Vanlieferinghen P, Gasq M et al. Fetal umbilical cord ligation under ultrasonic guidance. Ultrasound Obstet Gynecol 1994; 4: 399–401

373 Hecher K, Hackeloer B J, Ville Y. Umbilical cord coagulation by operative microendoscopy at 16 weeks' gestation in an acardiac twin. Ultrasound Obstet Gynecol 1997; 10: 130–132

374 Sebire N J, Sepulveda W, Hughes K S, Noble P, Nicolaides K H. Management of twin pregnancies discordant for anencephaly. Br J Obstet Gynaecol 1997; 104: 16–19

375 Lynch L, Berkowitz R L, Stone J, Alvarez M, Lapinski R. Preterm delivery after selective delivery in twin pregnancies. Obstet Gynecol 1996; 87: 366–369

376 Luks F I, Deprest J. Endoscopic fetal surgery: a new alternative? [Editorial]. Eur J Obstet Gynecol Reprod Biol 1993; 52: 1–3

377 Deprest J A, Lerut T E, Vandenberghe K. Operative fetoscopy: new perspective in fetal therapy? Prenat Diagn 1997; 17: 1247–1260

378 Albanese C T, Harrison M R. Surgical treatment for fetal disease. The state of the art. Ann NY Acad Sci 1998; 18: 74–85

379 De Lia J E, Cruikshank D P, Keye W R. Fetoscopic neodymium: YAG laser occlusion of placental vessels in severe twin–twin transfusion syndrome. Obstet Gynecol 1990; 75: 1046–1053

380 Ville Y, Hecher K, Gagnon A, Sebire N, Hyett J, Nicolaides K. Endoscopic laser coagulation in the management of severe twin–to–twin transfusion syndrome. Br J Obstet Gynaecol 1998; 105: 446–453

381 Quintero R A, Morales W J, Phillips J, Kalter C S, Angel J L. In utero lysis of amniotic bands. Ultrasound Obstet Gynecol 1997; 10: 316–320

382 VanderWall K J, Skarsgard E D, Filly R A, Eckert J, Harrison M R. Fetendo-clip: a fetal endoscopic clip procedure in a human fetus. J Pediatr Surg 1997; 32: 970–972

383 MacMahon R A, Renou P M M, Shekelton P A, Paterson P J. In utero cystotomy. Lancet 1992; 340: 234

384 Fortunato S J, Lombardi S J, Daniell J F et al. Intra-uterine laser ablation of a fetal CCAM with hydrops [abstract]. Am J Obstet Gynecol 1997; 176: S84

385 Hecher K, Hackeloer B-J. Intra-uterine endoscopic laser surgery for fetal sacrococcygeal teratoma. Lancet 1996; 347: 470

386 Bruner J P, Richards W O, Tulipan N B, Arney T L, Zaner R M. Endoscopic coverage of fetal myelomeningocele in utero. Presented at the 16th Annual Meeting of the International Fetal Medicine and Surgery Society, 1–5 June, Alyeska Resort, Alaska, USA, 1997

387 Trespidi L, Bischetto C, Caravelli E, Villa L, Kustermann A, Nicolini U. Serial amniocentesis in the management of twin–twin transfusion syndrome: when is it valuable? Fetal Diagn Ther 1997; 12: 15–20

388 Moore T R, Gale S, Bernischke K. Perinatal outcome of forty-nine pregnancies complicated by acardiac twinning. Am J Obstet Gynecol 1990; 163: 907–912

389 Ville Y, Hyett J A, Vandenbussche F, Nicolaides K H. Endoscopic laser coagulation of umbilical cord vessels in twin reversed arterial perfusion sequence. Ultrasound Obstet Gynecol 1994; 4: 396–398

390 Quintero R A, Reich H, Romero R, Johnson M P, Goncalves L, Evans M I. In utero endoscopic devascularization of a large chorioangioma. Ultrasound Obstet Gynecol 1996; 8: 48–52

391 Mychaliska G, Graf J, Filly R et al. Endoscopic fetal tracheal occlusion for treatment of CDH: technical innovations and clinical outcomes. Presented at the 16th Annual Meeting of the International Fetal Medicine and Surgery Society, 1–5 June, Alyeska Resort, Alaska, USA, 1997

Appendix; charts of fetal size

Lyn S Chitty and Douglas G Altman

Introduction

There are hundreds of published papers presenting charts (standards) of fetal size ([1,2] for references and review). Unfortunately, many of these have serious weaknesses in design or statistical analysis, or both. Some years ago the working group of the British Medical Ultrasound Society (BMUS) had difficulty identifying even one appropriate study for some fetal measurements.[3]

In this Appendix we consider the appropriate design and analysis of studies to derive reference centiles for fetal size. We describe a study that meets these requirements and present centile charts for various fetal measurements and dating charts. We also compare these new charts with those recommended in the BMUS Report.[3] Further details may be found in Altman and Chitty[4,5] and Royston and Wright.[6]

Study design

Selection of the sample

As with any research the choice of an appropriate sample is of great importance. A serious weakness of many published studies is that they use routinely collected data, so that multiple observations on the same fetus are included. However, it is likely that such fetuses are atypical, as multiple measurements are not taken unless there is some clinical concern. The best approach is to collect data expressly for the purpose of developing a reference range. The date of measurement for each woman can be chosen at random, to give about the same number at each week of gestation. Data can be collected at the time of a routine second-trimester scan, provided there is no selection for this examination, but each woman should be included only once. Later in pregnancy data should be collected only when examinations are performed specifically for the purpose of the study. Data collected from examinations performed later in pregnancy for some other clinical indication (e.g. ?small-for-dates) should not be included as they may bias the results. Some further sampling will be necessary to obtain sufficient numbers around term, because some women will deliver before the appointed ultrasound date.

A second problem relates to exclusions. Reference data should relate to normal fetuses: it is sensible to exclude data from fetuses subsequently shown to have had a serious congenital abnormality. The exclusion of neonatal deaths is questionable except for this reason. It may also be appropriate to exclude those with a condition that affects growth, such as maternal diabetes. With these exceptions it is wrong to make use of information not available at the time of the ultrasound measurement, most notably birthweight. It is reasonable, though, to exclude on the basis of data that are available when the measure-

ment is taken, but we favour as unselected a group as possible. We cannot see the justification for excluding smokers, for example.

Size of sample

It is not as easy to specify the appropriate sample size as, say, for a controlled trial. It should be remembered that attention is concentrated on the tails of the distribution – i.e. the extreme values – and so a large sample is necessary to get a good fix on the placing of, say, the 5th and 95th centiles. Without going into detail, it seems clear that several hundred observations are required. This issue is discussed further elsewhere.[6,7] The reference centiles should be calculated from single observations if that is the usual clinical practice. It is wrong to use the average of two or more measurements.

Analysis

There are two basic approaches to the calculation of reference centiles. We will illustrate these by considering the 5th and 95th centiles. The **non-parametric** approach involves calculating the observed 5th and 95th centiles at each week of gestation and joining these values. The resulting lines will not be smooth, although smooth curves can be obtained. The problem with this approach is that one needs a lot of data at each week of gestation to get a reasonable estimate of extreme centiles: at least 100 observations and preferably more. The total sample size would thus need to be several thousand. For this reason we think that this is not a viable method.

In the **parametric** approach we derive the 5th and 95th centiles as mean ± 1.645 SD, the value of 1.645 coming from the theoretical Normal distribution. The method is based on the strong assumption that at each gestational age the data have a Normal distribution. Most published centiles are constructed in this way, but most studies have deficiencies in the analysis.

Reference centiles should have the following properties:

1 they should change smoothly with gestation,
2 they should be a good fit to the data,
3 the statistical model should be as simple as is compatible with (1) and (2).

The most common problems with published reference centiles are:

1 there is no explanation of the statistical method used,
2 the centiles do not change smoothly across gestation,
3 there is no assessment of whether the data have a (nearly) Normal distribution,
4 there is no verification that the centiles are a good fit to the data,

5 the authors have failed to take account of changes in variability with gestation.

The last is an extremely common error. It has major consequences, because it leads to centiles that are too far apart early in pregnancy and too close later on. Most papers do not include a scatter diagram of the data with the centiles superimposed, and therefore the deficiencies may not be readily apparent.

When these aspects are considered in conjunction with design weaknesses it is clear that very few published studies can be considered statistically acceptable. This includes studies whose data are included in the BMUS report.[3]

Recommended approach to analysis

We will illustrate the suggested approach to the derivation of centiles by the analysis of 450 measurements of foot length (Fig. A1). This analysis follows the recommendations of Altman and Royston,[6–8] who give detailed explanations and discussion.

Step 1 – model the mean

A polynomial regression model is fitted to the data – a quadratic or cubic curve will usually give a reasonable fit. The 'linear–cubic' model seems to work well for fetal size data; this is given by

$$Y = b_0 + b_1 X + b_2 X^3$$

where X is gestational age and Y is the measurement. The model chosen is the simplest that gives a good fit to the data (see below). Figure A1 shows the linear–cubic model fitted to the foot measurements.

Step 2 – obtain residuals

Calculate the differences between the observed values and the fitted line (known as residuals). A plot of these values against gestational age will show how the variability changes with gestation.

Step 3 – check the distribution

Assess these for normality using a Normal plot, and perhaps also a formal test. If not Normal the data may require transformation.

Step 4 – model the variability

The standard deviation (SD) of the residuals is modelled as a function of gestation. For fetal size linear or quadratic regression is usually adequate. We have used the method described by Altman.[8] The values ±1.645 SD can be superimposed on the residual plot to see how well the SD has been modelled (Fig. A2). The numbers above and below the range should be close to the expected proportions. Here 4% of the observations lie above the 95th centile and 6% below the 5th centile.

Step 5 – calculate standard deviation scores

Calculate for each observation a standard deviation score (SDS) (also called a standardised residual) as

SDS = (observed value – fitted mean)/fitted SD.

Step 6 – check the distribution

Assess the SDSs for normality, as in step 3. Normally distributed data should lie on a straight line. Figure A3 shows the Normal plot for the foot measurements; and the associated Shapiro–Francia W′ test gives $P = 0.6$. Together these show that the model is a good fit to the data. Non-normality would indicate the need to transform the data.

Step 7 – derive the centiles

The required centiles are calculated and superimposed on a scatter diagram of the observations as a final check of the fit. Figure A4 shows the 5th, 50th and 95th centiles for

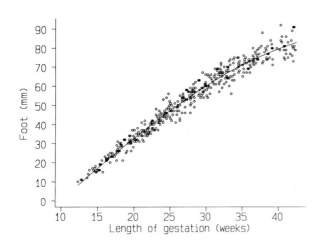

Fig. A1 450 measurements of foot length with fitted curve describing the mean.

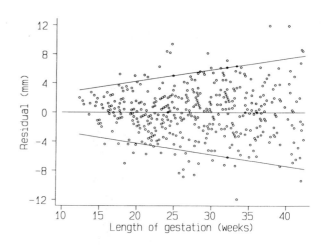

Fig. A2 Residuals from model describing mean with fitted 5th and 95th centiles.

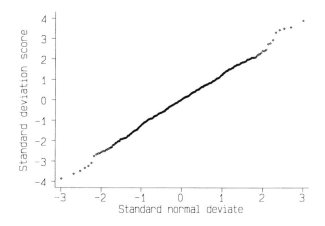

Fig. A3 Normal plot of standard deviation scores.

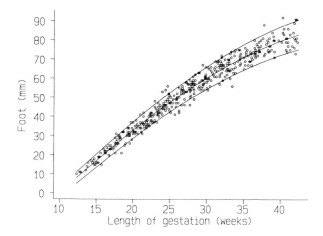

Fig. A4 Foot length measurements with fitted 5th, 50th and 95th centiles.

the foot measurements. The 5th and 95th centiles were obtained as mean ±1.645 SD. If a transformation has been used the mean and SD, and hence the centiles, are obtained in the transformed scale and need to be back-transformed to the original scale.

The approach described above meets all the previously stated requirements. A big advantage is that, because there are regression equations for the mean and SD, any observation can be converted into a standard deviation score. Thus we can obtain a precise centile for any measurement by reference to a table of the standard Normal distribution. Further, we can compare subgroups of fetuses or compare a new group with the reference group using simple *t* tests. For example, we can compare European and Afro-Caribbean groups.

The above method was used to produce the centile charts (Charts 1–22). For a few variables a transformation of the data was necessary.

Dating charts

There are many reports of the value of ultrasound in the prediction of gestational age. The literature has been comprehensibly reviewed by Geirsson.[9] The measurements found to be of most value in the second trimester are the biparietal diameter (BPD), femur length and head circumference. In the first trimester the crown–rump length is considered to be the most valuable measurement.[10] Charts for predicting gestational age from fetal size are produced in a similar fashion, except that they are based on regression of gestational age on fetal size.[3] Again, simple polynomial regression should suffice.

The dating charts[11] (Charts 23–29) were obtained using the same general approach as for the charts of fetal size. Only data up to approximately 30 weeks of gestation were included, i.e. BPD < 76 mm, head circumference < 281 mm and femur length < 56 mm. In each case it was found necessary to apply a logarithmic transformation to gestational age.

Construction of new charts of fetal size

Patient selection and recruitment

All the patients included in this study[11] were scanned by one of three operators using an Hitachi EUB-340 in the ultrasound department at King's College Hospital. As this was a cross-sectional study each fetus was measured once only between 12 and 42 weeks, for the purposes of the study. Women were recruited in one of four ways:

1 women scanned between 12 and 17 weeks were recruited prospectively at the time of booking for prenatal care and asked to attend for one extra examination before their routine second-trimester scan,

2 data were collected from women between 18 and 23 weeks at the time of a routine scan,

3 women were recruited prospectively in the ultrasound clinic at the time of their routine examination and asked to return for an extra scan at a randomly allocated gestation from 23 weeks,

4 as the study progressed it became clear that many of the women asked to return at 37 weeks or later had delivered prior to the study scan. Women were therefore recruited and studied between 37 and 42 weeks at the time of their visit to the antenatal clinic.

Only western European and Afro-Caribbean racial groups were included. All subjects had a known last menstrual period and the ultrasound and menstrual ages at 18–20 weeks agreed to within 10 days. Exclusion criteria were:

1 maternal disease or medication which was likely to affect the growth of the fetus (diabetes mellitus, renal disease, hypertension requiring treatment etc.),

2   multiple pregnancies,
3   the presence of a fetal malformation,
4   cases where the neonate was found to have a significant congenital malformation, abnormal karyotype, or other disease at birth.

A total of 669 fetuses were examined for the purpose of the study. There were two exclusions: one neonate who was scanned at 13 weeks gestation had trisomy 21; the other was scanned at 32 weeks, at which time marked asymmetrical intra-uterine growth retardation was noted. At birth the infant had dysmorphic features compatible with trisomy 18, a diagnosis confirmed by karyotyping.

We aimed to obtain 20 measurements for each variable for each week of pregnancy from 12 until 42 weeks. It was not possible to obtain every measurement from each fetus because of fetal position, and so this objective was not met in all cases. Only one measurement was taken of each variable.

Measurements

The BPD was measured in the axial plane at the level where the continuous midline echo is broken by the septum pellucidum cavum in the anterior third (see Ch. 9, Fig. 9.5 and Ch. 10, Fig. 10.2). The measurements were made from the proximal echo of the fetal skull to the distal side of the border deep to the ultrasound beam (outer–outer), or from the proximal edge to the proximal edge of the deep border (outer–inner). The head circumference was measured at the same level. The abdominal circumference was measured on a transverse section through the fetal abdomen, which was as close as possible to a circle and at a level where the umbilical vein was seen in the anterior third and the stomach was visualised in the same plane (see Ch. 10, Fig. 10.5). The head and abdominal circumferences were measured both directly by tracing around the perimeter and by derivation from the measurement of the diameters (OFD and BPD outer–outer for the head, and transverse and anteroposterior diameters for the abdomen).

All long bones (radius, ulna, humerus, tibia, fibula and femur) were measured in a plane such that the bone was orthogonal to the ultrasound beam. Care was taken to ensure that the full length of the bone was visualised and the view was not obscured by shadowing from adjacent bony parts. The radius and ulna, tibia and fibula were measured independently. The foot was measured in the plantar view, the measurement being made from the heel to the end of the longest toe.

The kidneys were measured in three planes. The renal length was measured from the upper to the lower pole. The anteroposterior and transverse diameters were both measured in a transverse section through the fetal abdomen. The level taken was at the height of the renal pelvis if visible or, if not, in a plane where the kidney

appeared largest. It was not always possible to visualise both kidneys well enough to obtain accurate measurements. We have therefore included measurements of only one kidney per fetus in the construction of the kidney size charts.

The size charts derived from these measurements, shown on pages 616–688, refer to exact gestational age. Half a week should be added if age is recorded in completed weeks. We have also derived a head circumference/abdominal circumference (HC/AC) ratio chart for use in the assessment of fetal growth, as described by Campbell and Thoms.[12]

These charts are based on cross-sectional data and should be used only for assessing size. Although serial measurements may show increasing or decreasing centiles for a fetus over time, these charts are not suitable for assessing how unusual such changes are.

Comparison with other published data

We have compared the data collected in the study described above with the published data selected by the BMUS working party on fetal biometry.[3]

Biparietal diameter

The data on the measurement of the BPD collected by Hadlock *et al.*[13] are only slightly different from our data[14] (Fig. A5), with the main difference occurring early in the second trimester, when the 50th centile derived from Hadlock's data is greater than ours. This may be a reflection of the very small numbers in the Hadlock study at these gestations: 2 at 12, 3 at 13 and 4 at 14 weeks, compared to

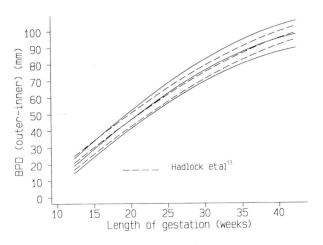

Fig. A5 Comparison of the authors' biparietal diameter chart with that of Hadlock *et al.*[13]

10, 18 and 18, respectively, in our study. Hadlock's curves show much tighter centiles, probably because they unreasonably excluded all fetuses with either head or abdominal circumference outside mean ± 2SD.

Head circumference

We compared the head circumference data from the same group[15] with our data.[14] The plane used for measurement was the same in both studies. As they used direct measurement around the outer perimeter of the calvarium we have compared their data with our data obtained by direct measurement (Fig. A6). The 50th centile derived from the Hadlock data shows a slightly greater decrease towards term. There are marked differences in the 5th and 95th centiles because of Hadlock's failure to take into account the increase in variability with increasing gestation.

Measurement technique is important, as we have found that there is a small but constant difference between the centiles derived from the data obtained by direct measurement around the perimeter of the head circumference and those obtained by derivation from the diameters. The latter are about 1.5% less across all gestations than the direct measurement.

Abdominal circumference

Comparison of our abdominal circumference data[16] with those from Hadlock's group[17] shows that there is no difference between the two 50th centiles (Fig. A7). As with the other studies, failure to model the standard deviation results in Hadlock's centiles being wider apart in early pregnancy and much narrower towards term. Deter *et al.*[18] do take the increasing variation into account, and the separation between their centiles is very similar to ours (Fig. A8). They used a straight-line regression model, and

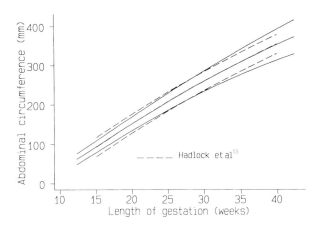

Fig. A7 Comparison of the authors' abdominal circumference (directly measured) chart with that of Hadlock *et al.*[17]

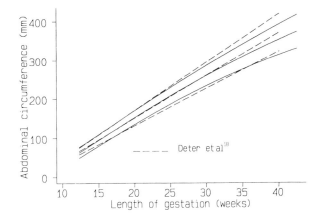

Fig. A8 Comparison of the authors' abdominal circumference (directly measured) chart with that of Deter *et al.*[18]

theretore their data do not show the customary decrease in abdominal circumference towards term seen in both our data and those reported by Hadlock *et al.*[17]

Technique is also important in the measurement of the abdominal circumference. The value derived from the measurement of the diameters is about 3.5% smaller than that obtained by direct measurement at all gestations. Jeanty *et al.*[19] derived their data from measurement of the abdominal diameters, and so we have compared their data with ours obtained using the same technique (Fig. A9). Jeanty *et al.* excluded fetuses who were below the 3rd centile for birthweight. If these babies were structurally normal we do not consider this to be a reasonable exclusion criterion. However, it does not account for the unusually marked fall in circumference from 30 weeks seen in their data. Difference in study design (i.e. longitudinal rather than cross-sectional) is unlikely to be the cause, as this fall is seen in both Jeanty's longitudinal and cross-sectional curves.

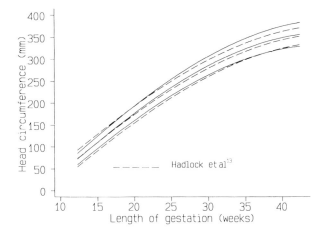

Fig. A6 Comparison of the authors' head circumference (directly measured) chart with that of Hadlock *et al.*[15]

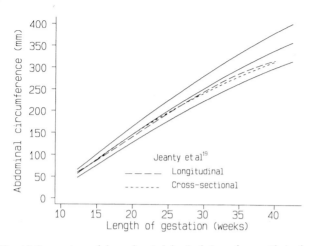

Fig. A9 Comparison of the authors' abdominal circumference (derived from the measurement of the abdominal diameters) chart with the cross-sectional and longitudinal data of Jeanty *et al.*[19]

HC/AC ratio

We have compared our HC/AC chart with that of Campbell and Thoms[12] (Fig. A10). Although Campbell and Thoms did not apply any mathematical smoothing, the two data sets appear similar overall.

Femur

The last comparison is that of our femur length chart,[20] which we have compared with the data collected by Warda *et al.*[21] There is a minimal difference in the 50th centiles (Fig. A11). Warda's derived line is straighter than ours. It is noteworthy that the authors state that all examinations in their study were performed because of a clinical indication unrelated to the study. Warda *et al.* modelled the standard deviation as a constant percentage of the mean, resulting in

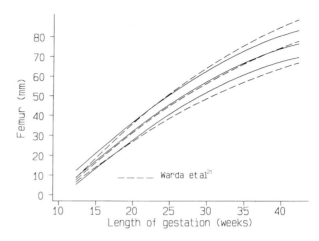

Fig. A11 Comparison of the authors' femur length chart with that of Warda *et al.*[21]

a very narrow separation earlier in pregnancy and a much wider separation at term.

Centile charts

The tables and charts attributed to Chitty *et al.* (or Chitty and Altman) in the following pages show 5th, 50th and 95th centiles for each measurement by exact gestational age. Dating charts, constructed using the same data,[5] are shown on pages 660–673 and give the best estimate of gestation with a 95% prediction interval. We did not study fetuses in the first trimester and so have included a dating chart of crown–rump length using the data from Robinson and Fleming.[10] We also include charts derived from other data sets. In some cases ideal study design has not been achieved. In these cases we have tried to include charts from studies with methodologies as close as possible to the optimum. Where appropriate we have added brief comments about methodological problems. For some measurements, because of inadequate documentation in published papers, we have been unable to produce suitable charts and tables, although some data exist in the literature.

Acknowledgements

LSC was supported by a Medical Research Council Training Fellowship. Thanks are due to Trish Chudleigh and Annabel Henderson for their help in scanning the fetuses included in the study described here.

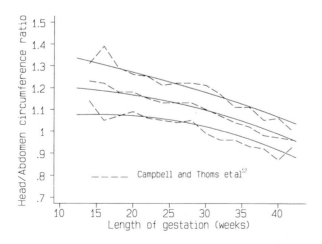

Fig. A10 Comparison of the authors' head:abdominal circumference ratio chart with that of Campbell and Thoms.[12]

REFERENCES

1 Deter R L, Harrist R B, Birnholz J C, Hadlock F P. Quantitative obstetrical ultrasonography. New York: John Wiley, 1986

2 Kurtz A B, Goldberg B B. Obstetrical measurements in ultrasound. A reference manual. New York: Mosby Year Book, 1988

3 British Medical Ultrasound Society Fetal Measurements Working Party Report. Clinical applications of ultrasonic fetal measurements. London: British Institute of Radiology 1990

4 Altman D G, Chitty L S. Design and analysis of studies to derive charts of fetal size. Ultrasound Obstet Gynecol 1993; 3: 378–384

5 Altman D G, Chitty L S. New charts for ultrasound dating of pregnancy. Ultrasound Obstet Gynecol 1997; 10: 1–18

6 Royston P, Wright E M. How to construct 'normal ranges' for fetal variables. Ultrasound Obstet Gynecol 1998; 11: 30–38

7 Royston J P. Constructing time-specific reference ranges. Stat Med 1991; 10: 675–690

8 Altman D G. Construction of age-related reference centiles using absolute residuals. Stat Med 1993; 12: 917–924

9 Geirsson R T. Ultrasound instead of last menstrual period as the basis of gestational age assignment. Ultrasound Obstet Gynecol 1991; 1: 212–219

10 Robinson H P, Fleming J E E. A critical evaluation of sonar crown–rump length measurements. Br J Obstet Gynaecol 1982; 89: 926–930

11 Altman D G, Chitty L S. Charts of fetal size: 1. Methodology. Br J Obstet Gynaecol 1994; 101: 29–34

12 Campbell S, Thoms A. Ultrasound measurement of the fetal head to abdominal circumference ratio in the assessment of growth retardation. Br J Obstet Gynaecol 1977; 84: 165–174

13 Hadlock F P, Deter R L, Harrist R B, Parks K. Fetal biparietal diameter: a critical re-evaluation of the relation to menstrual age by means of real-time ultrasound. J Ultrasound Med 1982; 1: 97–104

14 Chitty L S, Altman D G, Henderson A, Campbell S. Charts of fetal size: 2. Head measurements: Br J Obstet Gynaecol 1994; 101: 35–43

15 Hadlock F P, Deter R L, Harrist R B, Park S K. Fetal head circumference: relation to menstrual age. AJR 1982; 138: 649–653

16 Chitty L S, Altman D G, Henderson A, Campbell S. Charts of fetal size: 3. Abdominal circumference. Br J Obstet Gynaecol 1994; 101: 125–131

17 Hadlock F P, Deter R L, Harrist R B, Park S K. Fetal abdominal circumference as a predictor of menstrual age. AJR 1982; 139: 367–370

18 Deter R L, Harrist R B, Hadlock F P, Carpenter R J. Fetal head and abdominal circumferences: II. A critical re-evaluation of the relationship to menstrual age. JCU 1982, 10: 365–372

19 Jeanty P, Cousaert E, Cantraine F. Normal growth of the fetal abdominal perimeter. Am J Perinatol 1984; 1: 127–135

20 Chitty L S, Altman D G, Henderson A, Campbell S. Charts of fetal size: 4. Femur length. Br J Obstet Gynaecol 1994; 101: 132–135

21 Warda A H, Deter R L, Rossavik I K, Carpenter R J, Hadlock F P. Fetal femur length: a critical re-evaluation of the relationship to menstrual age. Obstet Gynecol 1985; 66: 69–75

22 Chitty L S, Campbell S, Altman D G. Measurement of the fetal mandible – feasibility and construction of a centile chart. Prenat Diagnos 1993; 13: 749–756

23 Aoki S, Hata T, Kilao M. Ultrasonic assessment of fetal and neonatal spleen. Am J Perinatol 1992; 9: 361–367

24 Merz E, Wellek S, Bahlmann F, Weber G. Sonographische Normkurven des fetalen knöchernen Thorax und der fetalen Lunge. Geburtsh Frauenheilk 1995; 55: 77–82

25 Arduini D, Rizzo G. Normal values of pulsatility index from fetal vessels: a cross-sectional study on 1556 healthy fetuses. J Perinat Med 1990; 18: 165–172

26 Bower S, Vyas S, Campbell S, Nicolaides K H. Color Doppler imaging of the uterine artery in pregnancy: normal ranges of impedance to blood flow, mean velocity and volume of flow. Ultrasound Obstet Gynecol 1992; 2: 261–265

27 Moore T R, Cayle J E. The amniotic fluid index in normal human pregnancy. Am J Obstet Gynecol 1990; 162: 1168–1173

28 Hadlock F P, Harrist R B, Sharman R S, Deter R L, Park S K. Estimation of fetal weight with the use of head, body, and femur measurements – a prospective study. Am J Obstet Gynecol 1985; 151: 333–337

29 Vintzileos A M, Neckles S, Campbell W A, Andreoli J W, Kaplan B M, Nochimson D J. Fetal liver ultrasound measurement during normal pregnancy. Obstet Gnecol 1985; 66: 477–480

List of tables and charts

Fetal size charts

Dating charts

Doppler charts

Others

1. Biparietal diameter (outer–outer)

Weeks of gestation	Centiles (mm)		
	5th	50th	95th
12	16.0	19.7	23.4
13	19.8	23.5	27.3
14	23.4	27.3	31.2
15	27.1	31.0	35.0
16	30.7	34.7	38.8
17	34.2	38.3	42.5
18	37.7	41.9	46.1
19	41.1	45.4	49.7
20	44.4	48.8	53.3
21	47.6	52.2	56.7
22	50.8	55.5	60.1
23	53.9	58.7	63.4
24	57.0	61.8	66.6
25	59.9	64.8	69.7
26	62.7	67.8	72.8
27	65.5	70.6	75.7
28	68.1	73.4	78.6
29	70.7	76.0	81.3
30	73.1	78.6	84.0
31	75.5	81.0	86.5
32	77.7	83.3	88.9
33	79.8	85.5	91.2
34	81.8	87.6	93.4
35	83.7	89.6	95.5
36	85.5	91.5	97.4
37	87.1	93.2	99.3
38	88.6	94.8	100.9
39	89.9	96.2	102.5
40	91.1	97.5	103.9
41	92.2	98.7	105.2
42	93.1	99.7	106.3

Source: Chitty *et al.*[14]

1. Biparietal diameter (outer–outer)

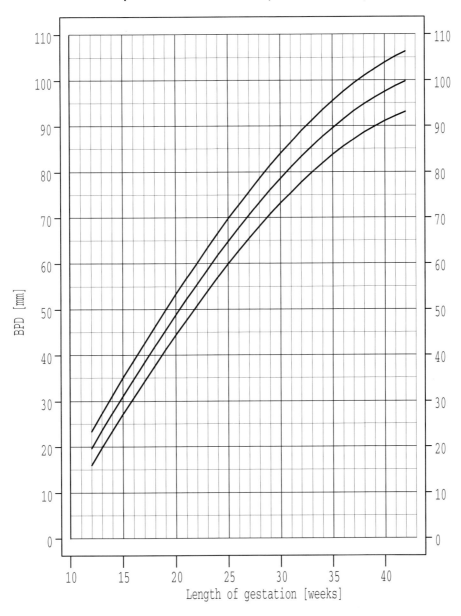

2. Biparietal diameter (outer–inner)

Weeks of gestation	Centiles (mm)		
	5th	50th	95th
12	14.9	18.3	21.7
13	18.5	22.0	25.5
14	22.0	25.6	29.2
15	25.6	29.3	33.0
16	29.0	32.8	36.7
17	32.4	36.3	40.3
18	35.7	39.8	43.9
19	39.0	43.2	47.4
20	42.3	46.5	50.8
21	45.4	49.8	54.2
22	48.5	53.0	57.5
23	51.5	56.1	60.7
24	54.4	59.2	63.9
25	57.3	62.1	67.0
26	60.1	65.0	70.0
27	62.8	67.8	72.9
28	65.3	70.5	75.7
29	67.9	73.1	78.4
30	70.3	75.7	81.1
31	72.6	78.1	83.6
32	74.8	80.4	86.0
33	76.9	82.6	88.4
34	78.9	84.7	90.6
35	80.7	86.7	92.7
36	82.5	88.6	94.7
37	84.1	90.3	96.5
38	85.6	92.0	98.3
39	87.0	93.5	99.9
40	88.3	94.8	101.4
41	89.4	96.1	102.7
42	90.4	97.2	103.9

Source: Chitty *et al.*[14]

2. Biparietal diameter (outer–inner)

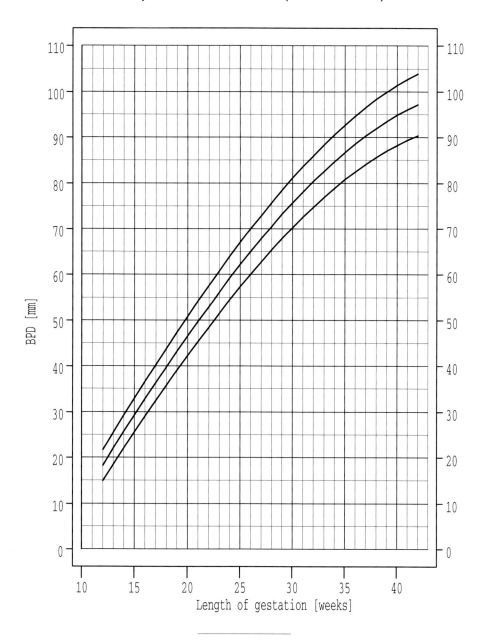

3. Head circumference (derived from diameters)
(a) using biparietal diameter outer–outer

Weeks of gestation	Centiles (mm)		
	5th	50th	95th
12	57.1	68.1	79.2
13	70.8	82.2	93.6
14	84.2	96.0	107.8
15	97.5	109.7	121.9
16	110.6	123.1	135.7
17	123.4	136.2	149.3
18	136.0	149.3	162.7
19	148.3	162.0	175.7
20	160.4	174.5	188.6
21	172.1	186.5	201.1
22	183.6	198.5	213.3
23	194.8	210.0	225.3
24	205.6	221.2	236.9
25	216.1	232.1	248.1
26	226.2	242.6	259.0
27	235.9	252.7	269.5
28	245.3	262.5	279.6
29	254.3	271.8	289.4
30	262.8	280.7	298.7
31	270.9	289.2	307.6
32	278.6	297.3	316.0
33	285.8	304.9	324.0
34	292.6	312.0	331.5
35	298.8	318.7	338.5
36	304.6	324.8	345.0
37	308.8	330.4	351.0
38	314.5	335.5	356.5
39	318.7	340.0	361.4
40	322.2	344.0	365.8
41	325.2	347.4	369.6
42	327.7	350.3	372.8

Source: Chitty *et al.*[14]

3. Head circumference (derived from diameters)
(a) using biparietal diameter outer–outer

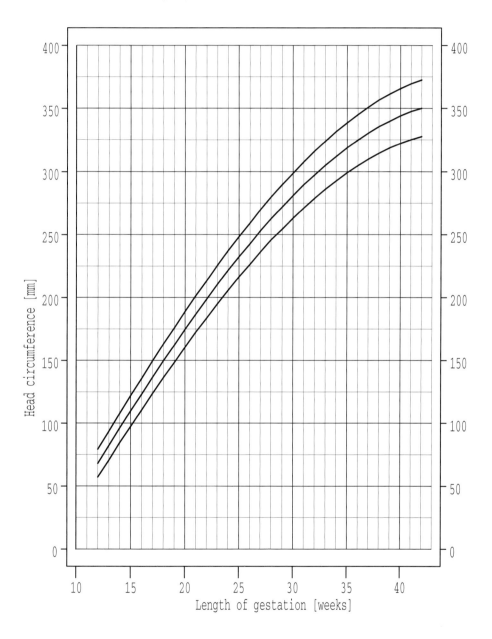

4. Head circumference (derived from diameters)
(b) using biparietal diameter outer–inner

Weeks of gestation	Centiles (mm)		
	5th	50th	95th
12	55.5	65.8	76.1
13	69.0	79.7	90.4
14	82.2	93.4	104.5
15	95.3	106.9	118.4
16	108.1	120.1	132.1
17	120.7	133.2	145.6
18	133.1	146.0	158.9
19	145.2	158.6	171.9
20	157.1	170.9	184.6
21	168.7	182.9	197.0
22	180.0	194.6	209.2
23	191.0	206.0	221.1
24	201.7	217.1	232.6
25	212.0	227.9	243.8
26	222.0	238.3	254.6
27	231.6	248.4	265.1
28	240.9	258.0	275.2
29	249.7	267.3	285.0
30	258.2	276.2	294.3
31	266.2	284.7	303.2
32	273.8	292.7	311.6
33	281.0	300.3	319.7
34	287.7	307.5	327.2
35	293.9	314.1	334.3
36	299.7	320.3	340.9
37	304.9	326.0	347.0
38	309.6	331.1	352.6
39	313.8	335.7	357.7
40	317.5	339.8	362.2
41	320.6	343.4	366.1
42	323.1	346.3	369.5

Source: Chitty and Altman (unpublished)

4. Head circumference (derived from diameters)
(b) using biparietal diameter outer–inner

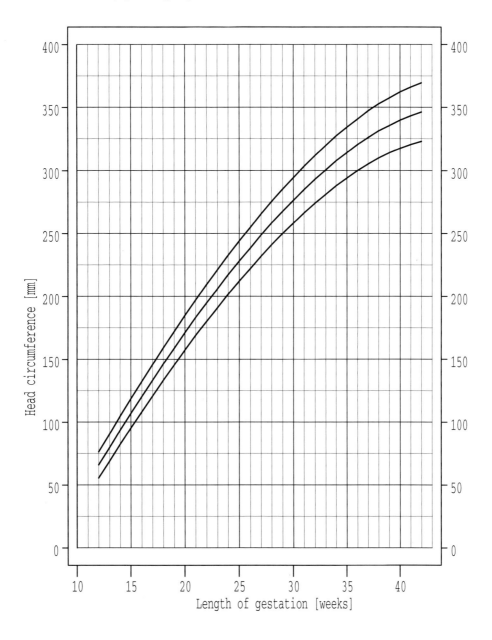

5. Abdominal circumference (derived from diameters)

Weeks of gestation	Centiles (mm)		
	5th	50th	95th
12	49.0	55.8	62.6
13	59.6	67.4	75.2
14	70.1	78.9	87.7
15	80.5	90.3	100.1
16	90.9	101.6	112.4
17	101.1	112.9	124.7
18	111.3	124.1	136.9
19	121.5	135.2	149.0
20	131.5	146.2	161.0
21	141.4	157.1	172.9
22	151.3	168.0	184.7
23	161.0	178.7	196.4
24	170.6	189.3	208.0
25	180.1	199.8	219.5
26	189.5	210.2	230.8
27	198.8	220.4	242.1
28	207.9	230.6	253.2
29	216.9	240.5	264.2
30	225.8	250.4	275.0
31	234.5	260.1	285.7
32	243.1	269.7	296.3
33	251.5	279.1	306.7
34	259.8	288.4	317.0
35	267.9	297.5	327.0
36	275.8	306.4	337.0
37	283.6	315.1	346.7
38	291.2	323.7	356.3
39	298.6	332.1	365.7
40	305.8	340.4	374.9
41	312.9	348.4	383.9
42	319.7	356.2	392.7

Source: Chitty *et al.*[14]

5. Abdominal circumference (derived from diameters)

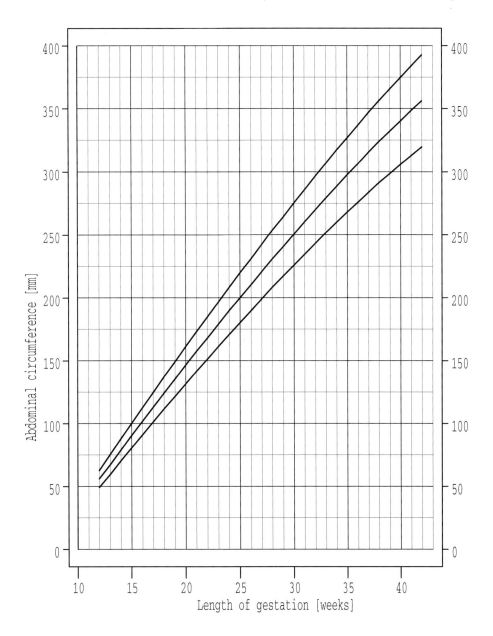

6. Head / abdominal circumference ratio

Weeks of gestation	Centiles		
	5th	50th	95th
12	1.13	1.23	1.33
13	1.13	1.23	1.33
14	1.13	1.22	1.32
15	1.12	1.22	1.32
16	1.12	1.21	1.31
17	1.11	1.21	1.31
18	1.11	1.20	1.30
19	1.10	1.20	1.30
20	1.10	1.19	1.29
21	1.09	1.19	1.28
22	1.08	1.18	1.28
23	1.08	1.17	1.27
24	1.07	1.17	1.26
25	1.06	1.16	1.26
26	1.05	1.15	1.25
27	1.05	1.14	1.24
28	1.04	1.13	1.23
29	1.03	1.13	1.22
30	1.02	1.12	1.21
31	1.01	1.11	1.21
32	1.00	1.10	1.20
33	0.99	1.09	1.19
34	0.98	1.08	1.18
35	0.97	1.07	1.16
36	0.96	1.06	1.15
37	0.95	1.05	1.14
38	0.94	1.03	1.13
39	0.92	1.02	1.12
40	0.91	1.01	1.11
41	0.90	1.00	1.10
42	0.89	0.98	1.08

Source: Chitty and Altman (unpublished)

6. Head/abdominal circumference ratio

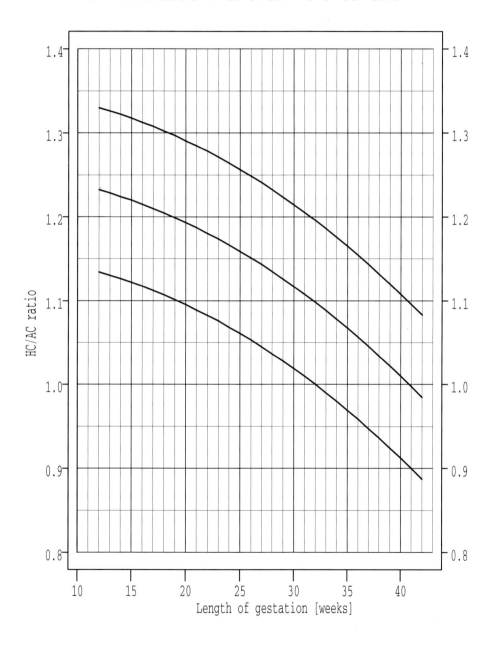

7. Femur length

Weeks of gestation	Centiles (mm)		
	5th	50th	95th
12	4.8	7.7	10.6
13	7.9	10.9	13.9
14	11.0	14.1	17.2
15	14.0	17.2	20.4
16	17.0	20.3	23.6
17	19.9	23.3	26.7
18	22.8	26.3	29.7
19	25.6	29.2	32.8
20	28.4	32.1	35.7
21	31.1	34.9	38.6
22	33.8	37.6	41.5
23	36.4	40.3	44.3
24	38.9	42.9	47.0
25	41.4	45.5	49.6
26	43.7	48.0	52.2
27	46.0	50.4	54.7
28	48.3	52.7	57.1
29	50.4	55.0	59.5
30	52.5	57.1	61.7
31	54.5	59.2	63.9
32	56.4	61.2	66.0
33	58.2	63.1	68.0
34	59.9	64.9	69.9
35	61.5	66.6	71.7
36	63.0	68.2	73.4
37	64.4	69.7	75.0
38	65.7	71.1	76.5
39	66.9	72.4	77.9
40	68.0	73.6	79.1
41	68.9	74.6	80.3
42	69.8	75.6	81.3

Source: Chitty *et al.*[20]

7. Femur length

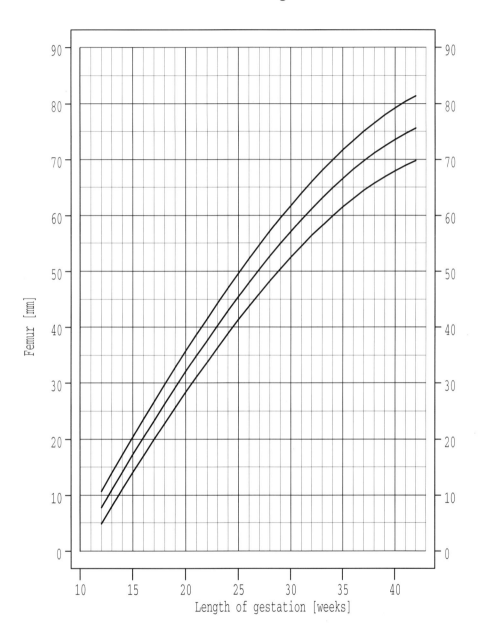

8. Humerus length

Weeks of gestation	Centiles (mm)		
	5th	50th	95th
12	4.1	7.1	10.1
13	7.6	10.7	13.8
14	11.0	14.1	17.2
15	14.1	17.3	20.6
16	17.2	20.4	23.7
17	20.1	23.4	26.7
18	22.8	26.2	29.6
19	25.4	28.9	32.4
20	28.0	31.5	35.0
21	30.4	34.0	37.6
22	32.7	36.3	40.0
23	34.8	38.6	42.3
24	36.9	40.7	44.6
25	38.9	42.8	46.7
26	40.9	44.8	48.7
27	42.7	46.7	50.7
28	44.4	48.5	52.6
29	46.1	50.2	54.4
30	47.7	51.9	56.1
31	49.2	53.5	57.7
32	50.6	55.0	59.3
33	52.0	56.4	60.8
34	53.3	57.8	62.3
35	54.6	59.1	63.6
36	55.7	60.3	64.9
37	56.8	61.5	66.2
38	57.9	62.6	67.4
39	58.9	63.7	68.5
40	59.8	64.7	69.6
41	60.7	65.6	70.6
42	61.5	66.5	71.5

Source: Chitty and Altman (unpublished)

8. Humerus length

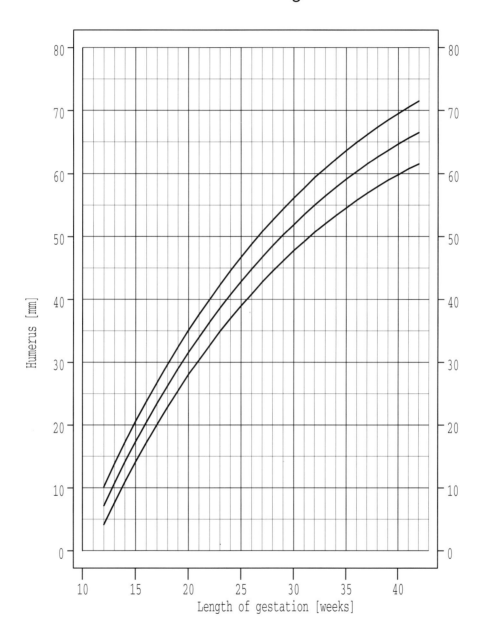

9. Radius length

Weeks of gestation	Centiles (mm)		
	5th	50th	95th
12	2.6	5.5	8.4
13	5.3	8.2	11.2
14	8.0	11.0	14.1
15	10.8	13.9	17.0
16	13.5	16.7	19.8
17	16.1	19.3	22.6
18	18.6	21.9	25.2
19	20.9	24.4	27.8
20	23.2	26.7	30.2
21	25.3	28.9	32.4
22	27.3	30.9	34.6
23	29.2	32.9	36.6
24	30.9	34.7	38.5
25	32.6	36.5	40.3
26	34.2	38.1	42.1
27	35.7	39.7	43.7
28	37.1	41.2	45.3
29	38.4	42.6	46.7
30	39.6	43.9	48.1
31	40.8	45.1	49.5
32	41.9	46.4	50.8
33	43.0	47.5	52.0
34	44.0	48.6	53.1
35	45.0	49.6	54.3
36	45.9	50.6	55.3
37	46.8	51.6	56.3
38	47.6	52.5	57.3
39	48.4	53.3	58.3
40	49.1	54.2	59.2
41	49.9	55.0	60.0
42	50.6	55.7	60.9

Source: Chitty and Altman (unpublished)

9. Radius length

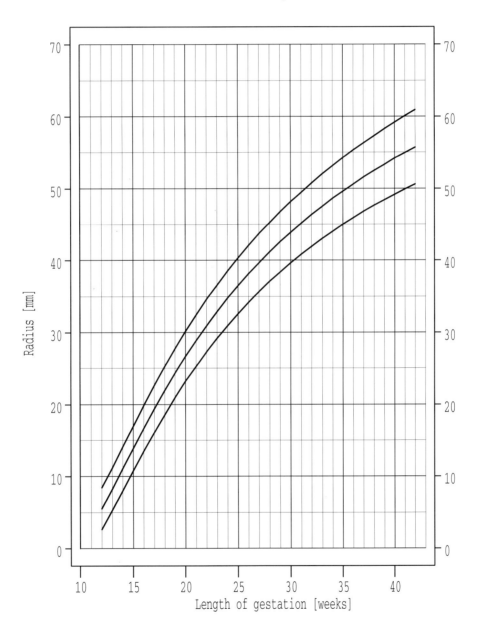

10. Ulna length

Weeks of gestation	Centiles (mm)		
	5th	50th	95th
12	4.4	7.3	10.3
13	6.6	9.6	12.7
14	9.3	12.4	15.5
15	12.1	15.3	18.5
16	15.0	18.2	21.5
17	17.8	21.2	24.5
18	20.6	24.0	27.5
19	23.3	26.8	30.3
20	25.8	29.4	33.0
21	28.3	32.0	35.6
22	30.6	34.4	38.1
23	32.8	36.6	40.5
24	34.9	38.8	42.7
25	26.9	40.9	44.9
26	38.8	42.8	46.9
27	40.5	44.7	48.9
28	42.2	46.5	50.7
29	43.8	48.2	52.5
30	45.3	49.8	54.2
31	46.8	51.3	55.8
32	48.2	52.7	57.3
33	49.5	54.1	58.8
34	50.7	55.4	60.2
35	51.9	56.7	61.5
36	53.0	57.9	62.8
37	54.1	59.1	64.0
38	55.1	60.2	65.2
39	56.1	61.2	66.4
40	57.0	62.2	67.5
41	57.9	63.2	68.5
42	58.8	64.1	69.5

Source: Chitty and Altman (unpublished)

10. Ulna length

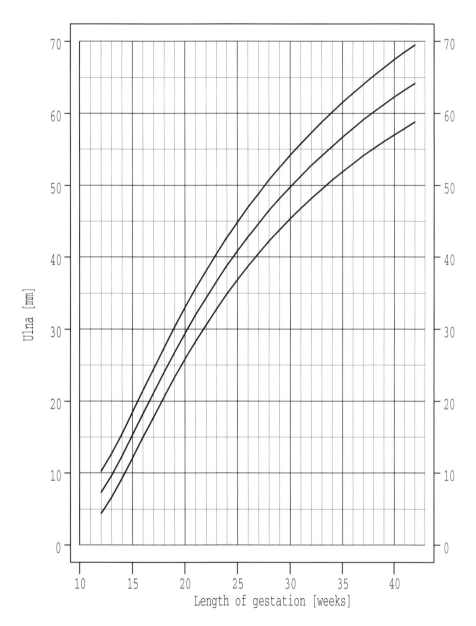

11. Tibia length

Weeks of gestation	Centiles (mm)		
	5th	50th	95th
12	4.8	7.6	10.4
13	6.3	9.2	12.0
14	8.4	11.4	14.4
15	11.0	14.1	17.1
16	13.8	16.9	20.1
17	16.6	19.9	23.1
18	19.5	22.8	26.1
19	22.3	25.7	29.1
20	25.0	28.5	32.0
21	27.7	31.2	34.8
22	30.2	33.8	37.5
23	32.6	36.4	40.1
24	35.0	38.8	42.6
25	37.2	41.0	44.9
26	39.3	43.2	47.2
27	41.3	45.3	49.4
28	43.2	47.3	51.4
29	45.0	49.2	53.4
30	46.7	51.0	55.3
31	48.3	52.7	57.1
32	49.9	54.4	58.8
33	51.4	55.9	60.5
34	52.8	57.5	62.1
35	54.2	58.9	63.6
36	55.5	60.3	65.1
37	56.7	61.6	66.5
38	57.9	62.9	67.8
39	59.0	64.1	69.1
40	60.1	65.2	70.4
41	61.2	66.4	71.6
42	62.2	67.4	72.7

Source: Chitty and Altman (unpublished)

11. Tibia length

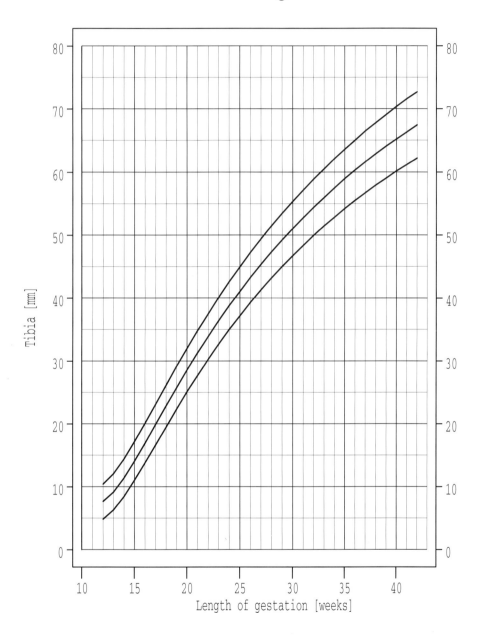

12. Fibula length

Weeks of gestation	Centiles (mm)		
	5th	50th	95th
12	4.0	6.8	9.6
13	5.6	8.5	11.4
14	7.9	10.8	13.8
15	10.5	13.5	16.6
16	13.3	16.4	19.5
17	16.1	19.3	22.5
18	18.9	22.2	25.5
19	21.7	25.1	28.5
20	24.4	27.9	31.3
21	26.9	30.5	34.1
22	29.4	33.1	36.8
23	31.8	35.5	39.3
24	34.0	37.9	41.7
25	36.2	40.1	44.0
26	38.2	42.2	46.3
27	40.2	44.3	48.4
28	42.0	46.2	50.4
29	43.8	48.0	52.3
30	45.4	49.8	54.2
31	47.0	51.5	55.9
32	48.5	53.1	57.6
33	50.0	54.6	59.2
34	51.3	56.1	60.8
35	52.6	57.5	62.3
36	53.9	58.8	63.7
37	55.1	60.1	65.1
38	56.2	61.3	66.4
39	57.3	62.5	67.7
40	58.4	63.6	68.9
41	59.4	64.7	70.1
42	60.3	65.8	71.2

Source: Chitty and Altman (unpublished)

12. Fibula length

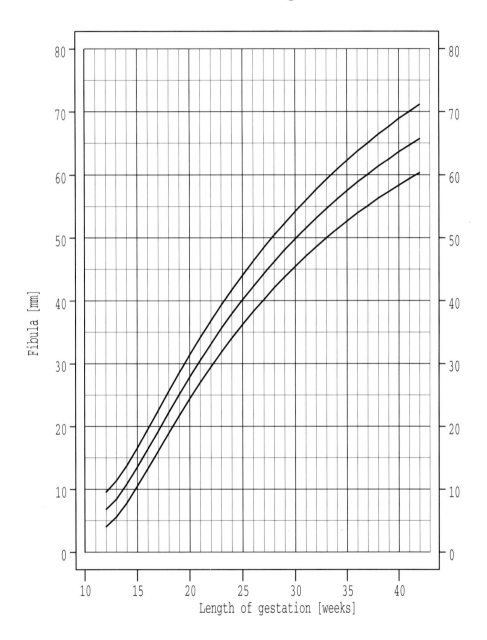

13. Foot length

Weeks of gestation	Centiles (mm)		
	5th	50th	95th
12	6.3	8.9	11.5
13	8.9	11.7	14.5
14	11.7	14.6	17.6
15	14.5	17.6	20.7
16	17.3	20.6	23.9
17	20.1	23.6	27.1
18	22.9	26.6	30.3
19	25.8	29.6	33.5
20	28.6	32.6	36.6
21	31.4	35.6	39.8
22	34.2	38.6	42.9
23	36.9	41.5	46.0
24	39.6	44.4	49.1
25	42.3	47.2	52.1
26	44.8	50.0	55.1
27	47.4	52.7	58.0
28	49.8	55.3	60.8
29	52.2	57.9	63.5
30	54.5	60.4	66.2
31	56.8	62.8	68.8
32	58.9	65.1	71.2
33	60.9	67.3	73.6
34	62.8	69.4	75.9
35	64.7	71.4	78.1
36	66.4	73.3	80.2
37	68.0	75.0	82.1
38	69.4	76.7	83.9
39	70.8	78.2	85.6
40	72.0	79.6	87.2
41	73.0	80.8	88.6
42	74.0	81.9	89.9

Source: Chitty and Altman (unpublished)

13. Foot length

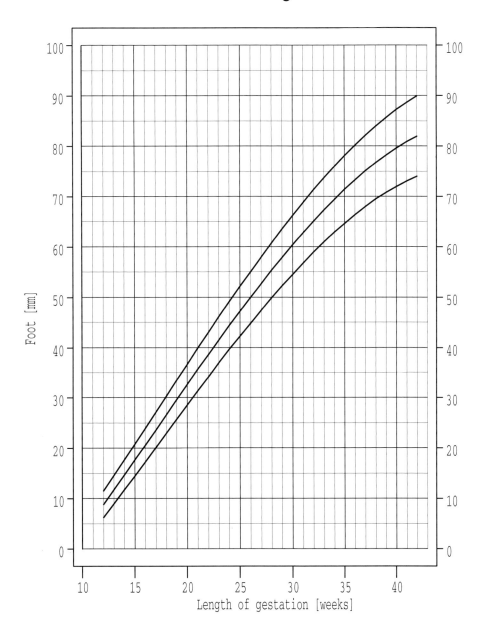

Length of gestation [weeks]

14. Mandible length

Weeks of gestation	Centiles (mm)		
	5th	50th	95th
12	6.3	8.0	9.8
13	8.2	10.3	12.3
14	10.1	12.4	14.6
15	11.9	14.4	16.9
16	13.7	16.4	19.1
17	15.3	18.3	21.3
18	17.0	20.2	23.4
19	18.5	22.0	25.4
20	20.1	23.7	27.4
21	21.5	25.5	29.4
22	23.0	27.1	31.3
23	24.4	28.8	33.2
24	25.7	30.4	25.0
25	27.1	32.0	36.8
26	28.4	33.5	38.6
27	29.7	35.0	40.4
28	30.9	36.5	42.1

Source: Chitty *et al* [22]

14. Mandible length

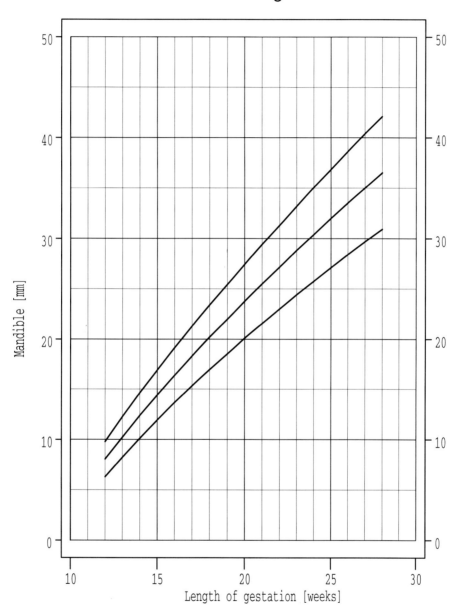

15. Transverse cerebellar diameter

Weeks of gestation	Centiles (mm)		
	5th	50th	95th
12	10.5	11.3	12.1
13	11.2	12.1	13.0
14	12.0	13.0	14.0
15	12.8	13.9	15.0
16	13.7	14.9	16.1
17	14.6	15.9	17.3
18	15.6	17.1	18.6
19	16.7	18.2	20.0
20	17.7	19.5	21.4
21	18.9	20.8	22.9
22	20.0	22.1	24.4
23	21.2	23.5	26.0
24	22.4	24.9	27.7
25	23.6	26.4	29.4
26	24.9	27.8	31.1
27	26.1	29.3	32.8
28	27.3	30.7	34.6
29	28.5	32.1	36.3
30	29.6	33.5	37.9
31	30.7	34.8	39.5
32	31.7	36.1	41.1
33	32.6	37.2	42.5
34	33.4	38.2	43.8
35	34.1	39.2	45.0
36	34.6	39.9	46.0
37	35.0	40.5	46.9
38	35.3	41.0	47.5
39	35.4	41.2	47.9
40	35.4	41.3	48.2
41	35.2	41.2	48.2
42	34.8	40.8	47.9

Source: Chitty and Altman (unpublished)

15. Transverse cerebellar diameter

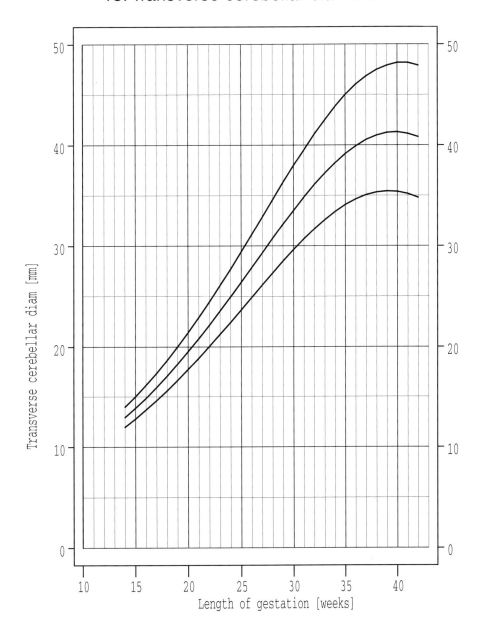

16. Internal orbit diameter

Weeks of gestation	Centiles (mm)		
	5th	50th	95th
12	4.8	5.7	6.9
13	5.6	6.8	8.1
14	6.4	7.7	9.3
15	7.2	8.7	10.5
16	7.9	9.6	11.5
17	8.6	10.4	12.5
18	9.3	11.2	13.5
19	9.9	11.9	14.3
20	10.4	12.6	15.2
21	11.0	13.2	15.9
22	11.4	13.8	16.6
23	11.9	14.3	17.3
24	12.3	14.8	17.9
25	12.7	15.3	18.4
26	13.1	15.7	19.0
27	13.4	16.1	19.4
28	13.7	16.5	19.9
29	14.0	16.9	20.3
30	14.3	17.2	20.7
31	14.5	17.5	21.1
32	14.8	17.8	21.4
33	15.0	18.0	21.7
34	15.2	18.3	22.0
35	15.4	18.5	22.3
36	15.6	18.7	22.6
37	15.7	19.0	22.8
38	15.9	19.1	23.1
39	16.0	19.3	23.3
40	16.2	19.5	23.5
41	16.3	19.7	23.7
42	16.5	19.8	23.9

Source: Chitty and Altman (unpublished)

16. Internal orbit diameter

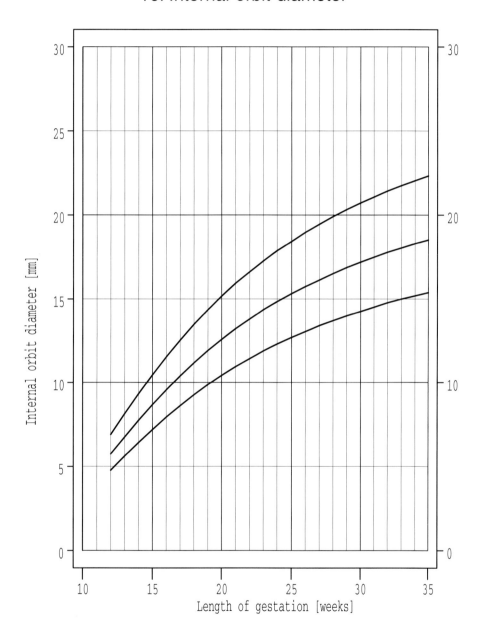

17. External orbit diameter

Weeks of gestation	Centiles (mm)		
	5th	50th	95th
12	12.0	13.3	14.7
13	14.2	15.6	17.3
14	16.3	18.0	19.9
15	18.4	20.3	22.4
16	20.5	22.6	25.0
17	22.5	24.8	27.4
18	24.5	27.0	29.8
19	26.4	29.1	32.1
20	28.2	31.1	34.4
21	30.0	33.1	36.5
22	31.7	35.0	38.6
23	33.3	36.8	40.6
24	34.9	38.5	42.5
25	36.4	40.2	44.4
26	37.9	41.8	46.1
27	39.3	43.4	47.9
28	40.6	44.8	49.5
29	41.9	46.3	51.1
30	43.2	47.6	52.6
31	44.4	49.0	54.1
32	45.5	50.3	55.5
33	46.6	51.5	56.8
34	47.7	52.7	58.2
35	48.7	53.8	59.4
36	49.7	54.9	60.6
37	50.7	56.0	61.8
38	51.6	57.0	62.9
39	52.5	58.0	64.0
40	53.4	59.0	65.1
41	54.2	59.9	66.1
42	55.0	60.8	67.1

Source: Chitty and Altman (unpublished)

17. External orbit diameter

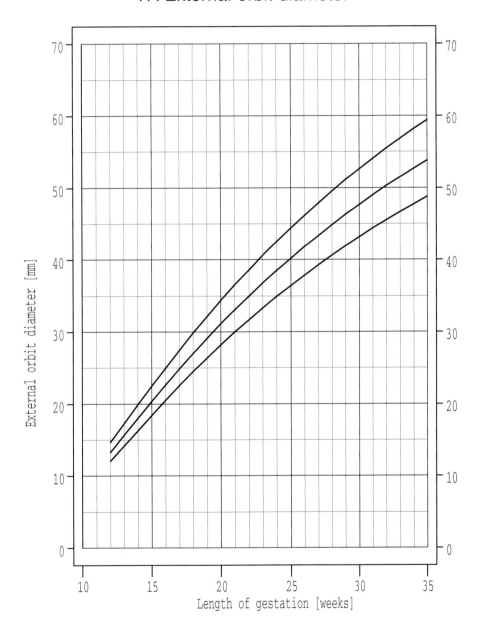

18. Posterior horn/hemisphere ratio

Weeks of gestation	Centiles		
	5th	50th	95th
12	0.50	0.61	0.71
13	0.46	0.56	0.67
14	0.42	0.52	0.63
15	0.39	0.49	0.59
16	0.36	0.45	0.55
17	0.33	0.42	0.52
18	0.30	0.39	0.49
19	0.28	0.37	0.46
20	0.25	0.34	0.43
21	0.23	0.32	0.41
22	0.21	0.30	0.39
23	0.20	0.28	0.37
24	0.18	0.26	0.35
25	0.17	0.25	0.33
26	0.16	0.23	0.31
27	0.15	0.22	0.30
28	0.14	0.21	0.28
29	0.13	0.20	0.27
30	0.12	0.19	0.26
31	0.12	0.18	0.25
32	0.11	0.18	0.24
33	0.11	0.17	0.23
34	0.10	0.16	0.22
35	0.10	0.16	0.22
36	0.10	0.16	0.21
37	0.10	0.15	0.21
38	0.10	0.15	0.20
39	0.10	0.15	0.20
40	0.10	0.15	0.20
41	0.10	0.15	0.20
42	0.11	0.15	0.20

Source: Chitty and Altman (unpublished)

18. Posterior horn/hemisphere ratio

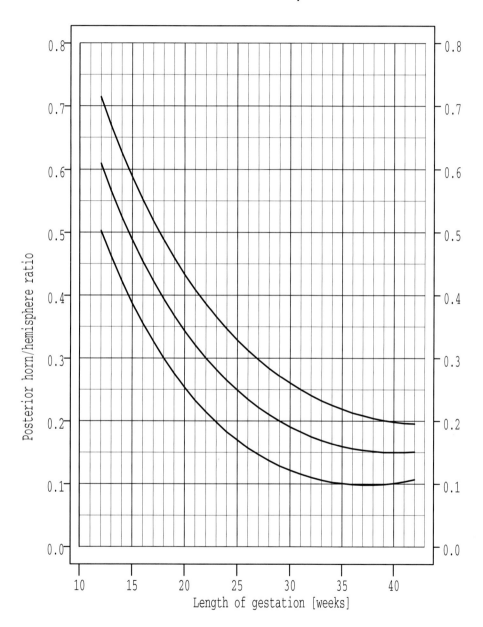

19. Kidney length

Weeks of gestation	Centiles (mm)		
	5th	50th	95th
12	5.2	6.3	7.7
13	6.4	7.8	9.4
14	7.7	9.3	11.3
15	9.0	11.0	13.3
16	10.5	12.7	15.4
17	11.9	14.5	17.6
18	13.4	16.3	19.8
19	15.0	18.2	22.1
20	16.5	20.0	24.3
21	18.0	21.8	26.5
22	19.5	23.6	28.7
23	20.9	25.4	30.9
24	22.3	27.1	32.9
25	23.7	28.8	35.0
26	25.0	30.4	36.9
27	26.3	31.9	38.8
28	27.5	33.4	40.5
29	28.6	34.7	42.2
30	29.7	36.0	43.8
31	30.7	37.2	45.2
32	31.6	38.3	46.6
33	32.4	39.4	47.8
34	33.2	40.3	48.9
35	33.9	41.1	50.0
36	34.5	41.9	50.9
37	35.1	42.6	51.7
38	35.6	43.2	52.4
39	36.0	43.7	53.1
40	36.3	44.1	53.6
41	36.6	44.5	54.0
42	36.9	44.8	54.4

Source: Chitty and Altman (unpublished)

19. Kidney length

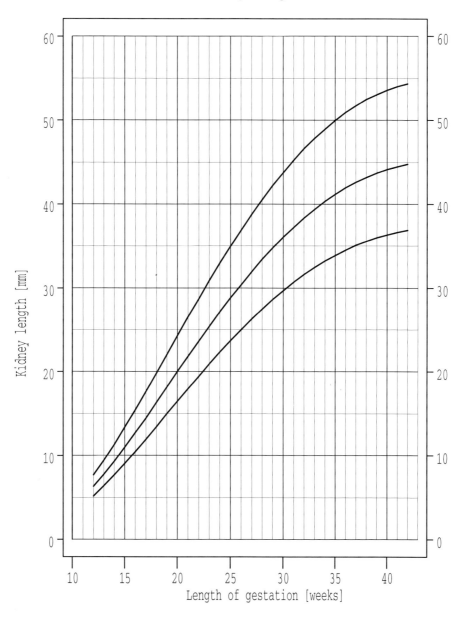

20. Spleen length

Weeks of gestation	Centiles (mm)		
	5th	50th	95th
20	11.1	15.2	19.2
21	13.0	17.0	21.0
22	14.8	18.8	22.8
23	16.6	20.6	24.6
24	18.4	22.4	26.4
25	20.2	24.2	28.2
26	21.9	25.9	30.0
27	23.6	27.6	31.7
28	25.3	29.3	33.3
29	26.9	30.9	34.9
30	28.4	32.5	36.5
31	29.9	33.9	38.0
32	31.3	35.3	39.4
33	32.6	36.6	40.7
34	33.8	37.8	41.9
35	34.9	38.9	43.0
36	35.9	39.9	44.0
37	36.8	40.8	44.8
38	37.5	41.6	45.6
39	38.1	42.2	46.2
40	38.6	42.6	46.7
41	38.9	43.0	47.0

Source: Aoki *et al* [23]
Comment: Excluded birthweight <10th or >90th centile; SD taken as constant

20. Spleen length

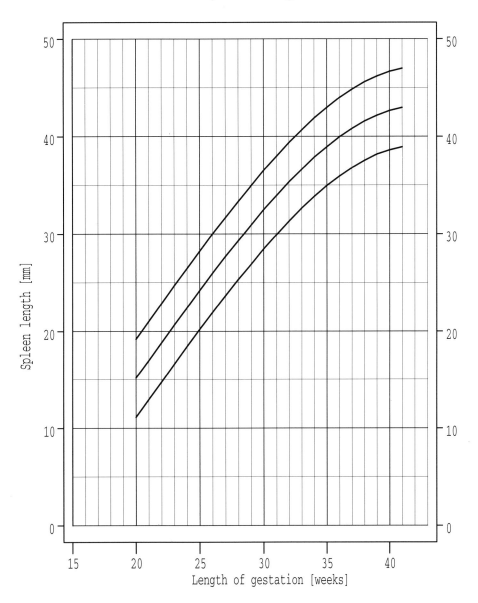

21. Liver length

Weeks of Gestation	Centiles (mm)		
	5th	50th	95th
20	22.9	26.7	30.6
21	24.2	28.1	32.0
22	25.5	29.5	33.5
23	26.8	30.9	35.0
24	28.0	32.2	36.5
25	29.3	33.6	37.9
26	30.6	35.0	39.4
27	31.9	36.4	40.9
28	33.2	37.8	42.3
29	34.5	39.1	43.8
30	35.8	40.5	45.3
31	37.0	41.9	46.8
32	38.3	43.3	48.2
33	39.6	44.7	49.7
34	40.9	46.0	51.2
35	42.2	47.4	52.7
36	43.5	48.8	54.1
37	44.7	50.2	55.6
38	46.0	51.6	57.1
39	47.3	52.9	58.6
40	48.6	54.3	60.0
41	49.9	55.7	61.5

Source: Vintzileos *et al* [29]
Comment: Excluded birthweight <10th or >90th centile and IUGR.
Fetuses included more than once
Data reanalysed from tabulated means and SDs

21. Liver length

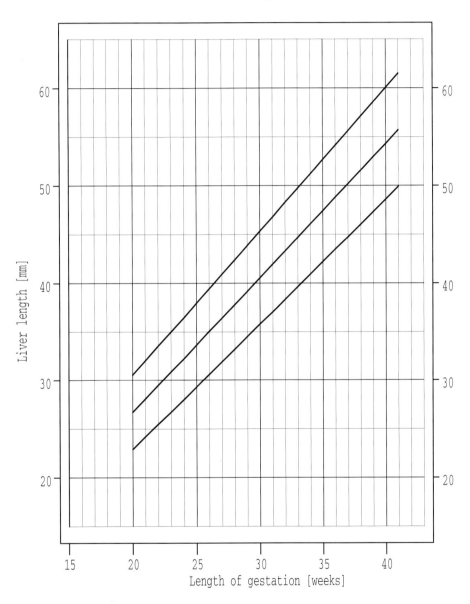

22. Thoracic circumference (derived from diameters)

Weeks of gestation	Centiles (mm)		
	5th	50th	95th
12	44	60	77
13	49	66	83
14	56	74	91
15	64	81	99
16	72	89	107
17	80	98	116
18	87	106	124
19	96	114	133
20	103	122	141
21	111	131	150
22	119	139	158
23	127	147	167
24	135	155	175
25	142	163	183
26	150	170	191
27	157	178	199
28	164	185	206
29	171	192	214
30	177	199	221
31	183	206	228
32	189	212	234
33	195	218	240
34	201	223	246
35	205	229	252
36	210	234	257
37	214	238	262
38	218	242	266
39	221	245	270
40	224	248	273
41	226	251	275

Source: Merz *et al.*[24]
Comment: Excluded IUGR

22. Thoracic circumference (derived from diameters)

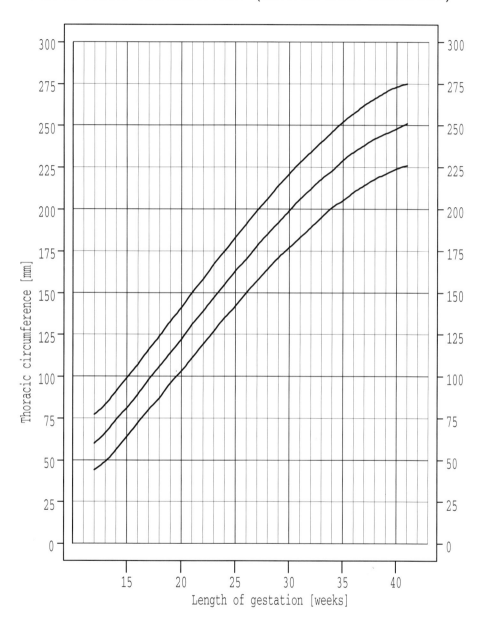

23. Biparietal diameter (outer–outer) – dating chart

BPD (mm)	Centiles (weeks + days)		
	5th	50th	95th
22	11 + 6	12 + 4	13 + 3
24	12 + 2	13 + 1	14 + 0
26	12 + 6	13 + 4	14 + 4
28	13 + 2	14 + 1	15 + 1
30	13 + 6	14 + 5	15 + 5
32	14 + 2	15 + 2	16 + 2
34	14 + 6	15 + 5	16 + 6
36	15 + 2	16 + 2	17 + 3
38	15 + 6	16 + 6	18 + 0
40	16 + 2	17 + 3	18 + 5
42	16 + 2	18 + 0	19 + 2
44	17 + 3	18 + 4	20 + 0
46	18 + 0	19 + 2	20 + 4
48	18 + 3	19 + 6	21 + 2
50	19 + 0	20 + 3	22 + 0
52	19 + 4	21 + 1	22 + 5
54	20 + 1	21 + 5	23 + 3
56	20 + 5	22 + 2	24 + 1
58	21 + 2	23 + 0	24 + 6
60	22 + 0	23 + 5	25 + 4
62	22 + 4	24 + 2	26 + 2
64	23 + 1	25 + 0	27 + 0
66	23 + 5	25 + 5	27 + 6
68	24 + 3	26 + 3	28 + 4
70	25 + 0	27 + 1	29 + 3
72	25 + 5	27 + 6	30 + 1
74	26 + 2	28 + 4	31 + 0
76	27 + 0	29 + 2	31 + 6
78	27 + 4	30 + 0	32 + 4
80	28 + 2	30 + 5	33 + 3
82	29 + 0	31 + 4	34 + 2
84	29 + 5	32 + 2	35 + 1
86	30 + 2	33 + 1	36 + 1
88	31 + 0	33 + 6	37 + 0
90	31 + 5	34 + 5	37 + 6

Source: Altman and Chitty[5]

23. Biparietal diameter (outer–outer) – dating chart

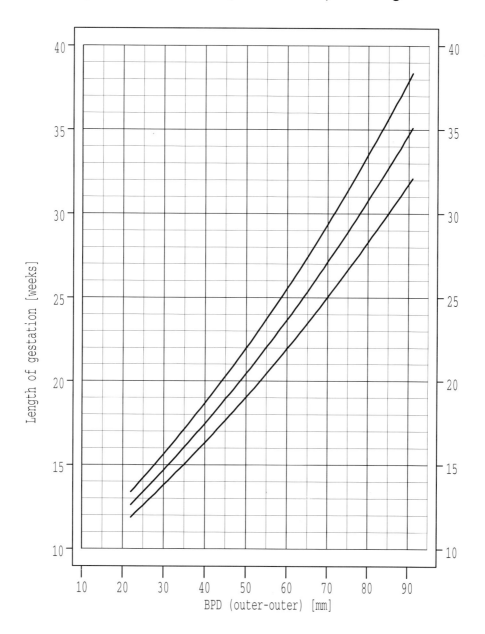

24. Biparietal diameter (outer–inner) – dating chart

Weeks of gestation	Centiles (weeks + days)		
	5th	50th	95th
22	12 + 2	13 + 0	13 + 6
24	12 + 5	13 + 4	14 + 3
26	13 + 2	14 + 1	15 + 0
28	13 + 5	14 + 5	15 + 4
30	14 + 2	15 + 1	16 + 1
32	14 + 6	15 + 5	16 + 5
34	15 + 2	16 + 2	17 + 3
36	15 + 6	16 + 6	18 + 0
38	16 + 3	17 + 3	18 + 5
40	17 + 0	18 + 1	19 + 2
42	17 + 3	18 + 5	20 + 0
44	18 + 0	19 + 2	20 + 5
46	18 + 4	19 + 6	21 + 2
48	19 + 1	20 + 4	22 + 0
50	19 + 5	21 + 1	22 + 5
52	20 + 2	21 + 6	23 + 3
54	21 + 0	22 + 4	24 + 1
56	21 + 4	23 + 1	24 + 6
58	22 + 1	23 + 6	25 + 5
60	22 + 5	24 + 4	26 + 3
62	23 + 3	25 + 2	27 + 1
64	24 + 0	26 + 0	28 + 0
66	24 + 5	26 + 5	28 + 5
68	25 + 2	27 + 3	29 + 4
70	26 + 0	28 + 1	30 + 3
72	26 + 5	28 + 6	31 + 2
74	27 + 2	29 + 4	32 + 0
76	28 + 0	30 + 2	32 + 6
78	28 + 5	31 + 1	33 + 5
80	29 + 3	31 + 6	34 + 5
82	30 + 1	32 + 5	35 + 4
84	30 + 6	33 + 3	36 + 3
86	31 + 4	34 + 2	37 + 2
88	32 + 2	35 + 1	38 + 2

Source: Altman and Chitty[5]

24. Biparietal diameter (outer–inner) – dating chart

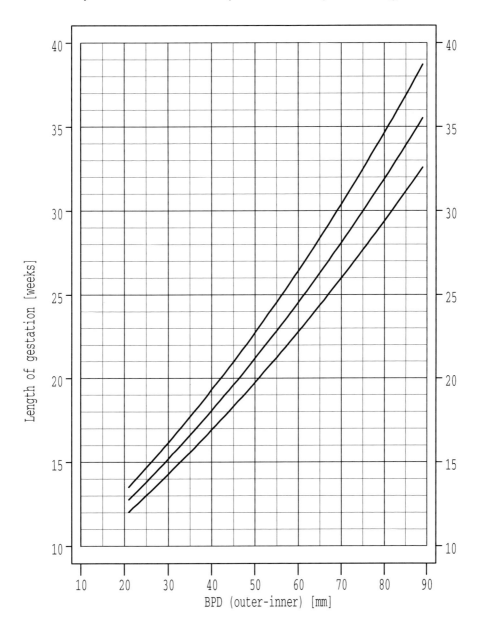

25. Femur length – dating chart

Femur (mm)	Centiles (weeks + days)		
	5th	50th	95th
10	12 + 2	13 + 0	13 + 5
12	12 + 6	13 + 4	14 + 2
14	13 + 2	14 + 1	15 + 0
16	13 + 6	14 + 5	15 + 4
18	14 + 3	15 + 2	16 + 2
20	15 + 0	16 + 0	17 + 0
22	15 + 4	16 + 4	17 + 4
24	16 + 1	17 + 2	18 + 2
26	16 + 6	17 + 6	19 + 0
28	17 + 3	18 + 4	19 + 5
30	18 + 0	19 + 2	20 + 4
32	18 + 5	20 + 0	21 + 2
34	19 + 2	20 + 5	22 + 0
36	20 + 0	21 + 3	22 + 6
38	20 + 5	22 + 1	23 + 5
40	21 + 3	22 + 6	24 + 4
42	22 + 1	23 + 5	25 + 3
44	22 + 6	24 + 3	26 + 2
46	23 + 4	25 + 2	27 + 1
48	24 + 2	26 + 1	28 + 1
50	25 + 1	27 + 0	29 + 0
52	25 + 6	27 + 6	30 + 0
54	26 + 5	28 + 5	31 + 0
56	27 + 4	29 + 5	32 + 0
58	28 + 3	30 + 4	33 + 0
60	29 + 2	31 + 4	34 + 1
62	30 + 1	32 + 4	35 + 2
64	31 + 0	33 + 4	36 + 2
66	32 + 0	34 + 4	37 + 3

Source: Altman and Chitty[5]

25. Femur length – dating chart

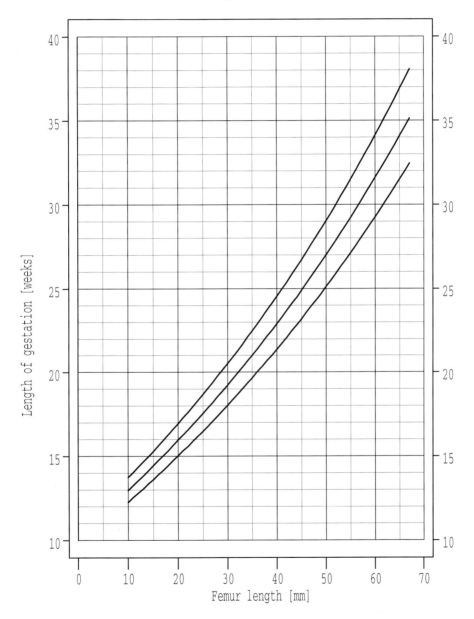

26. Transverse cerebellar diameter – dating chart

TCD (mm)	Centiles (weeks + days)		
	5th	50th	95th
13	13 + 2	14 + 3	15 + 5
14	14 + 1	15 + 2	16 + 5
15	15 + 0	16 + 2	17 + 4
16	15 + 6	17 + 0	18 + 3
17	16 + 5	17 + 6	19 + 2
18	17 + 3	18 + 5	20 + 0
19	18 + 2	19 + 4	20 + 6
20	19 + 0	20 + 3	21 + 5
21	19 + 6	21 + 1	22 + 4
22	20 + 4	22 + 0	23 + 3
23	21 + 2	22 + 5	24 + 2
24	22 + 0	23 + 4	25 + 1
25	22 + 4	24 + 2	26 + 1
26	23 + 2	25 + 0	27 + 0
27	23 + 6	25 + 6	27 + 6
28	24 + 3	26 + 4	28 + 6
29	25 + 0	27 + 2	29 + 5
30	25 + 4	28 + 0	30 + 5
31	26 + 1	28 + 6	31 + 5
32	26 + 4	29 + 4	32 + 5
33	27 + 1	30 + 2	33 + 6
34	27 + 4	31 + 0	34 + 6
35	27 + 6	31 + 5	36 + 0
36	28 + 2	32 + 3	37 + 1

Source: Altman and Chitty[5]

26. Transverse cerebellar diameter – dating chart

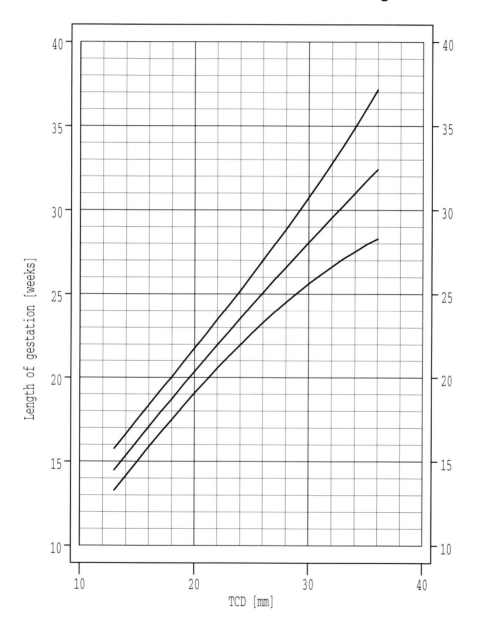

27. Head circumference (derived from diameters) – dating chart
(a) using biparietal diameter outer–outer

Head circ. mm	Centiles (weeks + days)		
	5th	50th	95th
80	11 + 4	12 + 4	13 + 4
90	12 + 3	13 + 2	14 + 2
100	13 + 2	14 + 1	15 + 1
110	14 + 0	15 + 0	16 + 0
120	14 + 6	15 + 6	16 + 6
130	15 + 5	16 + 4	17 + 5
140	16 + 3	17 + 3	18 + 3
150	17 + 2	18 + 2	19 + 2
160	18 + 1	19 + 1	20 + 1
170	18 + 6	19 + 6	21 + 0
180	19 + 5	20 + 5	21 + 6
190	20 + 3	21 + 4	22 + 5
200	21 + 1	22 + 2	23 + 4
210	22 + 0	23 + 1	24 + 3
220	22 + 5	24 + 0	25 + 3
230	23 + 4	24 + 6	26 + 3
240	24 + 2	25 + 6	27 + 3
250	25 + 1	26 + 5	28 + 3
260	26 + 0	27 + 5	29 + 4
270	26 + 6	28 + 6	30 + 6
280	27 + 6	30 + 0	32 + 1
290	28 + 6	31 + 1	33 + 4
300	29 + 6	32 + 3	35 + 2
310	31 + 0	33 + 6	37 + 0
320	32 + 2	35 + 3	38 + 6

Source: Altman[5] and Chitty

27. Head circumference (derived from diameters) – dating chart
(a) using biparietal diameter outer–outer

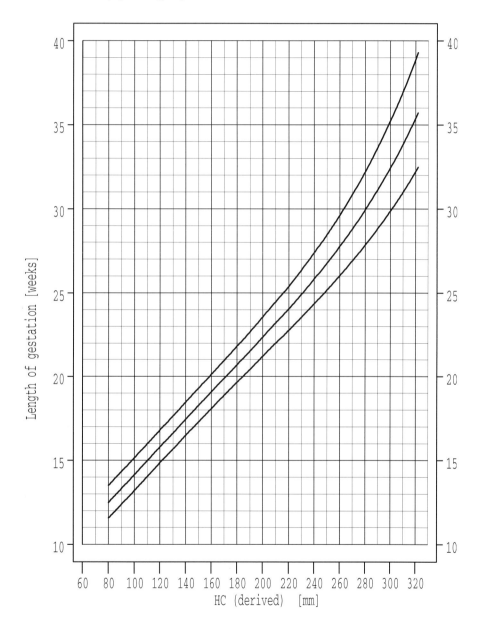

28. Head circumference (derived from diameters) – dating chart
(b) using biparietal diameter outer–inner

Head circ. (mm)	Centiles (weeks + days)		
	5th	50th	95th
80	11 + 4	12 + 5	13 + 5
90	12 + 3	13 + 4	14 + 4
100	13 + 2	14 + 3	15 + 3
110	14 + 0	15 + 2	16 + 1
120	15 + 6	16 + 0	17 + 0
130	16 + 5	16 + 6	17 + 6
140	16 + 3	17 + 5	18 + 5
150	17 + 2	18 + 4	19 + 3
160	18 + 1	19 + 2	20 + 2
170	19 + 6	20 + 1	21 + 1
180	20 + 5	21 + 0	22 + 0
190	20 + 3	21 + 6	22 + 6
200	21 + 1	22 + 4	23 + 6
210	22 + 0	23 + 3	24 + 5
220	23 + 5	24 + 3	25 + 5
230	23 + 4	25 + 2	26 + 5
240	24 + 2	26 + 1	27 + 5
250	25 + 1	27 + 1	28 + 6
260	26 + 0	28 + 1	30 + 1
270	26 + 6	29 + 2	31 + 3
280	27 + 6	30 + 3	32 + 6
290	28 + 6	31 + 5	34 + 2
300	29 + 6	33 + 0	36 + 0
310	30 + 0	34 + 3	37 + 5
320	31 + 2	36 + 0	39 + 5

Source: Chitty and Altman (unpublished)

28. Head circumference (derived from diameters) – dating chart
(b) using biparietal diameter outer–inner

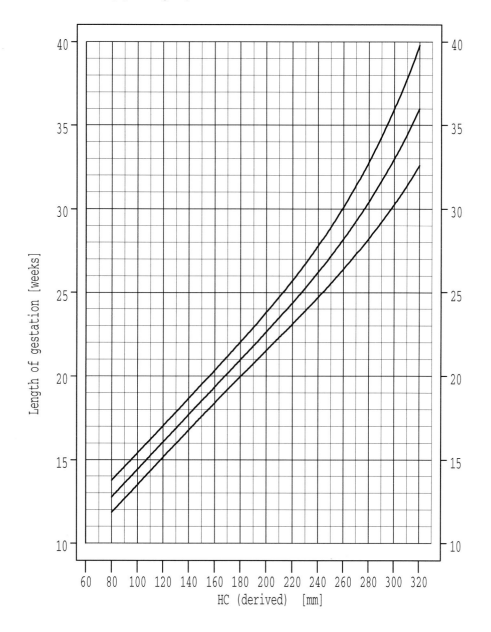

29. Crown–rump length – dating chart

Crown–rump length (mm)	Centiles (weeks + days)		
	5th	50th	95th
4	5 + 3	6 + 0	6 + 4
6	6 + 0	6 + 3	7 + 0
8	6 + 2	6 + 6	7 + 3
10	6 + 5	7 + 2	7 + 6
12	7 + 0	7 + 4	8 + 1
14	7 + 3	7 + 6	8 + 3
16	7 + 5	8 + 2	8 + 5
18	8 + 0	8 + 3	9 + 0
20	8 + 1	8 + 5	9 + 2
22	8 + 3	9 + 0	9 + 4
24	8 + 5	9 + 2	9 + 6
26	8 + 6	9 + 3	10 + 0
28	9 + 1	9 + 5	10 + 2
30	9 + 3	9 + 6	10 + 3
32	9 + 4	10 + 1	10 + 5
34	9 + 5	10 + 2	10 + 6
36	10 + 0	10 + 4	11 + 0
38	10 + 1	10 + 5	11 + 2
40	10 + 2	10 + 6	11 + 3
42	10 + 4	11 + 0	11 + 4
44	10 + 5	11 + 2	11 + 6
46	10 + 6	11 + 3	12 + 0
48	11 + 0	11 + 4	12 + 1
50	11 + 1	11 + 5	12 + 2
52	11 + 3	11 + 6	12 + 3
54	11 + 4	12 + 1	12 + 4
56	11 + 5	12 + 2	12 + 6
58	11 + 6	12 + 3	13 + 0
60	12 + 0	12 + 4	13 + 1
62	12 + 1	12 + 5	13 + 2
64	12 + 2	12 + 6	13 + 3
66	12 + 3	13 + 0	13 + 4
68	12 + 4	13 + 1	13 + 5
70	12 + 5	13 + 2	13 + 6
72	12 + 6	13 + 3	14 + 0
74	13 + 0	13 + 4	14 + 1
76	13 + 1	13 + 5	14 + 2
78	13 + 2	13 + 6	14 + 2
80	13 + 3	14 + 0	14 + 3

Source: Robinson and Fleming[10]

29. Crown–rump length – dating chart

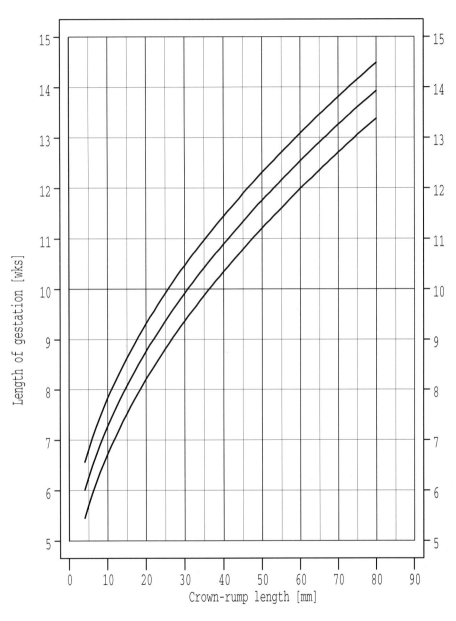

30. Umbilical artery pulsatility index

Weeks of gestation	Centiles		
	5th	50th	95th
20	1.04	1.54	2.03
21	0.98	1.47	1.96
22	0.92	1.41	1.90
23	0.86	1.35	1.85
24	0.81	1.30	1.79
25	0.76	1.25	1.74
26	0.71	1.20	1.69
27	0.67	1.16	1.65
28	0.63	1.12	1.61
29	0.59	1.08	1.57
30	0.56	1.05	1.54
31	0.53	1.02	1.51
32	0.50	0.99	1.48
33	0.48	0.97	1.46
34	0.46	0.95	1.44
35	0.44	0.94	1.43
36	0.43	0.92	1.42
37	0.42	0.92	1.41
38	0.42	0.91	1.40
39	0.42	0.91	1.40
40	0.42	0.91	1.40
41	0.42	0.92	1.41
42	0.43	0.93	1.42

Source: Arduini and Rizzo[25]
Comment: Excluded IUGR; SD taken as constant

30. Umbilical artery pulsatility index

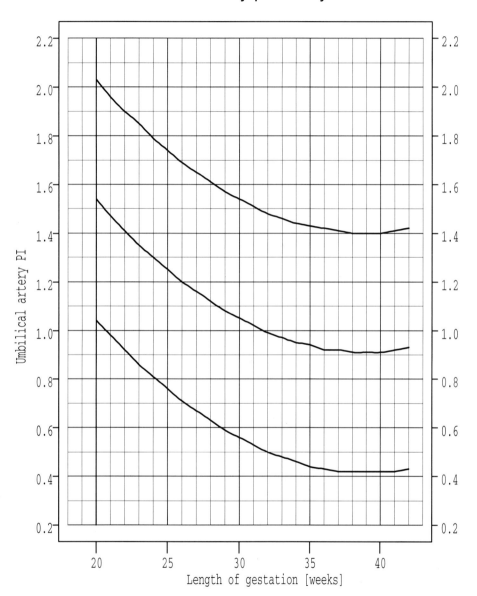

Umbilical artery PI

Length of gestation [weeks]

31. Descending aorta pulsatility index

Weeks of gestation	Centiles		
	5th	50th	95th
20	1.54	1.97	2.39
21	1.54	1.97	2.40
22	1.54	1.97	2.40
23	1.55	1.97	2.40
24	1.55	1.98	2.40
25	1.55	1.98	2.40
26	1.55	1.98	2.41
27	1.56	1.98	2.41
28	1.56	1.99	2.41
29	1.56	1.99	2.41
30	1.56	1.99	2.42
31	1.57	1.99	2.42
32	1.57	2.00	2.42
33	1.57	2.00	2.42
34	1.57	2.00	2.43
35	1.58	2.00	2.43
36	1.58	2.00	2.43
37	1.58	2.01	2.43
38	1.58	2.01	2.44
39	1.59	2.01	2.44
40	1.59	2.01	2.44
41	1.59	2.02	2.44
42	1.59	2.02	2.45

Source: Arduini and Rizzo[25]
Comment: Excluded IUGR; SD taken as constant

31. Descending aorta pulsatility index

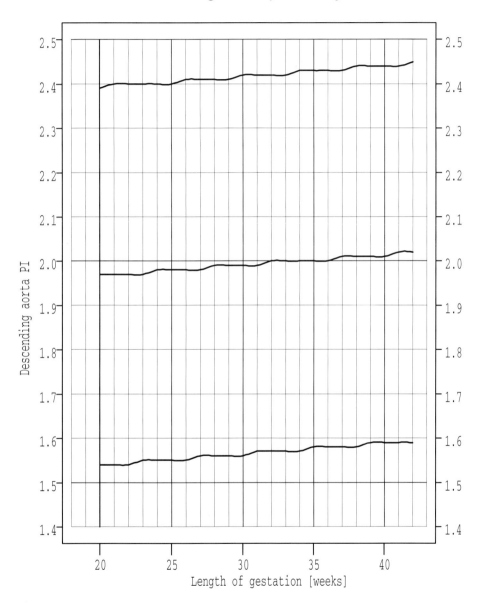

Length of gestation [weeks]

32. Middle cerebral artery pulsatility index

Weeks of gestation	Centiles		
	5th	50th	95th
20	1.36	1.83	2.31
21	1.40	1.87	2.34
22	1.44	1.91	2.37
23	1.47	1.93	2.40
24	1.49	1.96	2.42
25	1.51	1.97	2.44
26	1.52	1.98	2.45
27	1.53	1.99	2.45
28	1.53	1.99	2.46
29	1.53	1.99	2.45
30	1.52	1.98	2.44
31	1.51	1.97	2.43
32	1.49	1.95	2.41
33	1.46	1.93	2.39
34	1.43	1.90	2.36
35	1.40	1.86	2.32
36	1.36	1.82	2.28
37	1.32	1.78	2.24
38	1.27	1.73	2.19
39	1.21	1.67	2.14
40	1.15	1.61	2.08
41	1.08	1.55	2.01
42	1.01	1.48	1.94

Source: Arduini and Rizzo[25]
Comment: Excluded IUGR; SD taken as constant

32. Middle cerebral artery pulsatility index

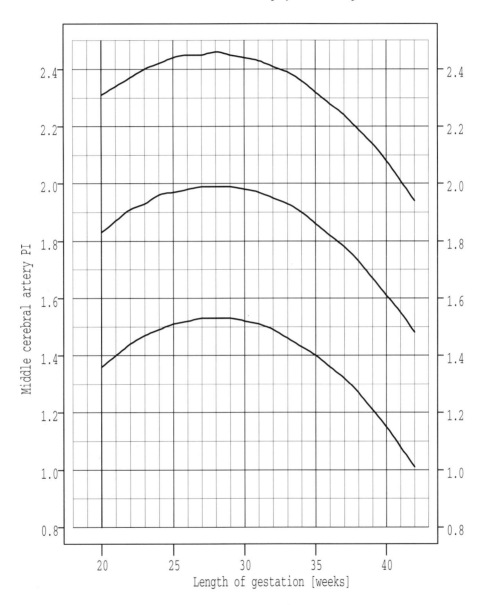

33. Non–placental uterine artery pulsatility index

Weeks of gestation	Centiles		
	5th	50th	95th
18	0.75	1.23	2.02
19	0.73	1.21	1.98
20	0.72	1.18	1.94
21	0.71	1.16	1.90
22	0.69	1.13	1.86
23	0.68	1.11	1.82
24	0.66	1.09	1.79
25	0.65	1.07	1.75
26	0.64	1.05	1.72
27	0.62	1.02	1.68
28	0.61	1.00	1.65
29	0.60	0.98	1.61
30	0.59	0.96	1.58
31	0.58	0.94	1.55
32	0.56	0.93	1.52
33	0.55	0.91	1.49
34	0.54	0.89	1.46
35	0.53	0.87	1.43
36	0.52	0.85	1.40
37	0.51	0.84	1.37
38	0.50	0.82	1.34
39	0.49	0.80	1.32
40	0.48	0.79	1.29
41	0.47	0.77	1.27
42	0.46	0.76	1.24

Source: Bower *et al.*[26]
Comment: Model not fully specified

33. Non-placental uterine artery pulsatility index

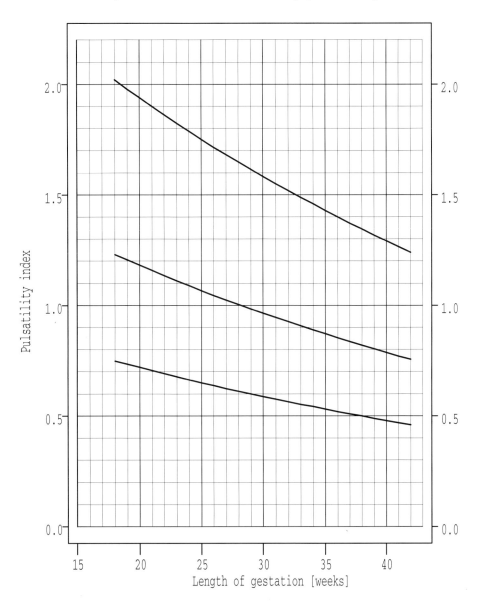

34. Placental uterine artery pulsatility index

Weeks of gestation	Centiles		
	5th	50th	95th
18	0.55	0.90	1.47
19	0.53	0.87	1.43
20	0.52	0.85	1.39
21	0.50	0.82	1.35
22	0.49	0.80	1.31
23	0.47	0.78	1.27
24	0.46	0.75	1.24
25	0.45	0.73	1.20
26	0.43	0.71	1.17
27	0.42	0.69	1.13
28	0.41	0.67	1.10
29	0.40	0.65	1.07
30	0.39	0.63	1.04
31	0.37	0.61	1.01
32	0.36	0.60	0.98
33	0.35	0.58	0.95
34	0.34	0.56	0.92
35	0.33	0.55	0.90
36	0.32	0.53	0.87
37	0.31	0.52	0.85
38	0.31	0.50	0.82
39	0.30	0.49	0.80
40	0.29	0.47	0.78
41	0.28	0.46	0.75
42	0.27	0.45	0.73

Source: Bower *et al.*[26]
Comment: Model not fully specified

34. Placental uterine artery pulsatility index

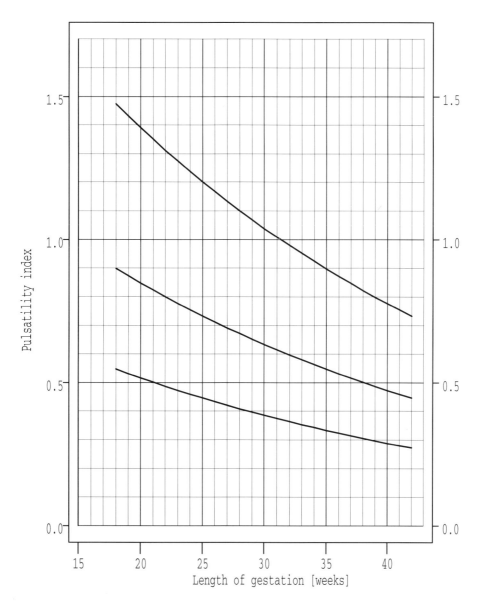

Pulsatility index

Length of gestation [weeks]

35. Amniotic fluid index

Weeks of gestation	Centiles (mm)		
	5th	50th	95th
16	79	121	185
17	83	127	194
18	87	133	202
19	90	137	207
20	93	141	212
21	95	143	214
22	97	145	216
23	98	146	218
24	98	147	219
25	97	147	221
26	97	147	223
27	95	146	226
28	94	146	228
29	92	145	231
30	90	145	234
31	88	144	238
32	86	144	242
33	83	143	245
34	81	142	248
35	79	140	249
36	77	138	249
37	75	135	244
38	73	132	239
39	72	127	226
40	71	123	214
41	70	116	194
42	69	110	175

Source: Moore and Cayle[27]
Comments: Excluded birthweight <10th or >90th centile. Model not fully specified.

35. Amniotic fluid index

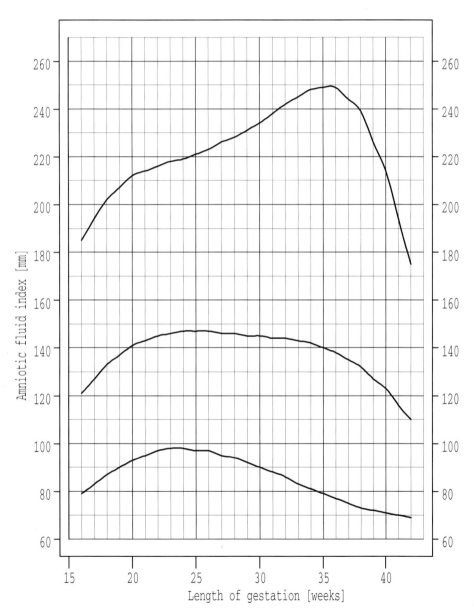

36. Fetal weight

From abdominal and head circumferences and femur length (in mm)

Weeks of Gestation	Centiles (g)		
	5th	50th	95th
16	122	143	164
17	151	177	203
18	186	218	250
19	227	266	305
20	274	321	369
21	329	386	443
22	392	460	527
23	464	544	624
24	545	639	733
25	635	745	854
26	735	862	989
27	845	991	1136
28	964	1131	1297
29	1093	1282	1470
30	1231	1444	1656
31	1378	1615	1852
32	1532	1796	2059
33	1692	1984	2275
34	1858	2179	2499
35	2029	2378	2728
36	2202	2582	2961
37	2377	2787	3196
38	2552	2992	3432
39	2726	3196	3665
40	2897	3396	3895
41	3063	3591	4119
42	3224	3779	4335

Source: Hadlock *et al* [28]
Comment: Related to gestation using Chitty *et al* [14,16,20]
Equation: Log_{10} weight =
$1.326 - 0.0000326 \times AC \times FL + 0.00107 \times HC + 0.00438 \times AC + 0.0158 \times FL$
SD = 7.5% of weight

36. Fetal weight

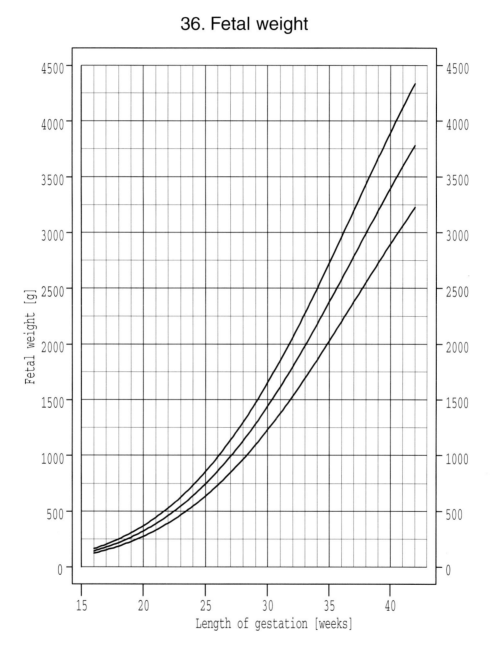

37. Fetal weight estimated from abdominal circumference and femur length

Femur length (mm)	Abdominal circumference (mm)										
	00	0	0	0	0	00	0	0	0	0	00
0	654	774	918	1087	:	:	:	:	:	:	:
	689	813	960	1133	:	:	:	:	:	:	:
	726	854	1004	1181	1389	:	:	:	:	:	:
	765	896	1050	1231	1442	:	:	:	:	:	:
	806	941	1099	1283	1497	1748	:	:	:	:	:
50	850	988	1149	1337	1555	1808	:	:	:	:	:
5	895	1037	1202	1393	1615	1871	2168	:	:	:	:
5	943	1089	1258	1452	1676	1936	2235	:	:	:	:
5	994	1144	1316	1513	1741	2003	2304	2650	:	:	:
5	1048	1201	1376	1577	1808	2072	2374	2721	:	:	:
0	1104	1261	1440	1644	1877	2143	2447	2795	:	:	:
	1163	1324	1506	1713	1949	2217	2523	2870	3265	:	:
	:	1390	1575	1786	2024	2294	2600	2948	3341	3787	:
	:	1459	1648	1861	2102	2373	2680	3027	3419	3861	4360
	:	1532	1724	1940	2182	2456	2763	3109	3498	3936	4428
0	:	:	1803	2021	2266	2540	2848	3193	3579	4012	4498
	:	:	:	2107	2353	2628	2935	3279	3662	4090	4568
	:	:	:	2196	2443	2719	3026	3367	3747	4170	4640
	:	:	:	:	2537	2813	3119	3458	3834	4251	4713
	:	:	:	:	2635	2910	3215	3551	3923	4333	4787
0	:	:	:	:	:	3011	3314	3647	4014	4418	4862

Source: Hadlock et al[28]

Equation: Log$_{10}$ weight = 1.304 + 0.005281 × AC + 0.01938 × FL − 0.00004 × AC × FL

Index

80025 75540